Arnulf Oppelt

Imaging Systems for Medical Diagnostics

Authors	Chapter
Lothar Baetz	2, 9
Detlef Becker	19
Heinrich Behner	12.1.5
Ralf Behrens	12.3.2
Jens Bernhardt	12.1.1
Siegfried Bocionek	21
Jan Boese	4
Gerhard Brinker	15.1.7.4
Herbert Bruder	13.4
Thomas Brunner	12.5
Dieter Cherek	13.3.1
Eduard David	1
Andrew Dewdney	15.1.2.1-15.1.2.4
Hendrik Ditt	4
Karlheinz Dorn	19
Martin Dugas	21
Thomas Flohr	13.2-13.6
Sven Fritzler	14.3, 17.2
Matthias Gebhardt	15.1.3.1
Rainer Graumann	5
Jan Grimm	18
Alok Gupta	20
Franz Hebrank	15.1.7.3
Bjoern Heismann	13.3.2
Arne Hengerer	18
Gert Hetzel	16.9
Peter Heubes	15.1.6.1
Dimitre Hristov	17.1
Hans Kaarmann	8.4
Stefan Kaepplinger	14.3, 17.2
Stephan Kannengiesser	15.2.3
Klaus Klingenbeck-Regn	14.1, 14.2
Wolfgang Knuepfer	6
Gerhard Kohl	13.5.4
Arun Krishnan	20
Wolfgang Kutschera	12.1
Gerhard Laub	15.2.4.5
Christine Lorenz	15.2.6.2
Thomas Mertelmeier	11, 12.6
Matthias Mitschke	5
Edgar Mueller	15.2.5.2-15.2.6.1
Ernst Neumeier	12.1.3-12.1.4
Hartwig Newiger	14.4, 17.2
Mathias Nittka	15.2.2
Wolfgang Nitz	15.2.1
Stefan Nowak	15.1.3.2
Niels Oesingmann	15.2.5.1
Bernd Ohnesorge	13.4, 13.5.1-
Arnulf Oppelt	7, 8, 10, 12.3.
Karlheinz Pauli	6.3
Paul Ponnath	12.1.3-12.1.4
Norbert Rahn	4
Bharat Rao	20
Rainer Raupach	13.1.4.4
Judith Regn	12.4
Wolfgang Renz	15.1.4.4
Arne Reykowski	15.1.4.4
Stefan Roell	15.2.7
Stefan Schaller	13.2, 13.6
Michael Scheuering	3
Wilfried Schnell	15.1.4.1-15.1
Christian Schultz	18
Eva Schwenzfeier-Hellkamp	15.1.7.1
Johann Seissl	17.3
Matthias Seufert	12.1.6
Hartmut Sklebitz	12.3.3
Karin Soeldner	12.1.2
Martin Spahn	12.3.4
Peter Speier	15.2.4.1
Eckart Stetter	15.1
Karl Stierstorfer	13.3.4, 13.3.5
Hans Stroehlein	12.1.5
Christoph Suess	13.3.6
Michelle Svatos	17.1
Stefan Thesen	15.2.4.2-15.2
Lewis J. Thomas III	16.1-16.8
Peter Tichy	12.2
Herbert Vestner	13.1.1, 13.1.2 13.1.4.1-13.1
Frank Wacker	15.2.6.3
Heinrich Wallschlaeger	13.1.3
Gerd Wessels	17.4
Karsten Wicklow	15.2.8
Karl Wiesent	10.6
Andreas Wunder	18
Zirao Zheng	17.1

Imaging Systems for Medical Diagnostics

Fundamentals, Technical Solutions and Applications for Systems Applying Ionizing Radiation, Nuclear Magnetic Resonance and Ultrasound

Edited by Arnulf Oppelt

Publicis Corporate Publishing

Bibliographic information from Die Deutsche Bibliothek
Die Deutsche Bibliothek lists this publication in the Deutsche Nationalbibliografie; detailed bibliographic data are available on the Internet at http://dnb.ddb.de

www.publicis-erlangen.de/books

ISBN 3-89578-226-2

Editor: Siemens Aktiengesellschaft, Berlin und München
Publisher: Publicis Corporate Publishing, Erlangen

Printed in Germany

Foreword

Twenty-five years ago, in 1980, the first edition of 'imaging systems for medical diagnostics' appeared as a German paperback. This was a time when computed tomography with X-rays had just made its way into clinical routine and when real time ultrasound replaced static B-scanners. Magnetic resonance imaging, single photon and positron emission tomography were still in their infancy. The rapid development of these methods has led to two further editions, the last having appeared in 1995. An English translation of the second edition came out in 1990.

Why is it time now for a new edition? Imaging technology has made tremendous progress. All imaging modalities are now capable of generating three dimensional information of the human body. In order to make this information accessible, sophisticated digital image processing is required. Methods for the exact spatiotemporal superposition of information from different modalities have to be applied. The drastically increasing importance of information technology is further emphasized by the need for a uniform platform with an identical user interface for all modalities. *Syngo* has been a pioneer in this field. Ultimately, information technology enables the optimization of clinical workflow and thus helps increase the quality of care while at the same time reducing cost.

A new edition of 'imaging systems for medical diagnostics', therefore, can no longer restrict itself to the physical basics and to the actual technology of imaging instruments. Because of their increasing significance, applications of image and information processing and distribution have to be included. Nevertheless, the importance of the physical principles of modern imaging systems persists, which has led to the well-known extraordinary technical solutions. The desire to convey this variety of technical knowledge explains the significant increase in the volume of the book.

In keeping with increasing internationalization not only in medical science but in all areas, this new edition appears only in English. The authors are active specialists in project management and development in the medical industry who drafted their contributions concurrently with their professional duties and were motivated by their devotion to the arena. A unique compendium of modern medical imaging technology has emerged which is useful for all parties, technically interested physicians as well as students, technicians, engineers and physicists.

Dr. Hermann Requardt
Executive Vice President, Siemens Medical Solutions

Preface

This book is intended to give an overview on medical imaging from the technical side. It starts by recapitulating the biological facts of the human visual system, presents the physics of the imaging process, portrays current technical designs and concludes with the last developments of software technology. It is composed of five parts: The first part is dedicated to images, how they are processed in the human eye, how they can be subjectively characterized, how they can be displayed and fused when obtained from different modalities, and how one can use them to navigate. The second part is devoted to the physics of the different imaging methods, applying X-rays and γ-rays, ultrasound or nuclear magnetic resonance. The third part gives an outline on system theory and image reconstruction. The fourth part deals with the technology of actual imaging instrumentation revealing some of their design secrets. Finally, the fifth part is devoted to the handling, evaluation and distribution of medical images. A uniform user interface, computer assisted detection of lesions and integration into the hospital workflow are becoming increasingly important matters.

To compile such a plentitude of information into a single volume is a challenging task. It is expected that the reader is familiar with basic mathematics and the fundamentals of Fourier transform theory. The editor wishes to thank the 85 authors and co-authors who have contributed with their professional knowledge for their cooperation. Thanks also go to the publisher for his patient willingness to respond to the suggestions of the editor and to bring the sometimes bumpy English manuscripts into readable form. In particular, the tremendous dedication of the publishing editor Gerhard Seitfudem warrants special mention. Finally, this book would not have been possible without the continuous encouragement and support of the members of the board of Siemens Medical Solutions.

May the 4th edition (i.e. 2nd edition in English) of 'imaging for medical diagnostics' be accepted as a handbook suited as well for students interested in biomedical engineering as for their teachers, for developers and experts, and for everyone interested in current medical technology.

Arnulf Oppelt

Contents

Part I – Principles of Image Processing

1 Physiology of vision 18
1.1 General considerations regarding sensory physiology 18
1.2 The eye 19
1.2.1 Adequate stimulusus 19
1.2.2 Anatomy 19
1.3 Functioning of the eye 21
1.3.1 The imaging mechanism 21
1.3.2 Aberrations in image production 21
1.3.3 Eye defects 22
1.3.4 The accommodation process 23
1.3.5 Eye movements 23
1.3.6 Depth of field 24
1.4 Conversion of light into neural impulses 25
1.4.1 Anatomy of the retina 25
1.4.2 Spatial resolution 26
1.4.3 Contrast resolution 27
1.4.4 Adaptation 29
1.4.5 Sensitivity to color 33
1.4.6 Temporal resolution 34
1.5 Neural processing 36
1.5.1 Anatomy of the visual pathway 36
1.5.2 Three-dimensional vision 36
1.5.3 Depth perception 37
1.5.4 Optical illusions 38
1.5.5 Visual memory 39
1.6 References 40

2 Subjective assessment of image quality 42
2.1 Introduction 42
2.2 ROC Methology 42
2.3 Contrast detail resolution 44
2.4 References 46

3 Image rendering 47
3.1 2D imaging 47
3.2 Planar reformation 47

3.3 Segmentation ... 48
3.4 Surface rendering ... 49
3.4.1 Extraction of isosurfaces and the marching-cubes algorithm ... 49
3.5 Volume rendering ... 50
3.5.1 Image-order techniques ... 50
3.5.2 Object-order techniques and the shear-warp-factorization ... 52
3.5.3 Compositing ... 53
3.5.4 Conclusion ... 56
3.6 Transfer-functions ... 56
3.7 Local illumination ... 56
3.8 Volume rendering on graphics adapters ... 59
3.9 References ... 60

4 Image fusion ... 62
4.1 Introduction ... 62
4.1.1 Clinical relevance ... 62
4.1.2 Image fusion steps ... 62
4.1.3 General challenges ... 64
4.2 Registration ... 65
4.2.1 Registration by calibration ... 65
4.2.2 Image-based, 3D-3D registration ... 66
4.2.3 Image-based, 2D-3D registration ... 78
4.2.4 Validation of fusion results ... 82
4.3 Visualization ... 83
4.3.1 Visualization of MPR slices ... 83
4.3.2 Fusion result visualization using volume rendering techniques ... 86
4.3.3 Visualization of fused projection images ... 88
4.4 Clinical applications ... 88
4.4.1 Nuclear medicine: fusion of CT/MR and PET/SPECT images ... 88
4.4.2 Surgery ... 89
4.4.3 Treatment planning in radiation oncology ... 91
4.4.4 Interventional radiology ... 92
4.5 References ... 93

5 Navigation ... 96
5.1 Introduction ... 96
5.2 Principles of navigation ... 97
5.3 Localizer technologies ... 99
5.3.1 Principles of optical tracking systems ... 99
5.3.2 Electromagnetic position tracking ... 101
5.3.3 Tool calibration ... 103
5.4 Registration ... 104
5.4.1 Point-pair matching using a 3D localizer ... 105
5.4.2 Surface matching ... 106

5.5 Navigation for image-guided surgery and intervention ... 107
5.5.1 CT/MRI-based navigation ... 107
5.5.2 2D mobile C-arm-based navigation ... 107
5.5.3 3D mobile C-arm-based navigation ... 109
5.6 Navigation accuracy ... 111
5.7 Clinical applications ... 111
5.8 Future prospects ... 113
5.9 References ... 113

Part II – Physics of Imaging

6 X-ray and γ-radiation ... 118
6.1 Generation of X-ray and γ-radiation ... 118
6.1.1 Properties of X-ray bremsstrahlung ... 119
6.1.2 Characteristic radiation ... 120
6.1.3 Intensity (energy flux density) of X-radiation ... 122
6.1.4 Target material ... 123
6.2 X-ray and γ-ray interaction with matter ... 124
6.2.1 Interaction effects and phenomenological description ... 124
6.2.2 The photoelectric effect ... 124
6.2.3 Compton effect ... 127
6.2.4 Coherent scattering ... 130
6.2.5 Interactions with real objects ... 131
6.3 Biological effects of radiation ... 135
6.3.1 Acute or deterministic radiation damage ... 135
6.3.2 Stochastic radiation damage ... 136
6.3.3 Estimate of radiation risk ... 136
6.3.4 Controversy concerning the effects of low radiation doses ... 140
6.4 References ... 141

7 Concepts in magnetic resonance imaging ... 143
7.1 Historical survey ... 143
7.2 The NMR phenomenon ... 144
7.2.1 Magnetization ... 144
7.2.2 Bloch equations ... 146
7.2.3 Relaxation ... 148
7.2.4 Magnetization transfer ... 151
7.2.5 Nuclear induction ... 152
7.2.6 Spin echoes ... 156
7.2.7 Steady-state free precession ... 158
7.2.8 Diffusion ... 161
7.2.9 Spectroscopy ... 165
7.2.10 Signal-to-noise ratio ... 168

7.3 Magnetic resonance imaging ... 170
7.3.1 NMR signal in a magnetic field gradient ... 171
7.3.2 Spatial resolution ... 173
7.3.3 Selective excitation ... 175
7.3.4 Pulse sequence and contrast ... 178
7.4 References ... 181

8 Physical principles of medical ultrasound ... 184
8.1 Introduction ... 184
8.2 Ultrasound field ... 185
8.2.1 Ultrasound field parameters ... 185
8.2.2 Ultrasound propagation ... 187
8.3 Imaging principles ... 197
8.3.1 Echo pulse method ... 197
8.3.2 Ultrasound transducer ... 199
8.3.3 Imaging methods ... 200
8.3.4 Methods of determining flow ... 202
8.4 Safety of diagnostic ultrasound ... 207
8.4.1 Acoustic output regulations ... 207
8.4.2 Bioeffects ... 207
8.4.3 Output display standard using thermal and mechanical indices ... 209
8.4.4 Summary – prudent use of ultrasound ... 210
8.5 References ... 210

Part III – Image Reconstruction

9 System theory ... 214
9.1 Introduction ... 214
9.2 Basic quantities for evaluating image quality ... 214
9.2.1 Contrast ... 214
9.2.2 Spatial resolution ... 216
9.2.3 Noise ... 224
9.3 References ... 228

10 Principles of image reconstruction ... 230
10.1 Introduction ... 230
10.2 Basic principles ... 231
10.3 2D Fourier reconstruction ... 233
10.4 Number of data ... 234
10.5 Filtered backprojection ... 235
10.6 3D projection reconstruction ... 237
10.7 Backprojection applying homogeneous coordinates ... 240
10.8 References ... 241

Part IV – Image Instrumentation

11 Image displays . . . 244
11.1 Advantages and challenges of soft-copy reading . . . 244
11.2 Impact of the human visual system on display design . . . 245
11.2.1 Contrast sensitivity and spatial resolution . . . 246
11.2.2 Contrast and dynamic range . . . 247
11.2.3 Color vision . . . 249
11.3 Medical display technologies . . . 249
11.3.1 Cathode ray tube monitors . . . 250
11.3.2 Liquid crystal displays . . . 252
11.4 Technical display performance values . . . 255
11.4.1 Display size . . . 255
11.4.2 Spatial resolution . . . 255
11.4.3 Luminance, contrast ratio, and veiling glare . . . 256
11.4.4 Dynamic range and display curve . . . 258
11.4.5 Noise . . . 258
11.5 Digital imaging display systems . . . 259
11.6 Referencess . . . 260

12 X-ray components and systems . . . 264
12.1 The X-ray tube . . . 264
12.1.1 Emitters . . . 265
12.1.2 Specifications for focal spot size and electron beam shape . . . 272
12.1.3 The anode assembly . . . 280
12.1.4 Anode load capacity . . . 289
12.1.5 X-ray tube vacuum envelopes . . . 292
12.1.6 Casing design . . . 296
12.2 X-ray generators . . . 300
12.2.1 General requirements . . . 300
12.2.2 Technical aspects . . . 303
12.2.3 Control circuits . . . 305
12.2.4 Exposure control in direct radiography . . . 309
12.2.5 Exposure control in indirect radiography . . . 312
12.3 X-ray image detectors . . . 315
12.3.1 Static detectors . . . 315
12.3.2 X-ray image intensifiers . . . 316
12.3.3 Processing the X-ray image intensifier's output image . . . 323
12.3.4 Flat detectors . . . 333
12.4 X-ray systems . . . 349
12.4.1 Classification of X-ray systems . . . 350
12.4.2 Intervention – a paradigm for a modern X-ray system . . . 357
12.5 Cone-beam CT with C-arm systems . . . 378
12.5.1 Introduction . . . 378

12.5.2 Acquisition protocols and system properties 380
12.5.3 Calibration 381
12.5.4 Reconstruction 384
12.5.5 Visualization 384
12.5.6 Advanced application tools 385
12.5.7 Image quality 386
12.5.8 Clinical applications and examples 389
12.5.9 Outlook 393
12.6 Mammography 393
12.6.1 System overview 394
12.6.2 Digital mammography 399
12.6.3 Other and new modalities 404
12.7 References 404

13 Computed X-ray tomography 413
13.1 Principles 413
13.1.1 Measurement principle 413
13.1.2 Basic image reconstruction 415
13.1.3 Single-slice axial CT and spiral CT 417
13.1.4 Image quality 422
13.2 From single-slice to multi-slice CT 434
13.3 Multi-slice CT (MSCT) 438
13.3.1 System design 439
13.3.2 Detector design for MSCT 447
13.3.3 The cone-angle problem 451
13.3.4 MSCT spiral scan and reconstruction techniques 453
13.3.5 Double z-sampling 466
13.3.6 Dose in MDCT 468
13.4 Multi-slice cardiac CT 470
13.4.1 Introduction 470
13.4.2 ECG-triggered MSCT imaging 471
13.4.3 ECG-gated MSCT imaging 471
13.4.4 Performance evaluation 477
13.5 Clinical applications 479
13.5.1 Quantification of coronary calcification 479
13.5.2 Cardiac and coronary CT angiography 482
13.5.3 Evaluation of cardiac function 484
13.5.4 Preventive care: CT of the lung and colon 486
13.6 The future of CT 488
13.6.1 From multi-slice to area-detector CT 488
13.6.2 Combined systems 490
13.6.3 Alternative system concepts 493
13.6.4 Maximum data volumes and theoretical CT limitations 494
13.7 References 495

14 Nuclear medicine 503
14.1 Introduction 503
14.2 Imaging with single photon emitters – measurement principles and devices 504
14.2.1 The scintillation detector 504
14.2.2 The gamma camera (Anger camera) 506
14.3 SPECT systems 514
14.3.1 General SPECT principle 514
14.3.2 Overview of current systems 516
14.3.3 Clinical applications 521
14.3.4 New detector technologies 523
14.4 PET systems 524
14.4.1 Principles of PET 524
14.4.2 Characterization of PET scanners 530
14.4.3 Clinical applications 532
14.5 References 536

15 Magnetic resonance imaging 540
15.1 MR systems and components 540
15.1.1 System overview 540
15.1.2 The main magnet 542
15.1.3 The gradient system 554
15.1.4 The RF system 563
15.1.5 System control 579
15.1.6 Image quality 579
15.1.7 MR safety 592
15.2 Methods and clinical applications 599
15.2.1 Sequences and contrast 599
15.2.2 Parallel imaging techniques (PAT) 619
15.2.3 Whole-body imaging 628
15.2.4 MRI and macroscopic motion 631
15.2.5 MRI and microscopic motion 669
15.2.6 Clinical examples 686
15.2.7 Clinical MR spectroscopy 698
15.2.8 Hyperpolarization 710
15.3 References 716

16 Ultrasound imaging systems 732
16.1 Introduction 732
16.1.1 Operation 732
16.1.2 Typical modes 733
16.2 System architecture 745
16.2.1 Beamformer 746
16.2.2 Mid-processor 758
16.2.3 Display 765

16.3 Transducer types (from a system perspective) 768
16.3.1 Sector and vector transducers 768
16.3.2 Linear transducers 769
16.3.3 Curved transducers 770
16.3.4 Intra-cavity transducers 770
16.3.5 Multi-row arrays (1.25 and 1.5 dimensional arrays) 770
16.3.6 Hanafy lens approach to control elevation beamwidth 771
16.3.7 Summary of different transducer types 772
16.4 B-mode imaging 773
16.4.1 Harmonics for clutter reduction 773
16.4.2 Transmit pulse coding 776
16.4.3 Compounding 779
16.5 Contrast agent imaging 782
16.5.1 Brief discussion of the physics of contrast agents 782
16.5.2 Destructive contrast agent detection techniques (disruption) 783
16.5.3 Pulse inversion as a nondestructive contrast agent detection technique . 784
16.5.4 Third order scattering for nondestructive contrast agent detection 785
16.6 Quantification 786
16.7 3D imaging 788
16.7.1 Wobblers 788
16.7.2 2D arrays 789
16.7.3 3D transesophageal imaging 790
16.8 Conclusion 791
16.9 Methods and applications in sonography 792
16.9.1 2D-imaging 792
16.9.2 Doppler imaging 794
16.9.3 Harmonic imaging 801
16.9.4 Compounding technologies and applications 805
16.9.5 Workflow-improvement and standardization technologies 814
16.9.6 Special cardiac transducers and evaluations 815
16.10 References 820

17 Special and hybrid systems 821
17.1 Imaging for radiation therapy 821
17.1.1 Introduction 821
17.1.2 The portal imaging beam 823
17.1.3 Portal imaging detectors 825
17.1.4 Advanced techniques 827
17.1.5 Summary 830
17.2 Hybrid systems: PET/CT and SPECT·CT 830
17.2.1 Clinical benefits of combined functional and morphological imaging . . 831
17.2.2 Design criteria for PET/CT systems 831
17.2.3 PET/CT applications 832
17.2.4 SPECT and CT 835

17.3 Combining imaging modalities for interventional procedures 836
17.3.1 Interventional angiography combined with CT imaging 837
17.3.2 Interventional angiography combined with MRI imaging 839
17.4 Imaging in the operating room 842
17.4.1 Intraoperative imaging 842
17.4.2 Integrated surgical workplaces 855
17.5 References 860

18 Molecular imaging 863
18.1 Introduction 863
18.2 Imaging probes 864
18.3 Signal amplification strategies 868
18.4 Imaging modalities 868
18.4.1 Nuclear imaging 869
18.4.2 Magnetic resonance imaging (MRI) 871
18.4.3 Optical imaging 873
18.4.4 Computed tomography 878
18.4.5 Ultrasound 878
18.4.6 Combined systems 879
18.5 Outlook 879
18.6 References 880

Part V – Information Processing and Distribution

19 Software platform for medical imaging 888
19.1 Overview 888
19.2 Introduction to medical imaging software domain 888
19.2.1 Aspects of a common style guide 891
19.2.2 A sample workflow 893
19.2.3 Analysis of the problem domain 905
19.2.4 From programming to software configuration 907
19.3 Software terminology 908
19.4 Application architecture 910
19.4.1 Three-tiered architecture model 912
19.4.2 Application architecture and component-runtime management 915
19.4.3 Presentation-logic containerware and componentware 918
19.4.4 Business logic containerware and componentware 918
19.4.5 Asynchronous communication: decoupling presentation and business logic ... 919
19.5 Business objects for medical imaging 920
19.6 Services for medical imaging 921
19.6.1 Data management services 921
19.6.2 DICOM work list, storage, query and print-management services 921

19.6.3 2D/3D/4D image processing services and framework ... 922
19.6.4 Security management services ... 923
19.6.5 Basic services ... 924
19.6.6 Systems management service ... 925
19.7 Tool support for *syngo*'s product-line architecture ... 926
19.8 Medical enterprise application integration (EAI) ... 928
19.9 References ... 929

20 Computer-aided detection and diagnosis (CAD) ... 931
20.1 Introduction ... 931
20.2 Performance measurement of CAD systems ... 934
20.3 Computer-aided detection dataflow ... 934
20.4 Development and validation of CAD systems – databases, training and testing of classifiers ... 937
20.5 Future directions in CAD ... 939
20.6 References ... 941

21 Hospital information systems ... 943
21.1 Information system basics ... 944
21.2 Introduction to hospital information systems ... 949
21.3 Purpose and classification ... 950
21.4 Hospital workflow and integration ... 953
21.5 HIS architecture ... 954
21.6 Patient administration and revenue management ... 958
21.6.1 Functionality ... 958
21.6.2 Technical realization of reimbursement workflow ... 961
21.7 The electronic medical record (EMR) ... 964
21.7.1 Functionality ... 964
21.7.2 User interface and technical realization ... 965
21.8 Clinical workflow applications ... 967
21.8.1 Functionality ... 967
21.8.2 Technical realization of system intelligence ... 971
21.9 Departmental information system: radiology ... 974
21.9.1 The radiology workflow ... 974
21.9.2 The radiology information system (RIS) ... 975
21.9.3 The picture archiving and communication system (PACS) ... 977
21.10 Integrated workplaces ... 979
21.10.1 Integrated workplaces in radiology ... 979
21.10.2 Integrated workplaces in cardiology ... 981
21.11 The digital hospital and beyond – a vision ... 983
21.12 References ... 988

Index ... 990

Part I – Principle
Image Proces

1 Physiology of vision

1.1 General considerations regarding sensory physiology

Over the last few decades much progress has been made in the area of imaging systems for use in medical diagnostics. New techniques, for example magnetic resonance tomography, have been developed, opening up new avenues in diagnosis. However, enormous improvements have also been made in conventional techniques, e.g. those using X-rays, in particular by the application of microelectronics: the amount of radiation to which the patient is exposed has been drastically reduced, and the quality of the images considerably enhanced.

Today industry is able to produce imaging systems which are to a large extent technically compatible with the biological needs of the human eye. In order to give a full account of these systems, it therefore seems appropriate to begin by giving some idea of the function of the eye as a sense organ.

The sense organs allow the organism to perceive its constantly changing environment. Depending on the physical dimension of the environmental change, the various sense organs are specialized for quite specific, adequate stimuli. Different sensory perceptions [1.1], also known as sensory modalities, arise in this way.

The amount of information received by all the sensory organs together is immense. It has been estimated at around 10^9 bits/s [1.2]. This flood of information, cannot, how-

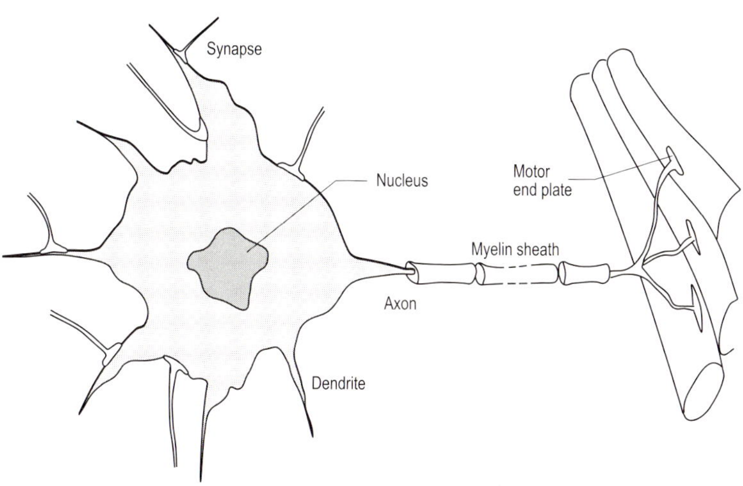

Figure 1.1 The neuron, the basic working unit of the central nervous system

ever, be transmitted by the nerves to the brain in its entirety. The nervous system therefore needs to select the most important information at any particular moment. This selection procedure cuts down the information received in the ratio of $10^7 : 1$. People vary greatly in the selection they make so that the same pattern of stimuli will be perceived and assessed differently from one person to another. In principle this information selection takes place in the nervous system by means of the excitation and inhibition of nerve cells. Thus the nervous system has the task of comparing information in terms of the degree of neural excitation and, where necessary, of passing it on to higher decision-making centers. In order to perform this task, the nervous system has two separate functional elements: nerve cell bodies for converting information and nerve fibers for stimulus conduction. Collections of nerve cells in the brain and in the spinal cord are known as gray matter and the fibers as white matter. The neuron is the basic working unit of the central nervous system (CNS). It consists of a cell body with several projections which increase its surface area, and a long fiber, the axon, which establishes the contacts (synaptic junctions) with other nerve cells. Figure 1.1 shows a diagram of such a neuron.

This method of transforming and transmitting information applies equally to all the sensory organs, including the *eye*. In this process, specific sensory perception is not generated by the nature of the impulse, but by the anatomy of the nerve connections between the relevant sensory organs and particular areas of the brain. Thus a distinction is made anatomically between a visual pathway, an auditory pathway, an olfactory pathway, a gustatory pathway and a pain pathway. Even the quality of sensory perception, which in the case of the eye constitutes the difference between color perception and light-dark perception, is governed by the finely-structured connections between individual nerve fibers and relevant sensory cells.

1.2 The eye

1.2.1 Adequate stimulusus

The eye is sensitive to certain electromagnetic waves. These waves can be divided up into various regions [1.3] which have quite different effects on the organism. As can be seen from fig. 1.2, the sensitivity range of the eye barely covers one octave (400 to 780 nm) of the electromagnetic spectrum. The frequency corresponds to the color (see fig. 1.17), the amplitude to the degree of brightness perceived.

In addition, the sense of vision can perceive objects in three dimensions. This is because of the parallactic shift of the image seen by the right eye relative to that seen by the left eye.

1.2.2 Anatomy

Like the camera, the eye has an optical imaging system. It consists of the cornea and the lens. In order to reduce chromatic aberration (color distortion), the lens is made

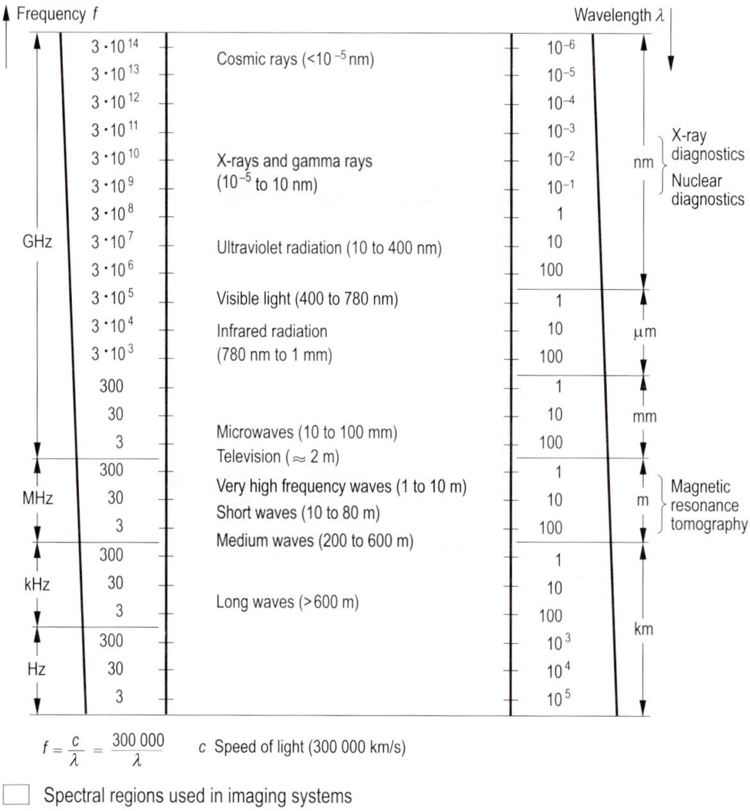

Figure 1.2 Regions of the electromagnetic spectrum

up of several layers, like an onion, each with a different refractive index. Anatomical details are shown in fig. 1.3 [1.4]. The space between the cornea and the lens (anterior chamber) is filled by the crystal-clear aqueous humor. The interior of the eye is occupied by the jelly-like vitreous body, which in common with all the other transparent parts of the eye does not contain any blood vessels, receiving nutrients by diffusion. Inside the sclera (the firm white outer membrane) lies the choroid (the brownish vascular membrane), followed by the retina. The retina contains the light-sensitive elements, the rods and the cones, which convert the electromagnetic waves into nerve impulses. The retina also contains nerve cells which carry out a preliminary processing of the information on the spot. This is also where the fibers of the optical nerve start. The lens is suspended in the ring-shaped muscle of the ciliary body. The iris, which covers the front of the lens, leaves only a small aperture (the pupil) open. Six muscles, stemming from the bone wall of the eye socket and attached to the outside of the sclera, are capable of moving and turning the eyeball in all directions.

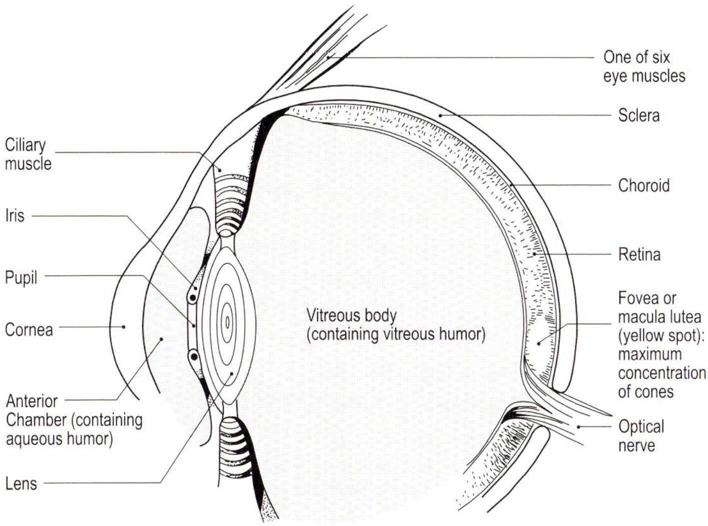

Figure 1.3 Anatomy of the eye

1.3 Functioning of the eye

1.3.1 The imaging mechanism

The projection of an image of the environment through the cornea onto the retina obeys the laws of geometrical optics [1.5, 1.1], as shown in fig. 1.4. The various optical media of the eye have the following refractive indices: cornea 1.38, aqueous humor 1.34, lens 1.44. Since the density of the eye roughly corresponds to that of water, the critical angle for total reflection can be calculated to be 48° 40'. In principle an image can be produced by the outer surface of the cornea alone. However, the lens in the eye permits light to be refracted to varying degrees, which in turn permits focusing on near and distant objects. The total refracting power of the healthy eye is about 48 diopters, and the capacity to vary this by means of the lens is known as the amplitude of accommodation. In young people the amplitude of accommodation is around 12 diopters; with increasing age (usually between 50 and 60) it approaches one diopter [1.6].

1.3.2 Aberrations in image production

As is generally the case in optics, the eye suffers from certain common lens aberrations. Spherical aberration, which leads to peripheral rays being more powerfully refracted than central rays resulting in a barrel-shaped distortion, is corrected to a large extent by the diaphragm action of the pupil. Chromatic aberration (color distortion), due to more powerful refraction of blue rays than red rays, is mitigated by the effect of the onion-like structure of the lens with its layers of different refractive index (the

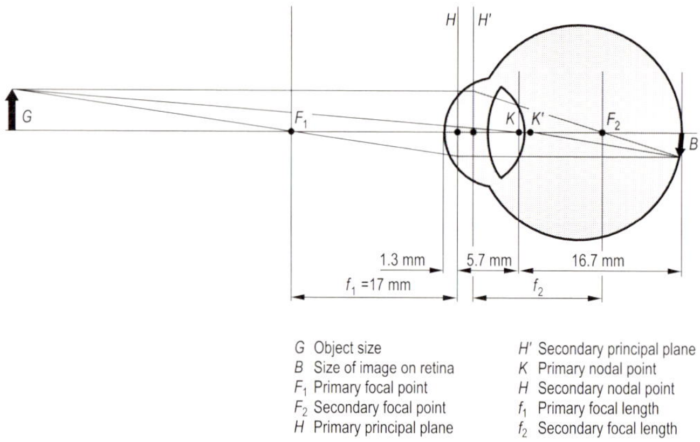

Figure 1.4 Geometrical optics of the eye

inner layers refract more powerfully than the outer layers). When colored objects are observed, difficulties in accommodation can occur if the object lies in a plane close to the eye, because the eye tries to accommodate in turn to the colors with shorter or longer wavelengths. When the object is further away, this effect does not arise because of the greater depth of field.

1.3.3 Eye defects

Figure 1.5 shows that a sharp image is formed on the retina of an eye with normal vision.

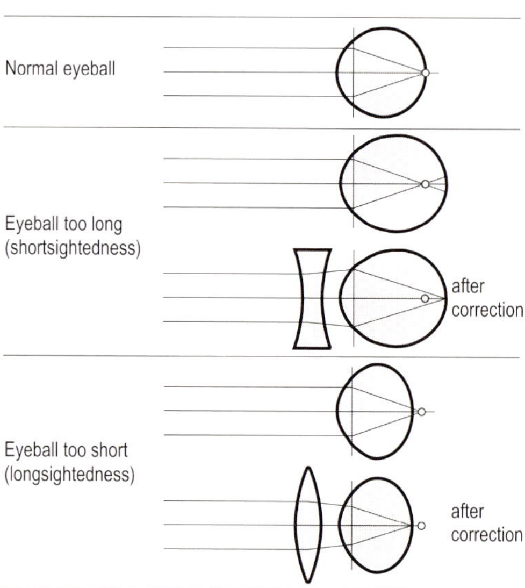

Figure 1.5
Visual defects produced when eyeball is too long or too short, and means of correction

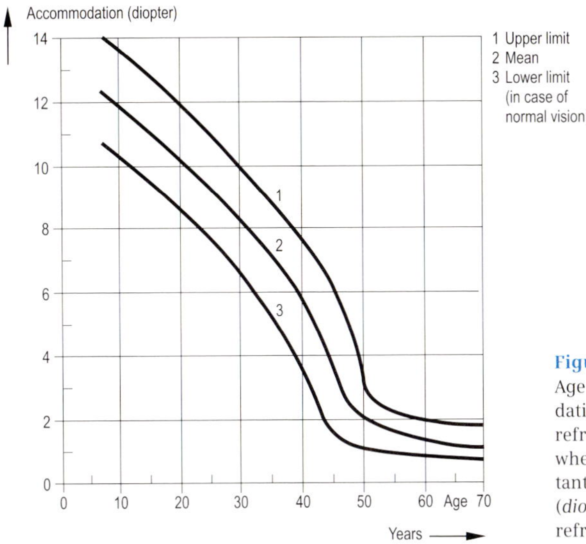

Figure 1.6
Age dependence of accommodation (difference between the refracting power of the lens when looking at near and distant objects) according to Graff (*diopter* = $^1/_m$ is the unit of the refractive power $^1/_f$ of a lens)

In the case of an eyeball which is too long (shortsighted) or too short (longsighted), the image is formed in a plane in front of or behind the retina. A sharp image can therefore only be achieved by means of correction with appropriate lenses (glasses or contact lenses). Apart from the decrease in amplitude of accommodation due to the loss of lens elasticity associated with increasing age (as illustrated in fig. 1.6), clouding of the lens or of the aqueous humor can cause sight to deteriorate.

1.3.4 The accommodation process

Focusing an image on the retina is achieved by changing the refractive power of the lens. This is done by contraction or relaxation of the ring-shaped ciliary muscle (see fig. 1.3) so that the lens is compressed or stretched radially. The process is controlled by the nerve cells of the oculomotor center in the brain which adjusts the refractive power of the lens until the size of the image reaches a minimum.

1.3.5 Eye movements

With the help of the eye muscles shown in fig. 1.7, the eye is moved until the image of the object to be observed is located at the point of maximum resolving power (smallest spatial resolution) on the retina (viz. the fovea: see fig. 1.3). As can be seen from fig. 1.10, this point has the highest cone density. The process is subject to continuous control, because the eye moves its optical axis in relation to the object observed until the number of stimulated cones reaches a maximum. As in any control process, there is permanent adjustment towards an optimum value, i.e. the axis of the eye is moving constantly to and fro. In order to maintain this maximum stimulation, the eye continually makes oscillatory movements (saccades) in all directions. Such movements are

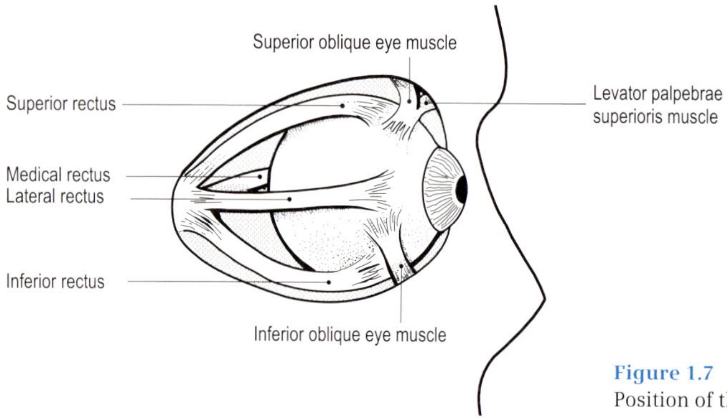

Figure 1.7
Position of the eye muscles

also carried out in a resting state (with the eyes open) at a frequency of approximately 10 Hz.

1.3.6 Depth of field

The eye's depth of field depends on the same parameters as does any ordinary optical apparatus. That is, it depends on the diameter of the pupil (aperture) and on the degree of accommodation (depth adjustment). As fig. 1.8 shows, in the case of medium

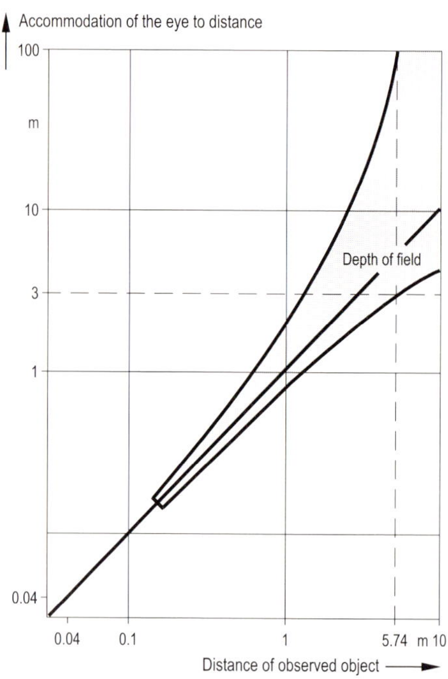

Figure 1.8
Depth of field of the human eye in relation to accommodation at medium pupil diameter. Accommodation to a distance of 5.74 m gives the ability to see in focus at distances between 3 m and infinity (fixed focus setting according to Ranke in [1.1])

pupil diameter and accommodation to a distance of 5.74 in, everything from 3 in to infinity is seen in focus [1.1].

1.4 Conversion of light into neural impulses

1.4.1 Anatomy of the retina

As fig. 1.3 shows, the retina lies on the inside of the rear half of the eyeball. It contains the photosensitive rods and cones as well as the nerve cells [1.4] which preprocess optical information. Figure 1.9 shows a diagram of a microscopic portion of the retina with all the optically active elements. From the diagram it is clear that the photosensitive outer segments of the rods and cones which contain the visual purple [1.7] are turned away from the light and are partially submerged in the pigment layer (not shown). This means that the effect of scattered light is reduced and that the sensitive elements are protected from overexposure to light by creeping into the pigment layer.

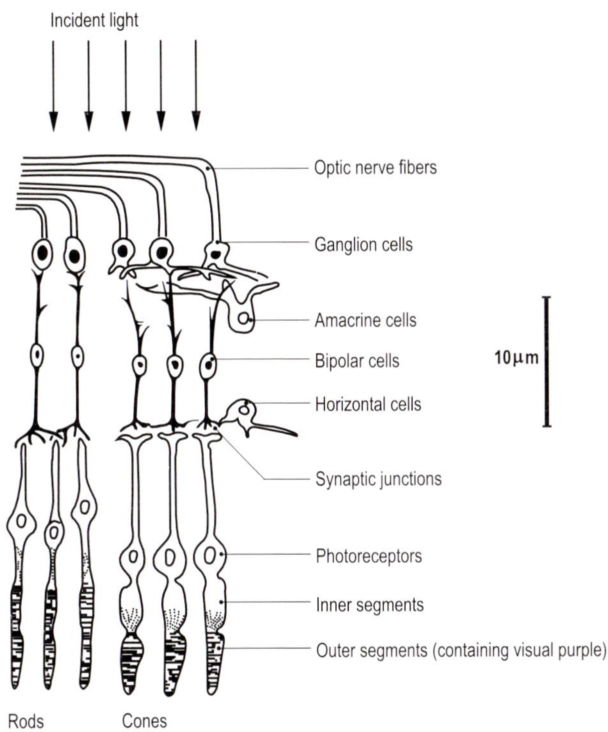

Figure 1.9
Diagrammatic representation of the structure and relative position of the active elements of the retina

The visual purple [1.8], a derivate from vitamin A, is stored in the outer segments of the cones; it is decomposed by the absorption of light, the cleavage molecules producing an impulse which is passed on by the photoreceptors to the bipolar cells via synaptic junctions. The connection of several photoreceptors to one bipolar cell forms the receptive field [1.9]. Every ray of light that hits one of the receptor cells in such a group stimulates the nerve cells connected to them in such a way that those at the edge have an inhibitory effect whilst those at the center have an excitatory effect (or more rarely, the other way round). With increasing light intensity, however, the activity changes in that the amount of inhibition becomes greater. In this way the difference between light (excitation) and dark (inhibition) is reinforced. The impulses travel from the bipolar cells via further synaptic junctions to the ganglion cells and optic nerve fibers, which transmit them to the brain.

1.4.2 Spatial resolution

Visual acuity

Two points are only recognized as being separate entities when the images on the retina are so far apart that an unstimulated cone or receptive field happens to be located between the two. The bigger the receptive elements, therefore, the greater will be the distance required between the two images in order for them still to be seen separately, and the spatial resolution of the eye will be correspondingly worse. In medicine

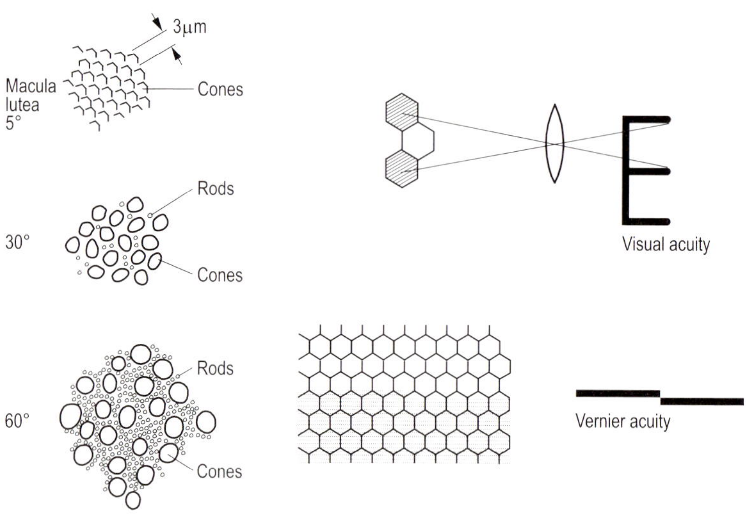

Figure 1.10
Diagram of the rods and cones at the fovea (macula lutea) and in sections of the retina separated by an arc of 30 and 60 degrees from the macula. In the macula lutea there are only cones; towards the periphery both rods and cones are found, with cones becoming progressively less numerous and rods more numerous. The diagram is copied from a microphotograph. Next to it are shown the mechanisms for visual acuity and Vernier acuity. See text for details.

this is called the visual acuity [1.1] and is related to the angle between two light rays which can still just be told apart. As is clear from fig. 1.10, the width of a cone in the macula lutea is about 3 µm, so that taking into account the laws governing image formation in the eye, there is a maximum possible visual acuity corresponding to 50 arc seconds. From fig. 1.10 it is also clear that the distance between cones in the outer regions of the retina increases giving the distribution of visual acuity over the retina shown. Only in a narrow range of 5°, corresponding to the extent of the macula lutea, can the maximal visual acuity therefore be achieved.

Vernier acuity

Whilst the visual acuity of the eye is already very high, an even greater resolving power is possible under certain conditions, namely when lines, rather than two points, have to be distinguished. As shown in fig. 1.10, the eye detects the break in a line due to a slightly offset continuation because the cones (or rather, the nerve cells connected to them) are all interlinked and can tell if on average more cones are being stimulated after the break (from the other half of the image) than before the break. By means of statistical evaluation of the distribution of the stimulated cones, the nervous system can recognize distances between lines which are even smaller than the distances detected in conditions of maximum visual acuity. This fact has long been known in engineering workshops and is used when reading the Vernier scale on measuring instruments, which has led to the name 'Vernier acuity'. In summary it should be emphasized that the nature of the neural processing mechanisms means that visual acuity also depends on the shape of the object perceived.

1.4.3 Contrast resolution

Differential sensitivity

In principle one might expect that a minimum increase in the brightness of an object exist which will produce a minimum increase in the magnitude of the eye's sensory experience. This assumption has proved to be correct, with one qualification: the minimal increase in the magnitude of the sensory experience depends upon the level of background illumination at the time. According to the Weber-Fechner law, the magnitude of the sensitivity E increases logarithmically with the strength of stimulus R according to the equation

$$E = K \ln \frac{R}{R_0}$$

in which, according to Fechner [1.1], K is a constant and R the original stimulus intensity. If, following the practice in technical fields [1.10], the logarithmic value of the light intensity is plotted on the ordinate and the magnitude of the sensitivity is plotted on the abscissa, the graph shown in fig. 1.11a is obtained. At the point where the graph climbs most steeply, the contrast sensitivity is high; where the graph is flat, the contrast sensitivity is low. In the top area glare is said to occur whilst in the bottom area the stimulus is said to be below threshold. Fig. 1.11b shows the differential quotient, i.e. the contrast sensitivity.

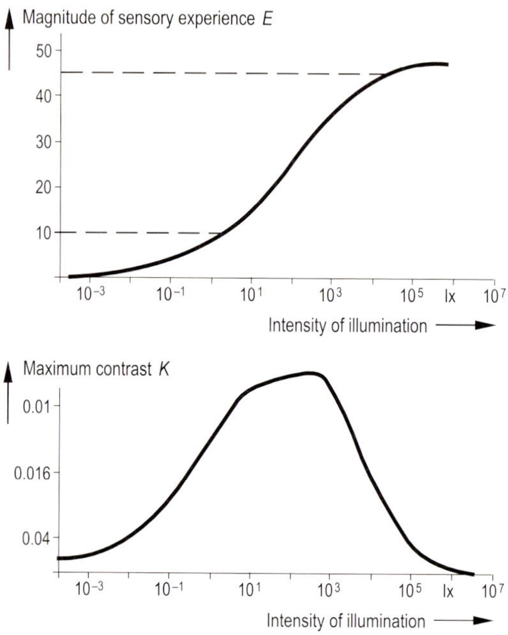

a) The sensitivity $E = K \ln {}^{R}\!/_{R_0}$ is plotted as function of the intensity of illumination. The eye can distinguish about 50 equally spaced levels of sensitivity. Of these roughly 35 lie in the linear region.

b) This graph shows the actual sensitivity to the eye to contrast (differences in brightness). If the Weber-Fechner law were to hold exactly (rising straight line in **a)**) the curve (taken from Ranke [1.1]) would be parallel to the *x*-axis.

Figure 1.11
Sensory experience of the eye according to Weber-Fechner **(a)** and actually measured contrast sensitivity **(b)**

Glare

As explained in the last paragraph, the term glare [1.11] means the reduction to zero of the contrast sensitivity as a consequence of being exposed to such great light intensity that one no longer sees anything but 'brightness'. This definition, however, fails to encompass all the phenomena and causes of glare. Glare also occurs locally, if next to a brightly lit portion of the retina the strongly stimulated cones there inhibit their weakly stimulated neighbors. In this way this area of the retina falls beneath the stimulus threshold and can no longer detect any differences in brightness. Such an effect is reinforced even more by the scattered light [1.12] emanating from a bright ray of light in the not completely clear media of the eye, especially of the vitreous body. This scattered light obscures the tiny differences in brightness of the weakly illuminated surroundings of a bright spot on the retina.

Simultaneous contrast

The mutual coupling of the rods and cones described previously, which is associated with a mutual promotion or inhibition of stimulation, is known as lateral enhancement or inhibition, as the case may be. It is the cause of the fact that a brightly illuminated spot on the retina inhibits the cells around it; by so doing the difference in brightness of the stimulus, and with it the sensory experience, is reinforced. The end

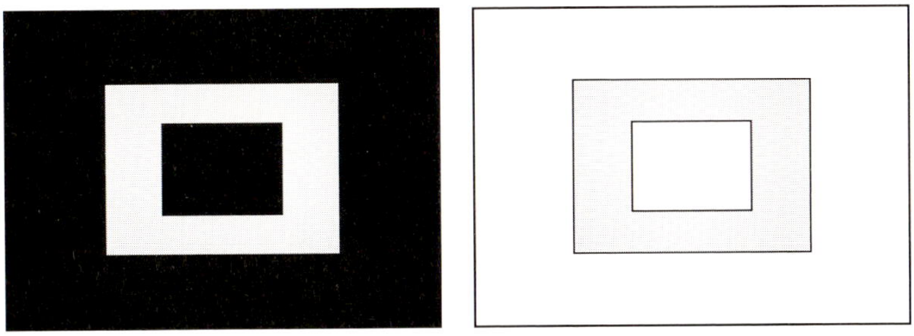

Figure 1.12
An example of simultaneous contrast. The same gray rectangle appears darker on a white background and lighter on a black background.

result is therefore always a neural enhancement in the perceived contrast, an effect which is demonstrated in fig. 1.12.

Successive contrast

Since in the case of pictures presented one after another the neural enhancement in the perceived contrast cannot occur because of the lack of inhibition, the contrast sensitivity is less than in the case of simultaneous contrast.

Contrast gradient (image definition)

The transition from a bright to a dark area of a picture normally takes place gradually so that a contrast gradient can be defined as the decrease in brightness over the appropriate distance in the image. Should this distance reach dimensions comparable to those of the diameter of a cone, it will lie beneath visual acuity and the physical contrast gradient can be ignored. In such a case it is only the physiological mechanisms for the perception of contrast which are involved, so that any further improvement in definition using technical means does not make sense. Besides these considerations, the problems mentioned in connection with glare play an important role, especially when the change in the level of brightness is very large.

1.4.4 Adaptation

Spatial resolution, the detection of contrast and the perception of definition, i.e. the mechanisms which are necessary for producing image quality, are extremely dependent on the eye's adjustment to brightness, known as adaptation [1.13]. This process can be described as follows: when bright light hits the eye, the visual purple in the cones is decomposed. The breakdown products give rise to stimulation. At the same time, however, the visual purple is reconstituted at a quite specific rate and is once more available for the visual process. When illumination starts, the breakdown process predominates, so that there is intense stimulation. With the onset of the reconstitution processes, a situation of equilibrium develops in which breakdown and reconstitution are exactly in balance. The breakdown products available at this stage are naturally smaller in number than during the initial illumination of the eye, which leads to a decrease in stimulation as shown in fig. 1.13.

This description is based on the assumption that a potential (the receptor potential) arises at the sensory receptors (see fig. 1.9) which is proportional to the intensity of the stimulus, if there is no adaptation. This receptor potential triggers the formation of the nerve action potential. Such potentials are temporary fluctuations in the electric potential of the nerve cell membrane with a duration of 1 ms and a constant amplitude of around 90 mV. The mechanism by which this potential is produced can be explained by the change in permeability of the membrane to sodium ions. These migrate from the region outside the cell into it, leaving behind a negative charge. This negative charge is, however, very quickly compensated by the exchange of potassium ions. Energy-consuming processes (sodium-potassium ion pump) finally ensure that the previous ion distribution is restored. By these means the intensity of the simulation is encoded into the frequency of the impulse train. The greater the stimulation, the more frequently action potentials are produced. This is the form in which the stimulation is conducted over long distances by individual nerve fibers.

The decrease in this stimulation is called adaptation. In this process the eye adapts itself to the average brightness of its surroundings. The process of adaptation is additionally reinforced by the mechanism of cone migration, by which cones which have been overexposed to light bury themselves in the pigment epithelium of the retina. These two processes take place in a time span of minutes, whereas the pupil reaction leads to fast adjustment. Here, depending on the total combined brightness of the retina, the amount of contraction in the sphincter muscle in the iris is varied so that the pupil narrows in bright light and dilates in darkness. Since when looking at nearby objects only a portion of the total brightness of the surroundings is observed, the

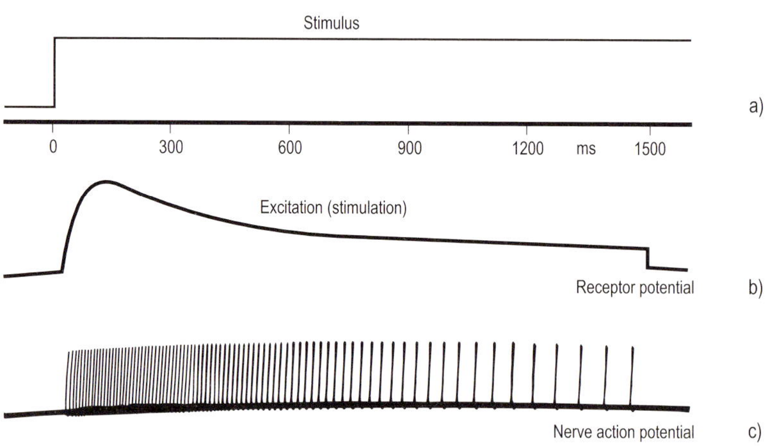

Figure 1.13
The receptor potential **(b)** and the number of nerve action potentials **(c)** as a result of stimulation **(a)**

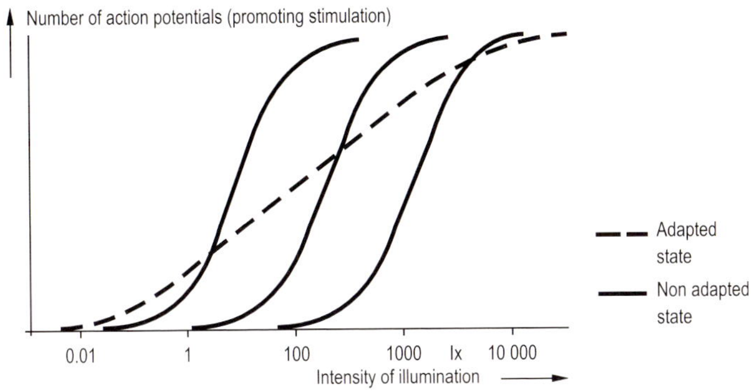

Figure 1.14
If one plots the value of the initial overshoot as a function of the stimulus strength, one obtains the dynamic characteristics (intensity functions) of the receptor (non adapted state). Entering the steady state values gives the static characteristics (adapted state). These are identical to the measurements of König and Brodhum. It can be seen that at the beginning of the adaptation process the characteristics steeply ascends, i.e. the contrast sensitivity improves. In this way the eye is able to detect 485 difference steps as opposed to 35 originally. The improvement shows the real importance of adaptation (from Ranke [1.1]).

amount of light which enters the eye is reduced. The pupil then dilates automatically, in conjunction with the process of accommodation. As previously indicated, adaptation must be understood as the eye's adjustment to the available brightness. Thus if one plots the intensity of nervous excitation as a function of the logarithm of the light intensity, the set of graphs shown in fig. 1.14 is obtained. It shows the relevant function as a function of brightness without adaptation and with adaptation (the latter is illustrated by the unbroken lines). The eye's contrast sensitivity is greatest where the curves are steepest. The figure shows clearly that by means of adaptation the contrast sensitivity is adjusted to the average brightness. The transition from one level of adaptation to another follows a particular pattern in time. This is illustrated in fig. 1.15 and shows that at least two processes must be involved. The first part of the curve corresponds to the adaptation of the rods, the second to that of the cones. The two together result in the shape of the curve. As already shown, visual acuity depends on the grid size of the photosensitive cells on the retina. Only at the spot where vision is sharpest, the so-called macula lutea, does every sensory cell have a nerve fiber leading away from it, and thus only here is the maximum visual acuity found. At all other places on the retina several sensory cells are connected to one nerve cell in order to improve the light yield. This group of sensory cells is called a receptive field. The field's peripheral elements generally have an inhibitive function, with the result that a stimulated central part comes to be surrounded by an inhibiting ring, enhancing the contrast. As the intensity of light diminishes the inhibiting ring gets narrower and narrower, i.e. the receptive field becomes larger and thus visual acuity progressively deteriorates. A very great decrease in visual acuity also occurs during the transition from cone vision to rod vision as a consequence of dark adaptation, caused by the lack of rods in the

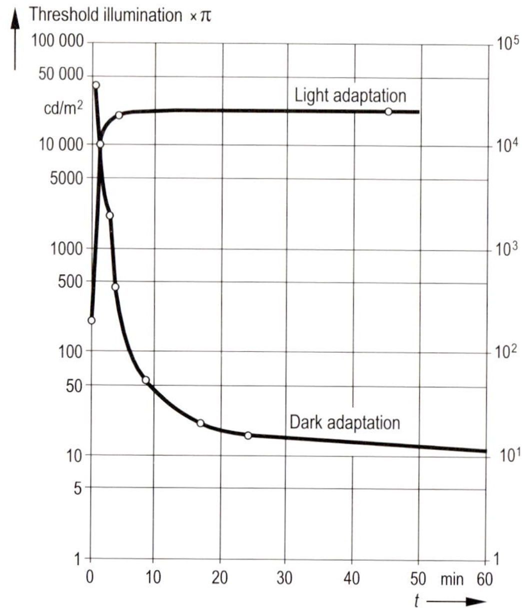

Figure 1.15
Dark-adaptation and light adaptation curves of the human eye measured with the Engelking adaptometer, with the threshold illumination (threshold stimulus intensity) along the *y* axis and the time elapsed after the initial change in illumination along the *x* axis. Notice the break in the dark-adaptation curve which is determined by the completion of the cones' adaptation (extra curve plotted). Evidence for the duplicity theory of visioning.

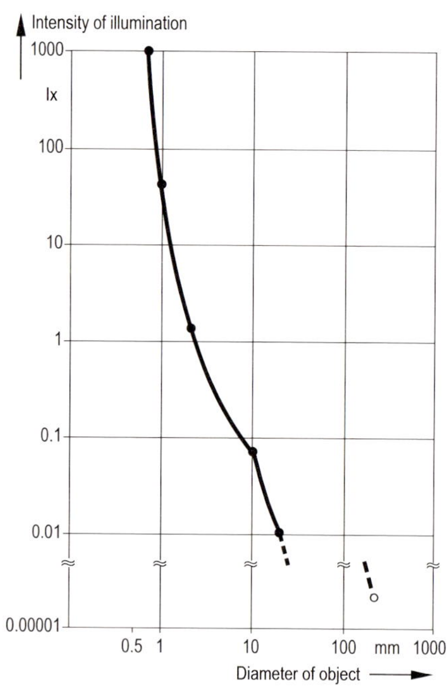

Figure 1.16
Curve of equal sensation of brightness. According to Ricco's law, in the area of low illumination the same experience of brightness does not correspond to radiation intensity, but to the product of intensity and test field size. This dependence on the test field diameter has a strong effect on visual acuity as shown in the figure. The break in the curve again corresponds to the transition from cone to rod vision. Distance of object 6 m, diameter of object in mm.

macula lutea. Thus the brightness of an object is also determined by its diameter. Fig. 1.16 illustrates this relationship between light intensity and object diameter.

1.4.5 Sensitivity to color

It is known empirically that the rods are responsible for the monochromatic light-dark sensitivity whilst the cones are responsible for color perception [1.14, 1.8]. The perception thresholds for the various colors can be read off from the graph in fig. 1.17, which shows the spectral sensitivity of individual rods and cones. The threshold energy indicated in fig. 1.17 is necessary in order to bring about the process of chemical decomposition of the visual purple. This relationship is consistent with the theory of color vision proposed by Helmholtz. This describes the presence of three different kinds of color receptors having maximum sensitivity in the red, yellow-green and green-blue bands of the light spectrum respectively. The individual color components

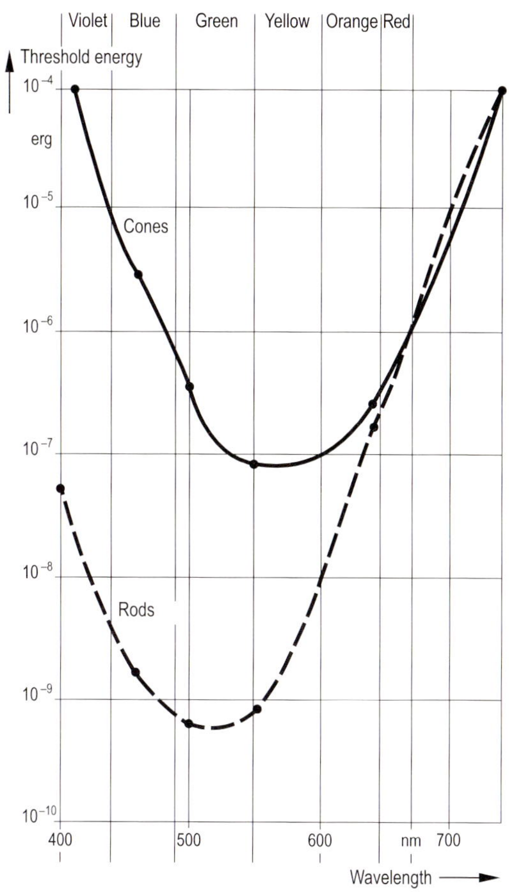

Figure 1.17
Graphs of threshold intensities of monochromatic light for the human eye. The lower graph relates to scotopic (rod) vision, the upper graph to photopic (cone) vision. The absolute threshold (with the eye completely adapted, at a wavelength of 507 nm in the yellow-green region) has a value of $1.3\text{-}2.6 \cdot 10^{-10}$ erg (plotted according to measurements by Trendelenburg [1.1]).

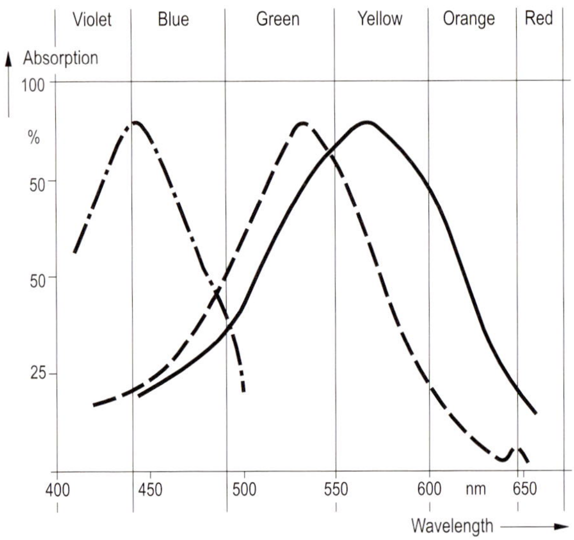

Figure 1.18
Young-Helmholtz three component theory of color vision. This assumes that there are three receptor substances which exhibit the displayed rates of absorption (*y* axis) for various wavelengths of light (*x* axis). The strongest evidence for this theory is the clinical observation of protanopia (malfunction of the first receptor (blue) red-green blindness or red-green deficiency), deuteranopia (second receptor, green) and tritanopia (third receptor, yellow). The spectral sensitivity of the human eye is in agreement with this representation.

are mixed in various ways to produce the familiar experiences of color. About 10 million shades of color can be distinguished. It should also be mentioned that equally intense stimulation of all three color components leads to the experience of white – or, if the stimulation is less, the various shades of gray. Following on from this, Granit has developed a second hypothesis of color perception in which he proposes that the experience of color is due to both stimulation and inhibition of the particular color receptors. Thus, inhibition will always yield the complementary color of the color receptors stimulated. This has a great impact on color contrast, since lateral enhancement and inhibition also apply to color perception. The eye's spectral sensitivity as shown in fig. 1.18 therefore only applies to large illuminated areas of the retina, in which the neural connections to neighboring cells do not play a role.

1.4.6 Temporal resolution

Absence of flicker (fusion frequency)

Talbot was able to establish that two flashes of light lead to a single sensory experience if the time period between them is so short that the impulses provoked by the first stimulus have not decreased by more than 10 percent by the time the second stimulus is given. Because of this, it is possible to show the eye series of individual

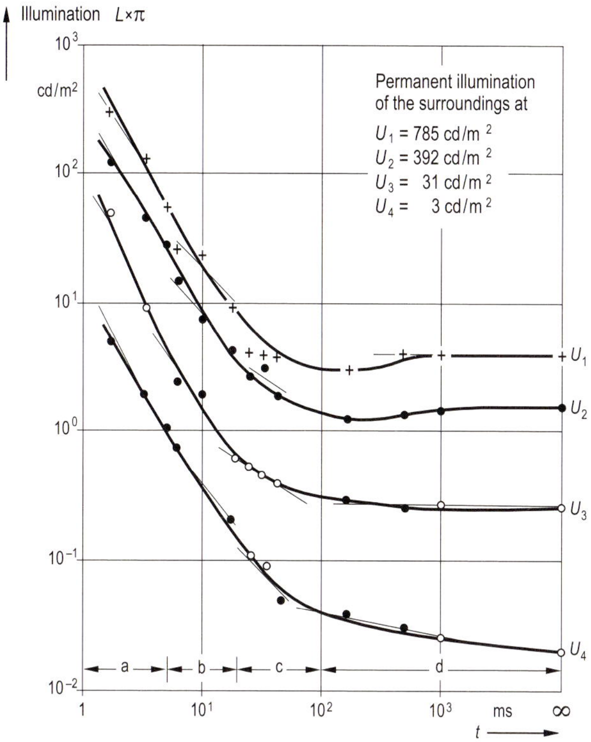

Figure 1.19
Curves of equal sensation of brightness as a consequence of the human eye's delayed response to brightness. The curves represent equal intensity sensation corresponding to permanent illumination with the specified luminance of surroundings (3 to 785 cd/m²). If the period of illumination is reduced (x axis), the intensity of illumination must be increased. The relationship is nonlinear. In region **a)** the quantities are related by $Lt^2 = k$, in region **b)** by $Lt = k$, in region **c)** for higher values of the luminance of the surroundings the relationship is $Lt_0 = k$, for lower values this only holds in region **d)**. Generally one has $Lt = f(t)$. Taking the average one arrives at a value of 50 ms for the response time of the human eye at average illumination intensities (according to Commichau [1.15]).

pictures which are experienced as continuously moving pictures, as in the cinema. The necessary frequency is about 16 to 26 pictures a second; it depends on the overall level of brightness and on the angle made with the optical axis. This is because the sensory cells on the periphery of the retina react more quickly to stimulation than the ones in the center. In addition, as fig. 1.19 shows, the delayed response to brightness is determined by the state of adaptation, which means that even fairly slow series of pictures merge into a smoothly moving picture if seen in a state of dark adaptation. Such a dependence of the temporal resolving power of the eye on the average intensity of the surrounding light is of great importance in the presentation of cinematographic images.

Integration time (response time) τ

Electrophysiological investigations have shown that, when the eye is illuminated, the neural excitation E caused by the decomposition of visual purple (see Sect. [1.4.1]) [1.8] increases exponentially according to the formula $E = 1 - e^{t/T}$ [1.13] and decreases according to the formula $E = -e^{t/T'}$. The time constants T and T' are of the same order of magnitude. After the time $t = 3T$, the degree of excitation reaches 95% of its final value, a value at which perception is practically complete. In about the same length of time $t = 3T'$ the stimulation has decayed. The integration time $\tau \approx 3T \approx 3T'$ is the length of time from the start of the stimulation up to attaining full perception, or alternatively from the termination of the light stimulus up to the cessation of the perception. The integration time τ depends upon the state of adaptation, the intensity of the light stimulus and the amount of visual purple available. The latter can be assumed to be constant in the healthy eye. τ can take values from 100 to 300 ms in the dark-adapted (scotopic) eye and from 15 to 100 ms in the light-adapted (photopic) eye.

Movement threshold

Closely connected with the response time and the decay time is the ability of the eye to perceive motion. For the experience of motion to occur the stimulation of a cone must have decreased by more than 10% of its total by the time the stimulation of the neighboring cone reaches its maximum. Apart from the decay rate of the degree of stimulation (which depends on the intensity of the illumination), the spatial threshold naturally plays an important role in relation to the movement threshold.

1.5 Neural processing

1.5.1 Anatomy of the visual pathway

Impulses from the retinal photoreceptors are led to the cerebral cortex by way of the path shown in fig. 1.20 (which includes several switching centers). Corresponding connections between the nerve fibers result in the above-mentioned receptive fields, which become more and more complex as the visual pathway progresses. The receptive field neurons located in the cortex are finally able to recognize objects independently of their location and orientation in space (constancy of visual objects). All these mechanisms provide the neural basis for the "perception of form."

1.5.2 Three-dimensional vision

The visual pathways of both eyes reach the visual centers in the cerebral cortex both directly and crossed over. Impulses from both eyes therefore enter both halves of the cerebral cortex. The image is of course somewhat different in the two eyes according to whether an object lies in front of the observed point object (fixation point) or behind it. As can be seen from the diagram (fig. 1.21), near points on an object give rise to a bitemporally displaced image (displaced on both sides towards the temples). Points further away on the other hand produce binasally displaced image points (i.e.

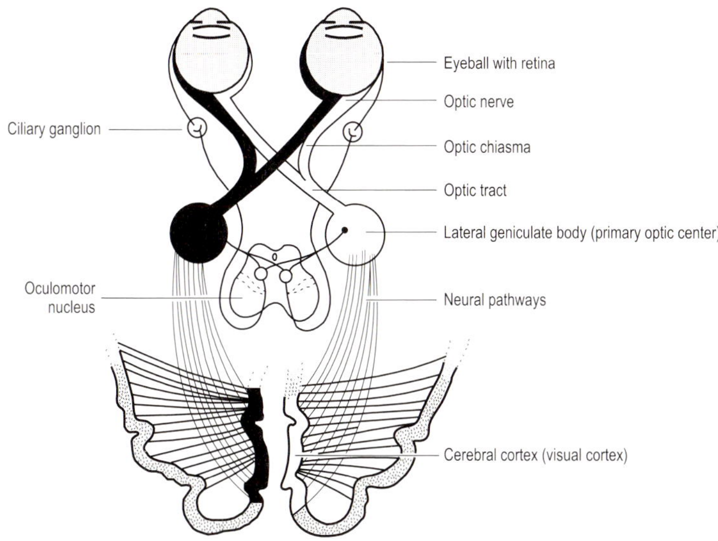

Figure 1.20
Diagram of the visual pathway. Left visual field back, right visual field white.
The nerve pathways are indicated by lines.

displaced on both sides towards the nose). Information about the displacement (binocular disparity) [1.1] is processed by the nerve cells in the visual cortex to give an impression of distance. Such an impression always relates to the point object actually focused on. The point object lies on the horopter plane, the geometrical locus of all point objects which, given a constant degree of accommodation, form a sharp image in the eye.

1.5.3 Depth perception

In the previous section the horopter plane for a fixed degree of accommodation was described. This corresponds to a fixed convergence angle, i.e. a fixed angle between the two optical axes. What two-dimensional shape the horopter plane takes at varying distances from the eye has not yet been established. Investigations by Kienle [1.19] and Hensel [1.20] indicate that the perception of size and the related constancy of visual objects depend on the shape of the horopter plane. In physiology, the constancy of visual objects means the recognition of the size of known objects irrespective of their distance from the eye. In the case of three-dimensional vision this causes the difficulty that on a two-dimensional surface a spatial image is produced in which the individual image points are no longer in accordance with the natural proportions.

1.5.4 Optical illusions

Neuronal connection and visual memory play an important role in image processing. Thus the eye is able to recognize known image patterns quickly and to classify them correctly irrespective of their size, position and intensity of illumination. Even in the case of incomplete information patterns, it is always complete pictures which are seen. Such complementary neural processes can lead to considerable illusions [1.17] and mistaken interpretations of reality. Fig. 1.22 gives an example of this; it shows in particular how the interpretation of the observed object is influenced by information about its surroundings [1.18].

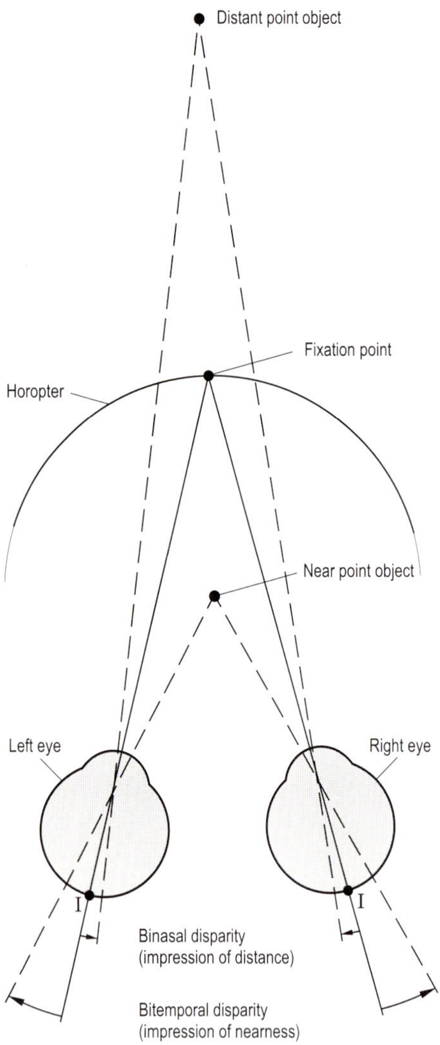

Figure 1.21
Principle of three-dimensional vision. Whilst convergence and accommodation of the eyes are aligned on a point on the horopter, the light rays from a near or distant object also form images which are laterally displaced in relation to the identical points *I* on the retina. This displacement (binocular disparity) is binasal in the case of distant objects and bitemporal in the case of near objects and is interpreted in the brain so as to give three-dimensional perception.

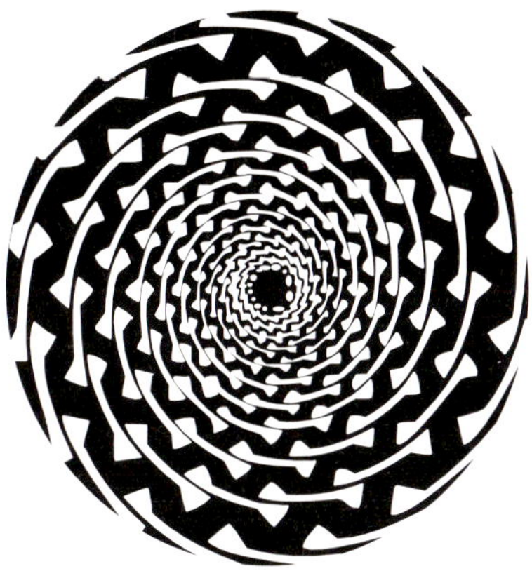

Figure 1.22
An optical illusion of the second kind. The concentric circles are seen as arithmetic spirals. This is a consequence of the oblique shading of the circles themselves and the sloping of the shading in relation to the radial-oriented background pattern. The example shows the influence of the surroundings on perception.

1.5.5 Visual memory

Afterimages

When a bright ray of light stimulates an area of the retina, visual purple is broken down at that point. When the illumination has finished the impulses produced die away gradually because of the prolonged decay time leaving behind a positive afterimage. On the other hand, fewer impulses are produced at the retina by the breakdown products of the visual purple when looking at a white wall, and the afterimage is therefore a negative one. Such afterimages are also features of color perception; in this case a negative afterimage always appears in the complementary color.

Short-term memory

Inside the higher processing centers there also exists an after-excitation (postexcitation effect) or continuation of the pattern of impulses, so that pictures can still be perceived up to several seconds later. This phenomenon, which is very marked in persons with photographic memory, is the short-term visual memory. It disappears after a short time but in certain circumstances causes the generation of memory contents which are distinctive in that they can, if necessary, be transformed into a consciously recognizable picture. The whole process is based upon a re-coding of impulse patterns into chemical changes located in the brain (long-term memory).

Recognition

In ways which still have not been investigated, the representation of an image causes the corresponding image pattern (stored in the long-term memory) to be transformed into a pattern of stimulation which, when compared with the new image, is recognized as being identical to it. Such recognition of images from the past is possible irrespective of other environmental parameters.

The nature of the images thus formed in the imagination has not yet been elucidated even though they appear to correlate with electrophysiological measurements [1.21].

1.6 References

[1.1] W.D. Keidel
Sinnesphysiologie
Heidelberger Taschenbücher, Bd. 97
Springer-Verlag, Berlin Heidelberg New York 1971

[1.2] W.D. Keidel
Kurzgefasstes Lehrbuch der Physiologie, 4. Aufl.
Georg Thieme Verlag, Stuttgart 1975

[1.3] W. Finkelnburg
Einführung in die Atomphysik
Springer-Verlag, Berlin Göttingen Heidelberg 1964

[1.4] J.W. Rohen
Handbuch der mikroskopischen Anatomie, Bd 3/4
Springer- Verlag, 1964

[1.5] W. Trendelenburg
Lehrbuch der Physiologie, 2. Aufl.
Springer-Verlag, Berlin Göttingen Heidelberg 1961

[1.6] Th. Graff
Die Akkommodation beim Sehen durch das Nahbrillenglas
Mbl. Augenheilkunde 121 (1952), 205

[1.7] M.G.F. Fuortes
Physiology of photoreceptor organs
in Handbook of sensory physiology, Vol. VII/2
Springer-Verlag, Berlin Heidelberg New York 1972

[1.8] H.J.A. Dartnall
Photochemistry of vision
in Handbook of sensory physiology, Vol. VII/1
Springer-Verlag, Berlin Heidelberg New York

[1.9] G. Baumgartner
Physiologie des zentralen Sehsystems
in Sehen Sinnesphysiologie III, S. 276 und 277.
Urban & Schwarzenberg, München Wien Baltimore 1978

[1.10] A. Gebauer, J. Lissner, O. Schott
Das Röntgenfernsehen, 2. Aufl.
Georg Thieme Verlag, Stuttgart 1974

[1.11] O.F. Ranke
Sinnesorgane
in G. Lehmann (Hrsg): Handbuch der gesamten Arbeitsmedizin, Bd. 1
Urban & Schwarzenberg, München Berlin 1961

[1.12] G. Stange
Rankes Streulichttheorie bei Blendung
Z. f. Verkehrssicherheit 9 (1963), 50

[1.13] W. Keidel
Rankes Adaptionstheorie.
Z. f. Biol. 112 (1961), 411-425

[1.14] W. Starkiewicz
Physiologische Grundlagen der Helligkeits- und Farbempfindungen.
VEB Georg Thieme, Leipzig 1970

[1.15] R. Commichau
Adaptionszustand und Unterschieds-Schwellenenergie für Lichtblitze
Z. f. Biol. 108 (1956), 145-160

[1.16] W. Rohen
Funktionelle Anatomie des Nervensystems
K.F. Schattauer Verlag, Stuttgart New York 1976

[1.17] H. Schober
Das Sehen.
Fachbuchverlag, Leipzig 1958

[1.18] L. Zusne
Visual perception of form.
Academic Press, New York London 1970

[1.19] G. Kienle
Wahrnehmungsstörung und die nicht euklidische Struktur des Sehraums
Georg Thieme Verlag, Stuttgart 1968

[1.20] H. Hensel
Allgemeine Sinnesphysiologie. Hautsinne, Geschmack, Geruch.
Springer-Verlag, Berlin Heidelberg New York 1966

[1.21] E. David (Hrsg.)
Grundlagen der Sportphysiologie
Perimed-Verlag, Erlangen 1986

2 Subjective assessment of image quality

2.1 Introduction

The fundamental requirement for an effective medical diagnosis based on images is that the signs of a disease or an injury are clearly visible. This property may be referred to as visualization capability or image quality of the applied imaging method.

Image quality can be objectively assessed by quantifying the physical parameters of the underlying image process or subjectively, simply by visual inspection and characterization of details in the image. Since the latter method is dependant on the individual observer stochastic methods have to be employed in order to come to representative conclusions. Imaging of phantoms with standardized details has been proven useful.

2.2 ROC Methology

Receiver operating characteristic (ROC) curve analysis is a tool applied to compare the diagnostic abilities of different diagnostic modalities. It assesses how well a certain diagnostic test discriminates between positive and negative results.

In an ROC test observers have to decide whether or not a detail (tumour, injury, phantom detail ...) is present in an image. There are four different outcomes for such a binary test commonly comprised in a 2×2 decision matrix:

	Detail really present	**Detail really absent**
Detail diagnosed as present	True Positive (*TP*)	False Postive (*FP*)
Detail diagnosed as absent	False Negative (*FN*)	True Negative (*TN*)

The sum $TP + FP + FN + TN$ is equal to the total number of cases in the study population. Notice that in order to fill in the matrix entries the 'truth' needs to be known. Hence, ROC studies on patients require independent confirmation of the 'true' diagnosis, e.g. based on biopsy tests, long-term follow-up, etc.

For the comparison of different studies the following quantities derived from the individual matrix element have proven useful:

Sensitivity is the probability that a detail present is correctly detected by the observer:

$$Sensitivity = \frac{Number\ of\ true\ positive\ decisions}{Number\ of\ actually\ positive\ cases} = \frac{TP}{TP + FN} \tag{2.1}$$

A synonym for sensitivity is true-positive fraction *TPF*.

The counterpart of sensitivity is specificity, which is the probability that a detail not present is correctly interpreted:

$$Specificity = \frac{Number\ of\ true\ negative\ decisions}{Number\ of\ actually\ negative\ cases} = \frac{TN}{FP + TN} \quad (2.2)$$

The specificity is sometimes also called true-negative fraction *TNF*.

A medical test for a disease having a high sensitivity but a low specificity means that in fact many cases are diagnosed correctly. However, also many cases will have been falsely assigned to the disease causing unnecessary or even harmful treatment.

In addition to eq. (2.1) and (2.2) two other performance indices, the false-positive fraction *FPF* and the false negative fraction *FNF*, are defined:

$$FPF = 1 - TNF = \frac{Number\ of\ false\ positive\ decisions}{Number\ of\ actually\ negative\ cases} = \frac{FP}{FP + TN} \quad (2.3)$$

$$FNF = 1 - TPF = \frac{Number\ of\ false\ negative\ decisions}{Number\ of\ actually\ positive\ cases} = \frac{FN}{TP + FN} \quad (2.4)$$

All quantities defined in eq. (2.1-2.4) are dimensionless with values in the range between zero and unity.

When the same test, e.g. looking for lesions in images, is performed by many observers, the result will be different for each observer. Plotting the individual pairs of true-positive fraction (sensitivity) and false-positive fraction in a diagram, this results in the so called receiver operating characteristic (ROC) curve (fig. 2.1) [2.1]. To obtain an ROC curve not necessarily several observers are required, a single person repeating the test several times may produce a comparable result. In order to get curve values also in the lower left (low values for *TPF* and *FPF*) and in the upper right (high values for *TPF* and *FPF*) the receiver might be asked to change his decision strategy, e.g. to be a little bit more or less critical.

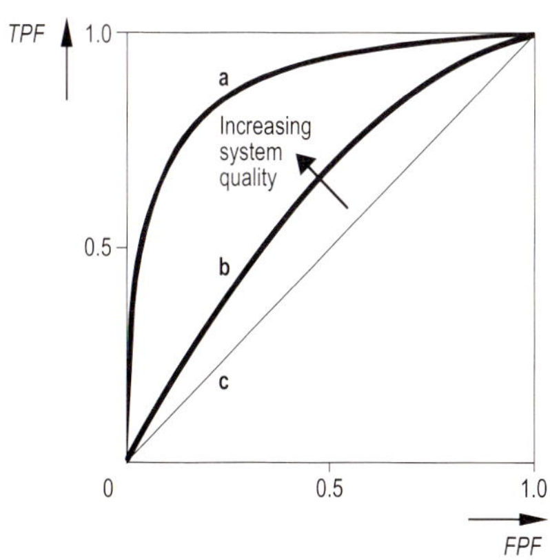

Figure 2.1
ROC diagrams for different hypothetical imaging systems: System **(a)** is better than system **(b)** for the specified imaging task. The diagonal line **(c)** denotes the lower limit of diagnostic performance, where decisions were done purely randomly. No diagnostic information can be obtained in this case.

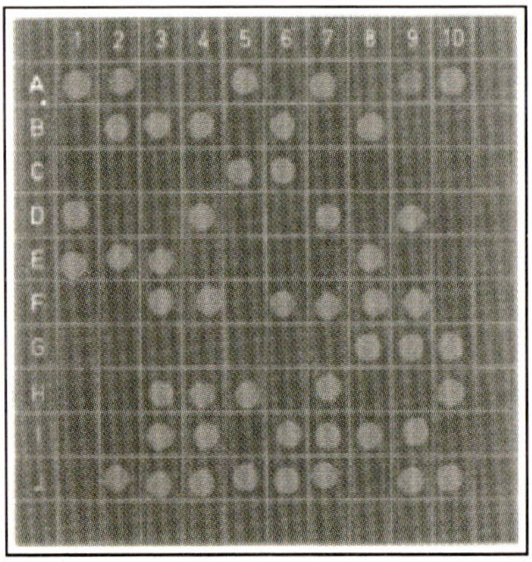

Figure 2.2
Image of an ROC phantom for X-ray systems: 50% of the fields have details inside (in this case Al discs of constant thickness and size).

ROC analysis provides a means to compare different imaging methods. An imaging method producing a diagonal i.e. as many true positive cases as false positive cases works at random and is useless. High values for the true-positive fraction and low values for the false-positive fraction are desired.

A simple model for obtaining an ROC curve is shown in fig. 2.2. 50% of the fields in a chequerboard phantom are occupied statistically with test objects of identical size and contrast. The human observer's task consists in deciding for each phantom cell whether or not an object is present inside. In this way e.g. it can be checked if image quality of an X-ray system has changed over time.

2.3 Contrast detail resolution

The detectability of individual details in images is governed by the combined effect of contrast, blur, and noise. As is demonstrated in fig. 2.3, in a noisy image large details

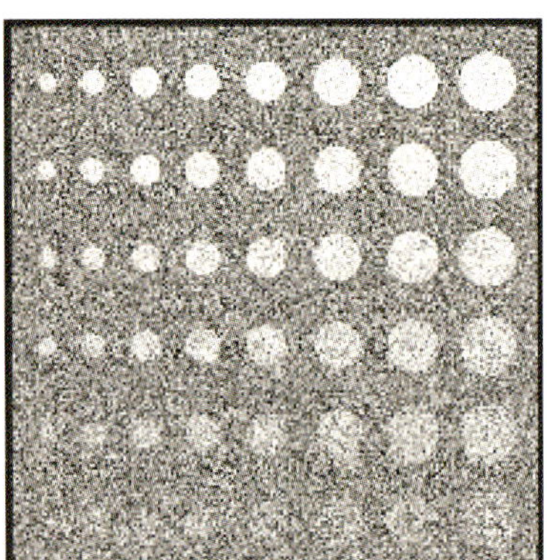

Figure 2.3
Simulation of a contrast-detail diagram by arranging objects in a rectangular matrix according to their physical contrast and their size and superposing noise

with low contrast can be easier recognized than small ones. It turns out that the quantity

$$\frac{C\,D}{N} \approx \text{const} \tag{2.5}$$

D: Object diameter, *C*: Contrast resolution, *N*: Noise level

for a wide range of object diameters is independent of the spatial resolution in the image [2.2].

The minimum recognizable contrast in an image with respect to the background is referred to as contrast resolution. Contrast resolution as function of detail size is a quality parameter of imaging systems that is evaluated with aid of contrast detail phantoms. These are designed for a specific imaging modality (X-ray, CT, MR ...) and consist of objects (e.g. discs) with different sizes that give various contrast levels when imaged. Plotting the contrast of the disc still just being visible as function of its diameter gives the contrast-detail diagram. Fig. 2.4 compares two CT scanners at different noise levels (characterized by the dose). The limiting value at small object sizes corresponds to the spatial resolution of the system. Contrast resolution for larger objects is independent of the spatial resolution of the scanner.

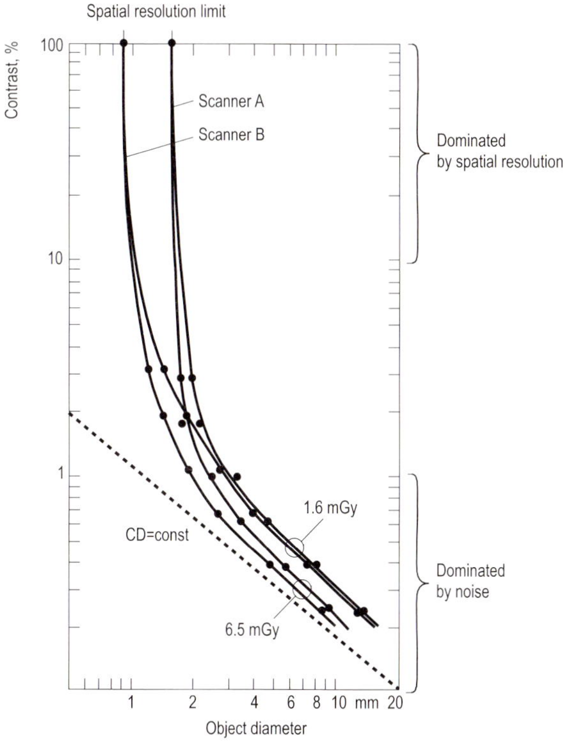

Figure 2.4
Contrast detail diagram comparing two CT scanners at different noise (dose) levels [2.3]. The *CD* = const line is given for comparison.

2.4 References

[2.1] C.E. Metz
ROC Methodology in Radiologic Imaging
Investigative Radiology 21 (1986), 720

[2.2] A. Rose
Vision: Human and Electronic
Plenum Press, New York 1973

[2.3] W.A. Kalender.
Computed Tomography
Publicis Corporate Publishing, Erlangen 2005

3 Image rendering

Modern imaging techniques like computed tomography (CT) or magnetic resonance tomography (MRT) produce an immense amount of data requiring advanced visualization techniques in order to process and display especially volumetric data. An example is the generation of multi-slice cardiac CT volumes at different heart phases, ranging from end-diastolic to end-systolic phase. Thus, in this chapter the basics of image rendering (or visualization) are introduced, and different possibilities of tomographic volume visualization techniques are discussed.

3.1 2D imaging

Before the introduction of 3D visualization techniques, which are becoming more and more important in the daily clinical routine, some basics of the standard 2D slice-based visualization have to be entailed.

The term zoom describes the possibility to scale up and down the image size which becomes necessary whenever the field of view of the image is not at optimum. The pan mode is mostly combined with the zooming mode and allows the translation of the image of interest. In most cases, this mode moves the center of the view rectangle to the current pointer position (e.g. of a mouse).

The ability to window is a necessary feature of all digital images. Windowing is the process of selecting some segment of the total pixel value range by the definition of a center and a window width (the wide dynamic range of the receptors) and then displaying the pixel values within that segment over the full brightness range from white to black. It is important to point out that contrast will be visible only for the pixel values that are within the selected window. All pixel values that are either below or above the window will be all white or all black and display no contrast. The person controlling the display can adjust both the center and the width of the window. The combination of these two parameters determines the range of pixel values that will be displayed with contrast in the image. A reason for that is based on the fact that standard computer display systems are only capable of displaying 8 bit grey values. Standard CT images for example contain grey values that are coded with 12 bit. Therefore, users have to reduce the information in order to visualize the data.

3.2 Planar reformation

Slice-based visualization of tomographic volume is still most important, when radiologists analyze image data.

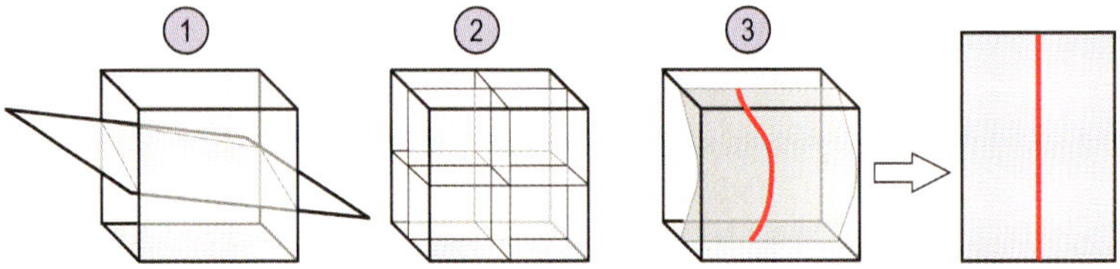

Figure 3.1
Planar reformatting techniques: the first image displays an arbitrary cut through the volume. The second one explains the MPR technique and the third image shows the curved MPR

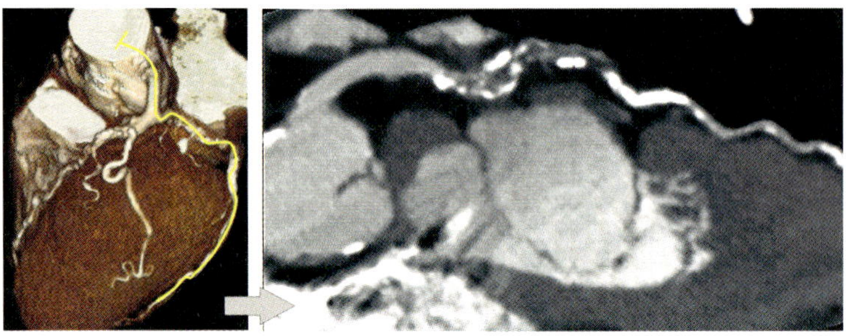

Figure 3.2 A curved MPR example is presented by the display of a coronary artery

Planar reformation (fig. 3.1) describes the possibility to cut the original stack of slices by arbitrary planes. In the first image in fig. 3.1 such a scenario is presented. A special case of this is orthogonal multi-planar-reformation (MPR), which is presented in the second image of fig. 3.1. Whenever the user moves the mouse in the 3D volume, three planes are cut off the volume whereby all three planes are orthogonal to each other.

In the third image, a special visualization is presented, which is referred as curved MPR. This type of rendering technique is often applied to volumes that contain vascular structures and straightens an arbitrary curve through the patient. In fig. 3.2 this technique is applied to a cardiac volume, whereas a coronary artery is straightened via a curved MPR. As can be seen from the image, a more detailed investigation of the vessel is possible.

A more detailed description of different planar reformation techniques is presented in [3.1].

3.3 Segmentation

In the analysis of the objects in tomographic images it is essential that we can distinguish between the objects of interest and "the rest". This latter group is also referred to as background. The techniques that are used to find the objects of interest are usually called segmentation techniques – segmenting the foreground from the background. However, in the context of medical images there is a variety of different types of applications and in consequence there is an even larger variety of different segmentation algorithms. For example, isolating the 3D heart from the rest of a 3D cardiac CT volume requires other algorithms than the extraction of the human brain from a 3D MRI volume. In addition, it is important to understand that:

- there is no universally applicable segmentation technique that will work for all images, and,
- no segmentation technique is perfect.

An outline of different segmentation techniques is illustrated in [3.2].

3.4 Surface rendering

Surface rendering (or indirect volume rendering) techniques do not process the whole volume data for visualization purposes. Contrary to direct methods (see 3.5) certain user-relevant information such as homogeneous regions of similar or equal attributes is extracted in a sometimes time-consuming pre-processing step. Such information reduction requires segmentation techniques (3.3). The data of interest will then be represented by polygonal surfaces, which can be visualized in an efficient manner by the use of hardware acceleration on standard graphics adapters. The classic example is a triangular representation of isosurfaces. In fig. 3.3, the ventricular system of a brain phantom is shown as an example. The image on the left shows the final rendering result. The image on the right displays the triangle mesh.

3.4.1 Extraction of isosurfaces and the marching-cubes algorithm

In order to extract isosurfaces, the most popular way is by the application of the marching-cubes algorithm that has been developed by Lorensen et al. [3.3]. In this algorithm the data volume is divided into a grid of cells, each cell consisting of 8 neighboring voxels. The user has to specify a threshold value that separates voxel values above from those below the threshold of the isosurface to be generated. In each grid cell that contains voxel values both above and below the threshold, polygons are generated connecting the interpolated points on the edges with the threshold value.

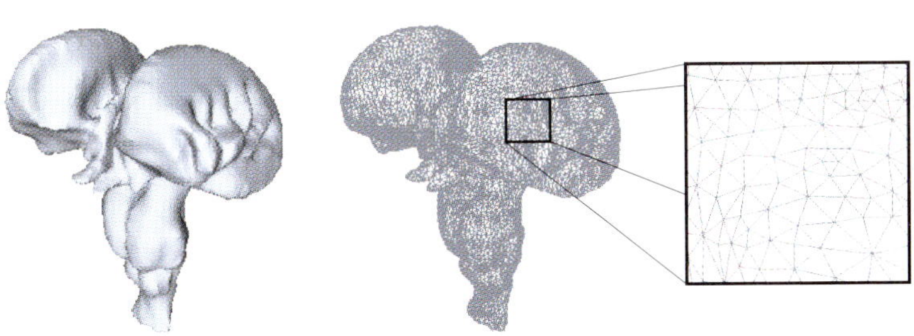

Figure 3.3 Visualization of an isosurface by the use of a triangle mesh representation

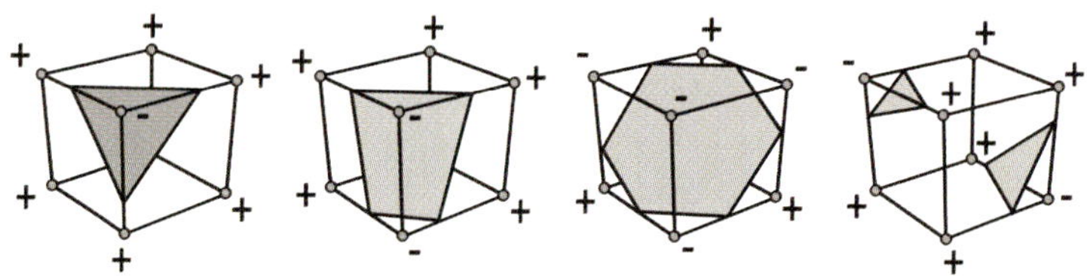

Figure 3.4
The images show four of the 15 possible intersection cases of the marching-cubes algorithm.

Each of the cell's 8 vertices can be either above or below the isosurface value, thus, there are $2^8 = 256$ possible ways in which a surface can intersect the cell. By symmetry these 256 ways can be reduced to 15 (fig. 3.4). Thus, the complete isosurface can be generated by elementary triangular planes that are obtained dividing the polygons in the single cells into triangles. Although the marching-cubes algorithm is often applied in order to extract triangular isosurfaces that can be efficiently rendered by the graphics hardware, a drawback of the method is the immense amount of polygons. Among those are very small and narrow triangles which can be removed with small loss of image and geometry quality.

3.5 Volume rendering

Volume rendering (or direct volume rendering) approaches map the scalar value of each sample point of a volume data set to physical quantities, describing the emission (color) and the absorption (opacity) of light. This mapping, also called classification, can be realized by the use of a transfer-function [3.4] that has to be set by the user, and which will be discussed in detail in 3.6. Also traditional rendering techniques such as MIP (maximum intensity projection) or SSD (surface shaded display) belong to this group of rendering algorithms. Their basics will be discussed in 3.5.3.

At first, we start by the introduction of the basic techniques of direct volume rendering techniques.

3.5.1 Image-order techniques

Taking into account every pixel on the image plane, a ray is sent into the volume data, and the final color of the pixel is calculated by integrating the emission/absorption values of each voxel of the data volume that is hit by the ray (fig. 3.5). The classic example is the ray-casting algorithm. Herein, the pixel's color value is defined by equidistantly resampling the volume along the ray using interpolation, and by mapping those values to emission-absorption coefficients [3.5]. Examples of standard implementations of such algorithms are proposed by Kajiya et al. [3.6] and Drebin et al. [3.7]. Since the voxel traversal has to be recalculated for each user interaction, high computational ef-

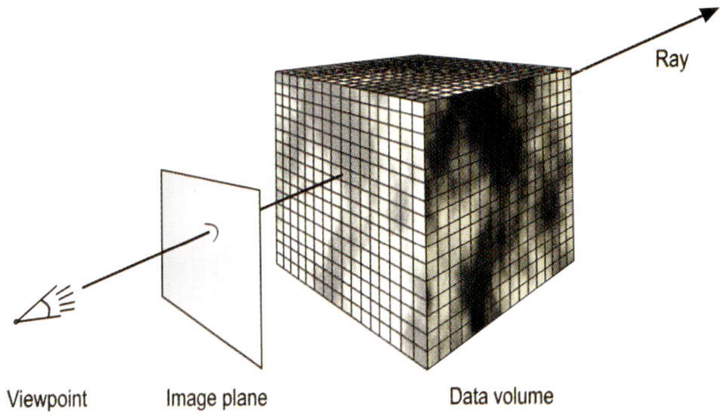

Figure 3.5
The image shows the basics of image-order techniques. A ray is sent from the viewpoint onto the image plane, whereby each ray traverses the data volume.

fort has to be invested. Therefore, different techniques for the reduction of computational costs have been introduced.

For acceleration purposes, Kajiya et al. used the early-ray termination that aborts the integration of emission/absorption values when the opacity reaches a value of one. Other examples for acceleration techniques are space-leaping [3.8], which excludes

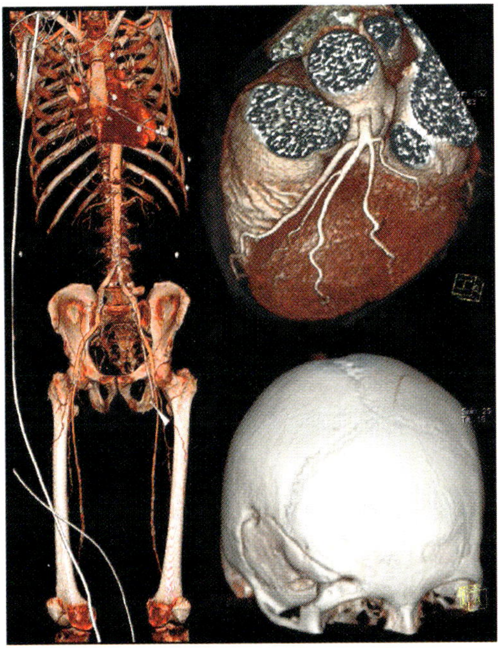

Figure 3.6
The image displays different visualizations of a human skeleton, a human heart and a human skull by the application of a ray-casting implementation (courtesy by Dept. of Neuroradiology, University of Erlangen-Nuremberg).

empty voxels during integration and hierarchical methods that progressively subdivide the volume, while rays are sent through the volume [3.9, 3.10].

Although ray-casting techniques are the chosen method for high quality images (fig. 3.6), computational costs caused by the large number of necessary interpolations for volume resampling demand a lot of calculation power.

3.5.2 Object-order techniques and the shear-warp-factorization

Contrary to image-order algorithms, object-order techniques start in object space and calculate a single voxel's contribution to a pixel on the image plane in recursive order. A famous example of this technique is the splatting-algorithm proposed by Westover et al. [3.11], where each voxel is interpreted as a radially symmetric kernel which is projected onto the image plane (splat). The final pixel's color on the image plane is composed by the contribution of all splats that hit this pixel.

A hybrid form of image-order and object-order techniques is the shear-warp-factorization proposed by Lacroute et al. [3.12]. The viewing transformation, which mathematically describes the relation between the viewer and the object (volume data) is decomposed into a shear transformation in 3D, a parallel projective mapping leading to a distorted intermediate image and a final 2D warping step for calculating the correct resulting image (fig. 3.7). The main advantage of the method is the interpolative reduction from trilinear to bilinear by cleverly placing the original sample points onto the image slices which eases the calculation immensely. In order to allow for perspective projection, an additional scaling of the image slices has to be introduced. As an example, fig. 3.8 (left) presents a rendering example.

Although this method reduces the interpolation costs, a drawback is the need for three copies of the volume in memory, one slice stack for each main slicing direction (x-, y-, z-direction). Depending on the angle between viewing direction and slicing normal, the correct slice stack has to be selected.

Another drawback is the slice artifacts that can arise due to this shear-warp visualization technique. Fig. 3.8 (right) shows such an example.

However, because of its rendering efficiency, the basic ideas of the shear-warp-factorization are adopted in 3.8 in the context of hardware-based volume rendering.

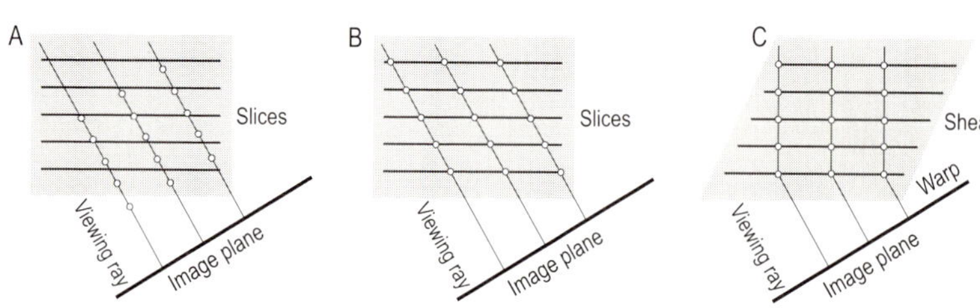

Figure 3.7 Principle of the shear-warp-factorization in conjunction with parallel projection

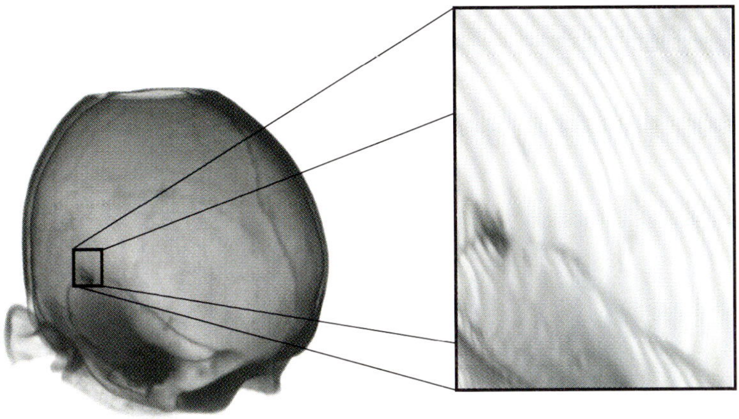

Figure 3.8
An example of the shear-warp-algorithm **(left)**: slice-artifacts generated by the algorithm **(right)** (courtesy by Dept. of Neuroradiology, University of Erlangen-Nuremberg)

3.5.3 Compositing

In the previous sections, the basic techniques in order to create 2D projections of 3D volumes have been introduced. Rays that are casted from the viewing point through the volume traverse different voxels along the viewing ray. These voxels determine the color of the pixels on the image according to e.g. an emission/absorption model. Alternatives are e.g. maximum or mean value along the ray. So the term compositing [3.4] is now introduced, which specifies, how each traversed voxel contributes to the final image pixels.

Fig. 3.9 presents different compositing possibilities that are often applied in the topic of medical volume visualization.

First of all, maximum intensity projection (MIP) detects the maximum value of all voxels along the viewing ray and sets the final pixel value on the image plane to this maximum value. Therefore, MIP is often applied in the context of the visualization of contrast enhanced vessels. In fig. 3.10 (left) such a scenario is presented, showing contrast enhanced vessels with MIP.

Alternatively to the maximum value along the viewing ray, also the mean intensity can be assigned to the final pixel value on the image plane, which then averages the projected voxels. Moreover, further different possibilities for compositing are thinkable such as the occurrence of the first local maximum or of a certain user-defined isovalue. In consequence, this provides an alternative possibility in order to create isosurface visualizations, compared to indirect volume rendering techniques such as the marching-cubes algorithm (see 3.4.1). Since the isosurface representation is given by voxel values and not by polygons, this type of isosurface visualization is referred as non-polygonal isosurface. An example is the surface-shaded-display technique (SSD) (fig. 3.10, right). In order to enhance the visual perception and realism, local illumination models can be integrated during this visualization. This topic will be discussed in 3.7.

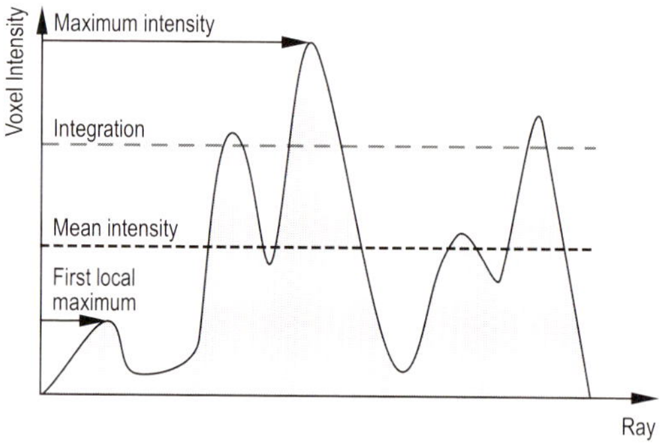

Figure 3.9
Different compositing possibilities including MIP (= maximum intensity projection) and mean intensity along the viewing ray that is casted through the volume

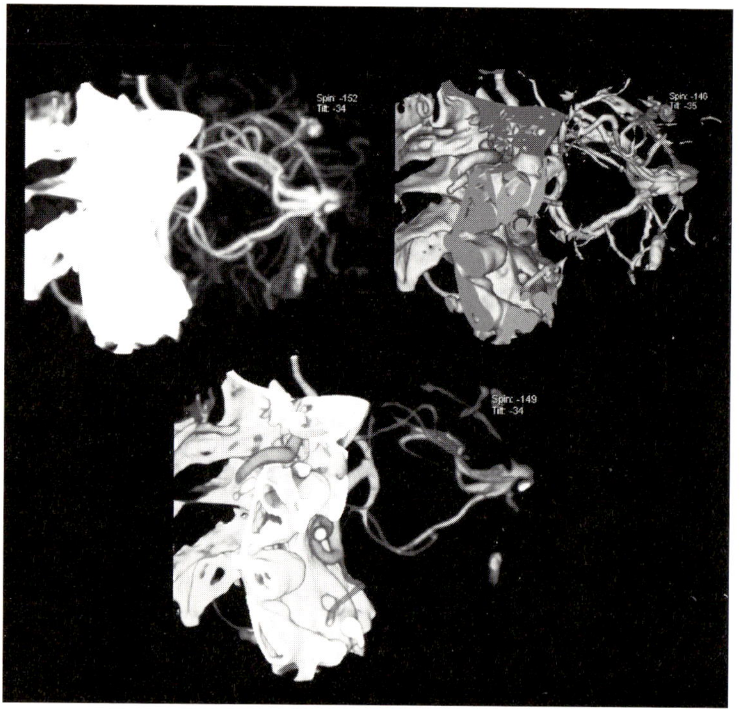

Figure 3.10
Comparison of MIP **(left)** and SSD (surface shaded display, **right**) and compositing by the OVER-operator **(bottom)**, showing vascular and osseous structures (courtesy by Dept. of Neuroradiology, University of Erlangen-Nuremberg)

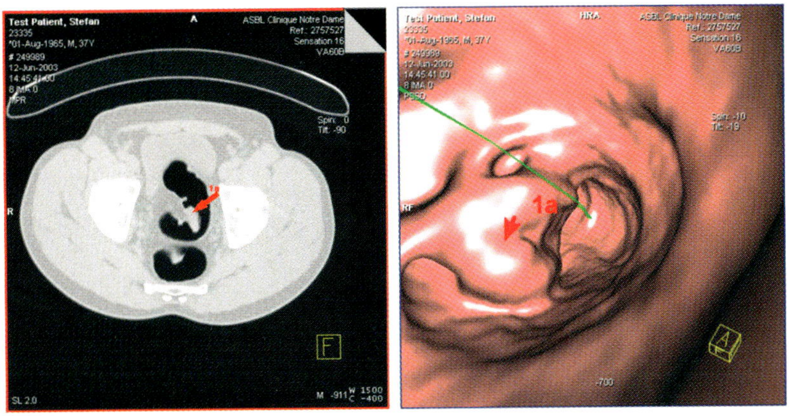

Figure 3.11
The image to the **left** shows the original CT slice of patient's colon. The arrow displays the position of the inspector's eye point in the virtual endoscopy application (**right**). The image has been generated by the use of a SSD algorithm (courtesy of Department of Radiology, Tournai, Belgium).

A very famous application for SSD algorithms is virtual endoscopy. Herein, the user's eye is placed directly into the patient's colon, which then allows the 3D inspection of e.g. polyps by the use of fly-through techniques. In fig. 3.11, such a virtual endoscopy scenario is presented.

Finally, voxel compositing can be realized via different integration steps in order to create semitransparent visualizations. For this purpose, mostly alpha-blending is applied via the *OVER*-operator according to Porter and Duff [3.13] (figs. 3.10, 3.1). Thus, if the emission and absorption coefficients ($q(s_i)$ and $A(s_i)$) are assigned by the user by the application of a transfer-function T (see 3.6), the integration is calculated in the following manner (back-to-front order):

$$I(s_{i+1}) = \alpha \cdot q(s_{i+1}) + (1 - \alpha) I(s_i) = q(s_{i+1}) \text{OVER } I(s_i) \tag{3.1}$$

$I(s_i)$: Ray intensity at position s_i. The blending factor α is defined as $A(s_{i+1})$.

Another integration possibility is given by digital reconstructed radiographs (DRR), which can be used e.g. in three-dimensional treatment planning for external beam radiotherapy [3.14].

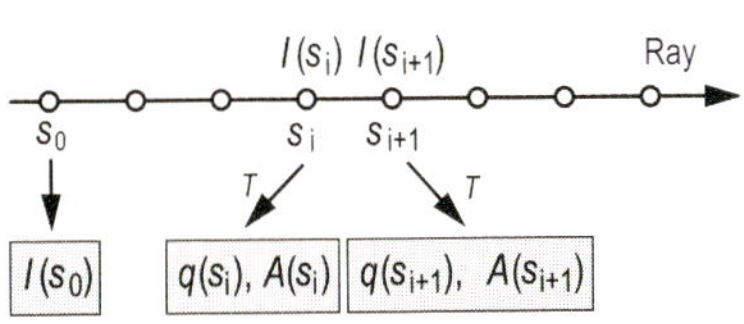

Fig. 3.1
Compositing via the *OVER*-operator

3.5.4 Conclusion

Summing up, although image-order techniques are the chosen methods in the context of image quality, they require immensely computational costs in order to calculate a final projection image. In order to keep manipulation possible during user interaction, the number of rays that are sent through the volume are often reduced which leads to intermediate low resolution images. Full resolution is finally calculated after the user interaction. However, direct volume rendering provides a big variety of different rendering possibilities, since different compositing schemes are possible (e.g. MIP or SSD or semitransparent visualization via the *OVER*-operator).

If a user wants to display isosurfaces, one has the possibility to choose between SSD (Direct Volume Rendering) and surface rendering using polygonal meshes (indirect volume rendering, 3.4). As far as polygonal representations are concerned, the generation of such meshes may be a time consuming process and hampers the flexible change of the desired isosurface. Furthermore, the final rendering can be performed very fast by the use of a graphics adapter. However, whenever high resolution images are required or the user performs high-level zooming (e.g. in the case of virtual endoscopy and polyp investigation), the triangle representation is visible which generates image artifacts, even by the use of local illumination (see 3.7). In order to tackle this problem, the number of the triangles has to be increased immensely, which then reduces the interactivity. Therefore, in the case of high resolution images, SSD algorithms are more favorable because of the more flexible possibility to change the isovalue and to change the image resolution.

3.6 Transfer-functions

By the application of a transfer-function

$$T : s \mapsto c \in RGBA \tag{3.1}$$

the user specifies the emission/absorption coefficients of each of the voxels within the volume that is to be visualized. To be more precise, each voxel with intensity value s is assigned a color value (RGB) and opacity (A) [3.4]. Thus, specific data that is contained within the 3D volume can be set to semi-transparent or opaque values. Furthermore, these values can be combined with color values in order to enhance visual perception. Fig. 3.12 visualizes this scenario. Herein, two transfer-functions T_1 and T_2 are applied to a human skull, whereas T_1 only emphasizes the bone structures. The function T_2 additionally visualizes skin structures in a semitransparent manner. However, due to the degree of freedom of such a transfer-function, the setting can be a time-consuming process, which strongly depends on the user's experience.

3.7 Local illumination

In order to enhance the perception of spatial relations and depth, local illumination techniques can be introduced in the context of direct volume rendering. Up until now

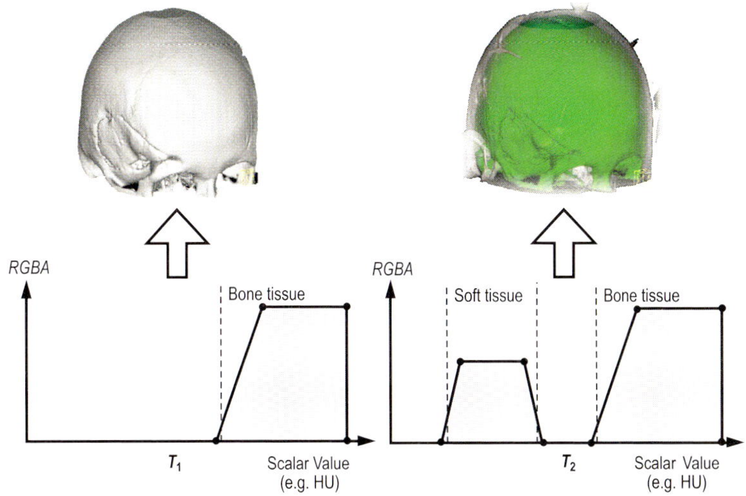

Figure 3.12
Basic principles of transfer-functions that map scalar values to emission values (*RGB*) and absorption coefficients *A*

it has been assumed, only volume elements were able to emit radiant energy. Now the possibilities of additional light sources are presented. It has to be emphasized that only local illumination models are focused on, which are easy to be calculated. Contrary, global models allow for indirect light or shadows, which increase the scene calculation time immensely.

A local illumination model allows the approximation of the light intensity reflected from a point on the surface of an object. This intensity is evaluated as a function of the orientation of the surface with respect to the position of a point light source and some material properties. In this context, the most applied local illumination model is the *Phong* model [3.15], which calculates the intensity by a linear combination of an ambient, diffuse and specular term (fig. 3.13):

$$I_{\text{Phong}} = I_{\text{ambient}} + I_{\text{diffuse}} + I_{\text{specular}} \tag{3.2}$$

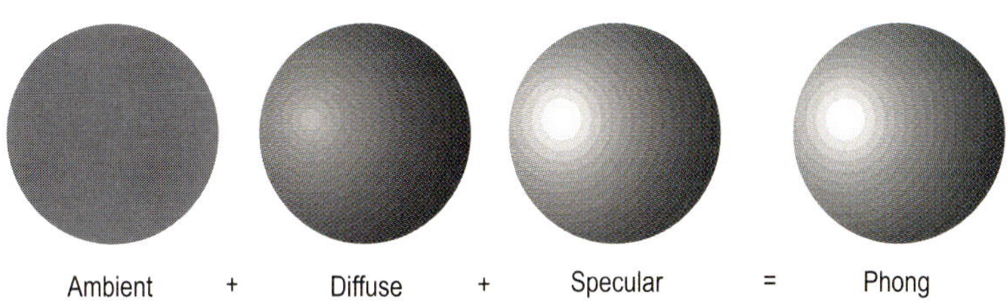

Figure 3.13 The Phong local illumination model

Ambient light

This light is represented by a constant term and illuminates parts of the surface that are not directly lit:

$$I_{\text{ambient}} = \kappa_{\text{amb}} = \text{const} \tag{3.3}$$

Diffuse reflection

The characteristic of diffuse (Lambertian) illumination is to reflect the light in all directions with equal intensity. Thus, the intensity depends only on the angle between the direction of the light source $\vec{l}$ and the normal $\vec{n}$ of the surface (fig. 3.14 (left)):

$$I_{\text{diffuse}} = I_{\text{diffuse}}\, \kappa_{\text{diff}}\, (\vec{l}\, \vec{n}) \tag{3.4}$$

Within this formula, I_{diffuse} represents the emitted intensity from the illuminating light source and the constant κ_{diff} denotes the property of the surface which has values between 0 and 1, specifying the amount of diffuse reflection.

Specular Reflection

Specular reflection is exhibited by every shiny surface including so-called highlights. Within this model, the viewer's position is taken into account. Thus, light is reflected in the direction of reflection $\vec{r}$ which is the direction of light mirrored about the surface normal $\vec{n}$. For efficiency purposes the reflection vector $\vec{r}$ can be replaced by the halfway vector $\vec{h}$, resulting in the Blinn-Phong illumination model [3.15] (fig. 3.14 (right)):

$$I_{\text{specular}} = I_{\text{Light}}\, \kappa_{\text{spec}}\, (\vec{h}\, \vec{n})^{d} \tag{3.5}$$

The parameter κ_{spec} denotes the amount of specular reflexion and the shininess d defines the size of the highlights.

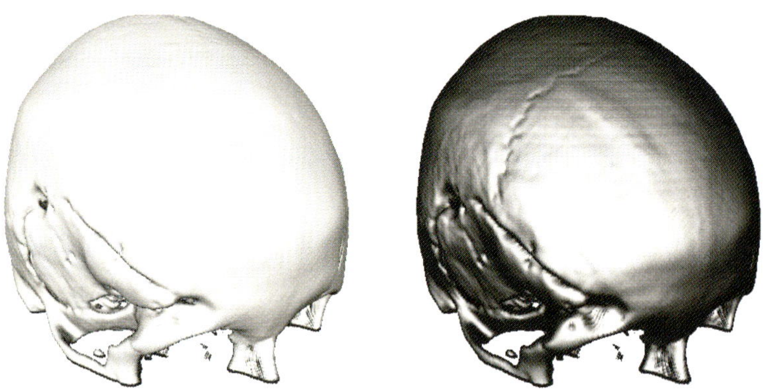

Figure 3.14
Application of the Phong illumination model: the **left** image displays diffuse illumination and the **right** image visualizes a CT head by the application of a specular illumination

The Blinn-Phong illumination model uses the normal vector to describe the local shape of an object and is primarily used for lighting of polygonal surfaces. To include the Blinn-Phong illumination model into direct volume rendering, the local shape of the volumetric data set must be described by an appropriate type of vector which substitutes the surface normal. In our concept of classification a single peak in the transfer function corresponds to an isosurface in the volume data set. We know that the normal direction of an isosurface coincides with the direction of the gradient vector of the underlying scalar field. In our illumination model, the gradient vector is thus an appropriate substitute for the surface normal.

3.8 Volume rendering on graphics adapters

In the previous sections, all fundamental basics have been discussed in order to understand the technique of direct volume rendering. However, this far all calculations for the creation of 3D image projections have to be done by the use of a computer's CPU. Thus, powerful machines can achieve high quality visualizations at high frame rates.

Nevertheless, the development of powerful graphics adapters advanced rapidly in the recent years, which is mainly driven by the increasing computer game market. However, these adapters are well suited also for the fast display of 3D tomographic volumes.

Since there is a very large variety of different applied techniques and since graphics adapters advance very fast and will allow therefore more and more rendering techniques in the future, only the very fundamental principles of hardware-based volume rendering will be mentioned [3.4, 3.16].

The basic principle of such a technique is texture-mapping by the use of 2D or 3D textures [3.4, 3.16], which is illustrated in fig. 3.15. In a first step, polygons (in this case quads) are defined for each of the original tomographic slices and placed within the 3D scene. In the second step, on each of the polygons the image content of the corresponding tomographic slice is 'glued'. Thus, each texture (= image) is mapped onto

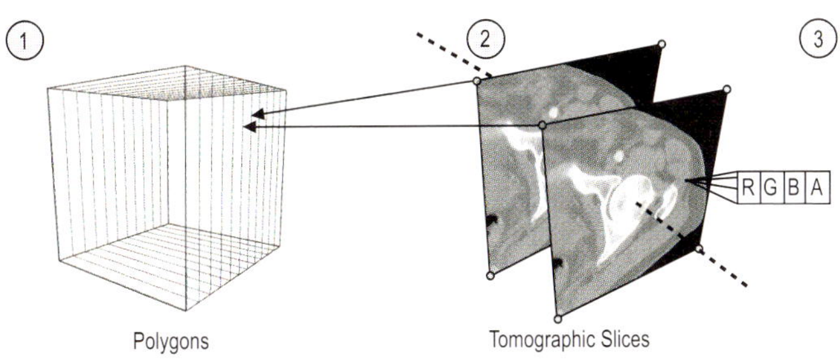

Figure 3.15
The image presents the basics of 2D-texture-mapping in order to perform volume visualization of tomographic volumes.

the correct polygon which is finally called texture-mapping. It has be to mentioned, that each texture is principally decomposed in *R*, *G*, *B* and *A* components which has to be defined by the application of a transfer-function.

Finally, after the definition of the textures, all the polygons have to be combined by the application of a compositing step (see 3.5.3). Since different compositing schemes (e.g. MIP or *OVER*) are also available in hardware, the final projection image can be calculated on the graphics adapter very efficiently which then allows high image quality at high frame rates. Whenever the user rotates the 3D volume onto the screen, a new projection image has to be calculated. In the case of 2D texture mapping, for each of the main slicing/polygon directions (x-, y- and z-direction) a polygon stack has to be generated which requires to have three copies of the volume in the memory. Whenever the angle between the viewer and the main slicing direction becomes too high, a new stack has to be permutated (see 3.5.2).

As far as the image quality is concerned, hardware-based volume rendering can be compared with software-based ray-casting techniques, but it is limited by the hardware's programmable possibilities. In the context of speed of display, the hardware-based techniques are generally superior to CPU-based approaches. Especially in the context of 4D visualizations, which allow the display of anatomy at different time steps, higher frame rates can be achieved, which is only limited by the available texture-memory on the graphics adapter.

3.9 References

[3.1] A. Kanitsar, D. Fleischmann, R. Wegenkittl, P. Felkel, E.G. Röller
CPR – Curved Planar Reformation
IEEE Visualization, 37-44 (2002)

[3.2] H. Niemann
Pattern Analysis and Understanding
Springer, Berlin Heidelberg 1990

[3.3] W.E. Lorensen, H.E. Cline
Marching cubes: a high resolution 3D surface construction algorithm
Proceedings of ACM SIGGRAPH, 163-170 (1987)

[3.4] C. Rezk-Salama
Volume rendering techniques for general purpose graphics hardware
Arbeitsberichte des Instituts für mathematische Maschinen und Datenverarbeitung (Informatik), Friedrich-Alexander Universität Erlangen-Nürnberg 2002

[3.5] H. Hege, T. Höllerer, D. Stalling
Volume rendering, mathematical foundations and algorithmic aspects
Technical Report TR93-7, Konrad-Zuse-Zentrum für Informationstech, Berlin 1993

[3.6] J. Kajiya, B. von Herzen
Ray tracing volume densities
Proceedings of ACM SIGGRAPH, 165-174 (1984)

[3.7] R.A. Drebin, L. Carpenter, P. Hanrahan
Volume Rendering
Proceedings of ACM SIGGRAPH, 65-74 (1988)

[3.8] J. Danskin, P. Hanrahan
Fast algorithms for volume ray tracing
ACM Workshop of Volume Visualization, 91-98 (1992)

[3.9] M. Levoy
Efficient ray tracing of volume data
ACM Transactions on Graphics 9(3), 245-261 (1990)

[3.10] R. Yagel, D. Cohen, A. Kaufman
Discrete ray tracing
IEEE Computer Graphics and Applications, 19-28 (1992)

[3.11] L. Westover
Footprint evaluation for volume rendering
Proceedings of ACM SIGGRAPH, 367-376 (1990)

[3.12] P. Lacroute, M. Levoy
Fast volume rendering using a shear-warp factorization of the viewing transformation
Proceedings of ACM SIGGRAPH, 451-458 (1994)

[3.13] T. Porter, T. Duff
Compositing digital images
Computer Graphics 18(3), 253-259 (1984)

[3.14] D. Sarrut, S. Clippe
Patient positioning in radiotherapy by registration of 2D portal to 3D CT images by a content-based research with similarity measure
Computer Assisted Radiology and Surgery, 707-712 (2000)

[3.15] J. Foley, A. van Dam, S. Feiner, J. Hughes
Computer Graphics, Principle And Practice
Addison-Wesley 1993

[3.16] M. Scheuering
Fusion of Medical Video Images and Tomographic Volumes
PhD thesis, University of Erlangen-Nuremberg 2003

4 Image fusion

4.1 Introduction

It has become common today for physicians to instruct their patients to undergo more than one imaging session, involving the same or different imaging modalities. Image fusion establishes an anatomical correlation between corresponding images derived from different examinations and thereby improves overall interpretability by more than the sum of the information gathered from the individual images. The goal of image fusion is to combine the results of different image acquisitions in order to generate additional information to support the various clinical stages, including diagnosis, treatment planning, treatment and follow-up [4.1]. Later in this chapter, fig. 4.14 shows an original computed tomography (CT) image of the human brain, an original magnetic resonance (MR) image of the human brain and a fusion of the two.

4.1.1 Clinical relevance

Image fusion is applied either to combine images of different modalities (multi-modality fusion) or images of the same modality (single-modality fusion).

Multi-modality fusion is used to combine complementary information provided by different modalities. Such information includes anatomical information derived from CT, MR, rotational C-arm angiography and ultrasound images (US) and functional information derived from functional MR, positron emission tomography (PET), single photon emission tomography (SPECT) and functional mapping modalities such as electro- (EEG) and magneto- (MEG) encephalography.

In contrast to multi-modality fusion, single-modality fusion is used to combine anatomical image data (e.g. MR-MR) or functional image data (e.g. PET-PET) to support follow-up examinations, i.e. to examine time-dependent variations of two or more images.

4.1.2 Image fusion steps

Registration versus visualization

The fusion of two images is performed in two steps: registration and visualization.

Registration refers to the spatial modification (e.g. translation, rotation, scaling, deformation) of one image (model image) relative to another image (reference image) in order to arrive at an ideal matching of both images.

Visualization refers to the display of both images in a manner relating to their current registration. Visualization updates allow one to see the progress that has been made in the registration procedure.

Categorization of registration techniques

Registration algorithms can be classified according to their operational characteristics. These include registration method, spatial transformation, distance measure and optimization strategy.

- *Methods:*

  Feature-based approaches require the extraction of corresponding features (e.g. pairs of landmarks, parts of extracted surfaces) from both model and reference image so as to provide a basis for calculating the spatial transformation. Intensity-based approaches compute ideal matching on the basis of the intensity information (voxel information) contained in both images.

- *Spatial transformation:*

  Irrespective of the selected approach (either feature or intensity based), registration techniques can be classified according to the type of the calculated spatial transformation that results from the registration process.

  Rigid transformations include rotations and translations of the model image relative to the reference image. Rigid (and affine) transformations assume that the model and reference images are not deformed in a non-linear manner relative to one another. The result of a rigid transformation can thus be stored in a single spatial transformation matrix.

  In contrast to rigid transformations, non-rigid transformations take deformations of the model image relative to the reference image into account. The result of a non-rigid registration is a calculated vector field that describes the deformations of the model image relative to the reference image.

- *Distance measure:*

  Various distance measures have been used to compute the ideal spatial transformation of the model image in order to arrive at a match of the reference image. These include mean square error (MSE), cross correlation, correlation ratio, joint entropy, mutual information (MI) and normalized mutual information (NMI).

- *Optimization:*

  The aim of the optimization strategy is to maximize or minimize a target function. The parameter of the coordinate transformation is determined in an iterative manner. This allows one to find the maximum/minimum of the target function.

  Many different optimization strategies are used to find an extremum of the distance measure so as to determine the ideal spatial transformation of the model image and thereby arrive at a match of the reference image [4.2].

Categorization of visualization techniques

Visualization is performed during or after the registration process. The goal of visualization is to depict the spatial relationship between the model image and the reference image in a single superimposed image or in two combined image displays. The main types of visualization include:

- *Side-by-side visualization:*
  Two displays contain visualizations of the model with respect to the reference image. Cursors are sometimes used to identify matching positions in the model and reference images.
- *Superimposed MPR visualization:*
  Corresponding renderings of model image and reference image are visualized in one superimposed display. Alpha blending allows one to assign different weightings and colors to model image voxels and reference image voxels in order to determine the correspondence of each voxel to the model or reference image.

4.1.3 General challenges

The following challenges arise in the context of applying various image fusion techniques:

- *Single generic registration algorithm:*
  Given that each imaging modality and each image registration/fusion application introduces its own unique challenges, there is no single generic registration algorithm. Therefore, it is often necessary to tailor registration algorithms (and visualization techniques used for image fusion) to application-specific requirements.
- *Non-rigid transformations:*
  The spatial transformation between model and reference image may vary considerably and may be highly non-linear. This non-linearity necessitates the use of various non-rigid registration algorithms. The causes of non-linearity in spatial transformations include different patient positioning when acquiring the model and reference images, organ activities (e.g. respiration and heart beat) and morphological changes (e.g. disease-related tumor growth).
- *Model and reference images with different information and resolution:*
  Images generated by different imaging modalities often differ significantly in terms of their information and resolution. CT-PET fusion, for instance, combines anatomical and functional information and CT image resolution is much higher than that of PET.
- *Model and reference images of different quality:*
  Imaging artifacts and noise present difficulties for registration algorithms. Furthermore, image distortions that are specific to the imaging modalities used tend to have an adverse effect on registration accuracy.
- *Performance issues:*
  Performance requirements are very important for registration applications for two reasons. First, registration algorithms (e.g. for 2D-3D registration) are sometimes applied in the context of surgical or interventional procedures that require real-time behavior. Second, non-rigid registration algorithms require exceptionally high degrees of computational power. These factors represent clear challenges for diagnostic and therapeutic applications.

  Such performance challenges can be taken into account via the parallelization of algorithm parts and running them on parallel hardware components. Another approach involves the implementation of multi-resolution strategies that enable a rough calculation of the spatial transformation based on lower image resolution. This is then compensated for at a later stage by refining the spatial transformation with the use of higher image resolution in an effort to arrive at an ideal spatial transformation.

- *Reliability, accuracy:*
  The use of image fusion applications in diagnostic and surgical contexts requires registration algorithms and visualization techniques that exhibit a high degree of reliability and accuracy. This makes the validation of registration algorithms and image fusion results in general a very important issue.

4.2 Registration

As mentioned above, registration refers to the spatial modification (e.g. translation, rotation, scaling, and deformation) of one image (model image) relative to another image (reference image) in order to arrive at an ideal matching of both images. Registration can be expressed symbolically as

$$\vec{x}_{\mathrm{M}}(i) \xrightarrow{T} \vec{x}_{\mathrm{R}}(i) \tag{4.1}$$

where $\vec{x}_{\mathrm{M}}(i)$ is a point in the model image, $\vec{x}_{\mathrm{R}}(i)$ is a corresponding point in the reference image and T is the spatial transformation of the model image M that is necessary to arrive at a match of the reference image R.

There are two distinct methods of achieving registration. First, if the image acquisition geometry defines a fixed relationship between M and R, registration can be determined by calibration (section 4.2.1). Second, if this is not the case, then the images themselves can be used for registration (section 4.2.2 and 4.2.3).

4.2.1 Registration by calibration

If there is a fixed geometrical relationship between two imaging devices, no image-based registration is required to fuse the images. Here, registration can be determined by calibration.

This fixed geometrical relationship can be achieved by mechanically combining the imaging devices, as is the case with current CT-PET devices.

Another option for establishing this fixed geometrical relationship is to track both of the imaging devices via the position sensors of an optic or electromagnetic tracking system. Here, handheld devices such as US transducers can also be used. Fig. 4.1 shows an example of the fusion of a 2D US image and a CT image where the registration is obtained by using tracking system position sensors (attached to both the US transducer and the CT gantry).

It will also be necessary to consider the problem of projection images when using X-ray images. Here, both the position and the projection parameters of the actual two-

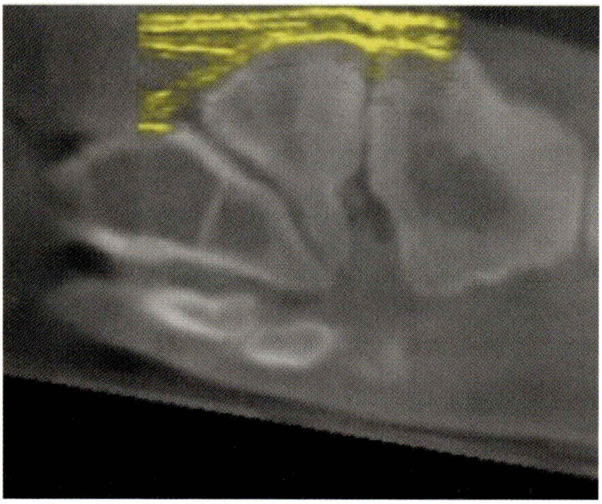

Figure 4.1
MPR rendering of a three-dimensional CT dataset of a pig's foot.
A US slice of the same region is overlaid in yellow.

dimensional image acquisition must be taken into account. Vessel intervention using a stationary C-arm system (section 4.2.3) represents an example. First, a 3D dataset is acquired using the C-arm. The position of the C-arm and therefore that of the 3D dataset is known. It is now essential that the patient remains stationary. The rotation of the C-arm is detected during the intervention. Given this position data and the known C-arm parameters, a calibration (and therefore a registration) can be calculated to overlay the three-dimensional dataset, for instance, as a volume rendering technique (VRT) display, with the two-dimensional projection X-ray images. Moreover, it is also possible to rotate the C-arm according to the rotations of the virtual VRT image. In this case, an X-ray image can be acquired that shows the patient in a position corresponding to the VRT display (section 4.4).

4.2.2 Image-based, 3D-3D registration

4.2.2.1 Rigid and affine registration

A spatial transformation T that transforms the location of a voxel of the model image M to a corresponding location in the reference image R is referred to as rigid transformation if the rotational and translational components are used in T only. The rigid transformation T contains 6 degrees of freedom and can be expressed as

$$T_{3D\text{-}3D} = \begin{pmatrix} \cos\beta\cdot\cos\gamma & \cos\alpha\cdot\sin\gamma+\sin\alpha\cdot\sin\beta\cdot\cos\gamma & \sin\alpha\cdot\sin\gamma-\cos\alpha\cdot\sin\beta\cdot\cos\gamma & t_x \\ -\cos\beta\cdot\sin\gamma & \cos\alpha\cdot\cos\gamma-\sin\alpha\cdot\sin\beta\cdot\sin\gamma & \sin\alpha\cdot\cos\gamma-\cos\alpha\cdot\sin\beta\cdot\sin\gamma & t_y \\ \sin\beta & -\sin\alpha\cdot\cos\beta & \cos\alpha\cdot\cos\beta & t_z \\ 0 & 0 & 0 & 1 \end{pmatrix} \quad (4.2)$$

where α, β, and γ represent the rotational components and t_x, t_y and t_z represent the translational components of the desired spatial transformation.

If shearing and scaling are contained in the spatial transformation T in addition to the rotational and translational parameters, then the spatial transformation in question is referred to as affine transformation. As with rigid transformation, the affine transformation T can be written as a 4×4 matrix. Moreover, it contains 12 degrees of freedom (3-dimensional rotation, 3-dimensional translation, 3-dimensional scaling and 3-dimensional shearing).

Both the rigid and the affine registration can be applied to one position x_M, y_M, z_M in the model image in order to calculate a position x_R, y_R, z_R located within the reference image:

$$\vec{x}_R = T_{3D\text{-}3D} \cdot \vec{x}_M \qquad (4.3)$$

The task of the registration process is thus to determine the parameters of the spatial transformation matrix T. While the following explanations of registration techniques presuppose rigid transformation, the concept described is also valid for affine transformation.

4.2.2.2 Visual alignment

One straightforward method of determining the parameters of the spatial transformation matrix T is to manually modify the spatial relationship (i.e. translation and rotation) between the model image and the reference image by interactively moving the model image by means of a graphical user interface.

4.2.2.3 Feature-based registration

In a pre-registration step referred to as feature extraction, corresponding pairs of features are extracted from both the model and reference image. Feature extraction can be performed manually or by using automatic feature extraction algorithms. Once feature extraction has been performed, the spatial transformation of one image relative to the other can be calculated in a manner that ensures that the corresponding features of both images match as closely as possible. Typical extraction features include:

- *Landmarks:*
  Landmarks include characteristic anatomical points (e.g. bone structures, vessel branches, etc.) and fiducial markers (artificial markers attached to the patient).
- *Structures:*
  Structures include anatomical surfaces (e.g. bone surfaces) and contours (e.g. vessel centerlines).

In what follows, landmark-based registration and surface-based registration techniques will be described using the classification just outlined.

- *Landmark-based registration:*
  Landmark-based registration is applied to cases involving the easy identification of

corresponding pairs of landmarks. The advantage of landmark registration centers on the fact that the desired spatial transformation can be calculated deterministically (i.e. without using iterative estimation methods). Nevertheless, landmark registration is the registration technique that demands the highest degree of user interaction. Landmark registration is thus used in cases for which surface-based or intensity-based methods can not be reliably applied.

Prior to registration, at least three corresponding pairs of landmarks are identified in both model and reference image. The landmarks can be identified by the user (e.g. located via an input device). Methods involving automatic landmark extraction and landmark pairing are sometimes applied as an alternative.

As soon as three corresponding pairs of landmarks have been identified, a non-iterative, least-squares method can be applied to calculate the desired spatial transformation. Here, an overestimated linear equation system can be formulated, which is then typically solved via SVD (singular value decomposition) as described in [4.9].

- *Surface-based registration:*

  Surface-based registration is especially helpful when it comes to image fusion applications that allow fast and accurate surface extraction in both model and reference image (e.g. CT-CT fusion by using surfaces of common bone structures).

  Prior to registration, the surfaces of corresponding image structures are extracted from both model and reference image. This surface extraction is performed by so-called segmentation algorithms. Segmentation can be performed in an interactive (e.g. by applying a lower and an upper intensity threshold), semi-automatic or automatic manner (e.g. region growing or watershed algorithms). For purposes of registration it is not always necessary to extract completely closed surfaces from the corresponding anatomical structures.

  As soon as the corresponding surfaces have been extracted from the model image and reference image, the parameters of the spatial transformation matrix T can be evaluated by minimizing the distance between both extracted surfaces. In other words, the position and orientation of the surface that was extracted from the model image is moved and rotated in order to minimize the distance between the model surface and reference surface. The evaluation of T is performed using an iterative optimization process. Various optimization strategies will be discussed later in this chapter.

Surface-based registration techniques can be broken down into the following categories: point-to-point matching, point-to-surface matching and surface-to-surface matching:

- *Point-to-point registration:*

  In contrast to point-to-surface and surface-to-surface registration, point-to-point registration approaches avoid the generation of mesh models. That being said, the accuracy of point-to-point registration is somewhat limited when compared to the other surface matching variants.

  Point-to-point registration, also known as the head-and-hat algorithm [4.3], involves the extraction of a surface contour from one of the images of one modality (e.g. the reference image). A set of surface points on the corresponding surface of the other modality (the hat) is matched to the contour (the head). Upon each iteration of the optimization process, the sum of the squares of the distances between hat and head is calculated and used as a distance measure for calculating the ideal spatial transformation T.

The hierarchical chamfer matching algorithm [4.4] is a variant of the point-to-point registration algorithm. A so-called distance image is calculated on the basis of the surface extracted from the reference image. This distance image reflects the distance of each reference image voxel to the extracted surface. The model is continuously transformed during the registration process and the distance image is used to score the individual transformations obtained so as to arrive at an ideal alignment of both surfaces.

- *Point-to-surface registration:*
  In the case of point-to-surface registration, one of the corresponding surfaces is represented by a set of surface points and the other is represented by a surface mesh model consisting of many (e.g. triangular) patches. The surface mesh model can be generated, for instance, by using the marching cubes algorithm. The closest patch is evaluated for each of the points and the distances between the points and surface model are minimized. A frequently used point-to-surface registration technique makes use of the iterative closest point (ICP) algorithm [4.5].
- *Surface-to-surface registration:*
  In the case of surface-to-surface registration, both of the corresponding surfaces are represented by surface mesh models consisting of many (e.g. triangular) patches. The distance of these models is minimized iteratively by applying an optimization strategy.

4.2.2.4 Intensity-based registration

By avoiding the task of identifying corresponding anatomical structures in both of the images, intensity-based registration techniques offer the highest degree of automation and require less user interaction (in some cases none at all) than landmark-based and surface-based approaches. Furthermore, intensity-based approaches are often more resistant to image-data noise and truncation effects caused by partially overlapping image volumes [4.5]. The normalized mutual information measure (see below), in particular, shows good results even when applied to images of complementary modalities (e.g. CT-PET fusion).

Intensity-based approaches use the voxel intensities of the model image in relation to the reference image as basic distance measures in order to arrive at an ideal matching of model and reference image. The parameters of the spatial transformation matrix T are evaluated by minimizing/maximizing distance measures that are derived from correlation computation or measures commonly used in the field of information theory. The evaluation of T is performed by applying an iterative optimization process, as described in the case of surface-based registration techniques.

The following distance measures have been used for intensity-based registration. The two distance measures mutual information and normalized mutual information currently enjoy wide acceptance.

Distance measures based on statistical parameters such as correlation, mean square deviation and ratio image uniformity assume the existence of similar intensity information in the model and reference image. Therefore, it makes more sense to apply these distance measures for single-modality fusion (e.g. CT-CT fusion) than for multi-modality fusion (e.g. CT-PET fusion).

The following distance measures have been used for single-modality fusion.

- *Cross correlation:*

$$Measure_{CC} = \frac{\mathrm{cov}(R, M) \cdot \mathrm{cov}(R, M)}{\mathrm{var}(R) \cdot \mathrm{var}(M)} \tag{4.4}$$

cov: covariance, var: variance

- *Mean square deviation:*

$$Measure_{MSD} = \frac{1}{N}\sum_{i=1}^{N}(R(x_i) - M(x_i))^2 \tag{4.5}$$

- *Ratio image uniformity:*
  Woods et al. [4.6] have defined ratio image uniformity (RIU) as a statistical similarity measure:

$$\text{Quotient image: } r(x) = \frac{M(X)}{R(x)} \tag{4.6}$$

$$Measure_{RIU} = \frac{1}{\mu \cdot N}\sum_{i=1}^{N} r(x_i) \tag{4.7}$$

N: number of voxels in quotient image, *μ*: mean value of *r*

$$\mu = \frac{1}{N}\sum_{i} r(x_i) \tag{4.8}$$

- *Correlation ratio:*
  Correlation ratio is an intensity-based distance measure introduced by A. Roche et al. Unlike the correlation coefficient, which measures the linear dependence between two variables, the correlation ratio measures functional dependence, with a value near 0 indicating low functional dependence.
- *Entropy and joint entropy:*
  The rationale behind entropy-based measures centers on the fact that matching images contain less information in their areas of overlap than unmatched images. Entropy-based registration techniques involve an attempt to minimize the joint information in the overlapping areas of model and reference image so as to better arrive at the ideal spatial transformation.

The entropy value H is a distance measure for the amount of information in a random distribution and is widely used in the field of information theory:

$$H_x = -\sum_{i=1}^{N} p_x(x_i) \cdot \log(p_x(x_i)) \tag{4.9}$$

$$H_y = -\sum_{i=1}^{N} p_y(y_i) \cdot \log(p_y(y_i)) \tag{4.10}$$

A further definition is required to the measure the similarity of two random distributions (images). The joint entropy of two distributions is defined as

$$H_{xy} = -\sum_{i=1}^{N}\sum_{j=1}^{M} p_{xy}(x_i, y_j) \cdot \log(p_{xy}(x_i, y_j)) \tag{4.11}$$

where $p_{xy}(x_i, y_j)$ is the probability that two corresponding voxels will have intensities x_i and y_i simultaneously.

While joint entropy represents a possible distance measure, it has the following disadvantage: by minimizing joint entropy an attempt is made to find the overlap containing the least information, and not necessarily the overlap containing the highest degree of correlation. This provides a reason for favoring mutual information and normalized mutual information over joint entropy as a distance measure for intensity-based registration for most intensity-based registration applications.

- *Mutual information (MI) and normalized mutual information (NMI):*
  Mutual information is probably the current most popular similarity measure for multimodal registration [4.5], [4.10]. It has been successfully applied to several modality combinations, including MR, CT, PET, and SPECT. The mutual information measure can be regarded as very general given that it makes very few assumptions about the relationship between image intensities. It assumes statistical dependence, but does not assume linear correlation and functional correlation.

  The mutual information measure is defined as

$$Measure_{MI} = H_x + H_y - H_{xy} \tag{4.12}$$

  H_x and H_y are the marginal entropies of the model and reference image respectively and H_{xy} is the joint entropy of all voxels in the spatial overlap between the model and reference image after applying a certain spatial transformation.

  Normalized mutual information is a variant of the mutual information measure introduced by Studholme et al. [4.5] in order to make the mutual information measure less sensitive to the number of common voxels in both model and reference image. In other words, the maximization of normalized mutual information permits the achievement of a spatial transformation involving a minimization of joint entropy with respect to the marginal entropies [4.5].

$$Measure_{NMI} = \frac{H_x + H_y}{H_{xy}} \tag{4.13}$$

4.2.2.5 Optimization strategies

The aim of the optimization process is to maximize or minimize a real-value target function (i.e. of the distance measure). The parameters of the spatial transformation *T* are determined in a manner that ensures that the distance measure will reach its respective maximum or minimum.

The following challenges arise for optimization strategies used to facilitate registration techniques:

- The ideal spatial transformation is typically represented by the global extremum of the distance measure. The possibility of arriving at erroneous local extrema represents a potential source of error for optimization strategies.
- Furthermore, the optimization should converge to the desired extremum as quickly as possible because the optimization loop will have to be repeated for each modification of each single parameter of the spatial transformation *T*.

Both challenges can be met by starting the optimization with an advantageous starting value, one that is as close to the desired solution as possible. Additionally, multiresolution approaches may be applied to accelerate the optimization process and to allow one to skip over erroneous local extrema. While the first optimization loop is run at reduced resolution for both model and reference image, the resolution is increased during subsequent optimization loops until the degree of resolution required for registration accuracy has been reached.

Fig. 4.2 offers an outline of the individual steps in the optimization loop when applying a multi-resolution procedure.

Optimization strategies can be classified as follows [4.4]:

- *Gradient-based optimization:*
  Gradient-based strategies use the derivative of the target function (i.e. distance measure) with respect to the parameters of the spatial transformation. Starting with an initial registration, the parameters of the target function are modified to ascertain the direction with the steepest gradient ascent. An additional parameter defines the step width of the modifications.

  Special optimization strategies such as resilient backpropagation and quickprop are variants of gradient-based optimization that involve an attempt to accelerate the convergence of the optimization strategy by adjusting the step width of the parameter modifications.
- *Nearest neighbor search:*
  When applying the nearest neighbor search, each parameter of the spatial transformation is increased/decreased by a given step width. The distance measure for all of these modifications is calculated by applying the modifications to the model image as a new spatial transformation. The transformation that results in the maximization of the metric is applied. The new transformation is then modified by the next optimization step, and so on, until no further distance measure improvements are possible. These optimization loops are performed using a multi-resolution strategy

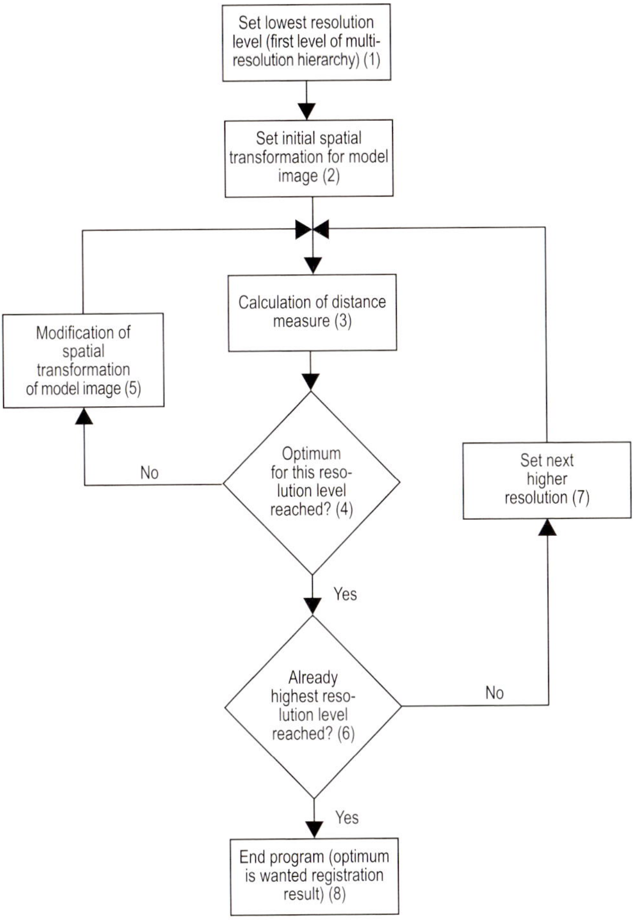

Figure 4.2
Flow chart showing the individual steps in the optimization loop. In box **(1)** the resolution is set to the lowest level in the multi-resolution hierarchy. This means that both (reference and model image) are sub-sampled at the first resolution level. **(2)**: An initial spatial transformation is set for the model image. **(4)** handles the inner loop for finding the optimum for the current resolution level. As long as the optimum for the current resolution level has not yet been found, **(5)** (modification of the spatial transformation) and **(3)** (calculation of the distance measure for the modified spatial transformation) will be executed within this inner optimization loop. As soon as an optimum has been found **(4)**, a check is made to determine whether any additional resolution levels are to be handled **(6)**. If so: **(7)** will set the resolution to the next highest level and the optimization loop **(3)**, **(4)**, **(5)** starts from the beginning. The optimization loop terminates as soon as the optimum has been found **(8)**.

according to which the step width of the parameter modifications is decreased from loop to loop.

- *Adaptive grid search:*
  The adaptive grid search strategy combines the properties of gradient-based optimization and the nearest neighbor search [4.2, p. 63]. A similar strategy, the Powell approach, is described in [4.11, p. 412].
- *Best direction search:*
  The best direction search strategy restricts itself to following the target function's steepest ascent [4.11, p. 61]. This approach requires a calculation of the target function's gradient vector. In contrast to the previously described approaches, the best direction search represents a one-dimensional search that can be applied in the context of optimization applications whenever many transformation parameters are involved (e.g. for non-rigid registration applications involving spatial transformations that consist of large vector fields).

4.2.2.6 Non-rigid registration

Our focus in the last chapter was on the rigid registration of two images, including the rotation and translation of the model image. In some cases, however, rigid registration is not sufficiently accurate. The reasons here include patient movement between scans, different scanning parameters, and different scanning times, as is exemplified by long lasting PET and fast CT scanning. Heartbeat and respiratory symptoms can also have effects on the accuracy of registration. Added to this are geometric changes that result from therapeutic intervention (e.g. in the context of open-skull neurosurgery or liver surgery). All of these cases may involve a significant lack of geometrical correspondence between the model and reference image.

Fusion of images from different patients and the fusion of patient data with atlas data also require non-rigid registration.

While the task of rigid registration is to find a global transformation matrix that includes rotation and translation, non-rigid registration uses global and local transformations to adapt the registration to local geometrical differences. The result is an *elastic* registration.

Fig. 4.3 shows examples of (a) rigid, (b) affine and (c) non-rigid registration. Rigid registration enables one to translate or rotate the model image only. Affine registration

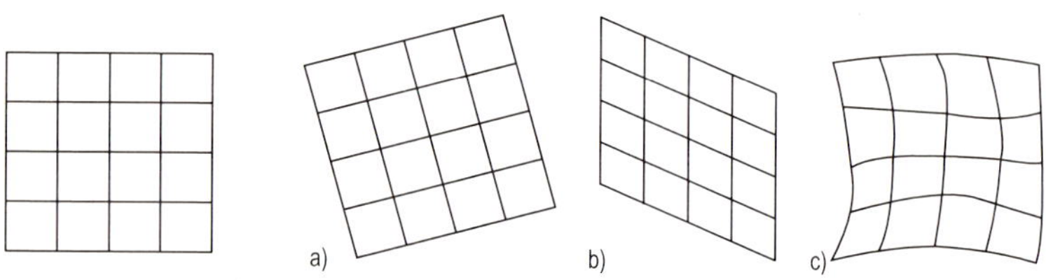

Figure 4.3 Example of a reference image: **(a)** rigid, **(b)** affine and **(c)** non-rigid registration

also enables one to correct for scaling and shearing. Non-rigid registration (also referred to as free-form deformation) enables one to correct other differences in the image as well.

Although non-rigid registration is more complex than rigid registration, it is nonetheless expected to be fast, reliable and accurate, especially when applied for therapeutic reasons. In the present chapter, we review various techniques of non-rigid registration that have been developed to meet these conditions. Still more about non-rigid registration can be found in [4.18, 4.19].

Like rigid registration, non-rigid registration can be divided into feature-based and voxel-based approaches.

4.2.2.7 Feature-based, non-rigid registration

The first step in the feature-based approach is to extract all of the corresponding features from the two images. These features may include landmarks or structures (section 4.2.2.3). The use of surface structures, for instance, enables one to model the movement of bones so that they do not change their shape (in contrast to the surrounding elastic tissue). In contrast to landmarks, contours and surfaces allow for a better simulation of elasticity. However, the tasks of feature extraction and interpolation are more difficult. For this reason, we will restrict our present discussion to landmarks.

The landmarks in the model image are exactly matched to the corresponding landmarks in the reference image. The position of all other points is calculated using interpolation. The tissue that lies between the landmarks is deformed in order to align the landmarks exactly. Interpolation is used to compensate for the deformations and to create a smooth image that is free of the edges that result from deformations.

In the context of medical image processing, thin-plate splines represent the most commonly used interpolative method for handling this task. Bookstein [4.13] and Rohr [4.14] offer a more detailed review of this topic. The physical analogy behind thin-plate splines is the following: The aim is to find the minimum energy for a bent thin plate. If forces are applied to several points on a thin plate, it is bent in a manner related to its material characteristics.

A thin-plate spline is a function $IR^2 \to IR$ where IR^2 is the thin plate and IR is the plate's deflection. Although forces are applied only to certain points on the plate, the plate's position at all remaining points can be calculated by interpolation.

The use of thin-plate splines forces landmarks into an exact match. However, due to the given image resolution and other sources of error, it would not be realistic to assume that one has a precise knowledge of the position of the landmarks. This is independent of the type of landmark extraction involved. Neither manual detection and nor automatic extraction are capable of giving exact results. For this reason, Rohr et al. [4.15] use approximating thin-plate splines. Here, the aim is not to force the landmarks to match exactly, but to create a thin-plate spline that is as smooth as possible.

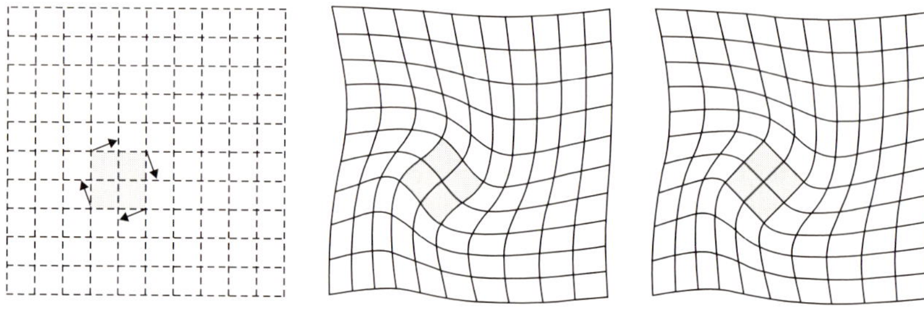

Figure 4.4
Use of contour orientation: **a)** original image, **b)** without contour data and **c)** with contour data.

Another way of improving the quality of the resulting non-rigid registration is to use the orientation of contours at extracted landmark positions, for example, the edges or surfaces of bones and inner organs. Fig. 4.4 offers an illustration of a case involving the use of eight landmarks: 4 at the edges of the square and 4 at the edges of the image. Fig. 4.4 shows a) the original image, b) the deformed images derived from the use of simple thin-plate splines and c) the deformed image derived from the use of thin-plate splines that incorporate the orientations of the contours at the edges of the square. Note that the edges of the square now match exactly because the use of contour splines has prevented their bending.

The detection of other features (e.g. edges, surfaces and volumes) in addition to landmarks enables one to generate more information for use in non-rigid registration. On the other hand, no matter whether one proceeds automatically or manually, it is not easy to ascertain these more general features. This topic is discussed further in [4.16].

4.2.2.8 Intensity-based, non-rigid registration

A lack of common image information may make it impossible in some cases to detect landmarks. If this is the case, one may wish to pursue the option of registering the images in non-rigid fashion using intensity-based approaches. Here, feature extraction will not be required because image intensity is considered directly.

Rigid, intensity-based registration, as introduced in section 4.2.2.4, does not sufficiently account for material elasticity. The present task is to establish good image matching with as few deformations as possible while also minimizing computational time.

First, global rigid registration is performed to get an initial alignment of the two images. This is then followed by a second step in which local adaptive deformations are used to achieve elastic registration.

A grid is usually placed over the model image for the sake of calculating the elastic registration. Each of the grid's vertices can be moved in any direction to improve the registration in terms of voxel values. Using a mass-spring model [4.17] each of the vertices can also be bound in order to facilitate smooth deformation. According to the

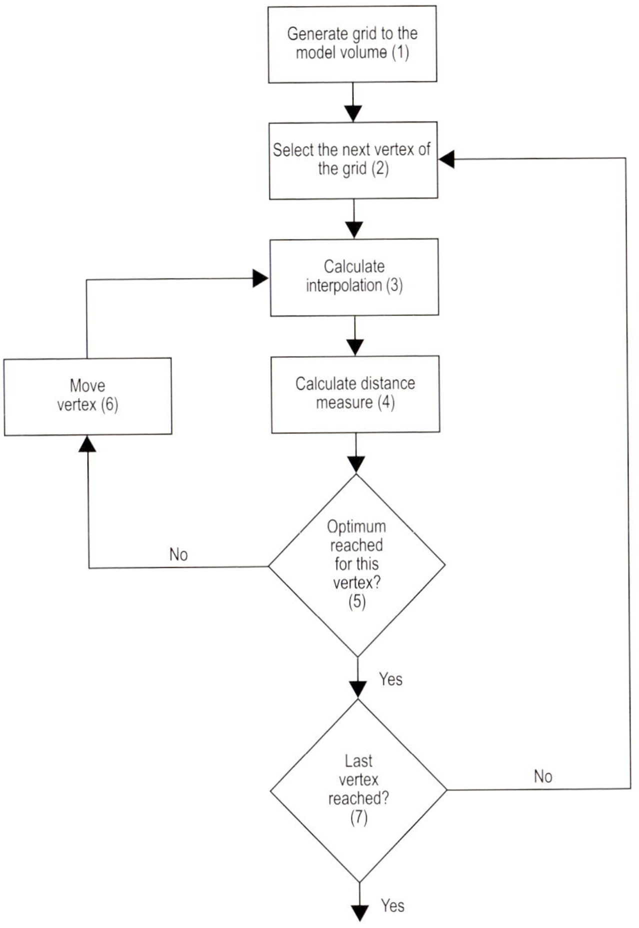

Figure 4.5
Calculation of a non-rigid registration by use of voxel values.
First, a grid is generated over the model volume. The grid vertices are then used to deform the model volume **(1)**. Given that it is not possible to change the position of all vertices simultaneously, they are selected one after another **(2)**. As we move a vertex, it becomes necessary to recalculate the voxels around it using an interpolation scheme **(3)**. Steps **(4, 5, 6)** can be compared to the search for the right transformation matrix used in rigid registration. In the case of non-rigid registration, this has to be done for each vertex in the grid. As soon as the optimum for the current vertex has been reached, the process is repeated for all other vertices until the whole volume is registered properly.

model, each voxel is represented by a mass that is bound to other masses via springs. In order to maintain a state of equilibrium, the moving of one mass must entail the moving of all other masses connected to it via springs.

It will be necessary to deploy non-rigid registration to calculate a new model image based on the positions of the vertices. All of the new voxel positions are calculated using a method of interpolation. This method is crucial because the calculation is performed repeatedly. Whenever moving a vertex, it is necessary to recalculate the volume parts around it. Simple trilinear interpolation and splines are commonly used to calculate the position of the voxels. Given that this task may be time consuming, it is advisable to use graphics hardware.

Fig. 4.5 shows a flow chart of the steps needed to calculate a non-rigid registration using voxel values.

A hierarchical image registration scheme can be used to speed up the calculation. At the beginning a low-resolution grid is used to calculate a best matching registration. The grid is refined with each step to increase the accuracy of the non-rigid registration. The advantage here is that it eliminates the need to move many grid-points at the beginning, allowing one to start with a few. The grid is then refined and the registration restarted for the image regions where the registration is not sufficiently accurate.

The use of rigid patches represents another option for reducing calculation time. Here, the whole model volume is divided into patches and each patch is registered using a rigid technique. This can be done quickly using rigid registration approaches for each patch. The resulting dataset may exhibit holes and overlapping volume parts following the rigid registration. A new continuous volume is created by performing interpolation using the center of each patch as a vertex. This process is repeated as one re-divides each patch to achieve better registration.

4.2.3 Image-based, 2D-3D registration

So far, we have considered image fusion between two 3D data sets. It is also possible, however, to fuse 2D images with 3D images via 2D-3D registration [4.18]. The most important application of 2D-3D registration involves the combining of 2D X-ray projection images with a 3D image. While it is in principle also possible to register 2D slices (such as US images) with 3D volumes, we refrain from discussing this special case in the present context.

4.2.3.1 Clinical applications for 2D-3D registration

The first 2D-3D registration algorithms were developed for radiation therapy. Planning usually takes place on the basis of 3D CT data sets. Using 2D-3D registration, these can be related to images that are acquired either in an X-ray simulator or directly via the radiation beam (portal images) used to test patient positioning [4.21].

Another important application of 2D-3D registration is the combining of X-ray images acquired during interventional or surgical procedures with 3D images that provide information not present in the X-ray images. Such 3D images may either be derived from another modality such as MR, CT or PET or from 3D rotational angiography images. The aim of registration in this context is to use X-ray imaging to show interventional or surgical devices such as catheters or guide wires while the 3D image shows detailed functional or morphological features [4.20].

With the use of an interventional X-ray imaging system capable of 3D imaging, registration can be performed using calibration, as described in section 4.2.1. However, the validity of such calibration is nullified as soon as any patient or organ movement occurs. 2D-3D registration can be used in such cases to update the calibration.

4.2.3.2 The 2D-3D registration problem

The main problem associated with 2D-3D registration centers on the task of finding a transformation T between a position in the 3D image (model image) and the corresponding position in the 2D image (reference image).

$$\vec{X}_{\mathrm{r}} = T \cdot \vec{X}_{\mathrm{m}} \tag{4.14}$$

In contrast to 3D-3D registration, this special case involving the 2D-3D registration of projection images is not represented by a one-to-one mapping. Instead, all points along a projection line in the 3D image are mapped to one point in the 2D image.

In the following, we consider cases of rigid transformation only. The transformation T, consisting of translation, rotation and projection, may be expressed as:

$$T_{\mathrm{2D/3D}} = T_{\mathrm{proj}} \cdot T_{\mathrm{rot}} \cdot T_{\mathrm{trans}} \tag{4.15}$$

$$T_{\mathrm{proj}} = \begin{pmatrix} f/d_{\mathrm{x}} & f*s & u_0 & 0 \\ 0 & f/d_{\mathrm{y}} & v_0 & 0 \\ 0 & 0 & 1 & 0 \\ 0 & 0 & 0 & 1 \end{pmatrix} \tag{4.16}$$

where the definitions of T_{rot} and T_{trans} correspond to those given in section 4.2.2.1. The parameters f, d_{x}, d_{y}, s, u_0 and v_0 define the projection geometry: f is the distance between the X-ray source and the detector plane, d_{x} and d_{y} define the pixel spacing on the detector, and s is a scale factor. In the general, we wind up with a total of 11 degrees of freedom, six from the translation and rotation (extrinsic parameters) and five from the projection geometry (intrinsic parameters).

The intrinsic parameters can sometimes be determined without registration. When using a calibrated C-arm imaging system, all of the intrinsic parameters are determined via calibration and only the extrinsic parameters remain to be determined via registration. In other cases (e.g. a mobile X-ray system that does not move in a reproducible manner), some of the intrinsic parameters have to be included (just like the extrinsic parameters) in the scope of the registration process. In some cases, however, their number can be reduced. For instance, the detector pixel size is known for flat-panel detector systems. The degrees of freedom are thus reduced to nine.

4.2.3.3 2D-3D registration methods

The methods used to perform 2D-3D registration are very similar to those used for 3D-3D image registration and described in section 4.2.2. Both feature-based and intensity-based registration can be used, and the optimization strategies for the latter are similar.

Corresponding points on the projection and 3D images can be selected when using landmark-based methods. Another common feature-based method is to fit surfaces extracted from the 3D images with the corresponding contours of the 2D images.

4.2.3.4 Intensity-based, 2D-3D registration

Intensity-based methods represent an interesting option whenever the 2D and 3D images contain similar information and the methods described in section 4.2.2.1 can all be used for 2D-3D registration. The general principle behind intensity-based, 2D-3D registration is shown in fig. 4.6.

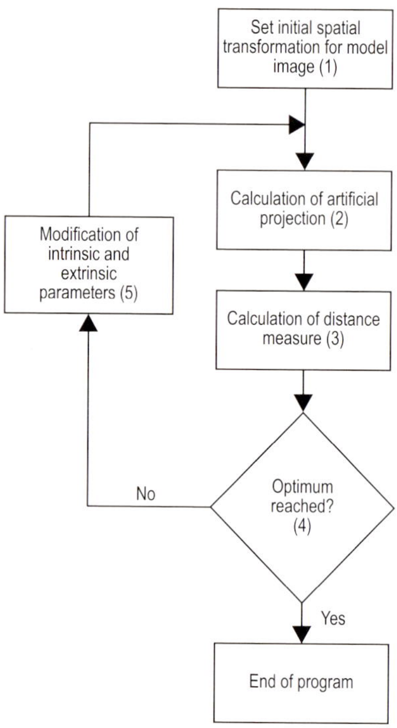

Figure 4.6
Flow chart for intensity-based registration: **(1)** The initial parameters for the spatial transformation are set. **(2)** The 3D model image *M* is rotated and translated according to the set of extrinsic parameters, and an artificial projection through the 3D volume *R'* is calculated with a projection geometry defined by the intrinsic parameters. **(3)** The 2D reference image *R* is compared to *R'* using a certain distance measure. **(4)** If the optimum distance is reached, the program ends. **5)** If not, the intrinsic and extrinsic parameters are modified according to an optimization strategy, and the process continues from step 2.

4.2.3.5 Projection generation and similarity measures

The projection step involves the mapping of all points along a line in M to one point in R'. Various options are available for combining the intensity values along the line into a single value in R'. These include summation and *maximum-intensity projection*. The physical projection process that results in the reference image R may be different from the artificial projection step. This can be taken into account by using a similarity measure that makes few assumptions about the relationship between the projections (e.g. mutual information).

The use of 3D CT images as model images represents a special case. Such data actually produce X-ray images when projected (digitally reconstructed radiographs or DRR) and are therefore perfectly suited for intensity-based 2D-3D registration.

However, an artificially produced projection of a CT image differs from an X-ray image on account of the different X-ray energy spectrum used. This is especially apparent when registering portal images that are acquired at energy levels of several MeV along with CT images acquired at around 100 keV. This can be corrected to some extent by using assumptions about the imaged material. Another option is to perform CT-image segmentation so that, for instance, only bone is used for projection.

Besides the similarities with 3D-3D registration, there are some important differences:

- If intrinsic parameters are to be included in the registration process, more degrees of freedom will have to be found in the registration process. The optimization of eleven parameters produces a very complex search space.
- Because of the additional step of generating projection images, 2D-3D registration algorithms are computationally demanding and therefore depend on an efficient search strategy. Another option is to apply sparse sampling for the projection step, which means that not all, but only a (usually randomly chosen) subset of the points in R are calculated and compared.
- Changes in one of the six parameters in 3D-3D registration cause similar changes to the 3D object. The effect of a parameter change on the projection image in 2D-3D registration depends significantly on the current configuration. In-plane and out-of-plane translations represent the most obvious example. Translations of the 3D data set that are parallel to the detector plane entail approximately identical translations of the 2D projection image. However, translations parallel to the central beam yield no more than minute translations and scaling of the 2D projection. It is thus very difficult to obtain reliable values for the translation from such projections.

4.2.3.6 2D-3D registration with calibrated projection geometry

Many of the problems associated with 2D-3D registration can be overcome by using a calibrated imaging system. Given that the intrinsic parameters are known, the number of parameters to be determined drops to six. Even more important, however, is the fact that calibrated projection geometry permits the use of more than a single projection image for registration. This can be very beneficial both for registration reliability and accuracy. If the projection angles are substantially different (e.g. orthogonal) then in-plane translations on one image are out-of-plane translations on the other. This makes optimization much easier.

The availability of two calibrated projection images also enables one to define a landmark using both images. A 3D position can then be found via back projection of the corresponding points. The corresponding landmarks in the 3D image can then be registered using the common 3D-3D registration methods.

4.2.4 Validation of fusion results

Possible sources of error

The following sources of error may adversely affect the accuracy of the registration process:

- Different resolution between model image and reference image
- Model and/or reference image limitations (e.g. artifacts, noise)
- Model image object deformations relative to the reference image (e.g. caused by different patient positioning, organ movements, disease processes)
- Problems involving the registration process itself (e.g. inaccurate feature extraction, hitting upon an erroneous local extremum)

Validation

A reliable and accurate registration algorithm is a prerequisite for the use of fused images in a clinical setting. Validation is therefore an essential part of the registration process. However, the lack of an exact reference makes it very difficult in practice to determine the accuracy of a given registration.

Two important requirements that apply to registration algorithms are:

- Accuracy (ability to calculate the spatial transformation as exactly as possible)
- Reliability/stability (registration results should be reproducible, irrespective of starting position and various aspects of image quality)

Various methods of validation are used in addition to visual verification to make sure that these requirements are met:

- Known anatomical or fiducial landmarks can be used to estimate the error of the calculated spatial transformation.
- Registration algorithms can be tested using synthetic data when the ideal spatial transformation to be calculated is known.
- Registration algorithms can be repeatedly applied to the same model and reference image while using different starting constellations. The different runs should yield identical registration results.

- A check can be made to determine whether the identity matrix is the result of the conjunction of individual registrations by serially registering several images via a chain of spatial transformations.

Study: benchmarking of registration algorithms

Various rigid, image-based registration algorithms developed by various universities, research institutes and companies have been benchmarked (using the same CT/MR/PET data sets) as part of a retrospective registration evaluation project [4.7] performed at Vanderbilt University in the United States. During the benchmarking project the different algorithms were run on the same data sets according to a blinded procedure (i.e. only certain independent Vanderbilt University staff members were informed of the true registration).

This enabled the project staff to examine and compare the accuracy of the various registration techniques as objectively as possible. The minimum registration error was less than 1 mm for CT-MR registration and 2 mm for MR-PET registration.

4.3 Visualization

The main subject of discussion in the previous section was the registration of two datasets. In the present section we turn our attention to the display and visualization of registration results and fused volumes.

A distinction is to be made when addressing the subject of visualization between two-dimensional (e.g. multiplanar reconstruction or MPR) and three-dimensional (e.g. volume rendering technique or VRT) presentation and the visualization of projection images and other two and three-dimensional images.

We begin with a discussion of planar reconstruction.

4.3.1 Visualization of MPR slices

One of the most common methods of visualizing two MPR renderings is α-blending. Every pixel in the resulting image is calculated as a weighted sum of the pixels in the two datasets at the corresponding positions. The weight is given by an α-value. The visualization procedure is thus referred to as α-blending.

$$G_{\mathrm{Sum}} = \alpha G_{\mathrm{Pic1}} + (1-\alpha)\alpha G_{\mathrm{Pic2}} \tag{4.17}$$

G_{Sum} is the resulting gray value, G_{Pic1} and G_{Pic2} are the gray values of picture one and picture two respectively. Changing the parameter α allows to cross-fade between the two datasets. Drawbacks associated with this method include lower contrast in both datasets due to the overlay of both images and an inability to draw a distinction between the shown datasets. A distinction between the datasets can, however, be achieved by using a color map for one dataset and a gray scale for the other (see fig. 4.7 left). Despite the low contrast, this visualization technique is widely used in clinical settings.

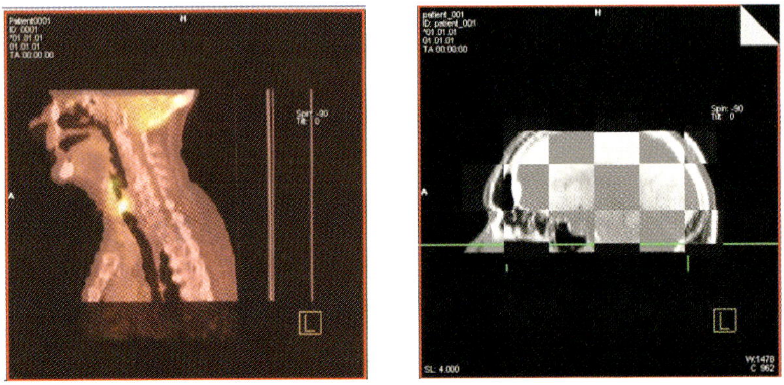

Figure 4.7
Left: CT-PET α-blending image of a patient with a head and neck tumor. CT shown in gray, PET shown in color. (Source: Dr. D. Townsend, University of Pittsburgh Medical Center).
Right: Checkerboard visualization of a human head. (Source: Vanderbilt University)

An obvious but not often used method is the checkerboard or chessboard method. Here, the two datasets are displayed on the board, with the white squares containing the first datasets and the black squares containing the second. An advantage of this method is the preservation of contrast in both datasets (see fig. 4.7 right). Using checkerboard visualization, relevant regions are only visualized by one dataset. A flip of the squares or continuous visualization movement is needed to obtain the full impression of the overlay of the two datasets.

The two datasets can also be displayed via side-by-side visualization. The result of the registration is displayed in two different windows lying side by side and showing the two datasets in the same size, orientation and displacement. Fig. 4.8 shows an exam-

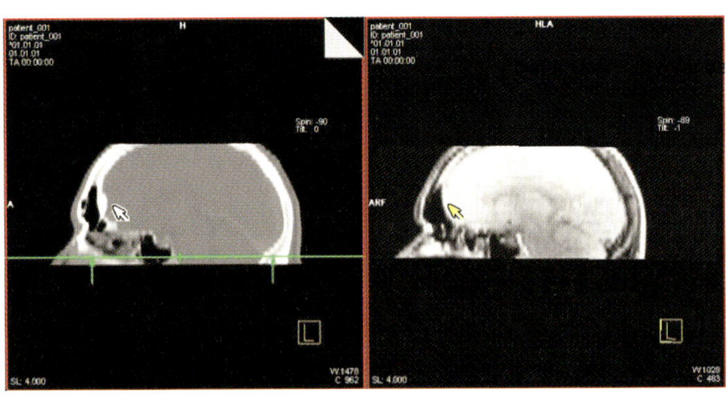

Figure 4.8
Side-by-side visualization for CT-MR fusion. Each position can be marked with the cursor. A corresponding "linked cursor" is inserted into the second image. (Source: Vanderbilt University)

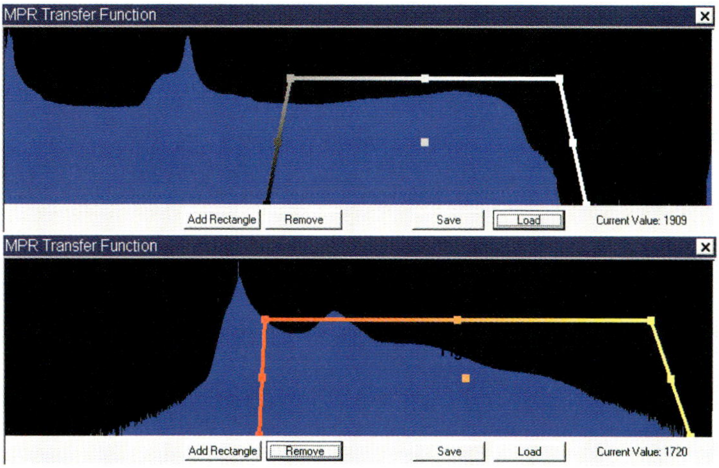

Figure 4.9
Transfer dialogs used for flexible α-blending. **Above:** CT transfer dialog showing the bones. **Below:** MR transfer dialog showing the soft tissue of the head. The corresponding rendering can be seen in fig. 4.14.

ple of registering CT and MR brain data. Corresponding positions in the datasets can be shown using the mouse cursor in the first dataset and a corresponding *linked* cursor displayed in the second dataset. Whenever the mouse cursor is moved across the first displayed image, the linked cursor in the second image is displayed at the appropriate position. Using side-by-side visualization the two datasets are displayed with full contrast owing to the fact that no overlay is applied.

The visualization of an overlay display of two datasets without losing contrast is referred to as flexible α-blending [4.12]. Individual image parts are weighted separately, depending on their specific clinical importance. The use of flexible α-blending enables one, for instance, to overlay two datasets (e.g. CT and PET) to show the hot spots in the PET dataset and all other information (bones, etc.) in the CT dataset without losing dataset contrast (see fig. 4.15). It is also possible to overlay MR and CT images of the brain: CT images yield high bone structure contrast and MR images yield high soft tissue contrast. The use of a flexible overlay enables one to display CT bone structures and MR soft tissue without losing contrast thanks to the fact that their gray values can be clearly distinguished (fig. 4.9).

This form of overlay can be expressed mathematically as follows:

$$G_{\mathrm{Sum}} = \begin{cases} \dfrac{\alpha_{\mathrm{Pic1}} G_{\mathrm{Pic1}} + \alpha_{\mathrm{Pic2}} G_{\mathrm{Pic2}}}{\alpha_{\mathrm{Pic1}} + \alpha_{\mathrm{Pic2}}} & \mathit{if}\ \ \alpha_{\mathrm{Pic1}} + \alpha_{\mathrm{Pic2}} \neq 0 \\ 0 & \text{in all other cases} \end{cases} \tag{4.18}$$

The α_{Pic1} and α_{Pic2} values describe discrete functions over the gray scales of the two image series. If $\alpha_{\mathrm{Pic1}} > 0$ for a gray value in one dataset, this gray value should be displayed in the overlaid visualization. These α-values can be explained using transfer dialogs known from volume rendering techniques: a trapezoid is generated and a color is assigned to this trapezoid for every gray scale that should be displayed. The height of the trapezoid at a distinct gray-value position indicates the α-value for this gray value. If a trapezoid exists only for the first dataset ($\alpha_{Pic1} > 0$, $\alpha_{Pic2} = 0$) for a given point in the output image, the color value of the trapezoid at the desired position is used for the output image. An overlay of the two datasets is calculated only in cases where trapezoids are defined for both datasets. The desired weight is calculated using the α-values at the appropriate positions.

These visualizations can also be used to overlay two-dimensional images (e.g. US images) with three-dimensional volumes. The displayed slice of the volume is calculated as described in section 4.2.

4.3.2 Fusion result visualization using volume rendering techniques

The volume rendering technique (VRT) represents a three-dimensional visualization of a volume. In order to visualize two registered volumes, one may proceed by displaying the first volume using a volume rendering technique while one slice of the second volume, either MPR or maximum intensity projection (MIP), is overlaid onto the rendered display as a cut plane (fig. 4.10). The cut plane can be moved within the three-

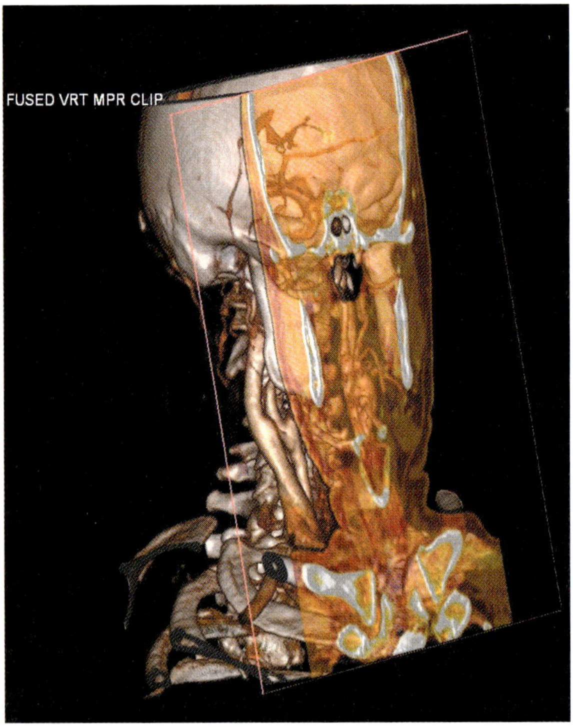

Figure 4.10
Fusion of a VRT volume with an MPR slice of a second dataset

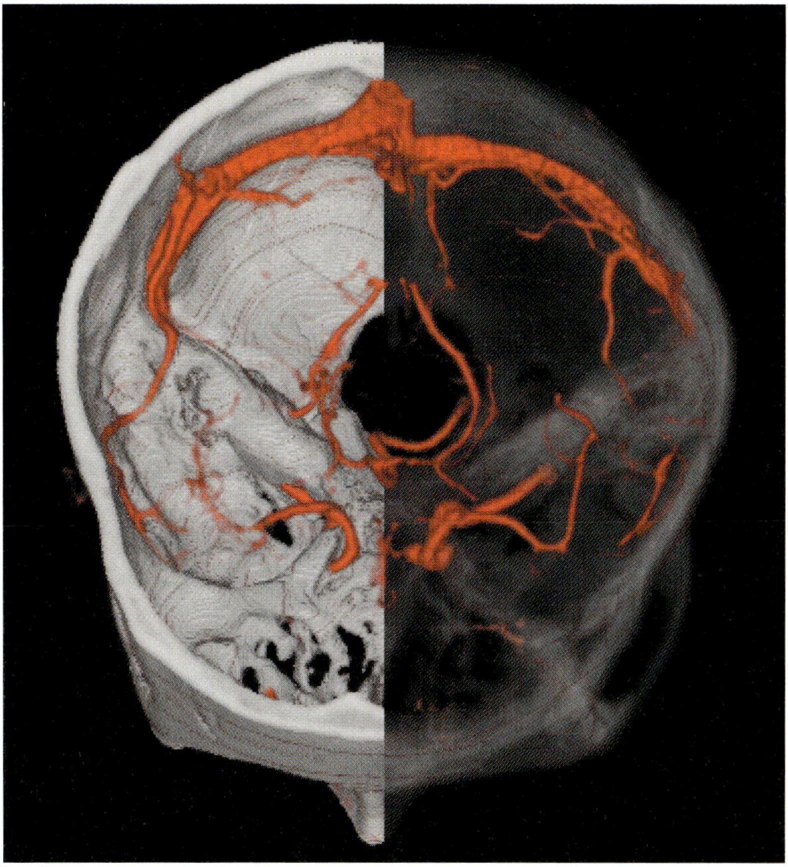

Figure 4.11
Fusion of two VRT visualizations, vessel tree and bones **(left)**, with semi transparent bones **(right)**. (Source: Dr. Tomandl, University of Erlangen)

dimensional display in any direction or it can be rotated. By using this visualization technique, the physician gains access to the three-dimensional information and the familiar two-dimensional slice visualization.

One can also use VRT displays for visualization by calculating VRT scenes from both reference and model volume and then overlaying them. As with the flexible blending of two MPR slices, the proportions of the visualization can be chosen separately for gray values of both image series. As an example, this enables one to visualize the vessel tree of a patient's brain together with the CT bone information (fig. 4.11). Moreover, one also has the option of looking through the bones (i.e. showing them in a semi-transparent way) to see the vessels lying inside of them.

4.3.3 Visualization of fused projection images

When overlaying projection images, it is first necessary to create a perspective projection of the three-dimensional dataset. The parameters of this projection must match the parameters used during the acquisition of the two-dimensional projection image. These projection images can be calculated using perspective MIP or a perspective VRT display. The calculated two-dimensional image of the three-dimensional dataset can be overlaid onto the projection image by deploying the methods used to overlay MPR slices (see section 4.4). Fig. 4.12 shows an example of such visualization.

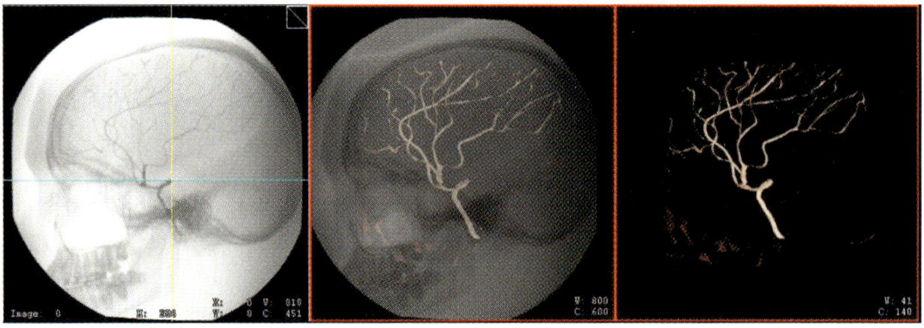

Figure 4.12
Left: X-ray projection image of a phantom. **Right:** VRT-rendered image of a volumetric dataset. **Middle:** fused image.

4.4 Clinical applications

In the present chapter, we offer some examples of diagnostic, interventional and intraoperative techniques as they are applied in clinical settings.

4.4.1 Nuclear medicine: fusion of CT/MR and PET/SPECT images

Nuclear medicine images (e.g. PET, SPECT) provide a description of metabolic functions in the body. The use of such images includes the detection and representation of metabolically abnormal tumors. While these functional images provide information about the size and the activity of the tumors, they contain very little information about patient anatomy and their spatial accuracy is limited.

Follow up studies using pre and post-treatment scans can be used to visualize treatment results. Tumor size and activity can be directly assessed in the fused image.

However, it is difficult to ascertain the exact location of the tumor using nuclear medicine images alone because the link to patient anatomy is missing. This link can be established by fusing the functional data with high-resolution morphological images derived from CT or MR. This high-resolution data can be used for planning of radiation therapy and surgery.

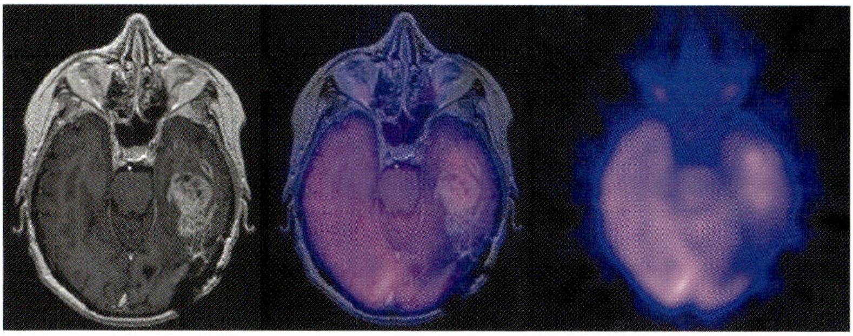

Figure 4.13
MR **(left)** and PET **(right)** visualization of a brain containing a tumor. The **center** image shows the fusion of the two images. (Source: Dr. Richter, Dr. Geworski, Charité Berlin)

Moreover, image data from nuclear medicine can help to improve target delineation in radiation therapy. Fig. 4.13 (left) shows an MR image of a brain tumor. It is difficult to distinguish between the active tumor and necrotic tissue. The fused MR-PET image can be used to ascertain the exact size and location of the active tumor. This information can be especially helpful when planning radiation therapy.

4.4.2 Surgery

Medical images are used not only for diagnostic purposes, but also for surgical planning and support. Registration and fusion also enhance the surgical environment by providing the surgeon with combined information generated by various modalities.

Neurosurgery

Fused images can be used to support navigation procedures during neurosurgery. Their use enables one to visualize functional areas of the brain (e.g. generated by FM-

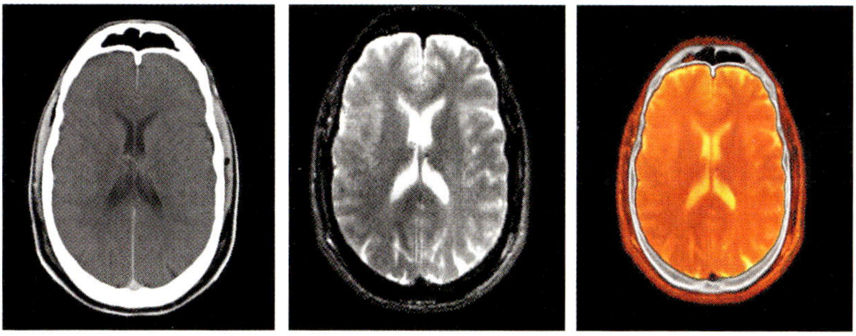

Figure 4.14
Left: CT image. **Middle:** MR image. **Right:** Superimposition with colorized MR information (soft tissue) and gray CT information (bone structures).

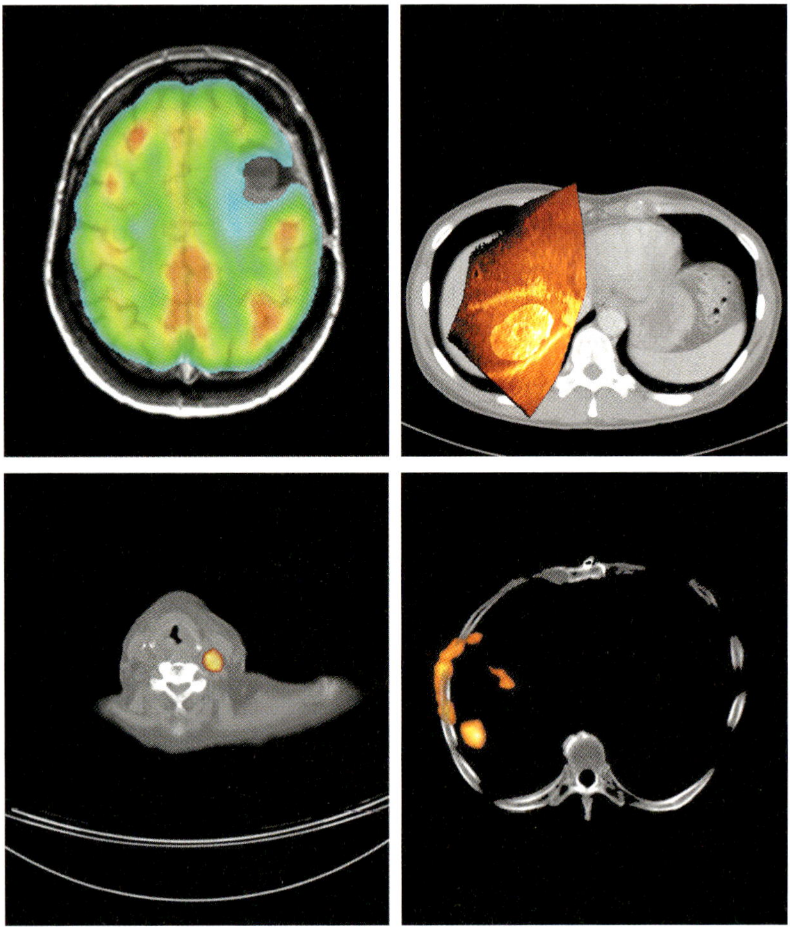

Figure 4.15
Upper left: MR-PET fusion. The post-treatment PET image shows missing PET uptake around the tumor, which is clearly visible in MR. (Source: Charité Hospital, Berlin, Germany) **Upper right:** CT-US fusion: the liver tumor (visible in 3D US) is superimposed onto the CT image. (Source: University-Hospital Klinikum, Munich, Germany) **Lower left:** CT-PET fusion: the head and neck tumor (PET) can be shown in the CT image. (Source: Dr. David Townsend, University of Pittsburgh Medical Center) **Lower right:** CT-PET fusion: the selective CT-PET superimposition enables an exact separation of tumor and bone structures. (Source: Charité Hospital, Berlin, Germany)

RI, PET, MEG, EEG) while visualizing surgical instruments within anatomical data (e.g. CT, MR, rotational C-arm angiography, US). An example of CT and MR image fusion is shown in fig. 4.14. Fig. 4.15 shows some examples of CT and PET fusion.

The so-called brain shift problem represents a special challenge for navigation procedures in the field of neurosurgery: Once the skull has been opened, the brain's form shifts away from its pre-surgical state. Preoperative images thus do not exactly reflect anatomical structure during surgery. Methods of non-rigid registration can be applied to the pre-surgical images (e.g. CT, MR) to compensate for any variance. Such methods transform the images according to known anatomical landmark positions or according to intra-operative real-time imaging (e.g. 3D US). Intra-operative MR can be used for brain shift compensation [4.8].

Another option is to overlay preoperative image information with optical images generated by the surgical microscope. For instance, the MKM system (manufactured by the German Zeiss company) enables one to superimpose pre-surgical image information (e.g. the boundary of a previously segmented tumor) onto microscope images in real-time during the surgery.

Spine surgery

The registering of preoperative spinal CT images to vertebral surface points can provide crucial support when it comes to the accurate placement of surgical tools or spinal fixation hardware during surgery. This registration can be achieved by surface matching the pre-operative CT images with intra-operative 3D-US images after extracting the surfaces of the vertebral structures from the CT and US images. The use of preoperative CT images for image-guided spine surgery allows the surgeon to determine the positions and orientation of surgical tools relative to vertebral anatomy with great accuracy.

Endoscopic and laparoscopic surgery

Image fusion can also provide crucial support in the context of minimally invasive laparoscopic and endoscopic surgery by combining optical information generated by the endoscope or laparoscope and preoperative anatomical images that are displayed according to the perspective and the position of the endoscope or laparoscope.

4.4.3 Treatment planning in radiation oncology

Three-dimensional planning for radiation therapy is conventionally performed using CT data. CTs offer the advantage of tremendous geometrical precision and CT data can provide information about tissue attenuation that is necessary for dose calculation. However, it may be helpful to include data from other modalities into the planning process. MR provides superior soft tissue contrast and is thus better suited when it comes to distinguishing diseased from normal tissue. PET data can be a helpful source of metabolic information. If MR or PET data are used to identify treatment targets, image fusion will be necessary to translate this data to the CT data set. One method of performing image fusion for this application involves the use of external markers. The patient is connected to a rigid stereotactic head frame (fig. 4.16). The frame contains interchangeable markers that may include either steel wires (CT imaging), plastic tubes filled with a contrast medium (MR imaging) or radioactive wires (PET imaging). The markers are identified via an automated procedure and the six degrees of rigid transformation can be calculated on the basis of their positions.

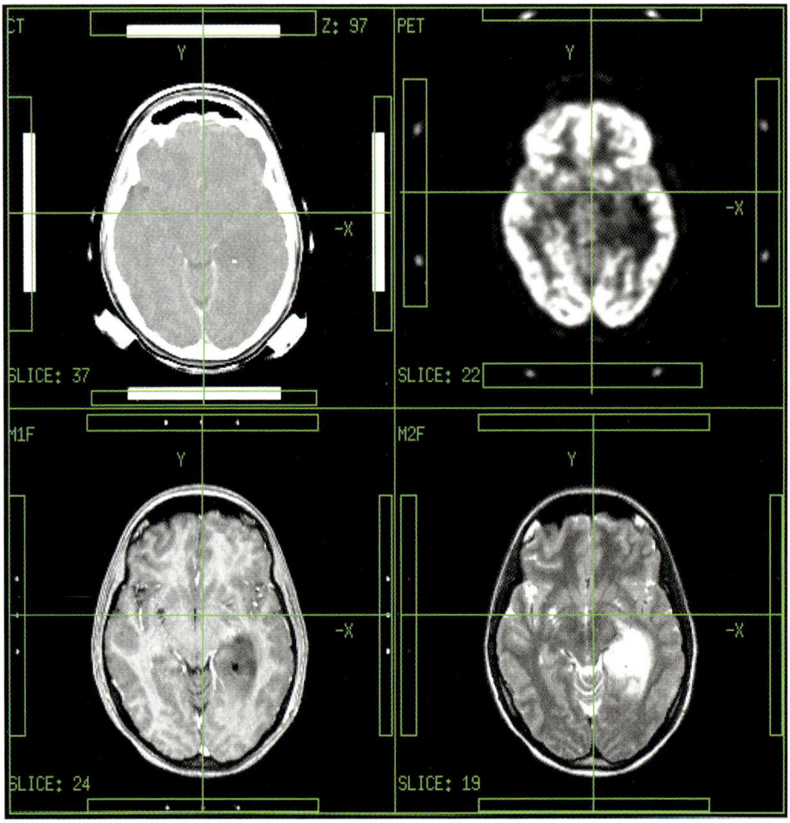

Figure 4.16
Example of marker-based multi-modality image registration. For this patient with an astrocytoma, a CT data set **(upper left)** is fused with PET data **(upper right)** and two different MR data sets **(lower row)**. The markers used for registration appear as small dots on the very borders of the upper right and lower left images. (Source: Professor L. Schad, German Cancer Research Center, Heidelberg, Germany)

4.4.4 Interventional radiology

Interventional radiology, including procedures performed using X-ray C-arm imaging systems capable of 3D imaging (3D angiography), represents another area of application for image fusion. Such procedures include various forms of neuro-radiological interventions performed for the sake of diagnosing and treating vascular and other diseases of the head, neck and spine. Such procedures are conceived to accurately steer an instrument or catheter through the patient's body. In certain situations, this can be a demanding task. In neuro-interventional procedures, for example, steering the catheter through the arterial system is made difficult by the various branches and tortuous arterial segments. The process is usually supported by monoplane or bi-

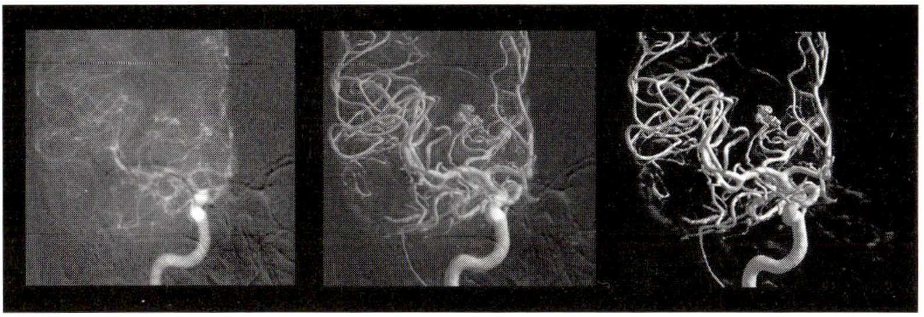

Figure 4.17
Example of image fusion during an interventional radiology procedure. **Left:** 2D DSA image. **Right:** 3D rendering of a 3D angiography reconstruction. **Middle:** blended 2D and 3D images.

plane X-ray imaging. While two-dimensional projection images generated by such systems can be used to visualize instruments, instrument orientation within patient anatomy is sometimes difficult. For this reason, 3D rotational angiography is performed using the same C-arm system and the user may combine information from the real-time X-ray projection images and the previously acquired 3D dataset. This can be achieved by overlaying the real-time X-ray image onto a rendering from a previously acquired three-dimensional dataset (fig. 4.17) or by translating the position of a relevant feature (e.g. catheter tip) from the 2D images to the 3D dataset or *vice versa*.

4.5 References

[4.1] B. Heigl, N. Rahn, H. Ditt
Imaging Fusion – State of the Art
The Neuroradiology Education and Research Foundation: ASNR (2003), 85-91

[4.2] T. Rohlfing
Multimodale Datenfusion für die bildgesteuerte Neurochirurgie und Strahlentherapie. Dissertation.
Tech. Univ. Berlin (2000), 57-68

[4.3] J.V. Hajnal, D.L.G. Hill, D.J. Hawkes
Medical Image Registration
CRC Press (2001)

[4.4] G. Borgefors
Hierarchical Chamfer Matching: A Parametric Edge Matching Algorithm
IEEE Transactions on Pattern Analysis and Machine Intelligence 10(6) (1988)

[4.5] C. Studholme, D.L.G. Hill, D.J. Hawkes
An Overlap Invariant Entropy Measure of 3D Medical Image Alignment Pattern Recognition 33(1) (1999), 71-86

[4.6] R.P. Woods, S.T. Grafton, C.J. Holmes, et al.
Automated Image Registration: I. General Methods and Intrasubject, Intramodality Validation
Journal of Computer Assisted Tomography 22(1) (1988), 153-165

[4.7] J.B. West, J.M. Fitzpatrick, M.Y. Wang, et al.
Comparison and Evaluation of Retrospective Intermodality Brain Image Registration Techniques
Journal of Computer Assisted Tomography 21(4) (1997), 554-566

[4.8] C. Nimsky, O. Ganslandt, S. Cerny, et al.
Quantification of, Visualization of, and Compensation for Brain Shift Using Intra-operative Magnetic Resonance Imaging
Neurosurgery 47(5) (2000)

[4.9] K.S. Arun, T.S. Huang, S.D. Blostein
Least-squares fitting of two 3-D point sets
IEEE Trans. Pattern Anal. Machine Intell., Vol. PAMI 9 (1987), 698-700

[4.10] W.M. Wells, P. Viola, H. Atsumi, S. Nakajima, R. Kikinis
Multi-modal volume registration by maximization of mutual information.
Medical Image Analysis 1(1) (1996), 35-51

[4.11] W.H. Press, S.A. Teukolsky, W.T. Vetterling, B.P. Flannery
Numerical Recipes in C: The Art of Scientific Computing
Cambridge University Press (1988)

[4.12] N. Rahn, H. Ditt, S. Wach
Ein neuer Visualisierungsansatz zur überlagerten Darstellung registrierter Bildserien
Bildverarbeitung für die Medizin 2002 (2002), 306-309

[4.13] F.L. Bookstein
Principle Warps: Thin-Plate Splines and the Decomposition of Deformations
IEEE Trans. On Pattern Anal. And Machine Intell. 11(6) (1989), 567-585

[4.14] K. Rohr
Elastic Registration of Multimodal Medical Images: A Survey
Künstliche Intelligenz (2000), 11-17

[4.15] K. Rohr, H.S. Stiel, R. Sprengel et al.
Point-Based Elastic Registration of Medical Image Data Using Approximating Thin-Plate Splines
Proc. VBC'96 (1996), 297-306

[4.16] D. Ruprecht, H. Müller
A Framework for Generalized Scattered Data Interpolation
Visualization in Scientific Computing, Springer Wien (1995)

[4.17] S. Cotin, H. Delingette, N. Ayache
Real-time elastic deformations of soft tissues for surgery simulation
IEEE Trans. on Visualization and Computer Graphics 5(1) (1999), 62-73

[4.18] J.B.A. Maintz, M.A. Viergever
A survey of medical image registration
Medical Image Analysis 2(1) (1998), 1-36

[4.19] D. Rueckert, L.I. Sonoda, C. Hayes
Non-rigid registration using free-form deformations: Applications to breast MR images
IEEE Trans. on Medical Imaging 18(8) (1999), 712-721

[4.20] J.H. Hipwell, G.P. Penney, R.A. McLaughlin, et al.
Intensity based 2-D-3-D registration of cerebral angiograms
IEEE Trans. Med. Imaging 22(11) (2003), 1417-26

[4.21] L. Dong, A.L. Boyer
An image correlation procedure for digitally reconstructed radiographs and electronic portal images
Int. J. Radiat. Oncol. Biol. Phys. 33(5) (1995), 1053-60.

5 Navigation

5.1 Introduction

Image-based surgical navigation can be defined as the tracking of moving instruments in space in relation to image data acquired prior to or during a surgical procedure so as to minimize access trauma and improve surgical outcomes. The origins of navigation lie in the introduction of stereotactic systems at the end of the 19th century [5.1]. The further development of such systems then led to the successful deployment of navigation procedures in several clinical areas. Modern imaging modalities such as CT and MR have introduced improvements in both radiological-diagnostic and surgical planning and today represent the foundation of modern computer-assisted surgery. Among the available computer-assisted methods, surgical navigation is the most established. While most current applications can be found in the fields of neurosurgery [5.2] and, more recently, orthopaedic surgery [5.3], the number of new applications and surgical areas is steadily increasing. An important element of surgical navigation is the precise planning of a procedure whose results are subsequently transferred to the operation room (OR) as the basis of the surgical procedure. Tracked instrument positions displayed in pre and intraoperative images in combination with planning results provide a kind of guiding script for the surgeon. This helps to make surgery more precise and safe (e.g. by reducing access trauma). It also opens the door to an array of novel surgical procedures.

Navigation systems are particularly well-suited to neurosurgery, given the relative immobility of the brain due to its encapsulation in the skull. Fixed stereotactic frame surgery [5.1] can be replaced by frameless navigation-based procedures [5.4]. After brain surgery, surgical navigation is most commonly used in orthopedic surgery (e.g. prosthetics and osteosynthesis) [5.5], craniofacial surgery [5.6] and dental surgery [5.7]. Research is currently underway involving the use of navigation in connection with soft tissue regions, for instance, in the context of abdominal, gastroenterological and thoracic surgery. Here, researchers are faced with the enormous challenge of treating deformable and moving organs [5.8, 5.9]. Although current navigation systems make use largely of pre-operatively acquired MR and CT images, the trend for future systems includes the use of intraoperative imaging methods that permit navigation on the basis of images displaying the patient's current anatomy (e.g. after patient repositioning or tissue removal).

Any organ movement or deformation that takes place between the moment of image acquisition and the navigation procedure itself will reduce surgical accuracy. This obstacle can be overcome to a large extent through the use of intraoperative imaging to display current patient anatomy (i.e. excepting cases of natural movement such as heartbeat, breathing and colon movement).

Although its technical realization is of fundamental importance, the clinical acceptance of surgical navigation strongly depends on a simple user interface and straightforward integration into the clinical workflow. While it seems clear that surgical navigation has improved surgical quality, the overall benefits of such procedures for patients, surgeons, clinics and healthcare institutions (such as insurance companies) are still in need of further verification via extensive clinical testing.

5.2 Principles of navigation

Image-related surgical navigation is based on the spatial correlation between actual patient anatomy in the OR and corresponding 2D or 3D image data sets (mainly MR or CT). This correlation is established intraoperatively by the registration procedure, which is usually performed by identifying corresponding anatomical landmarks or fiducial markers in both the image data set and the patient.

While images are usually acquired prior to surgery, methods have recently been introduced for navigating on the basis of intraoperative CT and MR images [5.10, 5.11]. However, given that the most prominent imaging modalities in the OR are still ultrasound, and 2D and 3D fluoroscopy [5.12] navigation has also recently been adapted for them. Among other advantages, intraoperative imaging enables the use of automatic registration procedures, thereby enhancing workflow.

System and workflow considerations

It is important to view navigation in a broader context that includes a variety of workflow steps (fig. 5.1). Surgical planning is based on pre-operative image data that are subsequently processed by the navigation system. The most important processing stage is registration. This enables one to display the actual position and orientation of instruments in the image, which enables the surgeon to track the progress of intervention on the basis of the planning data.

Navigation-based surgery is characterized by four major aspects: visualization, tracking, minimally invasive access and integration.

Visualization

The task of monitoring the surgical procedure depends on access to the patient imaging data. The deployment of intraoperative imaging equipment requires a system of real-time display, including the option of fusing current image data with pre-operative image and planning data. While multiplanar reformatted (MPR) images are usually sufficient, 3D rendering is preferable in some cases for reasons of orientation. It is necessary to superimpose the actual positions of the tracked instruments and the planned access paths. It is sometimes necessary to handle the images interactively, especially if changes in access paths become necessary on account of changes in patient anatomy, repositioning or other unanticipated findings.

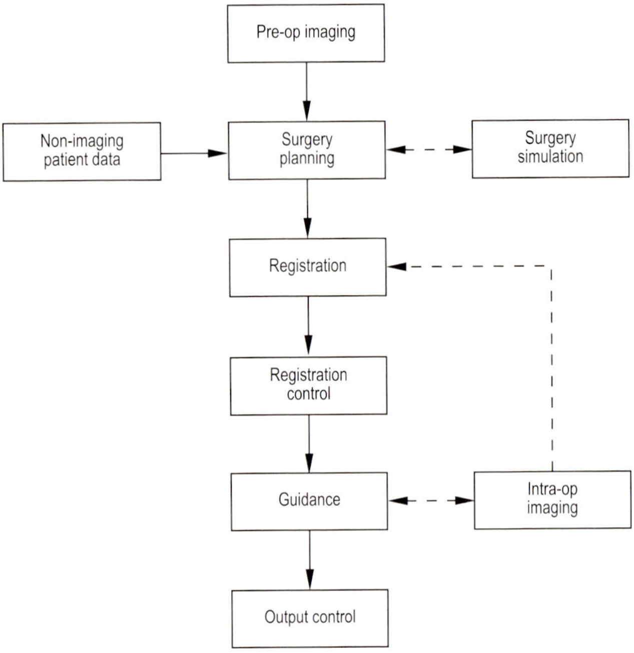

Figure 5.1 Clinical workflow in navigation-based surgery

Localization

Various technologies are applied for the sake of localizing the position of surgical instruments such as pointers, needles and microscopes and enabling their display in the image data sets after the registration procedure. These localization technologies include mechanical-arm, ultrasound [5.13], radar [5.14], electromagnetic [5.15] and optical systems [5.16].

Minimally invasive access

The minimization of the access trauma (tissue damage) that is caused during the approach to the target structure is the ultimate goal of minimally invasive surgery. Navigation systems enable one to optimally position surgical incisions, to identify and bypass critical structures and to visualize, approach and treat the target structure.

Integration

The integration of new intraoperative imaging and navigation takes place both with respect to the OR and the surgical workflow. An appropriate user interface is an important prerequisite, especially if interactive visualization or image processing is required. However, in addition to improvements in surgical quality, such systems can be expected to meet with wide acceptance only if they also demonstrate improvements in cost efficiency for the healthcare system.

5.3 Localizer technologies

Almost all of the navigation systems that are currently in use are optical or electromagnetic systems. In general, they consist of a signal transmission system and a sensor system rigidly attached to a surgical tool or to the patient. In the case of optical navigation, the signal transmission system consists of a camera system with 2 or more charge-coupled device (CCD) cameras, either in combination with infrared (IR) light emitting diodes (LEDs) attached to the tool or with IR illuminated reflecting spheres. Electromagnetic (EM) systems consist of an electromagnetic field transmitter combined with an arrangement of small induction coils as sensors. The dimensions involved in such coil systems permit the deployment of tracking probes inside the human body.

5.3.1 Principles of optical tracking systems

Position determination in the case of optical systems is achieved via geometric triangulation (fig. 5.2), using a stereo-camera system in combination with markers that are attached to the instruments being tracked (fig. 5.3). A marker plate with a fixed position (e.g. surgery table) is used as a dynamic reference so as to permit one to change the position of the camera without having to repeat the registration procedure.

Two types of systems are available, one applying active and the other passive markers. The markers are scanned using a CCD stereo camera whose base length usually ranges from about 50 to 100 cm, depending on the degree of accuracy required and the volume of interest [5.16]. The camera itself needs to be very well calibrated and temperature controlled in order to achieve a high degree of position-detection accuracy. During surgery an uninterrupted line of sight between instrument and camera is a precondition for optical tool tracking.

The active system makes use of IR emitting LEDs for localization while the passive system uses IR reflecting spheres. In the latter case, illuminating LEDs are positioned around the camera's CCDs.

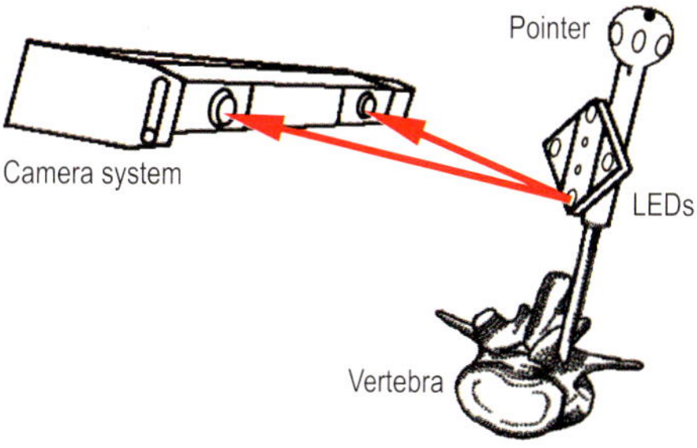

Figure 5.2
Geometric triangulation using a stereo-camera system and active LED sensors attached to a surgical tool

Active optical systems

The LEDs are used in pulse mode to enable one to identify the IR emitting LEDs attached to the instruments or reference frames and to differentiate with respect to ambient light. Localization is updated at a frequency of up to 60 Hz, allowing for real-time tracking. It is necessary to attach at least three LEDs (or more to improve accuracy) in order to determine both the position and the orientation of instruments. Assigning individual geometric LED patterns to individual instruments enables one to detect and track several instruments and reference markers simultaneously. While their brightness permits one to reliably localize active markers, electromagnetic radiation emitted by the cables may interfere with other sensitive equipment in the OR. Fig. 5.3 shows an example of an active optical system.

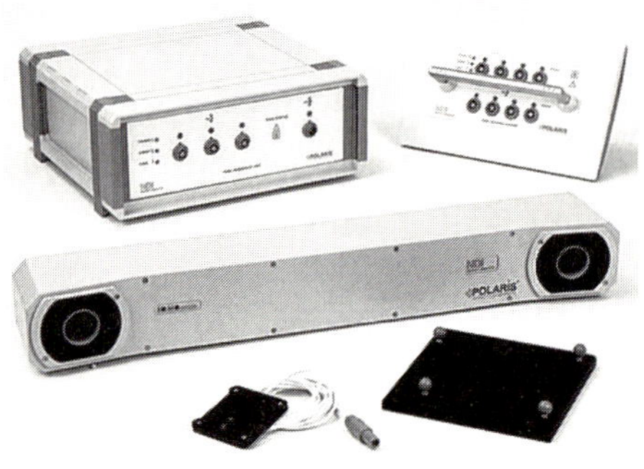

Figure 5.3
POLARIS® optical tracking system, including tool plates (NDI Waterloo, Ontario, Canada)

Passive optical systems

Passive optical systems are based on spherical markers that reflect infrared light. LEDs are arranged around the stereo camera's CCD sensors for purposes of illumination. The localization procedure is identical to that of an active system. In order to permit the simultaneous tracking of multiple instruments, it is necessary to establish a method of unambiguous instrument detection by attaching at least three markers to each instrument according to a unique pattern. However, pointers are sometimes equipped with only two markers when the information about the position and direction of the

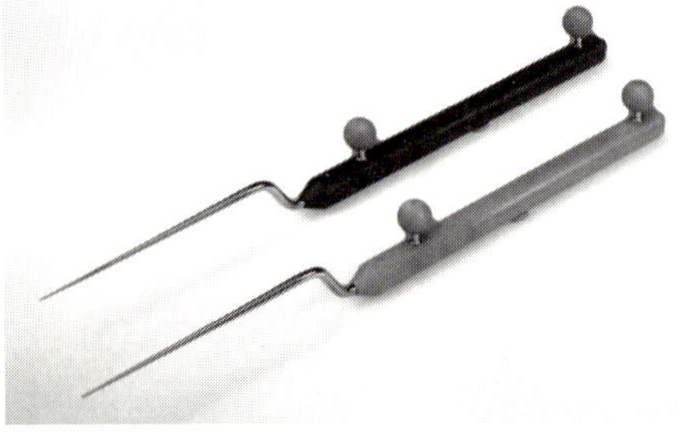

Figure 5.4
Two pointers, each with two reflecting marker spheres (VectorVision® pointer, BrainLab, Heimstetten, Germany)

pointer tip is sufficient and when the orientation around the pointer axis is not directly relevant (fig. 5.4). The essential advantage of passive systems is their cable-free design. Problems may occur when marker spheres cover each other in contexts involving the simultaneous deployment of several tracked instruments. Misdetection may sometimes occur due to illumination errors (infrared light from environmental sources or even scattered light).

The accuracy of optical systems ranges approximately from 0.1 to 0.4 mm (rms), calibrated in a measurement volume of approximately 1 m^3 for both active and passive systems. Having proven their effectiveness and reliability in many applications, optical tracking systems are far and away the most commonly used systems in surgical navigation today.

5.3.2 Electromagnetic position tracking

Electromagnetic tracking (i.e. at five or six degrees of freedom) is based on the application of electromagnetic fields (gradient or higher order fields, fig. 5.5). Such systems generally consist of a magnetic field transmitter, sensor coils and a processor unit (fig. 5.6). In its simplest form the field transmitter is made up of three orthogonal coils that are pulsed in a sequence to generate time and space-dependent electromagnetic fields, thereby allowing for unambiguous position measurements using induction coils in space. The measurement of six degrees of freedom requires a sensor with three orthogonal induction coils.

The calculation of the position and orientation of sensor coils can be performed in two different ways:

Applying a closed form solution and assuming a particular field distribution (e.g. a dipole field), the position of the transmitter field's origin can be derived directly from the measured field and gradient amplitudes at sensor position. However, this approach is limited to certain field transmitter geometries (e.g. three orthogonal transmitting coils with a common center of gravity).

Applying an iterative solution, the sensor signals can be optimally fitted (e.g. using the Levenberg-Marquardt algorithm) to values calculated for the transmitter's field distributions by varying the sensor coil position and orientation. A direct inversion of

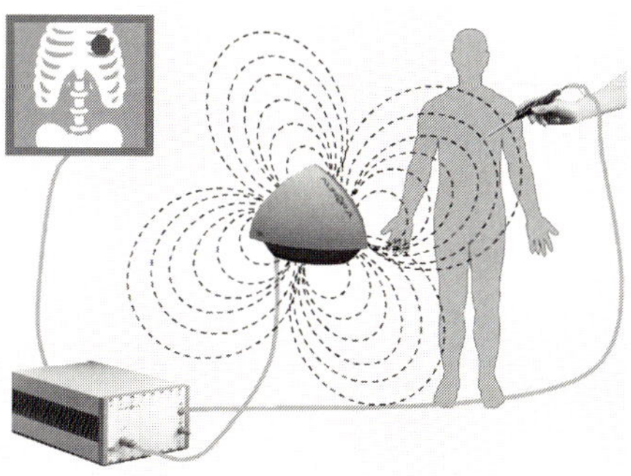

Figure 5.5
Electromagnetic tracking: a field transmitter generates an electromagnetic field that can be detected via sensor coils. The position and orientation of the sensor coils can be calculated on the basis of their measured field strengths. (NDI Waterloo, Ontario, Canada)

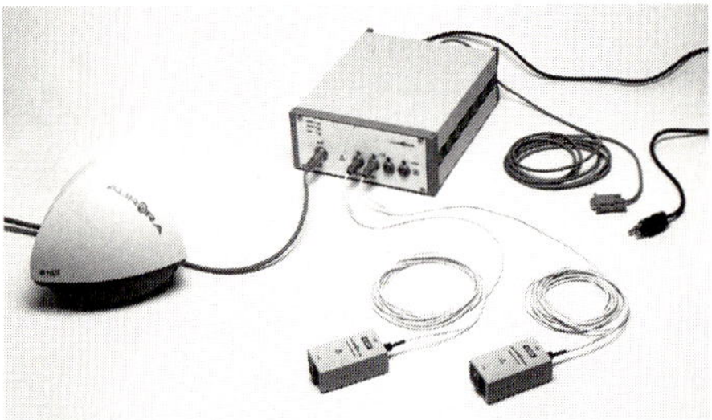

Figure 5.6
Electromagnetic tracking system AURORA®, consisting of a field generator, a system control unit and sensor interface units (NDI Waterloo, Ontario, Canada)

the transmitter field equations is not required. This approach is much more flexible with regard to field transmitter design and can therefore be better adapted to certain surgical requirements.

The sensor coils used in medical engineering are a couple of millimeters in size (fig. 5.7). Sensor coil systems of less than a millimeter have recently been developed. These utilize catheter and flexible endoscope applications for vessel and body-cavity tracking. Potential applications include the tracking of flexible endoscope tips in body cavities and catheters inside human vessels to permit certain surgical procedures (e.g. guidance of devices within complex cerebral vessels or within the human heart for radio-frequency ablation). However, there is a trade-off between sensor size, transmitter field strength and position detection accuracy. Common systems used in medicine have a measurement volume that corresponds to a 50 cm cube with a spatially dependent accuracy of approximately 1 to 2 mm (rms). Two different types of electromagnetic localizing systems are used in surgical navigation:

AC systems

Three mutually perpendicular magnetic fields are produced by an AC current distribution. These fields induce a voltage in the sensor coils that is then used to compute the sensor's location and orientation. The transmitter frequencies typically range from 5 to 15 kHz. The position detection is repeated at a rate of about 40 to 50 Hz.

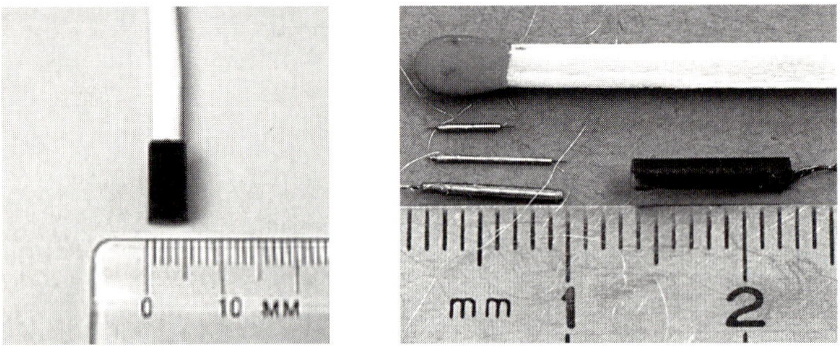

Figure 5.7
Miniaturized electromagnetic sensors: AURORA® sensors (NDI, Waterloo, Ontario, Canada)

Pulsed-DC systems

The magnetic field is produced by a sequence of rectangular pulsed DC currents that induce voltages in the sensor coils. These signals are recorded after a short delay to allow the eddy currents in surrounding metals to decay. Earth effects and those of other constant magnetic fields that arise when the sensor coils are moved are determined and subtracted from the measured signal. As in the case of the AC system, the sensor location and orientation are computed from the recorded signals. Pulsed-DC systems are designed for greater insensitivity to field distortions generated by eddy currents in nearby conductive materials.

Given that the localization principle depends on the local electromagnetic field at the position of the sensor coils, electromagnetic tracking systems are very sensitive to conductive environments. Conductive materials lead to field distortions and therefore to static and dynamic errors. These will require compensatory procedures. Examples of such environments include operation tables, imaging modalities and clamp systems. Dynamic sources include surgical equipment (e.g. nails or plates in orthopedic surgery), electro-coagulation equipment and even coils in monitors and nearby MR systems.

5.3.3 Tool calibration

The markers that are attached to surgical tools are either rigidly fixed or detachable. In either case, it is necessary to transform the actual position and orientation of the marker system to the position and orientation of the tip of the instrument. This instrument-dependent transformation (sometimes referred to as *tip transformation*) can be calculated by rotating the tool tip around a rigid pivot (fig. 5.8) and then tracking and recording the relevant positions and orientations to enable a subsequent calculation of the tip transformation. The transformation matrix itself is then stored at the navigation workstation and assigned to a specific tool. While fixed systems are calibrated once by the manufacturer, it is necessary to repeat the calibration procedure for detachable marker systems after each marker change.

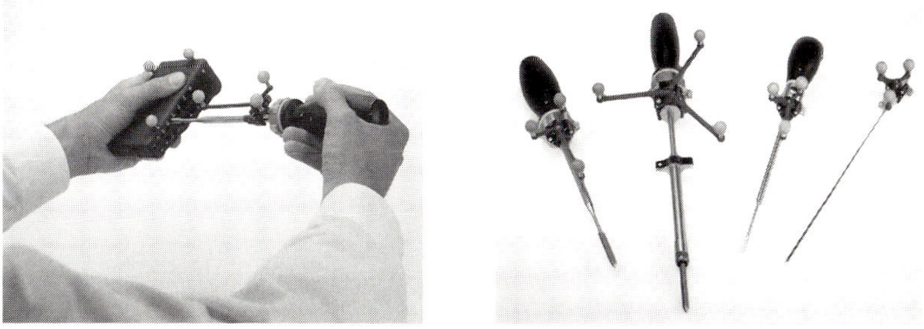

Figure 5.8
Left: calibration tool for spine instruments that compute tip transformation. **Right:** Various surgical spine tools equipped with passive optical markers (BrainLab, Heimstetten, Germany)

5.4 Registration

Image-related navigation is based on a calculation of the spatial relationship between the various coordinate systems involved in a specific application. These coordinate systems are defined by the following:

a) Pre-operative image data

b) Intra-operative imaging modality (if applied)

c) Tracking device

d) Fixed dynamic reference frame (if the tracking device is to be moved)

e) Tools to be tracked (fig. 5.9)

The relationship between the various coordinate systems can often be described as a rigid transformation that includes a rotation and a translation (it is sometimes necessary to consider scaling). While the parameterization of a rigid registration requires six parameters, it is important to bear in mind the procedure's limitations. Table movements and patient breathing and repositioning will diminish registration accu-

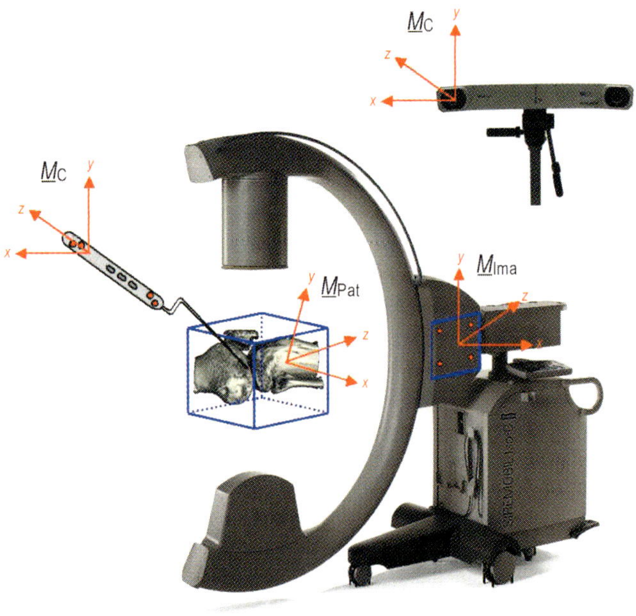

Figure 5.9
Representation of the various coordinate systems related to image-guided navigation. M_C: the stereo camera's coordinate system including that of the tools that are measured in the M_C camera system. M_{Ima} is the coordinate system of the pre- or intraoperatively acquired images and M_{Pat} is that of the patient or the dynamic reference frame attached to the patient. It is necessary to apply a registration procedure to transform all of these coordinate systems into a single system.

racy. Methods have therefore been developed to permit registration updates to handle cases of patient movement or deformation. These methods include the deployment of intra-operative imaging (e.g. ultrasound for the detection of brain shift in neurosurgery [5.17]), the deployment of attached sensors to detect global patient movement and the deployment of anatomical landmarks.

Rigid registration loses its applicability as soon as anatomic structures are deformed significantly during surgery. This fact introduces the necessity of more complex, non-rigid registration procedures. While the results of ongoing investigations of non-rigid (or deformable) algorithms show much promise, a sufficient degree of quality control, in particular, has not yet been established. Although non-rigid registration may help to reduce registration errors, the use of intraoperative imaging modalities for purposes of registration updating and quality control is preferable.

The registration methods used in surgical navigation are either voxel-based or feature-based. While voxel-based methods involve a point-to-point correspondence of fiducial markers or anatomical landmarks that are visible in both the imaging data set and the patient, feature-based methods rely on more complex image or object information (e.g. pertaining to surfaces and boundaries).

5.4.1 Point-pair matching using a 3D localizer

The most common registration procedure is point-pair matching using external markers. These markers can easily be identified in medical images (MR, CT) thanks to their high contrast. The spatial positions of the markers attached to the patient are measured using the localization system. The transformation between image space and object space can then be calculated by identifying the corresponding markers in the image data and on the patient. At least three non-coplanar points (3×3 equations) are required for a calculation of the six registration parameters. In practice, however, a larger set of corresponding points is used (10 to 15) in order to minimize registration errors due to inaccurate marker detection.

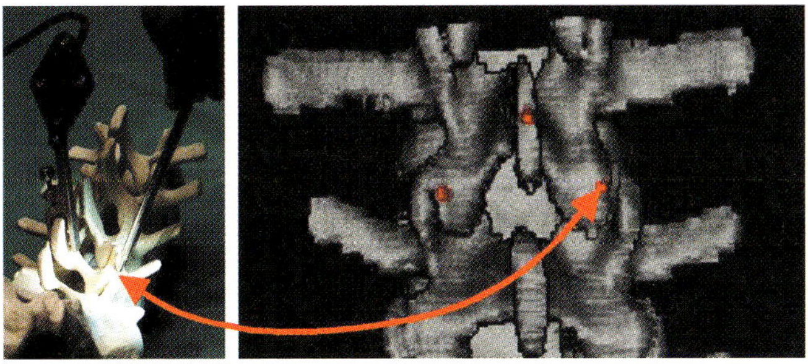

Figure 5.10
Registration procedure using point-pair matching. The corresponding points are localized in the patient using a navigation pointer **(left side)** and marked in the image data set **(right side)**. At least three non-coplanar corresponding points are required for rigid transformation.

Fiducials and anatomical landmarks (fig. 5.10) can be used for point-pair registration. It is necessary to attach fiducials to the patient prior to imaging so that the markers can also be detected in the image data set. Depending on the particular clinical application, the fiducial markers can be attached to the patient's surface or rigidly fixed in the patient's bone (e.g. for orthopedic or facial surgery). Compared to anatomical landmarks, fiducial markers offer the following advantages: they permit easier visual detection in image data sets, they enable a tailored spatial distribution across the patient's anatomy and their position is unambiguous because of their simple geometric structure. Procedures involving fiducials and landmarks both permit registration updating during surgery.

5.4.2 Surface matching

The surfaces of anatomical structures can be used for registration instead of a limited number of anatomical landmarks or fiducial markers. Dedicated image processing allows one to segment the surfaces or edges of 3D MR or CT image data sets as a basis for constructing a surface model. Matching this model to the anatomical surface provides the transformation matrix needed for registration. Various methods are available for digitizing the anatomical surface:

Surface registration using a 3D localizer

A localizer is used to randomly acquire a large number of points on the surface of the anatomical object. Registration involving 3D surface data (segmented from pre-operative CT or MR data) can be performed automatically. While this method of registration is reliable and more accurate than point-pair registration, it requires accessible surfaces of a sufficient curvature. The method has been used in spine surgery [5.18], robot-assisted total hip replacement and total knee arthroplasty.

Laser scanner

The surface of the anatomical structure that is to be registered can be digitized directly with a 3D laser scanner. A laser stripe projected across the object is viewed by a camera so that height variations in the object can be detected as changes in the shape of the line. Each viewed stripe forms a profile, with the total shape of the object being composed of several parallel profiles. The registration procedure is similar to that described above. This method has been primarily used in neurosurgery and facial surgery where the object is easily accessible, at least prior to the operation. While the procedure is fast, accurate and reliable, it presupposes anatomical structures that are accessible to an externally positioned laser source. Sterile covers used during surgery may hamper this method, i.e. at least with respect to the performance of registration updates during surgery.

Video imaging

In a procedure that is similar to that used with the laser scanner, the surface of the anatomical structure can also be rendered by projecting a fixed pattern onto the patient's skin and viewing this pattern with a stereo-video camera [5.19]. Beginning with the camera's exact geometry, a 3D model of the patient surface can be derived from the distortions in the projected pattern. The registration procedure and areas of application are similar to those of other surface-based methods.

5.5 Navigation for image-guided surgery and intervention

5.5.1 CT/MRI-based navigation

The capacity of MRI and CT to render 3D image data sets of high spatial and contrast resolution makes them indispensable in the context of image-based procedures. While CT is frequently used for orthopedic applications thanks to its excellent bone visualization, MR is predominantly used in neurosurgery thanks to its outstanding soft-tissue discrimination. At present, both CT and MR are frequently used in interventional procedures, such as needle biopsies [5.20] and tumor ablation [5.21], but seldom used as imaging modalities in the OR. Therefore image data sets are acquired pre-operatively and mainly used for surgical planning and navigation. Local anatomical changes (e.g. associated with patient movement or tissue removal) prevent navigation if the images cannot be updated.

Mobile C-arm-based navigation, as it has been applied increasingly in orthopedic surgery, represents an alternative to 3D MR and CT-based navigation in certain applications. Mobile C-arm systems are easy to use intraoperatively and in real time. The use of intraoperative X-ray images for navigation, however, requires a different registration process.

5.5.2 2D mobile C-arm-based navigation

C-arm-based fluoroscopic systems are frequently used in trauma and orthopedic surgery because they permit the real-time visualization of high contrast objects such as bones. Fluoro-based navigation was developed in order to reduce X-ray radiation times and to increase surgical accuracy. The principle is based on the registration of the C-arm system's position rather than on the position of reference points in previously acquired images.

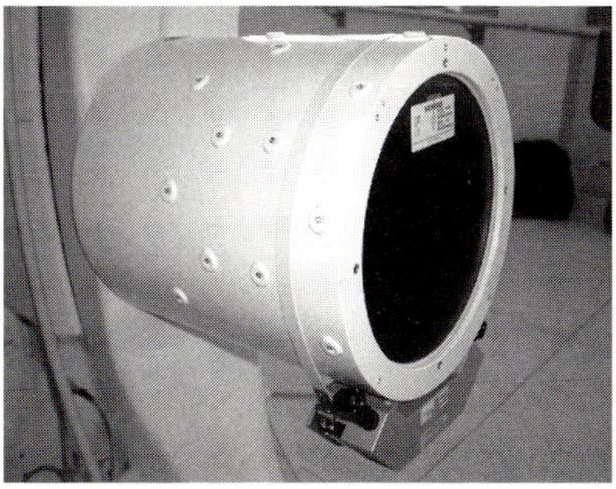

Figure 5.11
Image intensifier (Iso-C 3D®, Siemens Medical Solutions, Erlangen) equipped with LEDs for C-arm position detection in fluoroscopic navigation

A number of C-arm images is taken from various angles (5 to 10 different viewing positions) immediately prior to surgery. The respective C-arm positions are tracked by a navigation system in relation to a dynamic reference frame attached to the patient. A number of LEDs are fixed to the image intensifier for this purpose (fig. 5.11).

It is necessary to calibrate the C-arm with respect to intrinsic and extrinsic effects before proceeding with C-arm-based navigation.

The intrinsic calibration corrects for the spatially dependent geometric distortions caused by the image intensifier (I.I.). These distortions are mainly a matter of image translation, rotation and pincushion effects that are related to the actual position of the image intensifier in space on account of external magnetic fields. Such distortions can be corrected by imaging a rectangular, coplanar grid of steel spheres that is attached (parallel) to the I.I. image plane. Calibration matrices that can be used to correct the distorted I.I. images can be derived from the grid-frame geometry and the

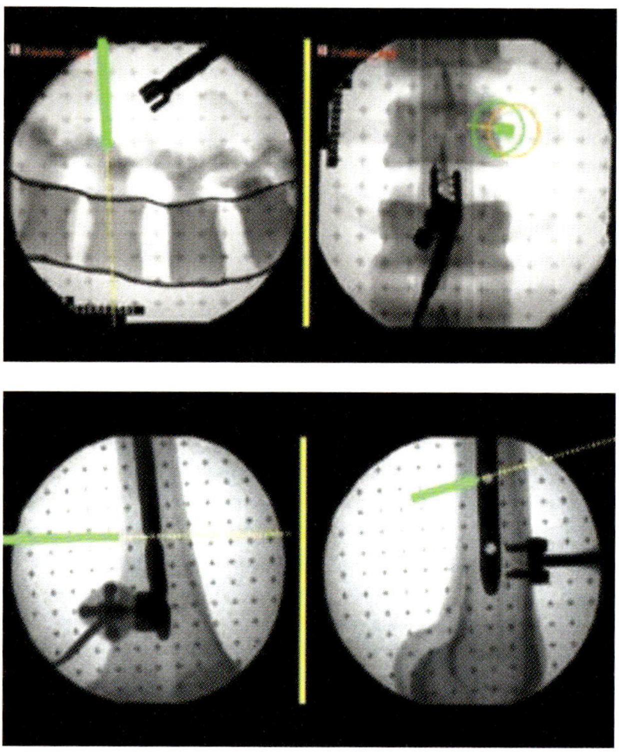

Figure 5.12
Examples of fluoro-navigated procedures. **Above:** two spine images acquired at two different projection angles, with the green line representing the actual position of the surgical tool and the yellow line representing that of the planned path. **Below:** similar images obtained in the context of an osteosynthesis procedure (M.E. Müller Research Center – Institute for Surgical Technology&Biomechanics, Bern)

measured grid distortions at different C-arm positions. Correction is possible with sub-pixel accuracy. It will also be necessary to measure the spatial relationship between X-ray source and camera via a phantom attached to the I.I. to correct for various mechanical deformations in the C-arm frame relating to the C-arm position.

The extrinsic calibration registers the C-arm positions during the acquisition of the images immediately prior to surgery with the reference frame attached to the patient. The C-arm can then be moved aside and the actual instrument positions can be displayed online in the acquired fluoroscopic images during surgery (fig. 5.12). Once the OR *situs* has been changed (e.g. by repositioning the patient), it will be necessary to repeat the image acquisition and registration procedure. These methods have proven to be very efficient in many surgical procedures [5.22].

5.5.3 3D mobile C-arm-based navigation

Recently developed mobile C-arm isocentric designs with I.I. technology enable 3D imaging. Image distortions related to the image intensifier can be minimized by using effective shielding materials against external magnetic fields and a tailored calibration procedure. Around 100 2D projection images of the patient are acquired during a continuous motorized orbital 190° rotation. A high-resolution 3D data cube with a side length of approximately 12 cm and an isotropic spatial resolution of around 0.5 mm can be reconstructed on the basis of these projections. Intrinsic calibration depends on a very precise knowledge of the C-arm acquisition geometry. However, due to limitations in the dynamic range of the I.I. and the number of projection images acquired, reconstruction is limited to high contrast images (e.g. bones and vessels filled with contrast agents) [5.12, 5.23]. Areas of application include orthopedic sur-

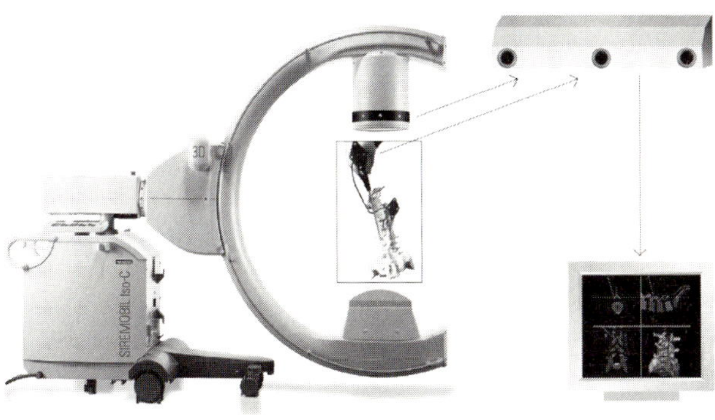

Figure 5.13
Navigation using the intraoperative imaging modality Iso-C 3D. The C-arm is equipped with a marker ring containing a number of active LEDs that are detected during image acquisition with the use of an optical localizer. The surgical tools are detected during surgery via the same localizer and appear in real-time in the reconstructed 3D data set either in reformatted slices or surface shaded displays.

gery, traumatology and facial surgery. Intraoperatively acquired 3D images can be used to guide and monitor surgical procedures and to support navigated surgery.

The use of such a system in combination with navigation requires the prior execution of a calibration procedure to calculate the transformation between a reference point attached rigidly to the C-arm and the image volume that is to be reconstructed [5.24]. This calibration procedure needs only to be carried out once by the manufacturer before system delivery. In the case of intraoperative image acquisition, the reference point attached to the C-arm is tracked by a 3D localizer. Given that the relationship between this reference point and the reconstructed volume has already been calibrated, the registration between the image volume, the camera system and the instruments with attached markers is also available (fig. 5.13). It therefore becomes possible to immediately display the tracked surgical instruments in the 3D patient data and to use this information for surgical guidance (fig. 5.14). Furthermore, a dynamic reference frame can be fixed to the surgery table to serve as a geometrical reference point during the procedure. This enables one to move aside the mobile C-arm after image acquisition and tracking of the position of the modality. The image acquisition proce-

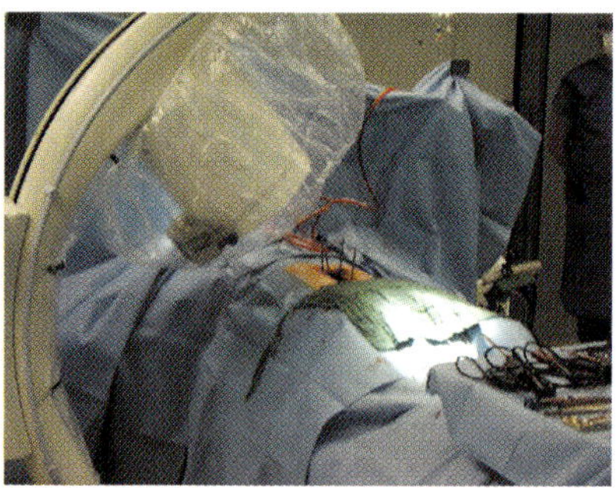

Figure 5.14
Top: Application of Iso-C 3D in spine surgery. The C-arm is wrapped in sterile drapes to fulfill OR sterilization requirements. **Below:** a reconstructed 3D cube displayed in the form of 3 reformatted slices that show the actual positions of the pedicle screws in the vertebrae.

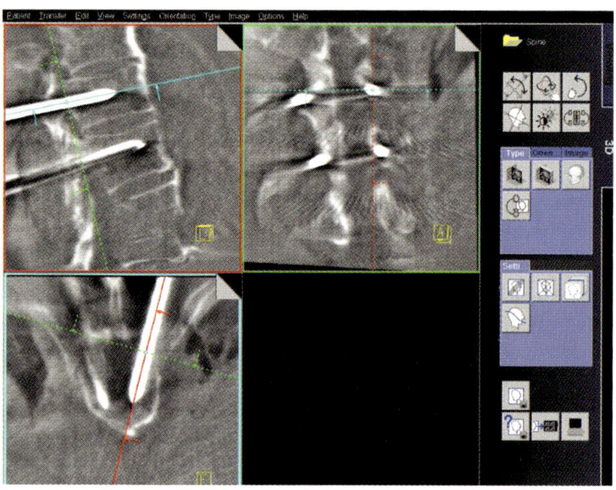

dure can be repeated as often as required (e.g. in order to update the registration after patient movement, tissue removal and the repositioning of bones or in order to control surgical results).

The obvious advantages associated with mobile 3D C-arm-based navigation center on the fact that it makes time consuming and error prone semimanual registration and additional pre-operative image acquisitions with attached markers unnecessary. However, the image fusion of pre-operative images (e.g. based on CT and MR) with the intraoperatively acquired 3D C-arm images is always an option. The benefits of this new technology have been amply shown in surgical practice. Even better results will be achieved as image quality improves and, even more importantly, as advances are made in the intraoperative 3D reconstruction of soft tissue objects [5.9].

It warrants mention that similar approaches involving the application of automatic registration procedures have also been developed for intraoperative MR (e.g. BrainSuite [5.11]) and CT.

5.6 Navigation accuracy

The task of determining the overall clinical accuracy of navigation is made difficult by its relationship to technical parameters and organ motion. From a technical point of view, registration error is related to the resolution of the image data sets, the accuracy of the tracking systems and the accuracy of marker detection (both in image data sets and patient). In the case of non-rigid objects, errors occur primarily in connection with object deformation and object movement. Image data set resolution ranges from 0.5 to 1.0 mm, depending on modality (CT, MR) and slice thickness. As mentioned, tracking system accuracy ranges from 0.1 to 0.4 mm (RMS) for optical and from1.0 to 2.0 mm for electromagnetic systems [5.25]. This results in an overall navigation error of 1 to 3 mm. Errors associated with object deformation may be even larger, making additional intraoperative image data and registration updating necessary.

5.7 Clinical applications

The critical structures in the brain make neurosurgery very demanding in terms of surgical accuracy. On the other hand, the brain is relatively fixed with respect to the skull, therefore allowing for accurate and stable reference. For these reasons, neurosurgery has historically been one of the main navigation-based applications. [5.26]. In addition to neurosurgery, applications have been developed in the area of surgical orthopedics and craniofacial surgery. This is mainly due to the relative rigidity and macroscopic nature of the skeletal system with the excellent rendering of bone structures in radiographic and CT images (figs. 5.15, 5.16).

The well-established applications include the placement of pedicle screws [5.27] in spine surgery, support for computer-assisted total hip replacement (THR), total knee arthroplasty (TKA) [5.28] and (more recently) reconstruction of the anterior cruciate

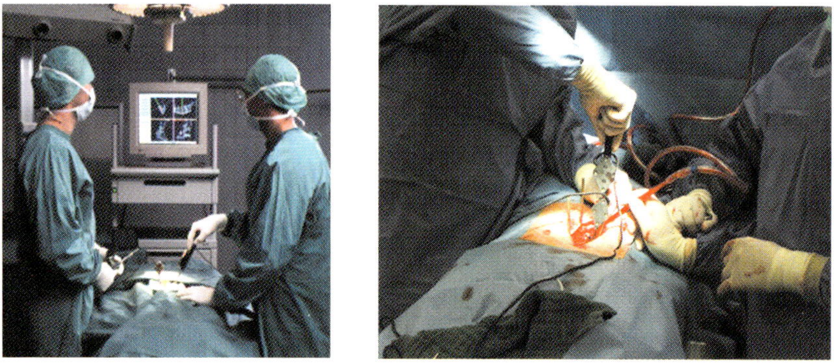

Figure 5.15
Navigation-assisted spine surgery. The positions of the tracked instruments are displayed in the 3D data sets to help guide the surgeon.

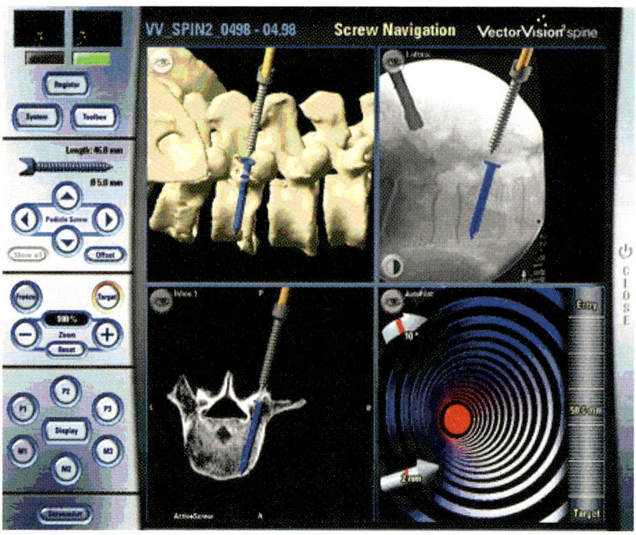

Figure 5.16
User interface of the BrainLAB VectorVision navigation system for spine surgery. The planned trajectories as well as the actual positions of the tools are displayed to help guide the surgeon.

ligament. Several applications have also been developed for the navigation-based placement of dental implants [5.7]. In the field of ear, nose and throat (ENT) surgery, applications have been developed for middle cranial fossa repair, temporal bone repair and paranasal sinus repair [5.29].

Initial attempts have been made to adapt navigation technologies and procedures to soft-tissue applications (e.g. gastroenterological procedures).

5.8 Future prospects

While clinical navigation is well-established in the areas of neurosurgery and orthopedic surgery, it is still a long way from being generally accepted for a wider range of applications. Further clinical evidence and further improvements in technology and user friendliness are required. Future developments will likely center on:

- More convenient user interfaces
- System control units that can be operated from the OR table
- Enhanced workflow integration (integration of diagnostic and therapeutic devices as well as networking)
- Simplification of the registration procedure and extension to non-rigid methods
- Open platform with customized application software and hardware
- Integration of new technologies (e.g. robotics)
- Improvement and integration of intraoperative imaging modalities
- Clinical evidence of benefits for patient and healthcare system

Navigation offers enormous potential for widespread surgical application. The full exploitation of this potential will require a multidisciplinary approach.

5.9 References

[5.1] L. Leksell
Stereotaxic apparatus for intracerebral surgery
Acta Chir. Scand. 99:229-233 (1949)

[5.2] P. Kelley
Computer-Assisted Neurosurgery: Needs and Opportunities in Computer-Integrated Surgery (Eds. R. Taylor, S. Lavallée, G. Budea, R. Moesges)
MIT Press (1995), Cambridge, MA

[5.3] P. Saulot, P. Cinquin, S. Lavallée, J. Troccaz
Computer-Assisted Spine Surgery: A first step towards clinical application in orthopaedics
Proceedings of the Annual International Conference of the IEEE 14, Engineering in Medicine and Biology Society (1992), 1071

[5.4] J. Gralla, C. Nimsky, M. Buchfelder, R. Fahlbusch, O. Ganslandt
Frameless stereotactic brain biopsy procedures using the stealth station: indications, accuracy and results
Zentralbl. Neurochir. 64 (2003), 166-170

[5.5] Joint Replacement Arthroplasty
in B.F. Morrey (Ed), Reconstructive Surgery of Joints,
Churchill Livingston (1996), 605.608

[5.6] S. Hassfeld, J. Mühling
Computer assisted oral and maxillofacial surgery – a review and an assessment of technology
Int. J. Oral Maxillofac. Surg. 20 (2001), 2-13

[5.7] R. Ewers, K. Schicho, M. Truppe, R. Seemann, A. Reichwein, M. Figl, A. Wagner.
Computer-aided navigation in dental implantology: 7 years of clinical experience
J. Oral Maxillofac. Surg. 62 (2004), 329-34.

[5.8] Ch. Nimsky, O. Ganslandt, S. Cerny, P. Hastreiter, G. Greiner, R. Fahlbusch
Quantification of, Visualization of, and Compensation for Brain Shift Using Intraoperative Magnetic Resonance Imaging
Neurosurgery 47 (2000), 1070-1080

[5.9] R. Marvik, T. Lango, G.A. Tangen, J.O. Andersen, J.H. Kaspersen, B. Ystgaard, H.E. Fjosne, R. Fougner, T.A. Hernes
3-D navigation in laparoscopic surgery
Tidsskr. Nor. Laegeforen 124 (2004), 617-9

[5.10] J.J. Froelich, N. Ishaque, B. Saar, et al.
Real-time CT-fluoroscopy for guidance of percutaneous drainage procedures
J. Vasc. Interv. Radiol. 9 (1998), 735.740

[5.11] BrainSuite,
BrainLAB GmbH, Heimstetten, Germany

[5.12] U. Linsenmaier, C. Rock, E. Euler, S. Wirth, R. Brandl, D. Kotsianos, W. Mutschler, K.J. Pfeifer
Three-dimensional CT with a Modified C-Arm Image Intensifier: Feasibility.
Radiology 242 (2002), 286-292

[5.13] R.D. Buchholz, K.R. Smith
Comparison of sonic digitizer versus light emitting diode-based localization
in R.J. Maciunas (Ed), Interactive image-guided neurosurgery
AANS Publications, USA (1993), 179-200

[5.14] J. Park, C. Nguyen
A new millimeter-wave step-frequency radar sensor for distance measurement
IEEE Microwave and Wireless Components Letters 12 (2002), 221-222

[5.15] D.D. Frantz, A.D. Wiles, S.E. Leis, S.R. Kirsch
Accuracy assessment protocols for electromagnetic tracking systems
Phys. Med. Biol. 48 (2003), 2241-2251

[5.16] Northern Digital Inc. (NDI), Waterloo, ON, Canada

[5.17] M.M. Bonsanto, A. Staubert, C.R. Wirtz, V. Tronnier, S. Kunze.
Initial experience with an ultrasound-integrated single-RACK neuronavigation system
Acta Neurochir. (Wien) 143 (2001), 1127-32

[5.18] D.V. Amin, T. Kanade, A.M. DiGioia, B. Jaramaz
Ultrasound registration of the bone surface for surgical navigation
Comput. Aided Surg. 8 (2003), 1-16.

[5.19] A.C. Colchester, J. Zhao, K.S. Holton-Tainter, C.J. Henri, N. Maitland, P.T. Roberts, G.G. Harris, R.J. Evans
Development and preliminary evaluation of VISLAN, a surgical planning and guidance system using intra-operative video imaging.
Med. Image Anal. 1 (1996), 73-90.

[5.20] R. Fahrig, G. Heit, Z. Wen, B.L. Daniel, K. Butts, N.J. Pelc
First use of a truly-hybrid X-ray/MR imaging system for guidance of brain biopsy
Acta Neurochir. (Wien) 145 (2003), 995.7

[5.21] S. Zangos, D. Kiefl, K. Eichler, K. Engelmann, M. Heller, C. Herzog, M.G. Mack, V. Jacobi, T.J. Vogl
MR-guided biopsies of undetermined liver lesions: technique and results
Röfo 175 (2003), 688-694

[5.22] L.P. Nolte, M.A. Slomczykowski, U. Berlemann, M.J. Strauss, R. Hofstetter, D. Schlenzka, T. Laine, T. Lund,
A new approach to computer-aided spine surgery: fluoroscopy-based surgical navigation
EuroSpine J. 9 (2000), 78-88

[5.23] D. Kotsianos, C. Rock, S. Wirth, U. Linsenmaier, R. Brandl, T. Fischer, E. Euler, W. Mutschler, K.J. Pfeifer, M. Reiser
Frakturdiagnostik am Kniegelenk mit einem neuen mobilen CT-System (Iso-C3D): Vergleich mit konventionellem Röntgen und Spiral-CT
RöFo 174 (2002), 82-87

[5.24] D. Ritter, M. Mitschke, R. Graumann
Markerless Navigation with the Intra-Operative Imaging Modality SIREMOBIL Iso-C^{3D}
electromedica 70 (1), 2002

[5.25] Ascension Technology Corporation, Burlington, VT 05402, USA.

[5.26] Ch. Nimsky, O. Ganslandt, B. v. Keller, T. Vetter, A. Oppelt, R. Fahlbusch
Erste Ergebnisse mit einem Hochfeld-MRT im OP
electromedica 70 (2002)

[5.27] Y. Kotani, K. Albumi, M. Ito, A. Minami
Improved accuracy of computer-assisted cervical pedicle screw insertion
J. Neurosurg. 99 Suppl. 3 (2003), 257-263

[5.28] S.D. Stulberg, P. Loan, V. Sarin
Computer-assisted navigation in total knee replacement: results of an initial experience in thirty five patients
J. Bone Joint Surg. Am. 84-A Suppl 2 (2002), 90-98.

[5.29] H.F. Zeilhofer, U. Kliegis, R. Sader, H.H. Horch
Video matching as intraoperative navigation aid in operations to improve the facial profile
Mund Kiefer Gesichtschir. 1 Suppl 1 (1997), 68-70

Part II – Physics of Imaging

6 X-ray and γ-radiation

6.1 Generation of X-ray and γ-radiation

X-ray and γ-radiation are electromagnetic waves of very short wavelength. Gamma radiation, with a wavelength of less than $1.25 \cdot 10^{-3}$ nm and energy levels above 1 MeV, arises as a product of radioactive decay and has its origin in the atomic nucleus. The energy of X-rays is mostly in the keV range, from 1 to 500 keV, and the wavelengths range from 0.006 nm to 1.25 nm.

Two processes are mainly responsible for X-ray production: the acceleration of charged particles (usually electrons) and the descent of electrons from one atomic or ionic energy level to a lower one. Examples of the first type are synchrotron radiation [6.1], which arises when relativistic charged particles are caused to travel in curved paths by magnetic fields and bremsstrahlung [6.2], which arises from the deceleration of electrons due to collisions with heavy nuclei. These normally yield continuous spectra, although it is possible to obtain quasi monochromatic lines from insertion devices (undulators) in storage rings (synchrotron sources).

The second emission process, which occurs when electrons bombard a target of a low atomic number or when a plasma is formed from a material of a low atomic number, yields discrete line spectra. Highly ionized plasmas can also be made to behave as X-ray lasers [6.3]. Other recently investigated emission processes, such as transition radiation [6.4], which occurs when a particle crosses an interface between two dielectric materials, and channeling radiation [6.5], which occurs when a particle moves along a channel formed by planes in a crystal, also give rise to X-ray. For the present, their use is limited to research [6.6].

Given that a well-controllable source is necessary for the application of X-ray techniques, we concentrate in the following on the emission process in which X-rays are produced by the deceleration of electrons in matter. This process is also the source of MeV γ-radiation in radiotherapy.

An electron emitted from a cathode in a vacuum tube (fig. 6.1) and accelerated in the electric field of an anode acquires kinetic energy according to:

$$E_{kin} = \frac{m}{2} v^2 = eU \qquad (6.1)$$

v: Velocity of electrons, U: Voltage between anode and cathode
$e = 1.6 \cdot 10^{-19}$ As: Electron charge

The electron then loses its energy as it penetrates the anode (or target). Here, two forms of interaction are possible. The first and more important form of interaction results from the electron's collision with the bound electrons of the atoms. These are

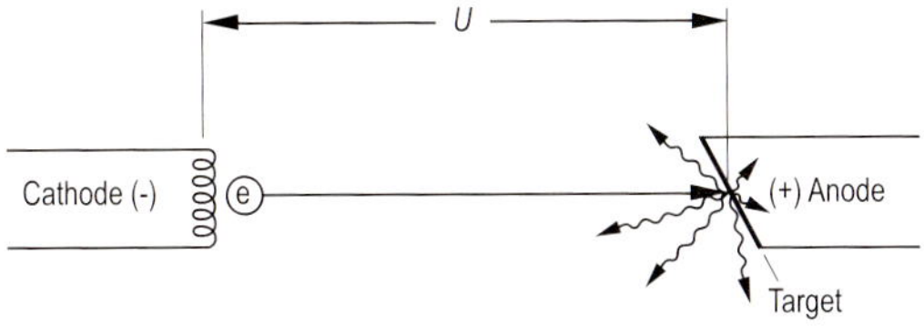

Figure 6.1
Principle of X-ray generation

raised to higher energy levels or ionized. The excited atoms then fall back to their state of equilibrium either via the emission of radiation or via radiationless processes. The electrons released by ionization may have enough kinetic energy to cause further ionizations. Finally, all energy transferred as a result of collisions is converted to lattice vibrations, i.e. heat. More than 99% of the kinetic energy produced by electron collisions is converted in this way.

The second form of interaction involves the deceleration of electrons colliding in the electric field of the nuclei in the anode material. This results in the emission of radiation (bremsstrahlung). The probability of radiative interaction or collision depends on the energy and the atomic number of the material. Less than 1% of the energy available in the energy range relevant for medical diagnostics is converted into X-ray energy.

6.1.1 Properties of X-ray bremsstrahlung

The closer the path of the electron to the nucleus and the higher its kinetic energy, the greater is the energy $h\nu$ of the X-ray quantum generated. At the upper limit, all of the electron's kinetic energy is transformed into radiation energy in the braking process. In this asymptotic case, the photon created has the greatest possible energy and frequency.

The slowing down of the electrons in matter takes place along their path of penetration into the target by a stepwise loss of kinetic energy. They travel through several layers of atoms until all of their energy is dissipated. The energies of the quanta from the multi-stage braking processes therefore assume arbitrary values below the maximum energy. Thus, X-ray quanta of every possible frequency below ν_{max} are generated. The spectral radiation intensity $\frac{\textit{Number of photons} \times h\nu}{\textit{Time} \times \textit{Frequency interval} \times \textit{Area}}$ (J/m^2) shows a linear dependence on frequency, with a slope proportional to the atomic number of the target (fig. 6.2).

$$\psi_\nu(\nu) \propto Z(\nu_{max} - \nu) \tag{6.2}$$

With respect to X-ray generation in the context of radiology, the intensity distribution of X-rays at the surface of the anode is nearly independent of the direction of emission (fig. 6.3). A reduced X-ray intensity distribution is observed only at very shallow angles due to the inherent absorption of the X-rays in deeper atomic layers (heel effect). This effect increases with the service life of X-ray tubes because the smoothness of the

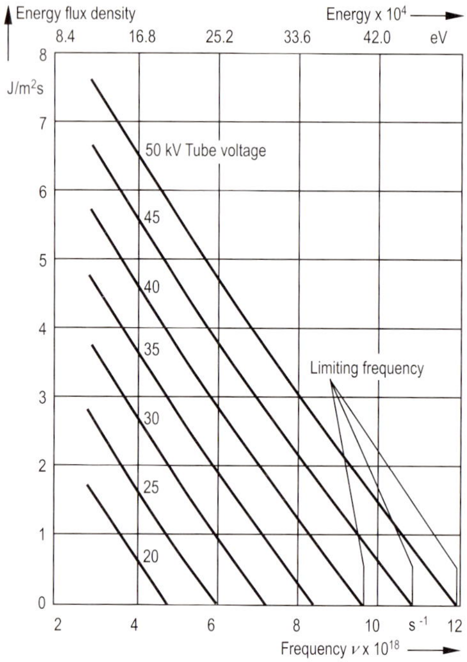

Figure 6.2
Unfiltered spectral intensity distribution (photon energy per time, frequency and area) for bremsstrahlung as a function of electron energy

anode surface tends to degrade, a condition that can lead to one-sided shading in X-ray exposures.

6.1.2 Characteristic radiation

Fig. 6.4 depicts the continuous bremsstrahlung spectrum of tungsten. This spectrum is overlaid by sharp peaks of characteristic radiation. In comparison to fig. 6.2, the low-energy X-ray radiation is strongly diminished. This is the result of absorption in the X-ray tube housing, the presence of additional filters and air filtration between the radiation emitter and the measuring device.

$$h\nu_{\max} = h\frac{c}{\lambda} = eU \qquad (6.3)$$

ν: Frequency, λ: Wavelength

$h = 4.135 \cdot 10^{-15}$ eVs: Planck's constant, $c = 2.998 \cdot 10^{8}$ m/s: Speed of light

Characteristic X-ray peaks are specific to the target material used. Electrons in atoms are bound in shells (K, L, M, N, O, P), their energy decreasing with increasing distance from the atomic nucleus. These shells are referred to by main quantum numbers (n = 1 to 6), with each shell filled by $2n^2$ electrons. By way of example, the energy levels for tungsten are shown in fig. 6.5. An electron penetrating the target with a kinetic energy higher than the binding energy of a given electron in the shell can knock the electron out of the shell. The shell is then no longer completely filled and the atom is in an ion-

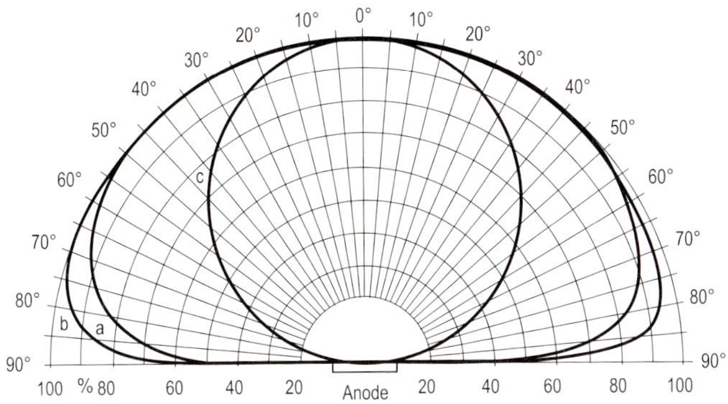

a Unfiltered radiation at 70 kV
b Filtered radiation (10 mm aluminium plate) at 70 kV
c Distribution according to the Lambert law

Figure 6.3 Angular intensity distribution of X-rays emerging from an anode

ized state. The hole created in the shell can be filled by an electron from an shell further outside, which then gives up the energy it gains by emitting a photon of characteristic frequency. Transitions to the K-shell generate X-ray lines of the K-series (K_α, K_β, K_γ, ...).

$$h\nu = E_{K\alpha} = E_K - E_L \tag{6.4}$$

The new hole in the L shell can be filled by an electron from the M shell or from a shell further outside, giving rise to radiation L_α, L_β, L_γ..., etc. However, the characteristic radiation from shells still further away from the nucleus (e.g. N, O or P shells) has so little energy that this is absorbed by inherent filtration.

The energy levels of the L, M and N shells are split further, according to their orbital and spin quantum numbers. Therefore, the transition of electrons from the L to the K

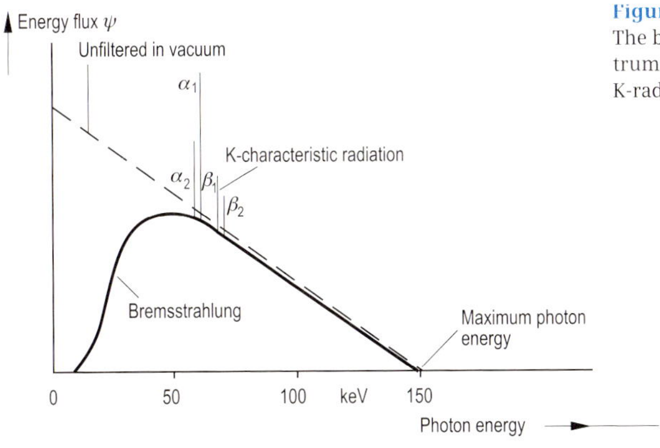

Figure 6.4 The bremsstrahlung spectrum and the characteristic K-radiation for tungsten

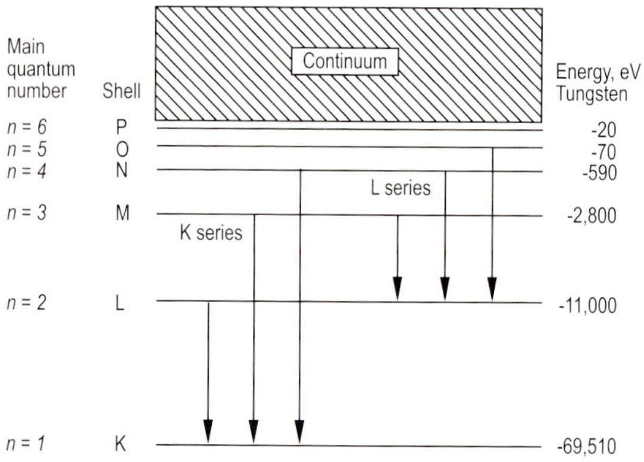

Figure 6.5
Simplified energy level diagram of tungsten

shell comprises two characteristic X-ray photons with energies (e.g. in Tungsten) of $K_1 = 59.3$ keV and $K_2 = 57.9$ keV. Further high-intensity characteristic radiation is produced as a result of the transition of an electron from the M to the K shell with energies of $K_1 = 67.2$ keV and $K_2 = 69$ keV, respectively.

6.1.3 Intensity (energy flux density) of X-radiation

The total energy flux density ψ of X-radiation (J/m²) generated by an X-ray tube is given by the area under the curves in fig. 6.2

$$\psi = \int \psi_\nu \mathrm{d}\nu \propto ZjU^n \tag{6.5}$$

j: Anode current density (A/m²)
U: Anode voltage
Z: Atomic number of the target material

While $n = 2$ for unfiltered radiation, this exponent may increase up to a value of 5, depending on the degree of filtration. Filtration is caused by the tube envelope and any additional filters, including the patient. Especially low energy X-ray is reduced, resulting in a shift of the spectrum's center of gravity towards higher energy levels, an effect called hardening.

In radiology, the quality of X-radiation is characterized by the half-value thickness (HVT) and homogeneity. The HVT is the thickness of an additional filter placed in the beam path to reduce the energy flux density by one half. Up to 150 kV, aluminum filters are used in preference to copper filters. The homogeneity coefficient is the ratio of the first HVT to the second HVT, the second HVT being the thickness of a further filter required for reducing the intensity by one half again.

Efficiency in X-ray generation is the ratio of the bremsstrahlung energy flux density ψ to the energy flux density of the incident electron beam jU. The following therefore applies for unfiltered radiation:

$$\eta = kUZ \tag{6.6}$$

k is a constant determined empirically to be 10^{-9} V^{-1}. For tungsten ($Z = 74$) at an anode voltage of 125 kV, it follows that $\eta \approx 1\%$. Since only a small solid angle of the total anode radiation field is used in radiology to generate an image, the yield is reduced once more to about one tenth of this value.

6.1.4 Target material

For the target material of an X-ray tube a large atomic number is preferable for more efficient X-ray generation. However, because the absolute efficiency is very low, thermal properties are of equal importance. Therefore, a high melting point, along with good thermal conductivity and high heat capacity, are the primary requirements for the target material.

For the optimal choice of materials it can be shown that for the case of a fixed anode for long-term operation (Z: atomic number, ϑ_{max}: maximum permissible temperature, c: specific heat, λ: thermal conductivity, ρ: density) the value $Z\vartheta_{max}\lambda$ must be as high as possible. In order to reduce the local thermal load at the target, where the electrons often impinge at an oblique angle, it is necessary to maximize the value $Z\vartheta_{max}\sqrt{\lambda\rho c}$.

In order to prevent degradation of the vacuum tube, the ϑ_{max} value is based on a maximum vapor pressure of $1.33 \cdot 10^{-2}$ Pa. As a rule, the maximum permissible focal spot temperature should be 20 to 30% lower than the melting point of the target material.

As indicated in table 6.1, tungsten emerges as an outstanding anode material for both short and long load times. This is due to its high atomic number, its high melting point and, compared to other materials with a high melting point, its good thermal properties. Because of the high thermal conductivity and heat capacity of copper, even better performance can be achieved by embedding a tungsten disk of an optimized thickness in copper [6.7].

Table 6.1 Anode materials used for fixed and rotating anodes

Element	Atomic number Z	Permissible temperature ϑ_{max} at $1.33 \cdot 10^{-2}$ Pa in °C	Thermal conductivity λ W/cm·K	Fixed anodes		Rotating anodes		
				$Z\vartheta_{max}\lambda$	Order of suitability	$\sqrt{\lambda\varrho c}$	$Z\vartheta_{max} \times \sqrt{\lambda\varrho c}$	Order of suitability
Cu	29	1032	3.98	119 113	8	3.68	110 135	10
Mo	42	2167	1.38	125 599	7	1.88	171 106	8
Ag	47	832	4.18	163 450	4	3.18	124 350	9
Ta	73	2587	0.55	103 868	9	1.13	213 402	6
W	74	2757	1.3	265 223	1	1.81	369 273	1
Re	75	2557	0.71	136 160	6	1.38	264 650	4
Os	76	2280	0.87	150 754	5	1.77	306 706	3
Ir	77	2220	1.46	249 572	3	2.06	352 136	2
Pt	78	1742	0.71	96 472	10	1.41	191 585	7
Au	79	(1063)	3.14	263 687	2	2.81	235 975	5
U	92	(1132)	0.25	26 036	11	0.75	78 108	11

Target materials other than tungsten (e.g. molybdenum, owing to the energy of its characteristic K_α radiation) are used only for special applications (e.g. in mammography).

6.2 X-ray and γ-ray interaction with matter

6.2.1 Interaction effects and phenomenological description

X-rays and γ-rays represent forms of electromagnetic radiation with very short wavelengths and high quantum energy levels. They are thus capable of passing through matter easily. Due to their interaction with atoms, part of the primary beam quanta is lost. This effect is used in radiology to generate images of organs within the body.

A thin layer (of thickness dx) attenuates the X-ray intensity in the following way:

$$d\Psi_v = -\mu \Psi_v dz \tag{6.7a}$$

$\mu = \mu(\nu, \rho, Z)$: Total attenuation coefficient (1/m)

For objects of thickness d, integration gives:

$$\Psi_v = \Psi_{v0} e^{-\mu d} \tag{6.7b}$$

The decrease in the number of quanta on passing through material can be explained by three effects: the photoelectric effect, scattering and pair production. Since however for the production of an electron/positron pair a photon energy level of at least 1.02 MeV is necessary, only the photoelectric effect and scattering are relevant in diagnostic X-ray radiology. Furthermore, given that scattering can be coherent (Rayleigh or Thomson, in which incident and scattered waves have the same frequency) or incoherent (Compton), the linear attenuation coefficient can be written as follows:

$$\mu = \mu_{\text{Photo}} + \mu_{\text{Compton}} + \mu_{\text{Coherent}} \tag{6.8}$$

μ_{Photo}: Photoelectric attenuation coefficient

μ_{Compton}: Compton coefficient and, μ_{Coherent}: Coherent attenuation coefficient

The attenuation is often expressed by the mass attenuation coefficient μ/ρ, where ρ is the density of the material used. Fig. 6.6 schematically illustrates the contributions of the different effects to X-ray absorption in soft tissue.

In the following, we will see that the attenuation coefficient depends on the wavelength or the energy of the X-rays and the atomic number of the material, independent of chemical bonding. PbS molecules thus exhibit the same absorption behavior as a homogenous mixture of elementary lead (Pb) and sulfur (S) atoms. The contributions to the absorption are superimposed on each other with no mutual influence.

6.2.2 The photoelectric effect

If an X-ray or γ-quantum is completely absorbed by a bound electron, the electron will be ejected from the atom with an energy E equal to the difference in energy between

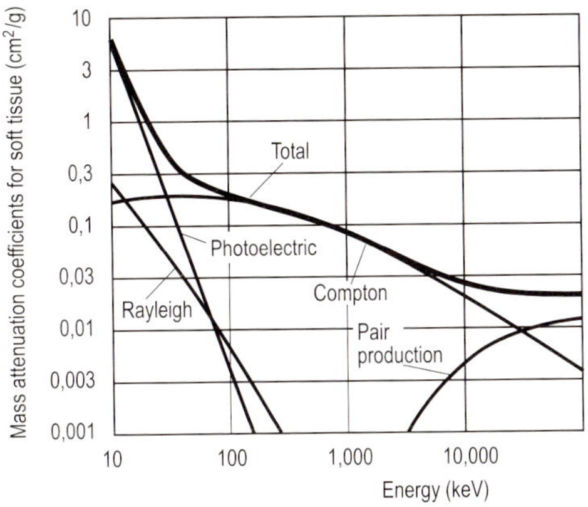

Figure 6.6
Mass attenuation coefficient of soft tissue as a function of X-ray energy

the colliding X-ray quantum and the binding energy of the electron (fig. 6.7). If the electron originates in an outer shell, with low binding energy, then it will assume – as a free photoelectron – virtually all of the quantum's energy. If the electron originates in the K or L shell, with high binding energy (this applies particularly in the case of atoms with a high atomic number Z), then its kinetic energy will be considerably reduced compared to that of the colliding quantum. The resulting vacancy in the relevant electron shell will then filled again, either by an electron from one of the outlying shells or, in the case of a solid, by an electron from one of the bands. The vacancies which are subsequently created are also filled successively in the same way.

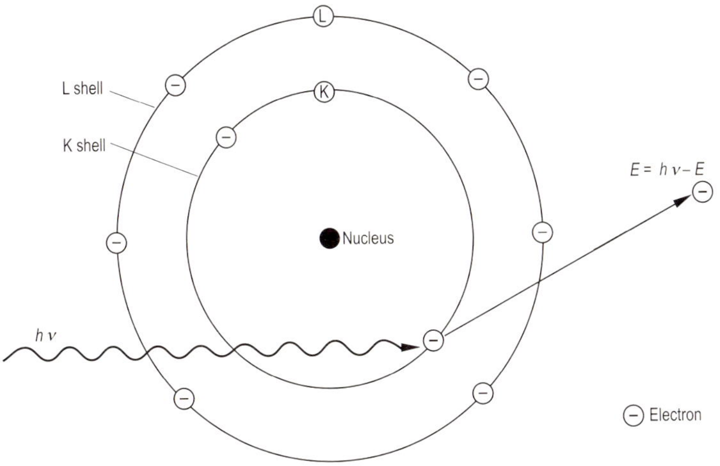

Figure 6.7
Photoelectric effect: a quantum with energy $h\nu$ collides with an atom, consisting of nucleus and electron clouds. An electron is struck and emitted with an energy equal to that of the quantum minus the binding energy.

Table 6.2
Example of X-ray fluorescence lines for xenon generated by electron transitions between various orbits

Transition	Name of line	Energy keV	Relative intensity
$L_{III} \rightarrow K$	$K_{\alpha 1}$	29.8	100
$L_{II} \rightarrow K$	$K_{\alpha 2}$	29.5	52
$M_{III} \rightarrow K$	$K_{\beta 1}$	33.6	20.2
$N_{II}/N_{III} \rightarrow K$	$K_{\beta 2}$	34.4	3.6

As outlined in 6.1.2, the discrete energies liberated in the process are emitted in the form of characteristic quanta. The discrete quantum spectrum ranges from very low energy values in the case of replacement by neighboring electrons from outer shells to a maximum value, corresponding to the difference between the energy of a photoelectron and the energy of a K-electron. This energy naturally increases as Z increases, as is the case with the maximum energies of the individual series (the edges). Here, *series* refers to the discrete energy values of all fluorescent quanta resulting from electron transitions into one particular electron orbit. By way of example, table 6.2 depicts a number of X-ray fluorescence lines for xenon, along with their relative intensities.

However, the energy released in the atom by an electron transition can also directly free another electron from the same atom. Since the creation of such *Auger* electrons is not accompanied by radiation, the process is also referred to as radiation-free transition or internal conversion. The probability of such a process is nearly 1 in the case of elements with a low atomic number Z and nearly 0 in the case of elements with high atomic number.

Absorption dependence on energy and atomic number

Fig. 6.8 depicts the mass attenuation coefficient for the photoelectric absorption of xenon as a function of photon energy as a log – log graph. The dependence of μ_{Photo}/ρ on $h\nu$ may be roughly described by an exponential law with an exponent of –2.7. The steep decrease that occurs along with increasing energy is interrupted by steps at energy levels corresponding to the binding energy of an atomic shell electron. The increase in absorption is larger than one would expect from the increased number of absorbing electrons. Thus, for example, at the K-edge of xenon, the number of absorbing electrons increases by 2, from 52 to 54, but μ_{Photo}/ρ increases by more than a factor of 5.

The dependence of μ_{Photo}/ρ on the atomic number Z can be roughly described by an exponential law, with an exponent of approximately 3.

Angular distribution of the photoelectrons

According to the classical picture, the electrons of the atom are accelerated by the field strength of the electric vector of the incident wave. Since the electric vector is always normal to the direction of incidence, one would expect the photoelectrons to be propelled outwards at an angle of exactly 90° to the direction of the incident X-rays. However, the X-ray quantum has a momentum, which it transfers to the atom and to the

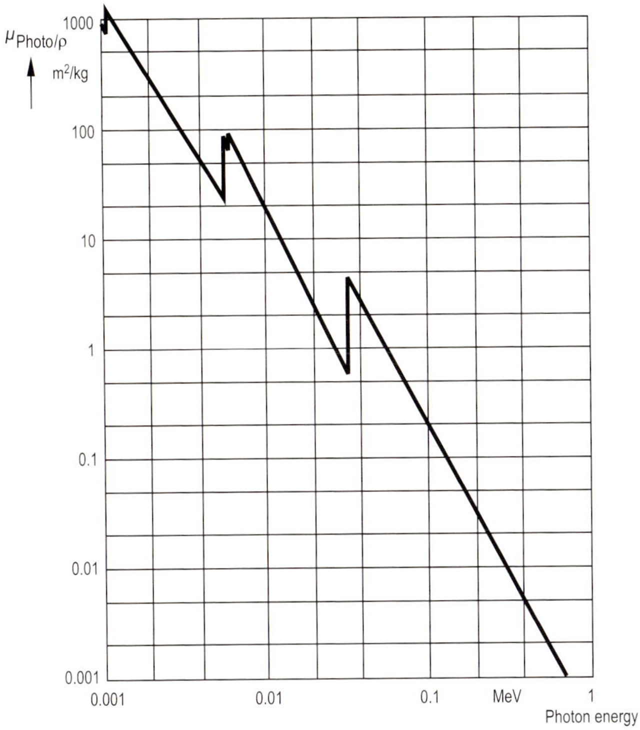

Figure 6.8
Mass attenuation coefficient μ_{Photo}/ρ for the photoelectric absorption process in xenon as a function of photon energy $h\nu$

photoelectron. Bearing in mind the law of conservation of momentum, this gives rise to the butterfly-shaped figures shown in fig. 6.9. It stands to reason that the more energetic the incident quanta, the more photoelectrons (on the average) will be catapulted out in the forward direction as a consequence of momentum conservation. This can be seen clearly in the polar diagram of the photoelectrons.

6.2.3 Compton effect

The Compton effect (incoherent scattering) offers clear evidence for the corpuscular nature of X-ray quanta. It provides a description, together with the laws of conservation of energy and momentum, of the interaction between high-energy quanta and the quasi-free electrons of the atoms. Given that the binding energy of electrons in atoms with low Z is very small compared to the energy of the incident quanta, one may treat these electrons as quasi-free. Extensive calculations exist for this case. Using the laws of energy and momentum conservation, one can calculate the energy E' of the recoil electron, for example, as a function of the energy $h\nu$ of the colliding quantum and the

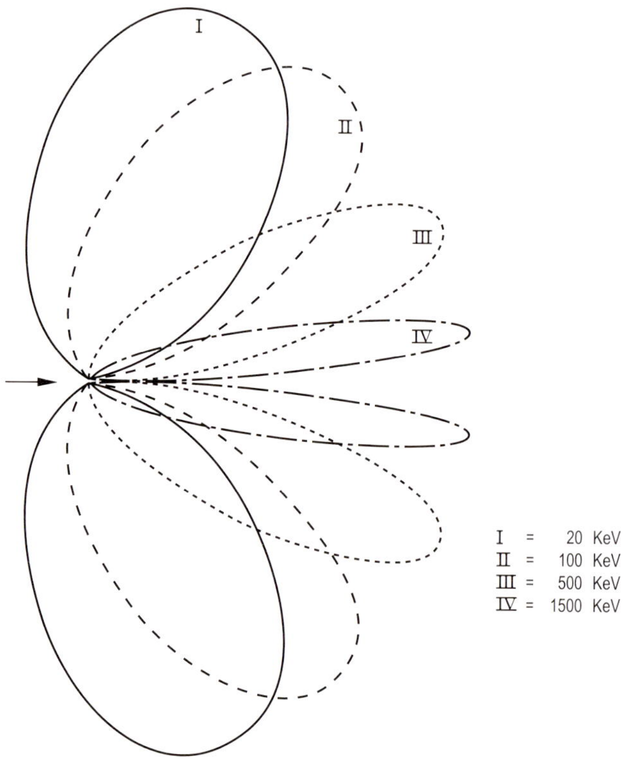

Figure 6.9
Angular distribution of the photoelectrons as a function of the incident X-ray quanta energy

angle ϕ through which the quantum is deflected from its original direction (fig. 6.8), as well as the energy $h\nu'$ of the scattered quantum or the angle θ of the recoil electron.

$$h\nu = h\nu' + T \qquad \text{(energy conversion)} \qquad (6.9)$$

$$\frac{h\nu}{c} = \frac{h\nu'}{c}\cos\phi + \sqrt{2mE'}\cos\theta$$
$$0 = \frac{h\nu'}{c}\sin\phi - \sqrt{2mE'}\sin\theta \qquad \text{(momentum conservation)} \qquad (6.10)$$

Defining $\alpha = \dfrac{h\nu}{m_0c^2}$ we find

$$E' = h\nu\frac{\alpha(1-\cos\phi)}{1+\alpha(1-\cos\phi)} \qquad (6.11)$$

$$h\nu' = \frac{h\nu}{1+\alpha(1-\cos\phi)} \qquad (6.12)$$

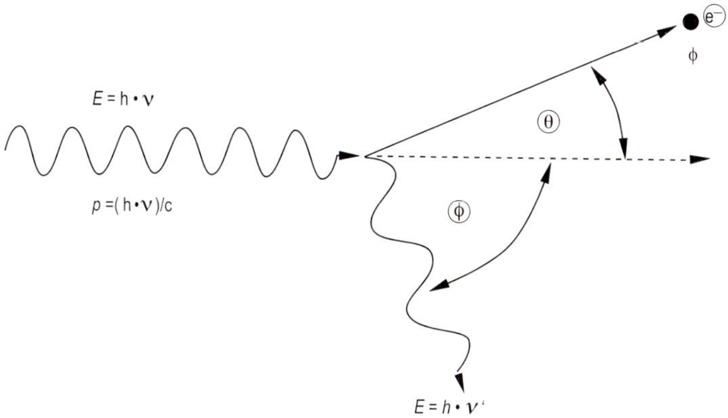

Figure 6.10 Kinematics of the Compton effect

Equation 6.11 shows that the energy transfer to the recoil electron is small when $h\nu$ is small and rises with increasing energy. The maximum transfer of energy occurs when $\phi = 180^\circ$ (i.e. $\cos\phi = -1$). This is shown in fig. 6.10. If we calculate the difference between the two wavelengths from equation 6.12, we obtain the following:

$$\lambda - \lambda' = \frac{h}{m_0 c}(1 - \cos\phi) \qquad (6.13)$$

Apart from its dependence on the scattering angle, the increase in wavelength is clearly independent of the incident quantum energy. The universal constant $h/m_0c = 0.0024$ is referred to as the Compton wavelength.

In 1928, Klein and Nishina derived the Klein-Nishina formula for the cross section per unit solid angle and per electron for non-polarized radiation scattered at an angle ϕ [6.8].

$$\frac{d\sigma^{e}_{Compton}}{d\Omega} = \frac{r_0^2}{2}\left(\frac{h\nu'}{h\nu}\right)^2\left(\frac{h\nu'}{h\nu} + \frac{h\nu}{h\nu'} - \sin^2\phi\right) \qquad (6.14)$$

$$r_0 = \frac{e_2}{m_0 c^2} = 2.818 \cdot 10^{-13}\ \text{cm: Classical electron radius}$$

In fig. 6.11 the differential cross section is plotted for different photon energies as a function of the scattering angle. Scattered photons tend towards the forward direction as their energy levels increase.

In the process of Compton interaction, the energy of the incident photon is shared between the scattered photon and the recoiling electron. In particular, with regard to dosimetric issues, it is important to know the fraction of energy carried by the primary photons that is transferred to the electrons. The total cross section for energy transfer to an electron is given by

$$\sigma^{Electron}_{Transfer} = \int \frac{d\sigma^{Electron}_{Compton}}{d\Omega}\frac{E}{h\nu}d\Omega \qquad (6.15)$$

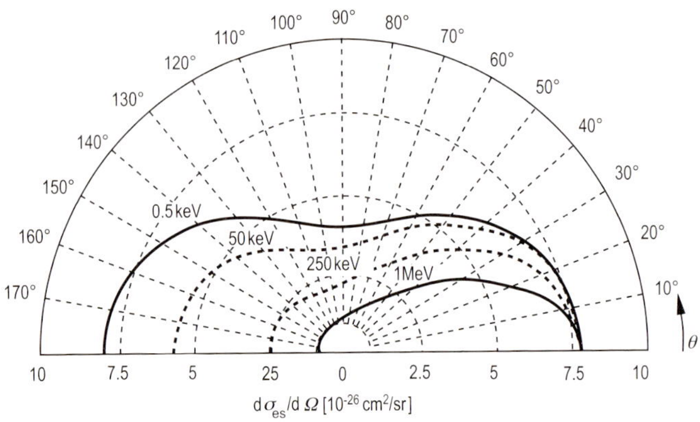

Figure 6.11
Differential Klein-Nishina cross section for photon energies of 0.5 keV, 50 keV, 250 keV and 1 MeV

This allows us to derive the Compton attenuation coefficient:

$$\frac{\mu_{\text{Compton}}}{\rho} = N_{\text{Avogadro}} \frac{Z}{A} \sigma_{\text{Transfer}}^{\text{Electron}} \tag{6.16}$$

$$N_{\text{Avogadro}} = 6.023 \cdot 10^{23} \frac{1}{\text{mol}} \text{: Avogadro's number}$$

Z: Atomic number, A: Nuclear number

Since $Z/A \approx 0.5$ μ_{Compton} is, to a good approximation, independent of Z.

Fig. 6.12 shows the total cross section for the Compton effect with free electrons $\sigma_{\text{Compton}}^{\text{Electron}}$, the cross section for energy transfer to the electrons $\sigma_{\text{Transfer}}^{\text{Electron}}$ and the cross section for the energy remaining with the scattered photons $\sigma_{\text{Scatter}}^{\text{Electron}}$ as a function of photon energy.

$$\sigma_{\text{Compton}}^{\text{Electron}} = \sigma_{\text{Transfer}}^{\text{Electron}} + \sigma_{\text{Scatter}}^{\text{Electron}} \tag{6.17}$$

As is evident, the energy transfer to the electron is small for low photon energies.

6.2.4 Coherent scattering

Coherent, or Rayleigh, scattering does not contribute to the transfer of photon energy to matter. In fact the photon loses no energy, since the recoil involves the entire atom, including the nucleus, rather than an individual electron as is the case in the Compton scattering process. An initial analysis by Thomson based on the classical theory of electromagnetic radiation yields the following for the differential cross section for coherent scattering at an angle ϕ per unit
solid angle Ω

$$\left.\frac{d\sigma_{\text{Coherent}}}{d\Omega}\right|_{\text{Thomson}} = \frac{r_0^2}{2}(1 + \cos^2\phi) \tag{6.18a}$$

r_0: Classical electron radius

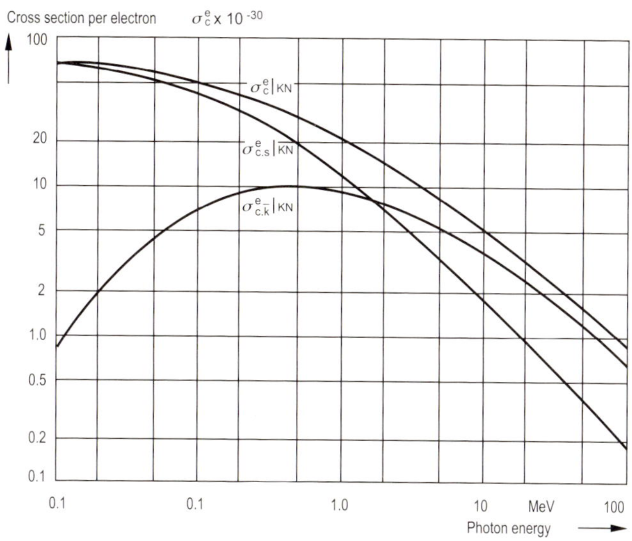

Figure 6.12
Klein-Nishina cross section per electron and corresponding energy transfer cross section per electron as a function of primary photon energy

This relation must be modified by an atomic form factor F [6.9]

$$\frac{d\sigma_{\text{Coherent}}}{d\Omega} = \left.\frac{d\sigma_{\text{Coherent}}}{d\Omega}\right|_{\text{Thomson}} \left| F\left(\frac{\sin\frac{\phi}{2}}{\lambda}, Z\right)\right|^2 \tag{6.18b}$$

The detailed analysis of the function F shows that the angular dependence of coherent scattering is highly forward-peaked, but rapidly decreases for energies above 10 keV. Coherent scattering is mostly negligible in radiology.

The total cross section for coherent scattering (after integration over Ω) is [6.10]

$$d\sigma_{\text{Coherent}} \propto \frac{Z^2}{(h\nu)^2} \tag{6.19}$$

This then yields μ_{Coherent} in accordance with equation 6.15.

6.2.5 Interactions with real objects

Up to now our approach has been to limit our discussion to interactions with individual atoms or the limiting case of infinitesimally thin layers. If we wish to quantitatively evaluate the effect of a real object (e.g. scattering in a real layer of thickness d) an integration over length (as in equation 6.8) is only possible if the expected contribution of multiple and secondary processes is sufficiently small relative to the precision required. If this is not the case, more accurate calculations are necessary.

6.2.5.1 Scattering and energy absorption

If we wish to have accurate information about the radiation which emerges behind a real object in terms of the number, direction and energy of its quanta or about the energy absorption in the object itself, it is necessary to examine the interactions of the relevant quanta and electrons in detail. This requires taking into account the multiple scattering of the primary quanta and the fluorescence quanta associated with the photoelectric effect. Furthermore, when calculating the energy absorption, it is necessary to consider the secondary processes of the photoelectrons, Compton electrons and Auger electrons. In a solid, the kinetic energy of these electrons is used almost exclusively for the creation of electron-hole pairs, while in gases and liquids it is used for the ionization and excitation of atoms or molecules.

While photoelectrons, Compton electrons and Auger electrons also cause other effects (e.g. bremsstrahlung, free-valence electron formation via the breaking of chemical bonds, crystal defects, photon creation), these account for no more than a very small part of the energy transfer and can usually be ignored (i.e. these electrons cause vibrations in molecular and lattice components).

Numerical calculations of single and multiple scattering in an object (phantom) had been carried out with the help of the Monte-Carlo method (e.g. [6.11]), as are calculations of the energy absorption in real receptor layers.

6.2.5.2 X-ray detectors

The detection of X-ray or γ-quanta must exploit the effects of their interaction with matter, since the quanta themselves move in empty space without changing their energy. Thus, their paths, for example, are not observable. Since photoelectrons, Compton electrons and Auger electrons generally possess a relatively high energy, they are used to detect high-energy quanta. In point of fact, these electrons are not used directly, but the products resulting from the electrons. In particular, the following conversion mechanisms are involved:

Chemical energy

Film: fast electrons activate a grain of silver, which is then developed as with ordinary photographic film.

Charge converters

Semiconductor detectors, high-pressure xenon gas detectors in computed tomography, xeroradiography: the electron-hole pairs or electron-ion pairs created by the fast electrons are separated by an external field and a current pulse is used to make a measurement. Xeroradiography involves the production of a surface charge relief.

Luminescence

Fluorescent screens for cassette recording and image intensification, Anger cameras, detectors in computed tomography: the fast electrons knock electrons in the crystal out of the valence band and into the conduction band. In general, the electron needs at least three times the energy of the band gap to produce one electron-hole pair.

$$N_{\mathrm{Electron\,/\,Hole}} \approx \frac{E_{\mathrm{kin}}}{3E_{\mathrm{Gap}}} \tag{6.20}$$

The electrons can then either recombine directly with their holes (crystal luminescence) or they can diffuse to the bottom edge of the conduction band and return from there via the electron traps to the valence band. Of course, some of the electrons may also recombine without emitting radiation (e.g. when defects exist in the crystal).

If light emission occurs immediately after excitation, the ensuing effect is referred to as fluorescence. However, some materials store excited electrons in metastable energy states for long periods of time. These electrons can be re-released, for example, by supplying thermal energy, whereupon luminescent light is emitted, or by raising them back into the conduction band by providing light of appropriate wavelength. Stimulated luminescence from the latter effect is utilized in storage phosphor X-ray image detector plates.

6.2.5.3 Dosimetric quantities

Ionizing radiation in the form of X-rays interacts with matter, transferring energy. Consequently its effect is characterized by the absorbed energy dose (Gy)

$$D = \frac{\mathrm{d}E_{\mathrm{abs}}}{\mathrm{d}m} \tag{6.21}$$

measured in Gray = J/kg. The term kerma (kinetic energy released in material, K) has been introduced to circumvent difficulties associated with the quantification of absorbed dose. Energy absorption usually occurs in two steps. Charged particles which can be quantitatively described are first generated by the photo effect and the Compton effect. These then undergo further interactions with matter. kerma is a measure of the primary effect. The fact that the released particles also dissipate their energy is not considered here.

$$K = \frac{\mathrm{d}E_{\mathrm{kin}}}{\mathrm{d}m} \tag{6.22}$$

where $\mathrm{d}E_{\mathrm{kin}}$ is the sum of the initial kinetic energies of all the charged ionizing particles liberated by uncharged ionizing particles (e.g. photons) in a material of mass $\mathrm{d}m$. The unit is again Gy.

The air kerma $K_{\mathrm{air}}(E)$ released by photons of energy E in air is related to the spectral radiation intensity ψ_{v} (J/m²) by

$$K_{\mathrm{Air}}(E) = \Psi_{\mathrm{v}} \frac{\mu_{\mathrm{Air}}(E)}{\rho_{\mathrm{Air}}} \tag{6.23}$$

Dosimetric measurements are usually carried out with ionization chambers. The charge liberated by the X-ray photons in the chamber air volume is recorded. The exposure (C/kg) is the ionization equivalent of the air kerma

$$X = \frac{dQ}{dm} \qquad (6.24)$$

where dQ is the value of the total ionic charge of one sign produced in air when all of the electrons created by the X-rays have come to rest. The ionization produced by Auger electrons is included, but the ionization due to photons emitted by radiative processes (e.g. bremsstrahlung and fluorescence photons) is not.

Exposure and air kerma are related via

$$X = \frac{e}{W} K_{\mathrm{Air}} \qquad (6.25)$$

where $W = 33.73$ eV is the mean energy expended in air per ion pair formed.

In diagnostic radiology the dose quantities describing the radiation field are essentially derived from the air kerma. The following quantities are in use.

The nominal air kerma rate K_{100} (Gy/h) is the air kerma rate in free air on the central ray for a focus distance of 100 cm. It is usually given for a tube current of 1 mA.

The radiation output of an X-ray tube assembly Y_{100} is the quotient of the air kerma K_{100} in free air on the central ray for a focal distance of 100 cm and the tube current exposure time product $I_R \cdot t$:

$$Y_{100} = \frac{K_{100}}{I_R \cdot t} \qquad (6.26)$$

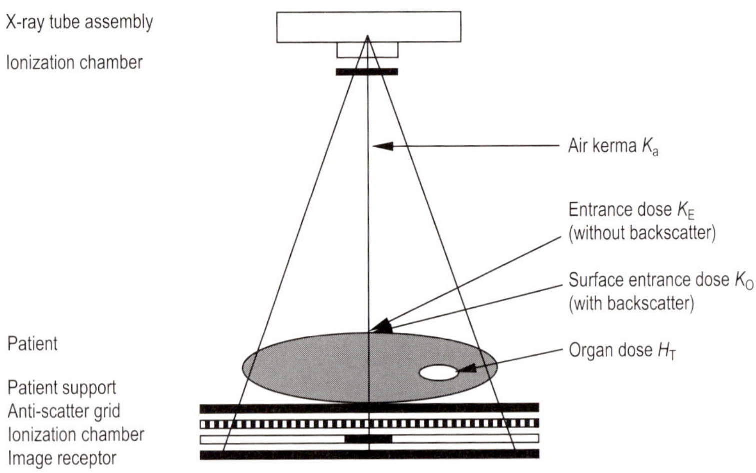

Figure 6.13 The dose quantities describing the X-radiation field

The entrance surface air kerma K_E and the entrance surface air kerma rate $\dot{K}_E$ relate to the point in the central beam on a plane corresponding to the entrance surface of a patient (without backscatter). The quantity K_E is also referred to as entrance *dose*.

The entrance surface dose K_0 and the entrance surface dose rate $\dot{K}_E$ is the air kerma (rate) with backscatter assessed at a point in the central beam on the entrance surface of a patient (or a phantom). In X-ray diagnostics the dose area product of surface dose and field of view is often taken as a measure of patient exposure.

In radiographic X-ray systems the image receptor or system dose K_B is the air kerma on the central ray at a point representing the position of the image receptor necessary for an optimized exposure of the image receptor (fig. 6.13).

6.3 Biological effects of radiation

The absorption of X-rays in matter leads to the ionization of single atoms and a modification of their chemical properties. While this may cause mutations in the DNA molecules in the nuclei of living cells, damage control mechanisms in the human body enable the repair of most of the DNA damage. Those cells for which damage is not correctly repaired will either be killed off or, with much lower probability, modified. The likelihood of successful repair depends on the time interval over which the dose in question has been applied. The probability of successful repair is greater when the application of a specific radiation dose is spread out over a very long period (thereby limiting concurrent damage) than when the same dose is applied over a very short interval. [6.12, 6.13, 6.14]

The dose equivalent H has been introduced in order to express the risk of deleterious effects associated with the application of different types of ionizing radiation in living organisms. It is given by the product of the absorbed dose D and a quality factor Q, representing the different types of ionizing radiation:

$$H = QD \tag{6.27a}$$

The unit of dose equivalent is the Sievert (Sv = QGy). The definition of the quality factor is based on the linear energy transfer (*LET*, kV/µm) of the charged particles generated by the primary radiation, which is a measure of the ionization density. The quality factor has the value one for photons and electrons of all energies. $Q = 5$ for alpha radiation and for neutrons the value of Q ranges between 5 and 20, depending on their energy. For a combination of different types of radiation with different quality factors, H is defined by

$$H = \sum_i Q_i D_i \tag{6.27b}$$

6.3.1 Acute or deterministic radiation damage

The term *acute* or deterministic radiation damage refers to the killing of cells. The death and replacement of cells is a natural process, which also occurs in the absence of radiation. Cell death and damage are dangerous only if the number of cells affected is large enough to prevent their replacement by undamaged neighboring cells. Therefore, deterministic radiation damage can be said to occur only if the dose exceeds a certain threshold. The value of this threshold depends on the type of tissue involved and decreases with increasing dose per time unit. The severity of the damage (number of cells killed) above this threshold increases with the radiation dose. If several different regions of the body are irradiated and the dose values do not exceed the individual threshold values of any region, the dose risk is not increased. Potential deterministic radiation damage includes nonhereditary teratogeneous damage (i.e. prenatal damage), especially between the 3rd and 25th week of pregnancy (above 100 mSv), skin erythema (above 0.25 Sv) and haematopoiesis impairment (above 1 Sv). Still higher doses are known to cause damage to the gastric and intestinal mucosa, with symptoms of diarrhea and nausea. The severity of the disease increases with increasing dose and mass of the irradiated tissue. Whole-body irradiation at more than 4 Sv can be lethal and whole-body irradiation at 20 Sv is known to cause instantaneous death. [6.12, 6.15]

Non-cancerous, post-treatment damage, such as fibrotic tissue alteration, cataracts and sterility may also occur. Survivors of deterministic radiation damage bear a dose-dependent increased stochastic risk for developing leukemia, cancer and genetic damage. Under normal working conditions diagnostic X-ray doses do not exceed the deterministic threshold levels.

6.3.2 Stochastic radiation damage

Even low X-ray doses may cause long-term damage such as leukemia, solid tumor formation and, if the gonads are affected, hereditary disease. Such cases arise when the effect is not cell death, but a modification of the cells' biological properties without impairing their capacity to reproduce. There is no threshold dose for stochastic damage. In contrast to deterministic damage, the probability and not the severity of biological damage increase with dose. The onset of diseases (leukemia and solid tumor formation) caused by stochastic damage develops only after a latency period of several years or decades.

6.3.3 Estimate of radiation risk

Due to the random effect of low radiation doses and the impossibility of establishing a causal link between low-dose X-rays and a specific form of cancer (which may not occur until a latency period of many years has elapsed) it is not possible to prove that any particular case of damage is related to any particular diagnostic investigation using X-radiation. Therefore, it is only possible to estimate a collective dose risk for a population using epidemiological-statistical methods. This means that a radiation risk can only be defined for a group of irradiated persons by comparing the number of cancers reported for this group with the number of spontaneous cancers that have occurred in a similar non-irradiated group. The main sources of information here are the studies of individuals who survived the atomic bombing of Hiroshima and Nagasaki. Between 1950 and 1985, dose values were calculated for 75,991 persons [6.16, 6.17]. For approximately 3050 persons the dose exceeded 1 Sv and for approximately 17,000 per-

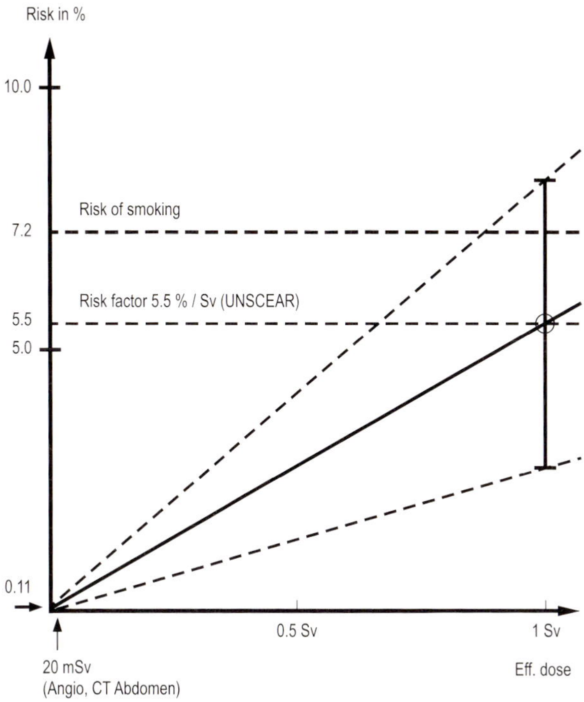

Figure 6.14
Estimate of the radiation risk for low doses by linear extrapolation based on a risk factor of 5.5% per Sievert. Even for examinations with relatively high effective doses (arteriography or CT), the risk is low (0.11%) compared with the risk of contracting disease as a result of smoking.

sons was between 0.1 and 1 Sv. Up to 1985, 202 persons had died of leukemia and 5,734 persons had died as a result of solid tumor formation. In a similar group of non-irradiated persons, 122 can be expected to die of leukemia and 5,474 as a result of solid tumors. It can therefore be assumed that 80 cases of leukemia and 260 cases of solid tumors were caused by radiation. Until now, the number of cases involving solid tumors and leukemia has increased to approximately 500 from a group of 85,000 [6.12]. Statistically significant cancer risks for this group can be demonstrated only above organ doses of approximately 50 to 100 mSv [6.15]. Lower dose risks must be estimated by extrapolation (fig. 6.14).

To estimate the potential risk at low dose levels, the International Commission on Radiological Protection (ICRP) has recommended the assumption of a linear relationship between dose and health risk. This means that the influence of repair mechanisms is not taken into consideration and effectively represents a worst case assumption, incorporating an additional margin of safety regarding the prevention of stochastic radiation damage. Based on this assumption, the ICRP has introduced the concept of effective dose. The effective dose converts the dose of a partial-body exposure to a whole-

Table 6.3 Numerical values of the tissue weighting factors *WT* according to ICRP 60 [6.18], [6.19]

Tissue or organ	*WT*	Tissue or organ	*WT*
Gonads	0.20	Liver	0.05
Bone marrow	0.12	Esophagus	0.05
Colon	0.12	Thyroid	0.05
Lungs	0.12	Skin	0.01
Stomach	0.12	Bone surface	0.01
Urinary bladder	0.05	Rest of body	0.05
Breasts	0.05		

body dose, taking into account the dose sensitivity of various organs. The effective dose is the sum of the organ-specific doses of a group of organs (as specified by ICRP), multiplied by organ-specific weighting factors. These weighting factors are also specified by ICRP and express the relative radio-sensitivity of the particular organs (table 6.3).

The lifetime risk of exposure-induced death can be estimated from the effective dose and a risk factor that depends on the age and sex of the irradiated persons, as well as on several other parameters.

One of these other parameters is the individual radio-sensitivity. It is estimated that 5 to 10% of the normal population suffers from congenitally enhanced sensitivity to radiation.

Based on the data from the survivors of Hiroshima and Nagasaki, the ICRP has established an overall risk factor of 5% per Sievert (0.5% for leukemia and 4.5% for solid tumors). This is largely confirmed by UNSCEAR [6.20]: for an acute dose of 1 Sv the risk factor is about 9% for men, 13% for women and 11% for the population at large. According to ICRP, these values can be reduced by 50% for low doses and chronic exposure, based on the assumption that low doses and frequent exposure are less dangerous than high doses and acute exposure. This means that a diagnostic X-ray risk factor of 0.0055% per mSv (5.5% per Sv) can be assumed for a normal population. The uncertainty of this value may be a factor of about 2 [6.20]. The specified risk factors are average values for all ages. However, due to the latency periods mentioned above, the risk of developing cancer increases with lifetime. The risk is therefore higher for younger persons and lower for older persons. To estimate the risk for an individual patient, it is necessary to take the patient's age into consideration. Here, a risk factor of 2 is recommended for persons below 18 years of age and a risk factor of 0.2 for persons at least 70 years of age.

The risk of exposure-induced leukemia over an entire lifetime is assumed to be 1% for an acute dose of 1 Sv [6.20]. Based on a linear-quadratic, dose-response relationship, it can then be assumed that decreasing the dose from 1 Sv to 0.1 Sv will reduce the lifetime risk by a factor of 20. The lifetime risk for leukemia is therefore estimated to be 0.05% per 0.1 Sv acute dose.

Table 6.4
Effective dose and the combined health risk of contracting leukemia and cancer for some typical X-ray examinations, using a risk factor of 5.5% per Sv. Note that a stochastic uncertainty, which may be a factor of about 2, also applies here.

Type of examination	Eff. dose in mSv [6.21]	Risk in % (eff. dose × 5.5%)
	Conventional X-rays	
Dental	0.01	0.000055
Thorax	0.03	0.00017
Mammography	0.5	0.0028
Colon	15.0	0.083
Arteriography	18.0	0.10
	Computed tomography	
Head	3.0	0.017
Thorax	10.0	0.055
Abdomen	20.0	0.11

For the assessment of the risks associated with diagnostic X-rays, it may be helpful to compare the values in table 6.4 with those associated with natural radiation and other everyday hazards.

Comparison with natural radiation: The greatest contribution to exposure arises from natural background radiation. The natural radiation dose is the sum of external exposure (cosmic rays and terrestrial gamma rays) and internal exposure (radon inhalation and ingestion). The worldwide average annual effective dose is 2.4 mSv and the typical range is 1 to 10 μSv [6.22]. Professional airline crews are exposed to a special natural radiation risk during long distance flights. Typical dose ranges are: Frankfurt -Gran Canaria 10 to 18 μSv and Frankfurt-San Francisco 45 to 110 μSv [6.23]. The variation range of the values is due to differences in flight altitude and solar activity. The dose for a typical dental or thorax X-ray examination (0.01 to 0.03 mSv) is therefore less than the dose of a long distance flight (0.045 to 0.110 mSv), and the dose of an annual mammography (0.5 mSv) is less than the average annual dose of natural radiation.

Comparison with other everyday hazards (average relative lifetime risks for Germany [6.21]): death rate due to all cancers 25%, due to smoking 7.2% and due to road accidents 1.1%. The hypothetical relative risk caused by X-radiation is 0.3% for diagnostic X-radiation and 0.9% for natural radiation. These figures show that the risk of cancer-related death caused by diagnostic X-radiation is relatively (very) low. At the same time, many people who voluntarily accept relatively high *lifestyle* risks tend to overestimate and otherwise react emotionally to involuntary low risks.

Multiplying the risk factor for mammography of 0.0028% (table 6.4) by the number of women in Germany ($40 \cdot 10^6$) yields 1,120 additional cancer-related deaths during lifetime (without considering the stochastic uncertainty). The verification of this apparently large number is not possible. Given that the probability of dying from cancer during one's lifetime is 0.25, the figures calculated for cancer-related death due to mammography should be compared to the 10 million women (out of 40 million) who die in Germany over a same period from cancer for other reasons, a figure which could be easily reduced by personal measures related to healthier living. Furthermore, when assessing the possible damage associated with medical X-rays, it is also necessary to consider the benefits. There is no doubt that X-ray examinations save lives by enabling the diagnosis of potentially lethal diseases.

6.3.4 Controversy concerning the effects of low radiation doses

The effect of low radiation doses is a source of controversy among experts and in the public eye. A low radiation dose means a dose below the deterministic threshold (approximately 200 mSv). While there is no doubt that radiation damage occurs above the deterministic threshold, scientifically sound claims about the effects of radiation can only be made on the basis of observed effects. However, even when drawing on the results of epidemiological studies, it is impossible to verify X-ray effects in the standard range of diagnostic doses (below 20 mSv). At the same time, it is equally impossible to prove that there are no effects. It is this lack of specific knowledge which is the actual source of the controversy.

The issue is therefore a matter of deciding how conservative the estimate of radiation risk must be in order to guarantee maximum safety. One proposal, advanced by the ICRP, involves a linear extrapolation from high doses down to zero. Nevertheless, not all experts agree with this linear description of radiation risk. In view of the body's capacity to respond by attempting to control damage, the existence of fundamental differences in the health-related impact of high dose radiation and long-term, low dose radiation can not be ruled out. The recommendation above, which would permit a reduction of the risk factor by 50% for low doses, thus represents a step in the right direction.

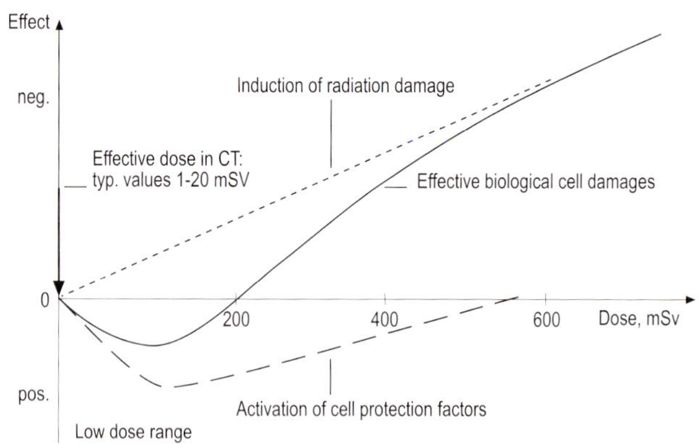

Figure 6.15 Possible biological effects at low dose ranges

Another matter of dispute is the existence of bio-positive effects due to low radiation doses. Several studies describe such effects as the terms *hormesis* and *adaptive response*. These effects include increased plant and animal vitality, cellular detoxification, reduction of DNA defects and increased resistance to radiation following irradiation with low doses. Luckey has given an overview of the relevant studies [6.24, 6.25] and suggests that bio-positive effects predominate in the dose range up to 200 mSv, the so-called zero equivalent point (ZEP), while radio-negative effects predominate above this range. In-vitro studies show that frequent and acute exposure can lead to an adaptive response. There is currently no general consensus in regard to how the results of such studies might be taken into account in assessments of radiation risk (fig. 6.15).

The public debate is characterized by a tendency to report the negative effects (bad news is more newsworthy!) of radiation rather than the positive effects. Nevertheless, a comparison of the relative risks presented in table 6.4 with other everyday hazards clearly shows that the health risk associated with diagnostic X-radiation is often exaggerated in lay circles.

6.4 References

[6.1] A.A. Sokolov, I.M. Ternov
Synchrotron Radiation
Pergamon, NY 1968

[6.2] S. Flügge
Handbuch d. Physik, volume XXX, Röntgenstrahlen
Springer-Verlag, Berlin Göttingen Heidelberg 1957

[6.3] M.H. Key
J. mod. Optics 35, 575 (1988)

[6.4] V. Bazyev, N.K. Zevago
Sov. Phys. Usp. 25, 565 (1982)

[6.5] M.A. Kumakhof, R. Wedell
Radiation of Relativistic Light Particles during interaction with Single Crystal
Spectrum Akad. Verlag Heidelberg 1991

[6.6] H. Genz, H.P. Graf, P. Hofmann, W. Lotz, V. Nething, A. Richter, A. Weickenmeier, W. Knüpfer, J.F.P. Sellschopp
Appl. Phys. Letter 57, 2956 (1990)

[6.7] K. Dietz
Altes und Neues über Röntgenröhren
S. Hirzel Verlag Stuttgart 1955

[6.8] F.H. Attix
Introduction to Radiological Physics and Radiation Dosimetry
Wiley, New York (1986)

[6.9] J.A. Hubbbel
Atomic form factors, incoherent scattering functions, and photon scattering cross sections
J. Phys. Chem. Reference Data 4, 431 (1975)

[6.10] E. Storm, H.I. Israel
Photon cross sections from 0.001 to 100 MeV for elements 1 through 100
Clearinghouse for Scientific and Technical Information
LA 3753 MC34, Physics TID-4500 (1967)

[6.11] W.A. Kalender
Determination of the intensity of scattered radiation and performance of grids in diagnostic radiology by Monte Carlo methods
Dissertation, University of Wisconsin, Madison (USA) 1979

[6.12] www.bfs.de/ion/wirkungen state of 2003

[6.13] H. Jung
Strahlenrisiko
Fortschr. Roentgenstr. 162, 91 (1995)

[6.14] F. Wachsmann
Über die Gefährlichkeit ionisierender Strahlungen
Arbeitsmedizin Sozialmedizin Präventivmedizin 21, 201(1986)

[6.15] www.bfs.de/ion/einfuehrung state of 2003

[6.16] Y. Shimizu, H. Kato, W.J. Schull
Life Span Study Report 11, Part 2. Cancer mortality in the years 1950-85 based on the recently revised doses (DS86)
Report RERF-TR5-88, Radiation Effects Research Foundation

[6.17] Y. Shimizu, H. Kato, W.J. Schull
Studies of the mortality of A-bomb survivors 9. Mortality, 1959-1985: Part 2. Cancer mortality based on the recently revised doses (DS86).
Radiat. Res. 121, 120 (1990)

[6.18] Recommendations of the International Commission on Radiological Protection.
ICRP Publication 26, Pergamon Press, Oxford 1977

[6.19] Recommendations of the International Commission on Radiological Protection
ICRP Publication 60, Pergamon Press, Oxford 1991

[6.20] Epidemiolocical Evaluation of Radiation induced Cancer
UNSCEAR (United Nations Scientific Committee on the effects of Atomic Radiation)
Report 2000, Annex 1

[6.21] Röntgendiagnostik – schädlich oder nützlich?
Bundesamt für Strahlenschutz, Strahlenthemen, Jan. 2003,

[6.22] Source of radiation exposure. Natural radiation exposures.
UNSCEAR Report 2000

[6.23] Überwachung der Strahlenbelastung beim Fliegen
www.bfs.de/druck/jahresberichte/jb2002.html

[6.24] T.D. Luckey
Hormesis with Ionizing Radiation
CRC Press, Boca Raton 1980

[6.25] T.D. Luckey
Radiation Hormesis
CRC Press, Boca Raton 1991

7 Concepts in magnetic resonance imaging

7.1 Historical survey

Magnetic resonance imaging (MRI) was introduced to clinical practice in the early nineteen-eighties. Thanks to its unparalleled soft-tissue contrast and its capacity to generate images of slices in arbitrary orientation and of entire volumes, MRI has become the imaging gold standard in many diagnostic areas.

Magnetic resonance (MR) is a physical phenomenon involving the precession of particles with an angular and a magnetic moment in a magnetic field where they absorb or emit electromagnetic energy. This effect is referred to as electron spin resonance (ESR) or electron paramagnetic resonance (EPR) for unpaired electrons in atoms, molecules and crystals, and nuclear magnetic resonance (NMR) for nuclei. Discovered in 1944 by the Russian scientist Zavoiskij [7.1], ESR has thus far gained no real significance in terms of medical application. NMR was observed independently in 1945 by Felix Bloch et al. [7.2] at Stanford University in California and Edward Mills Purcell et al. [7.3] in Cambridge, Massachusetts. The Nobel Prize for physics was awarded in 1952 to these two American groups.

The interaction of atoms and nuclei with magnetic fields has been a subject of investigation for much longer. In 1897 the Dutch scientist Pieter Zeeman discovered that the optical spectrum of sodium was affected by a strong magnetic field [7.4], a discovery for which he was awarded the Nobel Prize for physics in 1902. A classical interpretation of the Zeeman Effect was given by the Irish physicist Joseph Larmor in the year of its discovery [7.5]. Twenty-five years later, Otto Stern and Walter Gerlach [7.6] discovered that silver atoms were capable of aligning themselves either parallel to or antiparallel to an external magnetic field. Their experiment, which proves the quantization of angular momentum, represents a fundamental discovery in quantum physics. In 1937 Isidor Isaac Rabi [7.7] was able to precisely ascertain the magnetic moment of nuclei by investigating the exposure of a molecular beam in a homogeneous magnetic field to a radiofrequency (RF) magnetic field. The Nobel Prize for physics was awarded to Stern in 1943 and to Rabi in 1944.

NMR has proven to be an extremely valuable tool for investigating the structure of matter in the fields of physics, chemistry and biology. Richard Ernst at the Swiss Federal Institute of Technology (SFIT) in Zurich was awarded the Nobel Prize for chemistry in 1991 for his contributions to the method's development. Ten years later the Nobel Prize was awarded to Kurth Wüthrich, a colleague of Ernst at the SFIT, for his work in ascertaining the three-dimensional structure of biological macromolecules.

The first attempts to deploy NMR for medical purposes were made ten years after its discovery when Odeblad and Lindström [7.8] of the Karolinska Hospital in Stockholm used it to analyze proton line widths in biological samples. In 1960 Singer [7.9] reported on blood flow measurements using NMR nine years after the effect of flow on the NMR signal had first been observed by Suryan [7.10] in 1951. Based on his observation that relaxation times in tumorous tissue tend to be prolonged, Damadian [7.11] claimed in 1971 that NMR could be used for the detection of cancer. Although Gabillard [7.12] recognized the interrelation between magnetic field inhomogeneity, sample shape and NMR line profile (which yields what is referred to today as a projection) as early as 1952, it was not until 1973 that Lauterbur [7.13] of the State University of New York at Stony Brook demonstrated how linear magnetic field gradients can be employed to obtain images. Paul Lauterbur was awarded the Nobel Prize for medicine in 2003 together with Sir Peter Mansfield from the University of Nottingham, England, another pioneer in MR imaging.

The limits placed on spatial resolution by wavelength in wave-based imaging processes are circumvented in MRI by the superposition of two fields. With the aid of an RF field in the MHz range and a locally variable static magnetic field, the sharp resonance absorption of magnetic nuclei in biological tissue is used to obtain the spatial distribution of the nuclear magnetization. In particular, hydrogen atoms (which occur naturally in large numbers) allow for the production of medically meaningful images. While it is also possible to detect naturally abundant or artificially injected magnetic nuclei other than protons in biological tissue (e.g. ^{13}C, ^{19}F, ^{23}Na, ^{31}P, and hyperpolarized ^{3}He and ^{119}Xe), the value of the information gained using these nuclei does not approach that obtained via the resonance of hydrogen nuclei.

In what follows, we review a few basic physical principles that are important for gaining a better understanding of NMR and MRI. Readers may wish to refer to the relevant textbooks for a more detailed discussion [7.14-7.16].

7.2 The NMR phenomenon

7.2.1 Magnetization

All atomic nuclei with an odd number of protons or neutrons (i.e. roughly two-thirds of all stable atomic nuclei) possess an intrinsic angular momentum. This is always coupled with a magnetic dipole moment, which is proportional to the angular momentum. As a consequence, these particles possess potential energy in a magnetic field. As is known from quantum mechanics, particles cannot continuously change their angular momentum and their energy, but can only assume discrete values (fig. 7.1). In a magnetic field with flux density B_0 a nucleus with quantum number I (e.g. for ^1H $I = 1/2$ and for ^{23}Na $I = 3/2$) may assume $2I + 1$ discrete energy values

$$E_m = -\gamma \hbar B_0 m \tag{7.1}$$

γ: Gyromagnetic ratio (e.g. for the hydrogen nucleus $\frac{\gamma}{2\pi} = 42.577 \frac{\text{MHz}}{\text{T}}$)

$\hbar$: Planck's constant ($\hbar = \frac{h}{2\pi} = 1.055\ 10^{-34}\ \text{Ws}^2$), m: Magnetic quantum number $(-I \le m \le I)$

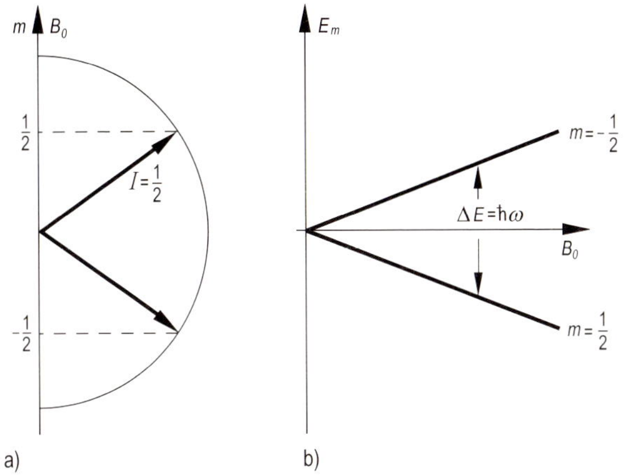

Figure 7.1
a) Orientations of a spin $I = 1/2$ in a magnetic field (the magnitude of the spin vector is $\sqrt{I(I+1)}$).
b) Energies of a spin $I = 1/2$ as a function of the magnetic field (B_0). For a quantum transition the difference energy has to be added or subtracted in the form of electromagnetic quanta $\hbar\omega$.

A change in such an energy level entails the absorption or emission of a photon:

$$\hbar\omega = E_{m-1} - E_m = -\gamma\hbar B_0 \tag{7.2}$$

Such processes were observed early in this century as hyperfine structures in the optical spectroscopy of fluorescent gases and correctly interpreted by Pauli [7.17] in 1924.

Atomic nuclei do not occur as individual entities in matter, but as part of an ensemble (e.g. 1 mm^3 water contains $6.7 \cdot 10^{19}$ hydrogen nuclei). In a magnetic field, the occupation of the energy states (fig. 7.2) described by eq. (7.1) conforms to Boltzmann statistics:

$$\frac{N_{m-1}}{N_m} = e^{-\frac{\hbar\omega}{kT}} \tag{7.3}$$

k: Boltzmann's constant ($k = 1.38\ 10^{-23}\frac{\text{Ws}}{\text{K}}$)

The result is thus a surplus of spins aligned parallel to the magnetic field (for the same reason that air density decreases with increasing height). For water in a magnetic flux density of 1 T (Tesla) at room temperature, the surplus amounts to $3.2 \cdot 10^{-6}$ of the protons. The result is therefore a small, but measurable angular momentum and an associated macroscopic magnetic moment. The exponential function in eq. (7.3) can be linearized to yield the nuclear magnetization

$$M_0 = N_V \frac{I(I+1)\gamma^2\hbar^2 B_0}{3kT} \tag{7.4}$$

N_V: Nuclear spin density

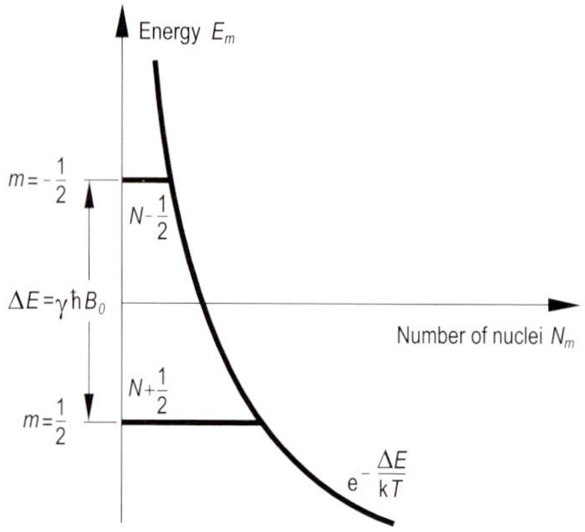

Figure 7.2
Occupation of the energy levels of a spin $I = 1/2$ ensemble according to the Boltzmann distribution.

7.2.2 Bloch equations

The phenomenon of MR can be treated both in the framework of classical physics and in that of quantum mechanics. The juxtaposition of the two representations – the quantum mechanical in which a spin can only assume discrete angles with respect to the direction of a magnetic field and the classical in which (as will be shown in the following exposition) a macroscopic magnetization conforming to eq. (7.4) precesses around the axis of an applied magnetic field at an arbitrary angle – can lead to difficulties of incommensurability. The reader should thus bear in mind Bohr's correspondence principle, which says that quantum mechanical systems reduce to classical physics in the limit of large quantum numbers (in this case many particles). Given that the mathematical formalism of classical physics is simpler, it will be used in the present context as the system of reference. Even if reference is occasionally made to single spins, such reference is merely a placeholder for many spins forming a local sub-magnetization.

In the case of thermal equilibrium, the magnetization of a probe with spins aligns itself parallel to an applied magnetic field. If this equilibrium is disturbed, for example, by suddenly changing the direction of the magnetic field, then a torque $\vec{M}\times\vec{B}$ acts on the magnetization of the sample. According to the law of angular momentum conservation, this torque causes a temporal change of the angular momentum (per volume unit).

$$\frac{\mathrm{d}\frac{\vec{M}}{\gamma}}{\mathrm{d}t} = (\vec{M}\times\vec{B}) \tag{7.5}$$

This results in the precession of the magnetization around the axis of the magnetic field with the resonance or Larmor frequency

$$\omega_{\mathrm{L}} = -\gamma B_0 \tag{7.6}$$

in a manner analogous to the precession of an obliquely orientated top around the normal (fig. 7.3). This precession (nuclear magnetic resonance) can be detected by

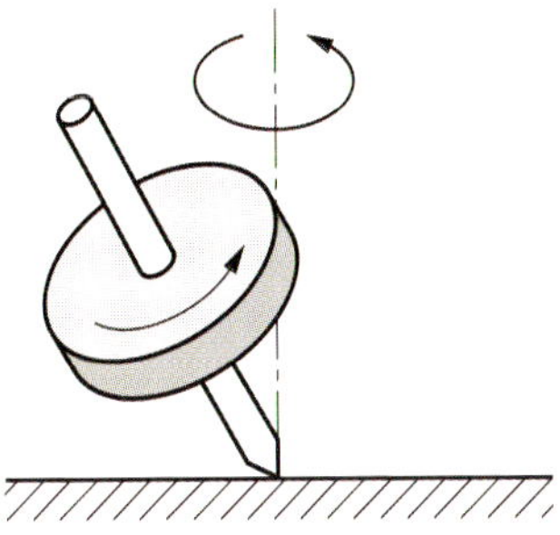

Figure 7.3
Precession of a top in the gravitation field

measuring the induced alternating voltage in a coil surrounding the sample (free induction decay or FID). It is the classical analog of the quantum transition expressed by eq. (7.2). The rotation direction of the precessing nuclear magnetization depends on the sign of γ. For hydrogen nuclei or protons, which are the most frequently occurring in nature, the gyromagnetic ratio is positive, thus resulting in a clockwise rotation. Protons yield a nuclear magnetic resonance frequency of 42.577 MHz in a magnetic flux density of 1 T. Table 7.1 lists the Larmor frequencies of other nuclei found in biological tissue together with their natural abundance.

Experience shows that the disturbed thermal equilibrium is reestablished after a finite interval. This process, referred to as relaxation, can be described phenomenologically by adding relaxation terms to eq. (7.5). Bloch [7.18] assumes that the components of the magnetization parallel and perpendicular to the magnetic field tend to their equilibrium states (M_0 and 0 respectively) at a rate proportional to their deviation from equilibrium:

$$\begin{aligned} \frac{\mathrm{d}M_z}{\mathrm{d}t} &= \gamma(\vec{M}\times\vec{B})_z + \frac{(M_0 + M_z)}{T_1} \\ \frac{\mathrm{d}M_\perp}{\mathrm{d}t} &= \gamma(\vec{M}\times\vec{B})_\perp - \frac{M_\perp}{T_2} \end{aligned} \tag{7.7}$$

M_0 denotes the equilibrium magnetization expressed in eq. (7.4), T_1 the time constant (longitudinal relaxation time) with which the magnetization component M_z along the direction of the applied magnetic field is restored, and T_2 the time constant with which the transverse component $M_\perp$ decays (transverse relaxation time); T_1 is always $\geq T_2$. Longitudinal relaxation is associated with the emission of energy to the surrounding space (e.g. in a solid state, the crystal lattice in which the atomic nuclei are embedded). It is thus often referred to as spin-lattice relaxation (although the probe does heat up as a result, this effect is hardly measurable). The disappearance of the transverse magnetization is due to the interaction of the spins that loosens the relationship between the phases of the individual spins. This case is thus often referred to as spin-spin relaxation. Given that the longitudinal component of the magnetization, which determines the energy of the spin ensemble, remains the same during transversal relaxation, T_2 can be considered an entropy effect, while T_1 is an energy effect.

Table 7.1
MR detection capabilities for various elements in biological tissue. The final column gives the relative edge length of the cube that would result in a constant signal.

Isotope	MR frequency in MHz (at 1 T)	Normalized detection sensitivity in tissue at constant frequency	Normalized resolution
^{1}H	42.58	100	1
^{2}H	6.53	0.006	25
^{13}C	10.71	0.025	16
^{14}N	3.08	0.31	7
^{17}O	5.57	0.049	13
^{19}F	40.06	0.006	25
^{23}Na	11.26	0.1	10
^{31}P	7.24	0.14	9
^{35}Cl	4.17	0.0084	23
^{39}K	1.99	0.011	21

7.2.3 Relaxation

The nuclear relaxation times express the mobility of the molecules in which the nuclei under consideration are located. Each nucleus is surrounded by other magnetic moments that are in constant thermal motion (Brownian molecular motion) and produce a continuously changing microscopic magnetic perturbation field. Spectral components corresponding to the Larmor frequency induce longitudinal relaxation. Transverse relaxation, on the other hand, is determined by the frequency of the collisions between the molecules as a whole.

The temporal behavior of molecular motion is described by the autocorrelation function $K(t)$ of the microscopic magnetic flux density $\vec{b}(t)$ that is transferred during a collision by the magnetic moment (nuclear or electron spin) of one molecule to the nuclear spin of another:

$$K(t) = \langle \vec{b}(t')\vec{b}(t'+t) \rangle = \lim_{T \to \infty} \frac{1}{2T} \int_{-T}^{T} \vec{b}(t')\vec{b}(t'+t)\mathrm{d}t' \tag{7.8}$$

This is a measure of how long a molecule can remember colliding with another. Given stochastic molecular motion with a mean or correlation time τ_c between two collisions one may assume an exponential decay for the correlation function

$$K(t) = K(0)\mathrm{e}^{-\frac{|t|}{\tau_c}} \tag{7.9}$$

If the magnetic field being transferred during two collisions changes by an amount of $\pm b_z$, the nuclear spin on which it acts precesses with an additional phase

$$\delta\varphi = \pm\gamma b_z \tau_c. \tag{7.10a}$$

Thus, after n collisions, an average squared de-phasing angle

$$\langle \varphi^2 \rangle = n\delta\varphi^2 = n\gamma^2 b_z^2 \tau_c^2 \tag{7.10b}$$

results (of course, for the average de-phasing angle $<\varphi> = 0$).

The time needed for a spin to de-phase by one angular unit can be regarded as transverse relaxation time

$$T_2 = \frac{n\,\tau_c}{<\varphi^2>} = \frac{1}{\gamma^2 b_z^2 \tau_c}. \tag{7.11a}$$

The decreasing of the reciprocal $1/T_2$ (termed transversal relaxation rate) along with the number of collisions is often referred to as motional narrowing. However, if the correlation time becomes larger than the time needed for one rotation around the transferred magnetic field (i.e. $\tau_c > \frac{1}{\gamma b_z}$) transverse relaxation ceases to be influenced by collisions. T_2 is then independent of τ_c and becomes

$$T_2 \approx \frac{1}{\gamma b_z}. \tag{7.11b}$$

The reciprocal $1/T_1$ of the longitudinal relaxation time or longitudinal relaxation rate is a measure of the probability of transitions between two adjacent energy levels that a magnetic nucleus may assume in the main magnetic field as per eq. (7.2). These transitions are induced at the Larmor frequency by the spectral components $b_x(\omega_L)$ and $b_y(\omega_L)$ of the microscopic magnetic flux density that is active during collisions between two molecules. The frequency distribution of the transferred flux density is given by the Fourier transform of the autocorrelation function expressed in eq. (7.9)

$$J(\omega) = 2K(0)\frac{\tau_c}{1 + \tau_c^2\omega^2} \tag{7.12}$$

The longitudinal relaxation rate is then proportional to the spectral density of the autocorrelation function at the Larmor frequency and twice the Larmor frequency (as linear polarized spectral components with $2\omega_L$ can cause a circular polarized field that is constant in the reference frame rotating with ω_L):

$$\frac{1}{T_1} \propto \left(\frac{\tau_c}{1 + \omega_L^2\tau_c^2} + \frac{2\,\tau_c}{1 + 4\,\omega_L^2\tau_c^2}\right) \tag{7.13a}$$

The longitudinal relaxation time T_1 approaches a minimum where τ_c equals the time for one Larmor precession $1/\omega_L$. Autocorrelation times smaller than the precession time yield

$$T_1 \propto \frac{1}{\tau_c} \quad (\omega_L\tau_c << 1) \tag{7.13b}$$

and larger times yield

$$T_1 \propto 2\,\omega_L^2\tau_c \quad (\omega_L\tau_c >> 1) \tag{7.13c}$$

The principal dependence of T_1 and T_2 on τ_c is plotted in fig. 7.4. Although the aim of the arguments for the derivation of T_1 and T_2 is no more than plausibility, the results are essentially correct. It should be mentioned that the finite lifetime T_1 of a spin in an energy level limits the intrinsic lifetime of the transversal magnetization. A term $2/T_1$,

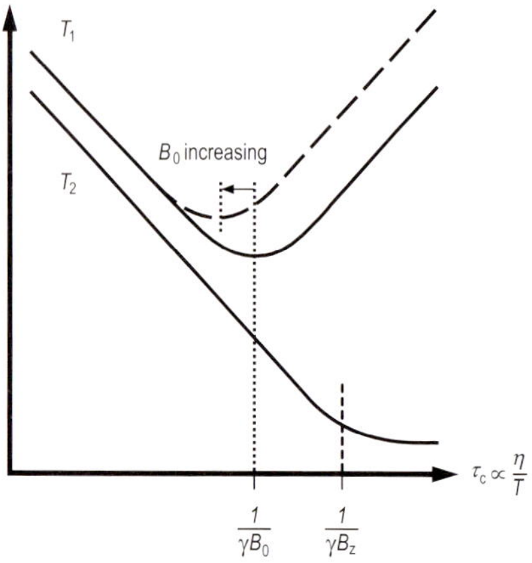

Figure 7.4
Relaxation times T_1 and T_2 as functions of auto-correlation time τ_c, which describes the time between the collisions of two molecules undergoing Brownian motion. In viscous fluids, τ_c can be varied by the ratio of viscosity η over temperature T. A minimum is observed when τ_c approaches the reciprocal Larmor frequency. T_2 increases along with collision frequency (motional narrowing).

therefore, has to be added to the reciprocal of eqs. (7.11). This does not alter the general dependence of T_2 on the correlation time as has been shown in experiments using viscous liquids for which, according to Bloembergen [7.19], the autocorrelation time is proportional to the ratio of viscosity η over temperature:

$$\tau_c \propto \frac{\eta}{T} \tag{7.14}$$

For nuclei with nuclear spin $I > 1/2$, e.g. ^{23}Na ($I = 3/2$), the electrostatic interaction of the nuclear quadrupole moment with the electric field gradient formed at the site of the nucleus (on account of the molecule structure) leads to additional relaxation. The relaxation times for such nuclei are therefore much shorter than those with spin $I = 1/2$.

Table 7.2 gives the order of magnitude for the relaxation times exhibited by protons in biological tissue [7.20]. The frequency dependence of T_1 for protons in tissue may be roughly expressed

$$T_1 \propto \omega_L^{0.3}. \tag{7.15}$$

Transverse relaxation is mainly independent of the Larmor frequency, as is indicated by eq. (7.11b).

It is the wide range of relaxation times in biological tissue that makes nuclear magnetic resonance so interesting in medical diagnostics. T_1 for protons is of an order of mag-

Table 7.2 Typical relaxation times T_1 (at 1 T) and T_2 [5.7]

Tissue	T_1 in s	T_2 in ms	Tissue	T_1 in s	T_2 in ms
Muscle	0.73 ±0.13	47 ±13	Spleen	0.68 ±0.19	62 ±27
Heart	0.75 ±0.12	57 ±16	Fat	0.24 ±0.07	84 ±36
Liver	0.42 ±0.09	43 ±14	Gray matter	0.81 ±0.14	101 ±13
Kidney	0.59 ±0.16	58 ±24	White matter	0.68 ±0.12	92 ±22

nitude of several 100 ms, while T_2 ranges from 30 to 100 ms. Imaging the nuclear magnetization of a biological object produces high levels of contrast and the different relaxation times involved enable one to clearly discern pathological areas. Furthermore, the fact that T_1 increases with temperature enables one to non-invasively monitor thermal tissue ablation using RF, lasers or high intensity ultrasound in real time.

Of special significance is the fact that relaxation times can be shortened dramatically by introducing small concentrations of paramagnetic ions, as these produce a much larger perturbation field during collisions than nuclear spins. Highly specific contrast agents have been developed for medical purposes [7.21]. These are injected intravenously and enable a variety of functional studies (i.e. involving blood flow and tumor perfusion).

7.2.4 Magnetization transfer

Tissue cannot be considered a viscous fluid in all respects. In general, tissue contains a large amount of mobile and a smaller amount of bound water molecules, the latter forming a hydration layer around macromolecules and proteins. Owing to the permanent mutual collisions (correlation time τ), the two systems are coupled via intermolecular, dipole-dipole interaction and chemical exchange so that, in addition to direct spin-lattice relaxation, an additional relaxation path between the more solid and the mobile protons exists [7.22]. This allows for the transfer of magnetic properties associated with water protons bound to biological macromolecules to free water protons. An averaged longitudinal relaxation time for the two is observed.

$$\frac{1}{T_1^{\text{obs}}} = \frac{c}{T_1^{\text{bound}}} + \frac{1-c}{T_1^{\text{free}} + \tau} \tag{7.16}$$

c: Fraction (<< 1) of immobile water molecules

T_1^{bound}: Longitudinal relaxation time of immobile water molecules

T_1^{free}: Longitudinal relaxation time of free water without coupling

τ: Collision time

The transfer of longitudinal magnetization between spins in the two pools can be influenced externally. The FID of bound water is so short that the bound water signals cannot be detected against those of free water. However, irradiating the broad line of immobile protons off-resonance from the narrow water line using a narrow bandwidth RF pulse before excitation and acquisition of the water signal, leads to an equal population of the two energy levels of the bound water without generating transversal magnetization, an effect referred to as saturation. During collisions with mobile water molecules, saturation is transferred to the water spins that adopt the longitudinal magnetization

$$M_z^{\text{sat}} = \frac{M_z^{\text{free}}}{1 + rT_1^{\text{free}}}. \tag{7.17}$$

r: Magnetization transfer rate

M_z^{free}: Longitudinal magnetization of the free water protons excluding coupling

The intensity of the water signal is thus reduced. In MRI, magnetization transfer contrast (MTC) furnishes a basis for contrast options [7.23] other than relaxation, diffusion and flow.

7.2.5 Nuclear induction

Precession of nuclear magnetization can be experimentally stimulated by disturbing the alignment of the nuclear magnetization parallel to the applied static magnetic field B_0 with a radio-frequency (RF) excitation pulse of a frequency similar to the Larmor frequency. The RF field is created by winding a coil around the sample so that its field axis is orthogonal to the static magnetic field. The linearly polarized RF field in this coil can be thought of as a superimposition of two circularly polarized fields rotating in opposite directions. Thus, there is always one RF field component rotating in the same direction as the Larmor nucleic precession. The reference frame (rotating frame) rotating at the Larmor frequency thus contains only the constant magnetic flux density B_1. This exerts torque on the nuclear magnetization, causing the spins to precess around the axis of the B_1 field in the rotating frame in the same manner as around the B_0 field in the laboratory frame. The combined rotational movement around the static B_0 and the RF-B_1 field in the laboratory frame causes the tip of the nuclear magnetization vector to run a spiral path on the surface of a sphere (fig. 7.5).

Having twice the Larmor frequency in the rotating frame, the contra-rotating RF field acts as a perturbation and averages out. The application of two crossed coils driven with RF currents 90° out of phase allows one to use a circular polarized field instead of a linear polarized RF field. The RF power required to tip the nuclear magnetization is thus reduced by a factor of 2.

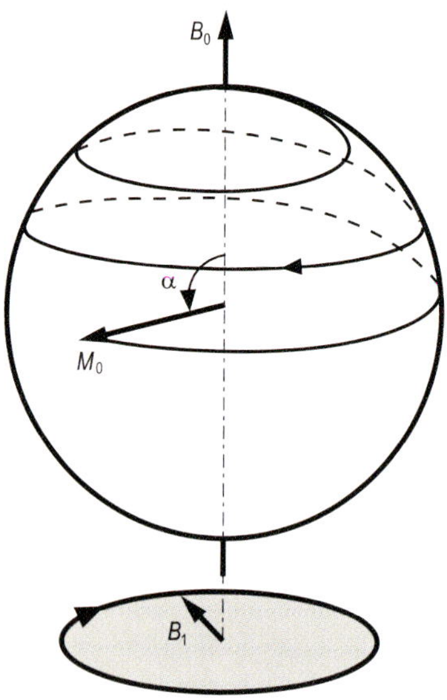

Figure 7.5
Motion of the nuclear magnetization vector M_0 under the influence of a static magnetic field B_0 and a circularly polarized RF field B_1 with a Larmor frequency of $-\gamma B_0$. The initial position of M is parallel to B_0. After time t_D, M_0 is oriented with an angle of $\alpha = \gamma B_0 t_D$ along the direction of B_0. (The direction of precession depends on whether the angular and the magnetic moment of the nuclei are parallel or antiparallel. For protons a clockwise rotation follows.)

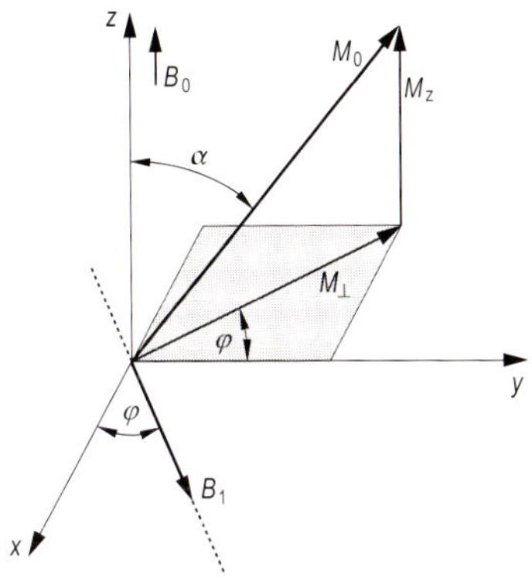

Figure 7.6
Influence of the B_1 field on the equilibrium magnetization in the rotating frame

Under the influence of the rotating RF magnetic flux density B_1, an angle α emerges between the static magnetic field and the nuclear magnetic moment. This angle is proportional to the duration t_D of the RF field:

$$\alpha = -\gamma B_1 t_D. \tag{7.18a}$$

In the more general case of a non constant B_1 field, α can be expressed as

$$\alpha = -\gamma \int_0^{t_D} B_1(t)dt. \tag{7.18b}$$

In the case of a B_1 field that confines an angle β with the x-axis of the rotating frame, the nuclear magnetization attains the following components (fig. 7.6):

$$\begin{aligned} M_x(0) &= -M_0 \sin\alpha \sin\beta \\ M_y(0) &= M_0 \sin\alpha \cos\beta \\ M_z(0) &= M_0 \cos\alpha \end{aligned} \tag{7.19}$$

Switching off the RF pulse leaves the nuclear magnetization precessing around the B_0 field, a case of free induction decay (FID):

$$M_\perp(t) = iM_\perp(0)e^{i\beta}e^{i\omega_L t}e^{-\frac{t}{T_2}} \tag{7.20}$$

The x and y-component of the transverse magnetization are combined here into the complex quantity

$$M_\perp = M_x + iM_y, \quad i = \sqrt{-1} \tag{7.21}$$

The longitudinal magnetization approaches thermal equilibrium as

$$M_z(t) = M_0 - [M_0 - M_z(0)]e^{-\frac{t}{T_1}} = M_0\left(1 - e^{-\frac{t}{T_1}}\right) \quad \text{for } \alpha = 90° \tag{7.22}$$

The FID can be detected by recording the voltage that is induced in a coil wound around the sample (e.g. which has already been used for RF excitation). Maximum signal is induced when the RF field is switched off after the magnetization has been tilted by 90° (90° pulse).

The transversal magnetization can be experimentally measured by mixing the voltage induced in the receiver coil with an AC voltage of frequency ω_0, which is roughly the same as or equal to the Larmor frequency ω_L. The signal at difference frequency

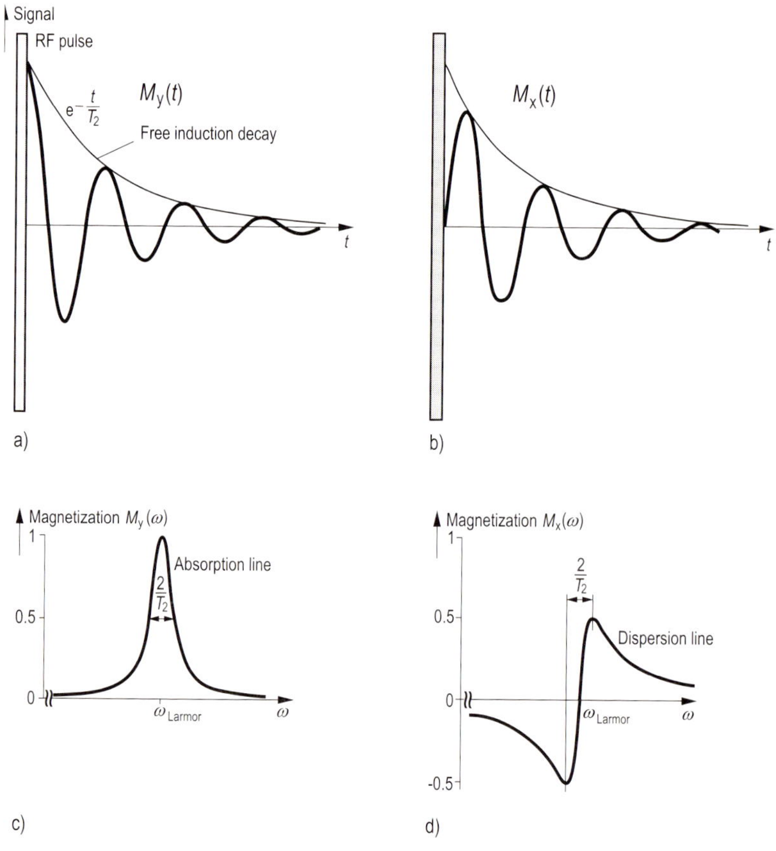

Figure 7.7
a) In-phase induction signal following a 90° pulse about the *y*-axis of the rotating frame: In order to evaluate the transverse magnetization as well as its absolute value, the induction signal is mixed with an alternating voltage of similar frequency and the same phase as the FID at $t = 0$ to give a signal with the difference frequency (phase-sensitive demodulation). **b)** 90° out-of-phase signal: The induction signal is mixed with an alternating voltage of similar frequency out of phase with the FID by 90°. **c)** Absorption signal: The imaginary part of the Fourier transform of the signal in the time domain represents the frequency dependence of the *y*-component of the precessing magnetization vector. **d)** Dispersion signal: The real part of the Fourier transform of the signal in the time domain represents the frequency dependence of the *x*-component of the precessing magnetization vector.

(phase sensitive detection) directly represents the magnetization in a reference frame rotating at frequency ω_0

$$\Omega = \omega - \omega_0 \tag{7.23}$$

In other words, if $\omega_0 = \omega_L$, then resonance occurs at $\Omega = 0$. In a reference frame rotating at a circular frequency of ω_0, the spins precess around a magnetic field of magnitude $B_0 - \left|\frac{\omega_0}{\gamma}\right|$.

The precessing x and y-component of the nuclear magnetization can be determined using two reference voltages, one shifted by 90° in phase. Instead of working with two reference signals, a circular polarized receiver coil assembly can be used. This provides an improvement in the signal-to-noise ratio by a factor of $\sqrt{2}$.

The complex Fourier transformation of the detected precession signal yields the distribution of the transverse magnetization as a function of frequency (fig. 7.7). When the RF field has tilted the magnetization around the x-axis so that it aligns with the y-axis after a 90° pulse, the imaginary part is referred to as the absorption line

$$M_y(\Omega) = M_\perp(0)\frac{T_2}{1+\Omega^2 T_2^2} \tag{7.24a}$$

and the real part is referred to as the dispersion line

$$M_x(\Omega) = M_\perp(0)\frac{T_2^2\Omega}{1+\Omega^2}. \tag{7.24b}$$

The full width at half maximum (*FWHM*) of the absorption line and the distance between the extreme points of the dispersion line are given by the transverse relaxation time T_2:

$$\Delta\omega = \frac{2}{T_2} \tag{7.25}$$

Protons in distilled water exhibit a line width of less than 1 Hz. Obtaining a measurement of T_2 when analyzing the free induction decay, however, is only possible in very homogenous magnetic fields. In practice, the magnetic field B_0 varies in space, resulting in different precession frequencies for the nuclear magnetization. A shortened FID is observed on account of destructive interference. This results in an inhomogeneously broadened resonance line. The line shape depends on the spatial distribution of the magnetic field deviations $\Delta B_0(x, y, z)$ across the entire sample. Reference is often made to an effective transverse relaxation time

$$\frac{1}{T_2^*} = \frac{1}{T_2} + \frac{1}{2}\gamma\Delta B_0 \tag{7.26}$$

However, given that the signal clearly ceases to decay exponentially, this is at best a coarse description of the effect of magnetic field inhomogeneities.

7.2.6 Spin echoes

The signal loss in an inhomogeneous field B_0 can be recovered by means of an RF pulse that tilts the magnetization by 180° [7.24]. The diverging transverse magnetization that is due to field inhomogeneities following a 90° pulse re-converges after a 180° pulse because the pulse reverses the order of the spins (fig. 7.8). The spins that have lagged behind move ahead after the second RF pulse and realign themselves with the spins that have been precessing at a faster speed. A spin echo is formed behind the sec-

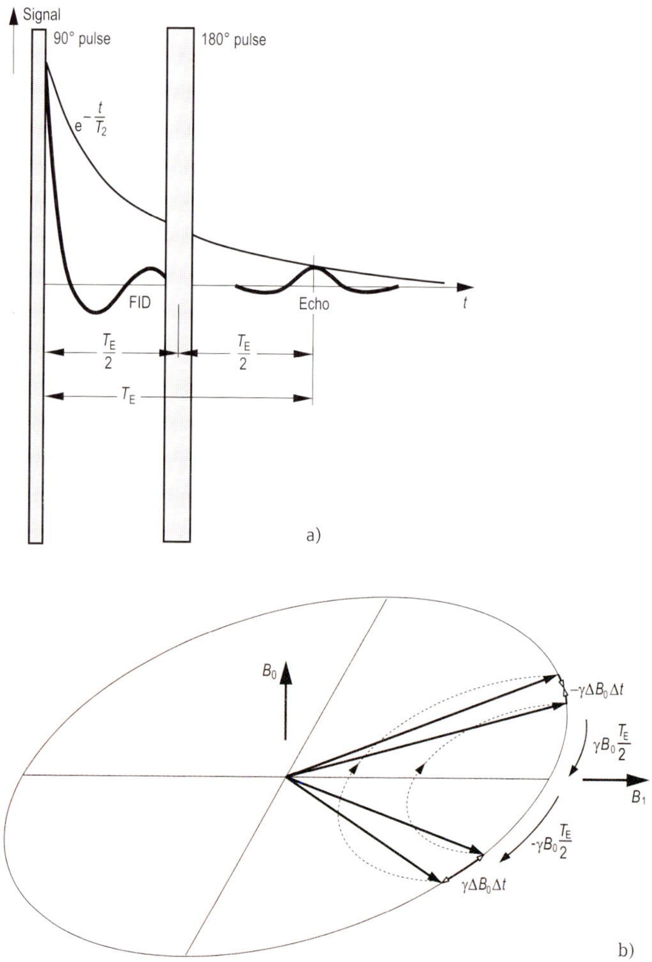

Figure 7.8
a) The FID decays rapidly following a 90° pulse on account of magnetic field inhomogeneities. It can be reestablished by means of a 180° pulse with reduced amplitude due to transversal relaxation. **b)** The de-phasing effect of an inhomogeneous field on the transversal magnetization can be reversed by means of a 180° pulse.

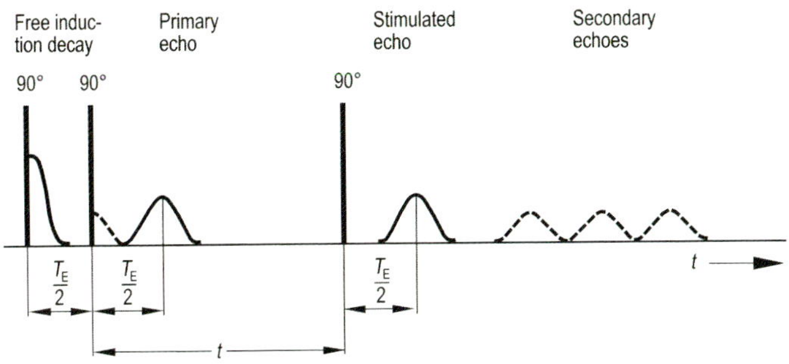

Figure 7.9
Sequence of three 90° pulses for generating a stimulated echo. Deviations from the 90° condition lead to the appearance of extra secondary echoes.

ond RF pulse at a distance that conforms to the pulse spacing. Its amplitude is determined by transverse relaxation (fig. 7.9)

$$|M_{\perp}(T_E)| = M_0 e^{-\frac{T_E}{T_2}} \tag{7.27}$$

An echo train with exponentially decreasing amplitudes can be generated by applying additional 180° pulses to provide a simple way of measuring T_2 [7.25].

The so-called stimulated echo also warrants mention in this context. Applying two 90° pulses instead of a 90°/180° pair produces an echo whose amplitude is only half of that produced by a 180° pulse. The missing magnetization is stored along the z-axis where it undergoes longitudinal relaxation. After a time period t, it can be re-tilted into the transverse plane by a third 90° pulse. It will then manifest itself as a stimulated echo with a distance from the third 90° pulse corresponding to that of the first two 90° pulses (fig. 7.10). The amplitude of the stimulated echo is determined by the longitudinal relaxation.

$$|M_{\perp}(t + T_E)| = \frac{1}{2} M_0 e^{-\frac{T_E}{T_2} - \frac{t}{T_1}} \tag{7.28}$$

Further echoes appear if the 90° condition is not met exactly. These can be explained as echoes that are generated by the third RF pulse from the FIDs following the first and second RF pulses and from the first echo.

Another method of determining T_1 consists in first inverting the magnetization by means of a 180° pulse and then probing the longitudinal magnetization (inversion recovery) after time t

$$M_z(t) = M_0\left(1 - 2e^{-\frac{t}{T_1}}\right) \tag{7.29}$$

by means of an FID produced by an interrogating 90° pulse (fig. 7.10).

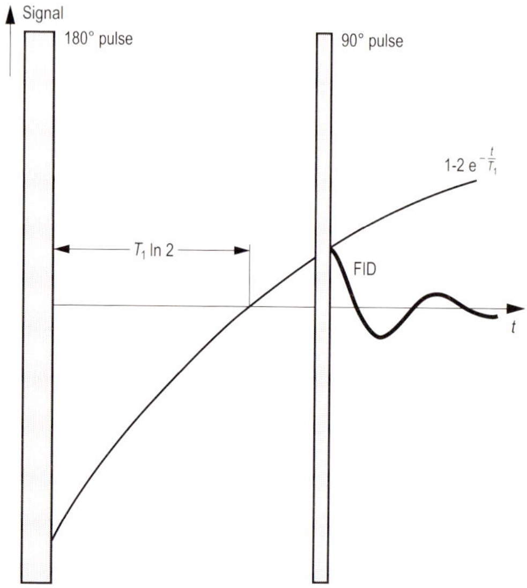

Figure 7.10
Inversion recovery sequence for determining the longitudinal relaxation time T_1. The magnetization is aligned antiparallel to the magnetic field by means of a 180° pulse. The magnetization tends to decay at time constant T_1. The momentary value of the longitudinal magnetization can be measured by flipping it with a 90° pulse into the transverse plane and evaluating the resulting FID.

Finally, longitudinal relaxation will manifest itself when 90° FIDs are repeatedly generated at repetition time T_R. After some transients the starting amplitude stabilizes at

$$|M_\perp(T_R)| = M_0\left(1 - e^{-\frac{T_R}{T_1}}\right). \tag{7.30}$$

The signal vanishes in the case of short repetition times, i.e. the spin system saturates (saturation recovery). T_1 can be determined by recording the FID amplitude as a function of repetition time.

7.2.7 Steady-state free precession

The dynamic equilibrium or steady state that is established in a train of RF pulses is characterized by the fact that the magnetization is the same after each RF pulse. One thus observes the following at a distance t from an RF pulse:

$$\vec{M}(nT_R + t) = \vec{M}((n+1)T_R + t) = \vec{M}(t) = \begin{bmatrix} M_x(t) \\ M_y(t) \\ M_z(t) \end{bmatrix} \tag{7.31}$$

n: Index of RF pulse, T_R: Repetition time

The magnetization immediately after the RF pulse $\vec{M}(0)$ follows from that immediately before $\vec{M}(T_R)$ from the rotation by tip angle α

$$\vec{M}(0) = \mathbf{Q}(\alpha) = \vec{M}(T_R) \tag{7.32}$$

with rotation matrix

$$\mathbf{Q}(\alpha) = \begin{bmatrix} 1 & 0 & 0 \\ 0 & \cos\alpha & \sin\alpha \\ 0 & -\sin\alpha & \cos\alpha \end{bmatrix}. \tag{7.33}$$

On the other hand, owing to the precession and relaxation between the RF pulses, $\vec{M}(T_R)$ and $\vec{M}(0)$ are related by

$$\vec{M}(T_R) = \mathbf{R}(T_R)\vec{M}(0) + M_0 \begin{bmatrix} 0 \\ 0 \\ 1 - e^{-\frac{T_R}{T_1}} \end{bmatrix} \tag{7.34}$$

where the matrix

$$\mathbf{R}(T_R) = \begin{bmatrix} \cos\Omega t\, e^{-\frac{T_R}{T_2}} & \sin\Omega t\, e^{-\frac{T_R}{T_2}} & 0 \\ \sin\Omega t\, e^{-\frac{T_R}{T_2}} & \cos\Omega t\, e^{-\frac{T_R}{T_2}} & 0 \\ 0 & 0 & e^{-\frac{T_R}{T_1}} \end{bmatrix} \tag{7.35}$$

(with $\Omega = \omega - \omega_0$) describes precession and relaxation in a reference frame rotating at frequency ω.

In the following, we analyze steady-state magnetization for two cases relevant to MRI. First, we assume that there is no residual transverse magnetization directly prior to the RF pulse:

$$\begin{aligned} M_x(T_R) &= M_y(T_R) = 0 \\ M_x(0) &= M_z(T_R)\cos\alpha \\ M_z(T_R) &= M_0 - (M_0 - M_z(0))e^{-\frac{T_R}{T_1}} \end{aligned} \tag{7.36}$$

The transverse magnetization immediately after the RF pulse then yields

$$M_y(0) = M_z(T_R)\sin\alpha = M_0 \sin\alpha \, \frac{1 - e^{-\frac{T_R}{T_1}}}{1 - \cos\alpha\, e^{-\frac{T_R}{T_1}}} \tag{7.37}$$

Adjusting $\alpha = 90^\circ$, eq. (7.30) follows, as it is used when measuring T_1 with saturation recovery. Maximum signal is reached for the so called Ernst angle:

$$\cos\alpha_{opt} = e^{-\frac{T_R}{T_1}} \tag{7.38}$$

Numerical example:

$$T_1 = 1\text{ s},\ T_R = 0.1\text{ s}$$
$$\alpha = 90^\circ \quad \rightarrow \quad M_y = 0.095\ M_0$$
$$\alpha_{opt} = 25.2^\circ \quad \rightarrow \quad M_y = 0.22\ M_0$$

The reduction of the excitation angle can thus result in a significantly larger MR signal. This principle is applied in MRI with the so called FLASH (Fast Low Angle SHot) sequence [7.26].

We shall next assume that the following relation obtains between $\vec{M}(0)$ and $\vec{M}(T_R)$:

$$M_y(T_R) = -M_y(0)\mathrm{e}^{-\frac{T_R}{T_2}} \tag{7.39}$$

This relation can either be assured by adjusting the frequency of the RF pulses in the rotating frame to

$$\Omega = \pm\frac{\pi}{T_R} \tag{7.40}$$

or (at resonant excitation, i.e. $\Omega = 0$) by alternating the phase between adjacent pulses by 180°.

The following then applies to the other magnetization components:

$$\begin{aligned} M_y(0) &= M_y(T_R)\cos\alpha + M_z(T_R)\sin\alpha \\ M_z(0) &= -M_y(T_R)\sin\alpha + M_z(T_R)\cos\alpha \\ M_z(T_R) &= M_0 - (M_0 - M_z(0))\mathrm{e}^{-\frac{T_R}{T_1}} \end{aligned} \tag{7.41}$$

Signal amplitude is determined by the transverse magnetization immediately following the RF pulse:

$$M_y(0) = \frac{M_0\left(1-\mathrm{e}^{-\frac{T_R}{T_1}}\right)\sin\alpha}{\left(1-\mathrm{e}^{-T_R\left(\frac{1}{T_1}+\frac{1}{T_2}\right)}\right)+\left(\mathrm{e}^{-\frac{T_R}{T_2}}-\mathrm{e}^{-\frac{T_R}{T_1}}\right)\cos\alpha}. \tag{7.42}$$

For $\frac{T_R}{T_{1,2}} << 1$

$$M_y(0) = \frac{M_0\sin\alpha}{\left(1+\frac{T_1}{T_2}\right)+\left(1-\frac{T_1}{T_2}\right)\cos\alpha} \tag{7.43}$$

is obtained, which then reduces for $\alpha = 90^\circ$ to

$$M_y(0) = \frac{M_0}{1+\frac{T_1}{T_2}} \tag{7.44}$$

Such a sequence is referred to as (true) FISP (fast imaging with steady precession) [7.27]. Signal intensity is determined by the ratio T_1/T_2. For fluids such as water, where $T_1 \approx T_2$, a signal equivalent to half of the maximum nuclear magnetization can be obtained using 90° pulses with rapid pulse repetition.

7.2.8 Diffusion

Relaxation is not the only mechanism that reduces spin-echo amplitudes. Molecules in liquids, in particular, move stochastically (diffuse) due to their thermal energy (Brownian motion) during the period between excitation and echo observation. If B_0 is not perfectly homogeneous, then local field differences will cause the nuclei to precess at different Larmor frequencies and destructive interference will reduce the echo amplitude.

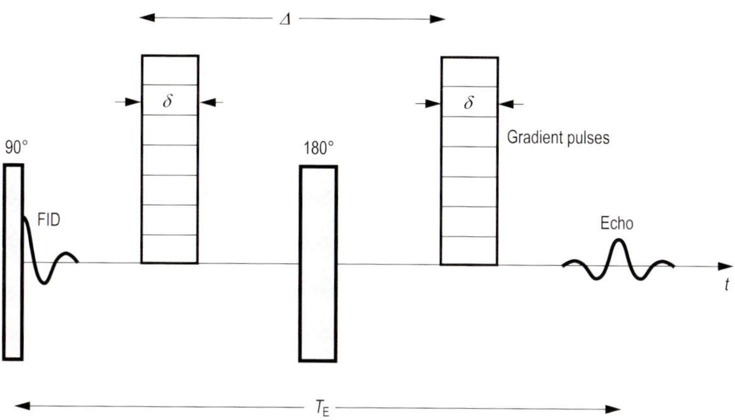

Figure 7.11
Pulsed gradient spin echo (PGSE) sequence. Recording the echo amplitude as a function of gradient amplitude gives the diffusion profile.

The influence of spin diffusion can be investigated using a spin echo experiment involving the application of strong magnetic field gradient pulses before and after the refocusing RF pulse (fig. 7.12) [7.28]. To avoid losing too much signal strength due to transverse relaxation between the two gradient pulses, the refocusing 180° pulse can be divided into two 90° pulses so that diffusion is probed via the stimulated echo. Such pulsed gradient spin echo (PGSE) experiments are of interest because they permit the investigation of microstructures.

Given that diffusion is a stochastic process, it is best described using a probability function [7.29]. The so-called displacement propagator $P_D(\vec{r}_0 \mid \vec{r}, t)$ gives the probability per volume unit of a single spin traveling from position $\vec{r}_0$ to $\vec{r}$ in time t.

It is strongly localized for $t = 0$:

$$P_D(\vec{r}_0 \,|\, \vec{r}, 0) = \delta(\vec{r} - \vec{r}_0) \tag{7.45}$$

In a confined environment (i.e. for restricted self-diffusion) at $t \to \infty$, the spin will have lost all of its memory at the starting position $\vec{r}_0$ so that the displacement propagator approaches a mean probability or relative spin density of

$$P_D(\vec{r}_0 \,|\, \vec{r}, \infty) = \rho(\vec{r}), \tag{7.46}$$

which is normalized as

$$\int \rho(\vec{r})\,d^3r = 1. \tag{7.47}$$

In the case of unrestricted self-diffusion, the Gaussian propagator

$$P_G(\vec{r}_0 \,|\, \vec{r}, t) = P_G(\vec{R}) = \frac{1}{\sqrt{4\pi D t}^{\,3}} e^{-\frac{R^2}{4Dt}} \qquad \vec{R} = \vec{r} - \vec{r}_0 \tag{7.48}$$

D: Diffusion constant

arises as a solution to Fick's second law, which is independent of the starting position $\vec{r}_0$ of the individual diffusing spin, and thus depends only on the dynamic displacement $\vec{R}$ over time t during which a spin travels the mean distance $\sqrt{2Dt}$. It is safe to assume that unrestricted diffusion occurs as long as the diffusing spins are not colliding with the wall of their confining compartment:

$$t << \frac{d^2}{D} \tag{7.49}$$

d: Compartment size

The echo amplitude in the PGSE experiment is derived by summing up the weighted phase shifts arising from the displacements $\vec{R}$ that occur in the time Δ between the two gradient pulses:

$$E(\vec{q}, \Delta) = \int \bar{P}_D(\vec{R}, \Delta) e^{i\vec{q}\vec{R}} d^3r. \tag{7.50}$$

The weighting factor $\bar{P}_D(\vec{R}, \Delta)$ (named ensemble average propagator) is given by

$$\bar{P}_D(\vec{R}, \Delta) = \int \rho(\vec{r}_0) P_D(\vec{r}_0 | \vec{r}, \Delta) d^3r_0 \qquad \vec{q} = \gamma \vec{G} \delta \tag{7.51}$$

G: Pulsed gradient strength, δ: Duration of pulsed gradient

The echo amplitude $E(\vec{q}, \Delta)$ in this context is a relative quantity because of the normalization in eq. (7.47).

In the case of free diffusion, the echo amplitude is derived by applying the Gaussian propagator (eq. (7.48)

$$E(\vec{q}, \Delta) = E_0 e^{-bD}, \quad \text{with} \quad b = q^2\left(\Delta - \frac{\delta}{3}\right). \tag{7.52}$$

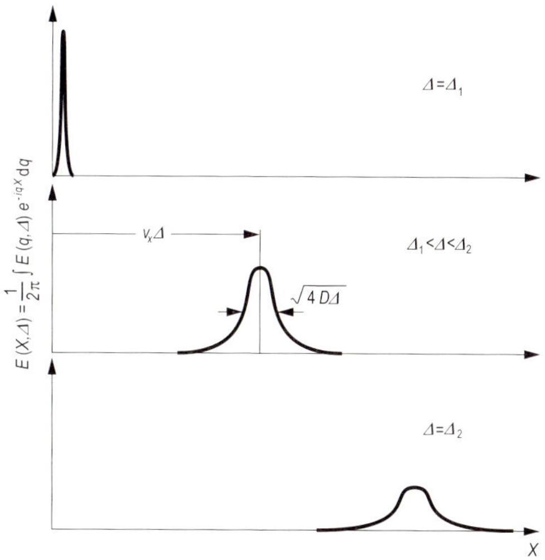

Figure 7.12
Diffusion profiles derived from the Fourier transform of the echo amplitudes as a function of gradient amplitude in a PGSE experiment. Increasing the time Δ between the gradient pulses broadens the distribution and shifts it along the gradient direction when flow is present.

The ensemble averaged propagator $\bar{P}_D(\vec{R},\Delta)$ can be obtained in a PGSE experiment by Fourier transformation of the record of echo amplitudes as a function of the *wave vector* $\vec{q} = \gamma\vec{G}\delta$ (i.e. as a function of gradient amplitude). It yields information on the dynamic behavior of the spin system not only with respect to diffusion, but also to flow. Assuming motion at velocity v_x along the x-axis leads to a Gaussian propagator along this axis of

$$\bar{P}_G(X,\Delta) = \frac{1}{\sqrt{4\pi D\Delta}}\,e^{\frac{(X-v_x\Delta)^2}{4D\Delta}} \tag{7.53}$$

When Δ is increased, the diffusion profiles broaden and shift in the direction of larger displacement values $X = x_0 - x$ (fig. 7.13). This method is well-suited to the investigation of very slow flow leading to displacements comparable to those exhibited by diffusion. More direct methods of analyzing the phase of the echo amplitude have been established to investigate larger flow velocities. See section 15.2.4.3 for a detailed discussion of flow.

While the diffusion constant increases strongly along with temperature, this effect is difficult to use for thermometry because of a living object's tendency to move. Experiments have also shown that diffusion in biological tissue (e.g. in fibers) is often not isotropic. Diffusion is apparently subject to different directional restrictions in such materials owing to their microstructures. It can thus be assumed that free diffusion has ceased to take place and the Gaussian diffusion model has lost its validity. While the quantity D in eq. (7.53) can no longer be regarded as a scalar, it is often approximated as the apparent diffusion tensor.

The case of restricted or bound diffusion is characterized by

$$\Delta \gg \frac{d^2}{D} \tag{7.54}$$

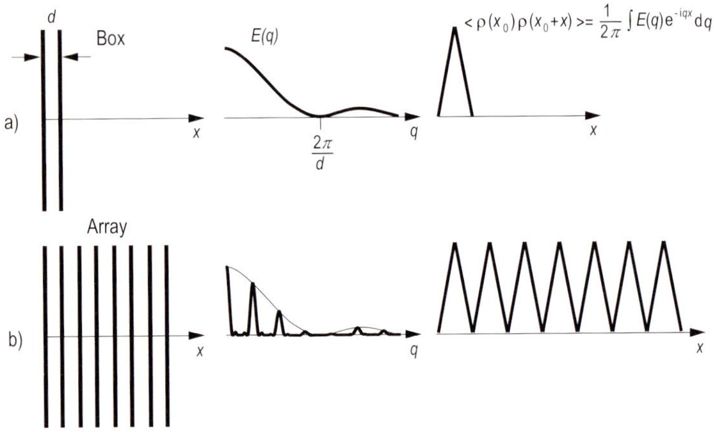

Figure 7.13
a) Diffusion profile of spins confined in a box. **b)** Diffusion profile of spins in an array. The Fourier transform of the echo amplitude as a function of gradient amplitude yields the autocorrelation function of the spin density.

In light of eq. (7.46), the average displacement propagator eq. (7.51) reduces to the autocorrelation function of the relative spin density distribution

$$\bar{P}_D(\vec{R},\infty) = \int \rho(\vec{r}_0)\rho(\vec{r}_0+\vec{R})d^3r_0. \tag{7.55}$$

According to the Wiener-Khintchine theorem, this means that the signal in q-space $E(q,\Delta)$, i.e. the echo amplitude as a function of the product of pulsed gradient strength multiplied by pulse duration in all three directions in a PGSE sequence, is the spatial frequency power spectrum of the investigated structure

$$E(\vec{q}) = \int \bar{P}_D(\vec{R},\infty)e^{i\vec{q}\vec{R}}d^3R = |\rho(\vec{q})|^2 \tag{7.56}$$

with

$$\rho(q) = \int \rho(\vec{r})e^{i\vec{q}\vec{R}}d^3r \tag{7.57}$$

as the Fourier transformation of the relative spin density.

Therefore, spins confined in a one dimensional box would yield a squared sinc signal in q-space from which a triangular autocorrelation function would be derived in R-space with the full width at half maximum (*FWHM*) being the compartment size (fig. 7.13a). A one-dimensional array of boxes would yield a signal pattern in q-space equivalent to the optical diffraction pattern of a grid (fig. 7.13b).

Various structures (e.g. fat globules in cream, yeast cells and water in an assembly of polystyrene spheres) have been investigated. These investigations provide structural information on a µm scale. See [7.16] for a more detailed discussion.

7.2.9 Spectroscopy

7.2.9.1 Chemical shift

The gyromagnetic ratio determining the Larmor frequency of nuclei in the main magnetic field is a fixed constant for each nuclear species. However, NMR experiments involving nuclei embedded in different molecules show slightly different resonance frequencies. This effect is caused by the molecular electrons responsible for chemical bonding. Bringing these electrons into a magnetic field induces diamagnetic ring currents (Lenz's law) that impair the magnetic field at the nucleus, with the result that the atomic nucleus sees different magnetic fields (chemical shift) depending on the nature of the chemical bond.

$$B_k = B_0 - \delta_k B_0 \tag{7.58}$$

One often observes several resonance lines attributable to individual groups of molecules in molecular complexes. Quantitatively, the chemical shift δ_k is usually given in ppm (parts per million) relative to a reference line. The chemical shift depends on temperature. For protons in water molecules

$$\delta_{H_2O} \approx -0.01 \text{ ppm} \frac{T}{K} \tag{7.59}$$

is observed, providing the possibility of linear thermometry in vivo.

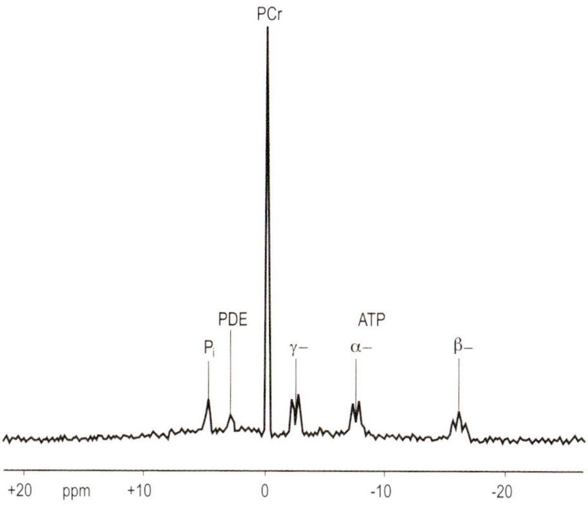

Figure 7.14
^{31}P-spectrum of a human thigh muscle recorded with a surface coil at 2 T. On the basis of their different chemical shifts the metabolites adenosine triphosphate (ATP), phosphocreatine (PCr), inorganic phosphate (P_I) and phosphodiester (PDE) can be distinguished. The three ATP lines correspond to three phosphorous atom locations in the molecule. The lines are split further because of the interaction of the nuclei with other nearby nuclei.

In biological tissue the NMR signal originates mainly from protons in water and in fat. These protons differ in their chemical shifts by 3.5 ppm. This corresponds to a frequency shift of 150 Hz in a magnetic field of 1 T. In MRI, the different chemical shifts of protons in fat and water can cause artifacts given that fat and water may be associated with different locations. Tissue contrast can be masked by the superimposition of fat and water signals. Various techniques have thus been devised to suppress either the fat or the water signal (see section 15.2.1). For instance, applying a narrow band RF pulse at the frequency of fat yields an equal population of the two proton energy levels in fat without generating transversal magnetization – an effect referred to as saturation (fat-sat). The succeeding NMR excitation affects only water-based protons and only these protons emit a signal. Another method of suppressing the fat signal involves the use of fat's much shorter relaxation times compared to water. Here, one applies a 180° pre-pulse to invert the nuclear magnetization of fat and water and then observes the water signal only at the zero crossing of the fat protons (approx. at 100 ms at 1 T).

7.2.9.2 Spin-spin coupling

Besides the chemical shift, one often observes a fine splitting of the NMR lines (fig. 7.14). This is caused by the magnetic interaction (spin-spin coupling) between nuclei either of the same or of different species, which again acts indirectly via the electrons of the chemical bonds. Such spectra can be explained by an energy function (Hamilton operator) that describes both the chemical shift and the mutual interaction energy of the spins $\vec{I}_k$ via the coupling constant $\boldsymbol{J}_{kl}$:

$$H = -\sum_k B_z(1-\delta_k)I_{zk} + \sum_{k,l} \boldsymbol{J}_{kl}\vec{I}_k\vec{I}_l. \tag{7.60}$$

The Eigenfunctions and Eigenvalues of a Hamilton operator compiled for a given molecular structure describe different spin configurations with different energies. Transitions between these energies are observed as NMR lines. For medical purposes, typical metabolites can be identified non-invasively by NMR (see chapter 15.2.7).

The coupling constant $\boldsymbol{J}$ is a scalar. Closely neighbored spins can also couple via the anisotropic dipole-dipole interaction, which normally does not cause line splitting because it is averaged out by the rapid thermal spin movements. Dipole-dipole interaction, however, is a preferred cause of relaxation.

7.2.9.3 Double resonance

Spin coupling (either of the same species ^1H at different sites in a molecule or of different species, such as ^{13}C, ^{31}P and ^1H) can be studied by double resonance. This means that one line in the spectrum is irradiated with RF energy and the effect of this on the resonance of the others is observed. Many variations of double resonance experiments have been designed that involve the application of continuous or pulsed irradiation to analyze the steady state or transient behavior of the nuclear magnetization. We mention only two variants in the present context by way of emphasizing the importance of double resonance in NMR spectroscopy. These include decoupling, and the nuclear Overhauser effect (NOE).

The effect of spin coupling can be eliminated by saturating a line applying a constant or pulsed RF field. This causes the number of spins in the excited and unexcited state to become equal so that no net magnetization is left. In the case of ^{13}C spectroscopy, the coupling of carbon and hydrogen nuclei leads to complex ^{13}C spectra; decoupling the protons (i.e. saturating the proton line(s)) greatly reduces the number of ^{13}C lines and increases their intensity because the integral intensity is distributed across fewer lines.

In fact, the degree to which intensities increase in a decoupled spectrum is often greater than one would expect from the collapse of the multiplet structures into single lines. The increases result from a redistribution of the energy level populations, which causes an enhancement of the polarization for the ^{13}C spins. First analyzed by Overhauser in the case of electron spin resonance saturation and its influence on nuclear magnetic resonance, this effect is now commonly applied to coupled nuclear spins (the nuclear Overhauser effect or NOE) to increase NMR detection sensitivity.

In what follows, we describe the nuclear Overhauser effect for an AX system of different species (e.g. A = ^{13}C and X = ^{1}H) where $I_A = I_X = 1/2$. The energy levels and the associated transition probabilities are depicted in fig. 7.15. By applying the general master equation of populations

$$\frac{d\boldsymbol{P}(t)}{dt} = \boldsymbol{W}(\boldsymbol{P}(t) - \boldsymbol{P}(0)) \tag{7.61}$$

$\boldsymbol{P}(t)$: Vector of populations of the spin levels at time t
$\boldsymbol{W}$: Matrix of transition probabilities

it can be shown [7.30] that the longitudinal magnetization of the A spins increases as follows upon the saturation of the X-transition:

$$\frac{M_z^A}{M_0^A} = 1 + \frac{W_2 - W_0}{2W_1^A + W_0 + W_2}\frac{\gamma_X}{\gamma_A}. \tag{7.62a}$$

W_1^A: Transition probability $|\frac{1}{2}, -\frac{1}{2}\rangle \leftrightarrow |-\frac{1}{2}, -\frac{1}{2}\rangle$
W_0: Probability for zero quantum transition $|\frac{1}{2}, -\frac{1}{2}\rangle \leftrightarrow |-\frac{1}{2}, \frac{1}{2}\rangle$
W_2: Probability for double quantum transition $|\frac{1}{2}, \frac{1}{2}\rangle \leftrightarrow |-\frac{1}{2}, -\frac{1}{2}\rangle$

The simultaneous flip of an A and an X spin, as described by the probabilities W_0 and W_2, is referred to as cross relaxation. Transitions between these states are forbidden for electromagnetic radiation on account of the law of angular momentum conservation. If the predominant pathway along which the A spins relax is an intramolecular dipole-dipole interaction with a very short correlation time $\omega_A\tau_C << 1$, the relation $W_2 : W_1^A : W_0 = 12 : 3 : 2$ holds so that eq. (7.62a) reduces to

$$\frac{M_z^A}{M_0^A} = 1 + \frac{1}{2}\frac{\gamma_X}{\gamma_A}. \tag{7.62b}$$

A ^{13}C resonance signal enhancement of 300% can thus be obtained for a ^{13}C-^{1}H spin system using NOE. An NOE enhancement of 150% can be reached for a spin system

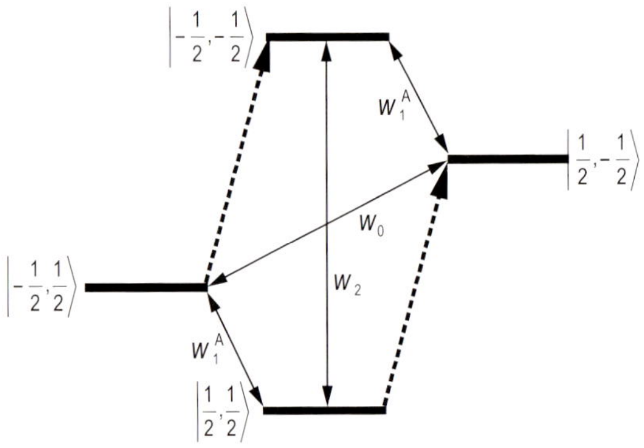

$$W_1^A \propto \frac{3\tau_C}{r^6(1+\omega_A^2\tau_C^2)} \approx \frac{3\tau_C}{r^6} \qquad W_0 \propto \frac{2\tau_C}{r^6(1+\omega_A^2\tau_C^2)} \approx \frac{2\tau_C}{r^6} \qquad W_2 \propto \frac{12\tau_C}{r^6(1+\omega_A^2\tau_C^2)} \approx \frac{12\tau_C}{r^6}$$

Figure 7.15
Energy level scheme of an AX spin system with transition probabilities when the X resonance is saturated. r denotes the distance between the two dipoles.

consisting of two protons. A close spatial distance r between the coupled nuclei is a prerequisite because the dipole-dipole interaction required for relaxation is inversely proportional to r^6. However, various alternative double resonance methods that involve the application of polarization transfer and that are more effective than the NOE are possible [7.31]. These include selective population inversion (SPI), selective population transfer (SPT), insensitive nuclei enhanced by polarization transfer (INEPT) and distortionless enhancement of polarization transfer (DEPT).

7.2.10 Signal-to-noise ratio

NMR in vivo is most meaningful when the magnetization can be measured in a manner that allows for spatial resolution. Before discussing such possibilities, however, it might be helpful to first analyze a fundamental restriction that applies to such mea-

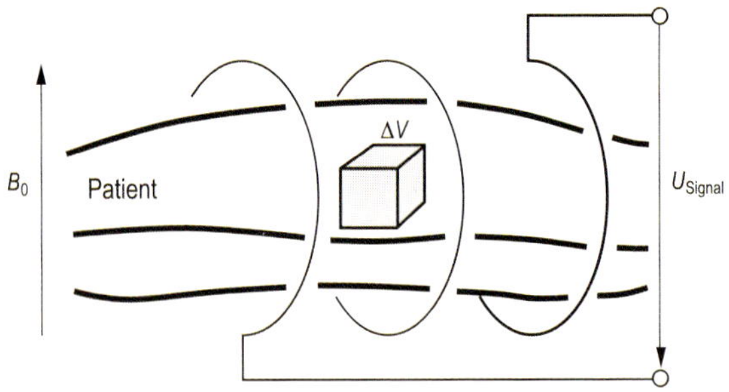

Figure 7.16
Volume element ΔV in a patient to be detected by an NMR RF coil

surements. This limit has its origin in the fact that the thermal motion of the electrons in the signal pickup coil and the Brownian molecular motion of change carriers in the object to be investigated (the human body) produce a noise voltage that competes with the NMR signal. An inferior signal-to-noise ratio (*S/N*) is observed when smaller volume elements (voxels) are to be resolved. Here, the measurement process is often longer on account of the need to average out the noise. However, given that nuclear magnetization increases with the applied magnetic field, rather large magnetic flux densities (in practice up to 3 T) are applied.

The voltage that is induced in the signal coil by the precessing magnetic moment of one volume element or voxel following a 90° pulse is expressed as

$$U_{\text{Signal}} = B_{\text{i}}\omega_{\text{L}}M_{\perp}\Delta V \tag{7.63}$$

B_{i}: Geometry factor of the signal coil (*field per unit current*)

ΔV: Voxel volume

$M_{\perp} \propto \sin\alpha \frac{B_0}{T}$: Transverse nuclear magnetization (eq. (7.4))

The noise voltage according to Nyquist is

$$U_{\text{Noise}} = \sqrt{\frac{2}{\pi}k_{\text{B}}(R_{\text{Coil}}T_{\text{Coil}} + R_{\text{Sample}}T_{\text{Sample}})\Delta\omega}. \tag{7.64}$$

$\Delta\omega$: Detection bandwidth for the signal, R_{Coil}: Resistance of signal coil without sample

R_{Sample}: Contribution of the sample to the resistance of the signal coil

T_{Coil}: Temperature of signal coil, T_{Sample}: Temperature of sample

While the noise contribution $R_{\text{Coil}}T_{\text{Coil}}$ dominates in the case of small samples of a few mm^3 (as is commonly verified by laboratory investigations), this is not true for samples as large as the human body. The signal coil resistance increases in the case of a conductive sample by a contribution [7.32]

$$R_{\text{Sample}} = \frac{1}{4}\sigma B_{\text{i}}^2\omega^2\int r_{\perp}^2\,\mathrm{d}v. \tag{7.65}$$

$r_{\perp}$: Radius coordinate orthogonal to the field axis of the signal coil

σ: Electrical conductivity of the sample, ω: Signal frequency, i.e. Larmor frequency

When the field per unit current B_{i} in eq. (7.65) is replaced by the alternating field B_1 that is used to excite the spins, the RF power distributed in the sample is given instead of its resistance.

Introducing the field distribution or filling factor

$$\eta = \frac{V_{\text{Sample}}B_{\text{i}}^2}{\int B_{\text{i}}^2\,dv}, \tag{7.66}$$

which is a measure of the ratio of the sample volume to the coil volume and the unloaded coil quality factor

$$Q_0 = \omega\frac{\textit{energy stored in coil}}{\textit{power dissipated in coil}}, \tag{7.67}$$

following a succession of steps omitted here yields the relation

$$\frac{U_{\text{Signal}}}{U_{\text{Noise}}} = \sqrt{\frac{\pi}{18k^3}}\, I(I+1)\hbar^2 \gamma N_V \frac{\omega_L}{T_{\text{Sample}}\sqrt{\frac{1}{\mu_0}\frac{T_{\text{Coil}}V_{\text{Sample}}}{\eta Q_0 \omega_L} + \frac{\sigma}{4}T_{\text{Sample}}\int r_\perp^2 \, dv}} \frac{\Delta V}{\sqrt{\Delta\omega}} \tag{7.68}$$

μ_0: Permeability in vacuum

The signal-to-noise ratio is proportional to $\omega^{3/2}$ for small values of the moment of inertia $\int r_\perp^2 dv$ (i.e. small samples) and for small filling and coil quality factors. In the case of a high coil quality factor or a low coil temperature, the signal-to-noise ratio is directly proportional to the Larmor frequency. One trick to improve the signal-to-noise ratio in large objects is to apply an array of small coils instead of a large receiver coil. Doing so ensures that each sub-coil receives less noise as it sees a smaller sub-object.

The most important parameter in MR, however, is the flux density of the applied magnetic field. B_0 is an important parameter in NMR experiments not only because of the signal-to-noise ratio, but because it determines the spectral resolution for distinguishing chemical compounds and because the longitudinal relaxation times T_1 of biological tissue depend on this value. Given that power absorption increases with Larmor frequency squared, RF heating is a limit to be considered when applying higher magnetic fields in MRI.

Once the NMR system has been set up (i.e. the main magnetic field and antennas have been selected), the signal-to-noise ratio may still be influenced by the voxel size and bandwidth. Repeating the NMR experiment n times and adding the individual signals together permits one to improve the signal-to-noise ratio by a factor of $\sqrt{n}$. However, since spatial resolution reductions are as undesirable as longer measurement times, these two choices are normally avoided.

7.3 Magnetic resonance imaging

In order to correlate an NMR signal from a large object to its spatial origins, at least one of the two fields (i.e. the main magnetic field or the RF field) required for the NMR measurement is made to vary over space. If it were possible to generate a sharp maximum or minimum in space for these fields, one would obtain signals only from that region [7.33]. In order to record information from other regions one would have to scan the object under investigation point by point. However, besides the technical difficulties of generating sufficiently sharp field extrema, this would not be an effective procedure. In the same time required to record the object point-wise, one can obtain the information necessary for reconstructing the object by measuring all points repeatedly under different conditions. Doing so dramatically improves the signal-to-noise ratio [7.34].

7.3.1 NMR signal in a magnetic field gradient

Use of the signal from the entire object (rather than from a single voxel) can be secured by deploying magnetic field gradients G in which the NMR resonance frequency varies linearly along one direction in space

$$\omega(r) = -\gamma(B_0 + Gr). \qquad (7.69a)$$

In the reference frame rotating at $-\gamma B_0$, NMR frequency varies as

$$\Omega = \omega(r) + \gamma B_0 = -\gamma Gr. \qquad (7.69b)$$

The amplitude of the NMR signal as a function of frequency then corresponds to the sum of all spins in the planes orthogonal to the direction of the magnetic field gradient [7.13], i.e. the projection of the nuclear magnetization (fig. 7.17a):

$$P(r) = \int M_\perp \mathrm{d}q\,\mathrm{d}s. \qquad (7.70a)$$

For the sake of simplicity we will restrict our present discussion to a two-dimensional (2D) object (fig. 7.17b). Following excitation with a 90° pulse, the observed NMR signal as a function of time t follows from the Fourier transform of the projection

$$P(r, \varphi) = \int M_\perp(x, y)\,\mathrm{d}s \qquad (7.70b)$$

as

$$P(t, \varphi) = \int P(\Omega, \varphi)\,\mathrm{e}^{i\Omega t}\,\mathrm{d}\Omega. \qquad (7.71)$$

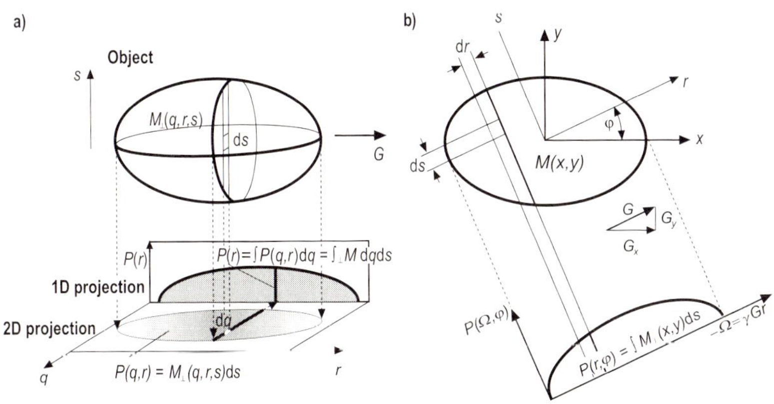

Figure 7.17
a) The NMR signal amplitude as a function of frequency for a 3D object in a linear magnetic field gradient represents the plane integral of the transverse magnetization in planes orthogonal to the field gradient. **b)** The MR signal as a function of frequency for a 2D object in a magnetic field gradient is its projection on the gradient direction.

Inserting eq. (7.69b) into eq. (7.70), it then follows that a measured set of signals $P(t, \varphi)$ in successively rotated gradients is the 2D Fourier transform of the magnetization

$$P(t, \varphi) = \int M_\perp(x, y) e^{i\Omega t} dq\,dr = \int M_\perp(x, y) e^{-i\gamma(G_x x + G_y y)t} dx\,dy \qquad (7.72)$$

Lauterbur's original suggestion was to collect a set of projections on different gradient directions φ and reconstruct an image of the nuclear magnetization with the same methods that are used in X-ray computed tomography. However, Kumar, Welti and Ernst [7.35] have presented a modification of this proposal that offers greater flexibility and simpler image reconstruction. Their method is now used routinely in MRI.

After the 90° pulse the phase of the magnetization is made to vary along the y-direction with a gradient G_y switched on for a time T_y so that a signal

$$P(G_y, T_y) = \int M_\perp(x, y) e^{-i\gamma G_y y T_y} dx \qquad (7.73a)$$

is obtained. Next, a gradient G_x is applied along the x-direction and the NMR signal is sampled over time t:

$$M_\perp(G_y, t) = \int P(G_y, T_y) e^{-i\gamma G_x x t} dy = \iint M_\perp(x, y) e^{-i\gamma G_y y T_y} e^{-i\gamma G_x x t} dx\,dy \qquad (7.73b)$$

A 2D set of signals as a function of G_y and the recording time t are obtained by repeating the encoding procedure with a variety of gradients G_y. One can regard this signal set as an interferogram or hologram. A 2D Fourier transformation yields the distribution of the local transverse nuclear magnetization:

$$M_\perp(x, y) = \frac{1}{(2\pi)^2} \int_{-T_X}^{T_X} \int_{-G_Y^{max}}^{G_Y^{max}} M_\perp(G_y, t) e^{i\gamma(y T_y G_y + x G_x t)} dG_y\,dt \qquad (7.74)$$

Since the spatial distribution of the transverse nuclear magnetization is given by the Fourier transformation of a 2D data set, it is common to view these data as having been acquired in Fourier or k-space (fig. 7.18) with spatial frequency coordinates

$$k_x = \gamma G_x t \quad \textit{and} \quad k_y = \gamma T_y G_y \qquad (7.75a)$$

or, in the more general case of time dependent gradients,

$$k_x(t) = \gamma \int_0^t G_x(t) dt \quad \text{and} \quad k_y(G_y) = \gamma \int_0^{T_y} G_y(t) dt. \qquad (7.75b)$$

The Fourier transformation of the amplitudes (real and imaginary part) along a line through the center of the Fourier space results in the projection (eq. (7.70b)) of the investigated object onto the direction of this line, a fact that is expressed by the central slice theorem. Collecting projections with rotated gradients is equivalent to the radial scanning of k-space.

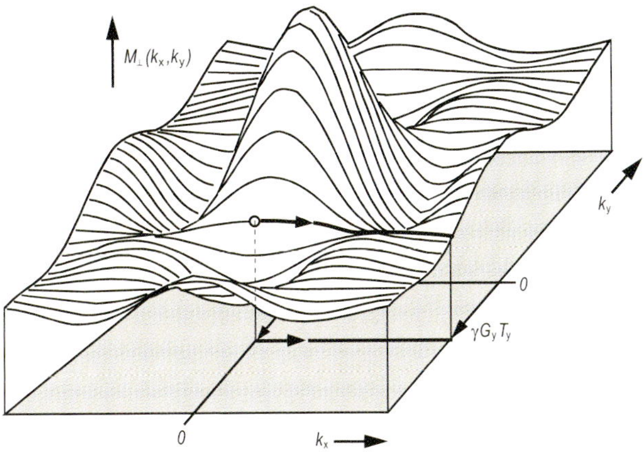

Figure 7.18
Rectangular scanning of a 2D Fourier space in magnetic resonance imaging: after encoding the k_y-direction, the NMR signal is recorded along the spatial frequency direction k_x. While only the real part of the k-space is shown, the imaginary part is sampled at the same time.

7.3.2 Spatial resolution

In digital imaging, an object is sampled with image elements (pixels) of size Δx, Δy corresponding to the spatial sampling frequencies

$$k_x^S = \frac{2\pi}{\Delta x} \quad \text{and} \quad k_y^S = \frac{2\pi}{\Delta y}. \tag{7.76a}$$

According to the sampling theorem, an object can then be completely reconstructed if it does not contain spatial frequencies higher than the (spatial) Nyquist frequency, which is half the sampling frequency

$$k_x^{max} \leq \frac{k_x^S}{2} \quad \text{and} \quad k_y^{max} \leq \frac{k_y^S}{2}. \tag{7.76b}$$

If the object contains information at spatial frequencies larger than the Nyquist frequency, truncation or aliasing will lead to typical artifacts (e.g. sharp intensity borders in an object are displayed with parallel lines, an effect referred to as Gibbs ringing). It follows that it is necessary to select pixel size according to the intrinsic spatial resolution (see below).

The spatial frequency interval necessary to image an object of size $\pm x^{max}$, $\pm y^{max}$ is accordingly expressed as

$$\Delta k_x = \frac{\pi}{x^{max}} \quad \text{and} \quad \Delta k_y = \frac{\pi}{y^{max}}. \tag{7.76c}$$

Hence, $N_y = \dfrac{2y^{max}}{\Delta y}$ phase encoding steps are necessary to image an object with a diameter of $2y^{max}$ in y-direction with the required pixel size Δy. The process involves stepping through the gradient $-G_y^{max} \leq G_y \leq G_y^{max}$ and taking $N_y = \frac{2x^{max}}{\Delta x}$ samples of the NMR signal each time. N_y and N_x are usually selected as a power of two to permit deployment of the fast Fourier transform algorithm for image reconstruction.

Spatial resolution achievable with MRI is limited by intrinsic factors such as transversal relaxation, diffusion, and magnetic field inhomogeneity. Let us assume two spins separated by a distance d. In order to distinguish the two points, the frequency difference due to the applied gradient must be larger than the frequency spread due to natural line width and magnetic field inhomogeneities (fig. 7.19):

$$\gamma G d \geq \frac{2}{T_2} + \gamma \Delta B_0 = \frac{2}{T_2^*} \tag{7.77}$$

To match pixel size Δ to intrinsic spatial resolution, *d* should at least be chosen as

$$\Delta \approx \frac{d}{2}, \tag{7.78a}$$

equivalent to a sampling duration of

$$T \approx \pi T_2^*. \tag{7.78b}$$

Much larger pixels (i.e. stronger gradients and shorter read-out times) are normally used in MRI than would be necessary to obtain the intrinsic spatial resolution limited by T_2^*. The reasons here center on restricting image acquisition time and improving the signal-to-noise ratio. According to eq. (7.68), an increase in resolution always entails a decrease in the signal-to-noise ratio, given that it is proportional to Δ^3. In order to compensate for this, the measurement time would have to be increased by a power of six! Thus, while aliasing artifacts could occur, they are not a problem in practice because noise buries the fine structures at high spatial frequencies. The intrinsic spatial resolution, however, is the limit for MR microscopy.

Limitation of spatial resolution is further restricted in MR microscopy by self-diffusion. The mean distance that spins diffuse during signal-read-out time (eq. 7.48) must

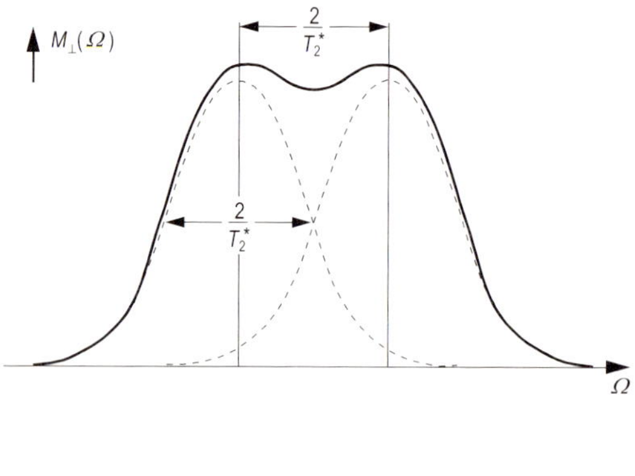

Figure 7.19
Minimum separation required to retain the distinguishability of two NMR lines

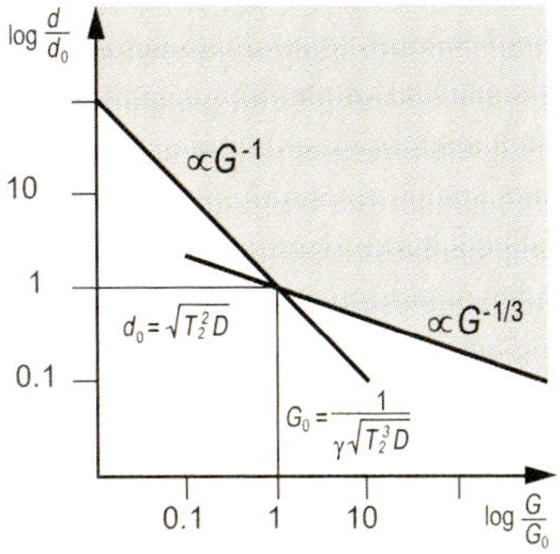

Figure 7.20
Spatial resolution as a function of gradient strength. The two asymptotes represent the limits due to natural line width and diffusion.

be smaller than the pixel size in order to avoid a destructive de-phasing of the magnetization in the gradient. This leads to the constraint

$$\Delta = 2d \geq \sqrt[3]{\frac{D}{\gamma G}}. \tag{7.79}$$

D: Diffusion coefficient

The diffusion coefficient in biological tissue is $D \approx 10^{-9}$ to 10^{-10} m²/s. Gradients on the order of magnitude of 1 T/m thus yield a spatial resolution on a µm scale. Indeed, single cells have been investigated by MRI [7.36]. Fig. 7.20 shows the principle dependence of the intrinsic spatial resolution on gradient strength. As long as the diffusion length is negligible with respect to pixel size, spatial resolution is determined by the product of gradient strength multiplied by T_2. As pixel size approaches the diffusion length, spatial resolution is determined by the $\sqrt[3]{\ }$ of this magnitude (i.e. it takes much more effort to increase resolution by stronger gradients).

The MR image principle described can be easily extended to three dimensions by adding and stepping through a gradient G_z during the encoding phase. However, this requires a longer measurement time. Given that the information for the complete 3D object is not always required, a 2D object is often generated from the 3D object by applying a gradient during RF-pulse excitation of the NMR (selective excitation). Doing so restricts the excitation of the spins to a plain perpendicular to the gradient where the precession frequency is identical to the pulse frequency (fig. 7.21).

7.3.3 Selective excitation

In what follows, we apply linear system theory [7.37] to analyze selective excitation. This represents only an approximation. In linear theory, the response of a system to excitation is given in the frequency domain by the transfer function multiplied by the excitation function. The transfer function (as a system response to δ-excitation) for a spin system in a gradient G_z is given by $P_0(z)e^{i\Omega t}$ in the rotating frame (excluding relaxation).

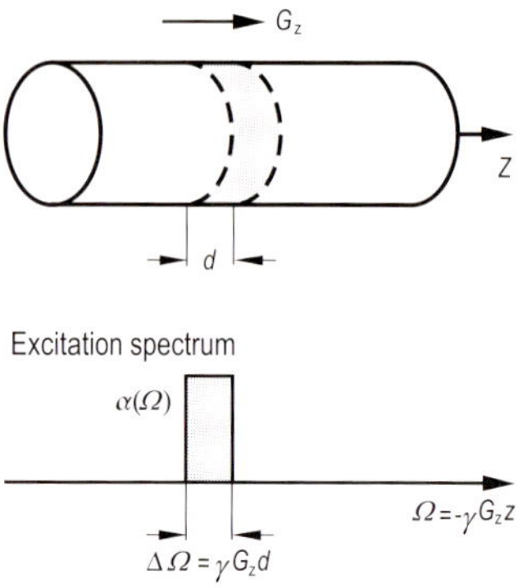

Figure 7.21
Selective excitation of a slice in a cylindrical object. A gradient along the object provides a spatial variation of the resonance frequency with the result that the spectrum of the applied 90° pulse determines the position and thickness of the slice.

$$P_0(z) = \int M_0(x, y, z)\mathrm{d}x\mathrm{d}y \tag{7.80}$$

is the projection of the magnetization on the z-axis. We will assume excitation function $i\sin|\alpha(\Omega)|e^{i\varphi}$ according to eq. (7.19).

The frequency dependant excitation angle $\alpha(\Omega)$ can be derived from the Fourier transform of the time dependant B_1 field used to excite the spins:

$$|\alpha(\Omega)| = \gamma\left|\int B_1(t)e^{-i\Omega t}dt\right| \tag{7.81a}$$

yielding the phase factor

$$\varphi = \beta + \arctan\frac{\mathrm{Im}(\alpha(\Omega))}{\mathrm{Re}(\alpha(\Omega))} \tag{7.81b}$$

β: Direction of the B_1 field

With an RF pulse of duration $2T_z$ the slice excited along the z-direction follows as

$$P_\perp(z, 2T_Z) = iP_0(z)e^{i\Omega 2T_z}\sin|\alpha(\Omega)|e^{i\varphi(\omega)}. \tag{7.82}$$

In order to obtain a rectangular distribution of the transverse magnetization along the slice thickness Δz at position z_0, the shape of the RF pulse must be selected so as to give a rectangular frequency distribution of spectral width $\Delta\Omega = \gamma G_Z d$ and a center frequency of $\Omega_0 = -\gamma G_Z z_0$ (recall that we are looking at the spins from the frame rotating at the Larmor frequency ω_L, so that a pulse of frequency $\Omega + \omega_L$ must be applied in the laboratory system to the coil surrounding the sample). Given that an RF pulse with the shape of a sinc (i.e. $\frac{\sin \pi x}{\pi x}$) function has such a rectangular spectrum, $B_1(t)$ is chosen to be a sinc function modulated with the center frequency Ω_0:

$$B_1(t) = B_1(T_z)\mathrm{sinc}\left(\frac{\Delta\Omega}{2\pi}(t - T_z)\right)e^{i\Omega_0(t-T_z)}. \tag{7.83}$$

$$0 \le t \le 2T_z$$

The sinc pulse is restricted here to a duration of $2T_Z$ in order to obtain a selective RF pulse of finite length. It is also shifted by the interval T_Z in order to expose the spins to the signal part left of the pulse maximum and is adjusted to extend over several sinc oscillations in order to approximate a rectangular slice profile. With the phase of the RF pulse selected for alignment along the x-axis in the rotating frame, the following applies to the transverse magnetization:

$$P_\perp(z) = iP_0(z)\sin\left(\alpha_0 \operatorname{rect}\left(\frac{z-z_0}{\Delta z}\right)\right)e^{-i\gamma G_z T_z}.$$

$$\alpha_0 \approx 2\pi \frac{B_1(T_z)}{G_z \Delta z} \tag{7.84}$$

$$\operatorname{rect}(x) = 1 \text{ for } \left(-\frac{1}{2} < x < \frac{1}{2}\right) \quad \text{and} \quad \operatorname{rect}(x) = 0 \text{ for } \left(|x| > \left|\frac{1}{2}\right|\right)$$

An oscillating function of the transverse nuclear magnetization along the slice thickness thus results (fig. 7.22). The selective RF pulse has flipped each spin in the slice addressed into the transverse plane, but in its own rotating frame. Since the resonance frequency changes across the slice width due to the applied gradient, the transverse nuclear magnetization is twisted. Given that the effective value of the spiral-shaped nuclear magnetization cancels out, almost no FID can be observed following

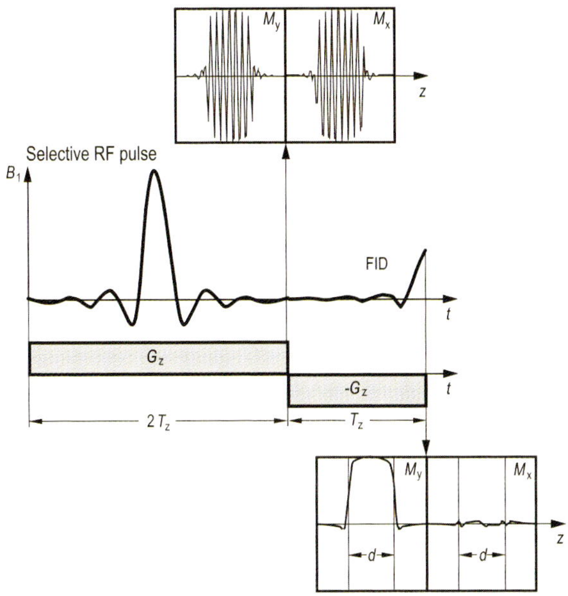

Figure 7.22
The x and y components of the transverse nuclear magnetization after excitation via an RF pulse of duration $2T_Z$ in a magnetic field gradient G_z that is applied along the y-axis: The twisted transverse magnetization resulting immediately after the selective pulse realigns in a refocusing interval of duration T_Z with a reversed gradient.

the selective RF pulse. Reversing the polarity of the field gradient during a period T_Z following the RF pulse [7.37] re-phases all of the spins and results in a signal corresponding to the full transverse magnetization in the excited slice. A 180° pulse and a gradient of equal polarity can be used as an alternative to a reversed re-phasing gradient.

As already mentioned, eq. (7.81) is only an approximation. It is assumed that the magnetization precesses around the $\vec{B}_1$ axis in the rotating frame instead of the $(\vec{B}_1 + G_z z\vec{e}_z)$ axis. Numerical methods can account for the Bloch equations exactly. It turns out that a residual nuclear magnetization $M_y(z)$ remains even after refocusing. This, however, can be minimized by tuning the re-phasing interval and modifying the RF pulse shape.

Selective excitation is not limited to slice selection. It is also used to obtain information about a single voxel (e.g. to record a spectrum). For this purpose, the FID in a z-gradient following a selective 90° pulse is first refocused via a selective 180° pulse in a y-gradient. This results in the selection of a line perpendicular to the z- and y-plain. A second 180° pulse in an x-gradient then generates an echo arising from a single voxel. A selective 90°/90°/90° sequence, yielding a stimulated echo, can be applied instead of a selective 90°/180°/180° sequence whenever a 90°/180°/180° sequence would fail to deliver a sufficient signal on account of a short T_2.

7.3.4 Pulse sequence and contrast

In order to obtain signals from which an image can be reconstructed, the nuclear magnetization must be exposed to a sequence of RF and gradient pulses. Many modifications of these pulse sequences have been designed to optimize the resulting image with respect to various parameters such as tissue contrast, flow display, diffusion, susceptibility and data acquisition time.

As a detailed discussion of pulse sequences is given in chapter 15.2.1, we will restrict ourselves here to the two main sequences. In general, one can distinguish between gradient echoes and spin echo sequences.

Fig. 7.23a shows an example of a 3D gradient echo or FLASH sequence. Nuclear magnetization is flipped by an RF pulse at a flip angle α into the transverse plane. Phase encoding gradients G_y, G_z and a reversed projection gradient $-G_x$ are then applied for an interval T. Next, the signal is recorded in $+G_x$ for an interval $2T$. Both positive and negative spatial frequencies are recorded during signal readout due to the signal conditioning of the magnetization via $-G_x$. The signal maximum occurs when the phases accumulated by the spins during $-G_x$ conditioning have been compensated. Consequently, this signal maximum is referred to as a gradient echo. The pulse sequence is repeated with different phase encoding gradients $-G_y^{max} \leq G_y \leq G_y^{max}$ and $-G_z^{max} \leq G_z \leq G_z^{max}$ until the Fourier space is filled with data. A 3D Fourier transformation reconstructs the image of the transverse magnetization. The signal in each voxel is given by eq. (7.37), i.e. by the local longitudinal relaxation time. FLASH images have a strong T_1 contrast.

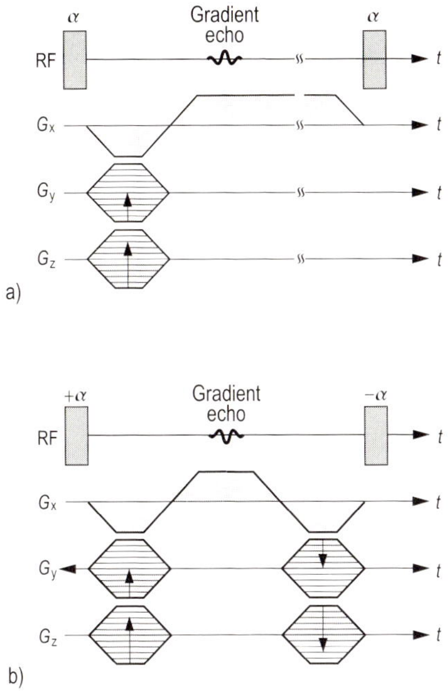

Figure 7.23
a) FLASH (fast low-angle shot)
b) True FISP (fast imaging with steady precession): examples of 3D gradient echo sequences.

When deploying FLASH imaging, it is assumed that the phase memory of the transverse nuclear magnetization will have been lost by the end of the repetition interval. However, given that this is not true when the repetition interval is smaller than the transverse relaxation time, spoiling gradient pulses must be applied at the end of each interval to prevent the emergence of coherent image artifacts. Alternatively, a stochastically varying jitter may be added to the repetition time [7.38].

However, instead of destroying the phase memory, one can put it to good use to obtain a stronger signal and information on the local transverse relaxation time. In true FISP, an interval is added after signal readout during which the effects of gradient encoding are reversed; RF pulses are alternated (fig. 7.23b). The signal in each voxel then follows from eq. (7.43), giving a contrast determined by the ratio T_1/T_2.

In order to avoid the de-phasing of the magnetization in the voxels, gradient echo sequences require very homogeneous fields, strong gradients and rapid signal-readout intervals. A 3D data set with a matrix of 128^3 voxels can typically be acquired in less than 1 s. The contrast with respect to tissues differing in their T_2, however, is generally low. While utilizing an additional 180° pulse in the case of spin echo sequences affords greater flexibility with respect to the manipulation of image contrast, doing so generally comes at the expense of acquisition time. The sequences are also much more stable with regard to B_0 inhomogeneities because of the refocusing RF pulse.

Slice-selective 90° and 180° RF pulses are applied together with a gradient pulse G_z to the standard spin-echo imaging sequence. The phase twist perpendicular to the excited slice is compensated and magnetization is encoded by gradients $-G_z$ and G_y between the two RF pulses. The echo signal is read out in the projection gradient G_x (fig. 7.24). Two parameters are available for signal manipulation, the repetition time T_R and the echo time T_E. Signal intensity in a picture element is given by

$$M_\perp(x, y) \approx M_0(x, y)\left(1 - e^{\frac{-T_R}{T_1(x,y)}}\right)e^{\frac{-T_E}{T_2(x,y)}}. \tag{7.85}$$

The repetition time and the echo time can be adjusted so that the image contrast (related to different types of tissue) is determined by either M_0, T_1 or T_2. Short T_E and T_R values yield T_1 weighted images, one long T_E and one short T_R value yield spin density or M_0-weighted images and long T_E and T_R values yield T_2-weighted images.

The standard spin echo imaging sequence can be modified in several ways. Given long repetition times, it takes no longer to acquire images of several different slices than images of a single slice when the different slices are addressed during the waiting interval. Information on diffusion can be obtained by adding strong gradient pulses before and after the 180° pulse. Images with increasing T_2 weighting can be acquired when the NMR signal is recovered several times by repeating the 180° pulses. Image acquisition time can be shortened by spatially encoding each echo differently in such a multi-echo sequence.

To conclude, MRI offers the capacity to generate images of very different tissue contrast. This is a unique feature and cannot be obtained via retrospective filter processes or post processing tasks. It is the variety of pulse sequences that has made MRI a flexible and universal diagnostic tool.

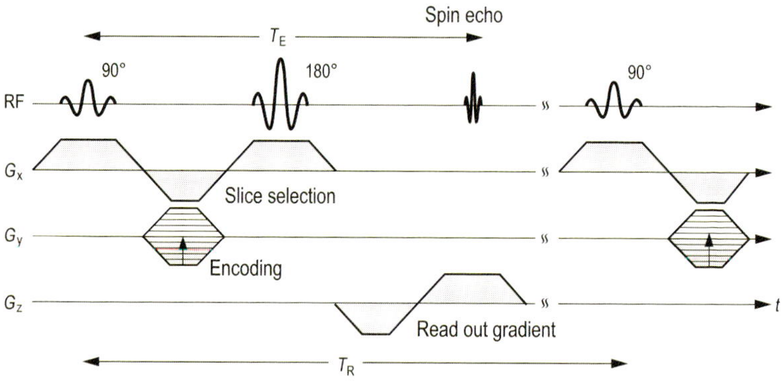

Figure 7.24 Principle of the standard spin-echo imaging sequence

7.4 References

[7.1] E. Zavoisky
Paramagnetic relaxation of liquid solutions for perpendicular fields
J. Phys. USSR 9 (1945), 211

[7.2] F.W. Bloch, W.W. Hansen, M. Packard
Nuclear Induction
Phys. Rev. (L) 69 (1946), 127

[7.3] E.M. Purcell, H.C. Torrey, R.V. Pound
Resonance absorption by nuclear magnetic moments in a solid
Phys. Rev. (L) 69 (1946), 37

[7.4] P. Zeeman
On the influence of magnetism on the nature of light emitted by a substance
Phil. Mag. 43 (1897), 226

[7.5] J. Larmor
The influence of a magnetic field on radiation frequency
Proc. Roy. Soc. 60 (1896-1897), 514

[7.6] W. Gerlach, O. Stern
Über die Richtungsquantelung im Magnetfeld
Ann. Physik 74 (1924), 673

[7.7] I.I. Rabi
Space quantification in a gyrating magnetic field
Phys. Rev. 51 (1937), 652

[7.8] E. Odeblad, G. Lindström
Some preliminary observations of proton magnetic resonance
in biologic samples
Acta Radiol 43 (1955), 469

[7.9] J.R. Singer
Blood flow rates by nuclear magnetic resonance measurements
Science 130 (1959), 1652

[7.10] G. Suryan
Proc. Indian Acad. Sci., Section A33 (February 1951), 107

[7.11] R. Damadian
Tumor detection by nuclear magnetic resonance
Science 171 (1971), 1151

[7.12] R. Gabillard
A steady state transient technique in nuclear resonance
Phys. Rev. 85 (1952), 694

[7.13] P.C. Lauterbur
Image formation by induced local interactions: Examples employing
nuclear magnetic resonance
Nature 242 (1955), 469

[7.14] A. Abragam
The principles of nuclear magnetism
Oxford University Press, New York 1961

[7.15] T.C. Farrar, E.D. Becker
Pulse and Fourier transform NMR, introduction to theory and methods
Academic Press, New York 1971

[7.16] P.T. Callaghan
Principles of magnetic resonance microscopy
Clarendon Press, Oxford 1991

[7.17] W. Pauli
Zur Frage der theoretischen Deutung der Satelliten einiger Spektrallinien und ihrer Beeinflussung durch magnetische Felder
Naturwiss. 12 (1924), 741

[7.18] F. Bloch, W.W. Hansen, M. Packard
The nuclear induction experiment
Phys. Rev. 70 (1946), 474

[7.19] N. Bloembergen, E.M. Purcell, R.V. Pound
Relaxation effects in nuclear magnetic resonance absorption
Phys. Rev. 73 (1948), 679

[7.20] P.A. Bottomley, T.H. Forster, R.E. Argersinger, L.M. Pfeifer
A review of normal tissue hydrogen NMR relaxation times and relaxation mechanisms from 1-100 MHz: dependence on tissue type, NMR frequency, temperature, species, excision and age
Med. Phys. 11 (1984) S.425

[7.21] H.J. Weinmann, R.C. Brasch, W.R. Press, G.E. Wesbey
Characteristics of gadolinium-DTPA complex: A potential NMR contrast agent
AJR 143 (1984), 619

[7.22] R.G. Bryant, D.A. Mendelson, C.C. Lester
The magnetic field dependence of proton spin relaxation in tissue
Magnetic Resonance in Medicine 21 (1991), 117

[7.23] S.D. Wolff, R.S. Balaban
Magnetization transfer contrast (MTC) and tissue water proton relaxation in vivo
Magn. Resonan. Med. 10 (1989), 135

[7.24] E. Hahn
Spin echos
Phys. Rev. 80 (1950), 580

[7.25] H.Y. Carr, E.M. Purcell
Effects of diffusion on free precession in nuclear magnetic resonance experiments
Phys. Rev. 94 (1954), 630

[7.26] A. Haase, J. Frahm, D. Matthaei, W. Hänicke, K. Merboldt
FLASH imaging: rapid nmr imaging using low flip angle pulses
J. Magn. Reson. 67 (1986), 217

[7.27] A. Oppelt, R. Graumann, H. Barfuß, H. Fischer, W. Hartl, W. Schajor
FISP – a new fast MRI sequence
Electromedica 54 (1986), 15

[7.28] E.O. Stejskal, J.E. Tanner
Spin diffusion measurements: spin echoes in the presence of a time-dependent field gradient
Chem. Phys. 42 (1965), 288

[7.29] J.E. Tanner, E.O. Stejskal
Restricted self-diffusion of protons in colloidal systems by the pulsed-gradient, spin echo method
Chem. Phys. 49 (1968), 1768

[7.30] I. Solomon
Relaxation processes in a system of two spins
Phys. Rev. 99 (1955), 559-565

[7.31] R.R. Ernst, G. Bodenhausen, A. Wokaun
Principles of nuclear magnetic resonance in one and two dimensions
Clarendon Press, Oxford 1987

[7.32] D.I. Hoult, P.C. Lauterbur
The sensitivity of the Zeugmatographic experiment involving human samples
J. Magn. Reson. 343 (1979), 425

[7.33] Z. Abe, K. Tanaka, K. Hotta, M. Imai
Noninvasive measurements of biological information with application of nuclear magnetic resonance in Biological and Clinical Effects of Low Magnetic and Electric Fields, 295-317
Thomas Springfield, Illinois 1974

[7.34] P. Brunner, R. Ernst
Sensitivity and performance time in NMR imaging
J. Magn. Reson. 33 (1979), 83

[7.35] A. Kumar, D. Welti, R. Ernst
NMR Fourier Zeugmatography
J. Magn. Reson. 18 (1975), 69

[7.36] J.B. Aguayo, J. Blackband, J. Schoeniger, M.A. Mattingly, M. Hintermann
Nuclear magnetic resonance of a single cell
Nature 232 (1986), 190

[7.37] D.I. Hoult
Zeugmatography: a criticism of the concept of a selective pulse on the presence of a field gradient
J. Magn. Reson. 26 (1977), 165

[7.38] R. Freeman, H.D.W. Hill
Phase and intensity anomalies in Fourier transform NMR
J. Magn. Reson. 4 (1971), 366

8 Physical principles of medical ultrasound

8.1 Introduction

Like electromagnetic waves, sound waves have the capacity to penetrate the human body. This capacity introduces a certain diagnostic and therapeutic potential. A distortion of the equilibrium in the molecules of a rigid body propagates as a transversal or longitudinal wave. Frequencies ranging from just a few Hertz to 15 kHz are accessible to the human ear. Higher frequencies are termed ultrasound.

Ultrasound plays an important role in various modern technologies. Sonar is used, for instance, to measure water depth and to detect underwater objects such as schools of fish and submarines. Ultrasound is used in the area of materials testing to detect the presence of cracks and cavities. It is also used in the area of material machining and cleaning. Ultrasound therapy has been in use since 1938. Acoustic energy applied to tissue is absorbed and transformed into heat. This leads to an enhancement of blood circulation that can counteract cramping, dampen pain and reduce inflammation. Pressure peaks can be generated via ultrasound shock waves to destroy kidney and gallstones, a procedure that has replaced elaborate surgical procedures. The use of high-intensity, focused ultrasound is currently being explored as a means of noninvasively destroying tumors via heat.

Ultrasound was first deployed for diagnostic purposes by Dussik in Austria [8.1] who used it to scan the human skull and thereby depict the ventricles of the brain. Progress in ultrasound in the areas of materials testing and sonar led to the application of the reflection principle to assist in the investigation of biological objects. Ludwig [8.2] recognized the capacity of sound waves to detect gallstones, Wild [8.3] investigated tissue, and Howry and Bliss [8.4] built an apparatus (an immersion tank system) to display anatomical details of objects placed in water.

In Sweden, Leksell [8.5] demonstrated the echo from the intracranial middle line, thus laying the foundation for echo encephalography. In the mid 1950s, Edler and Hertz [8.6] investigated the beating of the heart using ultrasound, thereby founding echo cardiography. At the same time, Mundt and Hughes [8.7] in the United States performed the first eye investigations using ultrasound. In Japan, Satomura [8.8] reported on the Doppler frequency shift of ultrasound reflected by the moving heart. The later introduction of real-time ultrasound imaging by Krause and Soldner [8.9] then led to a dramatic increase in the scope of ultrasound diagnostics and has proven to be an indispensable tool for the noninvasive examination of the human body.

In what follows, we offer a survey of the physical principles behind ultrasound and draw a link from these to current methods applied in medicine.

8.2 Ultrasound field

8.2.1 Ultrasound field parameters

Acoustic waves exist only in elastic matter. Given that molecules vibrate both parallel and perpendicular to the direction of sonic propagation, it is necessary to discern longitudinal and transversal waves. Owing to a lack in the shear force necessary for transversal movement, only longitudinal acoustic waves persist in fluids and gases. In this regard, biological tissue can be considered a viscous fluid.

Due to the elasticity and inertia of matter, a mechanical distortion will propagate in the form of a density and pressure wave (fig. 8.1) that can be mathematically represented by the following equation:

$$\frac{d^2\psi}{dt^2} = c^2\left(\frac{d^2\psi}{dx^2} + \frac{d^2\psi}{dy^2} + \frac{d^2\psi}{dz^2}\right) \tag{8.1}$$

c: Velocity of sound, ψ: Vibrating variable, e.g. mass density, acoustic pressure

A possible solution to this partial differential equation is the plane wave:

$$\psi = \hat{\psi} e^{i(kz - \omega t)} \qquad i = \sqrt{-1} \tag{8.2}$$

$\omega = 2\pi\nu$: Angular frequency, ν: Acoustic frequency

$k = \frac{\omega}{c} = \frac{2\pi}{\lambda}$: Acoustic wave number, λ: Acoustic wavelength

It can be shown (e.g. [8.10]) that the sound velocity

$$c = \lambda\nu = \frac{\omega}{k} \tag{8.3}$$

is given by

$$c = \sqrt{\frac{\partial p}{\partial \rho}}. \tag{8.4}$$

p: Acoustic pressure, ρ: Mass density

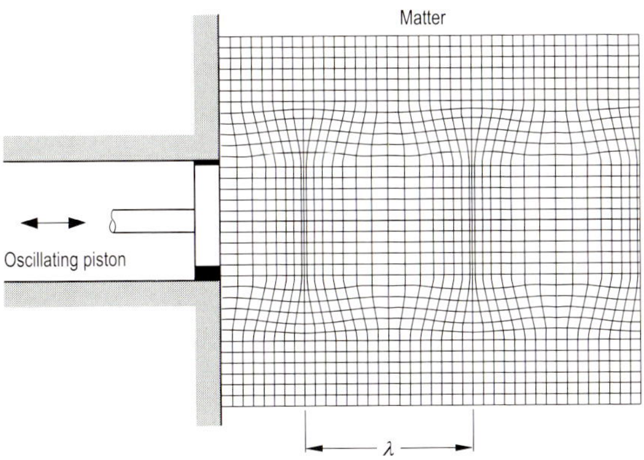

Figure 8.1
Pressure waves in elastic matter

Applying Hooke's law

$$p = -K\frac{\delta V}{V} = K\frac{\delta\rho}{\rho} \tag{8.5}$$

V: volume, *K*: compression module

yields

$$c = \sqrt{\frac{K}{\rho}}. \tag{8.6}$$

Sound velocity values for different types of matter are compiled in table 8.1.

The velocity and displacement of vibrating particles can be derived as further acoustic field parameters from the density and pressure variations that also propagate as waves. The particle velocity v_{P}, which is the speed at which a molecule oscillates and which should not be confused with the sound velocity c, emerges as

$$v_{\mathrm{p}} = \frac{p}{Z} \tag{8.7}$$

where Z is the acoustic impedance

$$Z = \frac{K}{c} = \hat{\rho}\,c = \sqrt{K\hat{\rho}}\,. \tag{8.8}$$

Z is measured in Rayl, an eponym deriving from Lord Rayleigh (1842-1919) who was the first to measure acoustic pressure (Rayl = $\frac{\mathrm{g}}{\mathrm{cm}^2\mathrm{s}}$). Typical values are given in table 8.1.

The displacement s of the vibrating molecule is given by

$$s = \mathrm{i}\frac{v_{\mathrm{p}}}{\omega}, \tag{8.9}$$

which is ahead of the particle velocity by a quarter wavelength.

Table 8.1
Typical values for the velocity of sound c, density ρ, acoustic impedance Z, and absorption

Substance	c in m/s	ρ in g/cm^3	Z in 10^5 Rayl	Absorption in dB/MHz·cm
Fat	1,470	0.97	1.42	0.5
Bone marrow	1,700	0.97	1.65	
Muscle	1,568	1.04	1.63	2
Liver	1,540	1.055	1.66	0.7
Brain tissue	1,530	1.02	1.56	1
Bone (compact)	3,600	1.7	6.12	4-10
Bone porous)			2.5	30-90
Water (20 °C)	1,492	0.9982	1.49	0.002
Air (NN)	331	0.0013	$43\cdot10^{-5}$	

A further important acoustic field parameter is the acoustic intensity

$$J = p v_{\mathrm{p}}, \tag{8.10}$$

which, being a quadratic variable, propagates as a wave at twice the frequency and half the wavelength of the linear variables pressure and particle velocity. The time-averaged value $\bar{J}$ is usually quoted. Typical parameter averages in diagnostic ultrasound include

$$\bar{J} < 100\ \frac{\mathrm{mW}}{\mathrm{cm}^2}; \qquad \bar{p} < 0.6\ \mathrm{Pa}; \qquad \bar{s} < 2 \cdot 10^{-6}\mathrm{mm}; \qquad \bar{v}_p < 3.5\ \frac{\mathrm{cm}}{\mathrm{s}}$$

In diagnostic ultrasound, the vibrating particles experience a considerable acceleration – on an order of magnitude of 10^5 of earth's gravity!

The medical application of ultrasound is based on its interaction with biological tissue. What follows is a summary of the physical principles involved in this interaction. You may wish to refer to the relevant textbooks for a more detailed description (e.g. [8.11]).

8.2.2 Ultrasound propagation

8.2.2.1 Absorption

The intensity of an acoustic wave decreases along its direction of propagation. In matter, the kinetic energy of the vibrating atoms is converted into heat (friction) and acoustic energy is absorbed as a result. In general, the attenuation conforms to an exponential law

$$J(z) = J(0)\mathrm{e}^{-\mu z}. \tag{8.11a}$$

Typical values for the absorption coefficient μ are listed in table 8.1. The absorption coefficient in biological tissue is roughly a linear function of the acoustic frequency ν. The following represents a good approximation for liver, kidney and brain tissue:

$$10 \frac{\mathrm{d}^2\left(\lg \frac{J(z)}{J(0)}\right)}{\mathrm{d}\nu\, \mathrm{d}z} \approx 1\ \frac{\mathrm{dB}}{\mathrm{MHz \cdot cm}}. \tag{8.11b}$$

In ultrasound diagnostics, it is the acoustic absorption that determines the order of magnitude of the frequencies used. While it is advisable on the one hand to use rather high frequencies or short waves because spatial resolution is inversely proportional to wavelength, longer waves are better suited when it comes to displaying deep-lying organs. Frequencies between 7 and 15 MHz (wavelengths of 0.22 to 0.1 mm) are thus used for superficial structures and a lower frequency of 2 MHz (a wavelength of 0.77 mm) is used for deeper-lying details (e.g. at an acoustic-wave penetration depth of 25 cm and a total propagation length of 50 cm).

8.2.2.2 Reflection and diffraction

The laws of wave optics are also valid for ultrasound. Reflection and diffraction occur on boundary planes between different materials (fig. 8.2). The pressure and the nor-

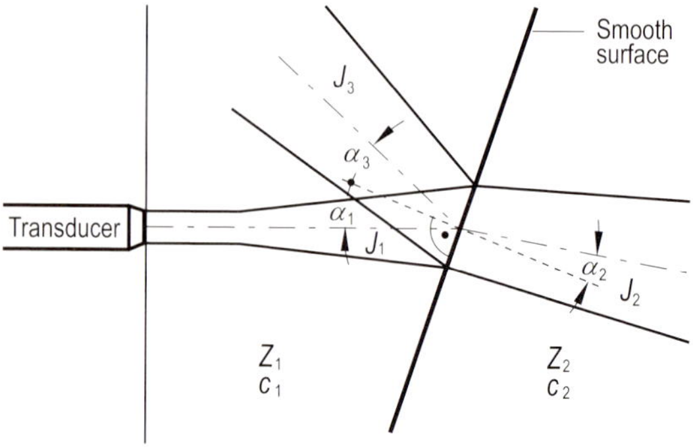

Figure 8.2
Refraction of an ultrasound wave on a smooth boundary surface

mal component of the particle velocity must remain constant when an ultrasound wave hits a boundary surface between two media of different acoustic impedances in order to avoid moving or tearing the plane. Splitting the incoming acoustic wave intensity J_1 into a reflected part J_3 and a passing part J_2 yields

$$p_1 + p_3 = p_2 \tag{8.12a}$$

and

$$v_1 \cos\alpha_1 - v_3 \cos\alpha_3 = v_2 \cos\alpha_2 \tag{8.12b}$$

α_1: Angle of incidence, α_2: Angle of diffraction, α_3: Angle of reflection

The law of reflection holds that

$$\alpha_1 = -\alpha_3 \tag{8.13}$$

and the law of refraction holds that

$$\frac{\sin\alpha_1}{\sin\alpha_2} = \frac{\lambda_1}{\lambda_2} = \frac{c_1}{c_2} \tag{8.14}$$

Taking into account eq. (8.9) and eq. (8.10), the intensity of the three waves can be derived from eq. (8.12) as:

$$\frac{J_3}{J_1} = \left(\frac{Z_1 \cos\alpha_2 - Z_2 \cos\alpha_1}{Z_1 \cos\alpha_2 + Z_2 \cos\alpha_1}\right)^2 \tag{8.15a}$$

$$\frac{J_2}{J_1} = \left(\frac{4 Z_1 Z_2 \cos\alpha_1 \cos\alpha_2}{Z_1 \cos\alpha_2 + Z_2 \cos\alpha_1}\right)^2. \tag{8.15b}$$

If one assumes that the incidence of the acoustic wave on the interface plane is perpendicular, then $\alpha_1 = 0$ and the following applies to the reflection coefficient

$$R = \frac{J_3}{J_1} = \left(\frac{Z_1 - Z_2}{Z_1 + Z_2}\right)^2 \tag{8.15c}$$

and the following applies to the transmission coefficient

$$R = \frac{J_2}{J_1} = \left(\frac{4 Z_1 Z_2}{Z_1 + Z_2}\right)^2. \tag{8.15d}$$

Reflection and diffraction allow one to modify acoustic fields using reflectors and lenses so as to redirect and focus an acoustic beam.

8.2.2.3 Scattering

The boundary planes between different types of matter are usually rough. Incident sound excites acoustic vibrations at every point on the plane, which then emits spherical acoustic waves. The superimposition of these waves leads to backscatter (diffuse reflection). The intensity of this backscatter is constant on conical surfaces (fig. 8.3). The total backscattered power can be derived on the basis of

$$P_S = \sigma_S J_E, \tag{8.16a}$$

J_E: Incident acoustic intensity, σ: Scattering cross section

with the scattering cross section depending on the structure of the boundary surface. The widening of the cone angles is a function of incident sound wavelength and surface roughness.

Rayleigh scattering occurs when sound passes through a medium containing stochastically distributed tiny particles whose radius is smaller than the acoustic wavelength:

$$J_S(r, \vartheta) = \frac{16}{9}\pi^4 J_E \frac{R^6}{\lambda^4 r^2}\left(1 + \frac{3}{2}\cos\vartheta\right)^2 \tag{8.16b}$$

J_S: Backscattered intensity, ϑ: Angle of scatter
r: Distance between locus of scattering and observing

The total reflected power

$$P_S = 2\pi \int J_S r^2 \sin\vartheta \, d\vartheta \tag{8.16c}$$

can be obtained by integrating eq. (8.16b). The scattering cross section then follows as

$$\sigma_S = \frac{112}{9}\pi^5 \frac{R^6}{\lambda^4} \tag{8.16d}$$

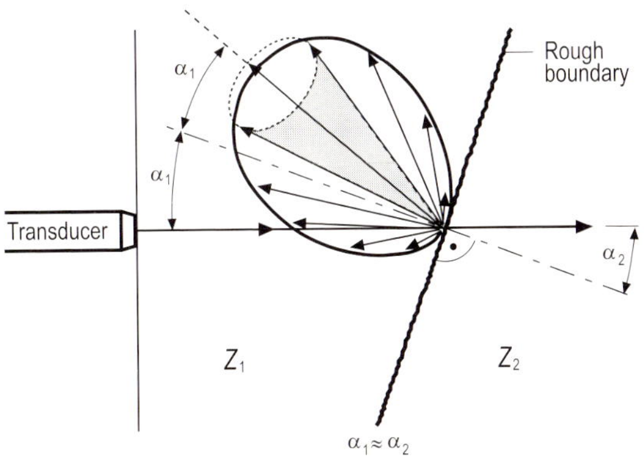

Figure 8.3
Ultrasound scattering on a rough surface

Acoustic scatter in tissue enables one to observe acoustic echoes, and thus forms the basis for diagnostic imaging with ultrasound.

8.2.2.4 Diffraction

Each boundary of an acoustic beam causes diffraction. A beam with a circular cross section of diameter D expands in a manner corresponding to

$$\alpha = 1.22\,\frac{\lambda}{D} \tag{8.17}$$

α: Angle between beam axis and first diffraction minimum

Narrow beams are applied in ultrasound diagnostics. The accurate scanning of an object presupposes a rapid dropping in the intensity of the ultrasound beam perpendicular to its propagation direction and the avoidance of excessive widening. Focusing acoustic lenses are often applied for this purpose. The diameter of an acoustic beam in the focus of an acoustic lens with respect to the first diffraction minimum is given by

$$d_F = 2\alpha f = 2.44\,\frac{\lambda f}{D} \tag{8.18}$$

α: Diffraction angle of the lens aperture
f: Focal distance of the lens, D: diameter of the lens (aperture)

The distance between diffraction minima in the direction of the ultrasound beam gives the longitudinal extension of the focus. Fig. 8.4 yields

$$l_F = \frac{\lambda}{1 - \cos\frac{\beta}{2}} \tag{8.19a}$$

where $\beta = \frac{D}{2f}$: Half the focusing angle (opening ratio), which reduces to the following for $\beta << 1$:

$$l_F \approx 16\lambda\left(\frac{f}{D}\right)^2. \tag{8.19b}$$

An acoustic beam with a large aperture can thus be focused very sharply. On the other hand, the field depth in focus is much larger for acoustic lenses with a small opening ratio D/f thus resulting in a larger sharpening depth.

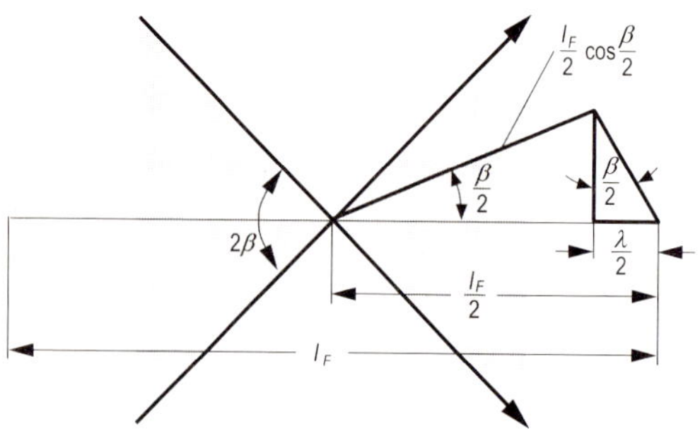

Figure 8.4
Diffraction-limited focal extension in the longitudinal direction of a focused ultrasound beam

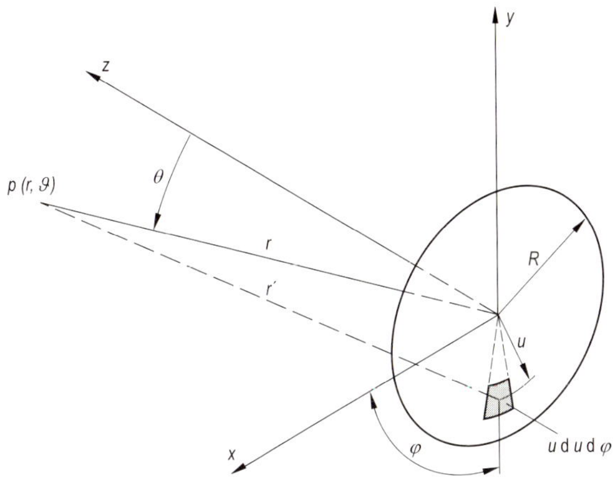

Figure 8.5
Diffraction-limited focal extension in the longitudinal direction of a focused ultrasound beam

Acoustic beams can be generated by moving a piston back and forth harmonically (figs. 8.1 and 8.5). The acoustic field can be calculated by superimposing the elementary spherical waves sent out by the single points on the surface of the piston. The pressure at a distance r from the center of a circular disc can be expressed as [8.12]

$$p(r,\vartheta,t) = \frac{\omega}{2\pi}\rho v_0 \int_0^{2\pi} \mathrm{d}\varphi \int_0^R \frac{i e^{i(kr'-\omega t)}}{r'} u \mathrm{d}u. \tag{8.20a}$$

ρ: Density of the acoustic medium, R: Piston radius
v_0: Maximum of the piston velocity, $r'^2 = u^2 + r^2 + 2ru\sin\vartheta\cos\varphi$

A natural focus forms at a distance

$$f = 0.75\frac{R^2}{\lambda}, \tag{8.20b}$$

which has a diameter with respect to the -6 dB point of pressure drop of

$$d_F \approx \frac{2}{3}R. \tag{8.20c}$$

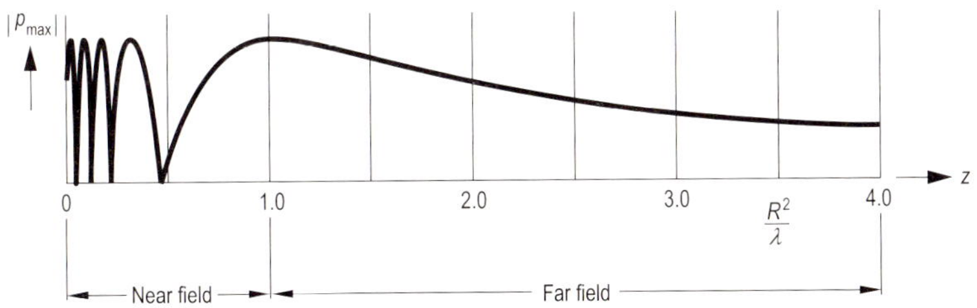

Figure 8.6 Pressure amplitude along the central axis of a circular piston oscillator ($R/\lambda = 5$)

The natural focus separates the near and far oscillator field zones. The acoustic intensity in the near field is subjected to strong fluctuations with R/λ pressure maxima. A diffraction-limited acoustic beam with a main lobe and side lobes is formed in the far field. The pressure decays approximately as

$$p \propto \frac{1}{z}, \tag{8.20d}$$

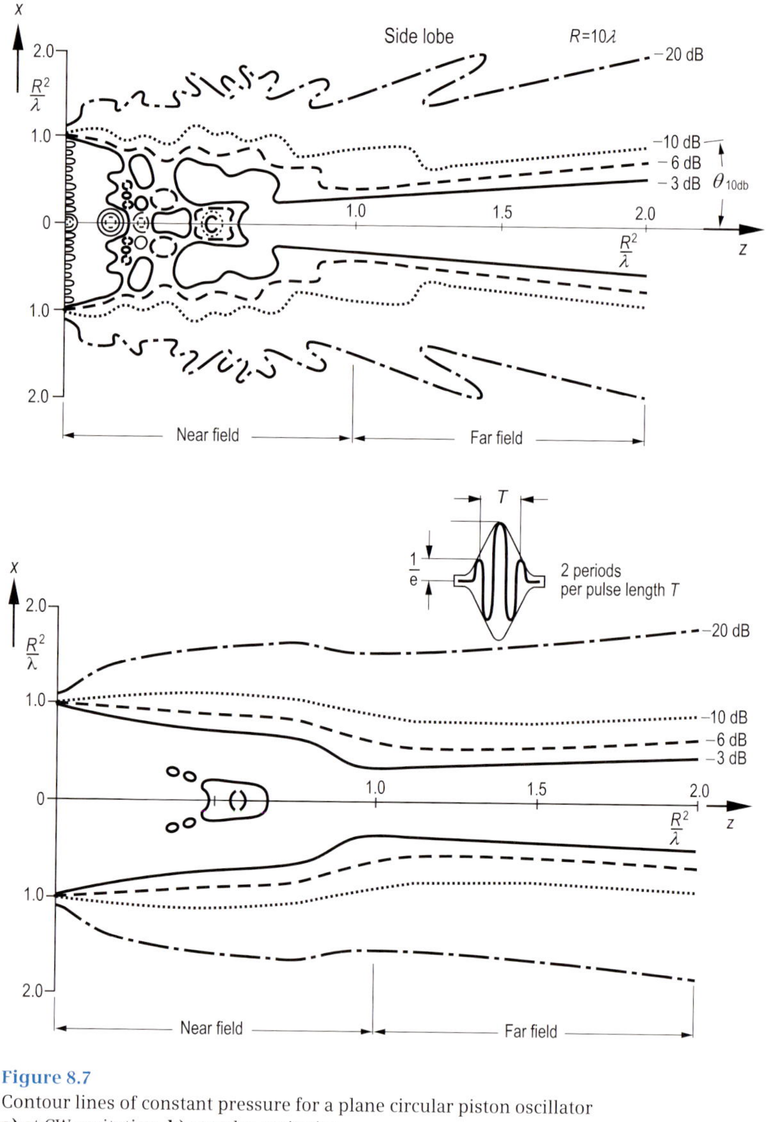

Figure 8.7
Contour lines of constant pressure for a plane circular piston oscillator
a) at CW excitation, **b)** at pulse excitation

Table 8.2
Focus diameter for unfocused and focused ultrasound transmission fields generated by a circular transducer

a) Non-focusing planar piston oscillator with diameter D

Pressure amplitude (dB)	Lateral distance in the focus at CW ultrasound	Lateral distance in the focus at 2 period pulse
−3	0.25 D	0.25 D
−6	0.35 D	
−10	0.4 D	0.4 D
−20		1.5 D
$-\infty$	0.6 D	

b) Focusing piston oscillator with diameter D and radius of curvature $R_C = 2f$ (valid so long as $\lambda \frac{R_C}{D} < \frac{D}{4}$ [8.18, 8.18a])

Pressure amplitude (dB)	Lateral distance in the focus at CW ultrasound	Lateral distance in the focus at 2 period pulse
−3	$1.00\lambda\frac{R_C}{D}$	$0.80\lambda\frac{R_C}{D}$
−6	$1.40\lambda\frac{R_C}{D}$	$1.20\lambda\frac{R_C}{D}$
−10	$1.72\lambda\frac{R_C}{D}$	$1.50\lambda\frac{R_C}{D}$
−20		$2.50\lambda\frac{R_C}{D}$
$-\infty$	$2.44\lambda\frac{R_C}{D}$	

It warrants mention that the acoustic wave field changes when the oscillator is driven intermittently instead of continuously to generate ultrasound pulses. The generation of elementary wave trains of a few wavelengths can only interfere if the difference in the time of flight permits a coincidence (fig. 8.7b).

Focal widths for continuous-drive or pulse-typed plane and curved oscillators are given in table 8.2 [8.13, 8.14].

8.2.2.5 Doppler effect

The frequency of acoustic waves reflected by moving targets changes in proportion to the velocity of the reflector or scatterer:

$$\Delta \nu = f_D = \frac{2\, v_F \cos\theta}{\lambda} \qquad (8.21)$$

$\Delta\nu = f_D$: Doppler frequency shift, v_F: Velocity of the reflecting or scattering target
Θ: Angle between the direction of the acoustic beam and the direction of target movement

In fluids containing scattering particles, the component of the flow velocity in the direction of an incident ultrasound beam can thus be determined by measuring the

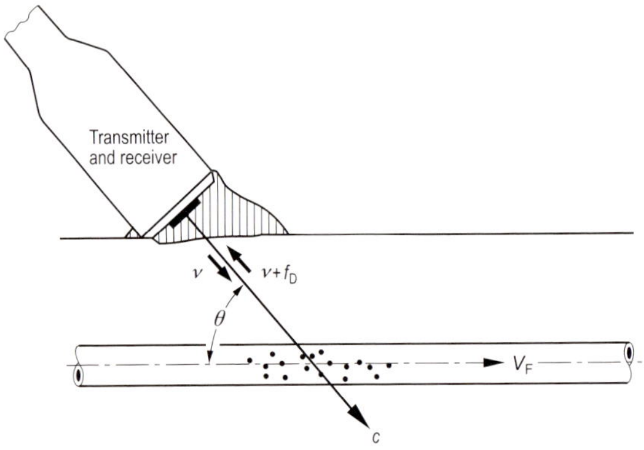

Figure 8.8 Measuring flow velocities using the Doppler Effect

Doppler frequency of the reflected beam. A shift to higher frequencies corresponds to flow towards the transducer. The Doppler effect has been broadly applied in medical ultrasound diagnostics to determine blood velocities in blood vessels and in the heart and to probe perfusion.

8.2.2.6 Shock waves

The linear relationship between pressure and volume or density that is assumed in Hooke's law (eq. (8.5)) ceases to apply when large acoustic pressure changes occur in biological tissue. What holds instead is the nonlinear relation

$$p = K\frac{\delta\rho}{\rho} + \frac{B}{2}\left(\frac{\delta\rho}{\rho}\right)^2, \tag{8.22}$$

K: Compression module, B: Nonlinear compression module

which [8.15] causes a non-constant sound velocity c conforming to eq. (8.4) where c depends on the momentary particle velocity speed v_p (eq. (8.7))

$$c = c_0 + \varepsilon v_p \tag{8.23}$$

c_0: Speed of sound at small pressure amplitudes

and where ε is a measure of the degree of nonlinearity

$$\varepsilon = 1 + \frac{B}{2K}. \tag{8.24}$$

An overview of the order of magnitude of ε is given in table 8.3.

Table 8.3 Numerical examples for nonlinear velocity of sound coefficients

Substance	ε
Water	3.5
Glycerine	5.4
Biological tissue	4-6

When looking at a plane wave in a nonlinear medium

$$v_p = \hat{v}_p \, e^{i\omega\left(\frac{z}{c_0 + \varepsilon v_p} - t\right)}, \tag{8.25}$$

one observes that the wave maximum moves $2\varepsilon\hat{v}$ times faster than the wave minimum and that the maximum catches up with the minimum after the critical interval

$$t_C = \frac{\lambda}{4\varepsilon\hat{v}_p} \tag{8.26a}$$

during which the wave travels the critical distance

$$d_C = \frac{\lambda c_0}{4\varepsilon\hat{v}_p}. \tag{8.26b}$$

A saw-toothed wave forms (fig. 8.9) and the inner friction of the medium then prevents further deformations.

While the present considerations concern only the continuous excitation of shock waves, the treatment of stone diseases requires the application of shock-wave pulses. The introduction of a strong ultrasound pulse into a nonlinear medium produces a shock wave exhibiting an asymmetric pressure distribution. A large compression amplitude forms at the shock front and a small negative pressure amplitude at the shock tail. Positive pressure increases as the shock front propagates faster than the shock tail, which loses intensity (fig. 8.10). In the end, however, the inner losses of the shock wave's higher harmonics account for the shock wave's degradation.

Pulsed shock waves are used in medicine to noninvasively shatter stones, including kidney, gall, pancreas and saliva stones (lithotripsy). Pulsed shock waves can be generated by a spark discharge, either piezoelectrically or electromagnetically [8.16]. The pressure amplitude can be further enhanced by focusing. Cracks are generated in the stone when it is hit by the shock wave. This allows for tissue-fluid penetration. Eventually, stone destruction is caused (mainly) by cavitation: The negative pressure part of the shock wave creates gas bubbles in the penetrated fluid. These implode, thereby smashing the stone [8.17].

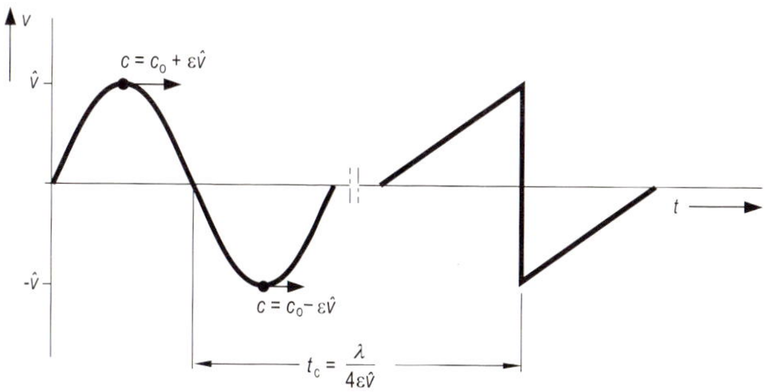

Figure 8.9 Formation of a CW ultrasound shock wave

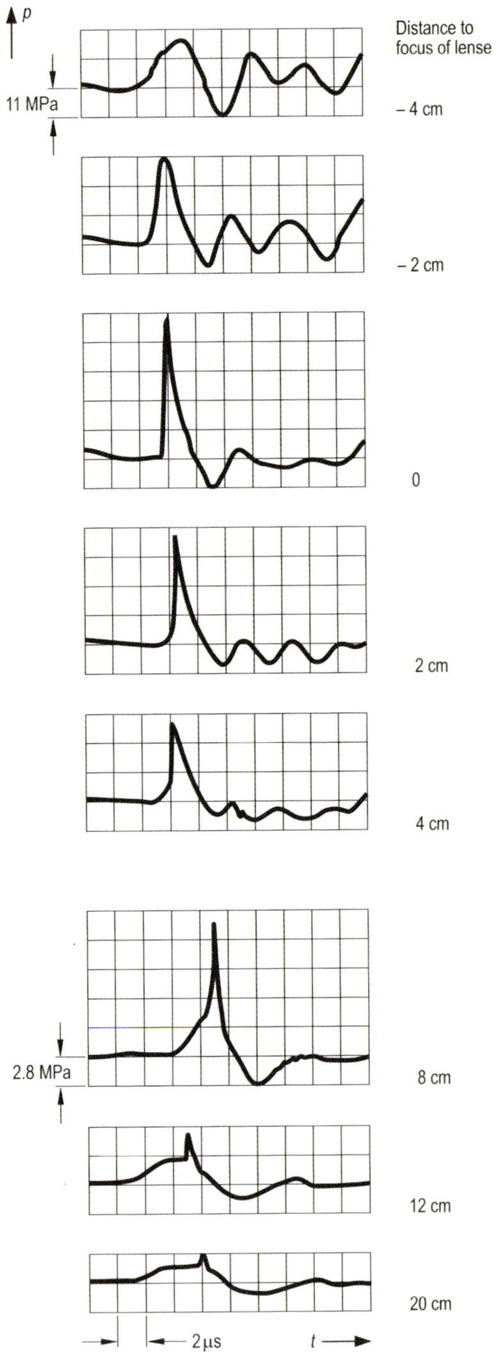

Figure 8.10
Shape of a shock wave pulse at different distances from the focus of a lens ($f = 12$ cm)

8.3 Imaging principles

8.3.1 Echo pulse method

Almost all ultrasound methods used today in medical diagnostics are based on the echo-pulse technique (fig. 8.11). A piezoelectric transducer converts an electric pulse into a sonic transmitter pulse, which penetrates the object under investigation. The sonic pulse is reflected by boundary surfaces within the object. The reflected energy that returns to the piezoelectric transducer causes the transducer to generate an electric voltage, which is then amplified and rectified. The simplest case of A-mode operation (A stands for amplitude) involves the use of the rectified echo pulses to vertically deflect a cathode ray tube's electron beam whose time-proportional horizontal deflection is triggered by the transmitter pulse. The experiment is repeated periodically to achieve a standing display.

Given that the differences in acoustic impedance are rather small, most of the ultrasound energy propagating into the object penetrates the object's internal boundaries so that the ultrasound echoes from the variously positioned organs are received in succession by the piezoelectric transducer. The distance of the boundary surfaces to the transducer can thus be derived on the screen of the oscilloscope from the echo pulses' time of flight. It has already been mentioned that rough surfaces cause backscattering. This explains the detection of planes that are tilted with respect to the direction of the sound beam.

The distance z of a boundary with respect to the transducer is derived as follows:

$$z = \frac{ct}{2}. \qquad t\text{: Time of flight} \qquad (8.27a)$$

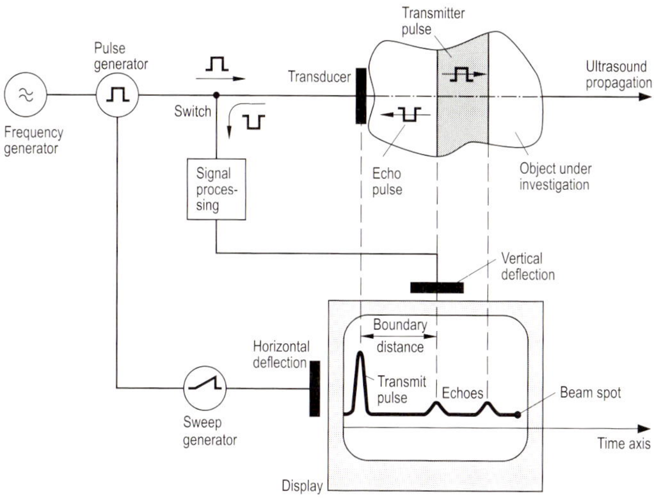

Figure 8.11 Basic scheme of an echo-pulse device

Two closely neighboring reflectors can be distinguished as long as two separate echoes are observed. Assuming that this is possible when the two echoes are separated by at least their half width, the spatial resolution Δz in axial direction to the ultrasound beam is expressed as

$$\Delta z \geq \frac{c\Delta t}{2}. \tag{8.27b}$$

Δt: Full width at the half maximum of the transmitter pulse

As the transmitter pulse lasts for at least one period of an ultrasound oscillation

$$\Delta t > \frac{1}{\nu} = \frac{\lambda}{c}, \tag{8.27c}$$

the axial resolution can be derived by

$$\Delta z \geq \frac{\lambda}{2}. \tag{8.27d}$$

Ultrasound absorption causes the echoes with a long time of flight to have a smaller amplitude than those with a short time of flight. For a uniform display of the echoes on the screen, the gain of the electronic signal amplifier is thus enhanced along with increasing time of flight (time gain control (TGC) or depth gain control (DGC)). However, this is only feasible if the echo signals are larger than competing noise. Current instruments have a dynamic range of about 110 dB. According to eq. (8.11b), this will yield different ultrasound penetration depths depending on frequency (see table 8.4).

The final lower limit for noise voltage is the thermal noise energy emitted by the object under investigation. Analogous to black body radiation, the noise sound intensity J_N received by the transducer is expressed as

$$J_N(\nu, t) = cD(\nu)\, kT\Delta\nu \tag{8.28}$$

J_N: Noise sound intensity received (e.g. in W/m^2), c: Speed of sound (e.g. in m/s)

$D(\nu)$: Density of vibration mode states in the investigated object at ultrasound frequency ν (e.g. in $\frac{1}{m^3 Hz}$)

T: Temperature of the object (e.g. in K), $\Delta\nu$: Receiver bandwidth (e.g. in Hz)

k: Boltzmann constant ($1.38 \cdot 10^{-23}$ J/K)

Table 8.4 Typical parameters in medical ultrasound

Frequency / MHz	Wavelength in mm	Penetration in cm (back and forth)	Lateral Resolution in mm	Axial Resolution in mm (2 period pulse)
2.0	0.78	25	3	0.8
3.5	0.44	14	1.7	0.5
5.0	0.31	10	1.2	0.35
7.5	0.21	6.7	0.8	0.25
10	0,16	5.0	0.6	0.2
15	0.10	3.3	0.4	0.15

Techniques have been developed to use ultrasound noise to noninvasively measure the temperature of objects (radiometry with ultrasound [8.18]).

8.3.2 Ultrasound transducer

The piezoelectric effect is used in medical technology to generate and detect ultrasound pulses. When exposed to mechanical stress, internal charges in certain ferroelectric ionic crystals (e.g. tourmaline, Rochelle salt and quartz) are displaced, a process that results in electric polarization. Conversely, these crystals deform when exposed to an electric field. A high frequency electric field can thus be used to generate ultrasound vibrations. Today, ceramic materials such as Ba-titanate and Pb-titanate/-circonate/-metaniobate are used to produce transducers. These materials have to be polarized before they can demonstrate their piezoelectric properties. To bring this about, electrodes are applied on opposite sides of the material in question and the transducer element is heated above its Curie temperature before being allowed to cool down with the application of electric DC voltage.

A simple ultrasound transducer assembly is shown in fig. 8.12. To obtain large vibration amplitudes, the geometrical dimensions of the piezoelectric disc are made in a manner that ensures that its mechanical resonance agrees with the desired ultrasound frequency. However, it is necessary to use a backing to dampen the intrinsic resonance, and to thereby enable the generation of short transmitter pulses without decaying tails and to avoid the reflection of ultrasound echoes from the backside of the piezoelectric disc.

While electronic noise emanating from the object itself represents the final limit for signal dynamics, a further noteworthy source of noise is the Nyquist noise that emanates from the transducer, which acts as a resistive load due to the backing and its capacitive coupling to tissue.

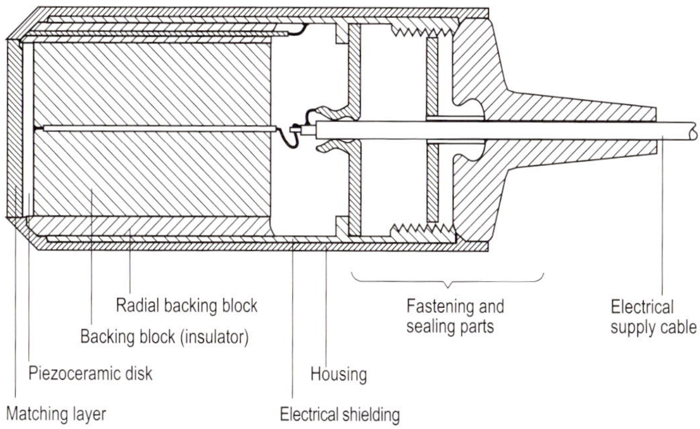

Figure 8.12 Design of a simple ultrasound transducer

The different ultrasound impedances Z_1 and Z_2 between the piezo-ceramic and biological tissue necessitate a matching layer to ensure the reflectionless transfer of ultrasound energy. Single layers have to have a thickness that is an uneven multiple of a quarter wavelength with an acoustic impedance of

$$Z = \sqrt{Z_1 Z_2}. \tag{8.29}$$

8.3.3 Imaging methods

Ultrasound A-mode imaging delivers one-dimensional information only. However, the temporal motion of boundary surfaces in the investigated object can be made visible by encoding the echo amplitude as the brightness of the display tube's cathode ray and writing successive echo lines next to one another instead of superimposing them (cf. time-motion mode (TM mode) in fig. 8.13). Even the rapid movement of heart valves can be analyzed in this way.

Brightness mode (B mode) is the most commonly applied mode. The scanning ultrasound beam is displaced on the body surface after each echo line. The echoes modulate the brightness of the display's electron beam. This is deflected in proportion to time in one direction, thereby yielding depth information. The displacement of the ultrasound beam positions the cathode ray orthogonal to its temporal deflection (fig. 8.14). This leads to the generation of a two-dimensional sectional image.

In B mode, spatial resolution in the ultrasound beam's direction of propagation is given by the pulse duration and lateral resolution is limited by diffraction. A focused ultrasound beam with a numerical aperture $f/D \approx 1$ has a width of approximately $2.4\,\lambda$ between the first two diffraction minima (eq. (8.18)). Thus, as with every imaging system that applies wave fields, the wavelength is the limiting factor for spatial resolution. The half width of the point spread function (as measured by scanning a point re-

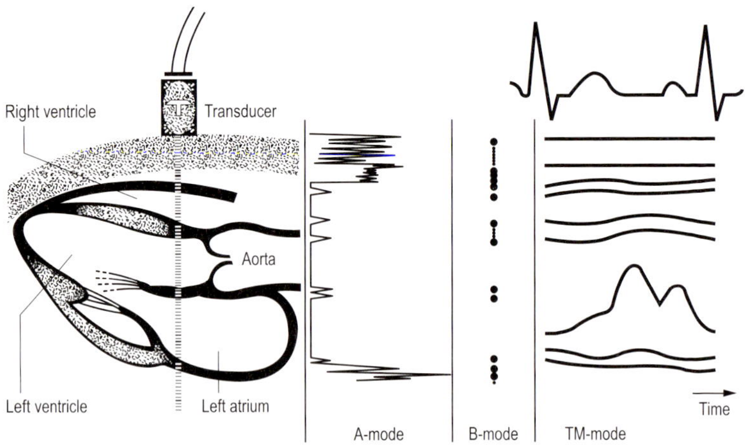

Figure 8.13 Principle behind A-mode and TM-mode methods

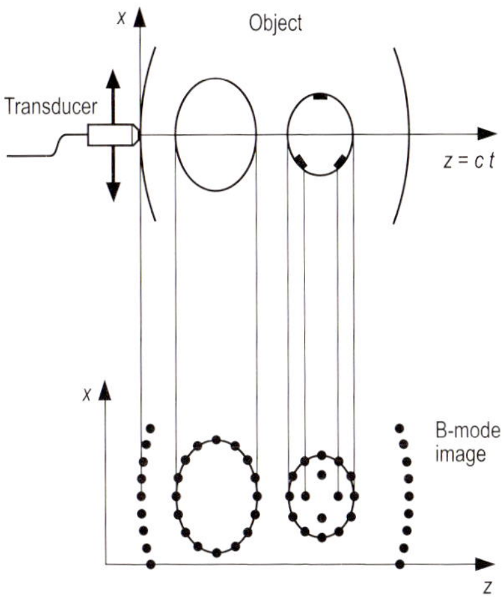

Figure 8.14
Principle of B-mode imaging

flector) is usually given as a measure of the spatial resolution. Given that the same transducer is used for transmitting and receiving, the point spread function is represented by the squared pressure amplitude of the scanning ultrasound beam. The figures in table 8.4 offer a rough guide for different ultrasound frequencies.

It has already been mentioned that backscatter plays an important role in the visibility of boundary surfaces in ultrasound than reflection. Ultrasound wave scattering also occurs directly in the tissue when several scatterers are present in a volume element that is smaller than that defined by the spatial resolution of the scanner. The waves that originate from this scattering interfere with one another, sometimes extinguishing and sometimes enhancing ultrasound intensity. What results is a speckle pattern that is typical for diagnostic ultrasound and that changes temporally due to stochastic fluctuations of the scatterers.

The transducer was originally moved over the body surface manually for B-mode imaging (compound scan). Real-time imaging emerged as a possibility only after it became possible to rapidly shift the scanning ultrasound beam laterally by applying a rotating transducer in the focus of an ellipsoid (Vidoson, [8.9]). Given that a successive ultrasound transmitter pulse is not to be sent until all of the echoes from its predecessor have been received, image formation requires the following temporal interval:

$$T = \frac{2XZ}{c\Delta X}. \tag{8.30}$$

X: Lateral image width, ΔX: Distance between image lines, Z: Image depth

An image acquisition time of 13 ms is needed (this corresponds to a frame rate of 75 Hz) for a 10 by 10 cm field of view with a line spacing of 1 mm.

Echoes no longer modulate the intensity of a cathode ray directly in modern ultrasound instruments. Instead, the image is stored in an electronic memory, read out independently of acquisition time and displayed on a monitor [8.19]. This enables the production of non-flickering images even in the case of slow scans. Applying interpolation, the number of image lines is not necessarily identical to the number of scanning lines.

Mechanical scanners have been replaced by electronic scanners. Instead of a single transducer, arrays are used, whose individual transducer elements can be activated as groups, thereby allowing one to displace and focus the ultrasound beam electronically. For details see chapter 16.

The deployment of three-dimensional ultrasound scanning methods is increasing. These methods involve the displacement of both the scanning line and the scanning plane. The generated data set is stored in memory, which allows for the reading out of three-dimensionally rendered images and arbitrarily selected planes. The term C-scan is used for planes parallel to the surface of the body.

8.3.4 Methods of determining flow

8.3.4.1 Continuous-wave Doppler

When a continuous ultrasound wave with a frequency of 5 MHz hits a target moving at 10 cm/s, the reflected sound is shifted in frequency by 650 Hz (eq. (8.21)). This difference frequency can be made audible with a loudspeaker when the signal from the reflected wave is heterodyned with the frequency of the transmitted wave. The heartbeat of a fetus can be verified in this way starting in the 12th week of pregnancy.

Blood flow in superficial vessels is also investigated using continuous-wave (CW) Doppler to localize strictures and stenoses. The flow velocity and its direction can be determined by deploying a quadrature demodulator to detect the phase of the reflected wave with respect to the transmitted ultrasound wave and applying a complex Fourier transformation to the two signal outputs. However, it is not possible to measure the depth of the vessel in this way.

8.3.4.2 Pulsed-wave Doppler

Pulsed ultrasound allows one to determine both the distance of a vessel to the transducer and the blood velocity when taking account of the phase of the echoes along an A-line. The echo signals that are detected phase-sensitively in quadrature can be considered the Doppler signal sampled at pulse repetition time (fig. 8.15)

$$T_R = \frac{1}{prf}. \quad prf\text{: Pulse repetition frequency} \tag{8.31a}$$

The transmitter pulses must be coherent, i.e. they have to be generated from a continuous RF signal.

According to the sampling theorem, the Doppler signals can be reconstructed unequivocally as long as the relation

$$f_D \le \frac{prf}{2} \tag{8.31b}$$

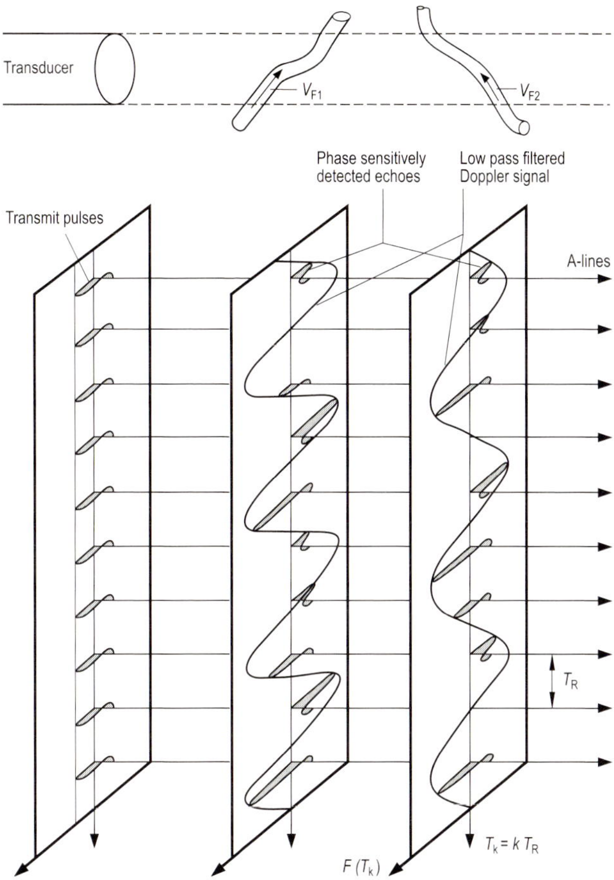

Figure 8.15 Principle behind the pulsed-wave Doppler technique

is valid for the Doppler shift. In keeping with eq. (8.21), this means that the maximum measurable flow component v_z^{max} in the direction of the ultrasound beam is limited to

$$v_z^{max} \leq \frac{\lambda}{4} prf. \tag{8.32a}$$

Given that the pulse repetition frequency also determines the field-of-view depth Z (eq. (8.30)), the following relation holds

$$v_z^{max} Z \leq \frac{\lambda c}{8}. \tag{8.32b}$$

The Doppler frequency resolution can also be obtained from the sampling theorem as

$$\Delta f_D = \frac{1}{T} \tag{8.32c}$$

where T is the total time during which the Doppler signal is sampled:

$$T = NT_{\mathrm{R}} = \frac{N}{prf}. \quad N\text{: Number of sampled echoes} \tag{8.33}$$

Of course, a signal observation time that is longer than the time the scatterer remains in the observation window would be meaningless. The observation window is given by the diameter of the ultrasound beam and by the length of the sampling gate at the selected depth. If this length is chosen according to the duration of the transmitter pulse (eq. (8.27b)), the dependency

$$T \leq \frac{c\Delta T}{v_{\mathrm{Z}}} = \frac{\Delta Z}{v_{\mathrm{Z}}} \tag{8.34}$$

Δt: Duration of the sampling interval, ΔZ: Length of the echo sampling gate

is valid provided the scattering particle has remained in the beam. The following relation thus applies to the pulsed-Doppler velocity resolution

$$\Delta v_{\mathrm{Z}} \Delta Z \geq \frac{\lambda v_{\mathrm{Z}}}{2} \tag{8.35}$$

(i.e. spatial and velocity resolution are inversely proportional).

Numerical example: A scatterer moving at a speed of $v_{\mathrm{Z}} = 10$ cm/s along the direction of the ultrasound beam stays in a sampling gate of length $\Delta Z = 2$ mm for the duration of 20 ms. Demanding a field of view with a depth of $Z = 5$ cm requires the selection of a pulse repetition time of $T_{\mathrm{R}} = 70$ µs (i.e. the Doppler signal can be sampled with $N = 285$ data points). At an ultrasound frequency of $v = 5$ MHz corresponding to a wavelength of $\lambda = 0.3$ mm, the velocity resolution amounts to $v_{\mathrm{Z}} = 7{,}5$ mm/s.

Doppler signal processing is normally performed by a complex fast Fourier transformation of the two output signals of a phase-sensitive quadrature demodulator, which gives the number of scatterers as a function of flow velocity at the selected depth (Doppler spectrum). Higher velocities v_{Z} than admitted by eq. (8.35) are backfolded to a value $(-v_{\mathrm{Z}}^{\max} + v_{\mathrm{Z}})$. The Doppler gate is usually marked in an independently acquired B-mode image and the Doppler signal is displayed in a separate graph showing the velocity as a function of time with the spectral amplitude encoded as gray level representing the number of scatterers at the particular speed.

8.3.4.3 Color Doppler

Given that it is not corrupted by phase variations, the power spectrum is normally evaluated instead of the complex Doppler spectrum. As illustrated in fig. 8.16, the Doppler power spectrum is characterized by three main parameters, including mean frequency (representing the average flow velocity), spectral width (indicating turbulence), and the area below the curve (representing a measure of the total number of moving particles in the sampling window).

Although all of these values can be deduced from the complex Doppler spectrum, time of measurement would become exceedingly long if one were to display them over a large field of view. Color Doppler provides methods of estimating the relevant spectral

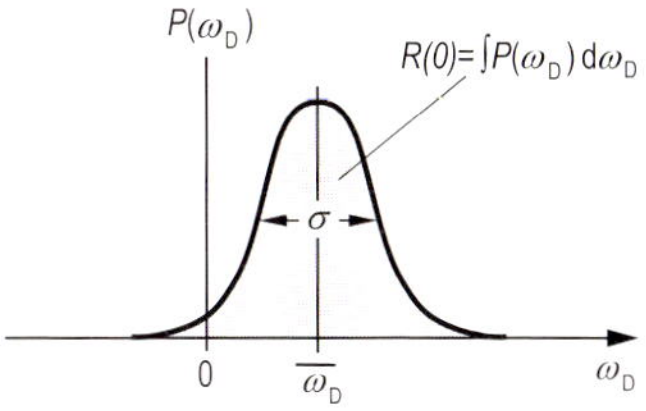

Figure 8.16
Ultrasound Doppler power spectrum

parameters on the basis of only a few measured samples obtained in real time from a few successive B-mode images.

The complex signal of the quadrature detector $F_D(t_k) = F_D(kT_R)$ evaluated in pulsed-wave Doppler corresponds to one echo along an A-line at a given time of flight repeated at repetition time T_R. The average Doppler angular frequency at this point is defined as

$$\bar{\omega}_D = 2\pi\bar{f}_D = \frac{\sum_{(l)} \omega_l P(\omega_l)}{\sum_{(l)} P(\omega_l)}$$

$$P(\omega_l) = F(\omega_l)F^*(\omega_l): \text{ Power spectrum} \tag{8.36}$$

$$F(\omega_l) = \sum_{k=0}^{N-1} F(t_k)e^{-i\omega_l t_k}: \text{ Fourier transform of } F_D(t_k)$$

The width of the power spectrum is defined by its standard deviation σ, with respect to variance

$$\sigma^2 = \frac{\sum_{(l)} (\omega_l - \bar{\omega}_D)^2 P(\omega_l)}{\sum_{(l)} P(\omega_l)} \tag{8.37}$$

It can be shown [8.20] that these quantities can be derived from the Fourier transform of the power spectrum, which is the autocorrelation function of the Doppler signal

$$R(T_R) = \frac{1}{N}\sum_{k=0}^{N-1} F_D^*(t_k)F_D(t_{k+1}) \tag{8.38}$$

and the area below it

$$R(0) = \frac{1}{N}\sum_{k=0}^{N-1} |F_D(t_k)|^2, \tag{8.39}$$

yielding

$$\bar{\omega}_D = \frac{1}{T_R}\arctan\frac{Im(R(T_R))}{Re(R(T_R))} \tag{8.40a}$$

and

$$\sigma^2 = \frac{2}{T_R^2}\left(1 - \frac{|R(T_R)|}{R_0}\right). \tag{8.41a}$$

While the mean Doppler shift can already be derived from two successive samples of the phase sensitive detector

$$\bar{\omega}_D \approx \frac{1}{T_R}\left\{\arctan\frac{Im(F_D(T_R))}{Re(F_D(T_R))} - \arctan\frac{Im(F_D(0))}{Re(F_D(0))}\right\}, \tag{8.41b}$$

more samples ($N = 5$ to 17) are typically used so as to achieve greater accuracy. Nonetheless, this still involves far fewer samples than are used in pulsed Doppler where $N = 128$ is typically the case.

(An estimate of the Doppler width derived from two successive samples would yield

$$\sigma^2 \approx \frac{2}{T_R^2}\left(1 - \frac{|F_D(0)||F_D(T_R)|}{|F_D(0)|^2 + |F_D(T_R)|^2}\right). \tag{8.41c}$$

However, this gives a correct value for a Gaussian distribution only. Again, it is necessary to collect more samples and to apply eq. (8.41b)).

If the Doppler angle Θ and the wave length of the ultrasound beam are known, the mean flow velocity and its spread can be calculated by applying eq. (8.21).

Color Doppler usually involves overlaying the flow velocity on the normal B image. Flow in the direction of the ultrasound beam is often encoded as red and flow in the opposite direction as blue, color saturation being a measure of the magnitude of flow velocity. The grade of turbulence is encoded by mixing in more or less green.

Doppler blood flow signals are up to two orders of magnitude weaker than echoes from stationary reflectors. In order to prevent them from exceeding the dynamics of the signal processing chain, stationary echoes are separated by a so-called wall filter. This suppresses the flow velocity zero. However, extremely slow moving reflectors such as vessel walls sometimes lead to the flashing up of artifacts.

8.3.4.4 Power color mode

In power color mode, the sum of all squared spectral amplitudes (i.e. the area below the power spectrum that can be calculated with eq. (8.39)) is color-coded and overlaid on the B mode image. However, the echoes from stationary boundaries first have to be removed by a wall filter. The number of moving particles is thereby displayed independently of the incident angle of the ultrasound beam and is undisturbed by aliasing. Given that only the squared output signal of the Doppler quadrature detector has to be averaged and no further processing steps are necessary, the signal-to-noise ratio is much better than that of the velocity distribution. However, all information about magnitude and direction of velocity is lost. Power-color Doppler is especially useful for investigating tissue perfusion.

8.4 Safety of diagnostic ultrasound

"Diagnostic ultrasound has proven to be a valuable tool in medical practice. An excellent safety record exists in that, after decades of clinical use, there is no known instance of human injury as a result of exposure to diagnostic ultrasound. Evidence exists, however, to indicate that at least a hypothetical risk for clinical diagnostic ultrasound must be presumed."

This statement is taken from the 1990 Radiological Health Bulletin [8.21]. Similar statements expressing somewhat different assessments of the potential risks have been issued by the European Committee for Medical Ultrasound Safety (ECMUS) [8.22] and the World Federation of Ultrasound in Medicine and Biology (WFUNMB) [8.23].

Why bother now with concerns regarding the safety of diagnostic ultrasound given its clean track record and the fact that many experts believe it is intrinsically safe? When responding to this question it is helpful to review both what is behind ultrasound's enviable safety record and the mechanisms that introduce the potential risks.

8.4.1 Acoustic output regulations

In 1976, the United States Medical Device Amendments were enacted, authorizing the Food and Drug Administration (FDA) to regulate all medical devices, including diagnostic ultrasound equipment. The FDA has required the manufacturers of diagnostic ultrasound equipment to keep acoustic output to levels below those of machines on the market before 1976. Manufacturers bringing new products to the market are required, in particular, to compare the acoustic output of their devices to those of devices previously approved for marketing. Within these limits, which are broadly applied throughout the world, ultrasound has proven to be a safe and effective diagnostic tool for medical application. However, it is important to recall that the pre-1976 output levels are based on experience and not on scientific safety evaluations.

The FDA guidelines have evolved since 1976. The upper limits are relaxed somewhat when safety information is provided by displaying thermal and mechanical indices according to an output display standard [8.24]. Providing these indices is an important step forward in helping users to avoid situations involving undue risk. The output display standard has also been incorporated into the international (IEC 60601-2-37:2001) standard [8.25].

8.4.2 Bioeffects

Two mechanisms are known to alter biological systems. These are the thermal mechanism, involving the heating of soft tissue and bone, and the non-thermal mechanism, involving the complex of mechanical phenomena associated with cavitation. (Please refer to [8.26] for a list of suggested readings.)

Thermal bioeffects

Much of the ultrasound energy that is emitted during an ultrasound examination is absorbed by the body tissue. The absorption of acoustic energy results in the generation of heat. If the rate of energy deposition in a particular region exceeds the body's ability to dissipate the associated heat (e.g. by perfusion), the local tissue temperature will rise. If this temperature rises too high, it will cause tissue damage. Exactly this effect is used, for instance, to destroy malignant tissue.

Increases in tissue temperature caused by the absorption of radiant energy are difficult to measure. Heat conduction equation models have thus been developed that take account of metabolic heat generation and heat transportation via perfusion [8.27]:

$$c\rho\frac{\partial T}{\partial t} = k\nabla^2 T + \omega\rho c_{Blood}\rho_{Blood}(T_{Blood} - T) + q_{Metabolism} + SAR \qquad (8.42)$$

ρ: Density of tissue ($\frac{kg}{m^3}$), ρ_{Blood}: Density of blood
c: Specific heat of tissue ($\frac{J}{kg\,K}$), c_{Blood}: Specific heat of blood
T: Temperature of tissue, T_{Blood}: Temperature of capillary blood
ω: Volumetric flow rate of blood per unit mass of tissue ($\frac{m^3}{s\,kg}$)
$q_{Metabolism}$: Rate of metabolic heat generation ($\frac{W}{m^3}$)
SAR: Local specific absorption rate ($\frac{W}{m^3}$)

This differential equation, often referred to as the bio-heat equation, can be solved using numerical means by taking into account a number of physical and physiological variables. The result is highly dependent on the organ or tissue type being investigated. Various models have been developed (e.g. centering on layered structures involving soft tissue and bone) to account for the variety of situations that might arise when deploying ultrasound for clinical purposes.

Non-thermal bioeffects

It has been known since the early days of ultrasound in the 1930's that biological cells in suspension can be lysed or otherwise damaged by ultrasound in the absence of significant heating. The primary mechanism here is linked to the generation of gas-filled cavities. This activity, referred to by the general term acoustic cavitation, has proven to have many aspects. These may involve violent implosions (which can generate very high temperatures and highly reactive chemical compounds), liquid jets (which can cause mechanical damage to interfaces), cavity growth and microstreaming. All of these phenomena are capable of affecting biological structures and processes.

Experiments and theoretical considerations have shown that cavity formation is related to the negative peak (or rarefactional) pressure and to the inverse of the square root of ultrasonic frequency. In the 2 to 20 MHz frequency range, a peak pressure of at least 15 MPa is required to cause cavitation in pure, degassed water.

Currently, there is no evidence to suggest that diagnostic ultrasound exposure has caused cavitation in humans during ultrasound examinations. However, special consideration needs to be given to the application of ultrasound contrast agents. These contrast agents typically consist of microbubbles that may introduce cavitation nuclei into the human body. Considerable work is currently in progress to outline the interaction of ultrasonic beams and contrast agents so as to assess the possible risks.

8.4.3 Output display standard using thermal and mechanical indices

Today's diagnostic ultrasound equipment offers a vast array of applications and capabilities, as well as a multitude of features for optimizing images. This degree of complexity can make it difficult for the user to arrive at an accurate assessment of acoustic output. The goal of the output display standard is to provide real-time indices relating to the potential for ultrasound-induced bioeffects and to make users aware of the actual output generated by their ultrasound equipment as it is being used. However, if the ultrasound equipment is not capable of exceeding an index value of 1 for a selected application, the index value will not be displayed. On the other hand, if the ultrasound equipment is capable of exceeding an index value of 1, the respective index will be displayed starting with an index value of 0.4.

Two types of indices may be displayed to account for the two main mechanisms of potential ultrasound-related bioeffects. These include the thermal index (TI) to estimate temperature increases and the mechanical index (MI) to estimate non-thermal bioeffects such as cavitation.

Thermal index (TI)

The purpose of the thermal index is to make the user aware of conditions that may lead to temperature increases. Since temperature increases are calculated by applying tissue models, three thermal indices are used in order to account for different combinations of soft tissue and bone: TIS, TIB, and TIC.

TI is proportional to the applied power. As heating is greatest in tissue immediately adjacent to the transducer, thermal indices indicate the maximum possible temperature increase at this location and not in the region being imaged, where it is lower.

The soft tissue thermal index (TIS) describes maximum possible temperature increases in homogeneous soft tissue at the applied US power.

The bone thermal index (TIB) indicates temperature increases in bone at or near the focus after the ultrasonic beam has passed through soft tissue.

The cranial bone thermal index (TIC) gives maximum possible temperature increases in bone at or near the surface (e.g. during a cranial examination).

The thermal indices are relative indicators of temperature increases. In the worst-case scenarios of the respective models, an index value of 1 means a temperature increase of 1 K. However, actual temperature increases are typically significantly lower and depend on a number of factors such as tissue type, blood perfusion, operation mode, and exposure time.

Mechanical index (MI)

The mechanical index is derived from the ratio of the maximum negative pressure amplitude and the square root of the frequency for the ultrasound power applied. The pressure amplitude cannot be measured directly in tissue, but only in water using hydrophones. Given that water shows nearly no ultrasound absorption when compared to tissue, measured pressure amplitude in water is de-rated by an average attenuation coefficient for tissue of $0.3\ \frac{\text{dB}}{\text{cm MHz}}$ to arrive at the mechanical index.

$$MI = \frac{\frac{p_-}{\text{MPa}}}{\sqrt{\frac{\nu}{\text{MHz}}}}\, 10^{-0.015 \frac{f}{\text{cm}} \frac{\nu}{\text{MHz}}} \qquad (8.43)$$

p_-: Negative peak power measured in pure water
f: Focal depth, ν: Ultrasound frequency

An ultrasound pulse of 5 MHz that creates a negative pressure peak of 2 MPa in water in the focal zone at 2 cm thus corresponds to $MI = 0.63$.

The higher the index reading, the larger is the potential for mechanical bioeffects. However, one needs to keep in mind that the mechanical index is intended to yield an estimate of the potential for mechanical bioeffects. Neither $MI = 1$ nor any other level indicates that bioeffects are actually occurring.

8.4.4 Summary – prudent use of ultrasound

In more than three decades of use, there have been no reports of patient injury stemming from medical diagnostic ultrasound equipment. In the past, the means of minimizing exposure centered on application-specific output limits and the user's knowledge of equipment controls and patient body characteristics. Providing safety information by displaying real-time indices in order to arrive at an estimate of the potential for bioeffects represents an important step in helping users to make individual benefit/risk decisions and to avoid situations involving undue risk while at the same time achieving the best possible images for their diagnostic goals.

8.5 References

[8.1] K.T. Dussik
Über die Möglichkeit hochfrequente mechanische Schwingungen als diagnostisches Hilfsmittel zu verwenden
Z. f. d. ges. Neurol. u. Psychiat. 174 (1942), 143

[8.2] G.D. Ludwig, F.W. Struthers
Considerations underlying the use of ultrasound to detect gallstones and foreign bodies in tissue
Naval Medical Research Institute Reports, Project 004-001 (1949)

[8.3] J.J. Wild
The Use of Ultrasonic Pulses for the Measurement of Biologic Tissues and the Detection of Tissue Density Changes
Surgery 27 (1950), 148

[8.4] D.H. Howry, W.R. Bliss
Ultrasonic visualization of soft tissue structures in the body
J. Lab. Clin. Med. 40 (1950), 479

[8.5] L. Leksell
Echoencephalography detection of intracranial complications following head injury
Acta Chir. Scand. 11 (1950), 301

[8.6] I. Edler and C.H. Hertz
The Use of Ultrasonic Reflectoscope for the Continuous Recording of Movements of Heart Walls
Kungl. Fysiogr. Sallsk i Lund Forhandl. 24 (1954), 5

[8.7] G.H. Mundt and W.F. Hughes
Ultrasonics in Ocular Diseases
Am. J. Ophth. 41 (1962), 488

[8.8] S. Satomura
Ultrasonic Doppler Methods for the Inspection of Cardiac Functions
J. Acoust. Soc. Am. 29 (1957), 1181

[8.9] W. Krause, R. Soldner
Ultraschallbildverfahren (B-Scan) mit hoher Bildfrequenz für medizinische Diagnostik
Electromedica 4 (1967), 8

[8.10] H. Morneburg (Hrsg.)
Bildgebende Systeme für die medizinische Diagnostik, 3. Auflage
7 Ultraschalltechnik
Publicis MCD Verlag, Erlangen 1985

[8.11] F.J. Fry
Ultrasound: its applications in medicine and biology
Elsevier Scientific Publishing Company
Amsterdam, Oxford, New York 1978

[8.12] J. Zemanek
Beam Behavior within Nearfield of a Vibrating Piston
J. Acoust. Soc. Amer. 49 (1971), 181

[8.13] A. Weyns
Radiation field calculations of pulsed ultrasonic transducers; Part 1: plane circular, square, and annular transducers, Part 2: spherical disc- and ring-shaped transducers
Ultrasonics July/Sept. 1980 IPC Business Press, 183-188 and 219-223

[8.14] A. Weyns
Studie en Optimalisatie van Elementaire Diagnostische Ultrasoonzenders en Ultrasoonontvangers
Promotion 1982 Katholieke Universiteit Leuven Faculteit van de Toegepaste Wetenschappen, Departement Electrotechniek

[8.15] R.T. Beyer
Nonlinear Acoustics
Naval Sea Systems Command 1976 Washington

[8.16] H. Reichenberger
Lithotripter Systems
Proc. IEEE 76 (1988), 1236

[8.17] W. Sass, M. Bräunlich, H.-P. Dreyer, E. Matura, W. Folberth, H.-G. Priesmeyer, J. Seifert
The mechanisms of stone disintegration by shock waves
Ultrasound in Med&Biol 17 (1991), 239

[8.18] Yu.V. Gulyaev, K.M. Bograchev, I.P. Borovikov, Yu.V. Obukhov, V.I. Passechnik
Passive thermoacoustic tomography: methods and approaches
Journal of Communications Technology and Electronics 43 (1998), 1061-1067 (In Russian)

[8.19] M.G. Maginess
Methods and Terminology for Diagnostic Ultrasound Imaging Systems
Proc. IEEE, 67 (1979), 641

[8.20] C. Kasai, K. Namekawa, A. Koyano, R. Omoto
Real Time Two-Dimensional Blood Flow Imaging Using an Autocorrelation Technique
IEEE Trans. Sonics. Ultrason, SU-32 (1985), 458

[8.21] Radiological Health Bulletin, Vol, XXIV, No. 8, August 1990

[8.22] 2003 Revision of the EFSUMB Clinical Safety Statement
EFSUMB, Copenhagen 2003

[8.23] S.B. Barnett (Editor)
WFUMB Symposium on Safety of Ultrasound in Medicine – Conclusions and Recommendations on Thermal and Non-Thermal Mechanisms for Biological Effects of Ultrasound
Ultrasound in Medicine & Biology, 24, SU 1 (1998)

[8.24] M.D. Laurel
American Institute of Ultrasound in Medicine/National Manufacturers Association: Standard for real-time display of thermal and mechanical acoustic output indices on diagnostic ultrasound equipment
American Institute of Ultrasound in Medicine (1992)

[8.25] International Standard IEC 60601-2-37: Medical Electrical Equipment
Particular requirements for the safety of ultrasonic medical diagnostic and monitoring equipment
International Electrotechnical Commission, Geneva July 2001

[8.26] M.D. Laurel
Medical Ultrasound Safety
American Institute of Ultrasound in Medicine, 1994

[8.27] H.H. Pennes
Analysis of Tissue and Arterial Blood Temperature in the Resting Forearm
Journal of Applied Physiology 1 (1948), 93-122

Part III – Image Reconstruction

9 System theory

9.1 Introduction

Medical imaging quality can be characterized in terms of contrast sensitivity, spatial resolution, noise, geometrical distortions and artifacts. In the present chapter, we concern ourselves mainly with a review of the first three characteristics, as these apply to all imaging modalities while the latter two are modality-specific.

While our discussion will focus on X-ray projection radiography, the basic concepts that we introduce can be applied also to other imaging methods, including CT and MRI, which are mainly based on image reconstruction algorithms, even though the nomenclature used for the image generation process differs to some degree.

9.2 Basic quantities for evaluating image quality

9.2.1 Contrast

In general, the term contrast refers to any reproducible differences in signals or intensities, regardless of their physical background:

$$C = q_2 - q_1 \tag{9.1a}$$

q_1, q_2: Intensities at two different sites

Beyond this absolute definition, various normalized quantities are used:

$$C_1 = \frac{q_2 - q_1}{q_1} \qquad C_2 = \frac{q_2 - q_1}{q_1 + q_2} \qquad C_3 = \frac{q_2 - q_1}{\frac{1}{2}(q_1 + q_2)} \tag{9.1b}$$

The clear rendering of individual image objects depends on their ability of exhibiting a contrast that is significantly higher than the statistical uncertainty in the recorded image intensities. The contrast-to-noise ratio (*CNR*) (see also fig. 9.11)

$$CNR = \frac{q_2 - q_1}{\sigma} \tag{9.1c}$$

σ: Standard deviation of the background signal (noise)

is thus often specified as a measure of contrast sensitivity.

Eqs. (9.1a, b, c) are purely phenomenological descriptions. Medical diagnosis requires a strong correlation between image brightness variations and properties of the irradiated objects. We will illustrate this using a simplified example of X-ray projection imaging (fig. 9.1). If a monoenergetic X-ray beam traverses a slab of absorbing matter

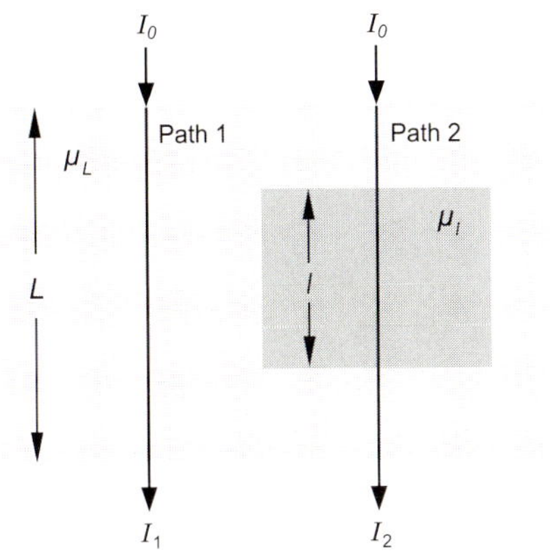

Figure 9.1
Irradiation of a slab with an enclosed detail as a model for X-ray projection imaging

with a linear attenuation coefficient μ_L enclosing a lesion with a different attenuation coefficient μ_l, the geometric arrangement depicted in fig. 9.1 yields the following beam intensities I_1 and I_2 along paths 1 and 2:

$$I_1 = I_0 e^{-\mu_L L} \tag{9.2a}$$

$$I_2 = I_0 e^{-\mu_L (L-l) - \mu_l l} \tag{9.2b}$$

Applying eq. (9.1a), the contrast that results in the radiation field behind the object amounts to

$$C = I_2 - I_1 = I_0 e^{-\mu_L L} (e^{-(\mu_l - \mu_L) l} - 1). \tag{9.3}$$

Eq. (9.3) indicates three options for increasing radiation field contrast:

- The primary X-ray dose I_0 may be increased. This, however, is not an option in medical imaging because it may lead to increased patient risk.
- The factor $e^{-\mu_L L}$ can be increased by reducing the irradiation path length L. The parts of the patient's body that are not of diagnostic interest should therefore remain outside the beam cone. In some medical examinations (e.g. mammography) the region under investigation is also compressed.
- Given that the linear attenuation coefficients $\mu(E)$ depend on radiation energy E, contrast can be optimized via the energy spectrum of the input radiation. This is achieved by appropriately setting the voltage of the X-ray tube, by selecting the proper anode material and by filtering.

Radiation field contrast is transformed by the imaging system into image contrast, which allows for medical diagnosis. Demands on the image detector cover the following two factors:

- Absorption performance: This has to be as high as possible so as to ensure the inclusion of information from every X-ray quantum.

- Response characteristic (as defined by sensitivity and dynamic range): The fact that X-ray film, for instance, shows little contrast at very low (fog) and very high (shoulder) exposure levels leads to reduced image contrast.

9.2.2 Spatial resolution

Imaging systems generally do not perfectly convert the physical parameter distribution of the imaging object into a signal distribution in the image. Some degree of blurring occurs. Furthermore, given the fact that some degree of blurring is present also in human vision, our capacity to detect small details and signs of pathology (e.g. calcification in the case of breast cancer and bone fractures) and to resolve closely adjacent objects remains limited.

Spatial resolution can be treated in a quantitative manner. In what follows, we restrict ourselves to a discussion of the image receptor's spatial resolution properties. Other features that contribute to blurring in X-ray images will not be considered. These include:

- The non-zero size of the emission focal spot
- X-ray scattering in the imaging object
- Geometric image distortions caused by the signal detector (e.g. image intensifiers)
- Lack of sharpness on account of object motion

9.2.2.1 Theory of linear and shift invariant systems

To use a mathematical characterization, the imaging detector may be regarded as a black box that maps an input field $q_{in}(x)$ to an output field $q_{out}(x)$ (fig. 9.2). The spatial coordinate is symbolized by x, generally a vector with three components. For the sake of simplicity, we will limit ourselves to one coordinate. For instance, $q_{in}(x)$ might be used to describe a spatial distribution of X-ray photons along one axis in the radiation field and $q_{out}(x)$ the resulting image brightness (gray level)

$$q_{out}(x) = S(q_{in}(x)). \tag{9.4}$$

The basis of linear-systems theory is that the response of the system to any input stimulus is linear

$$S(cq_{in}(x)) = cS(q_{in}(x)), \tag{9.5a}$$

c: Arbitrary constant

$$S(q_1 + q_2) = S(q_1) + S(q_2), \tag{9.5b}$$

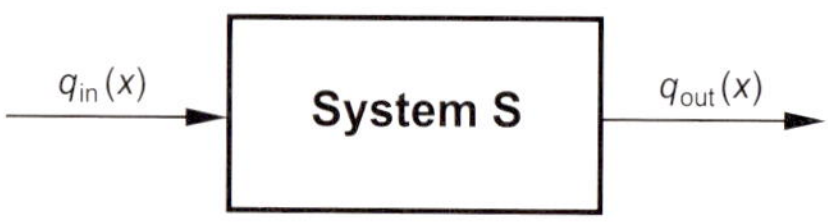

Figure 9.2
Input/output relation in an LSI model

and shift invariant

$$q_{out}(x - x_0) = S(q_{in}(x - x_0)). \qquad (9.5c)$$

x_0: arbitrary distance

A linear and shift invariant (LSI) system can be characterized by its response to a peak-shaped input function [9.1]:

$$LSF(x - x_0) = S(\delta(x - x_0))$$

$$\delta(x - x_0) = \begin{Bmatrix} 0 & \text{for } x - x_0 \neq 0 \\ \infty & \text{for } x - x_0 = 0 \end{Bmatrix} \quad \text{and} \quad \int \delta(x)\mathrm{d}x = 1 \qquad (9.6)$$

LSF(x) refers to line spread function in the one-dimensional case and point spread function (*PSF*) in two and three-dimensional cases.

Knowledge of an LSI system's *LSF* allows one to calculate its response to any input signal $q_{in}(x)$:

$$q_{out}(x) = \int q_{in}(x_0) LSF(x - x_0)\mathrm{d}x_0 = q_{in}(x) \otimes LSF(x) \qquad (9.7)$$

Applying the Fourier transform to eq. (9.7) yields

$$Q_{out}(u) = Q_{in}(u) TF(u), \qquad (9.8)$$

where $Q_{in}(u)$, $Q_{out}(u)$ and $TF(u)$ denote the Fourier transformed counterparts of $q_{in}(x)$, $q_{out}(x)$ and $LSF(x)$, respectively:

$$Q(u) = \int q(x) \mathrm{e}^{-\mathrm{i}2\pi ux}\mathrm{d}x \qquad \mathrm{i} = \sqrt{-1} \qquad (9.9)$$

u: spatial frequency

$TF(u)$ refers to system transfer function. To specify the resolution properties of an imaging detector, the modulation transfer function (*MTF*) is defined as

$$MTF(u) = \frac{|TF(u)|}{TF(0)}. \qquad (9.10)$$

$TF(0)$ can be considered the system gain.

As this leads to an alternative definition of the *MTF*, we shall investigate a system's response to a real-valued harmonic input function

$$q_{in}(x) = a + b\cos(2\pi u_0 x) = a + \frac{b}{2}(\mathrm{e}^{\mathrm{i}2\pi u_0 x} + \mathrm{e}^{-\mathrm{i}2\pi u_0 x}). \qquad (9.11a)$$

In the spatial frequency domain, this corresponds to

$$Q_{in}(u) = a\delta(u) + \frac{b}{2}(\delta(u - u_0) + \delta(u + u_0)). \qquad (9.11b)$$

The output function follows by multiplication with the Fourier transform of the *LSF*

$$Q_{out}(u) = aTF(u)\delta(u) + b\frac{TF(u)}{2}(\delta(u - u_0) + \delta(u + u_0)). \qquad (9.12a)$$

Given a symmetrical *LSF*, the inverse Fourier transform yields

$$q_{\text{out}}(x) = TF(0)a + TF(u_0)b\cos(2\pi u_0 x) \tag{9.12b}$$

so that the *MTF* at u_0 can be obtained from the contrast of the input and output harmonic images

$$MTF(u_0) = \frac{1}{TF(0)} \frac{\max(q_{\text{out}}(x)) - \min(q_{\text{out}}(x))}{\max(q_{\text{in}}(x)) - \min(q_{\text{in}}(x))}. \tag{9.13}$$

When passing through an LSI system, the amplitude of an input function is scaled to the system modulation transfer function at the corresponding frequency.

9.2.2.2 Evaluation of an X-ray imaging detector's modulation transfer function (*MTF*)

Experimental evaluation of the *MTF* is based on imaging of bar pattern grids (fig. 9.3). Drawing an intensity profile in the image perpendicular to the grid lines shows decreasing modulation coupled with increasing spatial frequency, which is indicative of a monotonically decreasing detector *MTF* (fig. 9.4). While the procedure for obtaining an intensity profile in the case of digital systems is obvious, one is required to use a scanning slot system for analog systems.

In order to extract the exact *MTF* values (fig. 9.6) from the patterns, one can compare (for each line group) the contribution of the first harmonic for the measured modula-

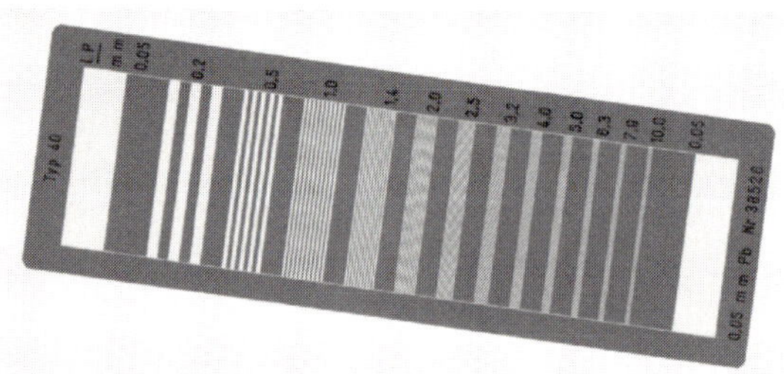

Figure 9.3
Digital image of a bar pattern grid recorded by a flat panel digital radiography detector with a pixel size of 0.143 mm

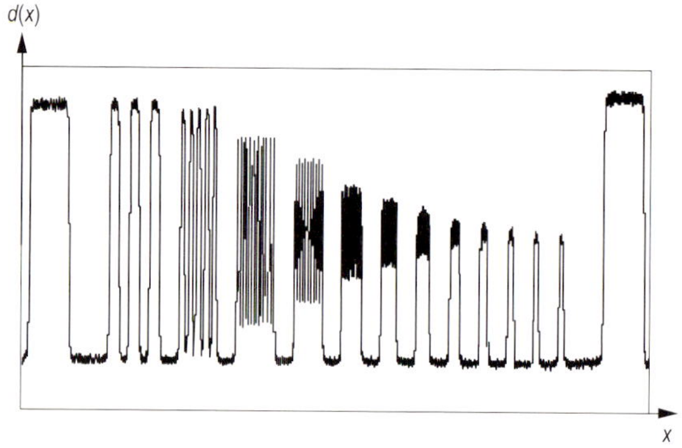

Figure 9.4
Profile across the bar pattern image shown in fig. 9.3. Modulation decreases (from left to right) along with increasing spatial frequency.

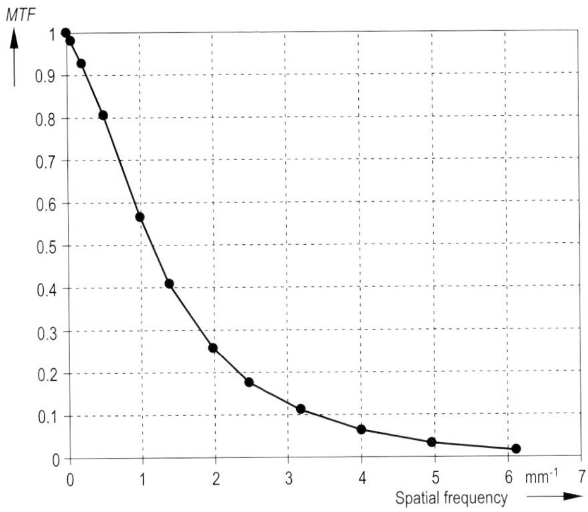

Figure 9.5
MTF derived from the bar pattern image shown in fig. 9.4

tion to the contribution of the first harmonic for the radiation field modulation. It will thus be necessary to take account of the resolution phantom's X-ray energy dependant absorption [9.2] to calculate the radiation field contrast.

Two additional methods are available for determining a detector *MTF*. The first of these is based on the numerical evaluation of line object images [9.3] and the second is based on edge phantoms [9.4]. The edge method has gained special relevance in the wake of its recent incorporation into the international standard [9.5] for determining the detective quantum efficiency (*DQE*).

If an imaging system consists of a series of several individual systems connected to one another (e.g. the image intensifier video chain in fig. 9.5), the total *MTF* is derived as the product of the individual *MTF*s

$$MTF_{\text{total}}(u) = MTF_1(u)MTF_2(u)MTF_3(u)\,... \tag{9.14}$$

However, it should be kept in mind that X-ray intensifier systems exhibit significant vignetting and distortion effects and therefore fail to satisfy the conditions of the LSI theory. This is also true for screen-film systems that show a non-linear response to incident X-rays. In such cases, the system response is linearized locally in order to apply linear system theory.

9.2.2.3 Digital signal sampling

Medical imaging systems that use digital signals have come to take precedence over other systems. The signals used by these systems to generate images as X-ray or ultrasound energy are transformed as early as possible after detection into binary values. Digital signals permit further processing that is not hampered by drift, linearity, fluctuation and reproduction problems and they permit the application of information technologies (IT) such as digital image processing, archiving and communication.

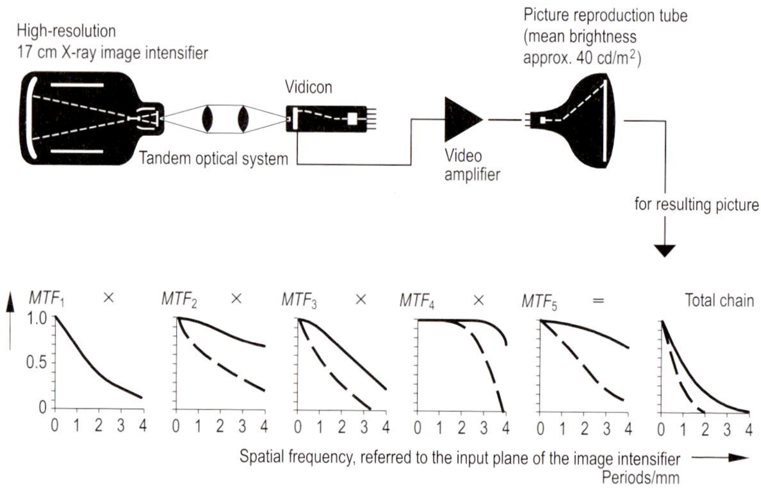

Figure 9.6
The total *MTF* of an image intensifier television chain is the product of the *MTFs* of the individual components (*MTFs* displayed on a logarithmic scale).

A digital imaging detector can be regarded as a two-dimensional regular lattice of picture elements or pixels. A digital value is assigned to each of these pixels so as to describe image brightness. The array of detector elements has two characteristic parameters: sampling interval (pixel pitch) p and pixel width (aperture) a. For the sake of simplicity, we will model a digital detector as a one-dimensional array (fig. 9.7).

Mathematically, the gathering of signal data by a pixel lattice can be represented as a two-step process:

- Integration of impinging photons (or secondary particles such as electrons) inside the discrete detector elements (presampling)
- Gathering of digital values for each detector element (sampling)

In the first step, the incoming X-photon fluence is absorbed (absorption coefficient α), blurred by the detector (line spread function $LSF(x)$) and then weighted according to the sensitivity profile of the pixel, which, ideally, is rectangular:

$$d(x) = q_{\text{abs}}(x) \otimes LSF(x) \otimes \operatorname{rect}\left(\frac{x}{a}\right)$$

$$\operatorname{rect}\left(\frac{x}{a}\right) = \begin{cases} 1 & \text{for } |x| < \frac{a}{2} \\ 0 & \text{for } |x| \geq \frac{a}{2} \end{cases} \tag{9.15a}$$

$d(x)$: Presampled detector output signal (dimensionless)
$q_{\text{abs}}(x) = \alpha q_{\text{in}}(x)$: Absorbed photon fluence (units in 1D: 1/m, in 2D: 1/m^2)
α: Absorption coefficient

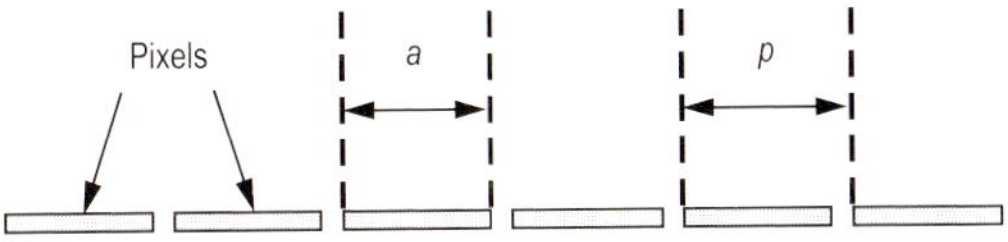

Figure 9.7 Pixel aperture width a and sampling pitch p of a pixel lattice ($a \leq p$)

In frequency space, Fourier transformation yields

$$D_u = aQ_{abs}(u)\,TF(u)\,\mathrm{sinc}(au). \qquad \mathrm{sinc}\,x = \frac{\sin \pi x}{\pi x} \tag{9.15b}$$

Thus, the pixel aperture acts as a gain factor in the presampling step and the spatial signal integration can be regarded in the framework of LSI system theory as an additional signal smoothing stage in a signal propagation cascade.

Data sampling in the second step means collecting values at equidistant increments p for the continuous presampled signal $d(x)$

$$s(x) = d(x)\,\mathrm{comb}\left(\frac{x}{p}\right).$$
$$\mathrm{comb}\left(\frac{x}{p}\right) = p \sum_{k=-\infty}^{\infty} \delta(x - kp) \tag{9.16a}$$

This set of grayscale numbers $s(kp)$ constitutes the final digital image data. The Fourier transform of the sampled data

$$S_u = pD_u \otimes \mathrm{comb}(pu)$$
$$\mathrm{comb}(pu) = \frac{1}{p}\int \mathrm{comb}\left(\frac{x}{p}\right) e^{-i2\pi ux}\,dx = \frac{1}{p}\sum_{k=-\infty}^{\infty} \delta\left(u - \frac{k}{p}\right) \tag{9.16b}$$

reveals that S_u consists of replicas of D_u arranged along the frequency axis and centered at multiples of $u = 1/p$. These multiples are commonly referred to as aliases of D_u.

The determination as to whether these aliases may constitute a problem for our imaging task depends on the result of a comparison between the frequency content of our presampled signal $d(x)$ (the broadness of the function D_u) and the precision of the sampling process (the sampling frequency or sampling bandwidth $1/p$). There are two possibilities:

- If D_u is equal to zero for all frequencies u where

  $$|u| \geq u_{Nyquist} = \frac{1}{2p}, \tag{9.17}$$

  then the aliases on the frequency axis remain disjoint and each individual replication can be regarded as an undistorted representative of the original, Fourier transformed and presampled signal D_u. No information about the continuous presampled function $d = d(x)$ is lost. Quantitatively stated, for any arbitrary argument x, the function value $d(x)$ can be restored from its set of sampled values $s(k\,p)$ by means of a sinc-interpolation:

$$d(x) = \sum_{k=-\infty}^{\infty} \mathrm{sinc}\left(\frac{x-kp}{p}\right) s(kp). \tag{9.18}$$

This conclusion is referred to as the sampling or Nyquist theorem [9.8].

- If D_u does not vanish for frequencies u where $|u| > 1/(2p)$, then some overlap will occur between the D_u aliases because the distance between adjacent replications is lower than their width. In general, this constitutes a considerable distortion and the

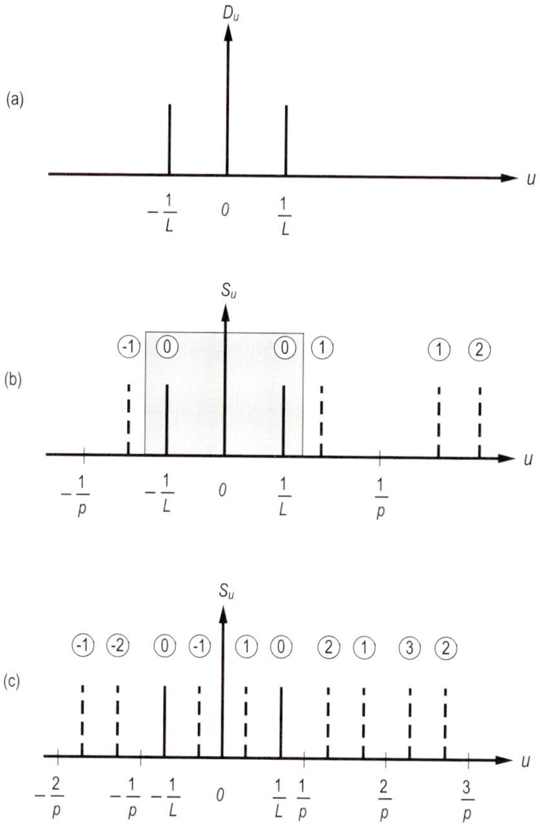

Figure 9.8
Sampling of a harmonic signal (periodicity L) in the frequency domain with different sampling increments. **(a)** Fourier transform of the original signal. **(b)** Sampling with distance $p = 0.375L < L/2$, the lowest frequency-aliased wave appears at $1/p - 1/L = 5/3L > 1/L$. **(c)** Sampling with excess distance $p = 0.75L > L/2$, the aliased-frequency appears at $1/p - 1/L = 1/3L < 1/L$. The same situations in the spatial domain is depicted in fig. 9.9.

function D_u cannot be recovered from S_u. Low frequency contributions with no correlation to structures in the irradiated body will appear in the spatial domain. These are referred to as aliasing artifacts or Moiré patterns.

Figs. 9.8 and 9.9 illustrate the sampling of a periodic signal with sufficient and insufficient sampling frequency.

Fig. 9.8b illustrates a case of uncritical sampling parameters: The replications of the original wave are so far away from one another that no overlap occurs. In principle, the cosine wave could be reconstructed by extracting the shaded frequency interval and then performing an inverse Fourier transform.

Fig. 9.8c shows a case of sampling with a sampling rate that is too low. Additional peaks appear inside the original frequency interval. Fig. 9.9 describes this situation in the spatial domain.

The pixel aperture blur, even though it constitutes a low pass filtering process to the image data, is not sufficient to avoid aliasing artifacts. The bandwidth $1/a$ of the pixel aperture is too broad to cut off frequencies above the Nyquist limit $1/2p \leq 1/2a$. Therefore, in order to avoid aliasing artifacts, the sampling frequency $1/p$ has to be larger than twice the highest spatial frequency in the object to be imaged. This can be estimated as the reciprocal diameter of the smallest detail in the object.

For instance, digital detectors used to detect very fine object details (e.g. microcalcifications in the human breast) have pixel sizes of 0.100 mm and smaller, whereas sampling increments between 0.125 mm and 0.200 mm are considered to be sufficient for chest radiography.

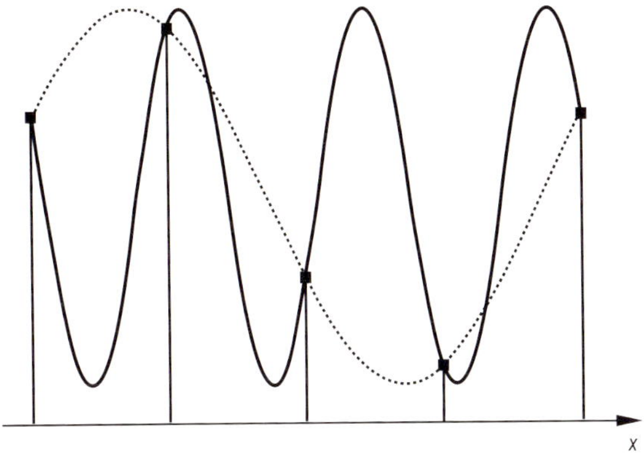

Figure 9.9
Aliasing due to the application of an excess sampling increment. An analog input signal (solid line) with a periodicity L is sampled with a sampling pitch $p = 0.75L$. A different harmonic with a higher frequency ($L/3$) (dotted line) would yield the same result.

9.2.3 Noise

9.2.3.1 Signal-to-noise ratio (*SNR*)

Images are usually corrupted by noise. The term noise can be broken down into stochastic and deterministic noise, with the latter also being referred to as fixed-pattern noise or image artifacts. Artifacts always retain the same appearance in repeated image recordings. Stochastic noise varies. In what follows, we restrict our discussion to noise as a stochastic phenomenon.

Fig. 9.10 shows an image of an objectless X-ray beam (flat field image) taken with a digital detector. A histogram displaying the frequency of (dimensionless) gray level occurrences caused by the number of absorbed X-photons in the detector as a function of the gray levels reveals that the gray levels are grouped around a mean value $<d>$ with a variance σ_d^2:

$$<d> = \alpha \frac{<N>}{A} TF(0) \tag{9.19}$$

α: Absorption coefficient of the detector
$<N>$: Average number of X-quanta impinging on the detector
A: Detector area, $TF(0)$: System gain

Given the Poisson statistics of the X-ray quanta, the variance of the gray levels can be expressed as

$$\sigma_d^2 = \alpha \frac{<N>}{A} TF(0)^2. \tag{9.20}$$

It follows that the mean signal intensity in an image has always to be seen in relation to the background noise. The signal-to-noise ratio is an important imaging-system performance parameter. In an ideal X-ray system (i.e. a system whose only noise

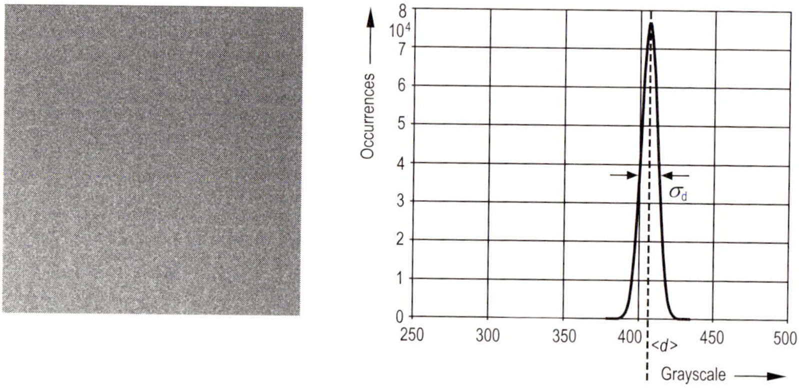

Figure 9.10
Flat field X-ray image from a digital flat panel detector and its histogram. The beam quality used to generate this image was RQA 3 (W anode/50 kV/10 mm Al), the applied input air kerma was 2.5 µGy.

source is the stochastic fluctuation of the X-ray photons), the signal-to-noise ratio amounts to (see fig. 9.11)

$$SNR = \frac{<d>}{\sigma_d} = \sqrt{\alpha \frac{<N>}{A}}. \quad (9.21)$$

9.2.3.2 Noise power spectrum (*NPS*)

Characterizing noise by its variance alone is not sufficient, as doing so provides no information about a possible spatial correlation between the noise pixels. This can be investigated by the autocorrelation function

$$r(x) = \langle f(x')f(x'+x)\rangle = \lim_{L\to\infty} \frac{1}{2L} \int_{-L}^{L} f(x')f(x'+x)\mathrm{d}x'. \quad (9.22)$$

The line noise $f(x)^2$ (measured in units mm) is a one dimensional signal that is generated from a two dimensional flat field image by summing up the gray level fluctuations along a long line

$$f(x)^2 = \int_{-Y}^{Y} (d(x,y) - <d>)^2 \mathrm{d}y. \quad (9.23)$$

A conclusion about the noise's spatial frequency dependence follows from the Fourier transform of the autocorrelation function, yielding the noise power or Wiener spectrum (typically measured in units mm^2)

$$NPS(u) = \int r(x)e^{-i2\pi ux}\mathrm{d}x = |F(u)|^2, \quad (9.24)$$

which is identical to the Fourier transform of the line noise (eq. (9.23)) squared (Wiener Khintchine relation).

By analogy to the case of discrete grayscale signal sampling, noise aliasing may also appear in digital detectors. This means that NPS contributions beyond the Nyquist border are folded back after the presampling step on account of a sampling rate that is too low (excess pixel pitch p). Hence, the same mechanism that generates Moiré artifacts in the image signal is also responsible for enhancing the final image noise [9.6]. It is therefore of interest to analyze the noise power spectrum's dependence on detector parameters such as gain and modulation transfer function. For this purpose, a modeling of the elementary processes in the detector is required. Here, it is essential

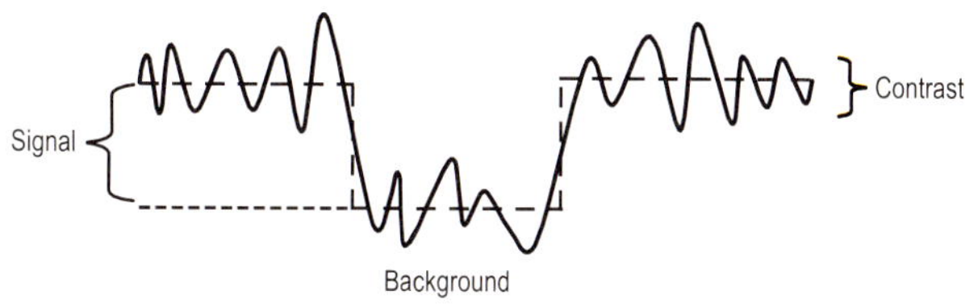

Figure 9.11 Scheme depicting the definition of the term contrast-to-noise ratio

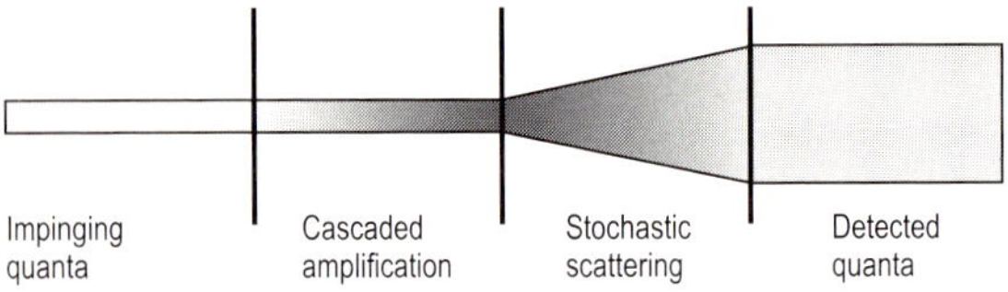

Figure 9.12 Cascaded quantum multiplication and scattering in an X-ray detector

to consider four basic processes, including deterministic blur, stochastic scattering, stochastic amplification [9.7] and noise generated by detector electronics.

In the framework of LSI theory, *NPS* transfer by the detector is given

$$NPS_{out}(u) = NPS_{in}(u)\, TF(u)^2 = NPS_{in}(u)\, MTF(u)^2 TF(0)^2. \tag{9.25}$$

TF(*u*): Transfer function, Fourier transform of the line spread function

TF(0): System gain

The input Wiener spectrum of the X-ray photons absorbed does not depend on spatial frequency and can be written as

$$NPS_{in}(u) = \alpha \frac{<N>}{A}. \tag{9.26}$$

A: Detector area

It follows that the noise power spectrum of an X-ray image can essentially be expressed as

$$NPS_{out}^{LSI}(u) = \alpha \frac{<N>}{A} MTF(u)^2 TF(0)^2. \tag{9.27}$$

While this deterministic model does not take into account additional stochastic noise sources in the detector that stem from quantum amplification and scattering, the function of an X-ray detector depends on the generation of many additional quanta by an absorbed X-ray quantum (fig. 9.12). Output fluence q_{out} and absorbed input fluence q_{abs} of quanta are linked by

$$q_{out}(x) = G q_{abs}(x). \tag{9.28}$$

Given the stochastic nature of this multiplication process, the gain G has a variance σ_G^2 so that the average noise at the output is larger than that of the amplified input

$$\sigma_{out}^2 = G^2 \sigma_{abs}^2 + q_{abs} \sigma_G^2.$$

The noise power spectrum after stochastic amplification is expressed as

$$NPS_{out}^{Gain}(u) = G^2 NPS_{in}(u) + \sigma_G^2 q_{abs}. \tag{9.29}$$

Given that the multiplied quanta in the amplification process are laterally scattered, thereby decreasing the detector's modulation transfer function, the noise power spectrum for stochastic scattering can be expressed as

$$NPS_{out}^{Scatter}(u) = (NPS_{in}(u) - q_{abs}) MTF(u)^2 + q_{abs}. \tag{9.30}$$

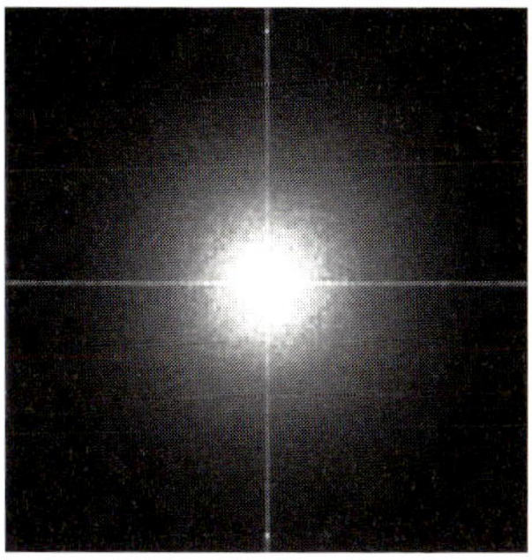
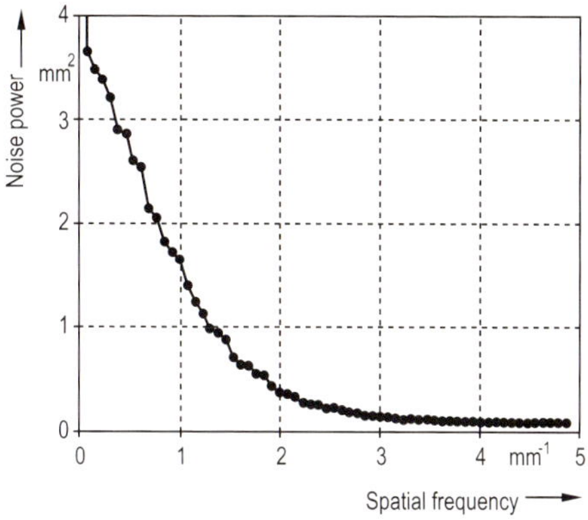

Figure 9.13
A flat-panel detector's two-dimensional noise power spectrum. 2D power spectrum of the signal distribution shown **left**. The 1D noise power spectrum **(right)** corresponds to a line through the center of the 2D spectrum.

Given that all three mechanisms (deterministic amplification, stochastic amplification, and lateral blur) are essentially present, the final Wiener spectrum is derived by cascading the individual spectra (i.e. each spectrum acts as an input noise power spectrum for its successor).

Noise generated by detector electronics is mostly of a thermal nature. The noise power is proportional to the (absolute) temperature and to the bandwidth of the signal processing path, which on the other hand is inversely proportional to the image read-out time. X-ray detectors are to be designed in a way that would permit one to disregard electronic noise with respect to quantum noise, although this noise may have to be considered in the case of very low quantum fluences.

Fig. 9.13 offers an example of a digital X-ray detector's noise power spectrum.

9.2.3.3 Detective quantum efficiency (*DQE*)

Although an imaging system is completely specified by its input signal, gain, *MTF* and output noise power spectrum, one would prefer to characterize it (at least in principle) in terms of a single function that is independent of the input signal. The notation of detective quantum efficiency was introduced for this purpose [9.8]

$$DQE(u) = \frac{SNR_{\text{out}}(u)^2}{SNR_{\text{in}}(u)^2}. \tag{9.31}$$

Given that the squared signal-to-noise ratio of an X-ray input field amounts to the average number <*N*> of X-ray quanta (eq. (9.21), one also defines a number of noise equivalent quanta (*NEQ*) for the output signal [9.9]

$$SNR_{\text{out}}^2 = NEQ. \tag{9.32}$$

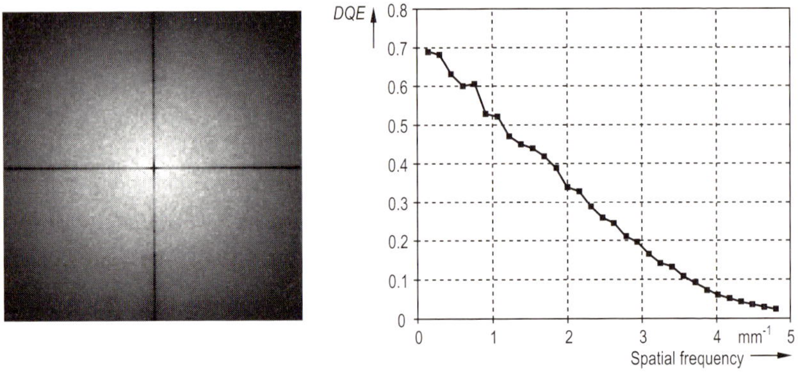

Figure 9.14
Two-dimensional *DQE* image taken from fig. 9.10 and corresponding *DQE* profile plotted in a diagonal direction

The *NEQ* depends on spatial frequency and has to be considered in the spatial frequency domain (with unit $1/\text{mm}^2$). One obtains

$$NEQ(u) = \frac{\langle d \rangle^2 \, MTF(u)^2}{NPS(u)}. \tag{9.33}$$

$\langle d \rangle$: Average output gray level

The detective quantum efficiency can thus be expressed as

$$DQE(u) = \frac{NEQ(u)}{q_{\text{in}}} = \frac{\langle d \rangle^2 MTF(u)^2}{q_{\text{in}} NPS(u)} = \frac{(\textit{signal transfer factor})^2}{(\textit{noise transfer factor})^2}. \tag{9.34}$$

$q_{\text{in}} = \frac{\langle N \rangle}{A}$: Input quantum fluence

This equation also yields the basis for the measurement of the *DQE*. An example is given in fig. 9.14. If stochastic noise sources were absent, the detective quantum efficiency would amount to the absorption coefficient α of the quanta in the detector (see eqs. (9.19, 9.27)).

9.3 References

[9.1] D.C. Champeney
Fourier transforms and their physical applications
Academic Press 1973, London and New York 1973

[9.2] W. Hillen, U. Schiebel, T. Zaengel
Imaging Performance of a Digital Storage Phosphor System
Medical Physics 14 (1987), 744-751

[9.3] H. Fujita, D.Y. Tsai, T. Itoh, K. Doi, J. Morishita, K. Ueda, A. Ohtsuka
A Simple Method for Determining the Modulation Transfer Function in Digital Radiography
IEEE Transactions in Medical Imaging 11(1992), 34-39

[9.4] E. Buhr, S.Günther-Kohfahl, U. Neitzel
Accuracy of a Simple Method for Deriving the Presampled Modulation Transfer Function of a Digital Radiographic System from an Edge Image
Medical Physics 30(2003), 2323-2331

[9.5] International Electrotechnical Commission
Medical Electrical Equipment – Characteristics of Digital X-Ray Imaging Devices – Determination of the Detective Quantum Efficiency
IEC 62220-1, 2003

[9.6] J.T. Dobbins III, D.L. Ergun, L. Rutz, D.A. Hinshaw, H. Blume, D.C. Clark
DQE(f) of Four Generations of Computed Radiography Devices
Medical Physics 22(1995), 1581-1593

[9.7] I.A. Cunningham, R. Shaw
Signal to noise optimization of medical imaging systems
J. Opt. Soc. Am. A 16 (1999), 621

[9.8] H.H. Barrett, W. Swindell
Radiological Imaging – The Theory of Image Formation, Detection, and Processing
Academic Press, San Diego 1981-1996
Lippincott Williams & Wilkins, Philadelphia 1990

[9.9] I.A. Cunningham
Applied linear systems theory
in Handbook of Medical Imaging 1. Physics and Psychophysics
SPIE Press, Bellingham (WA) 2000

10 Principles of image reconstruction

10.1 Introduction

The aim of medical diagnostics to obtain detailed information from within the body of a patient is only partially achieved by classic X-ray imaging. The X-ray image represents a silhouette or a projection of the object under investigation. Details from a region of the body that the physician is interested in may remain obscured by structures above or below the region. The art of radiology includes the skill of aligning the X-ray beam with respect to the patient in a manner that ensures that as little unwanted organ superimposition as possible will appear in the image.

Methods were developed as early as the 1930s to blur the structures above and below the plane of interest, for instance, by shifting the X-ray tube against the detector during image exposure so that an X-ray beam would hit the same point only in a single plane of the investigated object (fig. 10.1). While this method, commonly referred to as planigraphy or tomography, is still in use today, it does not bring about the complete removal of structure superimposition and the resulting X-ray images are still

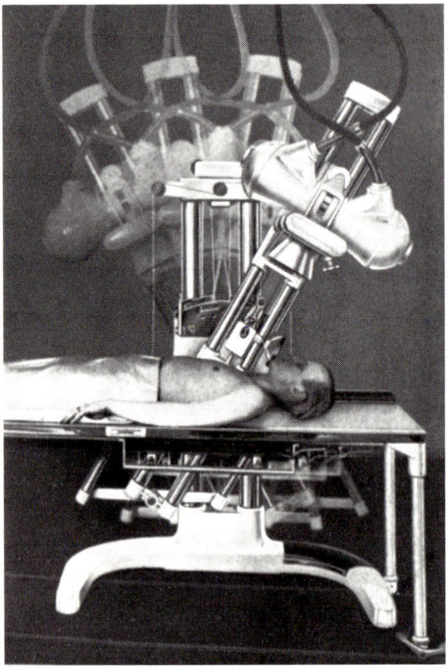

Figure 10.1
Linear tomography apparatus developed by Grossmann (1938)

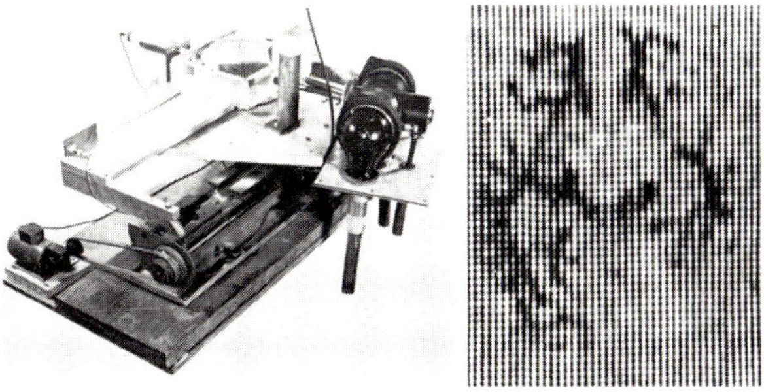

Figure 10.2 Hounsfield's experimental setup for computed tomography [10.3]

lacking in sharpness. Small X-ray attenuation differences in soft tissue that may be indicative of tumor formation remain hidden.

Introduced in the early 1970s, computed tomography (CT) has revolutionized not only diagnostic radiology, but the whole field of medicine. CT enables one to avoid blurred contours altogether via a mathematically exact reconstruction of the image derived from digital projection data. The mathematical principles behind the procedure were already established in 1917 by the mathematician Johann Radon who introduced the concept of reconstructing an object on the basis of its line integrals [10.1]. Unaware of the work of his predecessor, the South African nuclear physicist Alan M. Cormack developed a method of obtaining the distribution of X-ray attenuation coefficients for body tissue in 1963 in the context of attempting to improve upon existing methods of radiation treatment planning [10.2]. Cormack's discovery remained largely unnoticed. It was not until the late 1960s that Sir Godfrey Hounsfield developed the first clinically useful X-ray CT scanner (fig. 10.2) [10.3]. In 1979, Hounsfield and Cormack were awarded the Nobel Prize in medicine for their work.

Image reconstruction is now routinely used in several areas of medical imaging, including nuclear medicine, magnetic resonance imaging and volume CT. In the present chapter, we offer a brief summary of the basic principles behind image reconstruction. Readers may wish to refer to the standard works [10.4, 10.5, 10.6] for a more comprehensive discussion of the Fourier transform as the basis of image reconstruction. For the sake of simplicity, we forgo extensive mathematical precision and refer instead to the other chapters in this book that address specific imaging modalities. Further details are also available in the relevant standard works [e.g. 10.7] and in the scientific literature.

10.2 Basic principles

CT is based on the rectilinear propagation and attenuation of X-rays. Fig. 10.3 offers an example of a simple scanning geometry. The connection line L between the focus of an X-ray source and an X-ray detector is moved over the object at various projection

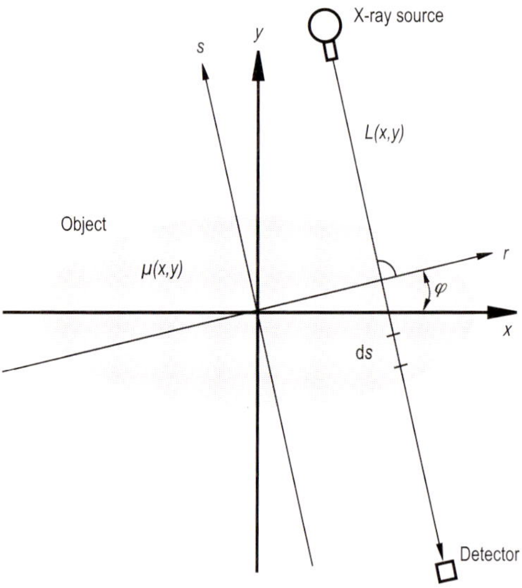

Figure 10.3
Basic CT scanning geometry

angles φ. The very first CT scanners applied such a geometry, which is why they were referred to as dual motion scanners. Today, complete projections are taken using fan or cone beams generated by the X-ray tube and deploying row or area detectors. By way of exemplifying the reconstruction principle, we restrict our frame of reference to parallel beam geometry, which is also applied in the fields of nuclear medicine and magnetic resonance imaging.

The intensity measured by the detector can be expressed as follows:

$$J(r,\varphi) = J_0 e^{-\int \mu \mathrm{d}s} \tag{10.1a}$$

J_0: Intensity of the X-ray source, μ: Attenuation coefficient

Taking the logarithm enables one to eliminate the exponential function and directly derive the line integrals of the spatial distribution of the attenuation coefficients μ. These are referred to in this context as the one-dimensional projection of a two-dimensional object:

$$P(r,\varphi) = \ln \frac{J_0}{J(r,\varphi)} = \int \mu \mathrm{d}s \tag{10.1b}$$

Given that the projection is carried out along lines

$$L(x,y) = r - x\cos\varphi - y\sin\varphi = 0, \tag{10.2}$$

it can also be expressed as

$$P(r,\varphi) = \iint \mu(x,y)\,\delta(r - x\cos\varphi - y\sin\varphi)\,\mathrm{d}x\,\mathrm{d}y. \tag{10.1c}$$

δ: Dirac function

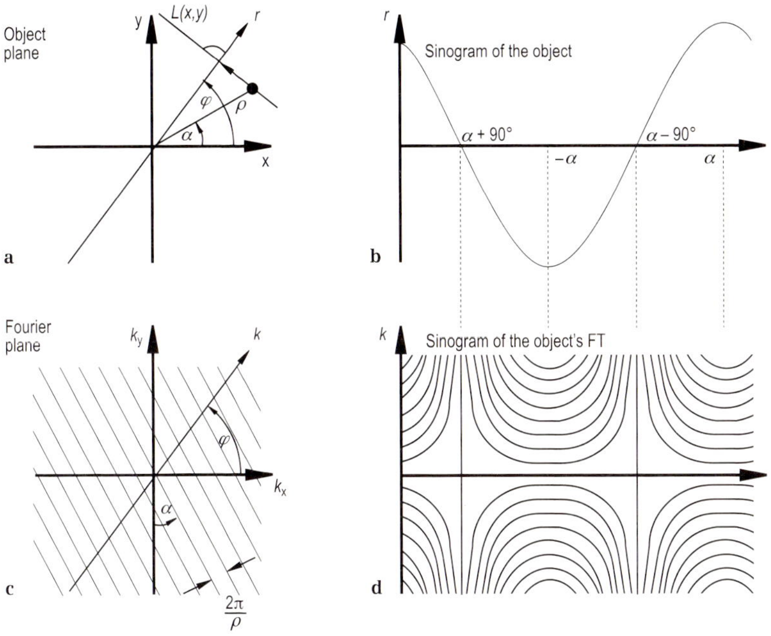

Figure 10.4
Sinogram **(b)** of a single point in the x,y plane **(a)**. The 2D Fourier transform of this point yields a plane wave **(c)**. The FT of the sinogram **(d)** is identical to the sinogram of the object's 2D FT.

This relation is commonly referred to as Radon transformation. A representation of P as a function of the rotation or projection angle φ and the distance between the center of rotation and beam r is referred to as a sinogram (fig. 10.4).

10.3 2D Fourier reconstruction

The task is now to reconstruct the physical property $\mu(x,y)$ (called density) of a 2D object from its set of projections $P(r,\varphi)$. We begin by taking the Fourier transform of eq. (10.1b):

$$p(k,\varphi) = \int P(r,\varphi)\mathrm{e}^{-ikr}\mathrm{d}r \tag{10.3}$$

k: Spatial frequency

to arrive at

$$p(k,\varphi) = \iint \mu \mathrm{e}^{-ikr}\mathrm{d}s\mathrm{d}r. \tag{10.4a}$$

If we now express the above equation in Cartesian coordinates, we wind up with the following result:

$$p(k_x, k_y) = \iint \mu(x,y) e^{-i(k_x x + k_y y)} dx dy. \tag{10.4b}$$

This result reveals that the 2D Fourier transform of the density distribution $\mu(x,y)$ (eq. (10.4b)) is identical to the 1D Fourier transform of the measured projections or line integrals (eq. (10.3)), a fact that is explained by the Fourier slice theorem.

The density distribution can be obtained from eq. (10.4b) via an inverse Fourier transformation:

$$\mu(x,y) = \frac{1}{(2\pi)^2} \iint p(k_x, k_y) e^{i(k_x x + k_y y)} dk_x dk_y \tag{10.5}$$

One method of computing the density $\mu(x,y)$ is to convert the Fourier transform projections $p(k,\varphi)$ into Cartesian coordinates so that the algorithm of a fast Fourier transform (FFT) can be applied. Such a process is referred to as regridding.

Regridding is commonly performed in nuclear medicine and magnetic resonance imaging. In the case of CT, the task of interpolation that is necessary for regridding is largely avoided because interpolation inaccuracies may lead to artifacts during the 2D FFT. Filtered backprojection (FBP) represents an alternative method of reconstruction.

10.4 Number of data

It is necessary to fill the spatial frequency domain also called Fourier space (figs. 10.4c, 10.5) with data according to the sampling theorem (see chapter 9). This means that the maximum spatial sampling frequency k_{max} determines the size Δr of the reconstructed picture element (pixel):

$$k_{max} = \frac{\pi}{\Delta r} \tag{10.6a}$$

On the other hand, an object with maximum diameter $2A_{max}$ requires a sampling width in Fourier space of

$$\Delta k = \frac{\pi}{A_{max}}. \tag{10.6b}$$

It follows that the increment necessary to change the projection angle is

$$\Delta\varphi = \frac{\Delta r}{A_{max}} = \frac{\Delta k}{k_{max}}. \tag{10.6c}$$

The minimum number of projections N_φ that is necessary (half a rotation) can thus be expressed as

$$N_\varphi = \frac{\pi}{\Delta\varphi} = \frac{\pi A_{max}}{\Delta r}, \tag{10.7a}$$

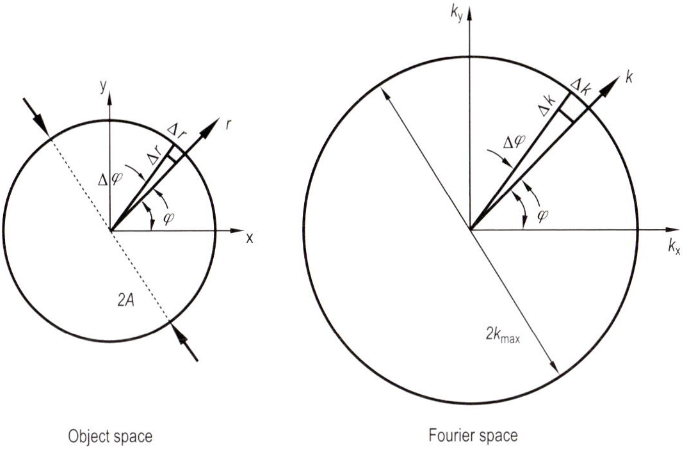

Figure 10.5 Comparison of object (*r*-) and Fourier (*k*-) space

with the number of samples N_r required for a projection being

$$N_r = \frac{2A_{max}}{\Delta r}. \tag{10.7b}$$

It follows that for isotropic resolution

$$N_\varphi \geq \frac{\pi}{2} N_r. \tag{10.7c}$$

10.5 Filtered backprojection

In order to continue with polar coordinates, eq. (10.5) can be rewritten as

$$\mu(r,\varphi) = \frac{1}{(2\pi)^2} \int_0^\pi \int_{-\infty}^{\infty} p(k,\varphi) e^{ikr} |k| \, dk \, d\varphi. \tag{10.8}$$

However, no fast algorithm (such as the FFT in Cartesian coordinates) is known for the 2D Fourier transform in polar coordinates. Therefore the quantity

$$P^*(r,\varphi) = \frac{1}{(2\pi)^2} \int_{-\infty}^{\infty} |k| p(k,\varphi) e^{ikr} dk \tag{10.9}$$

is 'backprojected' into the imaging plane giving

$$\mu(x,y) = \int_0^\pi P^*(r,\varphi) d\varphi. \tag{10.10}$$

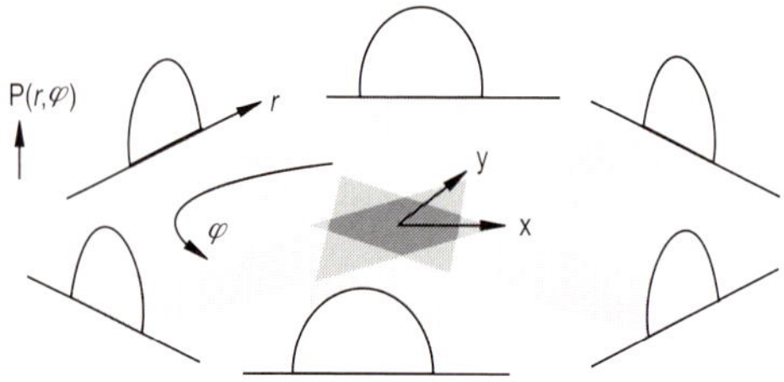

Figure 10.6
Principle of backprojection. The intensity of a projection is added to all points lying on rays perpendicular to the projection.

in order to obtain the density distribution in Cartesian coordinates. In other words, the quantities $P^*(r,\varphi)$ are superimposed according to their projection angles φ in the image (x,y) plane (fig. 10.6).

The variable P^* is referred to as a filtered projection because it can be derived from the measured projection P via convolution with a filter kernel $H(r)$:

$$P^*(r,\varphi) = \int H(r')P(r-r',\varphi)dr' = H(r) \otimes P(r,\varphi). \qquad (10.11)$$

Fourier transformation theory gives rise to the law that a convolution in space is equivalent to a multiplication in the Fourier domain. The spatial filter $H(r)$ thus corresponds to the Fourier transform of $H(k) = |k|$ for $k \le k_{max}$ and $H(k) = 0$ for $k > k_{max}$, where the cut-off frequency k_{max} is determined by the maximum sampling frequency π/d given by the detector separation d:

$$H(r) = \frac{1}{(2\pi)^2}\int_{-k_{max}}^{k_{max}} |k|\mathrm{e}^{ikr}\mathrm{d}k = \frac{2}{(2\pi)^2}k_{max}^2\left(\frac{\sin k_{max}r}{k_{max}r} - 2\left(\frac{\sin\frac{k_{max}r}{2}}{k_{max}r}\right)^2\right). \qquad (10.12)$$

The filter kernel for a linear ramp that is cut off[1)] at spatial frequency k_{max} has been developed by Ramachandran and Lakshminarayanan. A modified filter kernel developed by Shepp and Logan is often applied. This filter kernel multiplies the linear ramp that is cut off by a sinc function (fig. 10.7), thereby accounting for the finite length of the detector element.

If one were to backproject the unfiltered projection P, one would obtain a modified density μ^*, also referred to as a layergram:

---

1) Continuous sampling of the projections corresponding to $k_{max} = \infty$ would give

$$H(r) = \frac{1}{(2\pi)^2}\int_{-\infty}^{\infty} |k|\mathrm{e}^{ikr}\mathrm{d}k = \lim_{\varepsilon \to 0}\begin{cases} -\frac{1}{r^2} & r > \varepsilon \\ \frac{1}{\varepsilon^2} & r < \varepsilon \end{cases}$$

with a singularity at $r = 0$ arising from the requirement that

$$\int_{-\infty}^{\infty} H(r)\mathrm{d}r = H(k=0) = 0 \quad .$$

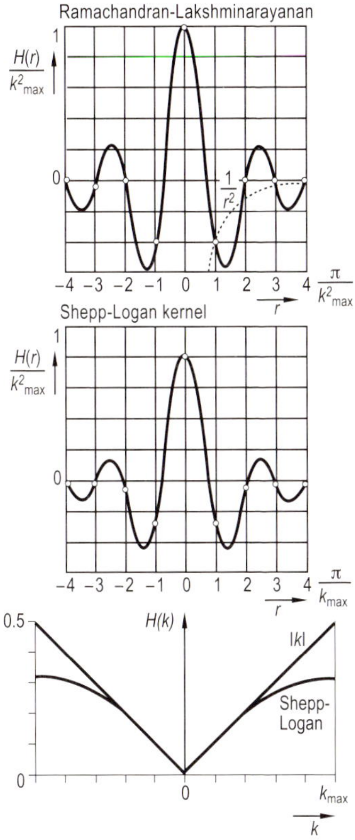

Figure 10.7
Filter kernels commonly used for backprojection. The Ramachandran-Lakshminarayanan kernel is the Fourier transform of the linear ramp with a cutoff at spatial frequency k_{max}. The Shepp-Logan kernel is shallower than the linear ramp at cut-off frequency k_{max}.

$$\mu^*(x,y) = \int P(r,\varphi)\mathrm{d}\varphi = \frac{1}{2\pi r} \otimes P(r). \tag{10.13}$$

The kernel $\frac{1}{2\pi r}$ represents the point spread function of a single (unfiltered) object point. The above relation is referred to as a Hilbert transform. Fig. 10.8 offers a comparison of backprojection and filtered backprojection.

10.6 3D projection reconstruction

The image reconstruction that has been described so far is limited to 2D objects. However, it can also be extended (also on the basis of line integrals) to 3D objects. A sufficient condition for an exact reconstruction, according to which all of the planes that intersect the object are required to intersect the source path at least once, has been derived by Tuy [10.8].

One straightforward method of reconstructing a 3D object is to separate it into several parallel slices, as is done, for instance, in nuclear medicine. In the case of CT, the pa-

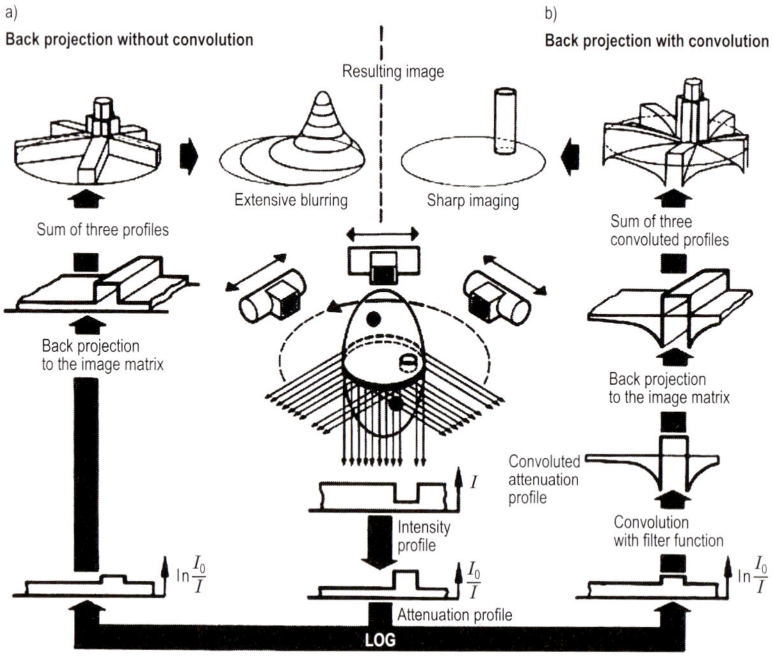

Figure 10.8
Basic concept of image reconstruction via backprojection in CT. A superimposition of attenuation profiles according to their projection direction causes considerable blurring **(a)**, which can be removed via convolution with a filter kernel $H(r)$ **(b)**.

tient is moved continuously through a rotating source detector arrangement and is thus scanned according to a spiral scheme (fig. 13.4, cf. chapter 13). The relevant geometry would involve a 3D reconstruction derived from parallel beams hitting a plane detector.

While digital area detectors have indeed been introduced to radiography (see chapter 12.4), X-ray sources that emit parallel beams are scarcely conceivable. Approximate algorithms have therefore been developed to reconstruct 3D objects on the basis of cone beams. The most widely used algorithm is one developed by Feldkamp, Davis and Kress (FDK) in 1984 [10.9]. Fig. 10.9 shows the basic geometry: a point-like X-ray source emitting a cone beam that hits an area detector.

Such a geometry would enable one to approximately reconstruct a cube (fig. 10.10) with the following edge length:

$$d \approx \frac{DR_0}{F + \frac{D}{2}} \tag{10.14}$$

D: Detector width, R_0: Source circle radius
F: Source detector distance

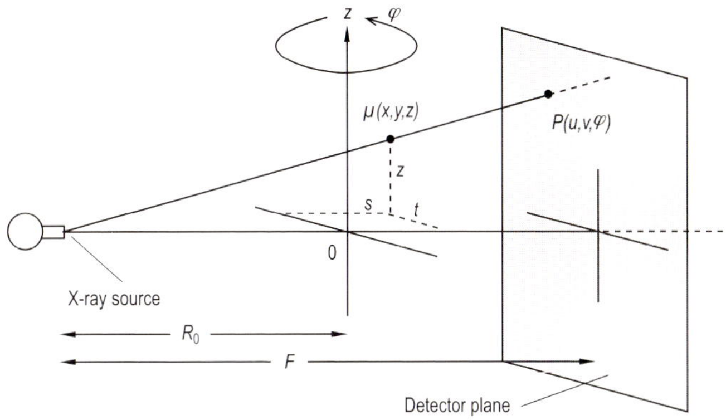

Figure 10.9 Cone beam geometry for scanning 3D objects

Clearly, Tuy's condition is not fulfilled, as planes that run through the object parallel to the source circle are not intersected.

Given that the relevant objects are larger than this cube, the projections are truncated. It is thus necessary to take account of this fact by applying approximations during the image reconstruction process (e.g. by extrapolating the missing data and using dedicated filter kernels).

The FDK approximation for the density that is to be reconstructed is a weighted back-projection

$$\mu(x,y,z) = \frac{1}{\pi}\int_0^{2\pi} w^2 Q_\varphi(u,v,\varphi)\,d\varphi \qquad (10.15)$$

$w = \frac{R_0}{(R_0 - s)}$: Weighting factor, R_0: Source circle radius

F: Distance between detector and source

s, t: Coordinates in the system rotating with the detector X-ray source (fig. 10.9)

$u = \frac{Ft}{(R_0 - s)}$: Abscissa on the detector for ray passing point (x,y,z) in the object

$v = \frac{Fz}{(R_0 - s)}$: Ordinate on the detector for ray passing point (x,y,z) in the object

of the quantity $Q_\varphi(u,v,\varphi)$, which is derived from a 1D filtering of the weighted line integrals $P_\varphi(u,v,\varphi)$

$$Q_\varphi(u,v,\varphi) = \frac{F}{\sqrt{F^2 + u^2 + v^2}} P_\varphi(u,v,\varphi) \otimes H(u) \qquad (10.16)$$

$H(u)$: Standard CT filter (eq. (10.10)), u,v: Coordinates on the detector

The detector coordinates u, v refer to the root point of a ray passing the point (x,y,z) in the object characterized by coordinates (s,t,z) with respect to the central beam and the center of rotation. The FDK algorithm for $z = 0$ is identical to the exact 2D fan-beam algorithm used in single slice CT.

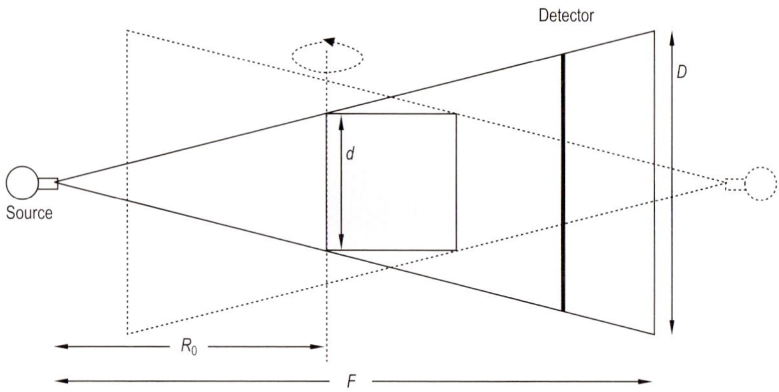

Figure 10.10 Object size that can be reconstructed with cone beam CT

10.7 Backprojection applying homogeneous coordinates

The necessary backprojection mapping between the coordinates x, y, z of the volume that is to be reconstructed and the detector coordinates u, v can be effectively computed by applying projection matrices. If we assume that $X = (x, y, z, 1)$ represents the projective or homogeneous coordinates of a volume element's (voxel) position in the object that is to be reconstructed from the line integral hitting a detector element at coordinates $U = (u, v, 1)$, then the 3 by 4 matrix Π_φ will map the voxel position X to the detector element's position U according to

$$U \propto \Pi_\varphi X \tag{10.17}$$

Using projective rather than Cartesian coordinates has the advantage of enabling one to describe a shift and a rotation between coordinate systems by a single matrix. This is ideal for a backprojection algorithm that sums up the quantity $Q(u_b, v_b)$ at each voxel x, y, z and at each projection angle φ. If we assume that Δx, Δy, Δz are voxel edge lengths, then a voxel numbered i, j, k will map to the corresponding detector coordinate as

$$U' = \Pi_\varphi(X_0 + (\Delta x\, i, \Delta y\, j, \Delta y\, k, 0)) = \Pi_\varphi X_0 + a\,i + b\,j + ck \tag{10.18}$$

The three-component vectors a, b, c correspond to the first three columns of the projection matrix Π_φ multiplied by the corresponding voxel sizes. Eq. (10.18) results in homogeneous detector coordinates (u', v', λ) that enable one to derive the coordinates of the detector element via renormalization: $u = u'/\lambda$, $v = v'/\lambda$. If we normalize $\Pi_\varphi(3{,}4) = 1$, the weighting factors for backprojection (eq. (10.15)) follow directly as $w = \lambda^{-1}$.

It is therefore necessary to perform exactly one matrix multiplication $(\Pi_\varphi X_0)$ for each projection.

To summarize, the algorithm for 3D backprojection can be formulated as follows [10.10]:

```
Loop1 over all projection angles φ
      compute reference point Π_φ X_0
      compute auxiliary vectors a, b, c
      Loop2 over all voxels i, j, k
            compute detector coordinate u_b, v_b on source voxel line
            add weighted and filtered projection
      End Loop2
End Loop1
```

We will refrain in the present context from offering an explicit description of the projection matrixes Π_φ in terms of parameters that describe the projection geometry (projection angle, source detector distance, center of rotation). These can be regarded as system properties that are either determined analytically or experimentally by scanning a dedicated phantom. 3D backprojection with projection matrices is applied in cone beam CT as it is in the case of a rotating C-arm used for interventional X-ray imaging in the operation room (see chapter 5) and 3D angiography (see chapter 12.6).

10.8 References

[10.1] J.H. Radon
Über die Bestimmung von Funktionen durch ihre Integralwerte längs gewisser Mannigfaltigkeiten
Ber. vor Sächs. Akad. Wiss. 69 (1917), 262-277
or
J. Radon
On determination of functions from their integral values along certain manifolds
IEEE Trans. Med. Imag., 1986; MI-5(4): 170-176

[10.2] A.M. Cormack
Representation of a function by its line integrals, with some radiological applications
J. Appl. Phys. 34 (1963), 2722-2727

[10.3] G.N. Hounsfield
Computerized transverse axial scanning (tomography), Part I. Description of system
Br. J. Radiol. 46 (1973), 1016
and
J. Lindsten
Nobel Lectures in Physiology or Medicine, 1971-1980
World Scientific Publishing Co.,
Singapore 1992

[10.4] D.C. Champeney
Fourier transforms and their physical applications
Academic Press 1973, London and New York 1973

[10.5] R.N. Bracewell
The Fourier transform and its applications, 3rd ed.
McGraw-Hill, Boston 2000

[10.6] E.O. Brigham
The fast Fourier transform and its applications
Prentice-Hall, Eaglewood Cliffs 1988

[10.7] F. Natterer, F. Wübbeling
Mathematical methods in image reconstruction
SIAM – Society for industrial and applied mathematics, Philadelphia 2001

[10.8] H. Tuy
An inversion formula for cone-beam reconstruction
SIAM J. Appl. Math. 43 (1983), 546-552

[10.9] L.A. Feldkamp, L.C. Davis, J.W. Kress
Practical cone-beam algorithm
J. Opt. Soc. Amer. A6 (1984), 612-619

[10.10] K. Wiesent, K. Barth, N. Navab, P. Durlak, T. Brunner, O. Schuetz, W. Seissler
Enhanced 3-D reconstruction algorithm for C-arm systems suitable for interventional procedures
IEEE Transactions on medical imaging 19 (2000), 391-403

Part IV – Image Instrumentation

11 Image displays

Somewhat more that one hundred years after the invention of the cathode ray tube (CRT) by Karl Ferdinand Braun in the year 1897, electronic image displays are a standard tool of primary diagnostic interpretation in the field of radiology. The increasing use of information technology, including the networking of radiology departments to provide remote and comprehensive access to critical information, has helped to bring about a surge in diagnostic productivity. This development has been accompanied by an opportunity to reduce healthcare costs. In an electronic and networked environment, the electronic display device represents the important interface between the image acquisition system and the medical user. What is lost during the acquisition or image reconstruction process can naturally not be recovered at the moment of display. The relevant information available in the image data need not be lost on account of the display process.

The digitization of imaging modalities began with the advent of computed tomography in the 1970s. At present, projection radiography – the modality that presumably meets the highest information content demands per image – is undergoing a transition to digital detectors. This development has lead to a similar digitization in the area of image display. Digital imaging has the advantage of enabling one to independently optimize image acquisition systems and output media (i.e. the display) so as to meet the requirements of the radiological diagnostic process.

An image displayed on an electronic display device is referred to as soft copy while the film image is referred to as hard copy.

In the present chapter, we offer a brief review of the human visual system (HVS) as it relates to soft-copy reading before moving on to present an overview of the most commonly used display technologies, including cathode ray tubes (CRT) and liquid crystal displays (LCD). We then venture a glance at a number of potential future technologies before concluding the chapter with a technical characterization of monitors.

11.1 Advantages and challenges of soft-copy reading

- *Digital image processing*
  Given that the data are provided in digital form by imaging acquisition systems, it is obvious that digital image processing methods can be applied directly to the images without first having to digitize them, as would be the case for film radiographs. Examples of such processing include contrast enhancement by applying look-up tables and edge enhancement by filtering. The image display can be customized to various applications, depending on the circumstances involved. For instance, the display can be designed for a specific task, for a specific user, for a specific organ, or

for specific ambient light conditions. Furthermore, the importance of electronic displays suited to the task of visualizing data from three-dimensional methods is likely to increase.

- *Elimination of film problems*
  Replacing film by soft-copy reading will also help to eliminate specific film problems. These include environmental problems associated with film chemistry, lost studies and incorrectly exposed films. Siegel [11.1] has reported that the rate of lost examinations dropped by more than a factor of 10 and the image retake rate dropped from 5% to around 0.8% following the introduction of picture archiving and communication systems (PACS).
- *Information technology*
  The replacement of film is only one aspect of the transition to the *filmless* hospital. A major additional aspect centers on the provision of access to crucial information via modern information technology. The simultaneous and instantaneous availability of images at different sites in a networked environment is one of the most important benefits. The healthcare process will include immediate access not only to images, but also to all relevant patient information.
- *User interface*
  The major differences in the handling of images on electronic displays of film radiographs will necessitate the creation of user interfaces for specific tasks. Strategies for the handling of images (e.g. their presentation and storage) will have to be developed. The transfer of images via networks will have to be fast enough to avoid time delays. Similarly, the reading process will have to be sufficiently quick for soft-copy interpretation to have a clear value. All of these challenges will have to be addressed as health care professionals make the transition to primary soft-copy reading in radiology.
- *Image quality*
  The crucial prerequisite, however, for the acceptance of soft-copy diagnosis is image quality. Do electronic displays provide sufficient image quality to render all of the information necessary for a safe diagnosis? Which technical approaches should be applied to provide and secure the best possible image quality in clinical practice? To answer these questions, it will be helpful to first have a look at the human visual system (HVS).

11.2 Impact of the human visual system on display design

An overall optimization of the imaging chain presupposes a consideration of the human visual system because this system is a part of the entire system. In order to optimize reading performance, it will be necessary to understand how the HVS is influenced by specific reading circumstances and ambient light conditions (cf. chapter 1). The technical parameters of display devices will thus have to be matched to the characteristics of the HVS, which comprises the optical system of the eye and the information processing that takes place from the receptor cells in the retina to the visual cortex [11.2]. In what follows, we review some of the most relevant properties of the human visual system, including contrast sensitivity, spatial resolution and dynamic range [11.3].

11.2.1 Contrast sensitivity and spatial resolution

Contrast sensitivity is defined by the smallest perceivable difference ΔL in the luminance of an object of luminance L in front of a background or surround luminance L_0. It can be expressed as the inverse threshold contrast:

$$\text{Contrast sensitivity} = \frac{L_0}{\Delta L} = \frac{L_0}{L - L_0}. \tag{11.1}$$

Contrast sensitivity is usually determined via observer experiments involving certain test targets such as a square in the center of a screen in front of an area of constant luminance. It is the measure of the probability that a standard observer will be able to perceive this object. The task of experimentally determining contrast sensitivity is rather complicated because the result depends on the test pattern, its size, its shape and its spatial frequency content. Furthermore, contrast sensitivity depends on the particular background signal, the noise in the image itself and the observer.

The model introduced by Barten [11.4] seems to offer an appropriate description of contrast sensitivity as a function of the luminance and spatial frequency of a test pattern consisting of a square with sinusoidal modulation in front of a uniform background. Fig. 11.1 shows the calculated contrast sensitivity for this test pattern [11.5] of 2 degrees extension.

The curves are parameterized by background luminance values ranging from 0.1 cd/m^2 to 1,000 cd/m^2. The situation illustrated in fig. 11.1 represents the ideal case because it is valid for adapted observers who are not subject to threshold elevation on account of insufficient adaptation to a certain luminance, masking effects [11.6] or irritating extraneous light. The graph demonstrates that the contrast sensitivity of the HVS reaches its maximum for spatial frequencies between 3 cycles/degree and 6 cycles/degree. Assuming a viewing distance of 0.4 m, these values correspond to image object sizes of 1.2 mm and 0.6 mm, respectively.

Contrast sensitivity for higher spatial frequencies rapidly decreases depending on luminance. The resolution limit is approached at roughly 30/degree, which corroborates the claim that the eye can resolve approximately 1 arc minute.

Contrast sensitivity for low spatial frequencies is independent of luminance in the case of medium to high luminance values. This is known as the Weber-Fechner law [11.7]. Contrast sensitivity decreases roughly according to $L^{1/2}$ as the luminance is lowered below a few cd/m^2. This dependency is known as the de Vries-Rose law [11.7]. This range marks the transition from photopic vision with cone receptors to scotopic vision with rods – where visual acuity is strongly impaired.

Contrast sensitivity can also be ascertained as a function of temporal frequency [11.6]. Contrast sensitivity for frequencies above a certain limit falls below the threshold of

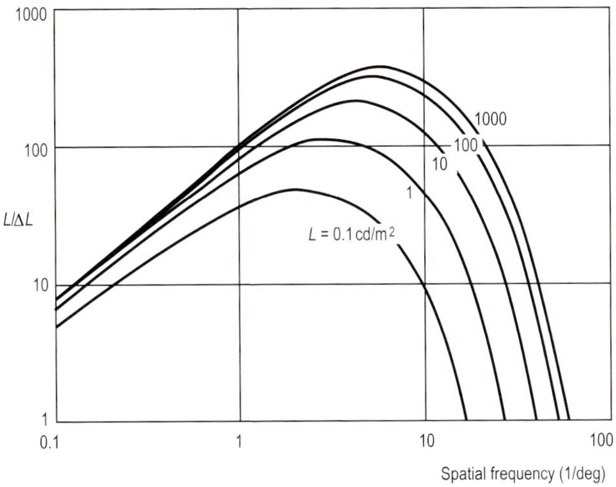

Figure 11.1
Contrast sensitivity as a function of spatial frequency for the perception of an object of 2° diameter and sinusoidal modulation for different background luminance levels L, computed according to the Barten model [11.4]

flicker perception. This critical flicker frequency amounts to approximately 70 Hz for commonly used luminance [11.8]. The frame rate of radiological monitors must exceed this limit in order to be flicker free.

11.2.2 Contrast and dynamic range

The HVS is capable of adapting to extremely different light situations, covering an absolute range in luminous intensity of several orders of magnitude. What is important for the diagnostic process, however, is the local dynamic range that can be perceived within a single radiograph [11.9]. Measuring the hyperpolarization potential V in vertebrate cone cells, Normann et al. [11.10, 11.11] showed that this photoreceptor response to a stimulus of luminance L can be expressed by the function

$$\frac{V}{V_{\max}} = \frac{L}{(L + 12.6\, L_{\mathrm{a}}^{0.63})}, \qquad (11.2)$$

where $V_{\max}$ is a normalization constant and L_{a} approximates the adaptation luminance. In this equation, it is necessary to measure the luminance in units of cd/m^2. These curves are plotted in fig. 11.2 for different adaptation luminance values.

Fig. 11.2 can be interpreted as follows: If the HVS is adapted to a certain luminance level, only a stimulus in the neighborhood of the adaptation level will cause the maximum response. Excitations either at the lower end or at the upper end of the adaptation range evoke a reduced response signal due to the smaller slope of the curves. Thus, contrast can be simultaneously perceived in a limited range of stimuli only.

Light scattering in the eye, expressed by the point-spread function [11.12, 11.13], and permanent involuntary eye movements known as microsaccades [11.11] lead to a further reduction in perceivable contrast.

In summary, the perceivable contrast will be much smaller than expected in the ideal case. The phenomenon of adaptation to a complex image scene represents an essential consideration. Based on the model and experimental data underlying fig. 11.2, it is obvious that the contrast ratio (the ratio of maximum to minimum stimuli luminance that can be experienced in a single nonuniform image) will be hardly above 100. This contrast ratio value is smaller than the estimates of the best-case scenarios [11.5]. These indicate contrast ratio values of 200 to 300. However, the exact value naturally depends on the specific image and adaptation process.

The dynamic range (i.e. the number of perceivable gray levels) is closely related to contrast ratio. The dynamic range is largely determined by the characteristic display curve that transforms the digital driving level or digital code value into luminance on the screen. The dynamic range can be maximized via a so-called perceptual linearization of the gray scale in order to provide equal luminance differences for equal input driving level differences over the full intensity range. However, this linearization process also depends on the image, image noise, the observer, the image's surroundings and ambient conditions. Although several methods of perceptual linearization have been discussed [11.14, 11.15, 11.16], the DICOM [11.17] grayscale function can be expected to become the accepted standard. However, it should be pointed out that the objective of such a standard is only to establish a common image appearance on various display devices and not to optimize image quality.

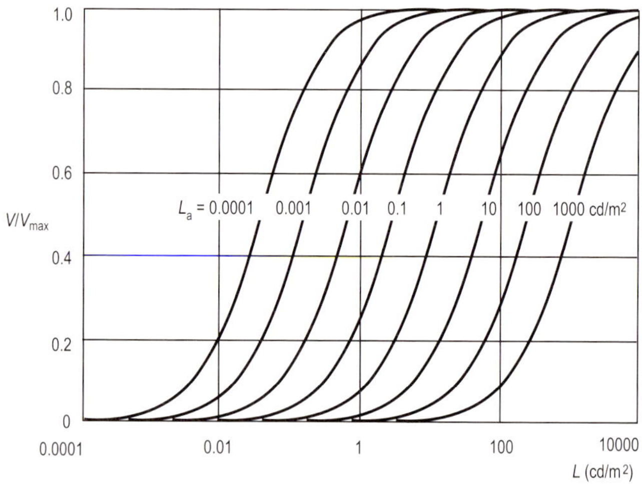

Figure 11.2
Calculated normalized model cone response as a function of the stimulus luminance L for different adaptation luminance levels L_a

11.2.3 Color vision

Although digital radiographs are generally black-and-white (B/W) images, it is also important to consider issues relating to color. B/W medical images can also be displayed on color monitors. Furthermore, some imaging modalities generate color images (e.g. ultrasound and nuclear medicine) and additional physiological and functional information can be overlayed in color on B/W images.

Color vision is provided by the cone cells, a phenomenon that also offers the highest degree of spatial resolution. The eye is sensitive to light at wavelengths between 400 nm and 700 nm, with maximum sensitivity at 555 nm. The perceived image will therefore depend on the type of the display (i.e. on the type of the CRT phosphor or the color of the LCD backlight).

A blue-tinted backlight or a bluish phosphor (e.g. P45) has been found to be advantageous for perceived sharpness. This phenomenon can be explained by the higher sensitivity of the rod cells that control pupil size in the presence of green-blue light [11.18]. A slightly blue background leads to a smaller pupil diameter, and therefore higher acuity.

11.3 Medical display technologies

As shown in fig. 11.3, the electronic display technologies currently in use for direct viewing include cathode ray tubes (CRT) and flat-panel displays (FPD). Not included in this overview are projection view displays and head-mounted devices.

The classical device is the cathode ray tube (CRT). Unlike most consumer television sets, which are based on color tubes, high-fidelity CRTs (i.e. monitors offering high luminance and high spatial and contrast resolution) are based on black-and-white

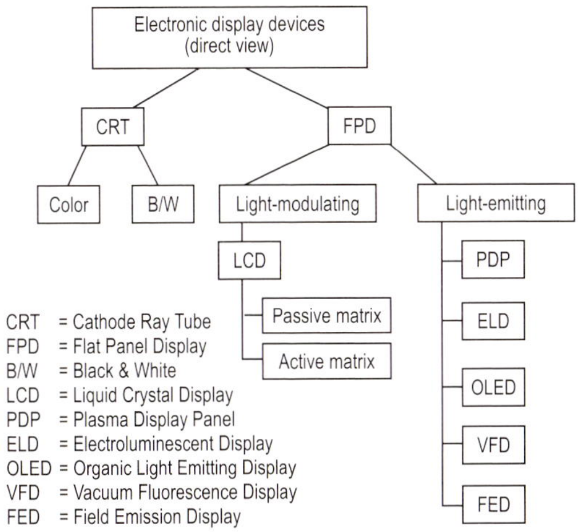

Figure 11.3
Overview of electronic display device technologies for direct view

(monochrome) tubes. However, the high price of monochrome monitors has led to an increase in the use of color CRTs to display B/W medical images. This trend has also been fueled by the widespread use of the Internet to make images available on networked office computers.

Several flat-display technologies are currently in development. The most advanced of these is the liquid crystal display (LCD). Owing to its superior image quality, the active matrix LCD (AMLCD), which involves the addressing of each pixel via a separate switching element, is virtually the only liquid crystal display currently used. In contrast to the emissive CRT, this display is transmissive (i.e. the image is controlled by a backlight modulated by the liquid crystal layer according to the image information and not by a light-emitting substance).

In the remainder of the present section, we describe how the two most widely used electronic display types (cathode ray tubes and liquid crystal displays) work. The AMLCD is the CRT's biggest rival and is set to become the most widely used electronic display type, also in the area of medical imaging. This development has been sparked by the nearly ubiquitous use of computer and mobile-computing technologies. In the meantime, LCDs have come into use as large-screen televisions. That being said, the CRT represents a virtually perfect form of electronic display and qualifies as the benchmark for all new display technologies. The main drawbacks of a CRT compared to an LCD include low energy efficiency and bulkiness [11.19].

Several emissive flat panel display technologies are currently in development. Plasma display panels (PDP) provide full color and high contrast [11.20] for very large display areas (up to 60-inch diameter), but only a relatively limited resolution (approximately 1 million pixels). Electroluminescence and vacuum fluorescence displays (flat CRTs) [11.20] are not currently used in medical imaging because they suffer from technical problems and do not offer sufficient image quality.

In the middle of the 1990s, field-emission displays (FED) were thought to be a candidate to replace CRTs because they seemed to possess the attributes of both CRT and flat displays. These displays are based [11.21] on the field emission of an electron beam from Spindt-type Mo microtips, diamond-like carbon nanotubes and carbon nanotubes. However, progress with these flat displays has been slower than expected and they still suffer from basic reliability problems.

Organic light-emitting diode displays (OLED) based on small-molecule or polymer light-emitting materials represent a very promising recent technological development with regard to their potential for high-fidelity medical application. This technology promises superb display performance coupled with relatively low manufacturing costs. However, technological challenges remain and one will have to wait and see whether this technology proves successful.

11.3.1 Cathode ray tube monitors

The CRT monitor consists of a vacuum tube (fig. 11.4) and electronic circuitry [11.22]. The digital image transmitted by the storage device represents the input for the digi-

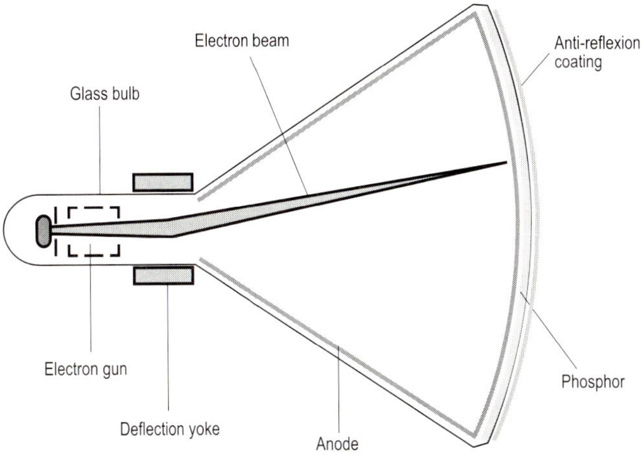

Figure 11.4 Schematic drawing of a cathode ray tube

tal-to-analog converter that is responsible for converting the digital code values (digital driving levels) into a temporal voltage signal that is then amplified by the video amplifier.

The electron gun emits an electron beam driven by the amplifier output voltage $U_A(t)$. The time-dependent beam current $I(t)$ is approximated by

$$I(t) = const(U_0 + U_A(t) - U_c)^{\gamma}, \tag{11.3}$$

where U_c is the cutoff voltage of the electron gun and the offset U_0 is given by the brightness setting of the monitor. The contrast setting controls the video amplifier gain. The exponent γ is referred to as the *gamma* of the monitor.

The tube's electron optics, which deploy electrostatic focusing, magnetic deflection and a high-voltage anode (25 to 30 kV), shape the electron beam that impinges on the phosphor layer. In the phosphor that can be characterized by a luminous efficiency between 15 and 25 lm/W, the energy of the scanning electron beam is converted into light that exits the faceplate and forms the visible image.

A detailed view of the faceplate structure is given in fig. 11.5. The faceplate is structured to suppress the influence of ambient illumination caused by reflected and scattered light and of internal scattering as much as possible without excessively reducing luminance due to the use of low transmission glass. These unwanted scattering (and reflection) processes in the faceplate reduce local contrast and increase the minimum luminance. This phenomenon is referred to as halation haze or veiling glare [11.23].

The final luminance L on a screen position can be approximated as a function of the digital driving level G by

$$L(G) = a_1 + (a_2 G + a_3)^{\gamma}, \tag{11.4}$$

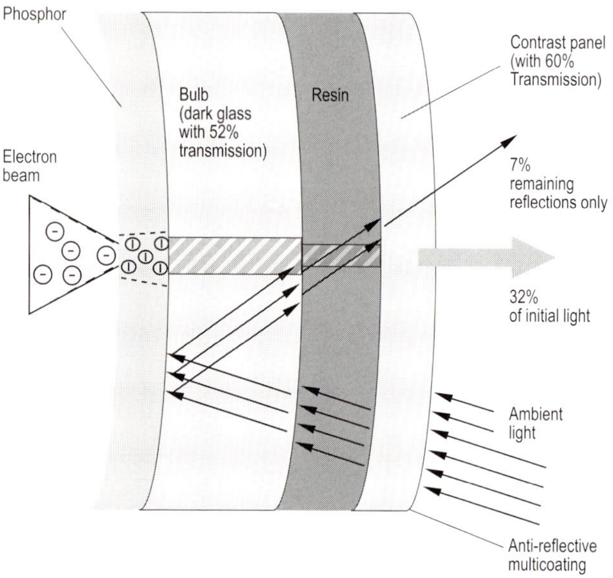

Figure 11.5 CRT faceplate structure (Source: Siemens A&D SE DT, Karlsruhe)

where a_1 is the veiling glare, a_2 is the video amplifier's gain (monitor contrast control) and a_3 is the video amplifier's offset voltage (monitor brightness control). The gamma of the monitor (eq. 11.3) is again denoted by γ, which usually takes on values between 2.2 and 2.5.

Color CRTs use the principle of additive color mixing [11.16]. They are accordingly outfitted with three electron guns and three electron beams (one for each color) that have to be focused onto a red, a green and a blue phosphor element from which the HVS constructs the composite color as a superimposition of the basic colors. The spatial resolution is defined by a shadow mask or an aperture grill in front of the phosphor that ensures that the right beam hits the right phosphor.

11.3.2 Liquid crystal displays

Liquid crystals are materials that exist in a partially liquid and partially solid physical state. When sandwiched between two glass plates, their optical properties can be altered by applying an electric field. This effect enables one to modulate the light that traverses the structure.

Nematic liquid crystals are the most common type of liquid crystal to be used in display technology [11.24, 11.25]. The molecules of the crystals change their orientation in the electric field. A liquid crystal cell can be switched from the off state to the on state by employing polarization filters (fig. 11.6). The transmission factor depends on the voltage applied. This enables one to display intensity and thus gray scale.

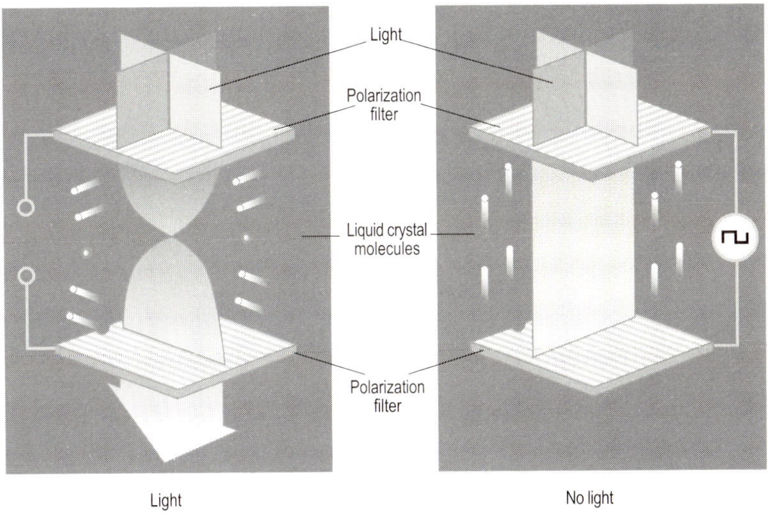

Figure 11.6 Principle of a twisted nematic LCD (Source [11.28])

The first pixel-array LCDs used to display images relied on simple-matrix or passive-matrix addressing schemes based on row and column lines. These had inherent limitations [11.26] in terms of the number of pixels and frame rates they could support. Super twisted nematic liquid crystals (STN) were developed to optimize performance. This development was then followed by the development of dual super twisted nematic liquid crystals (DSTN) to enable reliable color pictures.

Today, practically all LC displays designed to provide high spatial resolution, grayscale capacity and a high frame rate to enable motion pictures are operated by active-matrix addressing [11.27]. This principle is also used for large-area, solid-state detector read-

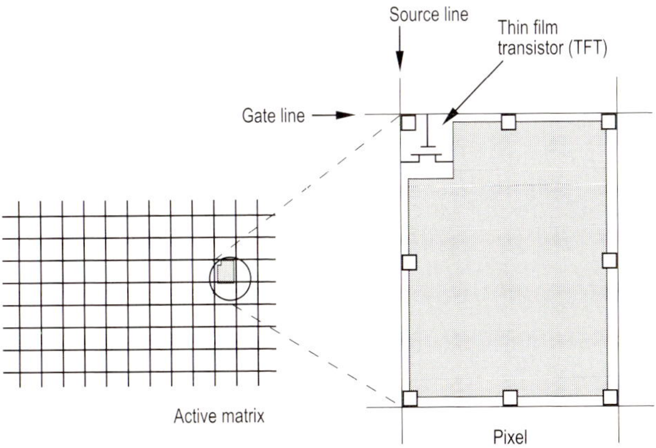

Figure 11.7 Active-matrix addressing scheme

a) b)

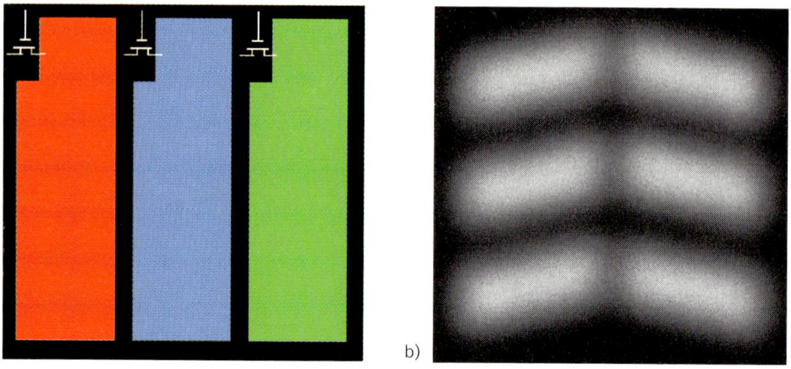

Figure 11.8
Pixel substructure of **(a)** a color LCD and **(b)** a dual domain B/W LCD in so-called Chevron structure.

out, as described in section 12.3. The liquid crystal layer is deposited on a glass substrate with an amorphous silicon (a-Si:H) thin-film transistor (TFT) array. Each pixel has a TFT switch connected to the gate line for switching and to the source line where the image (video) information is applied (fig. 11.7).

Each pixel of a color LCD has a substructure (fig. 11.7 illustrates a case without substructures) and three color filters (RGB) (fig. 11.8a). The pixel substructure naturally influences the spatial resolution. Monochrome LCDs for medical use do not have color filters, and their substructure pixels are usually addressed separately, so as to increase the number of gray levels (fig. 11.8b).

The typical structure of an AMLCD includes the following components:

- Backlight
- Diffuser
- Rear polarizer
- Rear glass plate with TFT array, electrodes and control lines
- Front glass plate with color filters
- Front polarizer

Given that the transmission of light through these layers is rather low (around 10% to 25%), it is necessary to use a strong backlight as a light source. Recent developments make use of flat discharge Xe light sources that provide bright and very uniform illumination, as well as a longer life cycle than conventional fluorescence backlight tubes.

Whereas CRT screens involve a nearly Lambertian emission of light, the emission characteristics of LCDs strongly depend on the viewing angle owing to the optical anisotropy of the liquid crystals. Modern LCDs are thus expressly designed for a large viewing angle and uniform emission. The so-called in-plane switching (IPS) feature is illustrated in fig. 11.9 [11.36]. Other techniques used to increase the viewing angle include vertical alignment (VA), multiple domains (MD), optical compensation birefrin-

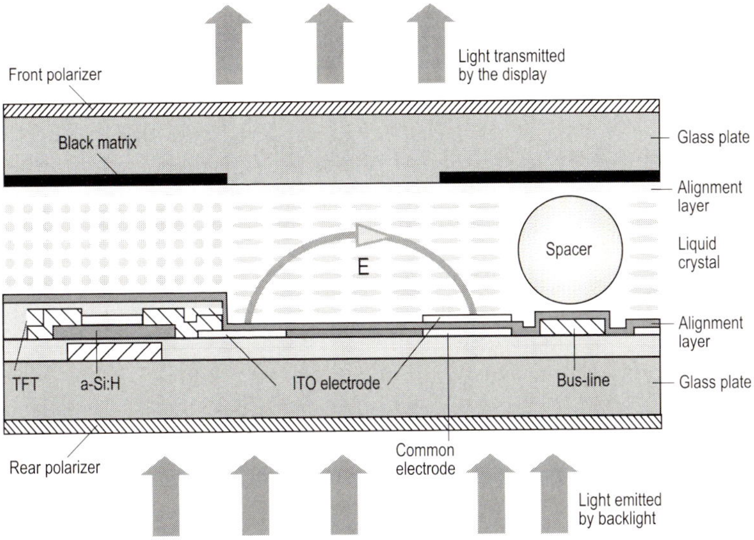

Figure 11.9 In-plane switching increases the viewing angle (Source: A. Badano and RSNA [11.36])

gent (OCB) films and combinations of these three. An example of the pixel substructure of a dual domain LCD operated in B/W mode is shown in fig. 11.8b.

11.4 Technical display performance values

Having presented various display technologies, we turn in the present section to a discussion of the most important design specifications for ensuring monitor image quality.

11.4.1 Display size

The standard-sized film radiograph is 14" × 17" (35 cm × 43 cm). The screens of common 21" monitors are slightly smaller, namely 30 cm × 40 cm. Given that bigger CRT displays are heavier and are less energy efficient, the 21" screen size is considered to be a good compromise between desirable image size and other considerations. However, this could change with the introduction of space-saving flat-panel displays. The limiting factor today is the cost of a large-area LCD.

11.4.2 Spatial resolution

The assumption that contrast sensitivity (fig. 11.1) is also relevant to medical image viewing and diagnosis enables us to draw conclusions about what one can reasonably expect from a monitor with regard to spatial resolution. If the resolution limit of the HVS is considered to be 30/degree, the minimum object size Δx that can be perceived

Table 11.1
Typical image formats (number of pixels in vertical and horizontal direction, column 2, and total number of pixels, column 3)

XGA	1,024 × 768	786 432
SXGA	1,280 × 1,024	1 310 720
UXGA	1,600 × 1,200	1 920 000
QXGA	2,048 × 1,536	3 145 728
QSXGA	2,560 × 2,048	5 242 880

from a viewing distance of 0.5 m is 0.145 mm. This applies to the just discernable object for a standard observer. The corresponding number of TV lines is about 2,600 for an image height of 0.38 m, which is typical for a 20" portrait CRT or an 18" LCD. On the other hand, the monitors that offer the highest number of addressable pixels available today have 2,560 × 2,048 pixels, a quantity that fairly well matches what the HVS can perceive.

All of this assumes that the user is optimally adapted and that the monitor's resolution, defined by the modulation transfer function, corresponds approximately to one display pixel or, in the case of a CRT, to one TV line. The latter is not a trivial requirement because the beam spot size on the screen, and thus the MTF, is different in horizontal and in vertical directions. It depends on the electron optics, on the phosphor spreading of the light generated by the impinging electron beam, on halation effects in the glass faceplate and additionally (in the horizontal direction) on the frequency response of the electronic circuitry [11.22].

Typical image formats used for medical displays are listed in table 11.1. The first column in this table gives the international format name, the second column lists the addressable pixels in each direction and the third column shows the total number of pixels.

11.4.3 Luminance, contrast ratio, and veiling glare

Given that the beam spot is broader for higher beam currents [11.22], it is necessary to limit the maximum luminance of a CRT display to maintain spatial resolution. The maximum luminance (L_{max}) of almost all currently available medical CRT monitors is between 200 and 600 cd/m^2, depending on the transmissivity of the glass faceplate and on the luminous efficiency of the phosphor. To the extent that the highest spatial resolution is required for the diagnostic task at hand (e.g. for the primary diagnosis of digital radiographs), practical experience with common medical monitors indicates that the luminance should not be set to values higher than about 300 cd/m^2.

The situation is different for LCDs. Here, the maximum luminance depends on the backlight and on the transmission coefficients of the various layers (cf. section 11.3.2).

It follows from the above considerations that the lowest luminance (L_{min}) should not be too low. One approaches the scotopic region (where vision is gradually impaired, threshold contrast increases, and detectability is reduced compared to the photopic region) at around 1 cd/m^2.

In the case of CRTs, there are several reasons that prevent L_{min} from becoming very low in practical circumstances. Applying realistic images, light traversing the faceplate is reflected at the interfaces and scattered inside the system, consisting of glass, phosphor and aluminum layer. Light originating from bright parts of the image is thus scattered into adjacent dark parts (fig. 11.5). A similar effect occurs with respect to the backscattering of electrons inside the tube [11.29]. These effects lead to the phenomena of veiling glare and halation haze [11.30] and tend to increase the actual L_{min}, depending on the image involved. The minimum luminance L_{min} is furthermore increased by ambient light reflected from the boundaries of the faceplate and scattered [11.31]. Reducing these effects through the use of darkened glass and anti-reflection coating unfortunately reduces the transmissivity of the glass faceplate. The use of higher beam currents is therefore required to generate the same luminance. This, however, increases the engineering challenge and electron-optical design task of keeping the beam spot size small. Fortunately, modern state-of-the-art CRT monitors are equipped with these faceplates and high-performance electron tubes. Nevertheless, it is necessary to keep the ambient light to an appropriately low level in order to achieve a high contrast ratio. The tradeoff between resolution and maximum luminance for state-of-the-art CRT monitors is illustrated in fig. 11.10.

The increase in electron scatter due to the shadow mask makes the situation regarding glare even worse for color CRTs.

In the case of LCDs no electrons are scattered and less internal light scattering occurs. LCDs thus offer the advantage of low veiling glare. Here, minimum luminance is de-

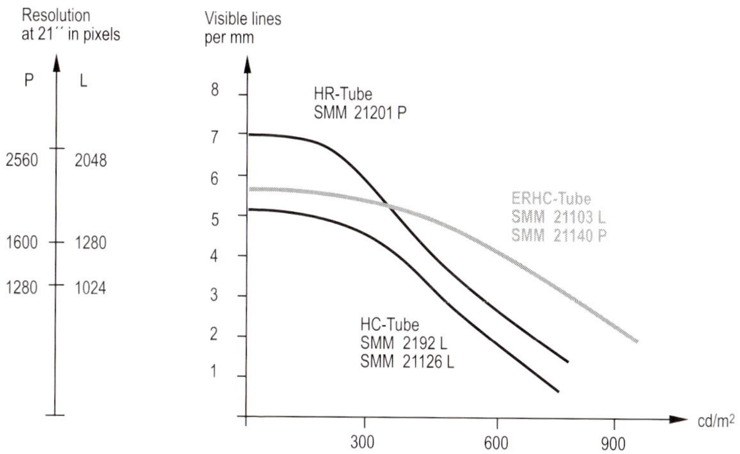

Figure 11.10
Spatial resolution as a function of a CRTs luminance. *P* indicates portrait format, *L* is landscape format. (Source: Siemens AG A&D SE BT, Karlsruhe)

termined by the non-zero transmission in the off-state of a liquid crystal cell and by the reflected ambient light, as no anti-reflection coating is applied in most cases.

Measurements show that the contrast ratio L_{max}/L_{min} in realistic situations is usually lower than 300 and lower than what can be obtained under ideal conditions [11.31]. While the contrast ratio for LCDs is often specified as 600:1, this value can only be achieved in very dark rooms and for viewing directions that are perpendicular to the screen surface. Nevertheless, a contrast ratio of 200 to 300 well matches the contrast ratio that the HVS is able to process (cf. section 11.2.2). Regarding an X-ray film radiograph hanging in front of a light box, only those image parts whose optical density is between 0.4 and 2.4 can be recommended for diagnosis [11.5, 11.32]. Given the logarithmic relation between optical density and luminance, this corresponds exactly to a luminance contrast ratio of 100. The range of recommended optical densities for less demanding applications [11.32] is between 0.5 and 2.1 (corresponding to a luminance contrast ratio of 40).

11.4.4 Dynamic range and display curve

The term dynamic range refers to the number of just noticeable gray levels. Assuming ideal conditions, the number of discernible gray levels in the luminance range under consideration should be larger than 500. It is unlikely in most realistic viewing situations – in which the threshold of the HVS is elevated by noise, surround luminance and ambient light – that smaller luminance differences than those corresponding to 256 gray levels will be perceivable in a complex radiological image [11.33].

The characteristic curve of a CRT monitor is essentially given by the voltage-to-current relationship of the tube's electron gun. While this relationship is highly nonlinear, it is similar to a perceptually linearized display curve. However, one cannot expect the intrinsic monitor curve to yield exact perceptual linearization. It is thus necessary to maximize the dynamic range by choosing a proper display curve to achieve perceptual linearization.

In digital systems, this can be done by applying a look-up table (LUT) to the digital driving levels. The application of a LUT may reduce the number of gray levels. Here, care has to be taken to avoid losing gray levels and thus generating artifacts. The application of LUTs, as with any other image processing steps, has to take place in the component with the highest available bit depth in order to avoid a loss of dynamic range.

The image look has to be optimized to the specific task and user so as to provide optimal softcopy diagnostic capability. In general, this can be regarded as a kind of dynamic range maximization in the luminance range under consideration, and may also include spatial frequency processing.

11.4.5 Noise

The electronic circuitry for the DAC and video amplifier in a CRT is the main contributor to temporal noise. The major source of spatial noise comes in the form of phosphor grain noise. Roehrig et al. [11.34] have shown that temporal display noise plays a role only in the case of very low luminance and that spatial noise dominates in the case of higher luminance values.

The phosphor grain noise power spectrum (NPS) can be estimated on the basis of measurements. Its impact on image quality has been assessed by the use of simulations and observer experiments [11.35]. Image display noise is of great interest and importance because it can mask small details, and thus elevate the detection threshold. The use of a low-noise phosphor (e.g. P45) is thus recommended when it comes to designing high-resolution monitors. Doing so helps one to avoid compromising image quality and to achieve the expected high spatial resolution [11.35].

LCD noise can also be generated by driving electronics, luminance variations in the liquid crystal cell caused by variations of the electric field and cell thickness. The pixel substructure represents the most obvious contribution to spatial noise in an LCD (fig. 11.8). The noise behavior of modern flat-panel displays is still in need of clinical investigation.

11.5 Digital imaging display systems

In order to secure optimized image quality, it is necessary to consider the display unit in the context of the entire imaging chain. The display is only one component in the system and is required to provide the user with all of the information acquired by the imaging system. When making the transition from acquisition space to display space, image size, magnification ratio, spatial resolution and contrast can all be modified.

Image size and magnification can usually be manipulated by software. These processes are referred to as zooming and panning. It is important for the display software to offer one the option of displaying the image (or perhaps a subsection of it) at full resolution, i.e. in a manner such that one pixel of the acquisition matrix corresponds to one pixel of the display matrix. Furthermore, in the interest of gaining an overall image impression, it should also be possible to display the whole image on a single screen (perhaps at reduced spatial resolution). The mathematical methods underlying these processes center on interpolation algorithms.

Image processing is not only applied to the acquired image (raw data processing), but also to the displayed image. For instance, in order to compensate for limited spatial resolution in the display, one can deploy a form of spatial frequency processing such as edge enhancement.

The contrast of the displayed image may be altered by a process referred to as contrast windowing or window and level (W/L) setting. In general, this process is carried out by applying a linear look-up-table (LUT) in the desired range. However, what is most important is tone scale optimization via nonlinear LUTs (see section 11.4.4).

The DICOM 3.14 standard [11.17] was established in the interest of providing a perceptual standard display curve, and thereby secures image similarity irrespective of

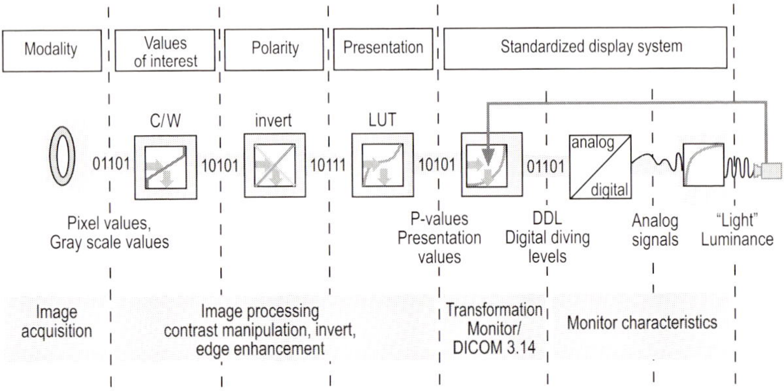

Figure 11.11 Standardized display system according to DICOM (Source: M. Wedel, Siemens)

display technology, manufacturer and absolute luminance range. To achieve this objective, the pixel values or gray scale values are transformed in accordance with the scheme illustrated in fig. 11.11. After accounting for modality, vendor and user-specific transformations that go into the generation of the presentation values (P-values), the standardized display system is required to transform the P-values to luminance according to DICOM PS 3.14. In the case of modern LCDs equipped with a digital interface, the last step of digital-to-analog conversion is skipped.

11.6 Referencess

[11.1] E. Siegel
Filmless radiology: How the Baltimore VA does it.
Diagnostic Imaging, June 1997, 54-66

[11.2] D.H. Hubel
Eye, brain and vision
W.H. Freeman, New York, 1988

[11.3] T. Mertelmeier
Why and how is soft copy reading possible in clinical practice?
J. Digit. Imaging 12 (1999), 3-11

[11.4] P.G.J. Barten
The effects of picture size and definition on perceived image quality
Proc. SID 30 (1989), 67-71

[11.5] E. Muka, H. Blume, S. Daly
Display of medical images on CRT soft-copy displays: A tutorial
Proc. SPIE 2431 (1995), 341-359

[11.6] B.A. Wandell
Foundations of vision
Sinauer Associates, Sunderland, MA 1995

[11.7] M.S. Chesters
Human visual perception and ROC methodology in medical imaging
Phys. Med. Biol. 37 (1992), 1433-1476

[11.8] J.E. Farrell, B.L. Benson, C.R. Haynie
Predicting Flicker Thresholds for Video Display Terminals
Proc SID 28/4 (1987), 449-453.

[11.9] E. Muka, B.R. Whiting
On the human visual system intrascene luminance dynamic range
Proc. SPIE 4686 (2002), 169-176.

[11.10] R.A. Normann, I. Perlman
The effects of background illumination on the photoresponses of red and green cones
J. Physiol. 286 (1987), 491-507

[11.11] B. Baxter, H. Ravindra, R.A. Normann
Changes in lesion detectability caused by light adaptation in retinal photoreceptors
Invest. Radiol. 17 (1982), 394-401

[11.12] G. Westheimer, F.W. Campbell
Light distribution in the image formed by the living human eye
J. Opt. Soc. Am. 52 (1962), 1040-1045

[11.13] G. Spencer, P. Shirley, K. Zimmermann, D.P. Greenberg
Physically-based glare effects for digital images
Computer Graphics Proceedings (1995), 325-334

[11.14] R.W.G. Hunt
The reproduction of colour in photography, printing & television
Fountain Press, Tolworth, England 1987.

[11.15] Sicherung der Bildqualität in röntgendiagnostischen Betrieben, Teil 57: Abnahmeprüfung an Bildwiedergabegeräten
DIN V 6868-57 (2000)

[11.16] D. Richter (editor)
Qualitätssicherung an Bildwiedergabegeräten
ZVEI-Fachverband Elektromedizinische Technik, Frankfurt, 05/2002.

[11.17] Grayscale Standard Display Function
DICOM PS 3.14 ed. NEMA, Virginia, 1998

[11.18] S.M. Berman, G. Fein, D.L. Jewitt, F. Ashford
Luminance-controlled pupil size affects Landolt C task performance
J. Illuminating Engineering Society, Summer 1993, 150-161.

[11.19] D. Theis
Displays – Schlüsselkomponenten der Informationsgesellschaft
Phys. Bl. 56 (2000), 59-63

[11.20] K. Blankenbach
Multimedia-Displays – von der Physik zur Technik
Phys. Bl. 55 (1999), 33-38

[11.21] S. Itoh, M. Tanaka
Current Status of Field-Emission Displays
Proc. IEEE 90 (2002), 514-520

[11.22] T. Mertelmeier, T.E. Kocher
Monitor simulations for the optimization of medical soft copies
Proc. SPIE Vol. 2707 (1996), 322-333

[11.23] M.J. Flynn, A. Badano
Image quality degradation by light scattering in display systems
J. Digit. Imaging 12 (1999), 50-59.

[11.24] M. Schadt, W. Helfrich
Voltage-dependent optical activity of a twisted nematic liquid crystal
Appl. Phys. Lett. 18 (1971), 127-128

[11.25] J.L. Ferguson, T.R. Taylor, T.B. Harsch
Liquid crystals and their applications
Electro technol, Jan 1970, 41-50

[11.26] P.M. Alt, P. Pleshko
Scanning limitations of liquid-crystal displays
IEEE Trans. Electron Devices, ED-21 (1974), 146-155

[11.27] H. Kawamoto
The history of liquid-crystal displays
Proc. IEEE 90 (2002), 460-500

[11.28] D. Theis
Flachbildschirme – das Fenster zum Informationszeitalter
Forschung und Innovation 2/1997

[11.29] E.B. Gindele, S.L. Shaffer
A Physical Optics CRT Faceplate Halation Model
SID 90 Digest (1990), 446-450

[11.30] J.J. van Oekel
Improving the Contrast of CRTs under Low Ambient Illumination with Graphite Coating
SID 95 Digest (1995), 427-430

[11.31] T. Mertelmeier, P. Scharl
Acceptance testing for softcopy displays
Proc. SPIE 4319 (2001), 525-535.

[11.32] H.-S. Stender, F.-E. Stieve
Bildqualität in der Röntgendiagnostik
Deutscher Ärzte-Verlag GmbH, Köln, 1990

[11.33] E. Muka, G.G. Reiker
Reconsidering bit depth for radiological images – is eight enough?
Proc. SPIE 4686 (2002), 177-188

[11.34] H. Roehrig, T.L. Ji, M. Browne, et al.
Signal-to-Noise Ratio and Maximum Information Content of Images Displayed by a CRT
Proc SPIE 1232 (1990), 115-133

[11.35] E. Muka, T. Mertelmeier, R.M. Slone, et al.
Impact of Phosphor Luminance Noise on the Specification of High-Resolution CRT Displays for Medical Imaging
Proc SPIE 3031 (1997), 210-221

[11.36] A. Badano
Principles of cathode-ray tube and liquid crystal display devices
In: E. Samei, M.J. Flynn (eds.), Syllabus: Advances in digital radiography – categorial course in radiology physics
Radiological Society of North America, Oak Brook, Ill 2003, 91-102

12 X-ray components and systems

12.1 The X-ray tube

The X-ray tube constitutes the source of radiation in an X-ray system and plays a decisive role in determining the degree of image quality produced by the system. The following factors are of primary importance:

- Variable radiation hardness (i.e. penetration capacity): the capacity to vary radiation hardness over a wide range by means of the magnitude of the voltage applied to the tube permits optimal adaptation to the object of examination and the method of examination.
- Variable radiation intensity (dose rate): the capacity to control radiation intensity over a wide range via the tube current offers the same adaptive advantages
- Focal spot size and energy distribution in the focal spot: these play a role in determining the radiation source's modulation transfer function (*MTF*) and thus contribute to contrast and resolving power.

Fig. 12.1 offers a sketch of an X-ray tube's basic design.

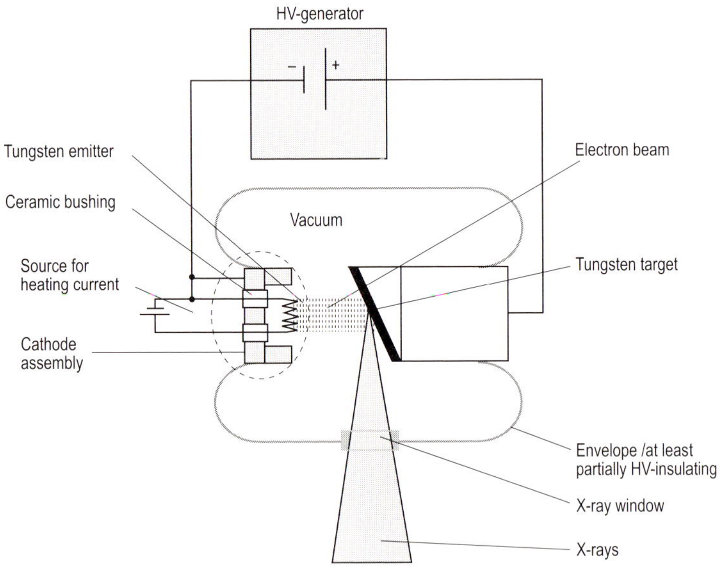

Figure 12.1 Cross section of an X-ray tube, illustrating its physical principle of operation

An evacuated envelope contains devices for high voltage insulation and the cathode assembly, including the emitter and the anode situated opposite one another. The electrons that are released by the emitter at low speed are focused by the shape of the cathode assembly and accelerated to 30 to 65% of the speed of light by the applied high voltage, as can be expressed by:

$$eU = m_0 c^2 \left(\frac{1}{\sqrt{1 - \left(\frac{v}{c}\right)^2}} - 1 \right) \tag{12.1}$$

e: Electron charge, U: Voltage between cathode and anode
m_0: Electron mass, c: Speed of light, v: Speed of electrons

The accelerated electrons abruptly decelerate as they strike the anode surface. As described in section 6.1, no more than 1% of the overall electron energy is converted into X-rays. A preponderance of the total energy is converted into unwanted heat, which needs to be dissipated by the anode.

In the following sections, we describe the function of the emitter, the formation of the electron beam and the resulting focal spot, the different types of anodes (including specific types of bearings used in X-ray tubes outfitted with rotating anodes), the calculation of maximum anode loads and their dependency on anode design, the function and the design of tube envelopes and the function and design of tube housings.

12.1.1 Emitters

The vast majority of X-ray tubes used today are equipped with a cathode assembly consisting of two parts: the electron source (emitter) and the auxiliary electrode surrounding it (Wehnelt electrode). While emitters generally consist of a helically wound tungsten wire with a diameter of 0.2 to 0.3 mm, flat emitters made of tungsten sheet are also used. Both kinds of emitters are heated directly by electrical current. In what follows, we offer a few basic principles of thermionic emission. Readers may wish to refer to the relevant textbooks for a more comprehensive discussion [12.1-12.3].

Thermionic emission

Electrons in metal are bound by a 3D potential constituted by their positively charged atomic cores (fig. 12.2). An electron has the capacity to leave the crystal as soon as it acquires sufficient energy (e.g. by means of heating or by the absorption of a photon). The height of the barrier is referred to as the work function W. Typical work function values for metals range from 2 to 5 eV and depend on the degree of crystallographic order, surface orientation and (critically) the purity of the surface (i.e. with regard to adsorbed species or coatings). An electric field E at the surface of the metal can lower the escape barrier by an amount ΔW. The quantum mechanical probability that an electron with an energy level of $< (\varepsilon_{Vac} - \Delta W)$ will tunnel through the wall (Schottky effect) increases as E increases. This process is referred to as field emission. Electric field strengths for field emission currents sufficient for technical purposes are obtained in the vicinity of kinks or tip-shaped metal surfaces.

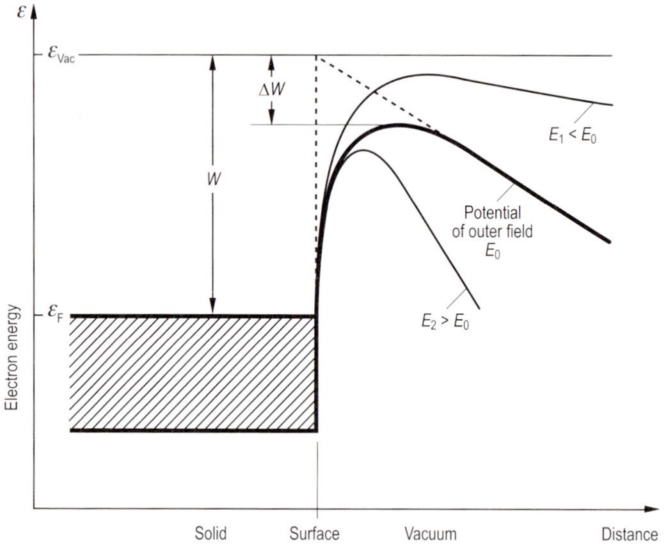

Figure 12.2
Energy diagram for electrons in a metal solid. ε_F: Fermi energy level (ε_{Vac}: vacuum energy level, minimum energy required by an electron to escape through the solid surface into the vacuum). The potential at the surface of a solid varies along with the strength of the external electrical fields $E_{1,2,3}$

Assuming that all of the electrons that leave the surface of the solid are removed by outer fields, the actual rate at which they leave the solid will equal the maximum achievable emission current density, i.e. the saturation current density. This density is given by the Richardson-Dushman equation (readers may wish to refer to the texts cited under [12.4, 12.5] for a more thorough discussion):

$$j_s = \frac{4\pi me}{h^3}(kT)^2 e^{-\frac{W-\Delta W}{kT}} \qquad (12.2)$$

j_s: Surface current density, h: Planck constant, W: Work function
k: Boltzmann constant, T: Temperature of the solid

where

$$\Delta W = \sqrt{\frac{e^3 E}{4\pi\varepsilon_0}} \qquad (12.3)$$

E: External electrical field strength, ε_0: Dielectric vacuum constant

The derivation of this equation relies on the assumption that every electron with an appropriate energy level and direction may pass the surface. Quantum-mechanical considerations indicate that this is not entirely accurate. When one takes the transmission and reflection probabilities of the metal electrons into account, the saturation current density is reduced to

$$j_s \rightarrow j_s \sqrt{\frac{\pi k T}{(\varepsilon_F + W)}} \qquad (12.4)$$

ε_F: Fermi energy

These equations offer detailed descriptions of the influence that the experimental parameters have on the saturation emission current. Indeed, the above outlined correlations have been used to experimentally determine the work functions of pure metal surfaces. However, it is important to bear in mind that these equations do not permit straightforward quantitative assessments of emitter emission currents in X-ray tubes. The reasons for this are outlined in our discussion of technical emitters below.

The direct proportionality of the tube current (i.e. the total electron current between cathode and anode) to the emitter's saturation current density holds as long as all emitted electrons are taken up by the electric field and accelerated towards the anode. However, a space charge region will form in the vicinity of the emitter surface as the number of emitted electrons increases (e.g. via an increase in the emitter temperature). This space charge modifies the electric field at the emitter surface and leads to a situation in which the tube current is no longer governed by the number of electrons escaping the cathode, but by the total voltage applied between cathode and anode (Langmuir-Child relation):

$$j_s = \frac{4\varepsilon_0}{9} \sqrt{2\frac{e}{m}} \frac{U^{\frac{3}{2}}}{d^2} \qquad (12.5)$$

U: Potential difference between anode and cathode
d: Distance between anode and cathode

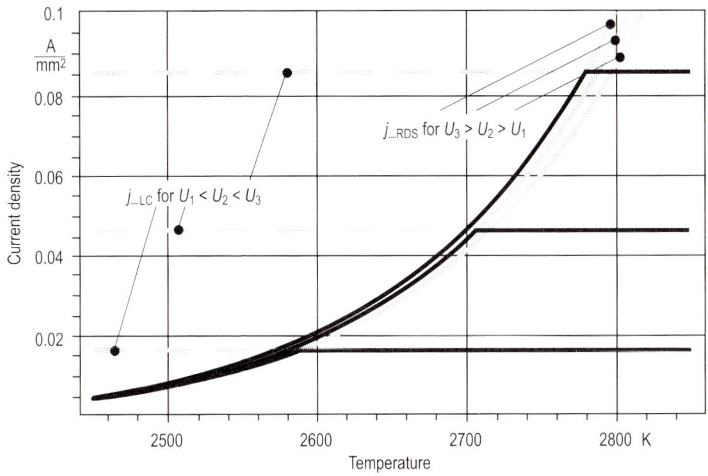

Figure 12.3
Saturation current density *j_RDS* and space-charge current density *j_LC*, plotted as a function of emitter temperature. Plots for three different tube voltages U_1, U_2 and U_3 are shown.

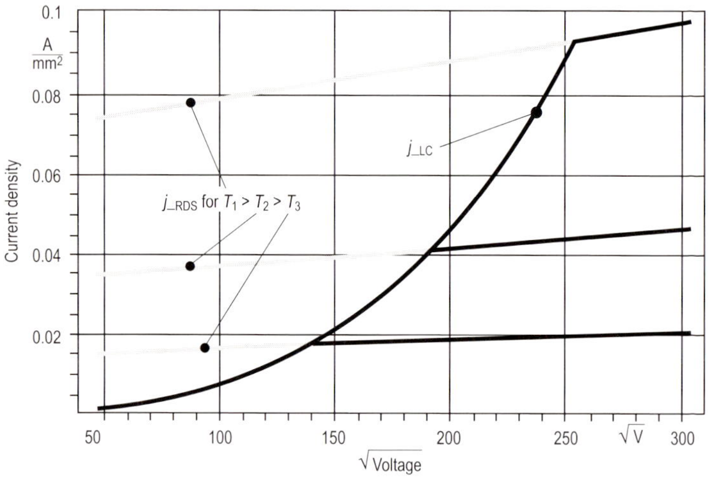

Figure 12.4
Saturation current density *j_RDS* and space-charge current *j_LC*, plotted as a function of tube voltage *U*. Plots for three different emitter temperatures T_1, T_2 and T_3 are shown.

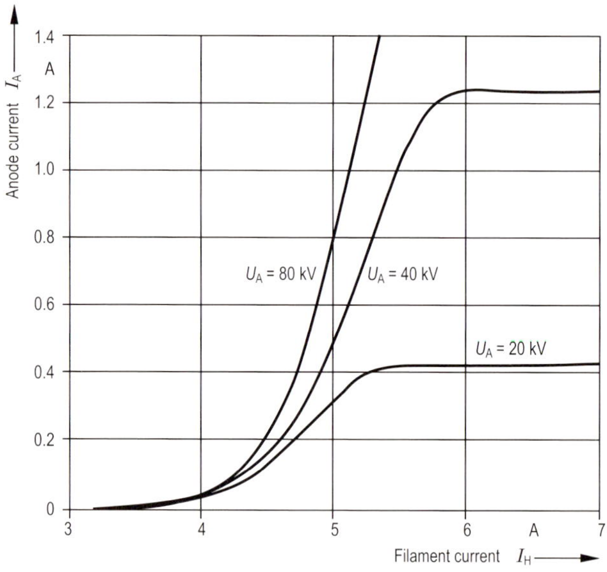

Figure 12.5
Tube anode current I_A, plotted against heating current I_H for three different tube voltages U_1, U_2 and U_3

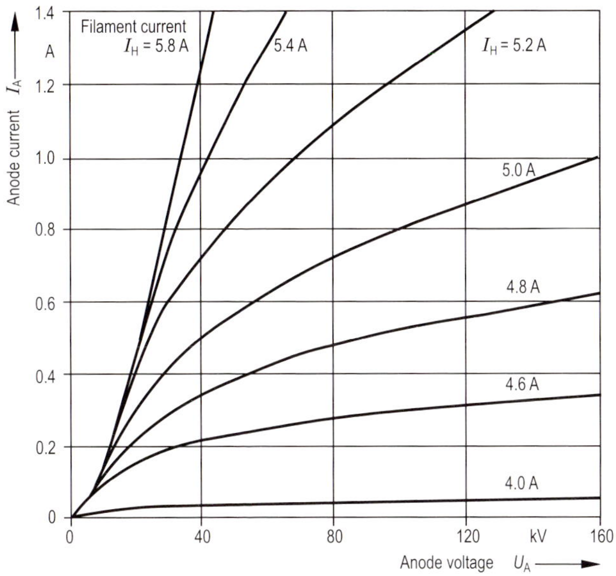

Figure 12.6
Tube anode current I_A, plotted against tube voltage U_A for multiple filament heating currents I_H ranging from 4.0 to 5.8 A

Space-charge and pure saturation current represent ideal conditions. Detailed investigations have shown that under common operating conditions some emitter areas operate in the saturation current regime while space-charge limit conditions apply to neighboring areas. Nevertheless, the characteristics of real X-ray tubes also reflect the dependencies described by the above equations, as can be seen in figs. 12.3-12.6.

Technical emitters in medical X-ray tubes

While many geometric configurations have been deployed to help bring about the emission of electrons from a heated solid, the most widely used emitter in medical X-ray applications is the helix-shaped tungsten filament (as depicted in fig. 12.7). A

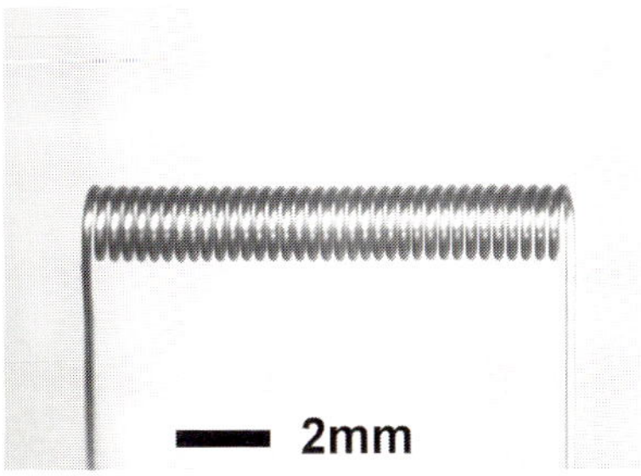

Figure 12.7
Helical heating filament made of tungsten wire

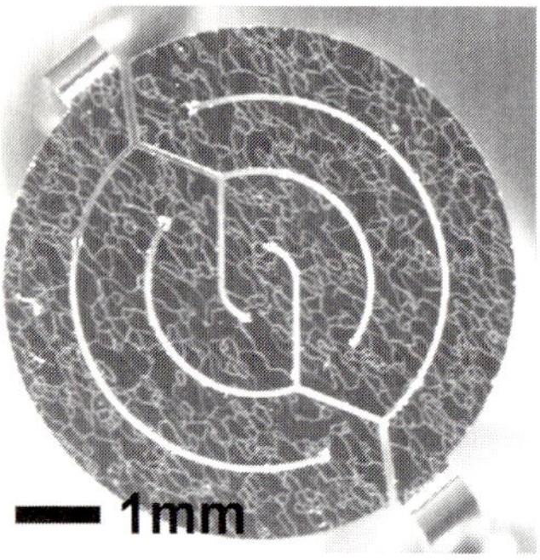

Figure 12.8
Flat emitter, manufactured from tungsten sheet using laser cutting technology

second type of emitter, the flat emitter (cf. fig. 12.8), has recently gained acclaim in connection with its application in mammography X-ray tubes and, even more recently, in connection with its application in high-end, rotating envelope X-ray tubes [12.6].

The following parameters are crucial for the maximum achievable tube current:

- Emitter area contributing to the emission
- Maximum applicable emitter temperature compatible with a sufficiently long tube service life
- Work function *W*
- Field gradient at the emitter surface

While the influence of the emitter area is straightforward, a point-like electron source (or at least a source with a homogeneous spatial distribution of emission) is required, especially for high resolution imaging. The concept of a flat emitter is suited to the task of increasing the emitting area. However, care must be taken to ensure uniform temperature distribution. Temperature distribution is not only crucial for emission homogeneity, but also for achieving a sufficient emitter configuration service life. The helix-shaped emitter exhibits a rather complex temperature distribution and does not allow for even a rough calculation of the emission current via the above formulas.

While X-ray tube currents may range up to 1.5 to 2.0 A, the electron emission surface area should not exceed around 20 mm^2 so as to ensure proper focusing across the whole current and voltage operation range. Given that this requires emitter temperatures as high as 3,000 K, tungsten is almost the only feasible material for use in the construction of emitters [12.7].

An emitter's work function *W* is mainly determined by the chosen material – pure tungsten shows 4.5 eV. However, the work function can be modified by the surface adsorption of other materials. The application of special coatings on the emitter (e.g. LaB_6) enables one to lower the effective work function and achieve a higher electron emission rate. Unfortunately, coating service life is often limited, which leads to a considerable decrease in emission performance as the emitter's service life increases. This problem has prevented broader use of coated emitters in medical applications.

The gradient of an external electrostatic potential at the emitter surface has a significant influence on the emission current. On the one hand, high field gradients amplify the saturation emission current due to the lowering of the potential barrier. On the other hand, they also lead to a depletion of the space-charge region and bring the emitter operation mode into the saturation current's current-limited regime. The steepness of the electrical field at the emitter surface is mainly governed by the design of the cathode cup, i.e. the elements surrounding the emitter that enable the focusing of the electron beam to the anode.

The helix-shaped tungsten wire filament represents a good compromise in that it accounts for the various – partly contradictory – emitter requirements. This filament combines, for instance, easy manufacturability, simple handling, long service life, reliable operation and the capacity to achieve high emission currents. Helix-shaped tungsten filaments provide good mechanical stability throughout the manufacturing process. The wires are usually treated with potassium to inhibit high temperature creep in the wire. The filaments are heated by an electric current flowing through the wire. Therefore, the emission temperature can be easily controlled via the applied heating current.

Slow emission-current response time represents a disadvantage associated with the helix-shaped tungsten emitter. For instance, in angiographic applications it is required to vary the emission current between "on" (100 mA) and "off" (0 mA) states in the ms time regime. Moreover, modern CT applications have led to a demand for fast tube current variations. While the latter can be achieved via fast heating current variations, this approach is no longer sufficient for requirements in angiography.

Emitter heating circuits are usually fed by medium-frequency power sources. This proves sufficient given the fact that the time dynamics are mainly governed by the wire's thermal inertia. The use of thinner filament wires in order to avoid the comparably high heat capacity is not feasible owing to mechanical instability and a shortening of operation time. While quick heating can be ensured by *pushing* the filament, the cooling process, inevitably determined by heat dissipation factors (mostly radiation), represents the speed delimiting factor. This is why all filament-operated X-ray tubes rely on fast tube current modulation, usually realized either via primary pulsing (i.e. modulation of the tube voltage) or electrode control (i.e. the cathode cup is set to a negative potential relative to the filament potential). In both cases, the filament is continuously heated during operation to the temperature required for maximum tube current.

However, given clear filament service life constraints, it would not be feasible to maintain a permanent maximum heating current. Fig. 12.9 offers an example of the relationship between filament service life and applied filament current. The limited filament service life can be explained in terms of wire evaporation, which – like the electron emission rate – depends exponentially on wire temperature.

Wire temperature surges cause tungsten to evaporate at an increased rate. The tungsten wire begins to thin at the highest temperature level. This thinning leads to increased electrical resistance at the same level, which, in turn, leads to a further in-

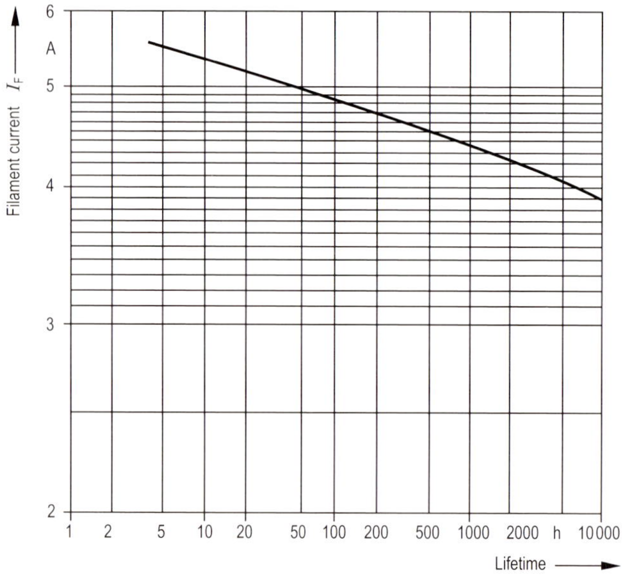

Figure 12.9
Service life plot for a helix-shaped tungsten heating filament with a diameter of 200 µm. Service life increases as the filament current I_F decreases.

crease in temperature – a self-accelerating process that quickly leads to the destruction of the filament. In order to ensure a sufficiently long filament service life, it is necessary to limit the application of high heating currents to short periods (e.g. whenever, as in the case of acquisition mode, high emission current is needed) and to reduce the heating current as soon as possible. This task requires active control: preventing the filament from exceeding the emission threshold when in standby mode and refraining from *pushing* to the desired operating temperature until immediately before the start of image acquisition.

12.1.2 Specifications for focal spot size and electron beam shape

When the accelerated electrons hit the anode surface, their energy is mainly transformed into heat. The amount and spatial density of power deposited onto the anode surface limits the anode's service life. Excessively high heat densities can exert a degree of thermomechanical stress that destroys (or even melts) the anode's structure. However, a small focus size with high power density is required for sharp images. To overcome these conflicting demands, Götze introduced the line focus already in 1918 [12.8]. This concept is still in use in almost every medical X-ray tube manufactured today. Fig. 12.10 offers a sketch of the principles behind the line focus.

A line focus enables the visible focal spot size to vary across the image and thus to influence image sharpness (fig. 12.11). A tube's effective focal spot size [12.9] is usually

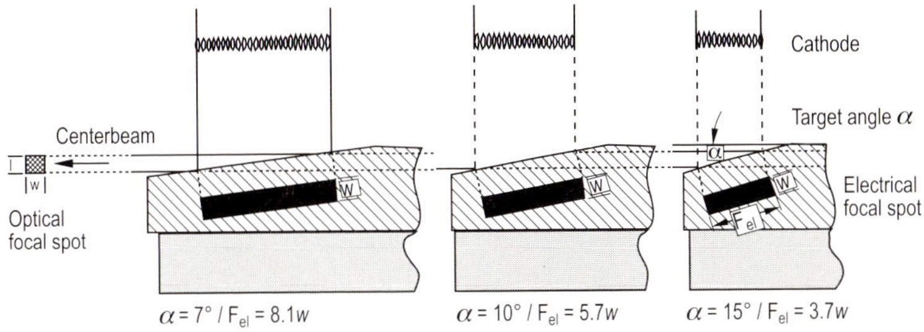

Figure 12.10
Principle behind the line focus with optical length l and width w. When the selected anode angle α is smaller than 45°, the length l of the optical focus visible to the detector corresponds to a greater length L of the electrical focus on the anode surface. This geometrical effect is used to further increase the optical X-ray power density beyond given technical limits so as to achieve the maximum anode power density.

measured using pinhole or slit cameras perpendicular to the tube housing assembly's axis at the height of the focal spot.

In addition to focal spot size, image quality is also influenced by the distribution of X-ray intensity across the entire focal spot and by the extra focal radiation that arises as electrons that have been scattered back from the anode surface in the direction of the cathode then fall back again onto the anode far from the desired focal spot area.

The relationship between the spatial X-ray intensity profile and achievable image quality is given by the modulation transfer function (*MTF*), as described in chapter 9.

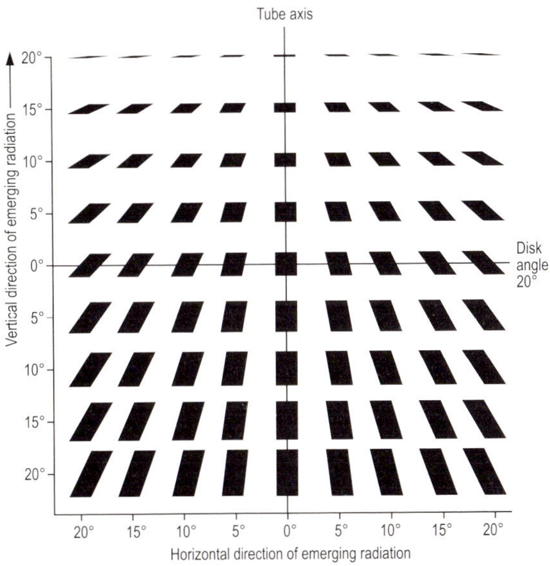

Figure 12.11
Geometry of the focal spot visible to an observer looking from different directions onto the same focal spot of a rotating anode X-ray tube

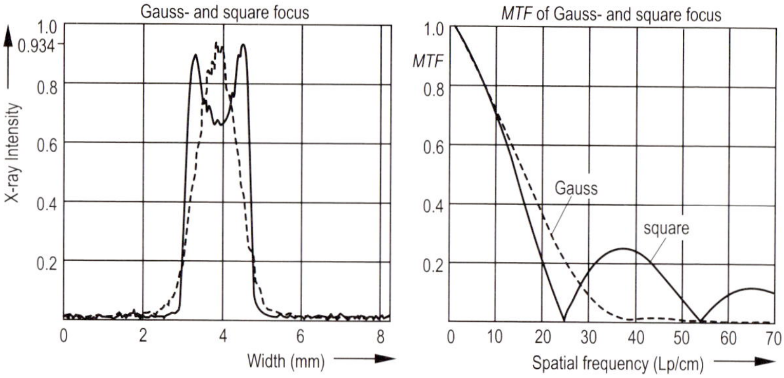

Figure 12.12
In addition to the absolute size of a focal spot, the shape of its intensity profile has an important impact on the achievable image quality. Given the same focal spot width, the modulation transfer function of a focal spot with a Gaussian intensity profile is superior to a focal spot with a rectangular intensity profile.

Fig. 12.12 offers an example of a typical intensity profile and its corresponding *MTF*. Given the same focal spot width, the modulation transfer function of a focal spot exhibiting a Gaussian intensity profile is superior to a focal spot exhibiting a rectangular intensity profile because the *MTF* of the Gaussian intensity profile offers a certain advantage at higher spatial frequencies. Moreover, the additional maxima at higher spatial frequencies may cause additional image quality problems due to aliasing. Fig. 12.13 shows the relationship between the focal spot width and the *MTF*.

Focal spot size and focal spot intensity distribution are crucial factors when it comes to image quality and anode service life. A given emitter design enables one to influence both spot size and intensity distribution via the electric and magnetic fields that form the electron beam.

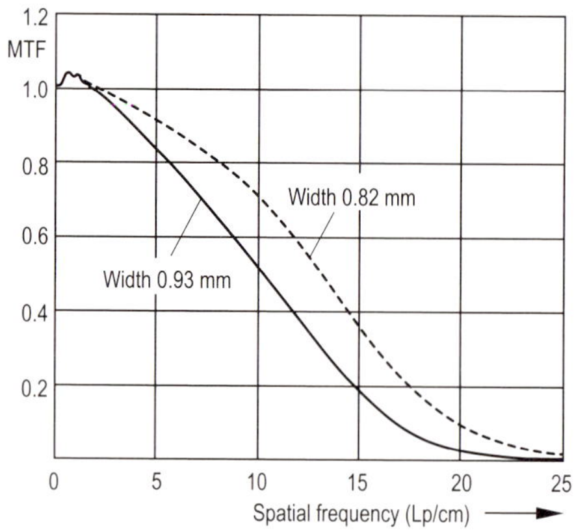

Figure 12.13
Modulation transfer function calculated for focal spots of different widths. Although the difference in focal spot width is small, the impact on the *MTF* is clearly visible.

Forming the electron beam

The movement of an electron in an electric and magnetic field is described by the Lorentz equation:

$$\frac{\mathrm{d}}{\mathrm{d}t}\left(\frac{\vec{v}}{\sqrt{1-\left(\frac{v}{c}\right)^2}}-1\right) = \frac{e}{m_0}(\vec{E}+\vec{v}\times\vec{B}) \tag{12.6}$$

$\vec{E}$: Electric field, $\vec{B}$: Magnetic field

The Poisson equation describes the relationship between the gradient of an electrical potential ϕ and a charge density:

$$\Delta\phi = \frac{-\rho(\underline{r})}{\varepsilon_0} \tag{12.7}$$

ϕ: Electric potential, $\rho(\underline{r})$: Charge density

Computer algorithms that have finite element methods and that apply these equations have been developed to iteratively calculate the electron paths of simplified cathode geometries. Unfortunately, a precise understanding of all of the boundary conditions has not yet been established, (e.g. the exact temperature at each point on the emitter surface, or the exact charge of insulating parts in the vicinity of the cathode). This and the required geometrical simplifications reduce the reliability of simulation results. Therefore, any computer calculation will require validation by experimental results and subsequent computer model adaptations until the results generated by both approaches converge (at least for a fixed set of parameters in a realistic scenario). Fig. 12.14 shows a computer simulation of a bifocal cathode with intertwining focal spots.

Fig. 12.15a-d shows the equipotential lines and electron trajectories for different cathode configurations. While the figures shown are based on the geometry of a helically wound tungsten filament, the following explanations are also valid for other types of emitters (e.g. flat emitters made of tungsten sheet).

Given that the electrons emerge from the emitter at different angles with thermal velocity distribution, a very wide electron beam would reach the anode (fig. 12.15a). Small focal spots are achieved by using an additional electrode that has the same potential as the emitter (Wehnelt electrode) and that surrounds the emitter. The Wehnelt electrode changes the equipotential lines and presses the electron trajectories together (fig. 12.15b). This leads to a crossover of the outer trajectories, and thereby focuses the electron beam. Electrons from the back of the emitter are avoided by placing the emitter into a narrow slot. The shape of the whole assembly resembles that of a cup. Focusing is influenced by the position of the emitter in relation to the inner surface of the focal cup, the width of the slot and the elevation of the cup. The focusing parameters are selected in a way that ensures that the crossover is near the surface of the anode.

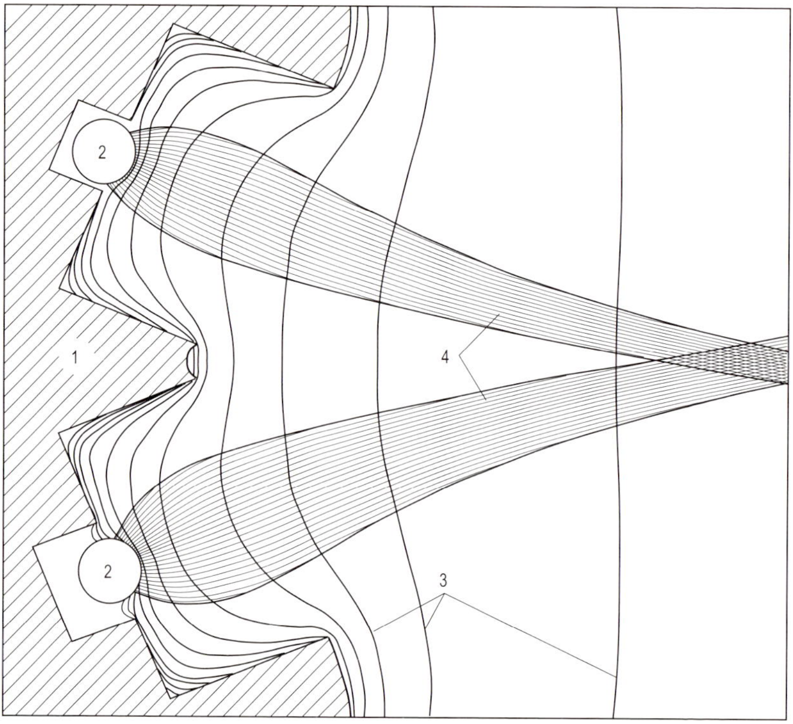

Figure 12.14
Computer simulation of electron trajectories in the electric field of a bifocal cathode assembly. The upper electron beam is optimized for a minimal focal spot width. The lower electron beam maximizes tube power at the price of a larger focal spot width.

One distinct disadvantage associated with the Wehnelt electrode is the reduction in the anode potential (fig. 12.15b). The equipotential lines move away from the emitter as the depth of the focal cup increases and as its width decreases.

Additional focusing capacity can be achieved by applying a grid potential that is slightly more negative than the emitter's potential (fig. 12.15c). This effect can be used to create very small focal spots, which are necessary in some angiographic applications.

If the difference in potential between emitter and focal cup is increased (fig. 12.15d), the electric field near the emitter changes its sign and the tube current comes to a stop. This effect can be used to switch the tube current on and off quickly (i.e. by quickly changing the gating voltage) without having to heat or cool the filament. This technology was widely used before recent developments in high voltage generation enabled primary pulsing, i.e. the direct modulation of tube voltage.

The use of an additional focusing lens is necessary in some applications to achieve the desired focal spot geometry. When a focal cup is positioned near an insulating ceramic

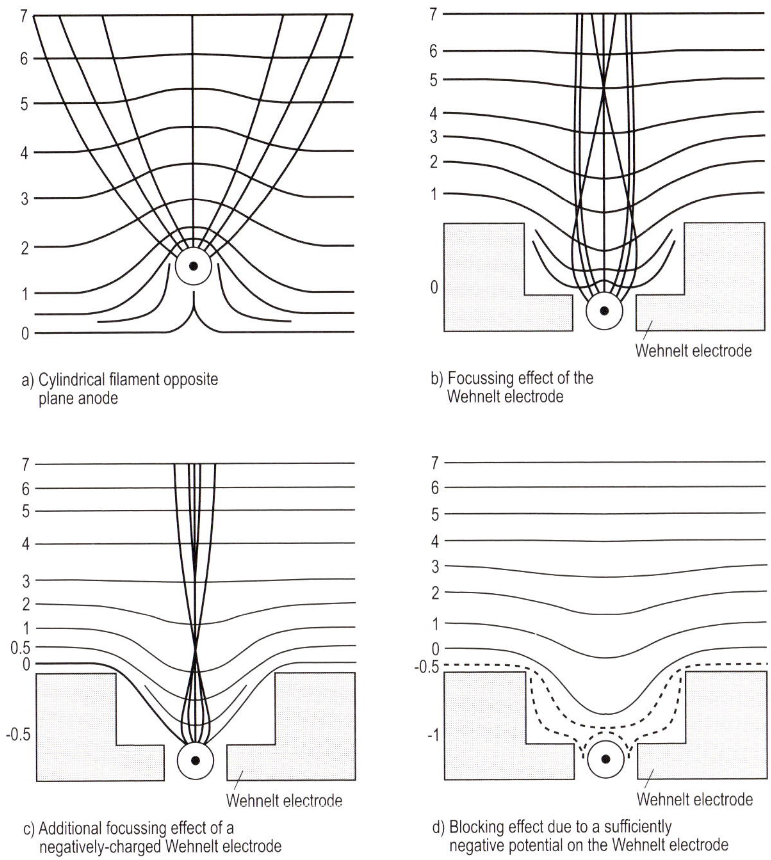

Figure 12.15
a) Cylindrical cathode filament opposite a plane anode (basic configuration). **b)** Basic configuration as in fig. 12.15a with an additional Wehnelt electrode focusing the electron beam (Wehnelt configuration). Wehnelt electrode at the same potential as the cathode filament. **c)** Wehnelt configuration as in Fig. 12.15b. This time the Wehnelt electrode is charged negatively compared to the cathode potential. This leads to a stronger focusing of the electron beam compared that shown in Fig. 12.15b. **d)** Wehnelt configuration as in fig. 12.15c. If the negative potential applied to the Wehnelt electrode reaches a critical level, the electron beam loses its focus and is entirely blocked. This effect can be used to switch an X-ray tube almost instantaneously.

part, it may also be necessary to use an additional potential sheet to avoid interference from ceramic charging effects. If the anode is positioned at a large distance to the cathode, an additional focal lens of anode or ground potential is placed between anode and cathode to ensure that a sufficiently strong electrical field reaches the surface of the emitter.

In such a configuration, the electrons move in a potential free area after passing the focal lens. An expansion of the electron beam vertical to the trajectory is observed due

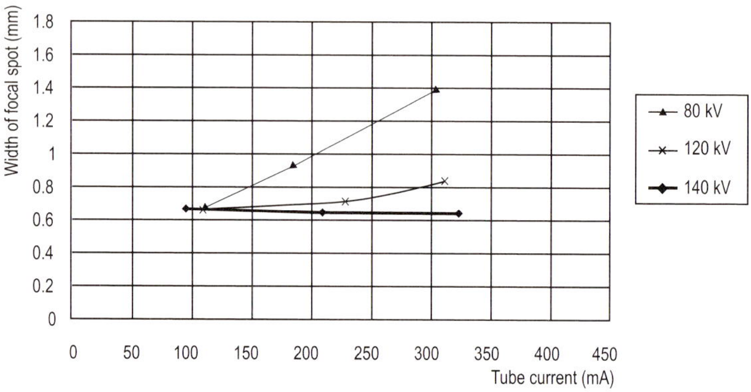

Figure 12.16
Focal spot width plotted against tube current I_A for different tube voltages. The focal spot's minimum width increases along with the tube current I_A.

to electrostatic repulsion. This effect increases as the tube current increases and the tube voltage decreases. Before passing the focal lens near the cathode, the same electrostatic rejection that is exhibited by the electrons influences the focusing effect of the focal lens and moves the position of the focal crossover point. This effect also has an impact on the dimensions of the focal spot at the anode. The selection of an appropriate focusing configuration can lead to a balancing out of both effects for a wide range of tube currents. Fig. 12.16 shows the variation of focal spot width in relation to tube current and tube voltage for a typical CT tube. A noticeable increase in the focal spot width is observed only at high tube currents and small tube voltages (80 kV).

Versatile electron beam deflection

It became necessary to increase the distance between anode and cathode in certain X-ray tubes in order to enable the introduction of additional components designed to actively control the focal spot on the target. Controlled deflection of the electron beam can be achieved by deploying a horseshoe electromagnet or a capacitor plate between the tube's anode and cathode.

Such flying focal spot tubes enable one to quickly switch the electron beam between two different points on the same anode radius in circumferential direction. The CT-system detector thus gathers information from two different focal spots at nearly the same time, an increase in information that enables improved image quality. Fig. 12.17 shows the technical assembly of a high-end CT tube with magnetic flying focal spot technology.

The electromagnetic forming and deflection of the electron beam in the latest generation of X-ray tubes is a prerequisite for the whole principle of tube operation: the rotating envelope X-ray tube has a cylindrical design that is invariant to rotation and built around a single emitter in the rotation center (fig. 12.18). The anode is an inte-

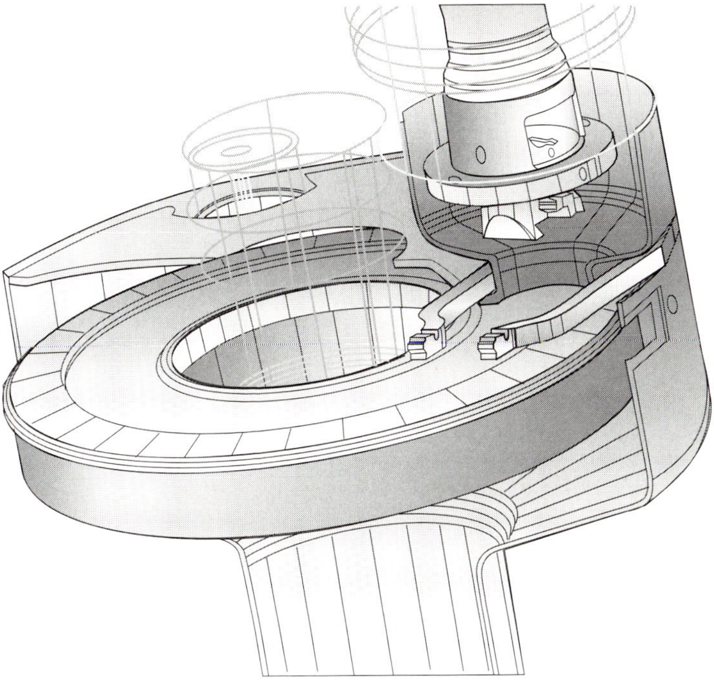

Figure 12.17
Cross section of a modern rotary anode X-ray tube configuration (Siemens Akron). Coils for controlled deflection of the electron beam are incorporated between cathode and anode. A *flying* focal spot can be created by means of alternating magnetic fields. This technique is used to further improve image quality.

gral part of the tube envelope and is directly exposed to the surrounding cooling oil [12.10, 12.11]. The whole tube rotates around its symmetry axis, while the electron beam is continuously deflected to a fixed spot in space on the anode plate by means of an external magnetic deflection unit that is positioned around the constriction in the tube envelope (fig. 12.19) [12.12, 12.13].

Two R-coils in the magnetic deflection unit are responsible for radial deflection. This enables adjustments in the focal spot path. Two additional Phi-coils (mounted vertically to the R-coils) enable deflection in the phi-direction. This is required in order to position the focal spot relative to the X-ray window of the housing and to create a flying focal spot [12.14]. Finally, the four Q-coils are quadruple coils used to influence the focal spot geometry. Their field is used to change the originally round focal spot geometry to an oval shape. This changes the important ratio of focal spot width to length. An additional electrical increase in focal spot length can be achieved by fast-wobbling deflection in the R-direction [12.15]. In this case, the wobble frequency needs to be sufficiently faster than the image sampling frequency in order to avoid image distortion.

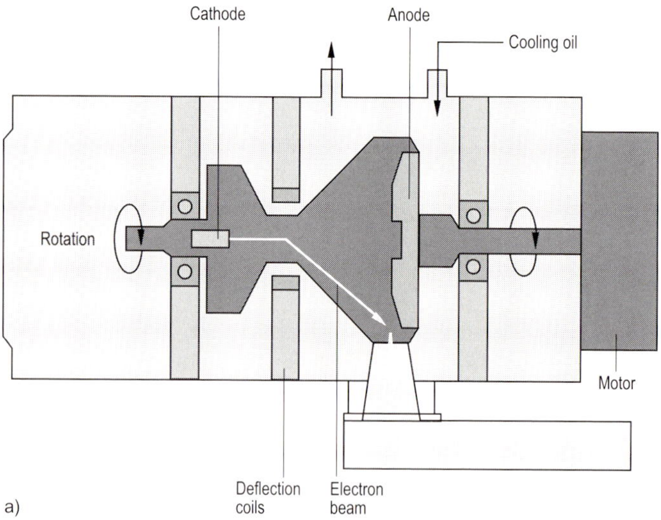

a)

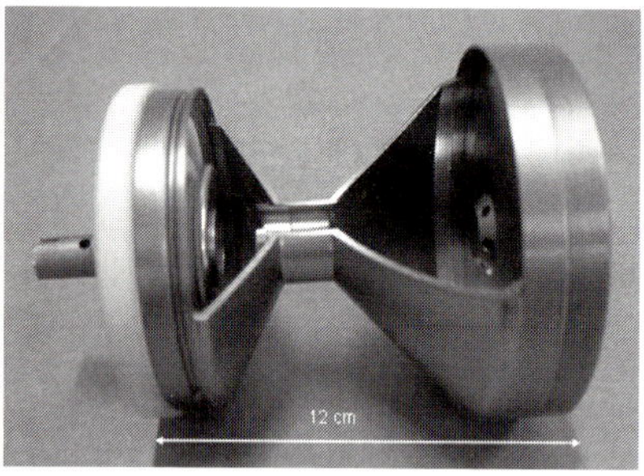

b)

Figure 12.18
Rotating envelope X-ray tube (Siemens Straton 120). **a)** Principle: Electrons generated at the cathode on the left are accelerated through a narrow channel surrounded by a magnetic deflection system (see fig. 12.19) onto the anode plate on the right. **b)** Technical realization: The envelope has been cut open for demonstration.

The entire magnetic deflection system is driven by a microprocessor-controlled electronic deflection unit.

12.1.3 The anode assembly

As has been mentioned in various contexts, more than 99% of the power applied to an X-ray tube is converted into heat (3.1). Efficient heat dissipation represents one of the greatest challenges faced in the development of high power X-ray tubes. Given its importance with respect to the functioning and service life of an X-ray tube as a whole, the anode is usually the prime subject of tube design [12.16, 12.17]. Medical X-ray tubes can be divided into three categories:

- Tubes with stationary anodes
- Tubes with rotating anodes
- Rotating envelope tubes

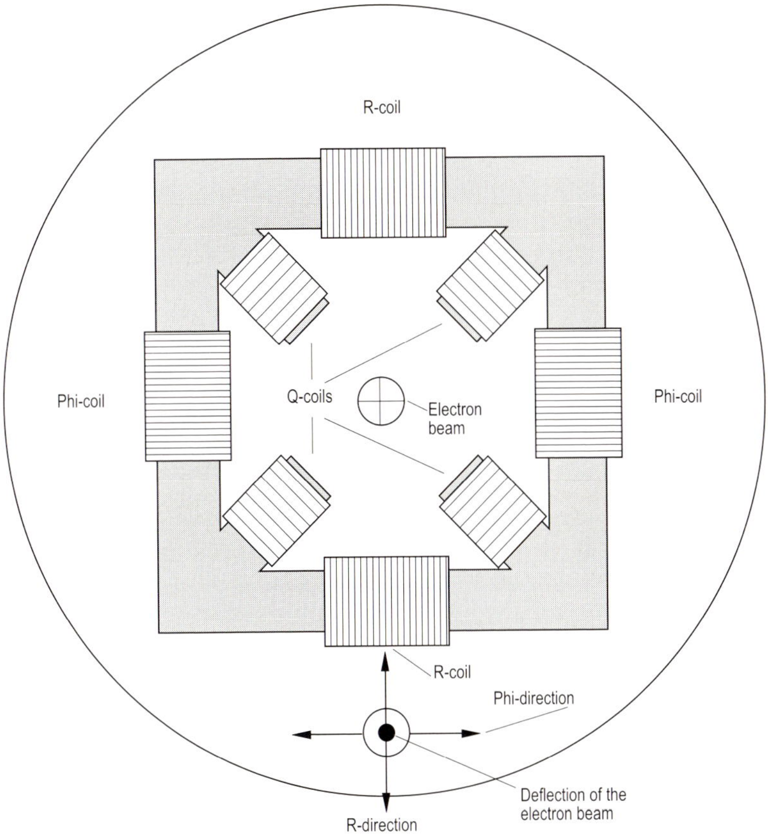

Figure 12.19
Magnetic deflection system deployed by the Straton 120 rotating envelope X-ray tube. The electron beam is shaped and deflected by means of R-, Phi- and Q-coils.

In the remaining sections of this chapter, we discuss these three tube types with respect to their specific anode designs, offer an overview of various bearing systems applied in rotating anode tubes, describe motor configurations for the driving of rotating anodes and present various schemes and methods for calculating design-specific anode load capacities.

Tubes with stationary anodes

Fig. 12.20 offers an illustration of a stationary anode. A tungsten rhenium target is embedded in a copper block. The electrons are focused onto a focal spot on the target surface. The deposited thermal energy is carried away from the heated focal spot via thermal conduction through the copper block towards its stem and hence to the outside of the tube. The copper block is connected (vacuum-tight) to the tube envelope.

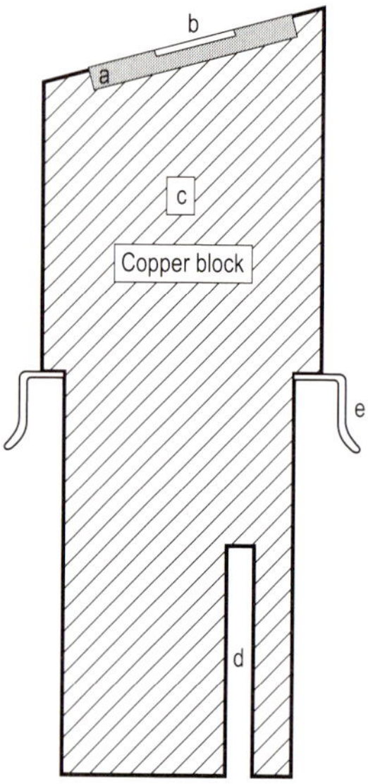

Figure 12.20
Stationary anode (**a:** Tungsten rhenium target; **b:** Focal spot; **c:** Copper block; **d:** Copper block socket. Channels for the circulation of cooling agents are drilled into the socket for some applications; **e:** Vacuum-tight connection between tube envelope and copper block).

One way of increasing the admissible tube power (although hardly ever used for diagnostic X-ray tubes) is to improve anode stem cooling by creating additional convection between the copper stem and the surrounding cooling medium by means of cooling boreholes in the anode block [12.18]. Water or oil is then pumped through these boreholes to improve cooling.

The anode is often outfitted with an electron capture hood with a beryllium window (fig. 12.21). While X-rays can pass the beryllium window without sustaining a substantial decrease in intensity, electrons reflected at the anode surface are prevented from reaching the glass envelope and are thus prevented from reducing the disruptive strength of the tube envelope. Due to the cup-shaped geometry of the capture hood, a

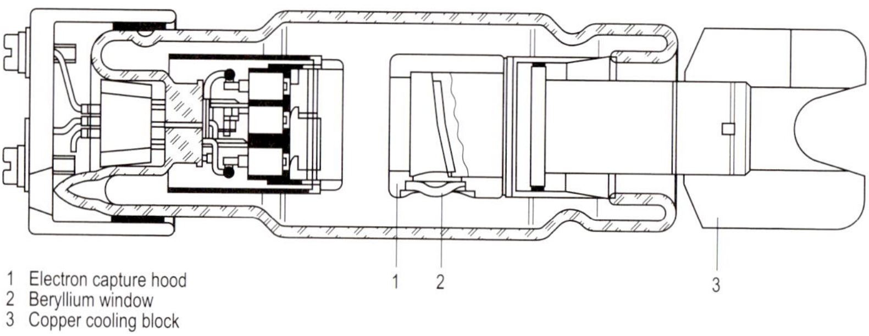

Figure 12.21
Tube with stationary anode
(**1:** Electron capture hood; **2:** Beryllium window; **3:** Copper cooling block)

field-free space is created in close proximity to the target surface. This design is thus also effective at stopping reflected electrons from falling back to the target surface and thereby helping to reduce undesired extra-focal radiation.

Due to their simple and robust design, stationary anode X-ray tubes distinguish themselves in terms of their high reliability and long service lives. However, their low power makes them unsuitable for many applications. In radiographic applications, the upper power limit is mainly determined by the maximum admissible temperature at the boundary between the tungsten target and the copper block. Temperature surges that exceed the melting point of copper will destroy the anode.

Tubes with rotating anodes

The first tubes with rotating anodes were built in 1933 [12.19]. Compared to stationary anodes, they offer the advantage of enabling one to distribute the thermal energy that is deposited onto the focal spot across the larger surface of a focal ring. This permits an increase in power for short operation times (fig. 12.22). However, as the anode is now rotating in a vacuum, the transfer of thermal energy to the outside of the tube envelope depends largely on radiation, which is not as effective as the liquid cooling used in stationary anodes. Rotating anodes are thus designed for high heat storage capacity and for good radiation exchange between anode and tube envelope. Another difficulty associated with rotating anodes is the operation of a bearing system under vacuum and the protection of this system against the destructive force of the anode's high temperatures. Appropriate designs for minimized heat flux into the bearing system are required.

In the early days of rotating anode X-ray tubes, the heat storage capacity of the anode was the main hindrance to high tube performance [12.20-12.22]. This has changed with the introduction of the following new technologies:

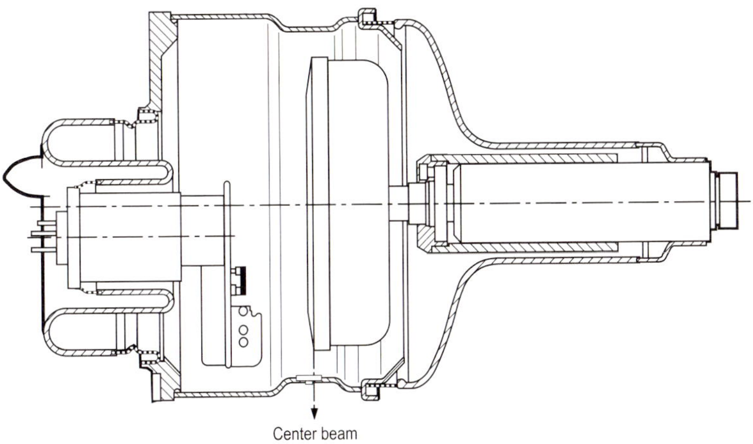

Figure 12.22 Typical tube with rotating anode

- Graphite blocks brazed to the anode dramatically increase heat storage capacity and heat dissipation.
- Liquid anode bearing systems (sliding bearings) provide heat conductivity to the surrounding cooling oil.
- Rotating envelope tubes allow direct liquid cooling for the backside of the rotating anode.

Materials for rotating anodes

Tungsten has been deployed as a target material in nearly all X-ray tube anodes designed for medical applications since 1909 (6.1.4). The anode plates of rotating anode tubes usually include a 1 to 2 mm thin layer of tungsten-rhenium alloy deposited onto a plate of molybdenum [12.23]. The rhenium increases the ductility of the tungsten, reduces thermomechanical stress and increases anode service life thanks to a slower roughening of the anode surface (always accompanied by a dose reduction) [12.24]. The ideal commercial and technological alloy has been determined to be composed of 5 to 10% rhenium and 90 to 95% tungsten (fig. 12.23).

As mentioned, the introduction of graphite blocks brazed to the backside of the molybdenum plate represents an advance in rotating anode technology. The graphite block in this design significantly increases the heat storage capacity of the anode, while requiring only a slight increase in overall anode weight. Furthermore, heat dissipation is accelerated by the larger anode surface and the superior emission coeffi-

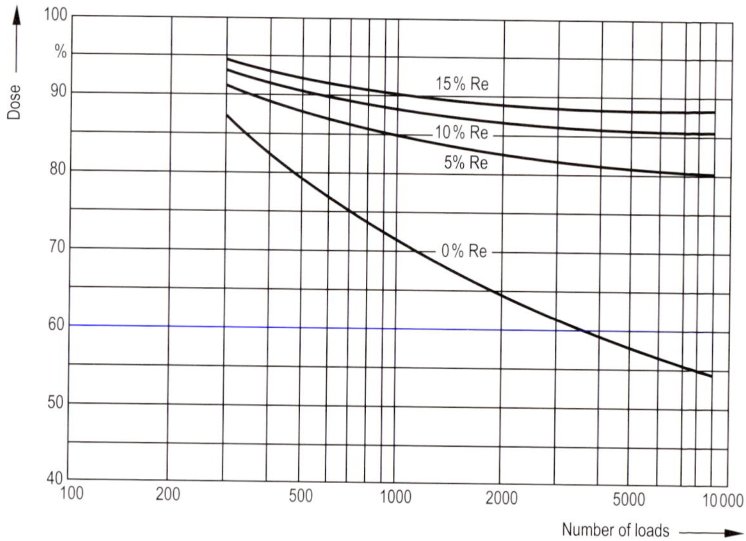

Figure 12.23
X-ray tube anode dose efficiency plotted against the number of tube loads. Plots are shown for different anode surface compositions containing between 0 and 15% rhenium in the tungsten layer. Resistance to wear and tear increases as the fraction of rhenium increases.

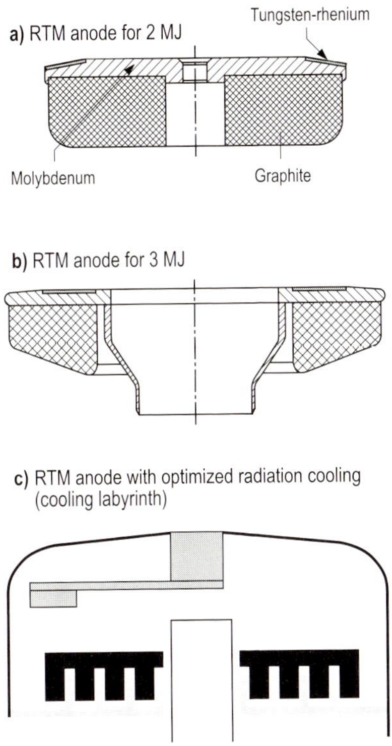

Figure 12.24
Various anode types. **a)**, **b)** Anodes with graphite rings that are brazed to the backside of the anodes. **c)** Anode with cooling labyrinth (Varian-specific)

cient of graphite compared to molybdenum [12.25]. Fig. 12.24a-c shows various anode designs offering different heat storage capacities.

Molybdenum and graphite are brazed together with zirconium or, for higher operating temperatures, with titanium or other specially designed brazing alloys.

Ball bearing systems

Ball bearing systems deployed in rotating anode X-ray tubes must be designed for operation under extreme conditions:

- They form a connection between the very hot anode plate and the cold environment.
- They need to operate under vacuum.
- They need to withstand high turning speeds of 100 to 150 Hz and substantial weight loads (e.g. a 10 kg anode plate in a typical CT machine equals a 100 kg effective load due to the centrifugal acceleration).

The lubricants need to fulfill certain specifications. For instance, they need to be constructed of soft deformable materials, resist alloy formation with the carrier material, remain stable at high temperatures and exhibit low vapor pressure under vacuum. These criteria limit the selection of lubricants to thin layers of lead or silver.

A sufficient reduction in the transfer of heat into the bearing system can be achieved by increasing the distance between the anode plate and the bearing and including materials of low heat conductivity. The bearing temperature must be kept below 400 °C to achieve good results.

In order to compensate for the wide operational temperature range and the high temperature gradients between the rotating and stationary parts of the bearing system, the bearings are designed with high degrees of axial and radial clearance, with special temperature compensation mechanisms and with a spring for preloading the system. Furthermore, only very small tolerances are accepted in the case of the individual bearing parts.

Liquid (sliding) bearings

The recent introduction of liquid metal bearings represents an innovation in rotating anode X-ray technology. These bearings use the aquaplaning effect of liquid metals and offer the following advantages:

- The bearing system is free of wear and tear.
- The generation of running noise is minimal.
- Additional anode cooling can be achieved by fast heat flux through the liquid metal in the bearing system.

The diagram in fig. 12.25 illustrates the principle. Two bodies are in motion relative to one another. The liquid between the bodies accumulates and forms a bow wave. This effect leads to a pressure buildup in the wedge between the two bodies. If the

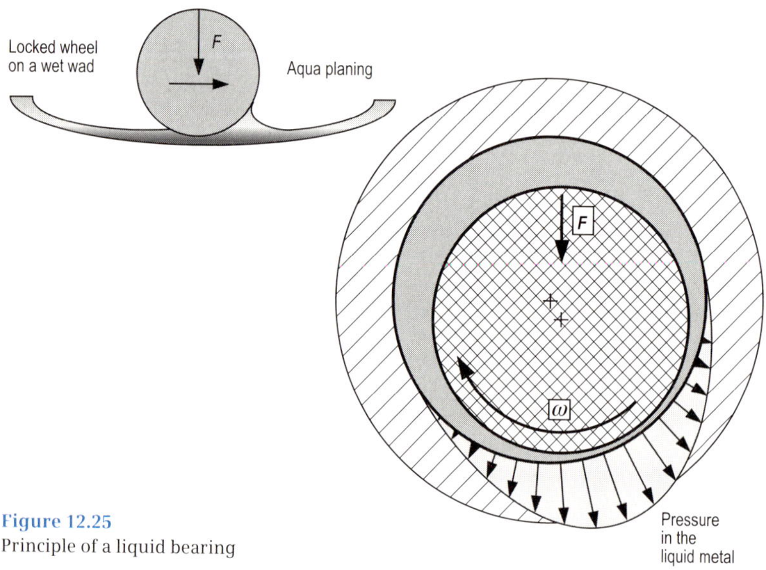

Figure 12.25
Principle of a liquid bearing

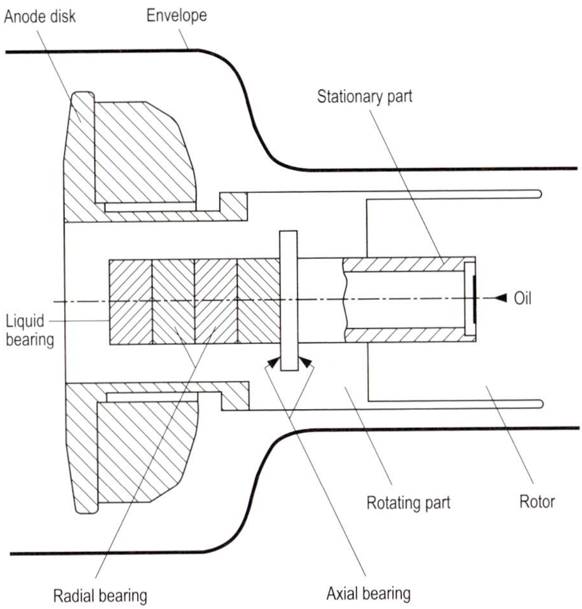

Figure 12.26
Typical assembly for an X-ray tube equipped with a liquid bearing. Due to the large contact surface between the liquid bearing's rotating and fixed parts, the heat deposited in the anode can be rapidly conducted to the cooling oil.

pressure exceeds a certain level, the liquid will enter the gap between the bodies until a film of liquid separates the bodies along their entire contact surface.

Fig. 12.26 offers an illustration of a liquid bearing used in X-ray technology. The bearing's stationary shaft is designed as a hollow body. This permits the active cooling of the bearing and thus also of the anode via the injection of a cooling agent. The thin ~20 μm gap between the stationary shaft and the rotating bearing body is filled with liquid metal. An eutectic of gallium, indium and tin with a melting temperature of between −10 °C and −11 °C is often used. In addition to the main radial bearing (i.e. formed by the stationary shaft and the rotating bearing body) an axial bearing is formed between the disk (with a larger diameter in the middle of the shaft) and the corresponding hollow ring in the bearing body (fig. 12.26). This construction enables one to achieve both radial and axial guidance and stabilization.

The load capacity of a liquid bearing depends essentially on the diameter and length of the design, on the rotation speed, on the viscosity of the liquid and on the size of the gap filled with liquid. It is necessary to ensure that the liquid metal does not escape from the bearing under any operating conditions and that the liquid metal does not form an alloy with other bearing parts. This can be achieved by selecting appropriate materials, using a surface coating and deploying accurate bearing parts. The anodes in commercially available X-ray tubes equipped with liquid bearings are typically run at a rotation speed of 150 Hz. The maximum heat transfer from the anode through the bearing into the cooling system is about 1 to 2 kW.

Tubes with rotating envelopes

A rotating envelope tube combines the advantages of stationary and rotating anodes:

- The backside of the anode is directly exposed to the cooling agent, as can be inferred from the stationary anode configuration. The anode thus cools down in a matter of seconds (fig. 12.27) and no additional heat storage capacity at the anode (e.g. graphite) is required.
- Given that the anode (together with the tube envelope) rotates in the manner of a conventional rotating anode, the thermal energy deposited at the focal spot is distributed across a focal ring (as with conventional rotating anode assemblies). The same performance thus results for brief high power X-ray generation, as is achievable with a (cold) rotating anode of the same diameter.

A number of mechanisms deployed in the development of rotating envelope tubes are protected by patents. One specific mechanism has recently been deployed in the development of a product currently sold under the brand name Straton. The most challenging task in the operation of this tube is the generation and stabilization of the focal spot relative to the non-rotating environment.

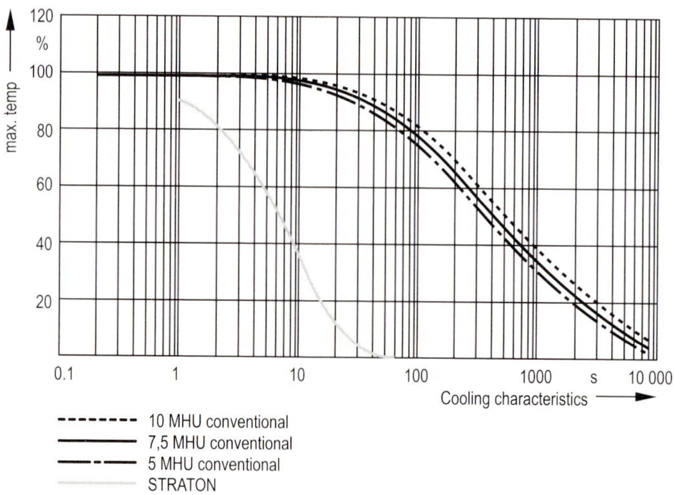

Figure 12.27
Cooling curves for different types of X-ray tubes. The cooling speed achievable via the direct cooling principle deployed in a rotating envelope tube (Straton 120) is several orders of magnitude faster than that of conventional X-ray tubes.

12.1.4 Anode load capacity

The impact of the electrons heats the anode. In order to avoid damage related to thermal stress and to prevent the evaporation of material, it is important to have access to information on the temperature of the anode base, the focal ring and the focal spot.

Anode disk temperature

The disk temperature is derived from the equilibrium of the power supplied by the electrons P and dissipated by radiation P_{Rad} and thermal conduction P_{Cond}

$$P - P_{\mathrm{Rad}} - P_{\mathrm{Cond}} = \frac{\mathrm{d}T_{\mathrm{Anode}}}{\mathrm{d}t} \sum_{\mathrm{i}} c_{\mathrm{i}}(T) m_{\mathrm{i}} \tag{12.8}$$

$c_{\mathrm{i}}\, m_{\mathrm{i}}$: Heat capacity of the single anode components (temperature dependent)

The subscript i in the formula is used to account for the various materials in anodes composed of several components (e.g. metallic disks, graphite rings and other materials).

The anode disk dissipates its heat power largely via thermal radiation, as described by the Stefan-Boltzmann law:

$$P_{\mathrm{Rad}} = \sigma (T^4_{\mathrm{Anode}} - T^4_{\mathrm{Envelope}}) \sum_{\mathrm{i}} A_{\mathrm{i\,Anode}} S_{\mathrm{i}}(T) \tag{12.9}$$

$A_{\mathrm{i}}(T)$: Anode absorption (temperature dependent) of component i

S_{i}: Surface area of anode component i

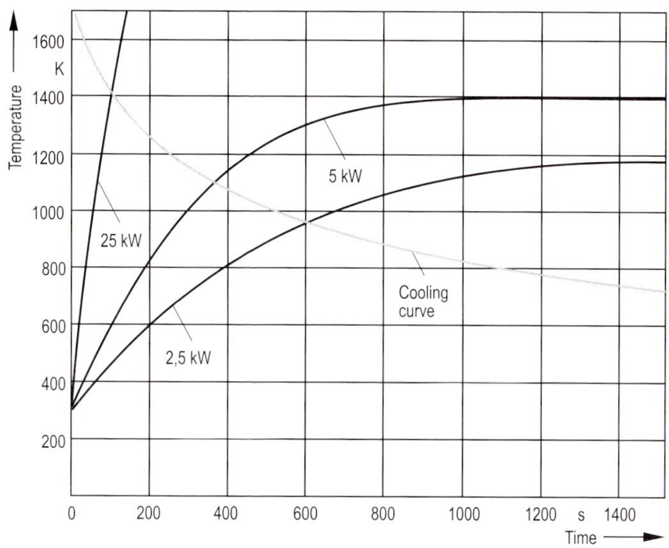

Figure 12.28
Anode plate temperature plotted against time for different scenarios: heating up during operation at 2.5 kW, 5 kW and 25 kW; cooling down without load

In the case of anodes with liquid metal bearings, a noticeable part of the anode heat is also dissipated by the liquid metal via thermal conduction. The efficiency of the dissipation depends on thermal conductivity κ, bearing surface S_B and the temperature difference between the anode and the cooling oil.

$$P_{\text{Cond}} = \kappa S_B (T_{\text{Anode}} - T_{\text{Oil}}) \tag{12.10}$$

κ: Thermal conductivity constant typical for the tube, S_B: Surface of the bearing

Fig. 12.28 shows anode disk heating and cooling curves for different loads P (fig. 12.28).

Focal spot and focal ring temperature rise

The temperature of the focal spot is significantly higher than the temperature of the anode disk. Fundamental work has been done on this subject by Bouwers [12.26] and Osterkamp [12.27] for stationary anodes. The rise in temperature ϑ for short load times (< 0.05 s for standard focal spot dimensions) can be approximated by

$$\vartheta = \frac{2P}{A_F}\sqrt{\frac{t}{\pi\lambda\rho c}} \tag{12.11}$$

P: Power input, $A_F = 2\delta l$ Area of focal spot, t: Load period
λ: Thermal conductivity, c: Specific heat, ρ: Mass density

and the rise for long loading times can be approximated by

$$\vartheta = \frac{P\delta}{A_F\lambda} \tag{12.12}$$

δ: Focal spot half width

The maximum permissible focal spot temperature in the case of stationary anodes is limited by the tolerable temperature at the boundary between the anode tungsten and copper and (during very long loading times) by the anode's thermal capacity and the heat dissipation to the surrounding oil.

While in the case of stationary anodes the time t in eq. (12.11) corresponds to the period during which the load is applied, it is necessary to replace this factor in the case of rotating anodes by an interval Δt in order to describe the duration the focal spot is hit by the electron beam at one revolution:

$$\Delta t = \frac{\delta}{\pi R f} \tag{12.13}$$

δ: Focal spot half width, R: Focal track radius, f: Anode rotation frequency

The temperature rise at the focal spot for a rotating anode is thus approximated by

$$\vartheta_{\text{Focus}} = \frac{2P}{A_F}\sqrt{\frac{\delta}{\pi^2 R\lambda\rho c f}} \tag{12.14}$$

The focal track on the target is formed by the multitude of all surface elements heated by the electron beam. The track is visible on used targets as a highly roughened circle (fig. 12.29). Focal track temperature ϑ_{Track} increases as the number of revolutions n increases (fig. 12.30):

$$\vartheta_{\text{Track}} = k\,\vartheta_{\text{Focus}}\sqrt{\frac{\delta}{\pi R}(n+1)} \tag{12.15}$$

k: Factor accounting for anode thickness, thermal radiation, radial heat diffusion
$n = t\,f$: Number of revolutions during time t

The focal ring temperature of an anode rotating at 100 Hz or 150 Hz increases during a 1-second load by a factor of 10 or 12, respectively. The reduction in the focal spot temperature that results from the increased rotation frequency is partially compensated for by the fact that the focal ring temperature increases as the frequency increases.

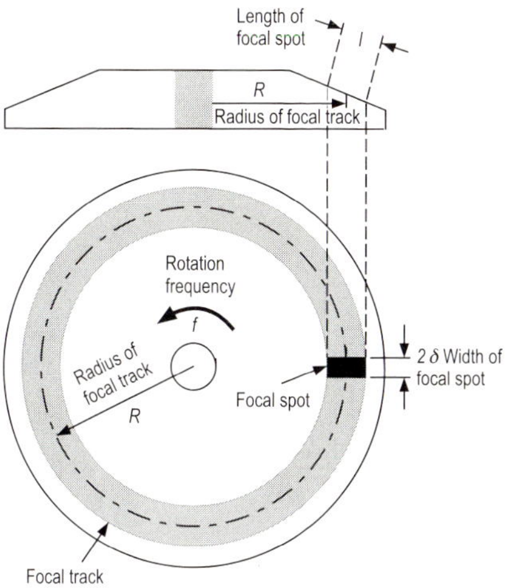

Figure 12.29
Anode plate geometry for a typical rotating anode X-ray tube

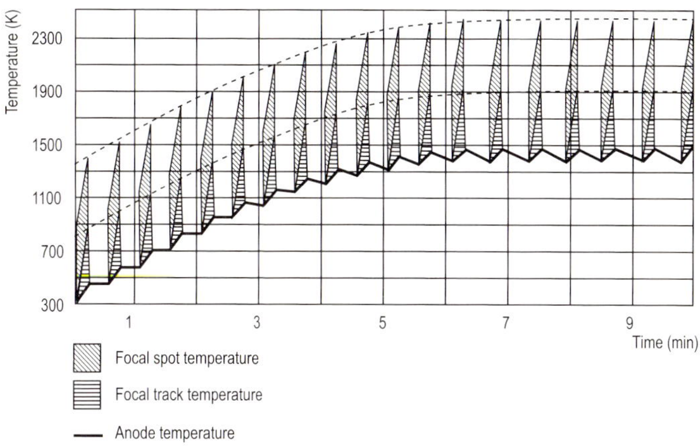

Figure 12.30
Temperature of the focal spot, the focal track and the target base of a rotating anode plotted against the number of revolutions or the elapsed time t during X-ray generation

By combining eqs. (12.14 and 12.15) one obtains the anode power necessary to achieve the total focal spot temperature rise:

$$\Delta T = \vartheta_{\text{Track}} + \vartheta_{\text{Focus}} \quad (12.16)$$

$$P = \frac{\pi \Delta T \sqrt{\lambda \rho c}\, l \sqrt{\delta R f}}{1 + k \sqrt{\frac{\delta}{\pi R}}\, f\, t} \quad (12.17)$$

l: Focal spot length

Temperature balance and time-related temperature changes

The absolute temperature in the focal spot T_{Focus} follows as

$$T_{\text{Focus}} = T_{\text{Anode}} + \Delta T = T_{\text{Anode}} + \vartheta_{\text{Track}} + \vartheta_{\text{Focus}} \quad (12.18)$$

The temperature rise in the focal spot takes place within milliseconds, the temperature equalization between disk and focal track takes some seconds. Each of the three quoted temperatures (focal spot, focal track and anode disk base temperature) is subject to specific limitations relating to the materials and processes used.

An upper temperature limit is reached when an arc discharge occurs between the anode and cathode or envelope as a consequence of the ionization of the evaporating metal. A second limitation in the maximum focal spot temperature is created by focal track wear and tear caused by thermomechanical stress and resulting in dose reduction. The maximum permissible focal spot temperature is set well below these limitations so as to safeguard the tube and secure an acceptable service life.

Anode temperature simulation

Calculating anode temperatures on the basis of the above described formulas is not sufficient to determine the dynamic spatial and temporal temperature distributions in complex tube designs. In such cases, the object can be physically and geometrically modeled via FEM (finite element-method) with the help of a dedicated computer simulation program. Here, the temperature is calculated for each small element, taking into account contributions from all neighboring areas. This enables one to obtain the spatial temperatures and the thermal mechanical stress for the whole object in relation to the applicable input power and time (fig. 12.31). Furthermore, it also yields parameters such as temperature rise, temperature gradients in the focus, temperature in the focal track, temperature in the brazing layer and stress in the target surface.

12.1.5 X-ray tube vacuum envelopes

Vacuum enclosure

Correct X-ray tube functioning depends on the capacity of the electrons to avoid collisions with gas particles as they move from the cathode to the anode. This requirement makes the establishment of mean free paths in the order of several meters necessary (corresponding to gas pressures smaller than 10^{-4} mbar). The key role of all tube en-

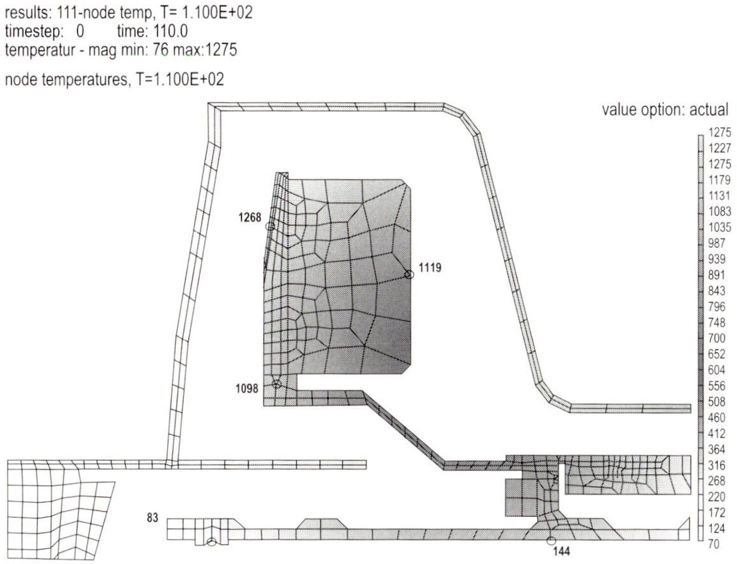

Figure 12.31
Theoretical calculation of the heat distribution in a rotary anode plate; calculation performed using a finite element approach.

velopes is to make such a vacuum possible and to maintain it for the entire service life of the tube.

The manufacturing process usually includes the deployment of turbomolecular pumps to evacuate the X-ray tube to an internal pressure of less than 10^{-6} mbar. The enclosure's maximum permissible effective leakage rate may not exceed 10^{-15} mbar l/s [12.28]. Operation at high power levels increases the initial internal pressure owing to the desorption of bound gasses caused by the increased temperature in the tube components. This process, however, is normally reversible. Furthermore, the rise in pressure can be counterbalanced by application of so-called getter materials (e.g. porous zirconium sinter bodies) in the tube [12.29].

In what follows, we discuss the design and the choice of materials.

X-ray tube envelopes used to be made exclusively of special glass materials (fig. 12.32a). As the technology developed, these were then replaced by so-called metal center-part tubes (fig. 12.32b) whose configurations were characterized by the use of glass only at the anode and cathode sites and the use of metals such as stainless steel, copper and Cu-Ni alloys for the center part of the tube. In the case of bipolar tubes, the center part is usually grounded in order to divert the high number of reflected electrons that originate from the anode focal spot and strike the tube envelope. Up to 15-20% of the original input power can be carried by these electrons to the tube envelope. The percentage of reflected energy is even higher (up to 30-35%) in the case of

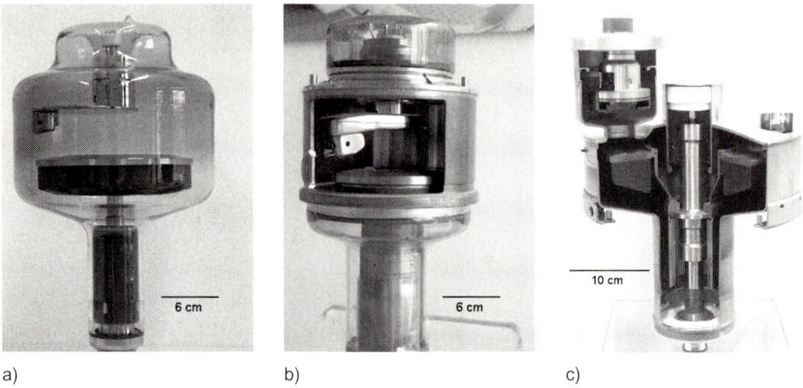

Figure 12.32
Different types of tube envelopes. **a)** Glass envelope, **b)** Metal-glass envelope, **c)** Metal envelope with ceramic insulators

an anode-grounded tube design. Modern tube envelopes are made almost entirely of metal (fig. 12.32c). Ceramic inserts of highly purified aluminum oxide are used at the anode and cathode sites (metal ceramic tubes) for purposes of insulation.

Mechanical and thermal stability

In addition to providing a vacuum enclosure, the tube envelope also serves as a backbone for the mechanical fixing of the individual X-ray tube components. Particularly high demands are placed on the mechanical stability of the envelope in order to maintain the stability of the focusing position on the anode. The highest forces acting on the tube enclosure are caused by the centrifugal acceleration of more than 20 g (g = earth acceleration) in modern CT scanners:

$$a = 4\pi^2 f^2 r \qquad (12.19)$$

a: Centrifugal acceleration, r: Gantry radius
f: Rotation frequency of the CT gantry

Typical values for the parameters are $r = 0.6$ m and $f = 1$ to 3 Hz.

The tube cover is also required to withstand the difference between the tube vacuum pressure and the pressure within the tube housing. This pressure difference may be higher than 3 bar in specific designs.

Metal enclosures also represent a safety feature in that they protect the patient from anode system bursting at high rotational speeds.

Finally, tube envelopes are also required to exhibit sufficient mechanical resistance to strong local stresses that arise in connection with temperature changes during tube operation. High temperature gradients in the envelope material are especially possibile in the vicinity of the focal spot, where the above-mentioned reflected electrons hit the tube envelope.

Electrical insulation

In addition to proper vacuum enclosure and mechanical stability, the tube envelope is also required to provide electrical insulation for the applied tube voltages relative to one another and to the system ground. Special glass or ceramic feed-through elements are used to connect the cathode and anode to the high voltage power supply. The high voltage potentials at the anode and cathode must remain reliably insulated throughout the tube's service life. The glass bulbs used in the past proved deficient in this regard on account of the formation of vaporized metal films on their inner surfaces. While production is currently dominated by metal ceramic tube envelopes, the introduction of this technology was also marked by certain drawbacks. For instance, the high specific resistance of the ceramic materials led to unwanted local charging effects and associated electrical breakdowns. This problem was finally resolved by the introduction of special shielding electrodes [12.30].

Heat dissipation

Nearly all dissipated heat is required to leave the tube during operation via the tube envelope so that it can be absorbed by the cooling medium circulating around the tube envelope in the tube housing. High performance X-ray tubes rely on the capacity of all tube envelope materials to deliver high heat conductivity and a high absorption coefficient for thermal radiation (at the vacuum side).

Maximum spectral intensity distribution for tubes designed for radiation cooling lies within a wavelength band of around 2 µm at a temperature of 1,500 K [12.31]. Optimal radiation transfer to the envelope depends on an optimization of the absorption coefficient for the inner surface of the tube enclosure, especially with respect to the regions of the main heat exchange in the vicinity of the anode. This can be achieved by mechanical roughening ($A \approx 0.5$) or the use of a coating ($A \approx 0.9$).

Heat dissipation in the case of directly cooled tubes (e.g. rotating envelope tubes) is dominated by heat conduction through the solid envelope material. The thermal conduction coefficients of the applied materials thus play a dominant role.

Magnetic properties

In order to increase image quality in CT applications, an external electromagnetic deflection system consisting of magnetic coils is sometimes used as a means of electronically controlling the focal spot position. In this case, the tube enclosure is required to be non-magnetic, at least in the relevant regions. Furthermore, the specific electrical resistance has to be large enough in order to avoid excessive eddy current losses. While glass offers ideal properties in light of the requirements, metals such as austenitic steel and Cu-Ni alloys can also be used [12.7].

X-ray absorption properties

Only a small fraction of the X-rays emerging isotropically from the focal spot contributes to imaging. All other X-rays need to be blocked to protect the operator and the patients. For this reason, envelope materials that offer high X-ray absorption rates are desirable, especially for the half space above the anode plate. Assuming that appropriate envelope materials are selected, a good proportion of the unwanted radiation will be absorbed close to its origin. This permits a reduction in the amount of shielding material that is incorporated in the tube housing to meet requirements relating to radiation leakage.

In contrast, the used X-ray beam should ideally remain uninfluenced when passing the tube envelope, unless a degree of modulation is desired (e.g. to harden the radiation). This contradiction is solved by incorporating X-ray windows into the tube envelope:

- In glass tubes, the thickness of the tube envelope is diminished in the region where the applied X-ray beam leaves the tube.
- In metal tubes, specially designed metal windows consisting of beryllium or titanium (also for radiation hardening) are used.

12.1.6 Casing design

The first X-ray tubes developed by Roentgen at the end of the 19th century had no additional casing besides the tube envelope. Today, the housing of an X-ray tube is an integral part of the system. It combines various functions necessary for the safe operation of the X-ray tube:

- X-ray shielding to protect the patient and operator
- High voltage tube connection and insulation
- Mechanical interface between tube and system environment

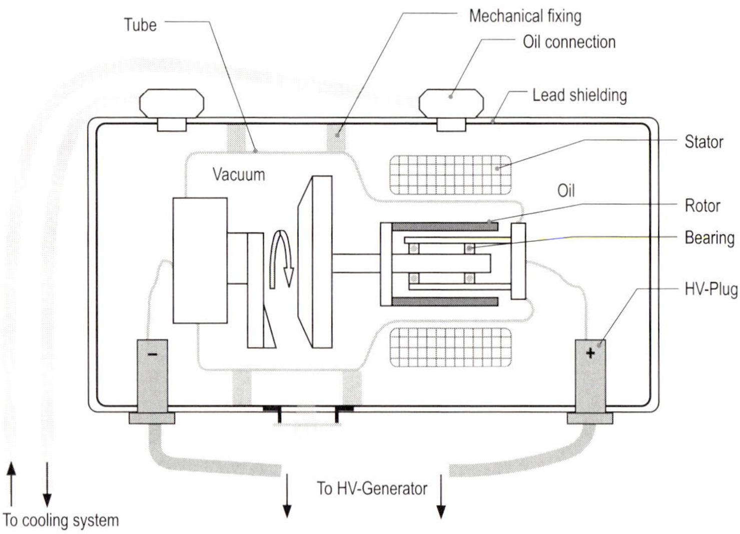

Figure 12.33 Housing and peripheral components around a typical rotating anode tube

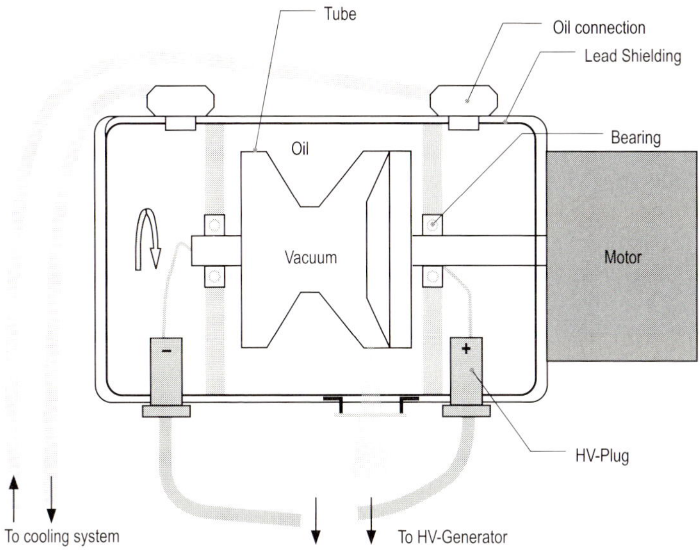

Figure 12.34 Housing and peripheral components around a rotating envelope tube (Straton 120)

While the current literature on X-ray generation and X-ray systems (e.g. [12.32]) centers mainly on tube design, engineers are increasingly faced by complex challenges in the area of housing design.

In general, two distinct casing designs are deployed in contemporary high performance tube systems:

- Classical, simple design used for rotating anode tubes (fig. 12.33)
- Complex design used for rotating envelope tubes (fig. 12.34)

X-ray shielding

In the early days of its clinical use, nothing was known about the harmful impact of X-radiation on the human body. Both tube operators and patients were left exposed to various degrees of X-radiation. Today, radiation doses for patients and tube operators are subject to strict regulations.

These regulations specify the precautions that are to be taken to prevent (scattered) X-rays from leaving the tube housing at any undesirable locations and from veering off in any direction away from the X-ray beam used for diagnostic image generation. This is achieved by deploying shielding in the tube housing. Apart from a small window in the direction of the X-ray beam, the entire housing is outfitted with a shielding envelope. The window usually contains collimators made of lead, which further limit and pre-shape the X-ray fan emitted from the tube focus through the X-ray window (fig. 12.35).

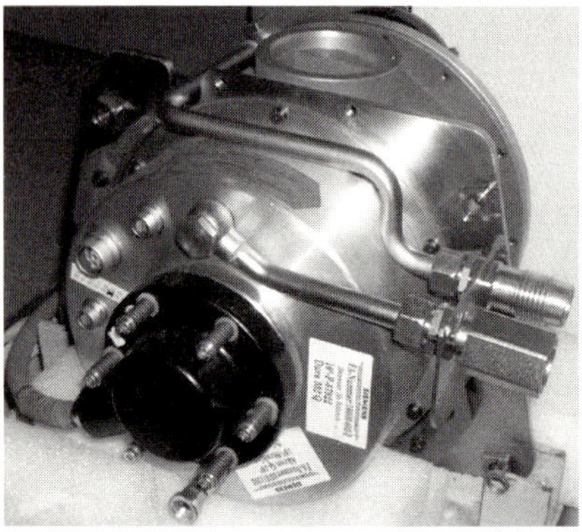

Figure 12.35
Siemens Akron tube in its housing. The X-ray window is clearly visible at the top.

Potential materials for shielding include heavy metals such as lead, molybdenum and tantalum. Lead is often used because it is cheap and easily available in sufficient quantities. Lead sheets are typically glued to the inner wall of the tube housing. Given that raw lead would have a negative impact on the quality of the cooling and insulation oil, all lead surfaces are usually coated.

High-voltage connection and insulation

The design of the tube housing assembly is required to guarantee a sufficient distance between the high voltage parts and the casing. Edges should be rounded off in order to avoid high electrical field strength. The risk of arcing can be reduced by spatially concentrating parts possessing high electrical potential towards the center of the tube housing and by introducing long insulation (creeping) distances (e.g. along roughened polymer or ceramic insulators). Furthermore, filling the space between the X-ray tube and the tube envelope with oil will provide both electrical insulation and cooling.

Most medical X-ray tube systems today are filled with mineral oil for purposes of cooling and insulation. However, air-cooled tube systems are also available. If oil is used for the sake of cooling, it is necessary to make sure that a sufficiently strong stream of oil is directed to the hot spots in the tube envelope.

A large portion of the heat that is generated during the operation of classical rotary anode tubes is stored in the anode plate and then slowly transferred to the tube envelope (and to the surrounding cooling oil) during the necessary cool-down phase following tube operation. The overall cooling system is required to provide continuous cooling of the average tube power (e.g. via the deployment of a heat exchanger connected to the primary oil circuit).

In the case of rotating envelope tubes, the generated heat is transferred almost instantaneously from the anode to the surrounding cooling oil during operation. This design relies on turbulent and significantly faster cooling oil streams and dramatically increased oil volumes per time period to fully support tube performance. A high performance cooling system with sufficiently high peak power is required. The introduction of an oil reservoir in the oil circuit represents an alternative. Here, the reservoir acts as a heat reservoir (~10 l oil have the same heat storage capacity as 1,000 cm^3 of the typical anode materials used in conventional rotating anode tubes). The use of latency heat reservoirs (as commonly used in automobiles) would also represent an option.

The only rotating envelope tube system that is commercially available today (Siemens Straton) uses an oil reservoir for the interim storage of thermal energy.

The cooling capacity of today's tube cooling systems ranges (depending on the throughput of cooling air) from around 7 to 10 kW. This amounts to a cooling capacity equal to the task of dissipating the heat emission from an open fire.

Mechanical interface

The housing is the mechanical interface between the tube and the X-ray system (e.g. a CT scanner or an angiography system). The rotation of the CT gantry in CT applications (fig. 12.36) generates centrifugal forces that act on the housing and the tube (up to 30 *g*). Both the tube envelope (as mentioned above) and the entire tube housing assembly with its weight of about 50 kg are required to resist these forces and the additional mechanical stress caused by temperature gradients.

In addition to the tube envelope, the tube housing is also required to guarantee the stability and the accuracy of the focal spot position when exposed to high centrifugal forces and thermal stress. Sophisticated design methods such as 3D-CAD systems and FEM (finite element method) simulations represent essential tools of modern tube housing design when it comes to fulfilling these complex requirements.

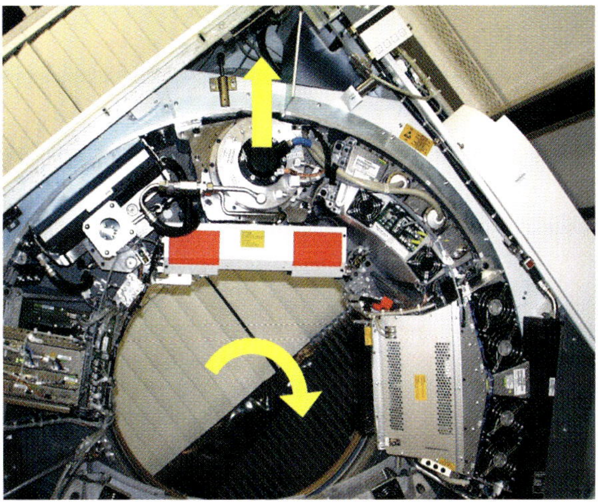

Figure 12.36
View into the open gantry (cover removed) of a CT scanner (rotation and centrifugal force indicated)

12.2 X-ray generators

12.2.1 General requirements

The X-ray generator numbers among an X-ray imaging system's crucial components because it effects and controls the setting of the exposure parameters. X-ray generator functioning thus has a direct effect on the contrast and detail perceptibility of the X-ray image. We will use in this paragraph the technical terms as are defined for medical equipment in [12.33].

Certain generator parameters, including X-ray tube voltage U (kV), X-ray tube current I (mA) and irradiation time T (s), determine the air kerma K (μGy) or the dose behind the patient that is detected by the image receptor. Dose and selected exposure parameters are empirically related by

$$K \propto U^n I \, T \tag{12.20}$$

The detected dose does not only depend on the irradiated object, but also on the beam quality or X-ray spectrum, which is determined by the tube's anode material, the filtration of the primary beam and the ripple in the X-ray tube voltage. The value of n is approximately 3 for X-ray tube voltages around 150 kV. The lower the X-ray tube voltage and the thicker the patient, the higher is the value of n, which will increase to values of 5 or more at voltages of around 50 kV [12.34].

The X-ray tube voltage determines the upper limit of the X-radiation's energy. When accounting for filtration and ripple, it determines the spectral distribution of the X-radiation, and thus image characteristics as well. The task of selecting the appropriate X-ray tube voltage is primarily a matter of answering specific diagnostic questions:

- What object is to be examined?
- What contrast ratio is important for the diagnosis? A radiograph of thoracic bone structure, for example, requires 66 kV, whereas a chest radiograph requires at least 125 kV (i.e. to permit a diagnosis of the lung tissue behind the ribs).

Ripple in the X-ray tube voltage causes an increase in the low energy part of the X-ray spectrum [12.35] (fig. 12.37). Given that this part of the spectrum is largely absorbed by tissue without contributing to image generation, it is essential to minimize ripple, with constant potential representing the ideal case.

While focal spot size determines the sharpness of the X-ray image, it also limits the X-ray tube's maximum electric power $P_{\mathrm{Tube}}(t)$. The maximum tube current $I_{\max}(t)$ is derived from the tube voltage U, which is selected on the basis of the image contrast criteria for the object under investigation:

$$I_{\max}(t) = \frac{P_{\mathrm{Tube}}(t)}{U} \tag{12.21}$$

The last parameter that has an effect on the dose is the irradiation time T. This time should be short enough to ensure sharp images of moving organs. Heart and lung tissue movements can reach velocities of up to 200 mm/s [12.36] and artery vessels pulse

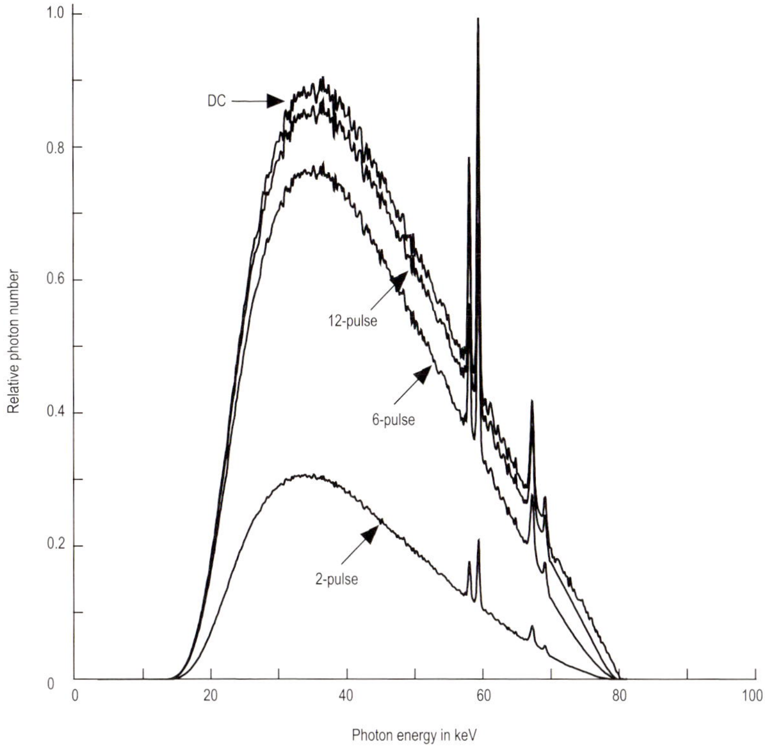

Figure 12.37 X ray spectra dependence on the waveform of the X-ray tube voltage

at similar velocities. X-ray examinations in children are particularly influenced by fast organ movements, as children exhibit faster heart-beat and breathing rates.

Given that dose at a given voltage is proportional to tube current and irradiation time, the value of the selected charge $Q = I\,T$ (mAs) as an exposure parameter should not exceed the tube's power limit.

The reproducibility of X-ray generator parameters is essential for obtaining constant image quality. Regular checks of generator parameters are therefore compulsory in many countries [12.37]. Restricting patient radiation exposure to values that are effective for image formation is a matter of basic X-radiation hygiene. The X-ray generator is required to quickly reach the nominal value of the X-ray tube voltage and then switch off immediately after achieving the right dose for an image of an appropriate brightness.

These requirements (i.e. optimal image quality and patient/operator safety) have led to a number of developments in the area of automatic exposure control (AEC) that can be applied to various kinds of X-ray examinations.

Operating range

The operating range of an X-ray generator is shown in fig. 12.38. The nominal electric power is defined [12.33] as the highest constant electric output in kilowatts that can be delivered for a single X-ray tube load of $U = 100$ kV at a loading time of 0.1 s:

$$P = f\,U\,I \tag{12.22}$$

The value of f depends on the voltage waveform. This value is 0.95 for six-peak and 1.00 for twelve-peak and constant potential high-voltage generators. Inverter generators (see below) are comparable to constant potential high-voltage generators.

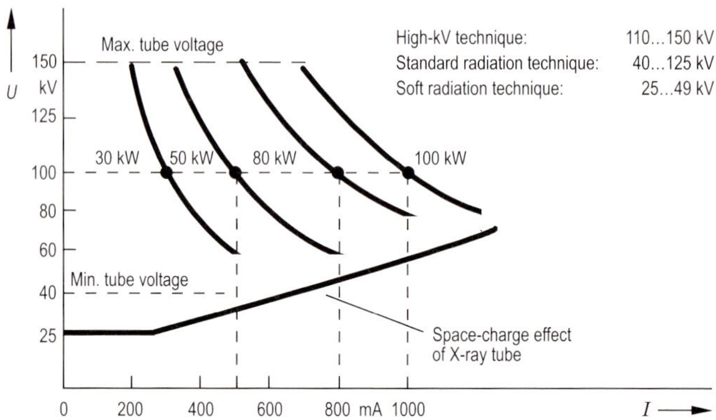

Figure 12.38 X-ray generator operating range

X-ray generators used in the area of dental diagnostics and mammography are outfitted for a maximum electric power of up to 5 kW. Mobile generators (sometimes battery-powered) are outfitted for a maximum power of up to 20 kW and fixed-installation generators used for general medical diagnostic purposes and CT are outfitted for a maximum power of up to 80 kW or more. Generators used for angiography, which involves very short irradiation times and high X-ray tube currents, exhibit a maximum electric power of up to 100 kW (fig. 12.38). Tube current I is usually around 0.1 mA for fluoroscopy and as high as 1,000 mA for radiography.

Exposure time and reproducibility

Fig. 12.39 illustrates the definition of exposure time as specified by the International Electrotechnical Commission (IEC) [12.33]. Standards have also been established for linearity and intermittent-mode constancy (switching tube current time product) as well as for system functions related to automatic exposure control (see section 12.2.4). Due to the discharge of high-voltage capacitors following switch-off, the actual current time product may be slightly larger than the pre-selected value. One exposure point in an exposure table [12.32] for X-ray diagnostics corresponds to a dose change of 25%, an easily discernable change in the density of an X-ray film.

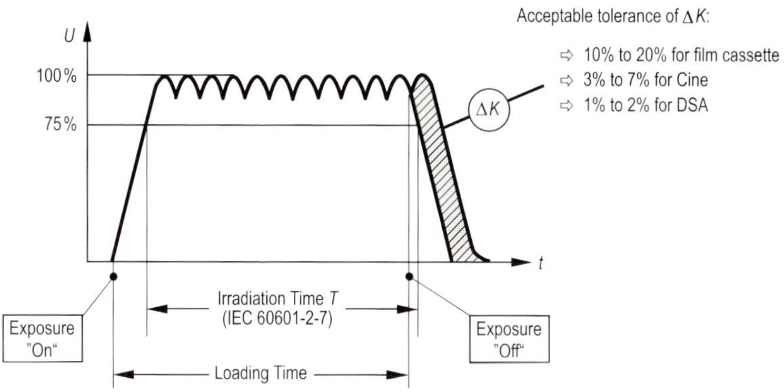

Figure 12.39
Loading and irradiation time of an X-ray exposure (frame-to-frame acceptable tolerance for dose ΔK)

Earlier generator technology based on thyristor inverters remained saddled with the problem of offering no way of influencing a charge amount ΔQ triggered just prior to the switch-off signal. The new high frequency inverter systems based on transistor technology represent a significant improvement in this regard. ΔQ is reduced thanks to the transistor inverter's higher frequency and the possibility of switching off a transistor at any time.

12.2.2 Technical aspects

In order to achieve constant image quality, the output characteristics of state-of-the-art generators, including power, tube voltage and current, should not exceed tolerances of more than 5%. Conventional six- and twelve-peak generators still in use show tolerances between 10% and 20% at best. These types of generators involve line-frequency feeding of a high-voltage transformer. The rectified voltage on the secondary side acts as anode voltage for the X-ray tube. This technology is quickly being replaced by inverter type generators.

Constant potential high-voltage generators use parallel capacitors and a control circuit between the rectified high-voltage and the X-ray tube. This control is based on triodes or tetrodes, and yields voltage tolerances as low as 0.1%. Although they are still in use for special applications (e.g. electron beam tomography, which depends on very constant potentials), constant potential high-voltage generators are also being replaced by inverter type generators owing to their high production cost and volume coverage.

The inverter type high-voltage generator (or high frequency X-ray generator) preserves the positive aspects of constant potential high-voltage generators with regard to reproducibility and tube voltage constancy and their principle of operation ensures that their output voltage remains largely unaffected by power-source voltage fluctuations and X-ray tube current. Further advantages include their small size and low production costs. All of these advantages have contributed to the establishment of the high frequency or inverter type generator's status as a standard component in all fields of X-ray diagnostics, including computed tomography, mammography and other areas where variable high-power DC voltage is required (e.g. gradient PSUs for MRI).

Fig. 12.40 shows the high frequency generator's principle components. The most important properties of these components include:

- Controlled or non-controlled intermediate DC voltage U_{DC} with more or less ripple generated by power source rectification. Although the electric output power will naturally differ, the same high-voltage quality can be obtained from a single-phase power source as from a 3-phase power source.
- The DC/AC inverter uses the intermediate DC voltage to produce a high frequency alternating current. This feeds a dedicated high-voltage transformer, which is connected on its secondary side to a high-voltage rectifier and smoothing capacitor. The high frequency inverter normally applies pulse width modulation or acts as a resonant circuit type [12.38], depending on the power switches used.
- Given that it allows for a reduction in the transformer core cross section, the transformation of high frequency AC voltage yields a very small high-voltage transformer volume.
- X-ray tube voltage and current can be controlled independently and are largely unaffected by power source voltage fluctuations.
- The electronic X-ray tube voltage control exhibits a response time of 0.1 ms or less.

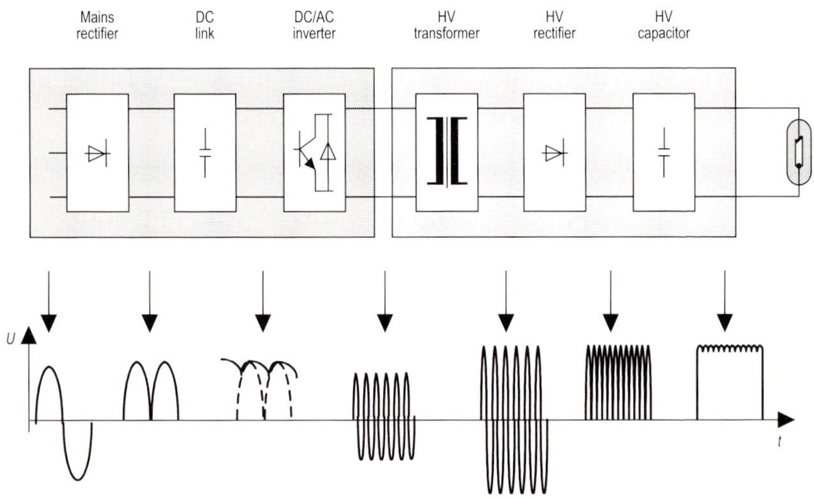

Figure 12.40 Principle behind the high frequency X-ray generator

12.2.3 Control circuits

Inverter system and X-ray tube voltage control circuit

The use of semiconductor power switch thyristors in inverter systems at the beginning of the 1980s led to dramatic changes in X-ray generator technology. This thyristor technology enabled one to design smaller systems with lower range kHz frequencies to achieve enhanced data reproducibility. Subsequent developments, including bipolar transistors and new power devices, such as metal oxide semiconductor field effect transistors (MOSFETs), then introduced the possibility of increasing frequencies above the hearing limit. Today, insulated gate bipolar transistors (IGBTs), which exhibit both the high impedance characteristic of MOSFETs and the low on-state voltage characteristic of bipolar transistors, are the devices of choice for use in inverters. Frequencies have increased up to 100 kHz or more, resulting in enhanced performance and smaller packaging.

Thanks to limitations of power losses of these silicon components, a further increase of the inverter frequency and with it generator performance has reached a limit. New devices with higher reverse voltage, smaller leakage current and reduced capacity are under development. Silicon carbide (SiC) is considered the most promising semiconducting material for this purpose [12.39].

- The principle behind the high-voltage closed loop control circuit is shown in fig. 12.41. The actual value of the X-ray tube voltage U_{act} is measured and compared to the nominal value U_{nom} selected by the operator at the control console in a comparator circuit. The comparator triggers the power switches in the inverter and these feed the high-voltage transformer with current pulses. The speed of this control

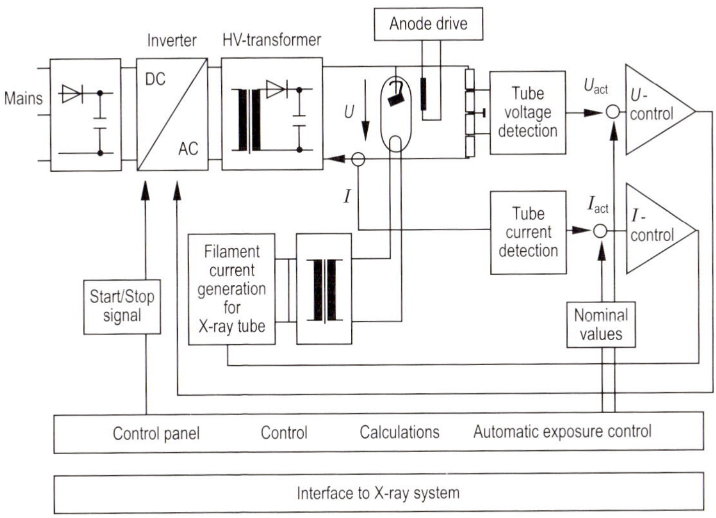

Figure 12.41 Principle behind X-ray tube voltage and tube current control circuits

system depends mainly on the inverter frequency. Although it is not quite as fast as constant potential high-voltage generators, the inverter easily exceeds the speed of conventional multi-peak rectifiers. The ripple in the resulting voltage on the secondary side of the transformer is influenced mainly by the inverter frequency, the internal smoothing capacity, the capacity of the high-voltage supply cables and the value U_{DC} of the intermediate DC voltage.

Filament circuit and current control

As shown in section 12.1, tube current I is mainly determined by the temperature of the cathode, and therefore strongly depends on the filament current I_F. Fig. 12.42 shows the correlation between I and I_F with anode voltage U as a parameter. I_F directly determines the maximum current I at voltage U and is therefore in need of careful control.

An X-ray generator usually deploys two different modes of operation for filament control:

1. Preheating: when the system is in stand-by mode, the filament control circuit holds the filament to a temperature that is low enough to prevent the generation of X-radiation and that permits a rapid return to operation temperature.
2. Heating during X-radiation: the filament current is set and controlled to a value that conforms to the required maximum current for the X-ray tube at the chosen anode voltage. The latter is derived in accordance with the selected application (continuous or pulsed fluoroscopy or radiography) from the tube's characteristic operating diagram.

Given the steepness of the curve $I = f(I_F)$, filament current control requires very high precision. A variation of a mere 1% of I_F will cause an unacceptable deviation in the X-ray tube current. The capacity to switch rapidly between fluoroscopy and radiography presupposes high filament current control standards.

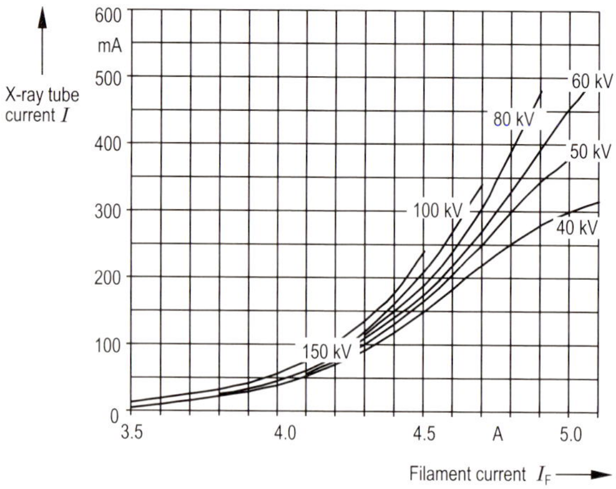

Figure 12.42
Filament current, tube current and tube voltage dependance

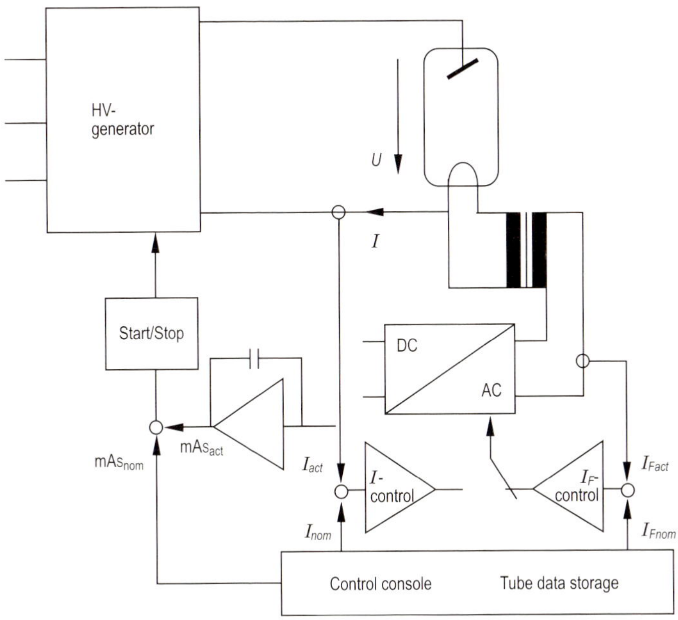

Figure 12.43 Filament and tube current control circuit

Fig. 12.43 shows a state-of-the-art filament current control circuit applying pulse frequency modulation. This control enables one to avoid low frequency power source ripple that can lead to the appearance of X-ray spectrum fluctuations in conventional filament circuits.

Filament current control in conformity with the required tube current permits two types of operation. Either tube current I is kept constant during exposure (constant load) or it is modulated along a given curve (continuously falling load). In the latter case, the tube's focal spot is allowed to remain at its maximum temperature. This results in a minimization of irradiation time and a reduction in motion-related blurring.

An internal microprocessor system updates the operating diagrams $I = f\,(I_F, U)$ for all connected tubes during the X-ray generator's set-up phase (service mode operation) and after X-ray tube changes. This is made necessary by cathode production tolerances. Finally, the independent control of tube voltage U, tube current I and irradiation time T by modern X-ray generators guarantees optimal image quality at minimum dose.

Rotating anode control

X-ray tubes outfitted with rotating anodes permit considerably higher tube loads than X-ray tubes outfitted with fixed anodes. Modern anode drives use 3-phase asynchronous motors connected to 3-phase inverter systems to provide application-specific drive frequency. Asynchronous motors require large air gaps on account of the need to isolate the rotor (anode potential) from the stator (ground potential). This reduces the degree of efficiency of these motors compared to ordinary asynchronous motors.

Ball bearings used in vacuum X-ray tubes have limited service lives owing to their exposure to high temperatures and a lack of lubricant. For this reason (and also because of acoustic noise) the anode is only rotated during the loading. The anode is accelerated at the beginning of the X-radiation period and is usually decelerated as soon as the period has ended. The anode disk's weight and torque define the acceleration time. This time can be minimized by continuously changing the drive frequency (the anode drive inverter's output frequency) that is applied to the stator.

Tubes with liquid bearings permit higher anode loads and generate minimal noise. Thanks to the automatic lubrication of liquid bearings the anode of such a tube type is accelerated once to nominal drive frequency and driven all day long. X-radiation can be generated at any time, with only a slight delay as the filament current switches from its stand-by value to its operating value.

Control console

User interfaces at the X-ray generator's control console provide access to all of the X-ray generator system's relevant data. The console permits one to set the nominal parameters, including X-ray tube voltage U, X-ray tube current I, irradiation time T and/or tube current time product. Depending on the radiological application involved, various adjustments are available:

- Selection of X-ray tube voltage U (kV)
- Selection of X-ray tube voltage U (kV) and tube current time product (mAs)
- Selection of X-ray tube voltage U (kV), X-ray tube current I (mA) (or tube current time product, mAs) and irradiation time T (ms)

Several other parameters (e.g. maximum power, focal spot, automatic exposure control (AEC), measuring electrodes, X-ray film speed, film density corrections) are also set at the control console. Fig. 12.44 offers an illustration of a modern control design. In special cases, however, the user interface for the X-ray generator data is also integrated into the examination unit's monitor, for instance, in CT systems or systems that apply digital image processing (e.g. DSA).

In order to optimize workflow and secure reproducible image quality, all of an X-ray investigation's important radiographic parameters may be set via a single program button. This is usually assigned to anatomic regions.

Actual data, including X-ray tube voltage and current and elapsed fluoroscopy time, are displayed in a dedicated area of the control console. If a special metering system is connected, the area exposure product $P_F (Gy \cdot m^2)$ will also be displayed.

Optic and acoustic information is issued during the X-radiation period signal to the operator and support staff when the X-rays are applied. The status of the X-ray thermal tube load also represents important information for the operator. The generator

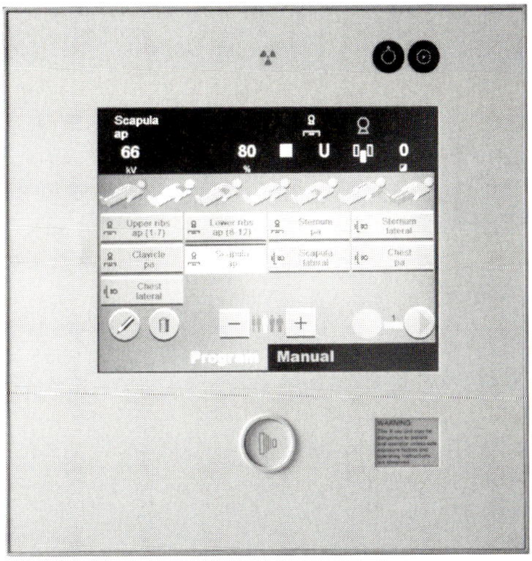

Figure 12.44
Modern control console with touch screen

system's internal microprocessor calculates this value on the basis of the loading and cooling times and displays it as a percentage of the maximum load or as a unit of waiting time for a subsequent exposure. In this case, power might be reduced automatically.

Finally, if use is not made of a foot switch or the release button on the examination unit, the operator has the option of releasing X-radiation by pressing a button on the console.

12.2.4 Exposure control in direct radiography

Fast control circuits for tube voltage and filament or tube current permit continuous dose adaptation during the exposure. Even rapid changes (e.g. pulsed fluoroscopy or cine operation, cf. section 12.2.5) can be applied during X-radiation. Several options are available for achieving correct exposure.

Primary timer

The manual selection of all three parameters (i.e. tube voltage U, current I and irradiation time T) when deploying the three-point technique has become an exception and is now used only for blurring effects (e.g. in planigraphy) or breathing technique exposures. These latter involve intentionally moving a part of the body during X-ray exposure so that it is blurred and does not superimpose the image of the stationary part under investigation. The time setting is made according to the mechanical movement of the radiographic table or of the body part that is to be blurred. The exposure is terminated at the moment the time has elapsed. Since electric charge $Q = \int_0^T I(t)dt$ determines image brightness and not tube current, modern X-ray generators are geared for the selection of the product of the tube current and irradiation time (mAs). The fast and accurate filament control system calculates and controls the X-ray tube current so as to ensure that the selected time is reached within small tolerances.

Tube current time product timer ("mAs timer")

If a long irradiation time is not explicitly required, the operator need only select the tube voltage and current time product for the organ or region of the patient to be imaged (two-point technique). The generator's control system automatically adjusts the tube current to tube and generator performance, integrates the current and then switches off so as to keep irradiation time to a minimum.

Automatic exposure control (AEC)

Users whose systems include automatic exposure control need only to set the tube voltage to the corresponding region of investigation (*one-point technique*). The dose at the image receptor is measured and the AEC terminates the exposure as soon as the correct image brightness has been reached. The image region of greatest interest is often referred to as the dominant. Automatic exposure control can be incorporated into all systems whose X-ray equipment allows for the alignment of the AEC sensor with the dominant and whose collimated X-ray fields are not smaller than the AEC sensor area. AEC is currently widely used for direct radiography (i.e. film-cassette, photostimulable phosphor imaging plate and flat-panel digital X-ray detector) and indirect radiography, including digital fluorescence radiography (DFR) and digital subtraction angiography (DSA).

Automatic exposure control operates on the basis of dose rate measurements (fig. 12.45). A signal is yielded (via integration) that is proportional to the actual accumulated dose K_{act}. X-radiation is terminated as soon as K_{act} coincides with a predefined nominal value K_{nom}. The latter is defined during system set-up.

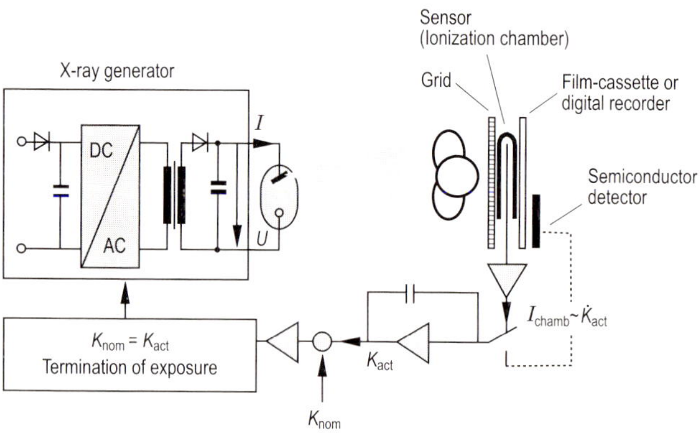

Figure 12.45
Principle behind dose rate measuring and AEC. The control circuit may either connect to an ionization chamber in front of the object or to a semiconductor sensor behind it.

Two types of AEC sensors are used in direct radiography:

- An ionization chamber is placed directly behind the anti-scatter grid in front of the image receptor. Current in the pA range proportional to the dose rate $\dot{K}$ is generated by the X-radiation in an air filled capacitor charged to 300-1,000 V_{DC}. Various sensor fields permit adaptation to the dominant. The ionization chamber is required to attenuate the imaging radiation as little as possible and to create no artifacts in the image.
- Semiconductor sensors have to be placed behind the image receptor because they are much more opaque to X-radiation than ionization chambers. This enables one to reduce image receptor dose, a requirement that applies especially to mammography and pediatrics. However, given that X-radiation quality is changed by the image receptor, the AEC signal from the semiconductor sensor will not necessarily correspond to the image receptor dose. This fact, as well as the energy dependent X-ray absorption for all of the image receptor system's components, must be taken into account in the context of exposure control.

The use of anti-scatter grids does not completely suppress X-radiation scattering. Thick objects cause more scattering than thin objects. The predefined dose for X-radiation termination is reached earlier in the case of thick objects, thus resulting in insufficient contrast. The operator can compensate for this by using the density correction switch on the control console to change the exposure by percentage points (plus or minus) [12.32] of the stored value.

Double-detector transparency correction in AEC mode

Given that X-ray absorption is energy dependent, the signal of an AEC sensor depends not only on the air kerma rate at the sensor position, but also on beam quality. This influence, referred to as voltage-response, can be corrected automatically with the use

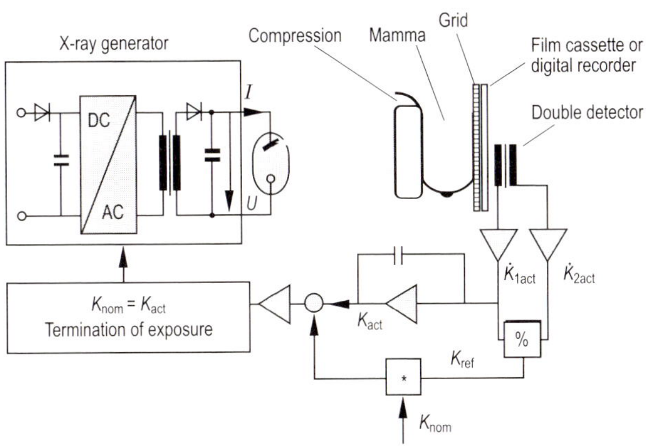

Figure 12.46
Principle behind AEC mode and double-detector correction for mammography

of a double detector. Such correction is of special importance in mammography, where the object dose has to be kept as low as possible and where beam quality depends on the thickness of the object (tube voltages used are 25 to 40 kV).

Beam quality can be estimated by measuring the dose behind the image receptor with two sensors placed in front of and behind a defined X-ray filter (fig. 12.46). Beam hardening can be estimated on the basis of the ratio of the two detector signals (i.e. the larger the ratio the higher the X-ray energy). Modern microprocessor-based automatic exposure control systems for mammography enable one to use the known energy dependence of the mammography image receptor to set the image dose automatically and precisely and thereby achieve optimal contrast.

12.2.5 Exposure control in indirect radiography

While automatic exposure control in the case of direct X-ray images (on a film-cassette or digital image receptor) presupposes the use of extra sensors, the exposure control signal in the case of indirect techniques is derived directly from the image sensor (image intensifier or flat-panel digital X-ray detector).

Automatic fluoroscopy control

Fluoroscopy is used to observe and diagnose dynamic events. Such examinations make use of long-term X-radiation at low dose. X-radiation is started and stopped via a foot switch. It is necessary to adjust the X-ray tube voltage and current according to the required contrast at the least possible dose for patient and operator. Automatic dose rate control systems unburden the operator by taking over the task of manual adjustment.

Fig. 12.47 illustrates the principle of automatic fluoroscopy using an image intensifier TV chain. The image is picked up by a CCD camera and displayed on a monitor. Average image brightness at the image intensifier is measured by a photodiode (formerly pho-

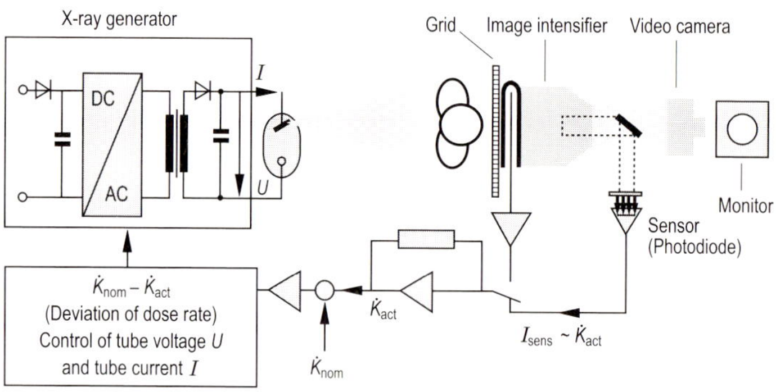

Figure 12.47
Principle of automatic fluoroscopy control. The sensor in front of the image intensifier is used only in single exposure.

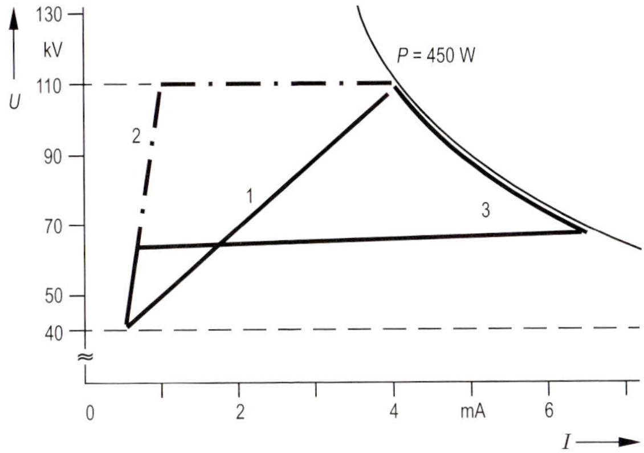

Figure 12.48
Characteristic operating curves in fluoroscopy

to multiplier) whose signal is used in the dose rate control loop. When photodiode arrays are used, the measurement region can be selected according to the dominant.

In fluoroscopy, tube voltages between 50 to 110 kV are meaningful. Larger values lead to poor contrast and lower values entail increased patient dose. Automatic dose rate control varies tube voltage and current along different characteristic curves (fig. 12.48), depending on the application involved, i.e. anatomic region and type of examination (e.g. deglutition, heart examination with catheter).

The linear characteristic (curve 1 in fig. 12.48) can be easily implemented and represents a good compromise between contrast and dose requirements for all fluoroscopic examinations. In pediatrics, however, minimum patient dose is of overriding importance and should be maintained even at the cost of contrast. Here, a characteristic corresponding to curve 2 is selected. This sets tube voltage to a constant high value over a wide range and controls only the tube current.

Thin catheters are made visible in interventional radiography by using adequate contrast. This task requires low tube voltages and high currents (curve 3). When the maximum tube load curve is reached in cases of very corpulent patients, the dose rate control will follow this curve.

Determination of single exposure data during fluoroscopy

It is often necessary during a fluoroscopic examination to obtain a single radiographic image of improved image quality. X-ray systems with image intensifier TV chains are therefore usually also equipped with static image receptors (film cassette, photostimulable phosphor imaging plate, flat-panel digital X-ray detector). While tube voltage and current are not the same for a radiographic exposure as they are in fluoro mode, an automatic exposure adjustment will make use of the values used during dose rate controlled fluoroscopy (*zero-point technique*).

When setting up a fluoroscopy system, dose rate at the entrance of the image intensifier is set (using a calibrated test setup) to a fixed value (e.g. 0.16 µGy/s). During fluo-

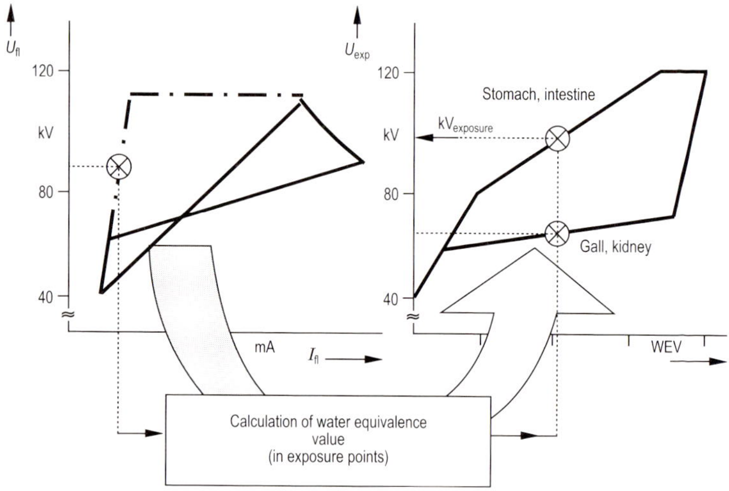

Figure 12.49 Determination of single exposure parameters on the basis of fluoroscopy

roscopic examination, X-ray absorption by the object (transparency, ratio of quanta leaving the object over quanta entering it) can then be calculated on the basis of the tube voltage and current applied, the distance between the source and image receptor and the anti-scatter grid used. Object transparency corresponds to a water equivalence value (WEV). Optimal exposure parameters with respect to organ-specific take-over curves (fig. 12.49) are automatically adjusted on the basis of the water equivalence value obtained.

The dose for the patient and operator can be further reduced by using pulsed instead of continuous fluoroscopy. Digital video systems store image data in a buffer. The data are then read out from the buffer at a constant frame rate for display that is independent of the image acquisition rate. Intermittent X-radiation can be applied without losing important information on the monitor, especially in the case of slow-moving or stationary objects. Pulse frequencies of 15, 7.5 and 3 frames/s result in dose reductions of up to 50%, 75% and 90%. Each single fluoro pulse is terminated by the AEC as soon as the nominal dose value has been reached.

Digital fluoro radiography (DFR)

DFR applies the same electronic image receptor (image intensifier, flat-panel digital X-ray detector) for single and series (up to 8 f/s) exposures. With respect to automatic exposure control, there is no technical difference between DFR and automatic fluoroscopy. All of the dose control modes already described (dose rate control, water equivalence value calculation, organ programs) are applicable and additional modes are possible.

In both single and series exposure, the exposure data, including X-ray tube voltage and tube current, are defined for the first frame by deriving the water equivalence value from the fluoroscopy. Each X-ray pulse is terminated at the defined nominal dose according to the characteristic of the organ program used. Subsequent frames may vary in terms of X-ray tube voltage, tube current and pulse width.

Any lack of geometrical sharpness can be reduced by deploying a control mechanism that automatically selects the smallest possible tube focal spot at tube voltages below the limit set for reasons of contrast. If the necessary image brightness requires exceeding this limit, the automatic exposure control switches to the next largest focal spot. This permits higher tube currents at lower voltages, and thus results in improved contrast.

The AEC function can be interrupted during examinations that include the use of contrast agents. The AEC adjusts the image brightness to a medium value before the contrast agent flow is initiated and then switches off automatically. Subsequent contrast agent flow is then clearly visible against a constant background.

In the case of single exposures, a fixed X-ray tube voltage is set according to the organ program. Tube current is reduced the longer the irradiation time is (*continuously falling load*) and the exposure is terminated at nominal dose. If subsequent images are taken (*serialography*), X-radiation is started at maximum tube current with shortest possible irradiation time according to the serialography table of the focal spot used, depending on frame rate, duration of the single exposure (pulse width) and the duration of the serialography.

Digital subtraction angiography (DSA)

Vessels are made visible in X-ray images by filling them with contrast agents. The quantity of a given contrast agent can be substantially reduced by applying digital subtraction angiography (DSA). According to the DSA technique, an image of the native vessels (the *mask*) is subtracted from an image of the vessels that have been filled with a contrast agent and obtained at the same dose. It results in the display of the vessels only (i.e. free of superimposition of other parts of the body such as bones).

While AEC is deployed in DSA in roughly the same manner as it is in DFR, it has to be adapted for the display of iodine contrast agents. Iodine has an absorption edge of 33.2 keV and is best imaged at an X-ray tube voltage of 63 to 66 kV. The tube voltage and tube current time product (mAs) of the mask image are used for all subsequent images of a series to receive constant background brightness for the images showing vessels during filling with contrast agent.

12.3 X-ray image detectors

12.3.1 Static detectors

The X-ray image depicts the spatial distribution of the X-ray quanta transmitted through the object on a plane perpendicular to an impinging X-ray beam. The conversion of an X-ray image into an optical image usually involves a luminescent screen that

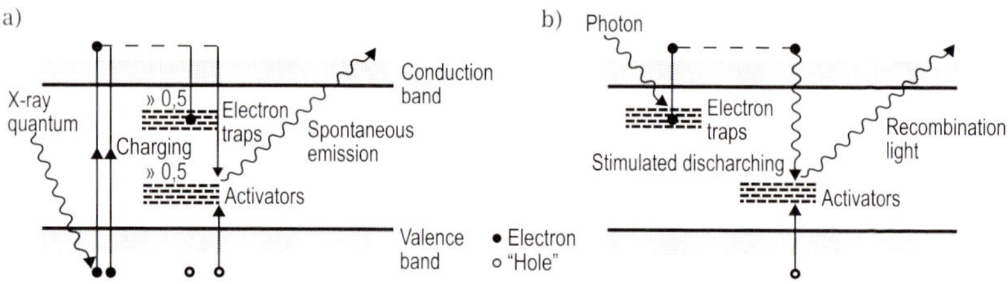

Figure 12.50 Principle of X-ray excitation **(a)** and optical readout **(b)** of a storage phosphor

absorbs X-ray quanta and converts them into visible quanta. As a rule of thumb, one absorbed X-ray quantum can generate up to 3,000 optical quanta.

In conventional radiography, high quality static images are first recorded and then observed. The placement of a film between two luminescent screens is still the most commonly used method for this purpose. Individual electronic images, which can be easily stored, copied and transmitted, can be generated either by scanning an X-ray film or by deploying photostimulable (or storage) phosphor imaging plates.

Storage phosphor screens are special luminescent screens that are capable of storing a latent image over a long period of time. Electrons generated in the screen during X-ray absorption dwell in metastable states or electron traps near the conduction band until they are released by low energy photons (fig. 12.50). Blue photons are released when the storage screen is scanned with a red laser beam following its exposure to X-rays. These blue photons are detected with an optical detector (e.g. a photo multiplier or PM). The PM's electric output is digitized and an image reassembled in computer memory.

Fluoroscopy involves the direct observation of the optical image supplied by an X-ray screen, and thus enables the real-time imaging of moving objects. However, given that current information and detector technologies provide a means of digitizing and storing not only single images, but also entire scenes, high-end fluoroscopic X-ray systems can also be used for radiological purposes, a duality that blurs the distinction between radiography and fluoroscopy.

12.3.2 X-ray image intensifiers

The direct viewing of a fluorescent screen is limited by the fact that not enough of the visible photons generated by an absorbed X-ray quantum can reach the eye so as to prevent a loss of information. While the mismatch between the flow of the X-ray quanta supplied (behind the patient) and the flow of visually recorded information was long recognized as a limitation, an effective remedy was not found until the introduction of the electron-optical X-ray image intensifier (I.I.) tube in 1948 [12.40].

Modern X-ray image intensifiers are manufactured with input field diameters ranging from 17 to 40 cm. Fig. 12.51 shows a modern 33 cm X-ray image intensifier. The X-ray input window in this case consists of a 1.2 mm thick aluminum sheet, the tube hous-

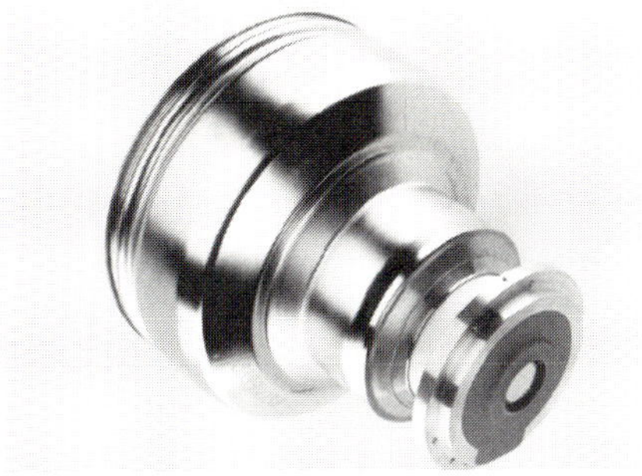

Figure 12.51
X-ray image intensifier tube with a 33 cm input diameter. Changing the focusing voltages while retaining the anode voltage of 30 kV enables one to switch to input field diameters of 22 cm, 17 cm and 13 cm. This process involves a decrease in the conversion factor (i.e. the output screen luminance relative to the dose rate in the input plane) and an increase in resolution.

ing is made of stainless steel and the insulating ring surrounding the output window is made of a ceramic material (aluminum oxide).

12.3.2.1 Principles of X-ray image intensifier operation

An X-ray image intensifier is a vacuum tube in which an X-ray image is transformed into a visible image of high luminance. Fig. 12.52 shows a longitudinal cross section of an X-ray I.I. tube in which only the essential components are depicted. The tube works as follows:

The X-ray radiation, which has been spatially modulated by the object under examination, penetrates the tube's radiolucent input window and strikes an X-ray fluorescent screen. This converts the X-ray image into an optical image. A very thin photosensitive layer, the photocathode, maintains optical contact to the fluorescent screen. This photocathode transforms the brightness distribution of the optical image on the screen into an electron flux density distribution. The photoelectrons are emitted in all directions within the half-space in front of the photocathode.

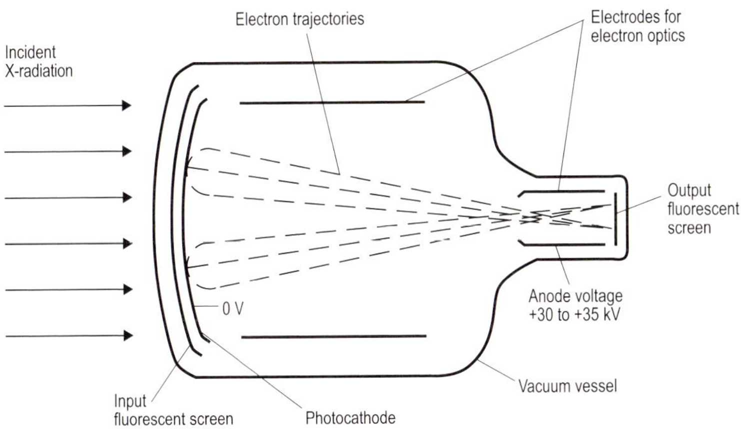

Figure 12.52 Longitudinal cross section of an X-ray image intensifier (schematic)

While every effectively absorbed X-ray quantum in the X-ray screen generates several thousand light quanta, only a small fraction of these reach the photocathode, and thereby lead to the emission of photoelectrons representing a quantum yield of a few percent. One obtains a total of around 300 photoelectrons per absorbed X-ray quantum.

The electrons that are emitted in various directions from a point in the photocathode are deflected by the electric field in the interior of the image intensifier in such a way that their combined trajectories form a lobar bundle that attains its greatest thickness near the photocathode and becomes progressively narrower towards the anode. The electron trajectories converge again at a point (the image point) on the output fluorescent screen. The electrons take on kinetic energy as they move in the externally applied electric field. After traversing a potential difference of around 30 to 35 kV, the energy of an electron is sufficient to generate roughly one thousand light quanta in the output screen.

The information in an X-ray I.I. image is thus passed through several conversion stages:

1 absorbed X-ray quantum $\rightarrow$ 3,000 light quanta
$\rightarrow$ 300 electrons
$\rightarrow$ $300 \times 1{,}000$ light quanta

The electric field in the X-ray I.I. has an effect on the photoelectrons that is similar to that of a focusing lens on light rays: an inverted (in this case substantially reduced) image arises. Given that all of the photo electrons emitted into the half-space are caught by the electron lens, electron-optical imaging qualifies as very efficient. The high luminance at the output fluorescent screen is achieved via the acceleration of the photoelectrons and via the concentration of the electron flux from the large photocathode area on the very much smaller output screen area. While the total luminous flux is not increased as a result of this second effect, the luminance is. The small, bright output image is very well suited for transmission to connected systems (e.g. CCD camera and imaging system with memory and monitor).

12.3.2.2 X-ray fluorescent screens (input screens)

The properties of the input phosphor have a major impact on the quality of the image transmission enabled by the X-ray image intensifier as a whole. The input phosphor determines the extent to which the X-ray quantum flux, which has to be kept as small as possible for reasons of radiation protection, can be exploited for image generation. Here, it is clearly necessary to find a compromise between the conflicting requirements of greater quanta absorption (large X-ray fluorescent layer thickness) and high resolution, which is diminished by excessively thick fluorescent layers due to the scattering of the generated light.

A breakthrough was made in this context as the X-ray fluorescent material zinc cadmium sulfide (ZnCdS: Ag) was replaced by cesium iodide (CsI:Na), an X-ray fluorescent material that combines several desirable properties in an almost ideal manner:

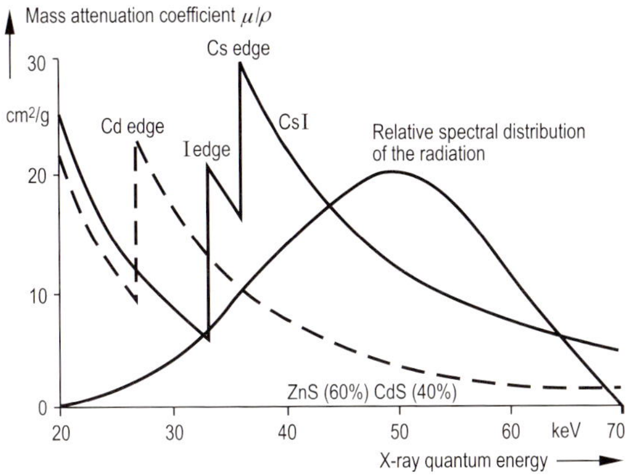

Figure 12.53
Mass attenuation coefficient μ/ρ for ZnCdS (dashed line) and for CsI as a function of quantum energy. By way of comparison: spectrum of the X-radiation behind a patient submitted to fluoroscopy, simulated by a 15 cm water layer, at an X-ray tube voltage of 70 kV.

- Favorable absorption values for X-ray quantum energies above the K-absorption edges of Cs (36 keV) and I (33 keV) (fig. 12.53)
- Good spectral matching to $SbCs_3$ photocathodes (fig. 12.54), chemical compatibility with this photocathode
- Good vacuum properties (capacity to withstand degassing temperature)
- Screen manufacture by vapor deposition
- Packing density almost equal to that of the bulk material (in contrast to sedimentation screens exhibiting substantially lower packing densities)
- Good adhesion of the vapor-deposited screen to aluminum sheet, enabling the easy production of any screen shape and narrow tolerances (important for the electron optics)

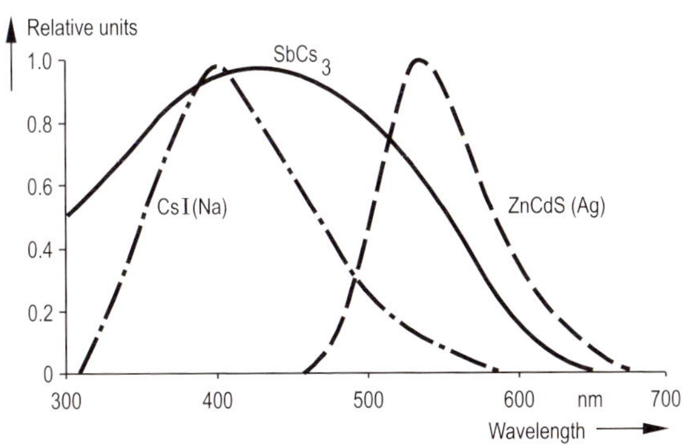

Figure 12.54
Spectral matching of ZnCdS:Ag and of CsI:Na to the sensitivity distribution of the cesium-antimony photocathode

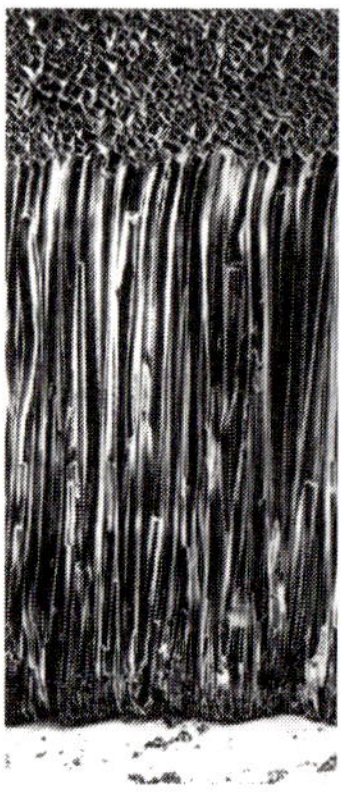

Figure 12.55
Picture of the broken edge of a CsI X-ray screen taken with a scanning electron microscope. Top: Surface of the X-ray screen. Middle: Broken edge of the CsI crystallites (height: around 450 μm). Bottom: Aluminum substrate

If the vapor deposition process is carried out in a suitable manner, the screen will consist of continuous crystallites partially separated by fissures that are perpendicular to the substrate and that help to conduct the light in the desired direction (fig. 12.55). This enables one to significantly increase the thickness of the layer and hence the quantum absorption without sacrificing spatial resolution. The optimization of manufacturing processes allows one to produce needle-shaped crystallites with diameters of less than 10 μm [12.41], and thereby achieve an improvement in *MTF*.

12.3.2.3 Photocathode

The transparent photocathode in the X-ray image intensifier is made of antimony and one or more alkali metals (preferably cesium), which are deposited simultaneously or sequentially by vaporization in a thin layer (around 10 to 30 nm) [12.42]. The photocathode's substrate is the X-ray screen (with or without a transparent intermediate layer). The spatial distribution of the photoelectron emission is thus a contact print of the instantaneous distribution of luminescent light in the X-ray screen.

The service life of the photocathode – and thus of the X-ray image intensifier tube – extends to many years where conditions include constant room temperature and a good vacuum of around 10^{-6} mbar (it may be necessary to re-getter the vacuum). Long-term exposure to temperatures above approximately 35 °C will have an adverse effect on the photocathode's longevity.

12.3.2.4 Electron optical imaging

The photoelectrons that are emitted from each point of the photocathode and move off in all directions in the vacuum space are accelerated in the X-ray I.I.'s electron-optical system and focused as sharply as possible onto a corresponding point on the output screen. This is possible only to a limited extent, especially given the fact that the photoelectrons, apart from the direction of their distribution, also possess an initial energy of between 0 and approximately 1.3 eV. This is small in comparison to the acceleration voltage of 30 to 35 kV, but not negligible. Furthermore, it is also necessary to keep pincushion-shaped distortions small and the length of the X-ray I.I. tube short.

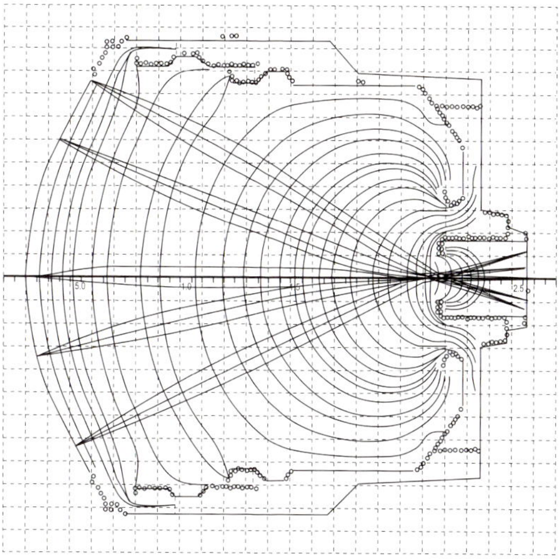

Figure 12.56
Numerically computed equipotential surfaces and electron trajectories in the meridian plane of an X-ray image intensifier with two focusing electrodes (initial photoelectron energy: 0.5 eV)

A planar output image is required for camera filming. A further requirement is the deployment of either a flat output screen or a fiber-optic plate with a hollow-ground inner surface coated with fluorescent material and a flat-ground outer surface.

Electron optical imaging takes place via axial symmetric electrostatic potential distribution, which is produced by the photocathode, several auxiliary electrodes and the anode with the output screen. Favorable imaging properties will result if the photocathode has the shape of a rotation hyperboloid whose contour deviates only slightly from that of a spherical cap. This enables one to achieve a nearly flat output image. Fig. 12.56 shows a computer-generated potential distribution involving just a few electron trajectories.

Deviations from the axially symmetric potential distribution lead to imaging errors (astigmatism). Electrode dimensional accuracy is therefore important. Fig. 12.57 shows the cross section of a 23 cm X-ray I.I. with the electrode system vapor deposited on enameled walls of stainless steel.

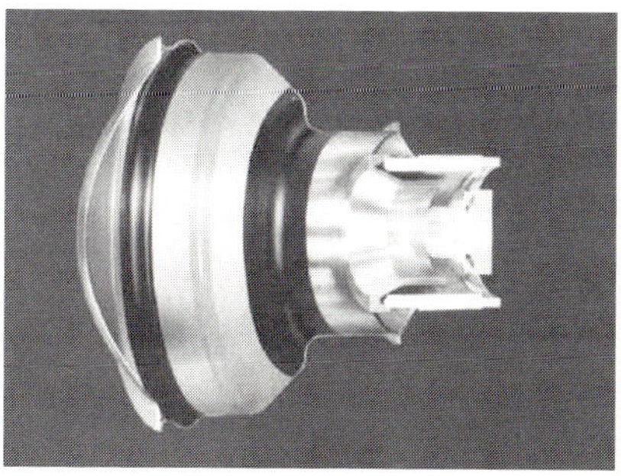

Figure 12.57
Cross section of a 23 cm X-ray I.I. made in enamel technology

Electron optical imaging is very sensitive to external electric and magnetic fields. X-ray I.I. devices are therefore surrounded by a protective housing that is made of highly permeable sheet metal and sealed as well as possible. While this effectively screens out the geomagnetic field, it is necessary to avoid exposure to electric coils, magnets and power lines.

Large format modern X-ray image intensifiers typically offer electron-optical format switching (zoom). Keeping the anode voltage constant and changing only the focusing voltages enables one to map a (concentric) part of the input field onto the output screen, i.e. the electron-optical diminution is lessened and the image resolution increased while the image brightness is also reduced.

12.3.2.5 Output screens

X-ray image intensifier output phosphors consist of a uniform fluorescent layer (generally ZnCdS:Ag) that is a few micrometers thick and that is applied to a glass base that can simultaneously serve as the vacuum envelope's image output window. The introduction of the finer and faster phosphor GdOS has led to an improvement in image quality. The feedback of light to the photocathode is prevented by covering the surface of the fluorescent layer with an aluminum skin that is opaque to light, but transparent to the high-energy electrons. The aluminum skin also serves as an equipotential surface and electrical connection to the anode.

Multiple reflections in the output screen's glass base cause stray light and diminished image contrast. Contrast can be improved using tinted glass for the screen base. Useful light that passes only once through the base is attenuated less than stray light, which goes through the glass base at least three times. The use of a fiber-optic disk for

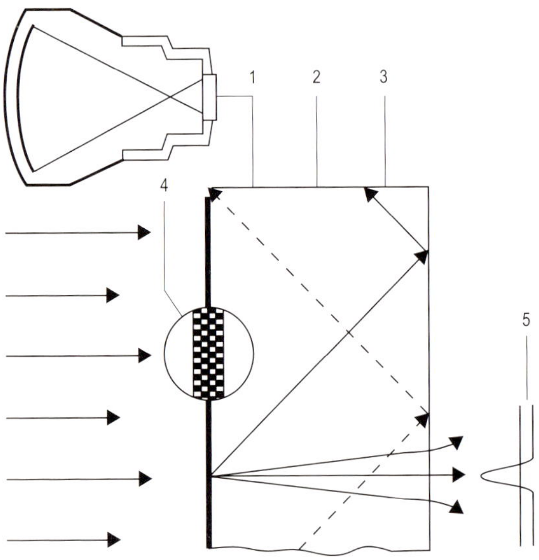

Figure 12.58
High resolution anti reflection output screen with stray light trap: **1:** Output screen; **2:** Absorption layer; **3:** Optical glass; **4:** Phosphor layer; **5:** Output light density distribution

the output screen's base represents an effective, but expensive measure to bring about the selective attenuation of stray light.

The best technical concept for stray light reduction involves making the output screen's glass base roughly as thick as its radius. The totally reflected part of the stray light, which is the largest part, is then not directed back towards the fluorescent layer, but to the blackened edge of the screen base, where it is absorbed (fig. 12.58).

12.3.2.6 Total gain factor, conversion factor

As mentioned above, one obtains around 100 light quanta at the output screen for every light quantum emitted by the input screen into the photocathode. This factor is referred to as the lumen gain, although the term is slightly dubious because of the different luminescence spectra involved. The luminance (cd/m^2) is increased additionally by the ratio of the areas of the input and output screens (i.e. 50 to 200 for a typical X-ray II). The total luminance gain is thus around 10^4.

It has become more common, however, to specify the conversion factor G_X (cd/m^2/μGy/s), which is the luminance at the output phosphor in relation to the dose rate of the incident radiation for standardized ICRU (International Commission on Radiological Units and Measurements) radiation quality, i.e. 20 mm Al-prefiltration and 7 mm first half-value aluminum thickness.

12.3.2.7 Resolving power, modulation transfer function (*MTF*), contrast ratio

The resolving power (characterized by the *MTF*) of an X-ray image intensifier is determined by the two screens and the quality of the electron-optical imaging – in particular, the electron-optical diminution ratio. The resolving power can thus be increased by electron-optical zooming (fig. 12.59).

In addition to its spatial resolution, an X-ray I.I. is also characterized by its contrast resolution at low spatial frequencies, which can be measured by imaging a disc of lead (fig. 12.60). It turns out that the disk's image brightness does not vanish altogether, even though it is entirely opaque to X-rays. The background brightness is referred to as veiling glare and is caused by the stray effects of X-ray quanta, photons and electrons in the X-ray I.I. tube.

A large amount of veiling glare leads to blurry images. This glare is characterized by the contrast ratio, i.e. the background brightness under an opaque disc related to the full brightness. Modern X-ray IIs have a contrast ratio of 35:1, measured using a lead disc that covers 10% of the input screen according to the IEC standard [12.43].

12.3.3 Processing the X-ray image intensifier's output image

12.3.3.1 Second quantum sink

The image intensifier (I.I.) provides a demagnified visible picture of the invisible X-ray image in real time. The size of this picture is too small to permit recognition of anatomic details with the naked eye and the picture's brightness is not sufficient for opti-

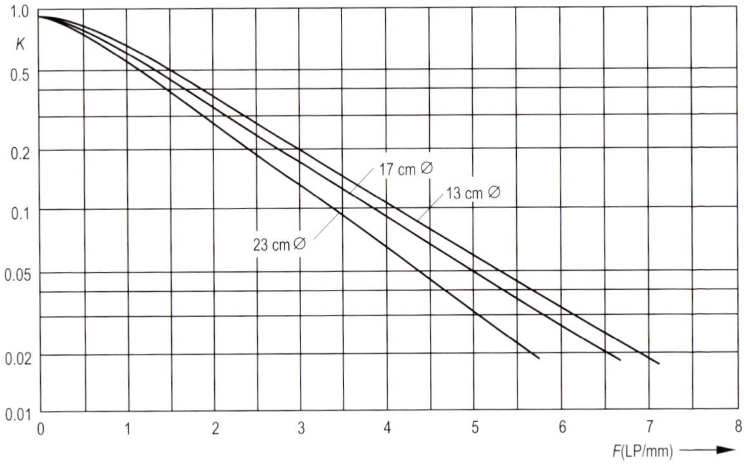

Figure 12.59
Modulation transfer function for a 23 cm X-ray image intensifier for the full input field and an input field switched electron-optically to 17 cm and 13 cm, respectively

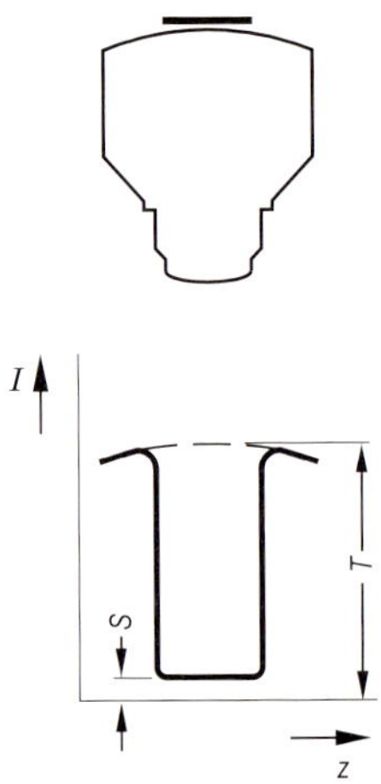

Figure 12.60
Schematic of the contrast ratio measurement. Manifestation of veiling glare (S) in the intensity distribution, if a lead disk is deployed to cover the center of the input screen.

cal magnification. The I.I.'s output screen is therefore recorded using a television (TV) camera and displayed as a large, bright and contrast-rich image on a TV screen. Furthermore, the fact that the electric signal of an electronic sensor can be digitized means that one can easily store, process and transmit the X-ray images.

The electrons generated by the impinging light in an electronic image sensor are the products of a multistage quantum process. This process is illustrated in fig. 12.61. The average total number of electrons generated in a pixel can be expressed by

$$Q = \alpha N g_1 g_2 g_3 \ldots \qquad (12.23)$$

α: Average absorption coefficient for the I.I. input screen
N: Number of X-ray quanta impinging on the I.I. input screen
g_i: Average gain factors for the generation of secondary quanta in conversion step i ($i = 1, 2, 3, \ldots$)

The fluctuations in the number of quanta in the pixel can be expressed by

$$\langle \Delta Q^2 \rangle = \left(\frac{\partial Q}{\partial N}\right)^2 \langle \Delta N^2 \rangle + \left(\frac{\partial Q}{\partial g_1}\right)^2 \langle \Delta g_1^2 \rangle + \left(\frac{\partial Q}{\partial g_i}\right)^2 \langle \Delta g_i^2 \rangle + \ldots \qquad (12.24a)$$

with average gain fluctuation at stage i

$$\langle \Delta g_i^2 \rangle = \frac{\sigma_i^2}{\alpha N g_1 g_2 \ldots g_{i-1}} \qquad (12.24b)$$

σ_i^2: Variance of the gain at stage i

For Poisson processes

$$\langle \Delta N^2 \rangle = N \qquad (12.25a)$$

and

$$\sigma_i^2 = g_i \qquad (12.25b)$$

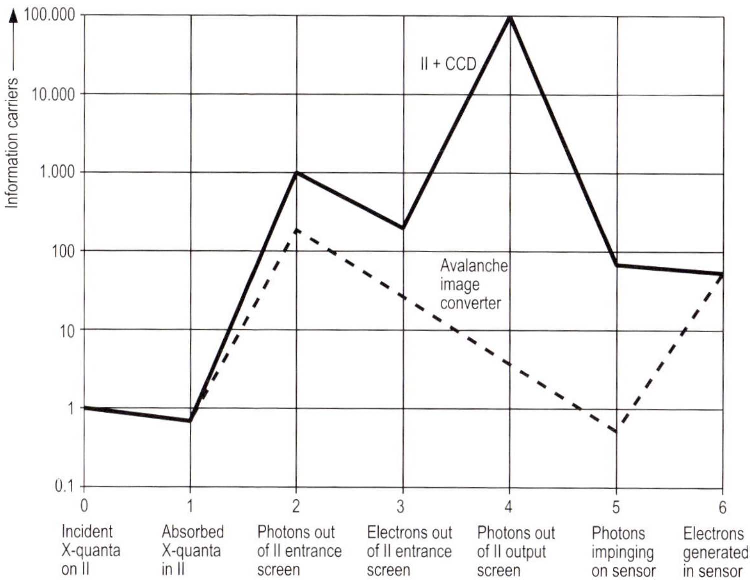

Figure 12.61
Quantum accounting diagrams for an X-ray imaging chain including an image intensifier and an optical sensor and for a hypothetical imaging system with a fluorescent screen and an avalanche image converter (without X-ray image intensifier), with both systems generating the same output signal

Hence, the total fluctuation of the electrons in the electronic sensor (also referred to as photon shot noise) can be expressed as

$$\langle \Delta Q^2 \rangle = Q(g_1 g_2 ... g_i ... + g_2 ... g_i ... + g_i ... + ... + 1) \tag{12.26}$$

and the detective quantum efficiency (*DQE*) (at spatial frequency $u = 0$) can be expressed as [12.44]

$$DQE = \frac{Q^2}{\langle \Delta Q^2 \rangle N} = \frac{\alpha}{1 + \frac{1}{g_1} + \frac{1}{g_1 g_2} + ... + \frac{1}{g_1 g_2 ... g_i}} \tag{12.27}$$

(Here, it would be necessary to replace g_i with the product $g_i MTF_i(u)^2$ to obtain the spatial frequency dependence of the *MTF*.) The denominator in eq. (12.27) has to be close to 1 in order not to degrade the *DQE*. The signal-to-noise ratio in a multistage conversion process is determined by the lowest number of quanta. As shown in fig. 12.61, if an optical sensor is coupled to the X-ray I.I., the number of subsequent quanta (following the conversion of one X-ray quantum) is always high enough to avoid degrading the information generated by the impinging quantum flux. However, if one were to use an avalanche image converter with an X-ray fluorescent screen, the *DQE* would decrease as a result of the insufficient number of photons reaching the light sensitive area, although the output signal has the same signal amplitude. An effect referred to as the second quantum sink (the first being the absorption of the X-ray quanta in the fluorescent screen) thus occurs in the absence of an I.I.

12.3.3.2 Lens systems

A lens system is used to match the size of the I.I.'s output to that of the optical sensor's input area. The relay optics for the X-ray I.I. are required to exhibit a large aperture and high optical transmittance in order to minimize the loss of photons. Image details are to remain free of blurring and distortion. Given that image sensors can only store a certain amount of electrons in their charge-integrating capacitors, it will be necessary to furnish the relay optics with a light control system. This enables one to reduce excess light (e.g. generated at high X-ray doses) before the occurrence of signal amplitude saturation. A combination of a motor driven iris and light absorbing filters in the light path is used for this purpose. The latter helps one to avoid excessively narrow iris openings in the case of bright objects that could cause disturbing optical effects (e.g. diffraction patterns or foreign-particle shadows in the image). Closing the iris will essentially reduce the *DQE*, however, doing so will have virtually no visual effect on the images.

The largest possible solid angle for light collection from the I.I. is provided by tandem optics (fig. 12.62). A telecentric beam configuration is usually applied with each of two individual lens systems focused to infinity. The magnifying ratio necessary to adapt the size of the I.I.'s output screen to the size of the sensor's light-sensitive area can be expressed by the ratio of the focal length of the two lenses. A mirror or prism can be placed between the lenses to provide an additional light channel for exposure control. The output lens with the charge-coupled device (CCD) may be rotated to provide upright images at all angulations.

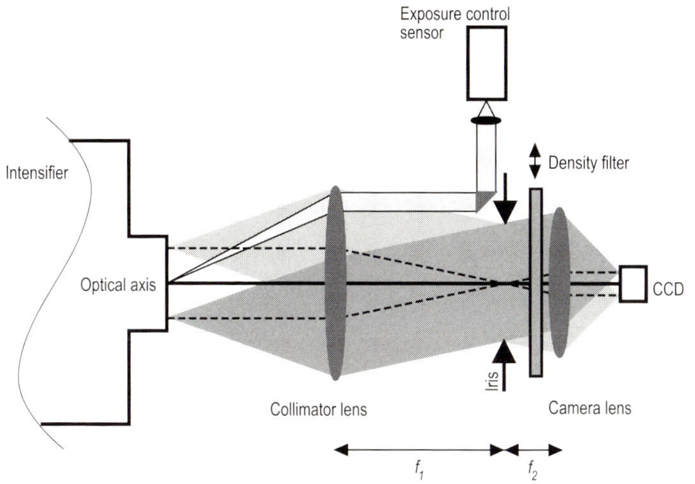

Figure 12.62
Double telecentric optical arrangement for an I.I.-CCD combination with iris for light control and channel for exposure control

12.3.3.3 Charge-coupled device (CCD) image sensors

The image pick-up tubes that used to be deployed as optical sensors with image intensifiers (e.g. the Vidicon) have been replaced by high resolution, charge-coupled devices (CCDs) that satisfy virtually all diagnostic imaging requirements, including digital spot filming and motion studies. Fig. 12.63 shows a typical example of such a camera system.

While the initial phases of their development date back to 1969, it was not until the late 1990s that charge-coupled devices (CCDs) had evolved to the point of meeting the rel-

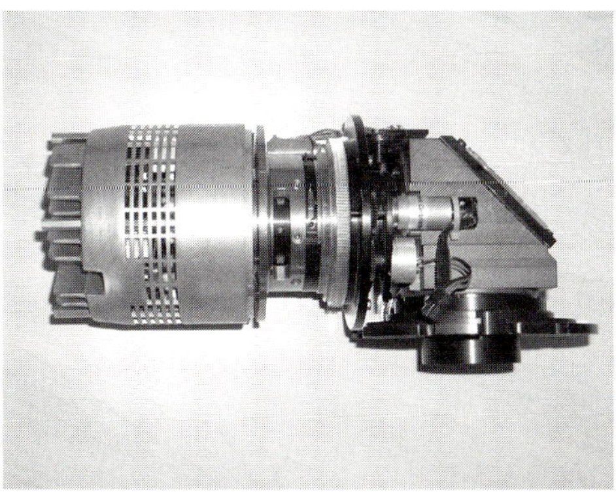

Figure 12.63
Angulated lens system with CCD electronics for X-ray image intensifiers

evant specifications (matrix size, signal-to-noise ratio) at production costs enabling their standard deployment as image sensors in X-ray TV chains. These devices are free of the typical disadvantages associated with image pick-up tubes, including temporal cathode degradation, dependence on several stabilized high supply voltages, high power consumption and large size.

Electron-hole pairs are generated in the depletion barrier of a silicon crystal when light photons impinge on the CCD's photo sensitive area. The raising of the electrons from the valence band to the conduction band leaves holes in the valence band. Both charges are separated by an applied electric field. The charges can be displaced from one location to another if one moves their potential well by changing the potential distribution with an array of electrodes. The charges trapped under a single pixel are shifted serially to an output capacitor that feeds a signal processing circuitry.

Fig. 12.64 offers an illustration of the basics of charge transport for a three phase CCD design. Three electrodes are placed above each pixel. In the first phase, only the left electrode over the pixel has a positive potential, causing all of that pixel's electrons to gather under that electrode. In the second phase, the middle electrode is also connected to the positive voltage and the charges are distributed under both electrodes. During the third phase, the left electrode is switched to negative and the electrons gather under the pixel's middle electrode. The charge has thus been moved by a distance of one electrode (a third of a pixel). Charge movement amounts to a space of one pixel when the described scheme is applied three times.

Many charge carriers are integrated into the pixel capacitors before read out. The voltage across the pixel capacitor increases during charge accumulation. If the voltage exceeds a certain level (full well capacity), charges can spill over to adjacent pixels, an effect called blooming. To avoid this, CCDs for X-ray imaging need to be furnished with an anti-blooming mechanism. A drain electrode is located in the substrate under each pixel. To protect against overload, the substrate voltage can be set to a potential

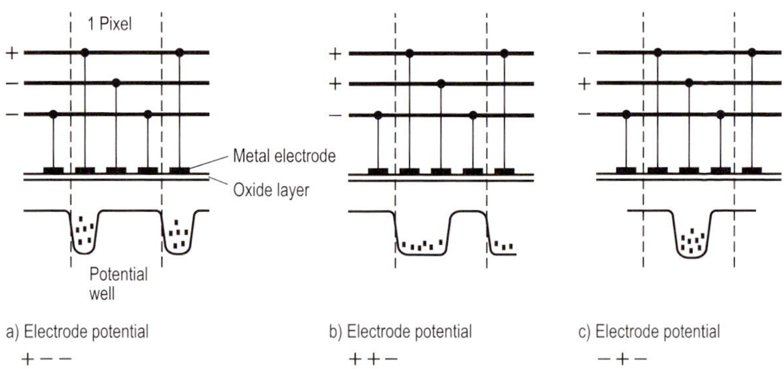

Figure 12.64
Part of a charge transfer cycle in a CCD element in the case of a CCD with three electrodes per pixel (three-phase CCD)

that will trigger the draining of surplus charges into the substrate during the CCD's integration period.

Given such a setup, the charge transport in the CCD can be performed until each pixel's charge reaches the output stage. The latest CCDs conserve more than 0.99999 of the total charge involved in the transfer across one pixel, with less than 1% of the signal leaking during transfer across 1,000 pixels.

After a short reset pulse, each pixel's charge is deposited into a small sense capacitor. The voltage across the capacitor is fed to an output amplifier that delivers its voltage to an analog-to-digital converter (ADC). The output signal as a function of time represents the serially scanned pixel charges that represent the average brightness at this pixel during the integration period.

12.3.3.4 CCD architecture

CCDs come in various architectures [12.45]. The simplest is the full frame (FF) CCD (fig. 12.65). Here, the integrated charges are shifted line by line into a horizontal read-out register after image acquisition. The FF-CCD is ready for a new image only after all the charges have been read out because smearing effects occur when light impinges on the photosensitive array during the charge transport. The frame transfer (FT) concept allows for a higher frame rate. The FT-CCD is divided into three areas: the image area, the storage area and the horizontal read-out register (fig. 12.66). The read-out register is shielded against light by an aluminum cover. Image signals can be read out while a new image frame is acquired as soon as the integrated charges have been moved to the storage area.

The interline transfer (IT) CCD design (fig. 12.67) enables one to avoid smearing effects to a very high degree thanks to the fact that no charge transport takes place across a photosensitive area. The charges of each photo site are transferred virtually instantaneously (i.e. within a few nanoseconds) into light-shielded vertical shift registers that then transfer the charges into the horizontal output register. However, as in the case of IT-CCDs of the same size, the light sensitive area is smaller than that of FF and FT-CCDs (i.e. they are less sensitive).

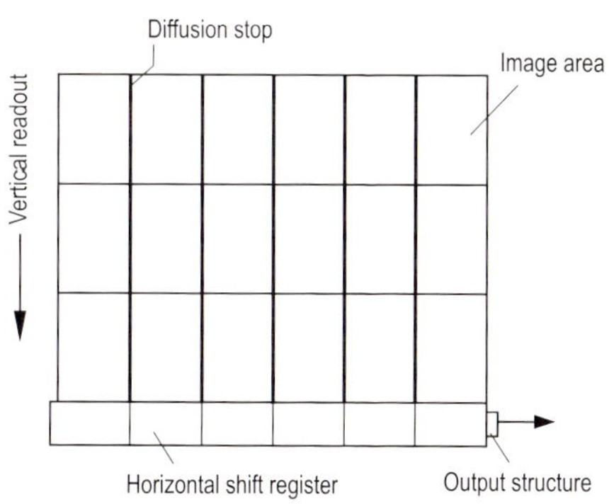

Figure 12.65
Principle design of a full frame (FF) CCD

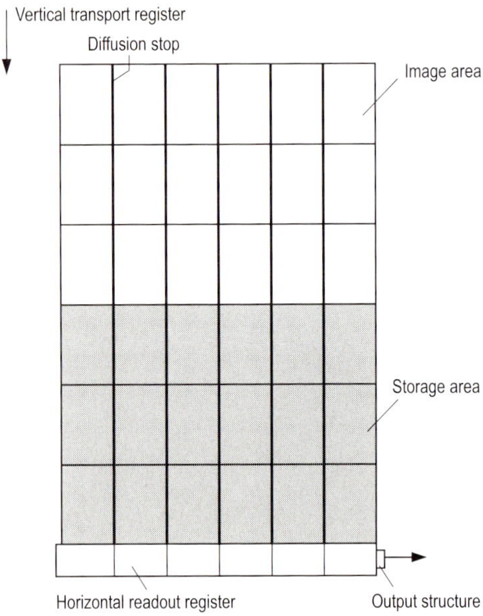

Figure 12.66 Principle design of a frame transfer (FT) CCD

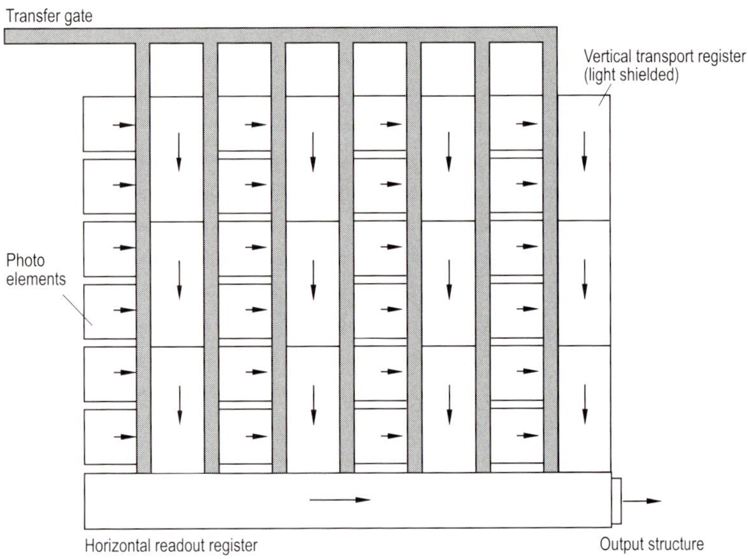

Figure 12.67 Principle design of an interline transfer (IT) CCD

12.3.3.5 CCD noise sources

When considering CCD noise it is important to draw a distinction between stochastic and systematic noise [12.46]. The composition of stochastically fluctuating noise charges can be expressed as

$$N_{Total}^2 = N_{Dark}^2 + N_{Transfer}^2 + N_{Shot}^2 + N_{Reset}^2 + N_{Amp}^2 \quad (12.28)$$

Dark noise $N_{Dark} = \sqrt{q_{Thermal}}$ stems from thermally generated electrons $q_{Thermal}$ in the light sensitive and storage areas. The value of $q_{Thermal}$ increases exponentially along with temperature.

Transfer-inefficient shot noise $N_{Transfer}$ results from the stochastically fluctuating loss of electrons during charge transfer from the light sensitive area to the read-out capacitor. This noise is generated by a multistage process that is similar to that described by eq. (12.23) and depends on signal intensity.

Photon shot noise N_{Shot} has already been explained (section 12.3.3.1). As has been shown, the number of electrons generated per optical photon in the CCD will have to be as high as possible and the CCD will have to be furnished with sufficient full well capacity.

Reset noise $N_{Reset} = \sqrt{kTC}$ (*T*: Temperature) is thermal noise generated by the channel resistance of the field effect transistor (FET) that resets the sense capacitor C. Reset noise can be avoided via correlated double sampling, a procedure that measures the difference between reset and signal level.

Output amplifier noise $N_{Amp} \propto \sqrt{\Delta f}$ arises from the analog signal processing circuits (1/frequency and resistive noise). It depends on temperature and on the bandwidth Δf, which is inversely proportional to the read-out time.

Dark noise in CCDs for X-ray imaging is very small, down to 5 equivalent electrons. The noise generated by all other noise sources can be as large as 75.

Regular disturbance structures extending across a uniformly illuminated CCD image are referred to as fixed pattern noise (FPN). These structures originate from small deviations in the CCD manufacturing process (e.g. nanometer-range errors in the alignment of the various photomasks deployed). These non-uniformities are usually so small that they do not hinder diagnostic procedures. Given higher requirements, however, image homogeneity can be augmented via flatfielding. Flatfielding involves acquiring and storing a zero image and then subtracting this zero image from the actual image during the image acquisition phase.

The same principle can also be applied to level out the small pixel sensitivity variations. Each pixel's actual signal will then have to be multiplied by its stored zero-image value to obtain homogeneous signal distribution at all illumination levels.

12.3.3.6 Other CCD properties

In contrast to some types of pick-up tubes, the amplitude response of a CCD is strictly linear. A deviation from signal linearity is to be expected only in the case of very high signals near the CCD's saturation point (where the anti-blooming mechanism begins to work).

Given that they involve a different scanning principle, CCDs offer a further advantage of being free of the ghost images that sometimes appear in connection with pick-up tubes. Therefore, CCDs do not limit overall temporal resolution when coupled with an X-ray I.I.

The imperfections in the scanning electron optics (as well as in the image itself) that are associated with pick-up tubes can degrade performance. In contrast to pick-up tubes, the *MTF* of a CCD is perfectly uniform across the sensor area. A CCD's *MTF* (when indicated in line pairs per picture height) is superior to a tube's *MTF* when operated at the same scanning matrix.

Given that virtually no charges are lost during transfer, the *MTF* of a CCD that is used in X-ray imaging is only dependent on the pixel aperture. A CCD thus enables the realization of an *MTF* at the theoretical limit established by the pixel size and the imaging matrix. However, if CCDs are deployed as digital detectors coupled to a scintillator layer (as is the case in mammography), the image quality in terms of *MTF* and *DQE* will largely depend on the scintillator and the optical coupling to the sensor.

12.3.3.7 Video signal digitization

Given that digital signals provide more freedom with respect to image processing, storage and display, the CCD's analog output signal is digitized using an analog-to-digital converter (ADC) that is usually integrated into the camera (fig. 12.68). Output signal filtering is necessary prior to digitizing the CCD so as to cut off all frequencies above half the sampling frequency and thereby avoid aliasing and additional noise.

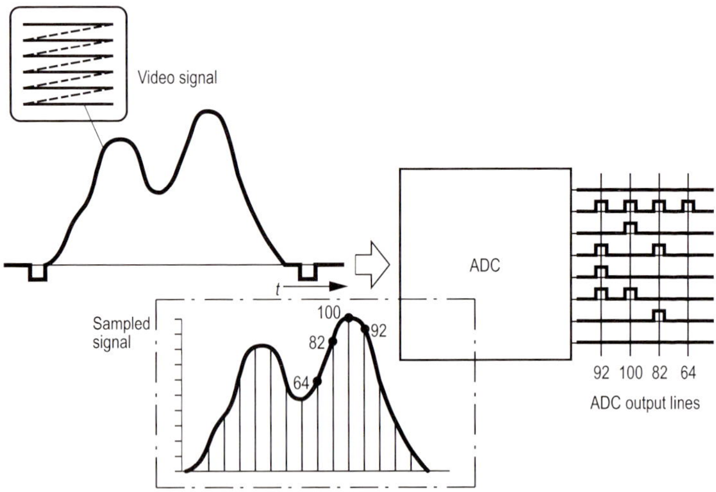

Figure 12.68 Digitizing an analog image signal

The ADC is usually a monolithic MOS circuit. The analog input signal is quantized into 2^N (N is the resolution of the ADC in bits) equal amplitude intervals. Each quantization level is assigned to an integer between 0 and 2^{N-1}. This number is turned into binary code by the ADC, which represents it on N separate output lines (fig. 12.68). In principle, one has to accept a loss of information (least significant bit or LSB) according to ±1/2 of the quantization step (least significant bit or LSB).

The number of necessary bits can be calculated by dividing the CCD's full well (e.g. 170,000 electrons) for a single scan by the electronic noise floor (e.g. 75 electrons). Here, a 12 bit ADC would be required for a low noise CCD camera. However, 10 bit ADCs are also used with CCD cameras for X-ray imaging.

12.3.3.8 CMOS sensors

The proven technology deployed in the latest CCDs offers a fully satisfactory solution for X-ray TV cameras. CMOS image sensors may become an interesting alternative in the future. These promise higher scanning speeds, lower noise levels, advanced circuit miniaturization and greater energy efficiency. The principle behind a CMOS image sensor is shown in fig. 12.69. The light sensitive area can be read out in an arbitrary order. This enables one to track rapidly changing details in a reduced image area via a significantly faster readout.

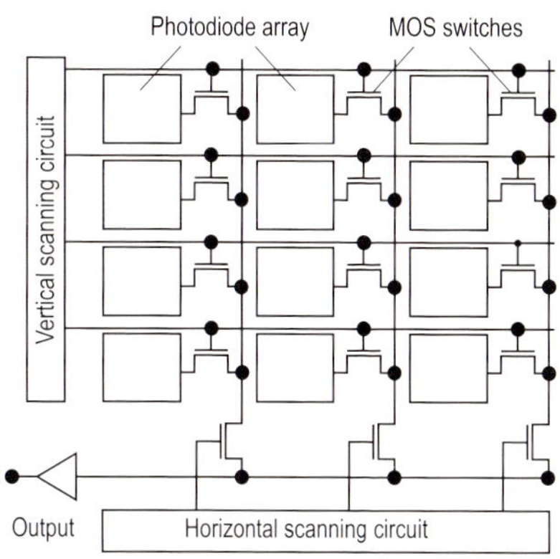

Figure 12.69
Device architecture for an x-y-addressable CMOS image sensor

12.3.4 Flat detectors

The flat detector (FD) established itself as the prime standard in digital X-ray imaging in the late 1990s. Flat detectors designed for use in projection radiography and mammography continue to replace analog screen-film combinations and digital storage-phosphor systems. In the areas of cardiac angiography and pediatric cardiac imaging, flat detectors offering real-time imaging of up to 30 frames per second (fps) or even 60 fps have become a popular replacement for the image intensifier. Similar changes are taking place in general angiography and in fluoroscopy. Flat detectors offer a tantalizing all-in-one potential: a single technology covering all diagnostic and interventional applications in X-ray imaging [12.47, 12.48].

In what follows, we introduce the subject of flat detector technology and its two basic designs: indirect conversion and direct conversion. After describing the required calibration and the steps involved in image processing, we present an overview of basic flat detector performance characteristics. We then turn to a discussion of the many advantages associated with flat detector technology and how these advantages relate to workflow and new applications. We conclude our discussion with a brief look at future developments.

12.3.4.1 Flat detector design and technology

The purpose of any medical imaging X-ray detector is to efficiently absorb the impinging X-ray flux and to convert this flux into a geometry-conserving digital image signal. In general, one should keep the unavoidable additional electronic noise generated during the numerous conversion and amplification steps to a minimum while maintaining the levels of spatial and contrast resolution that are required for the respective applications. Detective quantum efficiency (*DQE*) has become the fundamental physical parameter. This parameter describes a detector's ability to efficiently convert the X-ray radiation at its input into a useful image signal at its output. The objective of any developmental work in detector technology must be to either reach or surpass the established *DQE* levels. Besides *DQE*, the following design parameters are used to characterize detectors: a) dynamic range, b) maximum image acquisition rate, c) active area, d) pixel size, e) device size and f) weight. The values for all of these parameters need to be selected carefully so as to best match the detector's intended application.

Flat detector technology is the only detector technology available today that covers the various requirements of the entire application spectrum, ranging from general radiography to mammography, angiography and fluoroscopy.

Active readout matrices for flat detectors

The development of liquid crystal display (LCD) technology for the consumer market as a replacement for monitors based on cathode ray tubes has introduced a technology whose characteristics are also ideally suited to sensors in medical X-ray imaging. This technology is based on hydrogenated amorphous silicon (a-Si:H) that can be deposited in the form of a thin film. Amorphous silicon combines several favorable characteristics. First, it possesses the relevant semiconductor properties, including doping, photoconductivity and junction formation. This makes a-Si:H suitable for the manufacture of electrical components such as switching transistors (thin film transistors, TFT) and photodiodes, but not for amplification circuits. Second, the material permits large-format deposition and thus enables one to deploy large active matrices (exceeding 40×40 cm^2) of several million pixels (fig. 12.70). These active matrices represent the central component of flat detectors. Third, amorphous silicon exhibits high radiation hardness, making it suitable for applications in medical X-ray imaging.

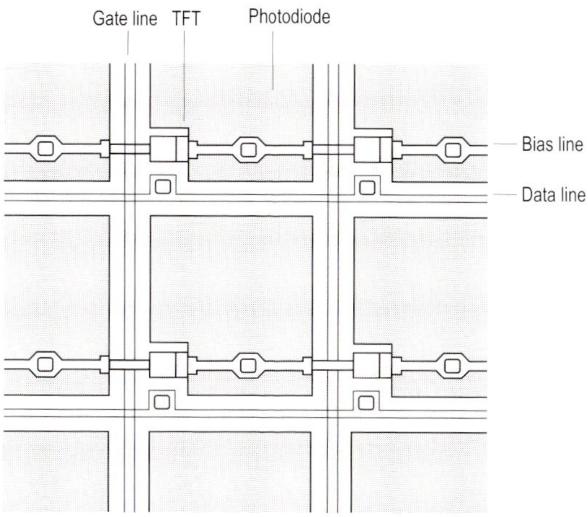

Figure 12.70
Microscopic image of the pixel structure of an a-Si active matrix sensor showing photodiode, TFT, gate, bias and data lines

Two different processes for converting X-ray radiation into electric charge are used. The first process (indirect) involves first converting the X-ray radiation into light and then using the absorption of this light to generate electric charge. The second process involves directly converting X-ray quanta into electric charge.

Flat detectors based on an indirect conversion process

The most widely used flat detector design today is based on a two-level, indirect conversion process (fig. 12.71). The photo absorption of the X-ray quantum generates a high energy electron. While losing energy in the scintillator material, the electron creates a large number of electron-hole pairs, which in turn recombine to produce photons in the visible range. This light subsequently strikes the photodiode where it is converted to electric charge. This two-step conversion process has the advantage of permitting one to optimize each step relatively independently of the other. Fig. 12.72 offers an illustration of such a detector.

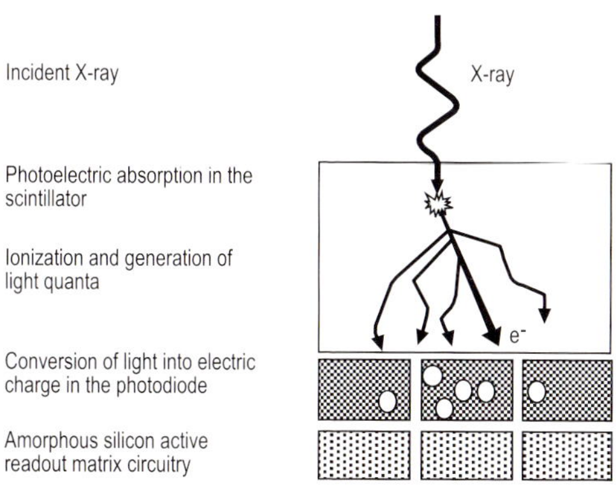

Figure 12.71
The indirect X-ray conversion process

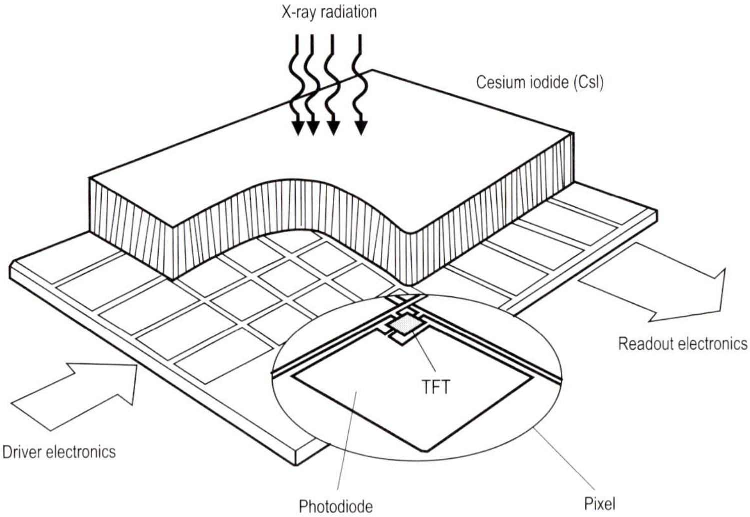

Figure 12.72
View of an indirectly converting flat X-ray detector based on CsI and an active read-out matrix with thin film transistors made of a-Si

Suitable scintillators for flat detectors include gadolinium oxysulfide (Gd_2O_2S) and thallium-doped cesium iodide (CsI:Tl) – CsI being the scintillator of choice. While CsI:Na is already well established in image intensifier technology, the alternative Tl doping substance used for flat detectors shifts the color of the fluorescent light from blue to green, thereby providing a better match for the spectral sensitivity of the photodiode. A thickness of about 500 µm yields absorption values of > 80% for a typical X-ray spectrum at 70 kV. The a-Si photodiode is designed for a large geometric aperture covering 70% of the pixel area (geometric fill factor) at a pixel size of about 150 µm. Taking all effects into account, an absorbed X-ray quantum with an energy of 60 keV will generate about 1,000 electrons in the a-Si photodiode.

Fig. 12.73 shows the electric circuit of a TFT-based pixel structure. The photodiode, which acts as a capacitor, is charged to full-bias voltage prior to X-ray radiation while the TFT remains in the off state. The absorption of the incident light that is generated in the photodiode during X-ray radiation creates electron-hole pairs. These pairs drift to opposite contacts and gradually discharge the photodiode. The readout is initiated when the TFT is switched on via the gate line. This causes charge to flow to the photodiode, thus leading to the restoration of the data-line voltage. The charge flow is measured in the external electronics and recorded as the signal. Given that this step resets the photodiode to full bias, the pixel is ready for the next acquisition.

The readout is performed row by row and addresses all pixels in a given row simultaneously. Optimized low-noise electronic circuits with high bandwidths are used to measure the charge and amplify the signal. Such application-specific integrated cir-

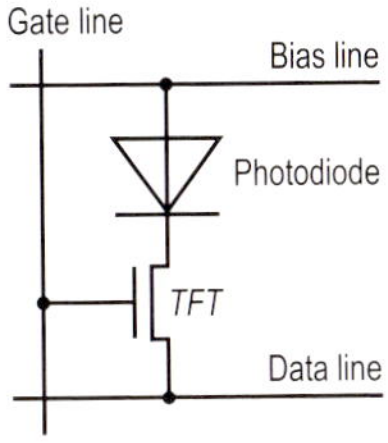

Figure 12.73
Pixel circuit of an active matrix with photodiode and TFT switch for data readout

cuits (ASICs) may be connected to as many as 120 or more individual readout channels. The readout chip also functions as a multiplexer that feeds the signals to an ADC. At this stage the signal is available for further processing in the image processing chain.

Flat detectors based on a direct conversion process

The direct detection process is depicted in fig. 12.74. The absorption of the X-ray in the photoconductor material generates a high energy electron. This electron loses its energy as it passes through the material, thereby creating many electron-hole pairs. An electric field applied across the detection material is used to collect the generated charge carriers.

The suitability of a material for use in direct converters is determined by the following basic characteristics: a) high X-ray absorption, b) generation of a large number of charge carriers for each absorbed X-ray, c) high charge-carrier collection efficiency and d) low dark current. The subjects of current research include photoconductor materials exhibiting high atomic numbers and densities and therefore good absorption characteristics (e.g. PbI, PbO, CdTe and HgI). However, the best understood and most frequently used material is amorphous selenium (a-Se). This material can be deposited directly onto an a-Si active matrix, with each pixel consisting of an electrode and a TFT, used for charge storage and charge readout, respectively.

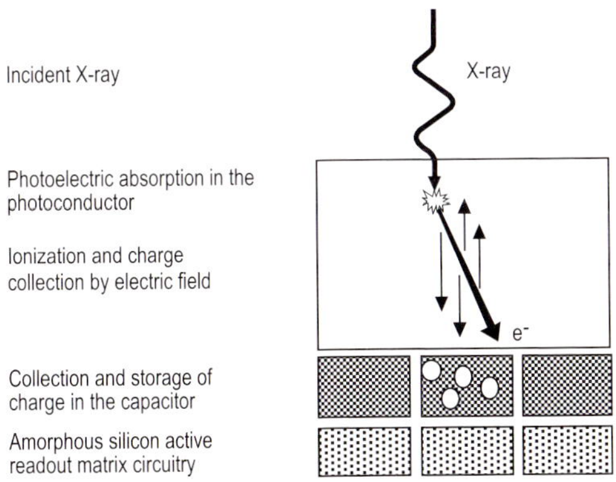

Figure 12.74
The direct X-ray conversion process

Due to its low-lying K-edge, a-Se is particularly well suited to the X-ray spectra used in mammography. A selenium thickness of 250 µm is adequate for mammography applications involving X-ray energy levels of around 30 keV. However, sufficient absorption can only be obtained in general radiography and fluoroscopy with a 'thick' a-Se layer of around 1 mm due to selenium's relatively low atomic number ($Z = 34$). Depending on the energy of the absorbed X-ray, anywhere from several hundred to more than a thousand charge carriers are generated and then transported to the electrode of the respective pixel via the applied electric field. A portion of the generated charge is lost via recombination and deep trapping as the charge carriers pass through the material to the storage electrode. A voltage of approximately 10 kV or more is applied across a 1 mm selenium layer to obtain sufficient charge-collection efficiency. This in turn requires special care in pixel design in order to protect the TFT against damage.

Charge readout is accomplished by addressing the TFTs line by line, recharging the electrodes via the data line and measuring the respective signals in the peripheral low-noise readout electronics. The amplified signals are sequentially converted to digital signals via one or more ADCs. The signal is then fed to the image processing chain for further processing.

12.3.4.2 Image pre-processing for flat detectors

Further data processing is required before the image data generated by flat detectors can be displayed for medical purposes. This further processing includes a) image pre-processing, b) image post-processing and c) final image processing at the display medium. While the first step is specific to a given flat detector whose characteristics need to be matched, the remaining two steps apply in general to all digital X-ray detector technologies, such as computed radiography and image intensifier CCD-camera systems.

Image pre-processing for flat detectors is usually required to generate artifact-free images from the generated raw data. The most common types of artifacts stem from a) pixel-to-pixel sensitivity variations, b) pixel-to-pixel dark-current variations, c) horizontal and vertical structures arising from channel-to-channel driver and readout-circuitry variations and d) inhomogeneous illumination of the radiation field.

Offset and gain corrections are carried out to remove such background patterns. Such flatfielding is applied for each individual pixel in the image matrix. The corrected image $I_{ij}(t)$ is calculated on the basis of the raw image $X_{ij}(t)$ acquired at time t for each pixel ij in row i and column j according to the formula

$$I_{ij}(t) = G_{ij}(t_2) \cdot (X_{ij}(t) - O_{ij}(t_1)) \tag{12.29}$$

where $O_{ij}(t_1)$ is the offset image taken at time t_1 and where

$$G_{ij}(t_2) = \frac{1}{X_{ij}^G(t_2) - O_{ij}^G(t_2)} \tag{12.30}$$

denotes the gain image derived at time t_2 from a set of X-ray and offset images, X^G and O^G, respectively. Here, the raw image X^G is generally acquired under conditions similar to those actually used in the application (with respect to X-ray spectrum, dose and geometry). Offset images, in contrast, are acquired without radiation.

Offset and gain images have to be calibrated. While gain images are typically required once every few months, new offset images need to be acquired every few hours or even minutes, as they depend strongly on temperature, which may change in the room or vary along with detector energy consumption (i.e. usage).

Flat detectors generally provide various modes of operation as defined by a) frame rate, b) effective pixel size, which is adjustable via analog or digital binning, c) dose range, which is determined by specific settings for the internal amplification stages, d) zoom factor and e) X-ray integration time. The values for all of these parameters are linked to specific applications. Each detector mode may need its own set of calibration data.

Furthermore, the linear approach to the flatfielding process described in eq. (12.29) may not be sufficient. A nonlinear approach to the gain correction (e.g. involving the acquisition of a set of gain images for different dose levels and appropriate interpolation techniques) may be required to obtain the best correction values.

Averaging techniques are often applied to reduce the noise contribution inherent to the calibration data. While standard averaging is typically used to generate the gain image, moving average methods may be required for offset images. These latter techniques reflect a compromise between adequate averaging and sufficient weight for the most recent offset image.

In addition to flatfielding corrections, other forms of image pre-processing may be necessary to correct for other common artifacts:

- Defective pixel interpolation: Owing to the huge number of pixels in an active matrix (as many as several million), defective pixels cannot be completely avoided if reasonable yields in the production process are to be obtained. The signal at the location of these defective pixels is restored by interpolation on the basis of the signal information from neighboring non-defective pixels.
- Image lag correction: Image lag derives primarily from deep traps in the detection material that may prevent the release of the charge until after normal readout. This effect presents two major drawbacks. First, it reduces the signal of the original image and second – and more importantly – it may contribute to the signal of the next image. In most cases, the interval between the images is long enough to negate the lag's contribution. If this is not the case – especially when switching from a high dose application to a low dose application (e.g. from DSA to fluoroscopy) – one can effectively compensate for the effect by correcting the next X-ray image with an offset acquired before or after that X-ray image.
- Line noise correction: Voltage fluctuations in the driving or readout circuitry may lead to line-correlated noise, i.e. small offset fluctuations from one line to the next. An effective way of removing this noise contribution is to measure the mean signal with the help of additional pixels positioned outside of the sensor's active area. Given that these pixels are not subject to X-ray radiation (dark reference zone), they

provide a measure of the line noise that can be used subsequently to perform the line-correlated noise correction.

Once the necessary pre-processing steps have been applied to correct for detector-specific artifacts, the images will be ready for further processing. A number of the post-processing techniques that help to reveal and improve the diagnostic content of the image will be addressed in section 12.3.4.4.

Final processing is required to actually view the image, either as a printout on film (hardcopy reading) or as an image displayed on a monitor (softcopy reading). This final processing includes grey-value mapping to the display device's grey-scale resolution and image-matrix rescaling to the display device's spatial resolution.

12.3.4.3 Flat detector performance

The main flat detector performance characteristics include a) dynamic range, b) modulation transfer function (*MTF*), c) detective quantum efficiency (*DQE*) and d) image lag. These performance parameters are fundamentally governed by a large set of detector design and material parameters.

Fig. 12.75 shows a flat detector specifically designed for general radiography applications [12.49, 12.50]. This detector uses CsI as a scintillator. Its active area of $(43\ \text{cm})^2$ – large enough to cover the most demanding sizes (thorax, pelvis) – and its pixel size of $(143\ \mu\text{m})^2$ yield a square matrix of around $9 \cdot 10^6$ pixels.

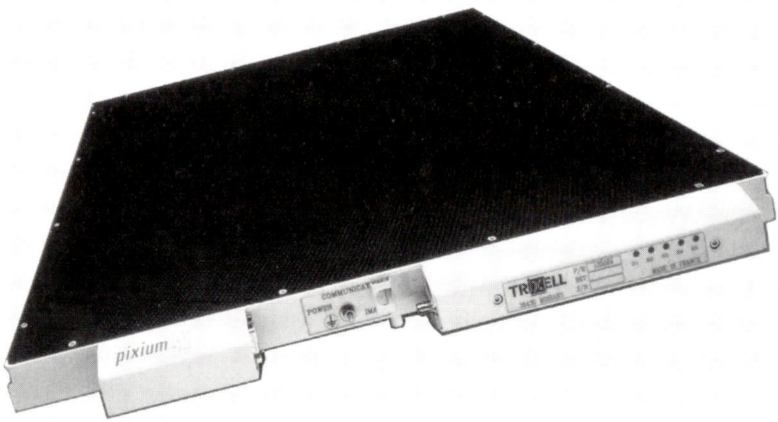

Figure 12.75
Flat X-ray image detector for radiographic applications with a sensitive area of $43 \times 43\ \text{cm}^2$ and a pixel size of $143 \times 143\ \mu\text{m}^2$

Dynamic range

Dynamic range is a key flat detector performance parameter. The low electronic noise (at the level of the least significant bit) of the flat detector shown in fig. 12.75, which uses several 14 bit ADCs, allows one to cover a large dose range without internal detector amplifier gain changes. Fig. 12.76 shows the signal response of this detector as a function of dose, indicating linear behavior over several orders of magnitude up to about 80 µGy, at which point the detector begins to saturate. This allows one to use the detector at the standard dose level of 2.5 µGy (equivalent to a screen-film combination speed of 400) and at higher (e.g. 5 µGy or a speed of 200) or lower (e.g. 1.25 µGy or a speed of 800) levels [12.51]. Even much lower doses have been demonstrated to be useful for specific purposes such as controlling implants and searching for foreign bodies. By way of comparison, fig. 12.76 shows a screen-film system's response function. The flat detector's much larger dose range nearly rules out the possibility of erroneous exposures, a particularly handy feature whenever dose sensing devices are not available (e.g. in the case of free exposures).

Given that it is necessary to address fluoroscopic and DSA (digital subtraction angiography) dose levels, an even broader dose range needs to be covered for applications such as vascular imaging and cardiac angiography. The need for a broad dynamic range to account for various applications can be met by selecting the appropriate detector mode (e.g. the right amplification level at the input stage).

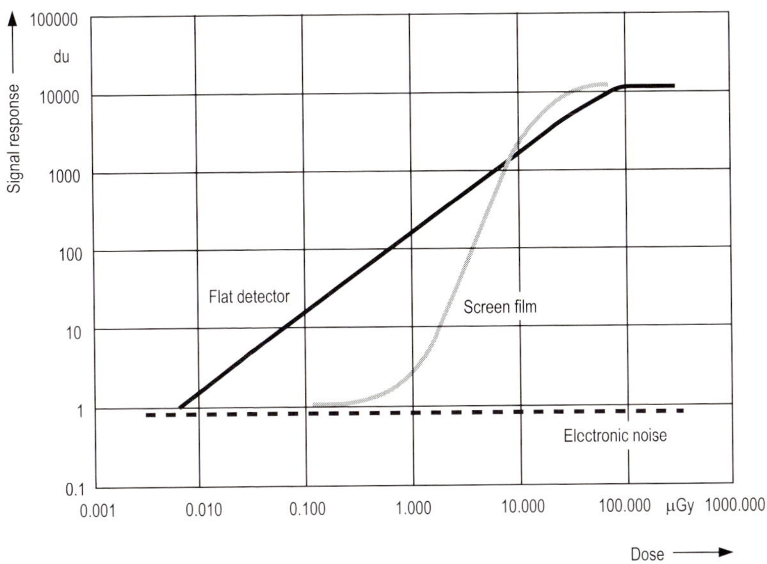

Figure 12.76
Signal response of a flat detector for radiographic applications with 14 bit ADC compared to that of a screen-film system. The flat detector's electronic noise level is also indicated.

Modulation transfer function

Measuring the *MTF* of a pixelized detector system with grids of different periodicity can lead to ambiguities owing to the fact that the output signal depends on the phase shift between the object and the pixel grid. One therefore defines the pre-sampling *MTF* (*MTF*) as the product of the Fourier transform of the line spread function present before sampling (MTF_{bs}) and the sinc function defined by the discrete sensor structure with pixel aperture a

$$MTF(f) = MTF_{bs}(f)\,\mathrm{sinc}(af) = MTF_{bs}(f)\,\frac{\sin \pi a f}{\pi a f} \qquad (12.31)$$

Fig. 12.77 shows typical pre-sampling *MTF*s for various technologies used in general radiography. The screen-film system and storage phosphor system exhibit similar curves across the spatial frequency range. Indirect converting flat detectors that are based on CsI show improved *MTF*, particularly at higher spatial frequencies. Light scatter in the CsI, however, leads to some spreading effects that prevent the *MTF* from reaching the theoretical maximum given by the sinc function. The *MTF* for direct, a-Se-based converting detectors comes closer to the theoretical limit because the applied electric field ensures that the charge generated in the volume above the pixel is collected almost completely in the one pixel below.

Flat detector spatial resolution is independent of the applied dose level (in the linear region). This represents an advantage over screen-film systems, where each dose range requires a different screen-film combination exhibiting reduced spatial resolution as the film speed increases.

Spatial resolution in digital imaging is not only limited by pixel aperture a, but also by pixel spacing $d \geq a$. Spatial Nyquist frequency is defined as $1/2d$, a level above which aliasing effects occur. This fact holds not only for the signal, but also for the noise.

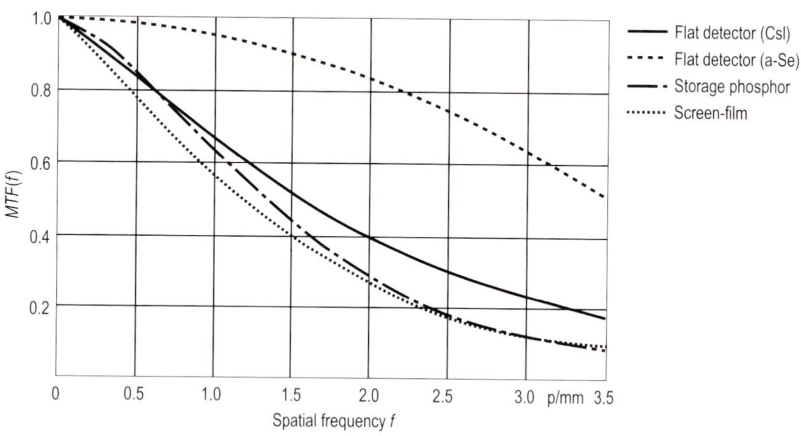

Figure 12.77
Comparison of typical pre-sampling *MTF* curves for various X-ray detectors applied in radiography

*MTF*s that do not reach the limit of the sinc function thus act as a kind of built-in, low-pass filter that reduces aliasing and thus the backfolding of noise from frequency regions beyond Nyquist. While this is the case for the most commonly used scintillators (CsI and Gd_2O_2S) due to light scatter processes in the scintillator layer, direct converting, a-Se-based detectors may exhibit this property to a lesser extend.

Detective quantum efficiency

A flat detector's detective quantum efficiency [12.52, 12.53] (*DQE*) is derived from the measurable quantities *MTF(f)*, noise power spectrum *NPS(f)*, detector gain *G*, and the calculated input quanta per unit area *q*.

$$DQE(f) = \frac{q^2 G^2 MTF^2(f)}{NPS(f)} \tag{12.32}$$

Fig. 12.78 offers a comparison of *DQE*s for different detector technologies in radiography for a typical X-ray spectrum of 70 kV. Indirect converting flat detector technology based on CsI shows the highest values, mainly due to the favorable absorption properties of the scintillator material. The advantage compared to a-Se is even more dramatic at higher X-ray energy levels (e.g. as occur in thoracic imaging). CsI is also superior to a-Se in fluoroscopic imaging where signal levels are low and electronic noise is not negligible.

Image lag

There are two potential sources of image lag and ghosting artifacts. The first potential source is the converter material (scintillator or photoconductor) and the second is the a-Si matrix. Traps in the a-Si photodiodes that are incompletely read out by the TFT constitute the main source in the case of indirect converting flat detectors (e.g.

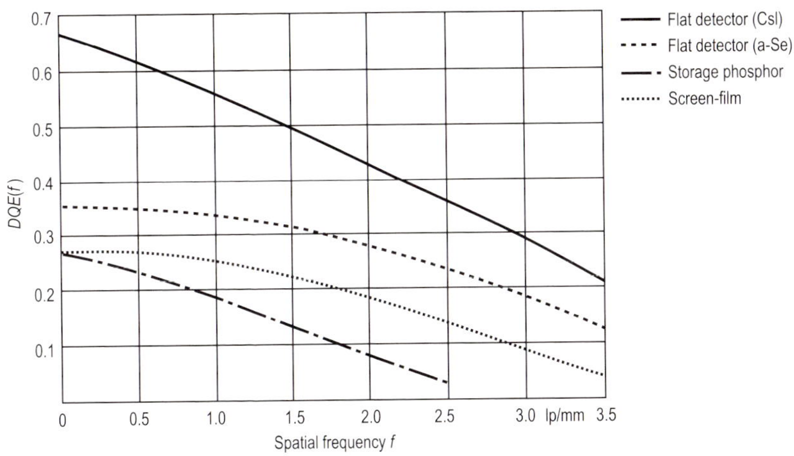

Figure 12.78
Comparison of typical *DQE* curves for various X-ray detectors applied in radiography

CsI/a-Si). The main source in the case of direct converter detectors (e.g. a-Se/a-Si) is the photoconductor itself. Indirect converting flat detectors based on CsI generally exhibit lower lag values than direct converting flat detectors based on a-Se.

Lag is defined as the ratio of the signal that remains in a dark image and of the signal of a previously exposed X-ray image. Lag strongly depends on the time that elapses after exposure. Indirect converting flat detectors based on CsI/a-Si, for instance, that are designed for real-time applications and that are running at 30 fps (frames per second) show values below 0.4% after 33 ms and below 0.2% after 66 ms. The intervals between images for general radiography applications are much longer. On the other hand, the integration time during the X-ray exposure is also much longer, giving way to the collection of more charges generated by thermally-induced de-trapping. The detector depicted in fig. 12.75 exhibits a lag of about 0.3% after 5 s and a lag of well below 0.04% after 20 s, which is a typical minimum time needed to reposition and prepare the patient for the next image acquisition. Intelligent offset acquisition techniques (see section 12.3.4.2) can be used to further reduce the remaining lag effect.

12.3.4.4 Flat detector advances for X-ray applications

Flat detectors have played a central role in the evolution of diagnostic and interventional techniques in X-ray imaging. The evolutionary process has included improved image quality, new image processing techniques, true workflow orientation and new interventional techniques based on the use of magnetic fields. In the sections to follow, we outline the advantages offered by digital imaging and workflow in radiography and present a number of new applications in real-time imaging (fluoroscopy and angiography).

Radiography

Radiography and mammography are still dominated by analog screen-film systems. These diagnostic fields stand to profit in two respects from the full integration of flat detector technology in the X-ray system and the connection of the X-ray system in turn to the RIS (radiology information system) and PACS (picture archiving system) data infrastructure of a hospital. First, digital image processing improves image quality and enables new applications. Second, the new technology enables workflow improvements within a given radiology department and provides connectivity within a medical services complex. In what follows, we discuss both areas in some detail.

Digital image processing can be broken down into three main areas: a) the optimized processing of single images to improve image quality, b) the fusion of several images to add new diagnostic content and c) the automatic extraction of diagnostically important features.

The capability to process images is a key feature of digital radiography and mammography. This capability allows one to extract diagnostic information not possible with analog screen-film systems. Flat detectors cover a dynamic range of up to 14 bits or even more. By way of comparison, the human eye is incapable of differentiating from among more than 7 to 8 bit grey levels. An adequate reduction in the dynamics of the

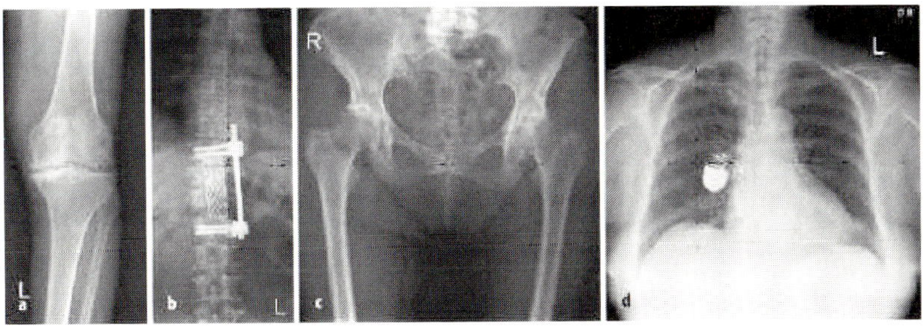

Figure 12.79
Images of a **a)** knee, **b)** spine, **c)** pelvis and **d)** thorax acquired with the Siemens AXIOM Aristos MX system for general radiography

image signal is thus required (fig. 12.79). Basic operations that meet this functionality include:

- Dynamic range rescaling by an appropriate setting of the grey scale window and level values: This function can be implemented automatically using the histogram of the image intensities. Additionally, image areas covered by the X-ray beam collimators can be removed.
- Nonlinear grey scale mapping to increase contrast in the region of interest
- Dynamic range or density compression via unsharp masking: This enables one to display a thoracic image of the lung and the mediastinum with the same high contrast. Similarly, this procedure lends itself to the simultaneous and optimal display of the breast wall and skin area of a mammogram.
- Edge enhancement to enhance fine details of objects via the application of a high pass filter
- Multifrequency filtering techniques used to combine contrast and resolution improvements with noise reduction: The image is divided into several spatial frequency domains that are separately filtered with optimized parameters. Furthermore, these parameters may adjust themselves to the local image's signal-to-noise ratio so as to enable an optimal presentation of the diagnostic image content to the eye of the radiologist.

Image stitching is a method deployed to create a new image that is larger than the detector area. A rapid examination is required in some applications (e.g. a full body scan of an elderly or weak patient in an upright position). The fast repetitive imaging capability of a flat detector allows one to take several consecutive X-ray exposures of the object with a minimal overlap between any two neighboring images. The overlapping areas of the X-ray exposures are used by the image stitching software to create seamless junctions. This enables one to display the complete spinal column or the entire skeleton in a single image.

The dual energy method makes use of the energy dependence of the mass absorption coefficient. Two X-ray images with very different spectra are gathered using different voltages and filters. Adequate linear superposition of the images permits one to selectively display different types of tissue. Flat detectors are ideally suited for this application because they allow one to acquire the two images rapidly and thus to reduce motion artifacts. In thoracic diagnostics, for example, soft tissue (lung parenchyma, mediastinum) or structures containing calcium (bone, calcifications) can be displayed separately, which may prove advantageous for displaying tumors. However, computed tomography is a well-established alternative to this kind of application.

The flat detector represents the missing link when it comes to integrating X-ray systems into RIS and PACS environments, in which several components are networked to generate an optimized workflow. The following is a sketch of the steps that are necessary to establish a smooth workflow for a general purpose radiography system: A work list provided by the RIS is automatically loaded at the system's acquisition station. As soon as a patient is selected from the work list, the system automatically selects the correct detector (if the system includes more than one detector), positions tube and detector to a predefined position corresponding to the first examination, sets the generator data, presets the tube collimator, and prepares the detector for acquisition. All of the necessary pre- and post-processing functions and parameters are also pre-selected. All of this takes place in the background before or while the patient is being positioned on the table or in front of the dedicated upright stand. As soon as the X-ray exposure has been taken the image is automatically processed and displayed immediately at the check monitor. In the meantime the system automatically selects the various predefined parameters for the next examination on the work list. Once all of the images have been acquired, they are automatically sent to the PACS and made available to all networked hospital departments or even to remote experts via teleradiology.

Workflow-oriented radiography systems based on flat detectors have been shown to substantially reduce the overall times required for nearly all examinations when compared to screen-film and storage-phosphor-based systems. They thus play a central role in improving radiology department productivity.

Angiography and fluoroscopy

Real-time X-ray imaging systems are used for a broad spectrum of clinical applications. Such systems range from mobile X-ray systems for surgery and over- and undertable fluoroscopy systems (e.g. for examinations of the gastrointestinal tract) to angiography systems equipped for the diagnosis of vessel pathologies and minimally invasive treatment. Moreover, the field of angiography includes special systems for cardiology and neurology.

Patient and user exposure to X-rays has been successively reduced along with the successive reductions in the X-ray doses required for examination and intervention. Much of this progress is due to improvements enabled by the X-ray image intensifier optical sensor combination, which still represents the gold standard for some areas in fluoroscopic X-ray imaging. All new detector technologies will have to be measured against this level of quality.

But it has to be pointed out that the image intensifier is not perfect, mainly because of its contrast (veiling glare) and spatial resolution limitations. Furthermore, its bulkiness limits both patient access and flexibility during angulation in C-arm X-ray systems. Large-format image intensifiers have not succeeded at replacing screen-film Bucky trays in fluoroscopy systems to cover radiography applications on account of their size, round image format and limited dynamic range at the high exposure levels required in radiography. Image intensifier-based systems are also very sensitive to magnetic fields and thus cannot be used in the vicinity of high magnetic fields.

Flat detector technology has the potential to eliminate or at least reduce some of the disadvantages associated with the image intensifier. In contrast to image intensifiers, flat detectors provide

- Homogeneous image quality across the entire image area, resulting in distortion-free images and position-independent spatial resolution
- High low-contrast resolution
- High *DQE* across all dose levels
- Square or rectangular image areas coupled with a flat and compact design, offering improved patient access
- Compatibility with environments that include the use of strong magnetic fields

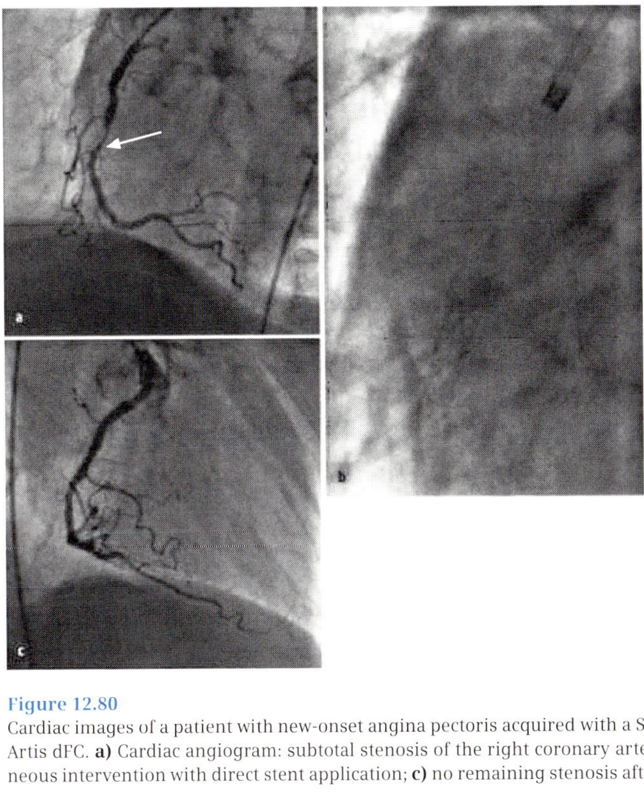

Figure 12.80
Cardiac images of a patient with new-onset angina pectoris acquired with a Siemens AXIOM Artis dFC. **a)** Cardiac angiogram: subtotal stenosis of the right coronary artery; **b)** percutaneous intervention with direct stent application; **c)** no remaining stenosis after intervention

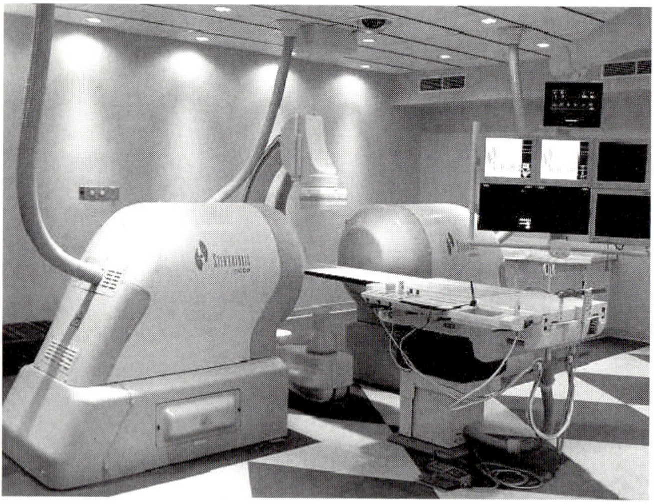

Figure 12.81
Magnetic navigation system with two steering magnets and a C-arm X-ray system with flat detector (Siemens AXIOM Artis dFC Magnetic Navigation)

These advantages suggest that X-ray systems with flat detectors may have the potential to further improve the existing applications and give way to new diagnostic and interventional techniques. The following three examples shall underline this statement.

The improved detectability of small structures such as the tip of the catheter (fig. 12.80) may lead to shorter examination times. This in turn should reduce the integrated applied dose. The improved visibility of stents in cardiac angiography allows one, for instance, to use hand injections of contrast media for left ventriculograms. This reduces the contrast medium load for the patient.

The rectangular image format, high spatial resolution, distortion-free images and excellent soft-tissue contrast resolution offer advantages when it comes to applying 3D image reconstruction techniques.

The flat detector's insensitivity to magnetic fields introduces a new technology for image-guided catheter navigation in the vascular system. The tip of a special catheter is equipped with a tiny permanent magnet. Two large magnets, positioned on both sides of the patient table (fig. 12.81), generate a magnetic field at the catheter tip whose gradient can be adjusted by moving or rotating the magnets. The catheter tip can thus be maneuvered into a pre-defined direction. Guidance is provided by acquiring two X-ray images from different projections that show the catheter and the vessel structure: by drawing the new intended direction of the catheter directly onto the projection images, the new required local magnetic field can be determined and set up by moving the magnets into their new position. Difficult navigation tasks can be accomplished such as changing direction at a bifurcation, moving along a vessel with a strong bending radius and navigating other difficult sections in the vascular or cardiac system.

The various applications of magnetic navigation center mainly on cardiac intervention. A chronic total occlusion of the cardiac vasculature, for instance, can be opened, thereby making it unnecessary for the patient to undergo cardiac surgery. Complex arrhythmia, such as fibrillation in the left atrium, can be treated via radio-frequency ablation of the arrhythmogenic tissue in the atrium. In the case of serious cardiac insufficiencies involving the use of pacemakers to stimulate both chambers of the heart, the surgeon can navigate the electrodes into optimal positions via the veins.

12.3.4.5 Future developments

Flat detector technology continues to develop and improve in fascinating ways. Higher bit depths of 16 or 18 bits promise improvements for 3D applications. Miniaturized electronics permit even flatter and lighter detectors for mobile and portable applications. External cooling systems, still required in some real-time applications today, may be made obsolete. Signal-to-noise ratio represents another area of improvement. Such improvements can be achieved, for instance, by extending the pixel structure into the 3rd dimension. This approach involves stacking the photodiode and switching transistors on top of one another instead of placing them next to one another in the manner of current and past designs. The active area of the photodiode is enlarged by such maximum fill-factor designs, thereby allowing one to detect nearly all of the generated photons and thus maximize the signal. The objective behind the development of new direct conversion materials (e.g. CdTe, PbI, and HgI) is to improve absorption characteristics and thus *DQE*.

Pixel arrays based on CMOS (complementary metal oxide semiconductor) technology may provide a basis for future progress. Several steps can be envisioned. Pixel structures in the integrating domain, including a photodiode and an amplifying transistor, help to increase the signal-to-noise ratio. A further step might involve the deployment of counting structures for the detection and individual registration of each absorbed X-ray quantum. Developments of this kind would introduce the possibility of detector systems in which noise is determined only by quantum statistics. If one were to expand the counting of quanta to include the detection of their energy levels, one would be close to the development of new X-ray image contrasts based on spectral tissue properties (color imaging).

12.4 X-ray systems

In the present section, we present a classification of X-ray systems that is based on the primary clinical applications of the various systems considered. The systems included in the classification range from standard single X-ray exposure systems to high-end systems for interventional procedures that include 3D imaging capabilities. In general, we discuss only the latest technical realizations (i.e. mostly based on modern digital imaging chains) in each system class. Readers may wish to refer other recent texts for a more general discussion of X-ray systems [12.54].

All of the systems in the classification are primarily geared to the acquisition of 2-dimensional projection images. The systems are used for skeletal, cranial, thoracic, body and vascular imaging, as well as for interventional procedures. The systems' basic components include an X-ray tube with a generator, a detection device for the X-ray transmission image (including an anti-scatter grid[1)]), an image processing chain, one or more display units and, depending on the clinical application, a patient table. Modern digital imaging systems also comprise connectivity to digital patient information systems, digital archives, multimodality/multipurpose workstations and post-processing functionality.

12.4.1 Classification of X-ray systems

12.4.1.1 Radiography systems

Radiography systems are used to acquire individual exposures. Typical applications include thoracic and skeletal imaging. For decades, the film-screen system was the only mechanism of recording X-ray transmission images. The introduction of storage phosphor plates in the 1980s represented a first step towards the digital imaging and processing of planar images. Today, digital flat panel detectors based on amorphous silicon technology (section 12.3.4) represent a core component in state-of-the-art digital radiography systems.

Recent studies and publications show that digital systems have made significant progress in the clinical environment compared to traditional film-screen systems. The reasons for this include an essential dose reduction of around 50% with equivalent image quality [12.55] as well as greater functionality and convenience. The production of digital data entails the immediate availability of images on the monitor for the sake of diagnosis. These data can also be immediately transferred to digital archives, workstations and hard-copy cameras.

The availability of digital data also opens up a number of image-processing applications, including orthopedic measurements, digital mirroring, zooming, windowing, edge enhancement, tissue harmonization and filtering. More challenging applications such as digital-image stitching in the area of spinal and long-leg imaging are now on the verge of becoming a matter of routine practice [12.56]. Recently developed algorithms for computer-aided detection (CAD) are also expected to soon support clinicians in their daily work [12.57].

Typical radiographic systems are equipped with X-ray tubes that provide electrical power of up to 80 kW and focal spot sizes of 0.6 and 1 mm. Tube power and the focal spot size are selected according to the specific imaging requirements. The large focal spot and high power are used to optimize image quality in the case of highly absorbing

[1)] The anti-scatter grid eliminates scattered radiation in the patient by permitting the passage of directly transmitted radiation only. Anti-scatter grids are used when scattered radiation threatens to significantly reduce contrast (i.e. for investigations involving the torsos of adults).

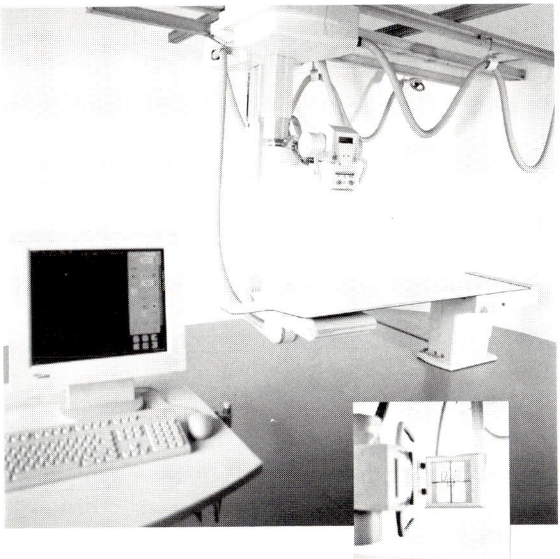

Figure 12.82
Multifunctional digital X-ray imaging system for applications involving the thorax, skeleton, skull, abdomen and the extremities (Siemens AXIOM Aristos FX). The insert shows a setting for standing patients.

body regions. Given that some structures in the body are affected by breathing and organ movement, it may be necessary to apply very short pulse durations in order to avoid image blurring. Only the large focal spot can tolerate the power needed in this application. The small focal spot is used when the highest spatial resolution is needed (e.g. fractures, lungs). Here, image quality is not that much affected by motion. This means that pulse durations may be longer and that less power is required.

The flat detectors that are currently used in such systems are 43 cm × 43 cm in size and produce images in a 3 k × 3 k matrix. This corresponds to a pixel size of 143 µm. This in turn corresponds to a spatial resolution of about 3.5 lp/mm, which is required for high resolution imaging. Digital filters can be applied in other applications to balance image noise and resolution. Automatic exposure control is implemented in all systems to eliminate over- and underexposure, and thereby ensure optimal image quality.

The X-ray tube and the detector can be deployed in various configurations. The full range of positions needed for whole-body imaging applications can be achieved with the use of ceiling supports (fig. 12.82). Wall and floor-mounted supports are available for special applications.

Modern digital radiography systems enable one to store the tube and detector positions as well as the imaging and post-processing parameters in organ programs for easy and efficient system operation.

12.4.1.2 Fluoroscopy systems

While fluoroscopy systems are primarily used for the imaging of dynamic processes, they can also be used to acquire individual exposures. Typical areas of application include the esophagus, stomach and colon, swallowing, phlebography (examination of the venous system using a contrast medium), myelography (imaging the spinal cord after the injection of a contrast agent into the subarachnoid space) and vascular and peripheral-vascular imaging. The detector is required to exhibit high temporal resolution in order to effectively render dynamic processes. The use of image intensifiers still represents today's standard. Standard radiographic detection devices (cassette films, storage phosphors, flat detectors) are used for individual exposures.

Given that current systems are equipped for digital imaging (fig. 12.83), they permit all of the post-processing and connectivity functions discussed earlier. These systems are normally operated via remote control in the case of noninterventional procedures.

X-ray tubes designed for radiographic systems can also be used in fluoroscopic systems. Image intensifiers for dynamic acquisition are used in various sizes. The most common sizes include entrance areas with diameters of 33 cm and 40 cm for a standard image size of 1 k × 1 k. Size selection is determined by the anatomical region and the patient group to be investigated. Typical frame rates used in fluoroscopy range from 0.5 to 15 frames/s in pulsed mode.

The X-ray tube and the image intensifier are mounted on a gantry together with the patient table (fig. 12.83). The source-image distance (SID) can be adjusted to achieve varying degrees of magnification. The tube angulations can be adjusted to avoid the overlapping of anatomical structures.

Special patient tables permit flexible angulations and tilting. This may be necessary to support the flow of the contrast medium into the body part that is to be imaged (e.g. in myelography and phlebography) or for the sake of examining the skeleton during load.

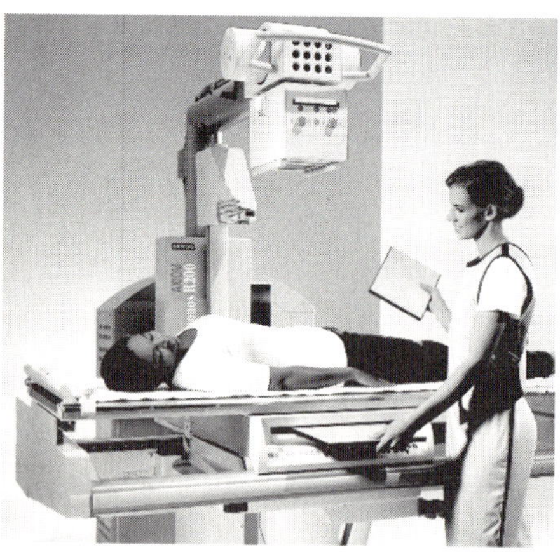

Figure 12.83
Digital fluoroscopy system. Applications include routine dynamic whole body imaging (Siemens AXIOM Iconos R200).

12.4.1.3 Multifunctional systems

Multifunctional systems are designed to meet the standard requirements that apply to examinations in areas ranging from radiography and fluoroscopy to angiography. System selection is often a matter of arriving at the right trade-off, i.e. the decision as to whether one should select a system with greater capacity in the area of radiographic and fluoroscopic investigations or in the area of angiographic/interventional procedures will depend on the frequency of the particular applications and the patient group.

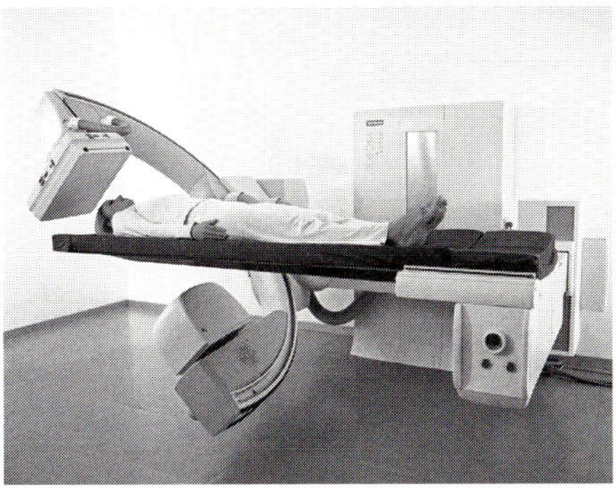

Figure 12.84
Multipurpose system: Applications include routine dynamic whole body imaging with a focus on angiography/intervention (Siemens AXIOM Artis dMP)

The X-ray imaging chain and the performance parameters in systems that are especially suited to angiographic/interventional procedures are very similar to those in the fluoroscopic system discussed above. In particular, the X-ray tube and the detector are mounted on a C arm to allow for the angulations necessary for angiography in all body regions except the heart. The system provides open access to the patient on the table so as to enable one to conveniently perform interventional procedures (fig. 12.84). A special control unit enables one to control all system functions from within the room. Moreover, the table can be tilted to achieve the upright positions that are necessary for examinations of the stomach and colon, as well as for myelography and phlebography.

12.4.1.4 Angiography systems

Angiography systems are dedicated systems for vascular imaging and intervention. Before CT angiography (CTA) and MR angiography (MRA) became clinically established, angiography systems were the only systems that enabled one to diagnose lesions of the vascular system. With the introduction of multi-slice CT and parallel acquisition techniques in MR, CTA and MRA established themselves as the standard procedures for diagnostic vascular imaging. Today, angiography systems are used primarily for the real-time guidance and control of interventional procedures, including percutaneous transluminal angioplasty (PTA), repair of vascular stenoses and aneurysms via stenting and coiling, placement of transjugular intrahepatic portosystemic shunts (TIPS), biopsies, and pain therapy.

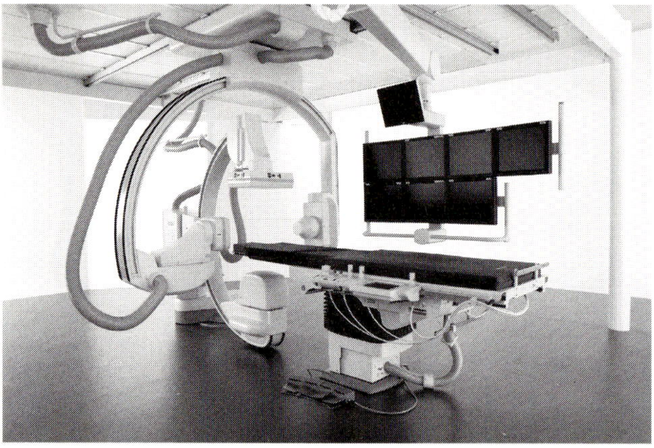

Figure 12.85
Biplane angiography system. Applications include vascular neuroradiology and neurological intervention (Siemens AXIOM Artis dBA).

Vascular procedures in angiography involve the guiding of catheters through the arterial or venous system to permit the injection of contrast media and/or the detachment of interventional tools (e.g. stents, coils) at specific locations. The femoral artery is usually punctured at the groin to allow for the insertion of the catheter. It is therefore necessary to perform these procedures under (semi) sterile conditions. This means that all of the controls for the stand and table and for the X-ray and imaging systems will need to be located in the room and operable under sterile covers.

The table top of an angiography system is designed for interventional procedures. This includes a manual floating function that enables greater flexibility with regard to the positioning of the catheter tip during fluoroscopy.

Angiography generally involves the deployment of two different system types: monoplane systems (one C-arm suspended from the ceiling or mounted on the floor) and biplane systems (one first-plane C-arm mounted on the floor and one *second-plane* C-arm suspended from the ceiling). Biplane systems are used to simultaneously acquire projections from two different angulations (fig. 12.85). Monoplane systems are mainly used in general angiography. Due to the complexity of the cerebrovascular tree, biplane systems are used for neuroradiology and neurological intervention.

3D-imaging of the vascular tree with a rotating C-arm represents a new application that has its origins in neuroradiology (section 12.5). In this case, the C-arm of the first plane is used to acquire the projection images from different angles. Cone beam algorithms as used in CT are then applied to reconstruct the 3D data set.

Angiography systems incorporate two different imaging modes: imaging with standard doses for diagnostic image quality and documentation (digital cine mode or DCM) and imaging with low doses to guide and control catheter movement in real time (fluoro mode). Fluoro modes apply about 1/10 of the dose of DCM. Frame rates used in angiography range from 0.5 frames/second to 15 (30) frames/second depending on the application. Image processing functions are applied in real time.

The X-ray tube provides electrical power of up to 80 kW and three focal spot sizes (0.3, 0.6 and 1 mm) to permit the viewing of different anatomical details. The large focal spot is used for body structures that might move. Such investigations require short pulse durations (and thus high power). The small focal spot is used for smaller structures and the micro focus (0.3 mm) is used for imaging very small details such as tiny vessels in the brain.

Image intensifiers are still used for dynamic acquisition. In the case of general angiography, they are commonly deployed in sizes of 33 and 40 cm. Image intensifiers with diameters of 40 cm are usually used for the first plane in biplane systems for neuroradiology while an image intensifier with a diameter of 33 cm is used for the second plane. Dynamic flat detectors with rectangular shapes of up to 40 cm in length currently represent the cutting-edge technology in angiography.

12.4.1.5 Cardiology systems

Cardiology systems are used for the diagnosis of cardiac diseases and for coronary intervention. Given that cardiac CTA and cardiac MRA are relatively new methods, cardiology systems still play a prominent diagnostic role in cardiac angiography. Symptomatic patients are usually admitted directly to the cath lab where diagnostic and subsequent therapeutic procedures are performed in a single session. The standard diagnostic elements include (1) the imaging of the coronary tree following the selective injection of a contrast medium through a catheter inserted from the groin and (2) a left-ventricular analysis of the heart function based on calculations of end-diastolic and end-systolic ejection fractions and an assessment of myocardial wall motion. In addition to imaging, special catheters are inserted to measure the hemodynamic and

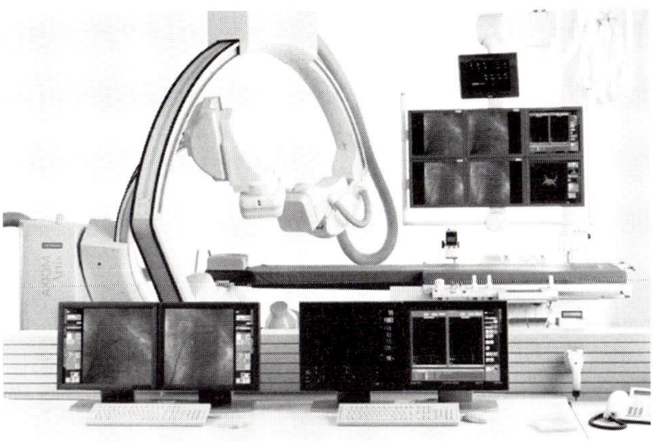

Figure 12.86
Biplane cardiology system with flat panel detectors for pediatric cardiology (Siemens AXIOM Artis dBC)

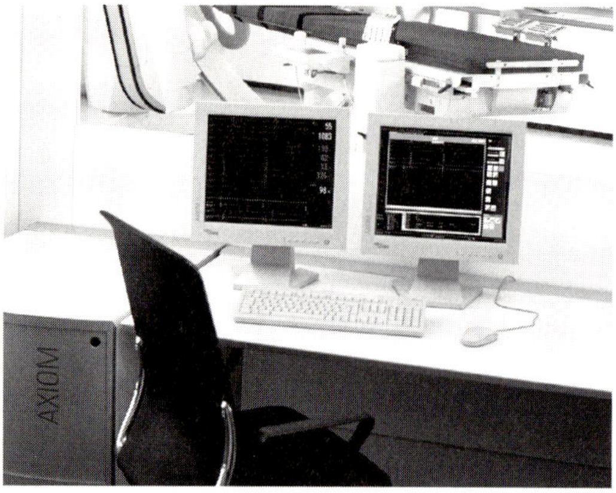

Figure 12.87
Hemodynamic and electrophysiology recording system in the control room of a biplane cath lab (Siemens AXIOM Sensis)

electrophysiologic parameters of the heart function. Examples of cardiac intervention include percutaneous transluminal cardiac angioplasty (PTCA) to reopen stenotic lesions via the inflation of balloons and insertion of stents, ablation of atrial fibrillations and the implantation of closure devices to repair cardiac defects.

As in general angiography, the cardiovascular system is accessed by inserting catheters from the groin. This means that the same requirements concerning the table and the operation of the system will apply.

Similarly, monoplane and biplane systems are also used in cardiology (fig. 12.86). Monoplane systems are mainly applied in adult cardiology and for electrophysiological procedures while biplane systems are applied in pediatric cardiology.

Dedicated cardiology systems were traditionally equipped with small image intensifiers (23 cm in diameter) in order to enable the steep angulations that are necessary to project the coronary tree without superimposition. Flat detectors of a comparable size (approx. 25 cm in diameter) have been routinely used for a number of years. Most cardiac systems today come with flat panel detectors because these detectors offer clear advantages with respect to signal linearity and extended dynamic range (i.e. improved visibility for small low contrast structures).

Patient monitoring systems to acquire and display the patient's vital signs (e.g. blood pressure, oxygen saturation, intracardiac electrograms) have become an integral part of cardiology suites. Functions that support electrophysiology include the stimulation and ablation of electrical propagation paths in various areas of the myocardium. These monitoring systems can be connected to cardiology information systems and to card-angio systems. They can also be used to track the administration of medication and the consumption of materials during interventional procedures and for purposes of reporting (fig. 12.87).

While it is essentially the case that the same imaging modes that are used in general angiography (fluoro and digital cine) are also used in cardiology, the motion of the heart makes it necessary to deploy higher frame rates in cardiology, with 15 to 30 frames/second in adult cardiology and up to 60 frames/second in pediatric cardiology.

The X-ray tubes used in cardiology systems are bifocal tubes with focal spot sizes of 0.4 mm and 0.8 mm and power of up to 80 kW.

As discussed in section 12.3, the flat panel's insensitivity to magnetic fields enables one to carry out a new application in the cath lab, the magnetic navigation of interventional devices. Magnetic catheter tips can be steered using externally applied magnetic fields. The direction of these magnetic fields can be varied arbitrarily in 3D space. The magnet controls and the imaging system are tightly integrated so that the anatomical information in the images can be used to define the targets of magnetic navigation. Clinical experience is currently restricted to the treatment of atrial fibrillation via targeted ablation (e.g. pulmonary vein isolation) and navigation through tortuous vessels. Preliminary data show significant reductions in fluoro times and lowered patient and clinician exposure.

12.4.2 Intervention – a paradigm for a modern X-ray system

As mentioned earlier, the clinical use of X-ray systems for vascular procedures has undergone a paradigm shift from diagnosis to intervention. This shift has been triggered by improvements in the vascular diagnostic capacities of noninvasive imaging modalities such as CT, MR and ultrasound in almost all regions of the body and by the ongoing replacement of open forms of surgery by minimally invasive procedures under X-ray control in angiography and cardiology suites. The design criteria for corresponding X-ray systems have accordingly changed to meet the needs of increasingly complex forms of surgical intervention. Moreover, diagnostic performance also needs to be included (e.g. for documentary purposes).

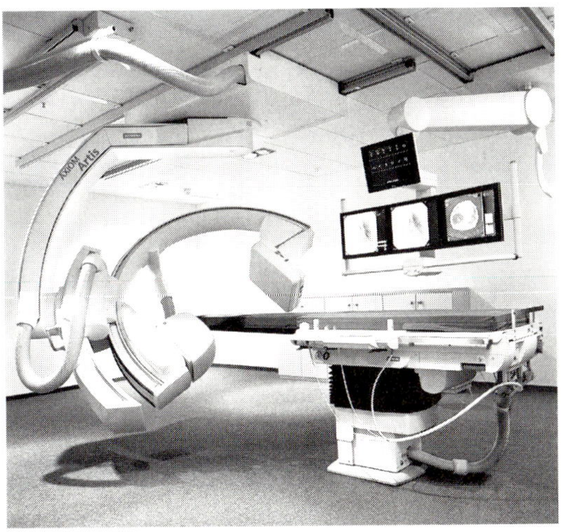

Figure 12.88
Dedicated interventional X-ray system with flat detector, integrated ultrasound, patient ECG monitoring and multimodality viewing (Siemens AXIOM Artis dTA)

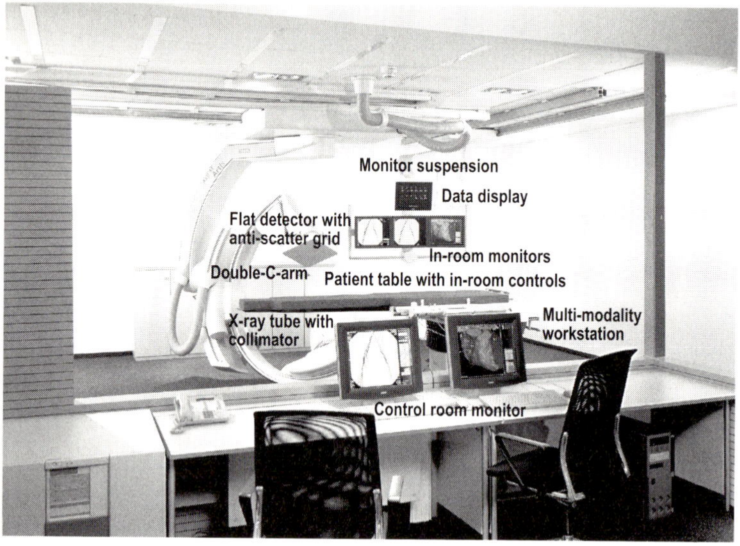

Figure 12.89
System components for a high-end interventional system (Siemens AXIOM Artis dTA)

In the following section, we are concerned to exemplify these requirements with reference to a state-of-the-art, ceiling-mounted monoplane angiography system (Siemens AXIOM Artis dTA) that is equipped with a flat detector (fig. 12.88).

12.4.2.1 System overview

The key system components include the C-arm with the flat detector, the tube and the collimator, the patient table with the in-room controls, a monitor suspension unit for the in-room monitors, a data display to show the C-arm and table position, the control room monitor with controls and a multimodality workstation (fig. 12.89).

Data and image-management system

The data and image-management system represents a key element in an interventional angiography system. It connects the various system components and functions as a link to all peripheral devices, including information systems, archives, networks, cameras and printers. Corresponding controls are available in the control room as well as inside the examination room.

The first step in a patient examination involves recording the patient's demographic data. These can be entered into the system manually or automatically via an information system such as HIS (hospital information system) or RIS/CIS (radiology/cardiology information system).

The protocols for the examination are selected and loaded into the system. The fluoroscopic or DCM images are displayed (in real time with the data acquisition) in the examination room and in the control room. The post-processing of acquired images can be performed using the imaging system either in the examination room or in the control room. In-room controls are available to enable one to control the imaging system from within the examination room. All of the images and scene data are stored on the system's hard disk and can be forwarded from this disk for printing, archiving and hospital network access. If necessary, the system also permits one to retrieve and display (in the examination room) previously archived patient data via the network for use as a reference during the current intervention.

C-arm

The X-ray tube and the detector are mounted on a C-shaped support (C-arm) that enables one to acquire images from a variety of viewing angles. The C-arm can be rotated around three mechanical axes to achieve the necessary angulations. One axis is parallel to the patient bed; the other two are perpendicular to each other and to the patient bed.

The detector should be positioned as close as possible to the patient so as to minimize patient dose and optimize image quality. The system enables one to vary the source-detector distance from 90 to 120 cm (i.e. by moving the detector up on the C-arm) to facilitate this positioning.

A minimum angular coverage of 180° + fan angle for the rotation on a circular orbit is necessary to permit one to use data acquisitions for purposes of 3D reconstruction. Angular coverage of up to around 300 degrees and a rotation speed of up to 60 degrees per second enable high quality volume imaging.

X-ray tube assembly

The X-ray tubes that are deployed for angiography typically meet the following specifications: 80 kW of electric power, various focal spot sizes between 0.3 and 1.0 mm (selection depends on the specific application and will influence maximum tube power), 2 MHU (mega heat units) of heat capacity and 3 kW of sustained power.

Typical voltages used in fluoroscopic and DCM investigations range from 60 to 125 kV.

A mechanical collimator is integrated in the tube assembly to permit one to adjust the X-ray beam to different fields of view. Various pre-filters (ranging from 0.2 to 0.9 mm of copper) are also integrated in the assembly for the sake of shaping the energy spectrum of the X-rays and achieving a minimum patient dose and optimal object contrast.

An automatic exposure control mechanism actively selects the appropriate kV, mA, pulse width and pre-filtration during standard fluoroscopic and DCM investigations so as to ensure the achievement of a pre-selected detector entrance dose (typically 20 to 40 nGy per pulse for fluoroscopy and 0.2 to 0.3 µGy per pulse for DCM).

Generator

The generator is a microprocessor-controlled high-frequency X-ray generator with automatic dose-rate control (fig. 12.90). The typical technical specifications are: max-

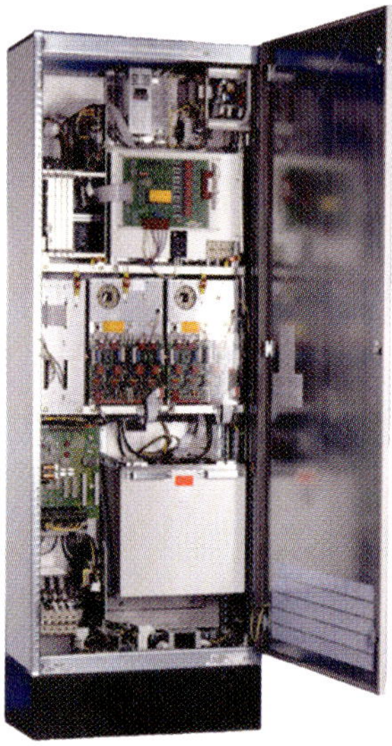

Figure 12.90
Typical X-ray generator used in interventional angiography (Siemens Polydoros IS)

imum electric power: 100 kW, tube currents: 0.5 to 1000 mA, continuous power: 3 kW, switching times: 0.5 to 800 ms and pulse frequencies: up to 60 frames per second.

Detector

Modern angiography systems like the one shown in fig. 12.88 deploy solid-state detectors to detect the X-rays transmitted through the patient. Current technology is based on amorphous silicon-diode matrices coupled to cesium-iodine scintillators. A size of 40 cm × 30 cm is appropriate in the case of general angiography to cover all of the anatomical areas that are to be imaged. The detector will need to be rotated to ensure proper anatomical coverage and patient access. Given a pixel size of 154 µm, the maximum spatial resolution is 3.25 line pairs per millimeter. The image is then represented in a 2,480 × 1,920 matrix. Neighboring pixels can be combined during detector readout to achieve an optimal balance of spatial resolution, image noise and contrast.

Patient table

To enable and facilitate proper interventional applications, the table construction makes provision for free access to the patient from both sides and head-to-toe imaging, a condition that presupposes a table top length of more than 2 m. The table top is made of carbon fiber so as to ensure radio translucence. It is also capable of tilting and cradling to enhance its deployability in a surgical environment. Angiographic tables provide for a manual positioning mode, i.e. the clinician has the option of moving or floating the table top manually to follow the catheter while it is advanced or to follow the contrast bolus. The control elements for the table functions are attached to the side of the table because the interaction with the table needs to take place in the examination room during the procedure.

In-room monitors

It is necessary for the physician to be able to see the patient images during interventional procedures in real time directly in the examination room while standing next to the table. The monitors are therefore mounted on a ceiling support unit inside the examination room. There are typically two monitors per plane, one live monitor showing the fluoroscopic or DCM images in real time and one reference monitor allowing one to display static images for the sake of comparison with the live images of the advancing catheter. If multimodality viewing or in-room 3D is required, an additional monitor is deployed to show the images of other modalities or the 3D reconstructions. Clinicians used to be restricted to the deployment of black-and-white diagnostic CRT monitors with X-ray systems. Today, the quality of LCD monitors is so good that they are used as the standard monitors for these systems (chapter 11). The fact that these monitors are less bulky than CRT monitors makes handling of their ceiling supports significantly more convenient.

In-room controls

As has already been pointed out, interventional procedures require that one be able to control the system from inside the room in a sterile environment. This is achieved via table-side controls that are mounted to an accessory rail attached to the table (fig. 12.91). The complete range of table movements (up/down, tilt, cradle) is controlled by push-buttons and a joystick (float, move). A second joystick is used to control C-arm motion and the source-detector distance. Modern systems permit one to store certain system positions for later retrieval. The collimators are controlled by the smaller joysticks depicted in fig. 12.91, with each joystick being assigned to a different collimator.

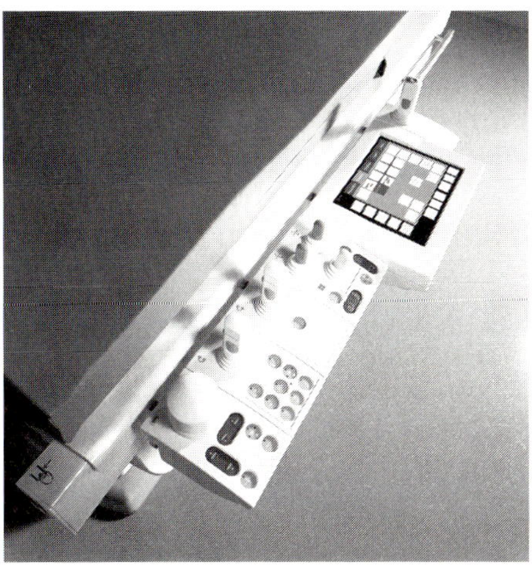

Figure 12.91
In-room controls (from left to right): table control module, stand control module, collimator control module, imaging system controls

The imaging system also needs to be controlled from within the examination room during interventional procedures. A separate control module (e.g. a touch pad) can be used to perform various functions, including image-sequence selection and looping, measurements in the images, reference image storage, examination mode selection, etc. The joystick next to the touch pad is used as an in-room mouse to control the imaging system.

A footswitch is used to release X-rays for fluoroscopy and DCM. The different examination modes are released by different pedals. Some footswitches enable one to program more functionality into the pedals (e.g. dim room light, release table brake).

Control room monitors and input devices

There is at least one imaging system monitor available in the control room for viewing live images when the X-ray system is in operation. When the X-ray system is not in operation, patient-related functions, viewing, post-processing, archiving, networking and printing can be performed in the control room using the system computer (usually a standard PC).

Workstations used for 3D imaging and post-processing are typically installed next to the system controls and are outfitted with a separate monitor, keyboard and mouse. A switch is available for multimodality viewing, i.e. to enable one to select from among the various input modalities for display in the control and examination room.

The components that are important for interventional system use include:

Multimodality viewing

As the use of volumetric data from CT and MR in the planning and guidance of interventional procedures increases, integrated solutions for the display and processing of these data are emerging as integral elements in interventional X-ray systems. Such solutions are realized by the installation inside the control room of a multimodality workstation that is connected to a multimodality monitor on the monitor suspension unit inside the examination room. This arrangement gives the user access within the examination room to the standard 3D visualization tools such as volume rendering and multiplanar reformation. The capacity to rotate the 3D representation of the patient data enables one to ascertain the optimal projection angle for the fluoroscopic control of the intervention. The reconstruction of the 3D data from a rotational acquisition of the C-arm enables one to use an automatic registration of the C-arm and the 3D volume to automatically align the C-arm to the appropriate projection angle for fluoroscopy.

The multimodality monitor can also be switched to other input sources for the sake of displaying data from other devices. The standard mouse operations for the corresponding workstation can be performed in the room by using a joystick available at the side of the table.

Patient monitoring

The system includes (at least) an ECG device mounted on the table accessory rails to monitor the patient's vital signs. The ECG curves and the oxygen saturation are usually monitored during the intervention.

Cardiology environments generally include a more sophisticated monitoring system that provides hemodynamic and electrophysiological capabilities. Additional functions used to assess vital signs include blood pressure measurements, invasive pressure measurements and intra-cardiac ECG (supporting up to 128 electrodes). Frequent applications in electrophysiology include the RF (radio frequency) ablation of atrial fibrillation and electro-anatomical measurements inside the heart chambers. Support of ablation and electrical stimulation is available for these applications in high-end patient monitoring systems.

Integrated ultrasound

The availability of real-time control in the form of ultrasound imaging in the examination room is advantageous in the case of some interventional procedures (e.g. puncture of the femoral artery at the groin and biopsies).

Various ultrasound probes (linear array, curved linear array, phased array) for B/M mode, Doppler, and color-flow imaging are available and can be selected according to the imaging task (fig. 12.92). The ultrasound images are displayed in real time in the examination room on the multimodality monitor. The ultrasound system can be completely controlled from the side of the table.

Compared to stand-alone ultrasound devices, the integration of the ultrasound system into the angiography system offers the advantages of immediate accessibility, a tidier examination room and image display at the location of the X-ray image display. The seamless management of patient data and images can be achieved by using standard DICOM connectivity.

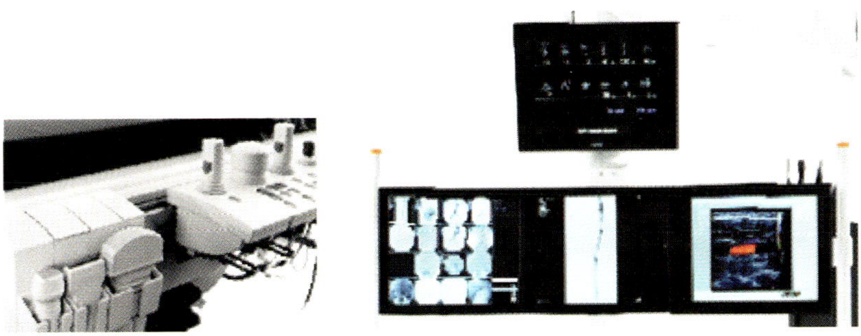

Figure 12.92
Integrated ultrasound in an angiography environment: **a)** linear, curved and phased array probes and table side control attached to the patient table, **b)** in-room display of the real-time ultrasound image on the multimodality monitor.

12.4.2.2 Imaging chain

The raw image as it is available at the output of the detector is determined by the physics of the imaging chain. The physical properties of the raw image are mainly determined as follows:

The spatial resolution is determined predominantly by the size of the focal spot and by the size of the detector pixels. The image contrast is determined by the energy spectrum of the X-ray beam and its noise is determined by the X-ray dose applied. In modern systems, the output signals of the detectors are digitized and calibrated. Calibration is necessary to correct for individual detector properties such as nonuniform sensitivity to the detector pixels, electronic offsets and scintillator afterglow. The image information is ultimately available in digital form. Here, digitization bit depth will also influence the achievable contrast resolution.

In the interest of enhancing image quality, one can bring about a further optimization in the relationship between image noise, spatial resolution and contrast by using dedicated image processing algorithms. These are applied after the digitization of the image content and are adapted for correspondence with the particular imaging applications (e.g. the algorithm will need to be optimized for low image noise when it comes to the visualization of low contrast).

In the interest of discussing some of these algorithms more explicitly, we will assume that the image information is available in digital form and at a digitization depth of 12 bits (i.e. the standard for modern angiographic systems). This means each pixel in the image is associated with a signal value (also referred to as a gray value) which corresponds to a number between 0 and 4,095.

Weighted averaging in the time domain is applied to reduce the noise in the images of a dynamic scene in fluoroscopy or DCM. This is of particular importance for the sake of dose saving in low-dose imaging modes such as fluoroscopy. In practice, a form of sliding weighted averaging is applied in a recursive manner. A motion detector is applied on an image-by-image basis to identify regions of fast motion in the images and to correspondingly decrease the weights for the averaging.

The nonlinear mapping of the original gray values (0 to 4,095) onto a new set of gray values (0 to 4,095) represents a standard element in image processing. The curve used for this mapping (a characteristic curve referred to as gamma curve) is usually selected so as to increase the contrast resolution in the dark areas (small gray values, high X-ray attenuation, bone and contrast-filled vessels) and to compress the contrasts in the bright areas of the images (high gray values, low X-ray attenuation, lung field). This is achieved by a steep slope in the gamma curve for small gray values and a flat gamma curve curvature for high gray values (fig. 12.93). As a result of this operation, the distribution of gray values within the image is redistributed such that the anatomically relevant regions are displayed with optimal contrast resolution. Look-up tables (LUTs) are used for the implementation so as to bring about the nonlinear transformation in real time (e.g. fluoroscopy at 30 frames per second).

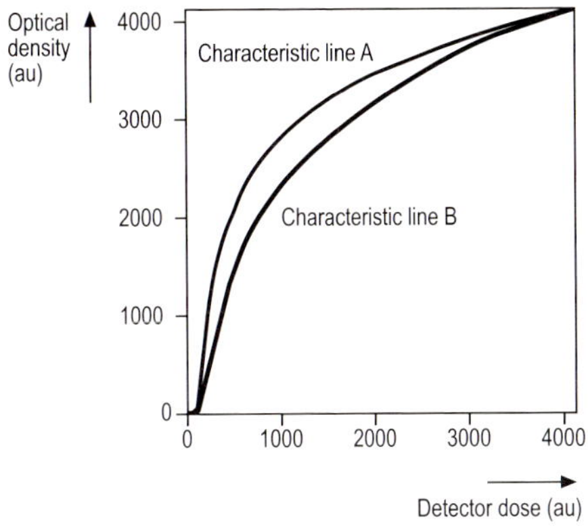

Figure 12.93
Gamma curve increasing the visual contrast in high attenuation areas and decreasing the visual contrast in low attenuation areas

Another standard element in image processing is windowing. Windowing is a different method of mapping the image's gray values. It is required for two reasons. First, the human eye is capable of distinguishing only around 35 gray levels. Second, display monitors are not capable of representing more than 256 gray values. Windowing usually involves the mapping of a certain subset of the image's 256 gray values onto the 256 gray values for the sake of monitor presentation. Fig. 12.94 offers an illustration of the basic principle. A window center *C* (within the 0 to 4,095 image data range) and a window width *W* are selected. The gray values within the range $C - W/2$ and $C + W/2$ are then linearly mapped onto the 0 to 255 scale of the monitor display. Apart from its technical aspects, windowing has an important practical consequence for viewing images. When using a wide window, several gray values from the original image are compressed into a single gray value at the monitor. As a consequence, both the contrast in the displayed image and the image noise are reduced. In contrast, narrow windows increase contrast while exaggerating the image noise. Fig. 12.95 shows the same image displayed in two different windows.

A further element in image processing is spatial filtering. Two common filter types (i.e. high pass filters and low pass filters) can be distinguished by their effect on the image's spatial frequency content. High pass filters enhance the high frequency content and therefore sharpen small details (e.g. edges). In practice, such filters are ap-

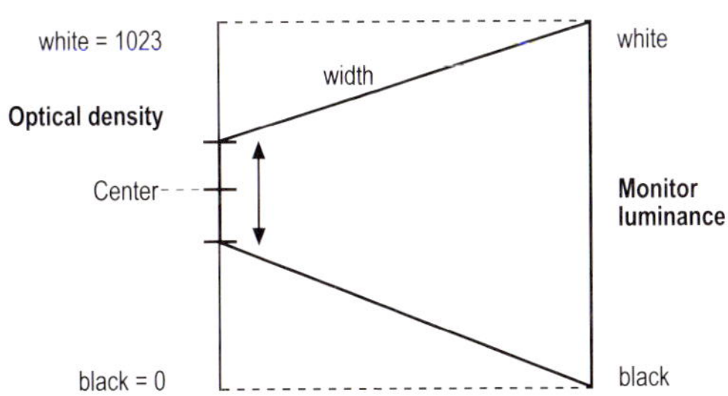

Figure 12.94
The windowing principle

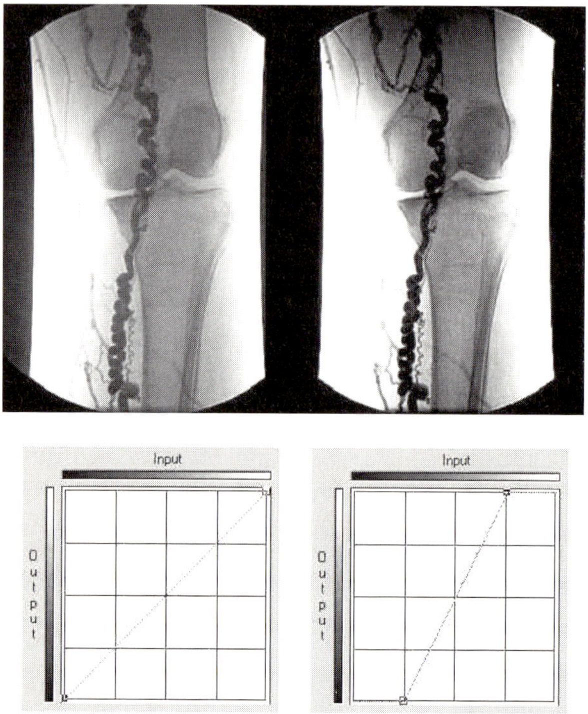

Figure 12.95
The same clinical image using different windows: **a)** wide window: the noise is decreased. **b)** narrow window: the contrast is increased.

plied to enhance the edge definition of contrast-filled vessels and to increase the reliability of diagnoses relating to arteriosclerotic changes in vessel walls. Edge-enhancing filters of this type are standard components in systems used for vascular intervention. Low pass filters smoothen images and reduce quantum noise, but also blur vessel edges. The most recent developments in filter technology have centered on advanced algorithms that allow for the detection of edges and homogeneous regions (i.e. edge definition is preserved and noise in homogeneous backgrounds is reduced). The implementation of these advanced filters was made possible by the introduction of high-end digital processors capable of performing several tens of billions of operations per second.

12.4.2.3 Modes of application

Fluoroscopy

The fact that fluoroscopy enables one to control the deployment of interventional devices in real time with lesser dose than DCM makes it the most important imaging mode in interventional cardiology and angiography. Its scope of application includes the advancement of guide wires and catheters and the placement of stents, coils and closure devices. Fluoroscopy is a low-dose imaging mode, typically involving a per-frame detector-entrance dose of 20 to 40 nGy. The automatic exposure control element is crucial to ensuring consistent image quality. This involves the optimization of the tube voltage (kV), the tube current (mA), the pulse width (ms) and the pre-filtration thickness so as to achieve a constant dose at the detector entrance, which in turn results in constant image noise. Internationally accepted rules of radiation protection limit the patient entrance dose rate to less than 100 mGy/min.

Fluoroscopy was previously based on the continuous emission of X-rays. Today's standard is based on an X-ray source in pulsed operation. The frame rates used for angiography range from 1 to 15 frames per second, those for cardiology range from 15 to 60 frames per second. A function is available for storing the last fluoro loop for immediate review and later archiving.

Digital cine mode (DCM)

In addition to fluoroscopy, a second imaging mode, referred to as digital cine mode (DCM), is needed to enable one to diagnose vascular lesions and to document the actual procedure. Higher doses than those used in fluoroscopy are used in DCM to obtain diagnostic image quality (mainly low noise images). Typical per-frame detector-entrance doses in DCM range from 200 to 400 nGy. The automatic exposure control described above is also applied in this imaging mode.

For the most part, the same frame rates that are applied in fluoroscopy are also applied in DCM. Single shots are sometimes performed for documentary purposes. DCM scenes are always stored on the system's hard disk so as to permit their review when selecting reference images and arriving at a diagnosis. These images can be automatically archived in the network or on a CD for the purpose of documenting the procedure.

Roadmapping

Roadmapping is a technique that is used to guide the advancement of guide wires and catheters while using as little contrast agent as possible (fig. 12.96). The technique consists of three steps:

1 – A short native scene is acquired using fluoroscopy. The last image of this scene is used as a mask for digital subtraction in step 2.

2 – Contrast medium is injected and the acquired fluoro images are shown as subtracted images using the mask from step 1. The subtracted images show the vascular tree. It is assumed that the last image shows the complete vascular tree with optimum contrast. Additionally temporal maximum intensity projection techniques can be applied (see below). The last unsubtracted image in this phase is inverted and used as a mask image for the following fluoro acquisitions.

3 – The catheter is advanced under fluoroscopy. The images shown on the monitor are images that have been subtracted using the mask as described in step 2. This means

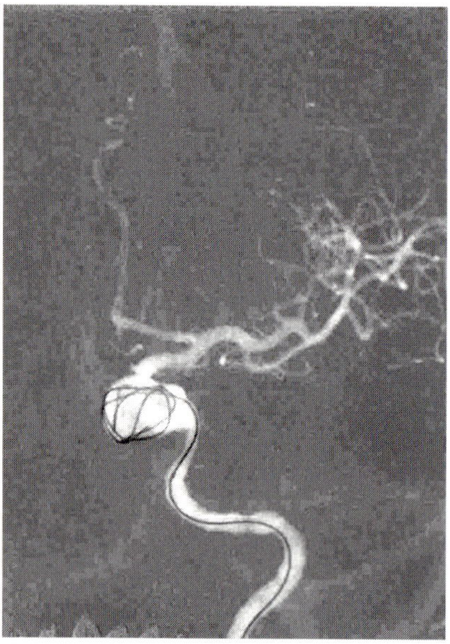

Figure 12.96
Roadmapping image

the appearance on the monitor of a black guide wire/catheter that is advanced in a white vessel.

Step 3 can be repeated without further injection of contrast medium so long as the patient has not moved in the meantime. If the patient has moved, the three steps will have to be repeated.

As described in step 2, the last image in phase 2 can be used as the mask for step 3 or the entire image stack from phase 2 can be searched pixel by pixel to identify the image for which the pixel under consideration has the maximum contrast. The corresponding gray value is attributed to this pixel of a new image that is used as a mask image for step 3. This procedure is equivalent to applying a temporal maximum intensity projection to the phase 2 images. An automatic pixel shift algorithm can be applied during the roadmapping procedure to adjust the mask image and the image that is to be subtracted if some small movement has occurred.

Digital subtraction angiography (DSA)

Digital subtraction angiography (DSA) is an imaging technique that enables one to show the contrast-filled vessels in the absence of an interfering anatomic background (e.g. bones and soft tissue) (fig. 12.97). This technique is used for diagnostic and documentary purposes in connection with angiographic procedures.

If this acquisition technique is selected, then the first image of a DCM scene (after the stabilization of the automatic dose control) will be used as the mask image. All subsequent images are shown in subtracted mode, which means that the mask image is subtracted from the acquired images. When a contrast medium is injected after the acqui-

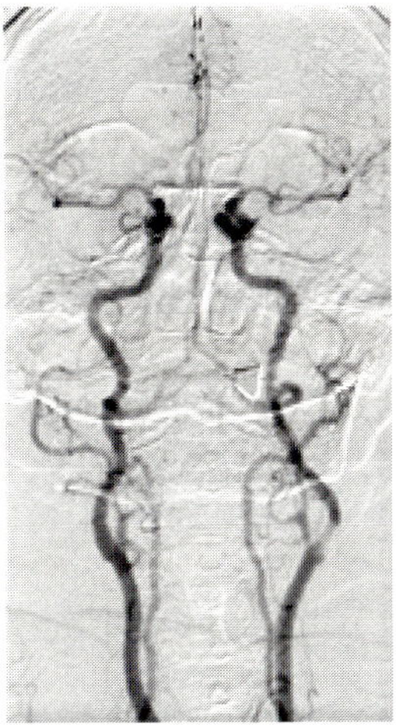

Figure 12.97
DSA image

sition of the mask image, a scene will appear on the monitor that includes only the contrasted vessels.

One will have an opportunity during post-processing to select a different mask image or to manually pixel-shift the images in the acquired scene to achieve an optimal subtraction of the anatomic background. An algorithm can be deployed in this context to analyze the two images that are to be subtracted with an eye to arriving at the best registration for these images. Referred to as auto-pixel shifting, this procedure can be applied online during data acquisition or later during post-processing.

Perivision and peristepping

Perivision is a DSA-like imaging mode that enables one to cover long anatomic areas (e.g. angiographic examination of the peripheral vasculature). In order to achieve the necessary range, either the C-arm or the table is moved automatically (step by step) between the corresponding imaging positions.

Three runs are necessary to complete the examination (fig. 12.98):

1 – Fluoroscopy is used during the first run to step from the initial to the final position so as to define the collimator and filter settings for each position (test run).

2 – The second run is performed in reverse direction in DCM to acquire the mask images at the various positions (mask run).

3 – The third run is started after the injection of a contrast agent. Images are acquired at each position in DSA mode (see previous page) using the mask images from the mask run. The stepping from position to position can either be initiated manually (based on a visual evaluation of contrast enhancement) or automatically.

The acquired images can be stitched during post-processing to display the long anatomy in a single image (fig. 12.99).

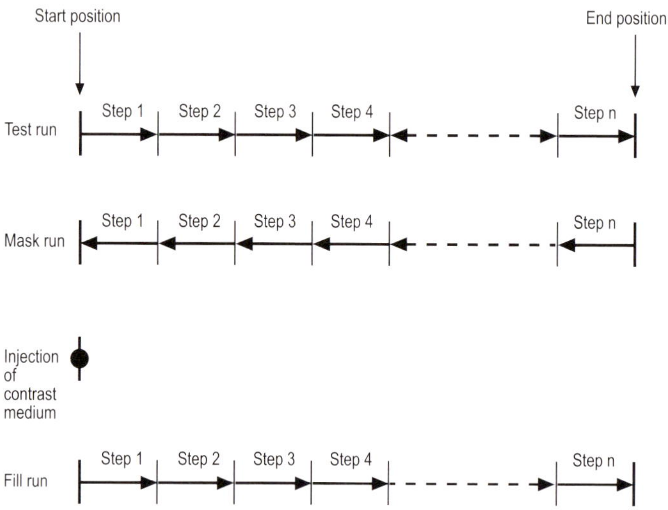

Figure 12.98 The principle of perivision

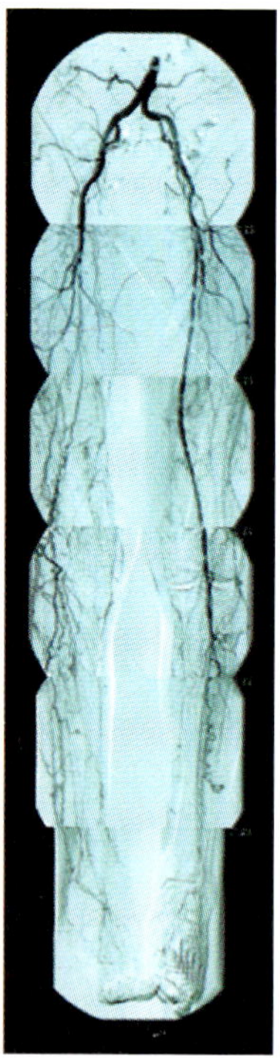

Figure 12.99
Perivision: clinical example

An imaging application referred to as DR stepping (or peristepping) represents a modification of the scheme shown in fig. 12.98: in this case the mask run is omitted and the images are shown in unsubtracted form during phase 3. This application is typically used to reduce dose when showing long bony structures and vessels.

Dynavision and DR dyna

Both dynavision and DR dyna imaging modes can be thought of as DCM scenes during which the C-arm continuously rotates around the patient. The C-arm usually rotates around the patient in a circular orbit with a constant angular increment. Images from dynavision and DR dyna scenes can be thought of as perspective views of the anatomy from different aspect angles.

Dynavision and DR dyna begin with a test rotation to make sure that there is no risk of collision for the C-arm. Fluoroscopy is possible, but not required during this test run.

In the case of dynavision, a rotation is then performed to acquire the mask images at each angular position. Another rotation is performed after the injection of a contrast agent to acquire the fill images at the same angular positions. The images ultimately displayed are the subtracted images at each angular position.

In the case of DR dyna, a single angular sweep is completed after the test run to view the anatomy from different angles.

Both imaging modes can be used to select optimal viewing angles for diagnostic purposes and to obtain optimal angulations for subsequent fluoroscopy. Replaying the scene creates a 3D impression for the user.

In the case of 3D imaging with a rotating C-arm, the dyna modes represent the basic acquisition modes for recording the two-dimensional projections that are used as input for the three-dimensional reconstruction of vessels (3D angiography) or other anatomical features.

Combined applications to reduce exposure (CARE)

The fact that complex forms of intervention may require fluoroscopic control over long periods of time makes it especially important to implement methods of reducing patient and staff exposure that do not compromise diagnostic information. Some methods are generally designed to make the user aware of the dose that has already been applied, to reduce the dose or to reduce the amount of contrast agent deployed.

The AXIOM Artis system includes the following functions:

CAREMATIC: The system automatically adjusts the system parameters (kV, mA, and pulse width) to achieve a constant detector-entrance dose and thus constant image noise. The mean brightness within a certain region of interest in the image is determined in real time and the result is used to determine the exposure of the subsequent image. This procedure enables one to avoid overexposure in slim patients and underexposure in obese patients. The system offers three different fluoro dose levels for each organ program.

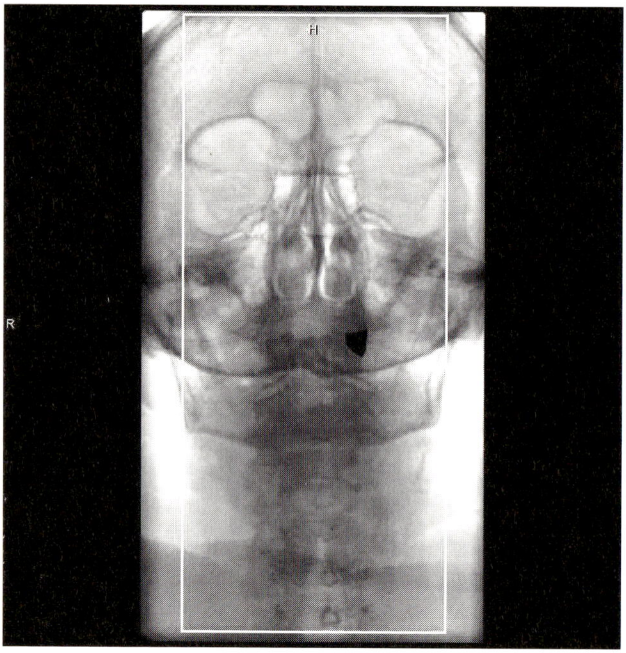

Figure 12.100 CAREPROFILE: position of the iris collimator in the image

CAREVISION: For fluoroscopy and DCM, the system offers frame rates ranging from 0.5 to 60 frames per second. A corresponding dose reduction can be achieved by adjusting the pulse rates to the particular application. In cardiology, for instance, one requires high pulse rates (e.g. 30 frames per second) on account of the rapidly beating heart. This is not the case in neuroradiology where the virtually stationary anatomy allows one to apply significantly lower frame rates (e.g. 3 frames per second). Assuming that the per-pulse dose rate is the same, one is in a position to reduce the dose by a factor of 10.

CAREFILTER: Pre-filtering the X-ray beam with copper filters of different thicknesses enables the optimization of image contrast with the lowest patient dose achievable. The CAREMATIC uses a real-time measurement of patient absorption as a basis for the automatic selection of the appropriate filter. The filter is then positioned in the beam path without user interaction.

CAREPROFILE: This function allows for the positioning of collimators and filters in the absence of radiation. When the user moves the collimator blades their actual position is shown in graphic form in a previously acquired image, which is usually the last image of the previous scene (fig. 12.100). This enables the user to adjust the filters to the desired positions. These adjustments are then applied to the subsequent image acquisition. Without this function, the user would be required to initiate fluoroscopy to adjust the collimators.

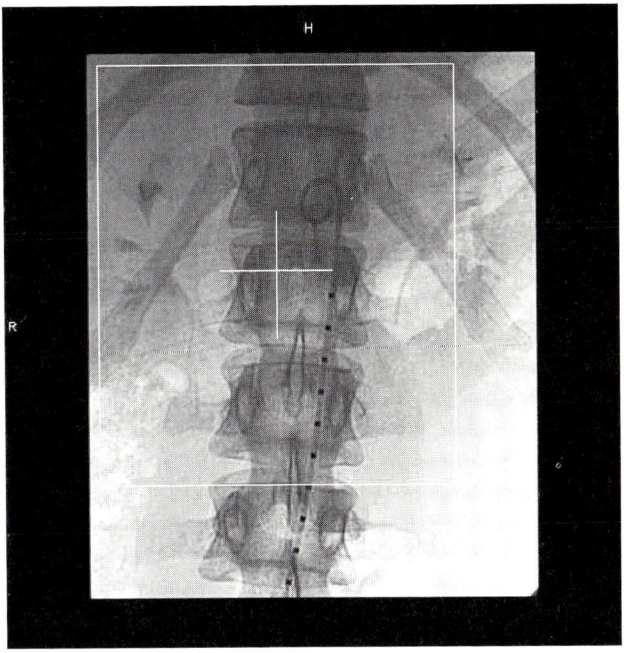

Figure 12.101 CAREPOSITION: the measurement field's position in the image

CAREPOSITION: The system shows the center of the measurement field graphically in the image currently on the monitor. When the patient table is panned, the center of the new measurement field is displayed on the current image (fig. 12.101). The measurement field can thus be repositioned without applying fluoroscopy.

Roadmapping: This function is described in detail in section 12.4.2.3. The use during the intervention of a previously acquired image that shows the vascular tree as a *map* to advance the catheter enables one to avoid the repeated injection of a contrast agent.

Reference image overlay: this function is a simplified version of the roadmapping procedure. A previous image that shows a fully contrasted vascular tree is selected as a reference image. If one then selects the overlay function, this reference image is inverted and any subsequent fluoroscopy scenes are superimposed onto it. As a result, the wire or catheter from the fluoroscopy is visualized in the contrast filled vessel of the reference image. As with roadmapping, this function allows one to save contrast agent.

Dose Display: To foster dose awareness, a dose display is available inside the examination room and at the control console. The dose values indicated include the actually applied dose rate during the acquisition, the accumulated dose area product and the skin dose. The skin dose can be displayed either as an absolute value or as a percentage of the 2 mGy threshold. The 2 mGy threshold is an internationally accepted standard representing the dose below which no X-ray-induced erythemia occurs. Observing accumulated patient dose values is of particular importance in the case of complex interventions (e.g. in neuroradiology) that can last up to several hours.

12.4.2.4 User interface

Angiography systems rely on two different kinds of user interfaces: the first relates to the operation of the system in the control room, the second relates to the operation of the system by the physician during the intervention in the examination room. While standard control elements (e.g. keyboard and mouse) can be used for control room operation, the user interface in the examination room is required to conform to sterility requirements, i.e. the control elements are normally covered by a transparent and sterile plastic sheet. Touchscreens and joysticks are therefore used instead of standard keyboard-and-mouse combinations.

The requirements for in-room controls and those for control room input devices are outlined in section 12.4.2.1.

The *syngo* software platform represents a unifying element in the design and implementation of user interfaces in systems manufactured by Siemens. This design provides modality-independent user interfaces and platforms for common functions such as patient registration, patient selection, post-processing, filming and archiving. Modality-specific functionality (e.g. the acquisition platform) is then added according to the same style guide, with the contents naturally differing from modality to modality. The main advantage of this platform approach is that it enables the operator to master different systems and modalities with a minimum of training. The *syngo* platform for Siemens modalities is analogous to the Windows platform for PCs (see chapter 19).

For systems with 3D imaging capability, the user interfaces in the examination room and in the control room enable one to display, process and manipulate the 3D data set as well as to synchronize the 3D view to the corresponding angulation of the C-arm for the following fluoroscopy/DCM system.

12.4.2.5 Post-processing

Post-processing is performed on individual images and scenes after their acquisition in order to enhance details quantify pathologies and optimize image appearance. This is done in the context of angiography either in the examination room using the table-side controls, in the control room or at a separate workstation. Technically speaking, the term image post-processing refers to any operation that can be performed on the digital image after it has been stored on the system's hard disk.

Windowing and edge enhancement have been described in detail in section 12.4.2.2.

A magnification of the region of interest can be achieved for the sake of a more effective presentation of the pathology in the images via image roaming and digital zooming. The electronic shutter is used to electronically collimate on the selected region.

It is also possible to flip images horizontally and vertically to achieve standard image orientations for easier viewing.

Image inversion constitutes a re-mapping of the gray-scale. Structures that were originally white become black and vice versa.

The most common purpose of annotation is to add text to the image so as to better inform the referring physician about the diagnostic findings.

Special post-processing functions are available for DSA scenes:

The scene can either be shown in native or subtracted form so as to provide information about the vasculature in relation to its anatomical background. Pixel shifting is used to register the mask image with the images of the scene to obtain an optimal view of the vasculature in the absence of its background. Various methods of pixel shifting are available: manual, automatic and flexible (i.e. corresponding to a warping of the mask image). If the mask image turns out to be less than optimal, then it can be changed (re-masking).

It is sometimes necessary to quantitatively determine the geometry of anatomic image details. The basic tools here include the distance measurement along a straight line and the measurement of angles. These measurement types are usually relevant to orthopedic applications, i.e. to enable one to plan surgical or minimally invasive forms of intervention involving the skeleton. While it is also important to know the length and width of the stenosis when stenting a stenosed vessel, the fact that vessels are generally more or less tortuous entails that measuring along a straight line will not yield accurate results. More sophisticated algorithms are necessary for evaluating vascular lesions (e.g. in the coronary and intracranial vessels).

Quantitative vessel analysis (QVA) and quantitative coronary analysis (QCA) are the corresponding tools: the user marks the beginning and the end of the stenosed vessel

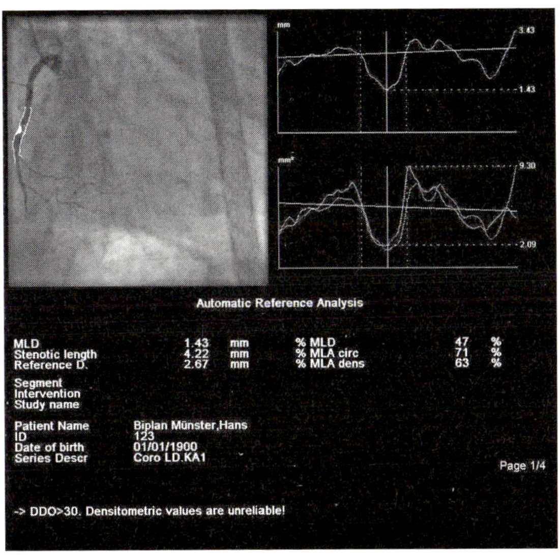

Figure 12.102 Screen shot of quantitative coronary analysis (QCA) (AXIOM Artis)

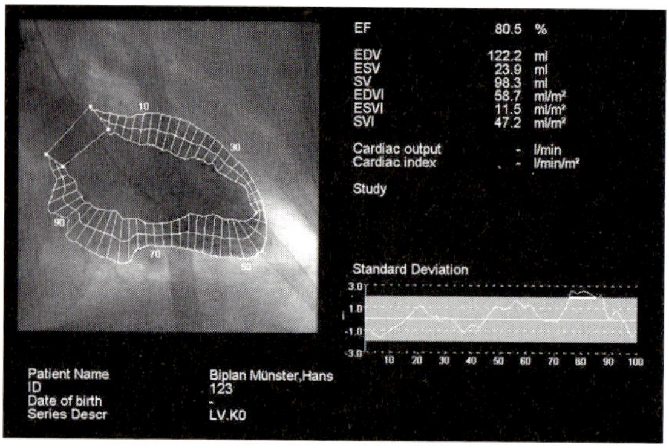

Figure 12.103
Left ventricular analysis (LVA) – screen shot with evaluated parameters

segment, and the stenosis itself. The algorithm then finds the vessel contours, measures the length of the midline in the vessel and determines the diameter and the cross sectional area of the stenosis (as absolute values or as percentages of the unstenosed part of the vessel segment) and plaque areas (fig. 12.102). The length of the stent or the size of the balloon can then be determined on the basis of these parameters.

In routine cardiac applications, the function is quantified by means of the quantitative left ventricular analysis (LVA). The system calculates ejection fractions, cardiac output, stroke volume and wall motion by comparing a scene's end-diastolic and end-systolic images. These represent the most important parameters for the cardiologist when it comes to diagnosing the functional behavior of a patient's heart (fig. 12.103).

The projection geometry causes structures at different depths within the object to be projected at different magnifications. The two-dimensional projection image, however, contains no information about depth. Calibration is therefore required to compensate for these projection effects. Various calibration methods are available:

Object calibration uses an image object of known size. The ratio of the true object size to the measured object size is used as the calibration factor. Calibration based on the diameter of the catheter in the vessel that is to be evaluated represents a special form of object calibration that is very accurate because the catheter is exactly within the depth of the vessel.

Another method involves calibration to the table-object distance. The system knows the location of the image intensifier, tube and table. Once the user enters the distance between the table and the object under consideration, the system will be able to calculate the true dimensions of the object according to the projection geometry.

An automatic version of this latter method begins with the assumption that the object of interest is positioned in the isocenter of the system and uses this assumption to calculate the true object dimensions.

All of the inaccuracies that are associated with the above calibration methods can be avoided if the object's true three-dimensional geometry is known. 3D angiography is a clinically established volumetric imaging method that is used today primarily in neuroradiology. The use in this context of precise 3D measurements of volumes, cross sectional areas and distances along curved lines represents a new standard. It is to be expected that these capabilities will be extended to other body parts.

3D reconstruction methods involving a limited number of views have recently been developed to enable quantitative evaluations of coronary artery segments. These methods are currently under clinical evaluation.

12.4.2.6 Reporting and documentation

The documentation of procedures prior to the introduction of digital techniques used to be a matter of recording scenes on 8-mm cine film. Film viewing, archiving and retrieval were obviously quite tedious compared to current methods.

Digital techniques enable one today to store scenes directly on the imaging system's hard disk. The images can be viewed directly and sent to workstations for purposes of reporting. Scenes can be automatically recorded on standard video film for later offline viewing.

After completing an interventional procedure, the physician usually begins to review the scenes and to select images for the report. These images represent the manner in which the procedure was performed and its final outcome.

There are various ways of documenting a procedure:

One way is to directly send the selected images to a laser camera for filming. Modern laser cameras conform to the DICOM (Digital Image Communication in Medicine) standard so that the user has a choice to choose from the variety of cameras available on the market. Although today's laser cameras avoid the lengthy wet processing of film, the film itself is still relatively expensive.

As the capacity of standard laser printers to resolve more gray levels and to provide enhanced spatial resolution continues to improve, the use of paper prints for purposes of documentation is on the rise.

The widespread availability of PCs facilitates the distribution of images on CDs. Computer systems can be equipped with image-copying capacities and DICOM viewers that start automatically as soon as a CD is loaded. This makes the viewing of images easy and convenient for the referring physicians as well as for the patients.

If the dynamic information in a scene is crucial, AVIs (Audio Video Interleave) of scenes or 3D scenarios can be created at the workstation. These movies can then be used for purposes of demonstration or distributed to referring physicians. Standard PC tools are available to replay these dynamic movies.

The standard approach used to be a matter of attaching film material to the patient record and to the report to document the pathology or the outcome of the procedure. Today, reporting tools are available that allow one to create reports from text templates in combination with an electronic copy of the images. The obvious advantage here is that the report and the images are tied together electronically. These reports can then be distributed within the hospital network either on a stand-alone basis or as a part of the electronic patient record.

The hemodynamic recording system is an integral part of the cath lab environment in interventional cardiology. AXIOM Sensis provides these reporting tools as a standard feature, thereby eliminating the need for a separate reporting workstation in the cath lab.

12.5 Cone-beam CT with C-arm systems

12.5.1 Introduction

Although more than 64 detector rows are routinely applied today in computed tomography (CT), large volumes are still scanned sequentially (see chapter 13). Two-dimensional detectors that collect data from a total volume within a single rotation of the X-ray tube detector system were first discussed for cardiac imaging in connection with the Dynamic Spatial Reconstructor [12.58]. This system consisted of 14 X-ray tubes and 14 TV camera systems that were mounted on a rotating gantry in order to acquire data from the beating heart in real time. Other prototypes such as the GE Morphometer [12.59] and the Hitachi SF-VA100 [12.60] were developed in the early 1990s. Both of these prototypes deployed image intensifiers mounted on CT gantries. Although technologically impressive, these systems were never made commercially available. In 1984, Feldkamp, Davis and Kress of Ford Motor Company introduced a CT volume image reconstruction algorithm for industrial non-destructive testing that takes account of the cone-shaped X-ray beam [12.61] when an area detector is applied. This algorithm remains the basis of most practical applications in medicine today. The breakthrough for cone-beam CT in medical applications came in the mid to late 90s in the form of the C-arm X-ray system routinely used in angiography.

The main differences between a C-arm CT system and a regular CT scanner include the following:

1. While the trajectory of the focal spot with respect to the patient is approximately planar on a C-arm system, it forms a spiral on a CT scanner. Given that it does not cover a full rotation, the trajectory is only a partial scan.
2. While standard CT scanning involves the application of a stack of row detectors (up to 64 rows with 700 to 800 columns) over which the patient is moved, the detector is two-dimensional (up to 1,920 rows × 2,480 columns). The broad X-ray cone in the case of C-arms enables enhanced use of X-ray quanta, but also leads to a higher degree of scattered radiation.
3. From a mathematical point of view, data acquisition in cone-beam CT necessitates the use of approximate reconstruction techniques such as the Feldkamp algorithm.
4. A C-arm CT system's field of view (FOV) in radial direction is more limited than that of a CT scanner. The FOV has a diameter of 25 cm (in the rotation center for a 40 cm detector, and less for smaller detectors) whereas the FOV of a CT scanner has a di-

ameter of 50 cm. An FOV with a diameter of 25 cm is usually too small for any parts of the anatomy except for the head (i.e. its use for other parts will involve truncated projections).

5. One partial rotation is sufficient to scan a volume of an axial extent of up to 20 cm. While a CT scanner needs more rotations, which are acquired in shorter times (see next item), it can cover any axial length as the patient is moved.
6. A partial scan with a C-arm usually takes 5 to 10 s (and longer for mobile C-arms). In contrast, a 360° scan on a CT scanner takes only 0.33 to 1.00 s. The frame rates on a C-arm system are 30 to 60 frames/s, whereas the readout frequency of a CT detector is much higher (several thousands per second). The number of projections ranges from 50 to 500 for a C-arm system and is more than 1000 on a CT scanner.
7. Modern two-dimensional X-ray detectors are optimized for the acquisition of 2D projection images. This is not yet the case for CT imaging, especially with respect to dynamic range.
8. The geometry of a C-arm system is not as well defined as that of a CT gantry. The geometrical calibration of a C-arm thus represents a technical challenge.

The first attempts to overcome the limitations of two-dimensional projection images for C-arm systems in angiography involved stereo X-ray tubes, biplane systems and, in particular, rotational angiography. Here, the C-arm is rotated between frames (i.e. one refrains from preserving constant C-arm angulation during a DSA acquisition). Rotational angiography usually consists of two rotational runs. The first run is a mask run without contrast injection. This is followed by the injection of a contrast agent. The second run is a fill run that involves image acquisition at the very positions where the mask images were acquired. Fill and mask images are subtracted. Projections of the vessel tree are seen from different directions, thus enabling a better evaluation of its geometry.

The following system properties are important for the technique of rotational angiography: (1) a high frame rate to enable the acquisition of many frames in a short amount of time, (2) fast rotation in order to cover reasonable angles in the short amounts of time that a contrast bolus can be held and (3) the capacity to drive the C-arm to identical positions. If mechanical reproducibility is not guaranteed and positions cannot be reproduced, the suppression of the mask in DSA will not be perfect and will require post-processing (pixel shift).

Although the implementation of CT reconstruction for C-arm systems was clear from a technical point of view, the actual introduction was rather late for the following reasons: limited C-arm system performance, the need to handle large data volumes and high computational needs. The first clinical prototypes exhibited frame rates of 7.5 to 10 frames/s, rotational speeds of around 30°/s and total scan angles of around 150 to 180°. A typical acquisition protocol involved the acquisition of only 50 frames (i.e. projections). Given that the scan geometry was not as stable as that in regular CT scanners (owing to mechanical instability and geometrical distortions in the image intensifier), tomography reconstruction presented a challenge. However, in the case of high contrast objects (such as vessels with arterial contrast agents offering a contrast resolution of a few thousand HU), the method proved clinically relevant [12.62], and then went on to establish itself as a successful procedure for interventional neuroradiology in the late 90s. Soon, the method was also applied in angiographic investigations for parts of the body other than the head. Then bone imaging became possible (with a contrast resolution of about 100 HU) [12.63], an application that is of special interest for mobile C-arm systems in surgical environments [12.64].

The original C-arm system detectors were image intensifiers with vidicon tubes. The tube cameras were then replaced by CCD cameras. Flat detectors are currently replacing the entire image intensifier camera system (see section 12.3.4). Thanks to flat detectors and other optimized system features, cone-beam CT systems with C-arms now permit one to visualize low contrasts in objects of 10 HU and lower.

CT gantry systems with large 2D detectors recently underwent a further revision, this time involving flat detectors instead of image intensifiers. Given their current status as pure research systems, we refrain from addressing them in this chapter.

12.5.2 Acquisition protocols and system properties

Cone-beam CT is an option for all stationary angio C-arm systems (floor-mounted, ceiling-mounted, general purpose) with any type of detector (large and small image intensifiers, large and small flat panel detectors). It is also an option on certain mobile C-arm systems. Fig. 12.88 shows a floor-mounted angio system with a large (30 cm × 40 cm) flat detector.

The total scan angle is typically 200 to 220° (180° plus at least the fan angle). Certain systems require one to accept a smaller angle and more limited image quality. For instance, while 150° on general purpose systems may be considered sufficient for high contrast applications (arterial contrast injection of several thousand HU), bone reconstructions will suffer considerably.

The C-arm can be rotated in both orbital and angular direction. The rotational speed of modern stationary C-arms ranges from 40 to 60°/s. Maximum frame rates reach up to 30 (or even 60) frames/s. A typical angio protocol may therefore involve: 200°, 5 s and 150 frames (with a short amount of time for holding the arterial bolus). A protocol involving more projections for improved low-contrast resolution might entail: 200°, 15 s and 450 frames (i.e. many frames). Given that mobile systems usually exhibit lower rotational speeds and lower frame rates, they take fewer projections in longer amounts of time (which is acceptable for bone imaging). Angio protocols are usually rotational DSA acquisitions with a mask run and a fill run. Low contrast acquisitions involve just one run.

Large detector sizes are preferable, especially for bone and low-contrast imaging because they minimize object truncation. Flat panel systems are superior to image intensifier systems. Mobile systems are outfitted with small image intensifiers. Mobile systems with flat detectors have entered the prototype stage.

The pixel size of the digital image is quadratic. It is typically 0.35 mm with large image intensifiers and flat panel systems (2 × 2 binning mode). Smaller pixel sizes can be achieved with image intensifiers by using the zooming capability. At flat detectors one can switch to the non-binned mode (giving half the pixel size), or detectors with smaller pixels have to be employed. Smaller pixel sizes require larger pixel matrices (meaning larger data volumes) or artifacts due to object truncation may occur.

Additional geometric quantities for C-arms include a distance of 70 to 80 cm between focal spot and isocenter and a distance of 115 to 120 cm between focal spot and detector. The geometric magnification is about 1.5.

The 2D projection images that are acquired on the C-arm system are usually transferred to a separate workstation for reconstruction and visualization. The time between acquisition and visualization of the reconstructed data set depends on the 2D image matrix size, the number of projections, the type of preprocessing steps being applied and the size of the 3D cuboid. The time value typically ranges from one to a few minutes.

12.5.3 Calibration

The system properties that are required for 3D reconstruction are established in the context of a calibration procedure. The most important properties include:

- Image distortion or distortion calibration (for image intensifier systems only)
- Acquisition geometry or geometry calibration
- Gain profile and monitor signal or intensity calibration

These properties are determined with calibration runs of dedicated phantoms. The runs are evaluated using special calibration software. The calibration information is stored in an appropriate (parameterized) form.

Calibration is an offline procedure that may be performed as often as once a month or once a year.

Initial factory calibration is not sufficient for image intensifier systems because it is the local magnetic field at the installation site that determines image distortion. However, factory calibration is conceivable for flat panel systems.

Distortion calibration

Image intensifier systems are 2D detectors that are not geometrically perfect (see section 12.4). In particular, the earth's magnetic field causes image distortions that change over a rotational run. The overall distortion is usually more complicated than pincushion distortion (e.g. S-shape contributions). Large fields are more affected than small fields.

Image distortion is calibrated by fixing a perfect 2D grid phantom (fig. 12.104) to the detector entrance screen and initiating rotational runs (as if it were a matter of patient acquisitions). The phantom defines the geometry of a virtually perfect detector without distortion. The calibration routine determines the deviation of real phantom pattern positions from ideal positions. The parameterization can be performed in different ways. A global fit of bivariate (x and y) polynomials up to the fourth order repre-

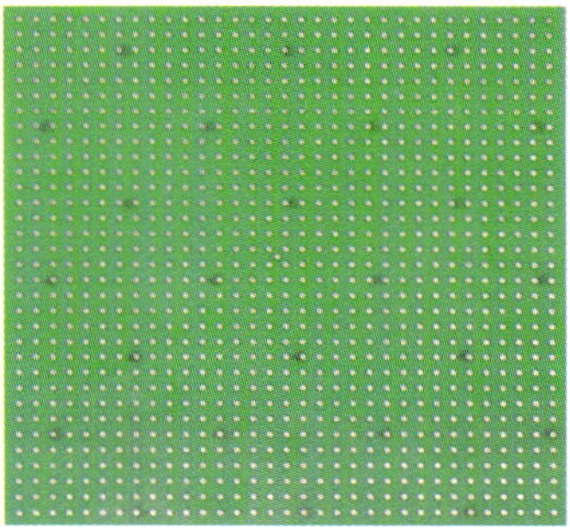

Figure 12.104
Phantom for calibrating the image distortion of image intensifier systems

sents a good balance of variables (number of free parameters, smooth instead of oscillatory behavior, overall accuracy).

Image distortion is the first effect to be calibrated in image intensifier systems, and also the first to be corrected, both in the context of other calibration procedures and during patient runs.

Mobile C-arms are outfitted with smaller image intensifiers that are less prone to magnetic distortion and are easier to shield effectively. Here, the correction of image distortion is less critical.

Geometry calibration

The mechanical setup of a C-arm system is more fragile and sensitive than the setup of a CT gantry. Heavy masses are moved using thin arms. This means that a semi-circular trajectory is not exactly planar and that the distance between focus and detector is not exactly constant (just to mention two imperfections). A reliable determination of all of the geometric degrees of freedom involved in the acquisition runs is essential for good spatial resolution in the reconstructions.

It turns out that the geometry – although far from ideal – is reproduced from run to run. This means that once it is performed in service mode, the geometry calibration will remain applicable for a long time. The online geometry determination systems based on markers in the image field or on external sensors have major disadvantages: image contents do not remain free of obscuring calibration patterns and the external sensors may not be reliable enough in a clinical environment or they may fail to achieve a sufficient degree of accuracy.

Geometry calibration or pose determination is performed with a special phantom (fig. 12.105) comprised of a plastic cylinder with metal balls of different diameters arranged in a specially designed spiral pattern. This phantom is placed in the isocenter and rotational runs are initiated. The calibration software detects the ball pattern points, associates each point with the corresponding point of the phantom, determines the respective pose and establishes a global coordinate system for all projections. The final result is a 3×4 projection matrix for each projection (homogeneous coordinates, see section 10.7 and [12.66]).

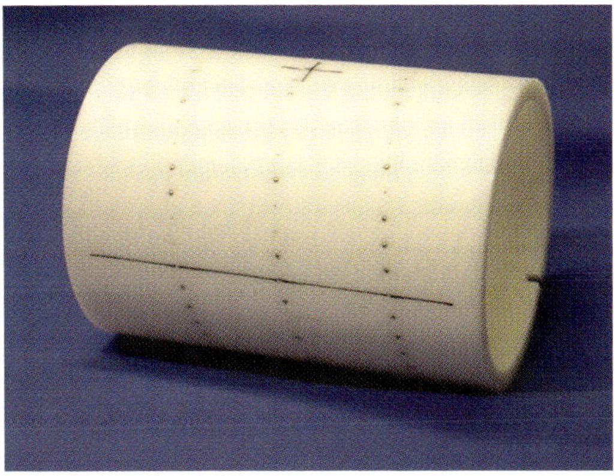

Figure 12.105
Phantom for calibrating the acquisition geometry in C-arm systems

The projection matrix describes the mapping between real space points *x*, *y*, *z* and detector pixels *u* and *v*. The 3×4 matrix has 12 elements. These 12 elements can be expressed in physical terms: *x*, *y*, *z* of the focal spot, *x*, *y*, *z* of the detector, 2 angles for the orientation of the detector rows, 2 angles for the orientation of the detector columns, detector spacing in row direction and detector spacing in column direction. One of these 12 elements is trivial for the pure projection part: if the detector spacing is multiplied by a certain factor and the distance between focal point and detector is multiplied by the same factor, then the projection values *u* and *v* will be identical. A projection matrix therefore has 11 degrees of freedom. This fact is conventionally used to set the right bottom element of the projection matrix to one. The 11 free parameters may be grouped into 6 extrinsic parameters (3 Euler angles for a rotation / 3 translation vectors for a transformation of the coordinate system) and 5 intrinsic parameters (describing the pure projection). If the detector rows and columns are orthogonal, there are only 10 degrees of freedom. If the pixel size is identical in both directions, then 9 degrees are left over.

Intensity calibration

The intensity calibration is needed to acquire gain (or flat-field) calibration data and to enable the $\log I_0$ determination (reference or monitor signal). The attenuation signals are transformed into line integrals using the reference or monitor signal (see eq. (10.1b) in chapter 10).

Gain calibration is important for larger image intensifier fields on account of the considerable vignetting. Given that flat detectors usually have a gain calibration of their own, one might regard an additional gain calibration as less important. However, a special gain calibration for purposes of reconstruction is altogether relevant in light of increasing demands for better image quality.

C-arm systems offer no physical way of determining the reference or monitor signal $\log I_0$ because there is no extra monitor detector. Nor is it possible to measure the unattenuated signal in some outside region of the detector, as the detector is usually fully covered by the object, and the detector dynamics are not sufficient for this purpose. Special calibration precautions can also be taken for this quantity.

Intensity calibration is performed with rotational runs of a homogeneous object that is put on the collimator.

12.5.4 Reconstruction

The transfer of the two-dimensional projection images to the reconstruction pipeline is followed by a series of initial preprocessing steps: distortion correction for image intensifier systems, gain correction and log I_0/I transformation. Advanced systems may also involve scatter, beam hardening and truncation correction as well as further correction steps.

Reconstruction is a convolution-backprojection procedure. Algebraic reconstruction techniques (ARTs) represent an interesting alternative only for very few projections and subtracted images.

The Feldkamp reconstruction formulas can be found in eqs. (10.15) and (10.16). It will be necessary to generalize these formulas in two respects. C-arm scans usually do not cover 360°. This will have to be compensated for by some type of Parker weighting [12.66]. Furthermore, real C-arm geometries are never ideal Feldkamp trajectories. One typical compromise for handling the geometric deviations from a perfect semicircular scan involves performing the convolution in detector row direction and then taking the real geometry into account during backprojection. Readers may wish to refer to a related work for more details [12.67].

12.5.5 Visualization

The reconstructed data sets represent large stacks of slices (256^3 to 512^3 voxels). All of the standard visualization and diagnosis techniques are applicable (see chapter 3).

The C-arm CT technique was initially used for high-contrast applications in the head region. A three-dimensional approach to analyzing and diagnosing data is very important in the case of the topologically complex vessel trees in the brain. At the time, however, the 3D visualization techniques for large data cubes were not yet very powerful (interactive rendering typically requires 3 frames/second, and 20 frames/s is desirable).

The maximum intensity projection (MIP) technique was initially one of the preferred ways of examining these data sets. MIP is very effective at showing high contrast objects (vessels with contrast or bones) and the associated computational task is manageable. The disadvantage of MIP is a loss of depth information (what is in front and what is on the backside). This loss can be partially compensated by interactively changing the viewing direction considerably or by applying stereo techniques (i.e. via shuttered glasses).

A second early technique was surface shaded display (SSD). This technique involves the use of a threshold gray value to visualize the surface of all voxels of a higher gray value. Once again, the computational demand is limited. SSD is complimentary to MIP. The shading shows depth information effectively, and is therefore helpful when it comes to analyzing three-dimensional objects. The disadvantage is the single threshold level. If the threshold is set too low, many disturbing objects or artifacts will become visible. If the threshold is set too high, clinically relevant objects may be lost. SSD depends on reliable gray values. This, however, could neither be guaranteed for the early reconstructions nor for the clinical applications (e.g. arterial contrast decreases in more distal branches).

Volume rendering (VR) represents the ideal technique for these data sets. It offers transparency, shows depth information through shading, and its soft transfer-function increase – as opposed to a unique threshold gray value – is far more tolerant with respect to gray values. Furthermore, it enables one to visualize several objects with several transfer functions (e.g. vessels and bone). While VR is computationally more demanding, advances in computer graphics have helped to facilitate its implementation. VR has become the method of choice for C-arm CT data set analysis.

The increased deployment of C-arm CT in low-contrast applications will have the effect of re-establishing certain traditional methods of two-dimensional data analysis (2D slices, MPR, i.e. multiplanar reformatting).

12.5.6 Advanced application tools

The capacity to generate volume data sets with C-arms enables one to execute a series of advanced applications. Task cards integrated into the user interface allow for the measurement of lengths, areas and volumes (e.g. for stenosis quantification and aneurysm volume measurement).

The subtraction techniques that are commonly deployed in DSA and roadmap imaging can also be applied to C-arm volume imaging. If the rotational runs are executed with the injection of a contrast agent (the majority of cases today), then mask and fill images will usually be available for each projection. These data enable one to reconstruct 3D data sets from the mask phase alone (bones, devices, clips, coils), from data sets based on the subtracted mask and fill phases (vessels filled with contrast only) and from fill-phase data alone (bone plus metal plus filling). The comparison of these data sets may yield important supplementary information (e.g. whether the coiling of an aneurysm has been successfully accomplished and the flow into the aneurysm has been stopped).

Virtual angio endoscopy applies volume rendering to allow for the visualization of vessel anatomy from the inside. Although the initial demonstrations of this tool have been very impressive, it has not yet gained relevance in routine clinical work.

Live fluoro and acquisition images are often compared with the reconstructed 3D data set (side by side) during interventional procedures. It is very helpful for this purpose to orient both data sets using identical angulations (3D automapping). The physician may find the ideal projection for guiding the interventional procedure when analyzing the 3D data set. In this case, the C-arm can be driven to this very angulation. On the other hand, if additional 3D information is needed in a given C-arm working position, the 3D data set can also be oriented in the same way.

The superimposition of 2D X-ray projection images and 3D data sets (3D road-mapping) represents a more advanced method that enables one to guide procedures with less contrast agent and/or less dose by using the 3D data set as a roadmap. However, the complicated problem of 2D/3D data fusion (involving more than 2 angles) necessitates the use of an advanced interface between the 2D X-ray system and the 3D image reconstruction system.

Direct interfaces to external tools (e.g. surgery tools) have been realized, especially as a support for mobile C-arm systems in a surgical environment (see chapter 5). Here, it is possible, for instance, to show the position of a tool in the 3D data set without further registration.

12.5.7 Image quality

12.5.7.1 Spatial resolution

High isotropic spatial resolution is the strength of C-arm systems.

The high spatial resolution is due to the small pixel size of the detectors (which can be further reduced by zoom capabilities at image intensifiers or non-binned modes at flat detectors). Limiting factors include object truncation and the accuracy of the geometric calibration. Very high spatial resolution can therefore be applied in the case of high-contrast objects, but not for low contrast imaging. Given that high spatial resolution and low contrast resolution are to some extent mutually exclusive, one is required to arrive at a reasonable balance of properties.

High spatial resolution in the isocenter is achieved in radial and axial direction: the spatial resolution is isotropic. This is no longer true for larger cone angles, i.e. for regions that are close to the very head or foot side of the detector. The spatial resolution can be estimated according to a simple procedure:

- Assume that the pixel size on the detector is 0.15 mm. Apply 2×2 binning (as is applied for a fast acquisition mode) for a detector pixel of 0.3 mm.
- Apply a resampling from the 1240 detector matrix to a 1024 matrix in overview format.
- The magnification factor between isocenter and detector is 1.5.

The effective pixel sizes in the isocenter are thus as follows:

- Overview format: 0.24 mm corresponding to a resolution of 2.1 lp/mm.
- Without resampling: 0.20 mm corresponding to 2.5 lp/mm.

Given that this estimate does not take account of the effects stemming from the focal spot size and the reconstruction process, one can expect the actual resolution to be a bit less favorable. Resolution is measured using dedicated phantoms (fig. 12.106, 12.107).

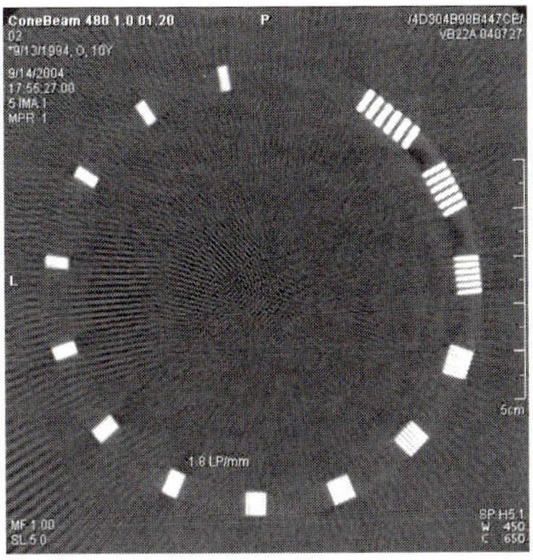

Figure 12.106
Overview reconstruction showing a series of multiline patterns in a phantom. Top right: the first group has 0.4 lp/mm. Successive groups: 0.6 lp/mm, ..., 1.8 lp/mm (7 o'clock), ... ending with 3.0 lp/mm (almost 12 o'clock). The phantom has a total diameter of 16 cm.

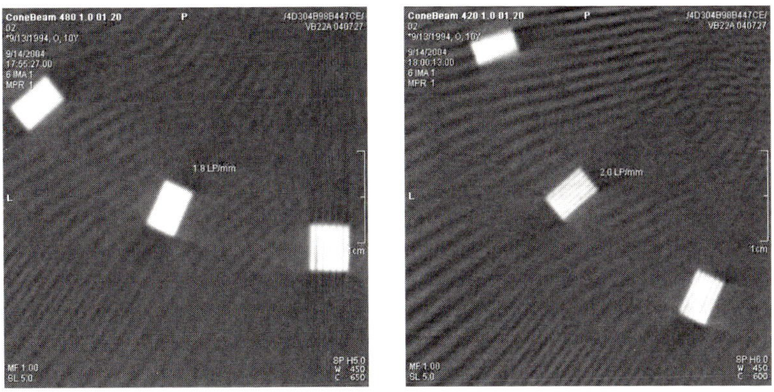

Figure 12.107
Overview reconstruction **(left):** 1.6 to 1.8 lp/mm can be resolved. Reconstruction without resampling **(right):** 2.0 lp/mm can be resolved.

12.5.7.2 Low-contrast resolution

Low-contrast resolution characterizes the capacity to image small test objects of low contrast that are embedded in a larger object, and is strongly influenced by the size of the small object, the size of the larger object and the applied dose.

Reconstructions based on 50 projections are dominated by streak artifacts. This number of projections permits no more than the reconstruction of high-contrast objects. The deployment of 150 projections allows one to resolve contrast differences of around 100 HU. The introduction of flat detector systems permits the achievement of improved low-contrast resolution. C-arm systems used in combination with the corresponding preprocessing and correction schemes then enable one to approach low-contrast regimes.

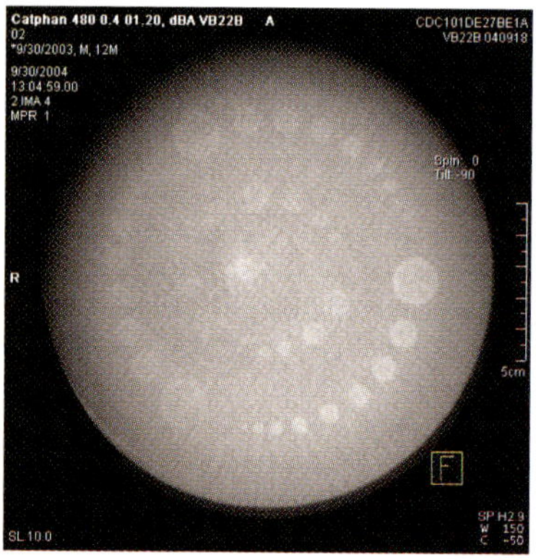

Figure 12.108
Reconstruction of a CATPHAN (The Phantom Laboratory, Salem, NY, US) CTP515 slice phantom, showing insets of 10 HU (3 o'clock to 6 o'clock), 5 HU (11 o'clock to 3 o'clock), and 3 HU. This data set was acquired with 538 projections and a CTDI dose of 40 mGy. The slice in the figure is an MPR of 10 mm thickness. Some image artifacts remain.

The use of Siemens DynaCT allows one to resolve 10 HU for an object with a diameter of 10 mm in a phantom with a diameter of 16 cm at a CTDI dose of 20 mGy. This is demonstrated with the measured data in fig. 12.108.

12.5.7.3 Dose

Dose in C-arm systems is set by the system-dose setting in the organ program, the system dose being the detector dose behind the anti-scatter grid in a central image area. This has two advantages for 3D applications: First, the dose is automatically adjusted for thicker objects. Second, the dose is automatically modulated according to the object's profile.

The typical C-arm CT system dose per frame is (far) lower than that of DSA, but much higher than that of fluoroscopy.

Patient exposure in interventional angiography is usually quantified in terms of entrance dose and dose-area product. The main problem in angio is dose accumulation at specific parts of the body owing to an ideal angulation that is not changed during the procedure (hot spots). C-arm CT is different in this respect and does not really cause problems because the dose is spread equally over a partial rotation. Nevertheless, if one were called upon to quantify a 3D dose in terms of entrance dose, one might use the following comparison: the dose per frame is a factor of 10 less than that of a DSA run. This means that 250 to 500 projections of a 3D run amount to around 25 to 50 DSA images, a number that can typically be reached with 2 DSA runs.

While entrance dose is not an issue in the case of 3D acquisitions, the applied dose and its statistical risk should be subject to quantification via an index of the sort used in CT (i.e. the CTDI). The CTDI quantifies the dose over the object profile. Plastic cylinders with diameters of 16 cm and 32 cm are used as phantoms to measure CTDI, with the first cylinder accounting for head acquisitions and the second for whole-body acquisitions. The phantoms are furnished with five holes (A to E) for the placement of a dose meter (fig. 12.109).

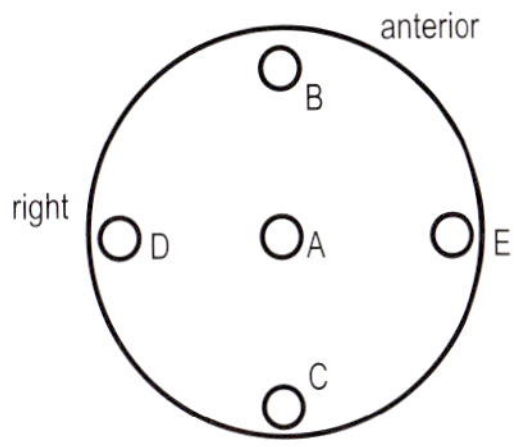

Figure 12.109
Profile of a CTDI phantom cylinder. The 5 holes A to E are used to measure dose.

A typical value for the axial CTDI (position A, 100%) in the 16 cm phantom for stationary angio C-arm systems is 2.8 mGy/100 mAs (at 70 kV). During the partial scan, the tube rotates more on the posterior side of the patient. The posterior dose is therefore higher (C: 220%) and the anterior dose is lower (B: 60%). The dose on the sides is somewhere in between the two (D and E: 150%). When using this asymmetric profile, the weighted CTDI is roughly equal to the axial CTDI (3.7 mGy/100 mAs).

The weighted CTDI for a neuro angio protocol with mask and fill runs (each of 150 projection images) is typically 11 mGy. It is around 16 mGy for a low-contrast protocol with 450 projections.

12.5.7.4 Advantages of flat detectors over image intensifiers

As has been discussed in section 12.3.4, flat detectors have advantages over I.I./CCD camera systems:

- *Dynamic range*
  Modern flat detectors deliver a digital signal of 14 bits. CCD cameras deliver a digital signal of only 12 bits.
- *Veiling glare*
  The effects of light and electron scatter in an image intensifier create an image background.
- *Field size*
  The larger flat detector areas reduce data truncation.
- *Geometric distortions*
  The absence of image distortion on flat detectors offers further advantages for applications such as 3D road-mapping.

Low contrast resolution under comparable conditions is limited in the case of an image intensifier to around 25 HU for 10 mm objects. Image intensifiers and flat detectors offer comparable spatial resolution.

12.5.8 Clinical applications and examples

The percentage of cases involving the use of angiographic C-arm systems for purely diagnostic reasons has decreased considerably over the last 10 years. Today such systems are predominantly used for interventional purposes. The sophistication of interventional techniques has also increased markedly. The C-arm CT represents an imaging tool that supports procedures in this environment.

Typical cases of interventional angiography include the treatment of aneurysms (e.g. embolization with coils), AVM (arterio-venous malformation, the shunt may be glued), stenoses (balloon angioplasty, stenting) and tumors (e.g. embolization of feeders, intra-arterial chemotherapy).

3D data sets are acquired before treatment to permit full diagnosis and intervention planning. A data set may be acquired after the intervention to determine therapeutic success and to document the outcome. It may also be necessary to acquire 3D data sets during the interventional procedure.

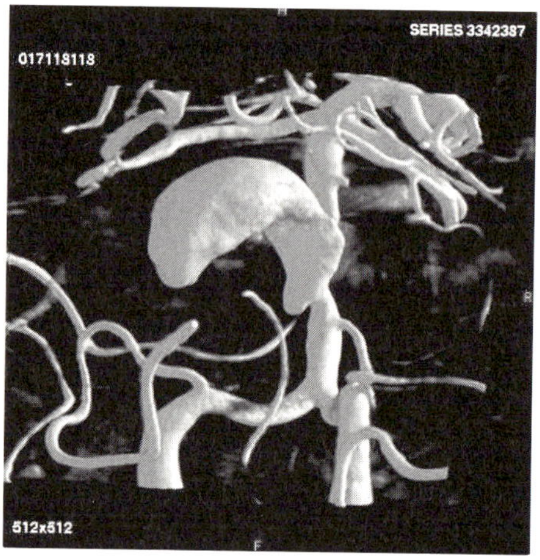

Figure 12.110
Huge aneurysm at the basilar artery (volume rendering)

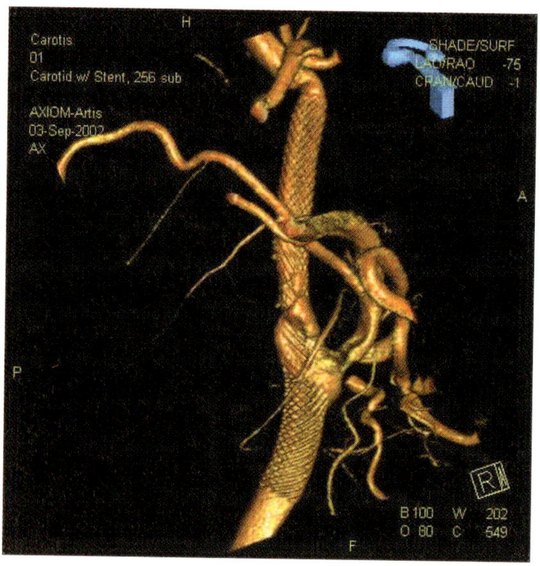

Figure 12.111
Carotid artery after stenting. The mesh of the stent wires can be easily identified (volume rendering).

Figs. 12.110 and 12.111 offer illustrations of volume imaging with C-arms for angiography.

Figs. 12.112 and 12.113 depict bone data sets that were acquired with an angiographic C-arm system and that demonstrate high spatial resolution. With the exception of spine work, these cases are not typical for angiographic C-arms. Bone imaging is more usual for mobile C-arm systems in orthopedic surgery.

The latest achievement in C-arm CT represents a considerable improvement in low-contrast resolution. Fig. 12.114 shows bleeding in the brain.

While the whole-body slice in fig. 12.115 still shows artifacts, it demonstrates the potential of low-contrast imaging with C-arms for areas other than the brain.

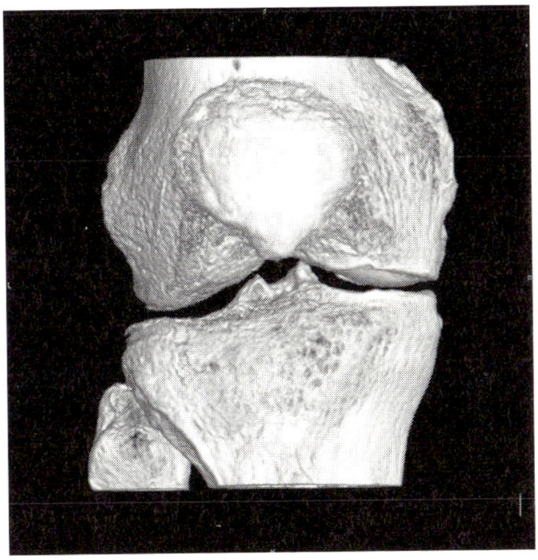

Figure 12.112
Reconstruction of a knee (volume rendering)

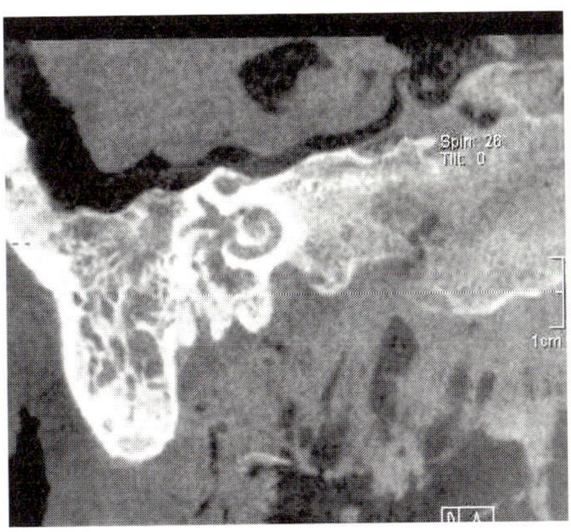

Figure 12.113
Reconstruction of the inner ear demonstrating excellent spatial resolution. The snail-shaped cochlea is easy to recognize (MPR).

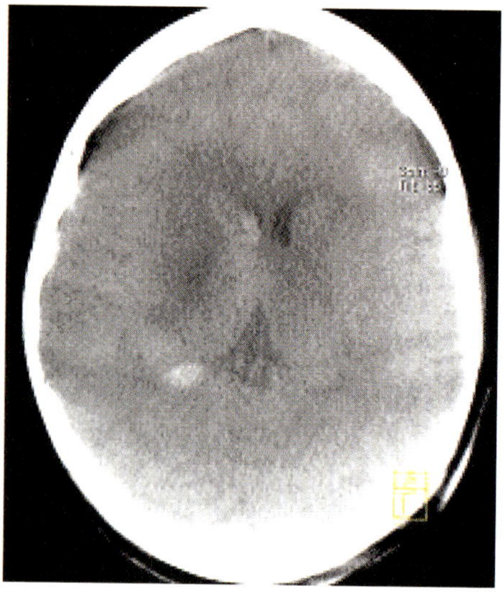

Figure 12.114
MPR image of a brain showing the ventricles and bleeding (lower left)

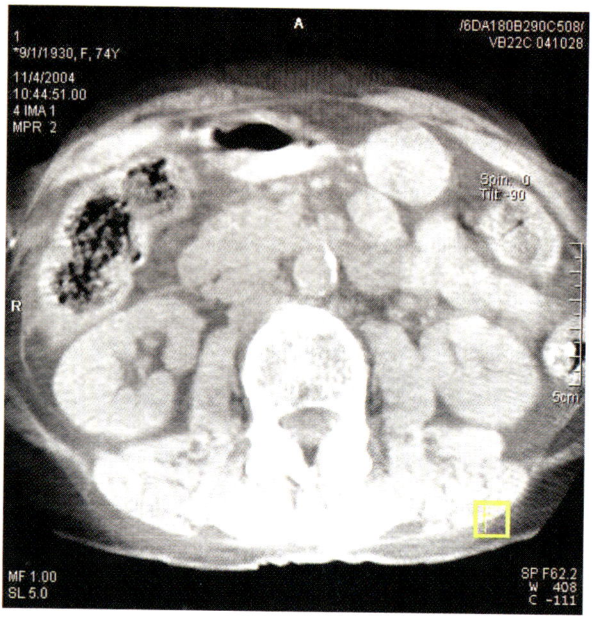

Figure 12.115
C-arm CT of the abdomen demonstrating good low-contrast resolution (thick MPR). Some artifacts are still visible.

12.5.9 Outlook

C-arm CT is well established now as an angio tool (in combination with arterial contrast injection). It has become a standard imaging technique, especially in interventional neuroradiology, with scans often being taken before and after interventional procedures and sometimes during the procedures. In general angiography for regions other than the head, C-arm CT is an advanced tool that helps facilitate special procedures. However, its use in other areas is lower because the vessel topology is simpler and can be easier assessed using 2D projection images. Although technically successful, the use of C-arm CT in bone imaging has not become the standard, except in the case of spine work (vertebroplasty, pain treatment). However, bone imaging is clearly a domain for mobile C-arm systems.

Low-contrast options such as DynaCT enable a whole new range of applications. While the purely diagnostic scan will continue to be done on a CT scanner, the option of deploying a CT-like scan during an interventional procedure enhances safety, supports clinical decision making, provides guidance, can effectively reduce contrast medium and dose levels and may introduce beneficial workflow changes in interventional radiology. Low-contrast capacity is also of interest in the case of mobile systems. Here, a mobile C-arm might be used as a mobile CT scanner.

From a CT standpoint, C-arm systems also have limitations. While the head is an ideal object (no truncation, total dynamics limited, no movement), whole-body acquisitions are in many respects more challenging. A 25 cm FOV will entail truncation, there is movement in the abdomen (heartbeat, breathing, peristalsis) and the total dynamic range is higher.

The main limitations that system engineers will have to deal with in the medium term in the case of low-contrast C-arm CT include:

- The limited field of view.
- The limited dynamic range of the detector (maximum/minimum signal and quantization – or bit depth).
- Timing and trajectory issues for advanced applications (e.g. cardiac applications).

C-arm CT promises to inspire a broad range of interesting and exciting developments and applications.

12.6 Mammography

Breast cancer is the most common malignant disease among women living in the western world. Approximately 180,000 new cases of breast cancer are diagnosed each year in the United States, where more than 40,000 women also die from the disease each year. After lung cancer, breast cancer is the second leading cause of death from cancer among women. The chance of getting breast cancer is around 1 to 8, i.e. more than 12% of all women develop breast cancer during their lifetime. These facts help to illustrate the dramatic human and economic costs associated with the disease. For the latest statistical information, readers may wish to refer to any of the various reputable sources [12.68, 12.69, 12.70].

The early detection and diagnosis of breast cancer is the main aim of breast imaging. The development of mammography, the X-ray imaging of the breast, began around 90 years ago when mastectomy specimens were X-rayed for the first time [12.71]. From there, breast roentgenology developed to modern mammography.

The assessment of a mammogram is primarily a matter of looking for masses (tumors) and microcalcifications. The detection and morphological assessment of masses requires high contrast resolution because such masses may have nearly the same density as their surrounding tissue. However, excellent spatial resolution is also required because some masses are detected via their subtle spicular structures. The detection and diagnosis of microcalcifications (i.e. detecting the shape of a single calcification or the geometrical distribution of a cluster of microcalcifications) requires extremely high spatial resolution. Other important indications of breast abnormality include architectural distortions and asymmetries between the left and right breast.

All of these features represent considerable challenges for imaging technologies. Mammography is probably the most demanding of medical imaging tasks when it comes to spatial resolution and contrast resolution.

Given the fact that it enables earlier medical intervention, the early detection of breast cancer is seen as playing a vital role. Recent studies show that the introduction of screening mammography (i.e. breast imaging of asymptomatic women) can indeed reduce mortality [12.70]. Besides this, studies have shown that the costs of overall treatment increase significantly when tumors are found at later stages. However, screening mammography is confronted by a considerable challenge in that the overall incidence of breast cancer among asymptomatic women is very low. Only 0.5% of the women in a given screening population will turn out to have cancer – and these cases have to be ascertained by the screening procedure without generating too many false positives.

In what follows, we describe the dedicated imaging equipment that has been developed to meet the challenges of detecting and diagnosing a disease with many different manifestations.

12.6.1 System overview

Breast tissue

The breast consists mainly of glandular tissue, adipose tissue (fat), connective tissue and blood vessels. The X-ray attenuation coefficient of these tissue types is very similar, and is also similar to that of cancerous tissue [12.72]. Only calcifications, one sign of the presence of breast cancer, show clearly higher X-ray attenuation coefficients than the other tissue types. It follows that one will have to reduce the applied X-ray energy to provide sufficiently high soft-tissue contrast. The penetrability of this lower X-ray energy is well-matched to the size of a compressed breast (between 2 and 8 cm).

X-ray spectrum and focal spot size

Molybdenum (Mo) is a very commonly used material for the anode of X-ray tubes that are used in mammography. The tube is usually operated in the range between 25 and 30 kV_p. The spectrum exhibits two strong characteristic lines (K_α at 17.5 keV and K_β at 19.6 keV) in addition to the bremsstrahlung spectrum [12.73]. Molybdenum or rhodium (Rh) filtration is employed to further reduce the low and high-end parts of the spectrum that contribute more to scattered radiation and patient dose than to image contrast (fig. 12.116).

The rhodium anodes and rhodium filtration that are also used yield characteristic lines at a slightly higher energy level. In addition to increasing the tube voltage, tungsten (W) anodes and rhodium filtration are often used for thicker and denser breasts, as these materials provide a spectrum with a higher mean energy. This substitution leads to adequate image quality at optimized dose levels. In particular in the case of digital detectors (see below), the spectrum of a W anode may be advantageous and may be better adjusted to the radiation response of solid-state detectors [12.75].

Mammography tubes operate with a small nominal focal spot value of 0.3 (IEC) in order to provide the necessary spatial information. When operating in magnification mode (i.e. the breast is positioned closer to the X-ray tube), it is necessary to reduce the focal spot size to below 0.15 (nominal focal spot value according to IEC) to meet the requirements for spatial resolution.

Advanced mammography tubes include two anode targets (e.g. Mo and W), three different filters (e.g. Mo and Rh in various thicknesses) and two focal spots for each target (one with a nominal spot value of 0.3 and the other with a nominal spot value of 0.15).

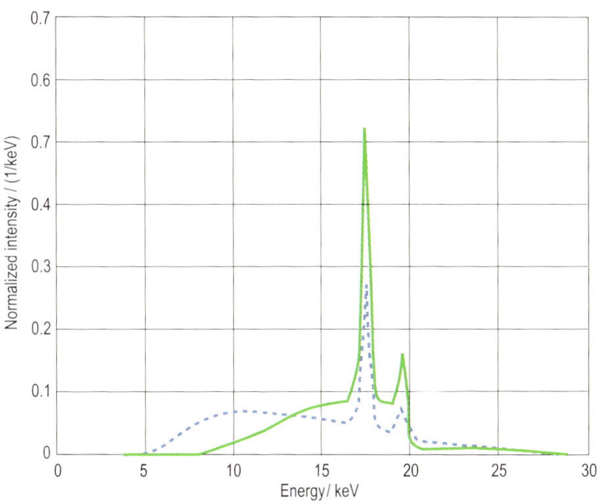

Figure 12.116
Normalized molybdenum spectrum at 28 kVp without (dashed) and with (solid line) 0.03 mm molybdenum filtration [12.74]

Compression

Image quality and thus detection capability can be improved by mechanically compressing the breast with a compression device. Compression leads to a more uniform breast thickness across the image field and to a smaller object thickness. This results in the generation of less scattered radiation and enables one to more clearly distinguish structures at different depths. It also helps one to largely avoid motion blurring.

Anti-scatter grid

An anti-scatter grid is used to further reduce scattered radiation. Given that the scatter fraction in mammography is moderate, grids of type 4/27 or 5/31 with approximately 75% primary transmission and a rather low Bucky factor[1)] (approximately 2) are usually employed in screen/film systems. While the role of anti-scatter grids in screen/film mammography has been clarified, their role in digital mammography remains to be investigated.

Automated exposure control (AEC)

A sensor is deployed under the screen/film cassette in order to control the exposure time automatically. This is because high-contrast mammographic screen/film systems require a very precise exposure due to their narrow exposure range. A feedback loop is used to determine the exposure needed to achieve the desired optical film density.

When using large-area flat-panel detectors in digital mammography, a very short pre-exposure is usually taken by the digital detector itself to compute and control the correct exposure. Together with the X-ray tube, the automatic exposure control (AEC) and the control software thus help to optimize image quality at the lowest possible average glandular dose in the individual breast.

Screen/film receptor

Screen/film systems have continuously improved with respect to dose and image contrast since the introduction of intensifying screens and their deployment in combination with highly sensitive film. Screen/film cassettes are available in two different sizes to cover a range of breast sizes: 18×24 cm^2 and 24×30 cm^2. Typical systems exhibit a detective quantum efficiency (*DQE*) of approximately 20 to 30% at a spatial frequency of close to 0, an efficiency that is thus inferior to that of digital detectors (fig. 12.120). However, given proper quality control, screen/film systems can be regarded as reliable and cost effective image receptors that offer very high spatial resolution (> 15 lp/mm).

Modes of operation

Both breasts are always imaged during routine screening and diagnostic examinations. This is because the comparison between left and right is an important diagnostic criterion. Breast images are usually taken in craniocaudal (CC) view and in me-

---

[1)] The Bucky factor of an anti-scatter grid is given by the ratio of the intensity of the total radiation without the grid to the intensity of the total radiation with the grid.

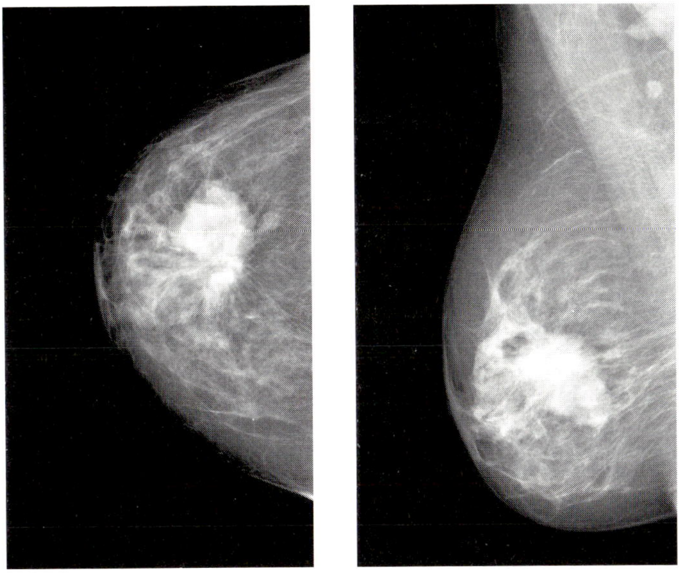

Figure 12.117
Mammograms: craniocaudal view **(left)** and mediolateral oblique view **(right)** (Siemens MAMMOMAT Novation^{DR})

diolateral oblique (MLO) view (fig. 12.117). This means that four images of each patient are acquired. It will be necessary to view these images together with the four images acquired during the previous examination in order to detect any changes in the breast that may have occurred. Other views (e.g. lateral views) may also be helpful when handling special diagnostic tasks and when preparing for surgery (e.g. involving wire positioning and localization). The magnification technique (i.e. deploying a magnification table) is frequently used to obtain a magnified image with an increased signal-to-noise ratio. Here, the breast is positioned closer to the X-ray focus.

Fig. 12.118 shows a full-field digital mammography system that looks very similar to an analog system. The cassette has been replaced by a digital detector that is operated from an additional acquisition workstation. A multimodality diagnostic workstation (including two high-resolution high-contrast monitors) is available for image viewing and reporting.

Any ascertainment of malignancy or suspicious lesions will need to be followed up by other imaging modalities (e.g. sonography) or by intervention. In the diagnostic workup often a biopsy is performed: fine needle aspiration (FNA) and core needle biopsy (CNB). Both of these techniques (i.e. particularly in the case of nonpalpable lesions) rely on image-based guidance, mostly involving ultrasound, but also involving mammography and, less frequently, magnetic resonance imaging. While special prone table systems are very common, biopsies are also often performed with patients

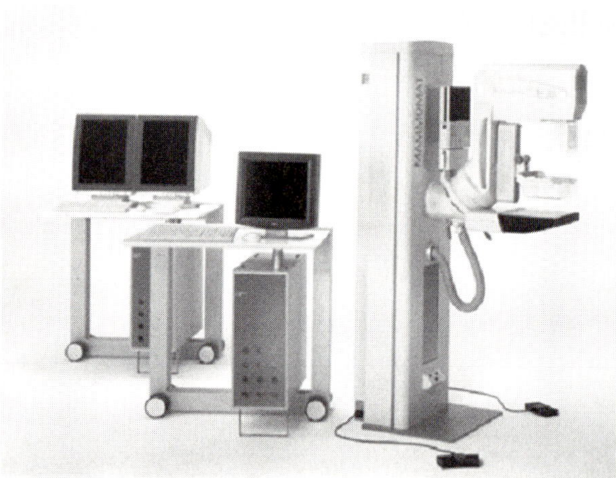

Figure 12.118
Mammography system (Siemens MAMMOMAT Novation^{DR}) **(right)**, acquisition workstation (center) and diagnostic workstation (MammoReport) **(left)**. Not shown is the radiation shield with its operator console. The MAMMOMAT has a pivoting bucky for rapid switching between two different film cassettes or between a digital full-field detector and a digital spot detector.

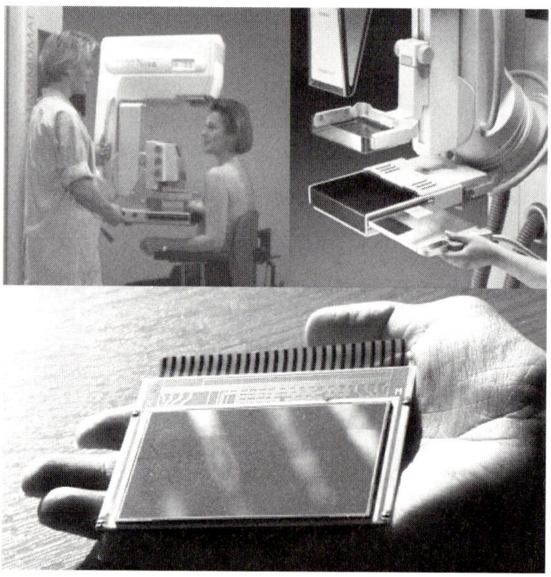

Figure 12.119
Stereotactic biopsy add-on **(top left)** for mammography: digital spot detector built into a screen/film cassette **(top right)**, CCD detector chip (4.9×8.5 cm^2) with spatial resolution of up to 20 line pairs/mm (Siemens OPDIMA).

in an upright position using a stereotactic add-on to mammography. This enables enhanced needle guidance based on 3-D information. Fig. 12.119 shows a typical digital spot-imaging system. This system provides support for the stereotactic biopsy in the form of a digital small-field-of-view detector that can be mounted on the second arm of the pivoting bucky table (fig. 12.118).

12.6.2 Digital mammography

12.6.2.1 Digital versus analog mammography

Digital mammography offers many advantages besides those associated with the digitization of radiology.

The linearity of the detector response curve offers a large exposure range. The system is thus insensitive to over and underexposure, quite in contrast to film, which requires a very precise amount of exposure for operation in the optimum optical density range. The total dynamic range, defined as the ratio of maximum signal to minimum signal, is larger than what can be rendered by screen/film.

While the film is simultaneously the recording medium and the display and archiving medium, the detector and the display in digital mammography can be optimized separately. This enables considerable potential for dose reduction and improvements in image quality involving methods of digital image processing.

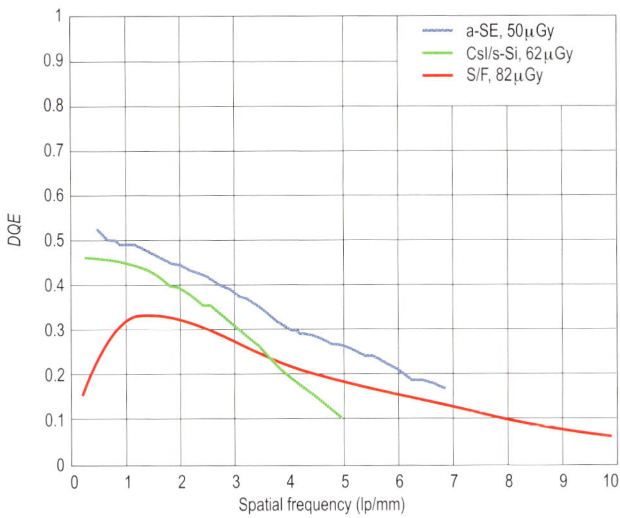

Figure 12.120
Comparison of *DQE* as a function of spatial frequency for direct conversion aSe detection (blue) [12.81], for indirect conversion CsI/a-Si detection (green) [12.79] and for screen/film (red) [12.84] using a comparable mammographic X-ray spectrum and similar detector exposure.

The detectors that are available today for full-field digital mammography (FFDM) have a pixel pitch between 0.05 and 0.1 mm (i.e. a Nyquist frequency between 5 and 10 lp/mm). This is lower than the limiting resolution of film. However, it is not the limiting resolution for high-contrast objects that counts, but the detective quantum efficiency (*DQE*), which also accounts for noise and thus low-contrast detectability. At low spectral frequencies, the *DQE* (i.e. the efficiency of signal and noise transfer through the detection chain) can be expected to be larger than that of a screen/film system by a factor of at least two (fig. 12.120). In other words, the high contrast resolution of a digital detector improves the perceptability of small details although its spatial resolution is not quite the same as that of film. Furthermore, one can also expect the higher *DQE* to translate into reduced dose. Screening studies that will permit one to compare analog and digital mammography from a clinical perspective are currently under way [12.76].

12.6.2.2 Detection concepts

Various detector technologies are applied in (full-field) digital mammography. All of these technologies involve the conversion of X-ray quanta into an electronic digital signal. Detectors used in digital mammography differ from those used in radiography and fluoroscopy in that they are required to provide higher spatial resolution with pixel sizes below 0.1 mm and they are optimized for the softer (i.e. lower) energy X-ray spectrum that is used in mammography.

Computed radiography (CR) was one of the earliest digital technologies available for mammography [12.77]. CR involves the storage of X-ray energy on a storage phosphor plate. This energy is read out in a CR reader using a scanning laser beam and then transformed into a digital image using photomultiplier tubes and analog-to-digital converters. Special CR systems offering high resolution (50 µm readout laser beam) and high sensitivity (double-sided readout) have been developed for mammography [12.78]. CR may represent a good and cost effective choice for a gynecology practice or a clinic that serves a relatively small number of patients.

However, in the case of hospitals and breast care centers that offer screening services for large numbers of patients, digital systems with solid-state detectors and efficient data flow are likely to be the technology of the future. This technology can be referred to as digital or direct radiography (DR).

The various DR detector technologies can be classified according to the following contrasting features:

- Indirect or direct conversion
- Crystalline or amorphous semiconductors
- Scanning (fan beam) or nonscanning (cone beam) mode
- Integrating or counting detection

In what follows, we discuss the various principles involved in these technologies and outline their specific advantages and disadvantages. While other detector variants are also subjects of current discussion in the scientific community, these are somewhat further from demonstrating clinical value.

Indirect conversion flat panel detector

The X-ray quanta are transformed into light quanta in a scintillator, either gadolinium oxysulfide (GOS) or CsI(Tl) [12.79]. The principle involved is described in section 12.3.4. The fill factor of a single pixel represents an important criterion for quantum absorption effectiveness. This is the relative area used for detection (photodiode) in relation to the area determined by the pixel pitch. Given that the electric lines for pixel readout, the separation gaps between pixels and the TFT readout switch all require some amount of space, the fill factor will always be smaller than one. The smaller the pixel pitch is, the smaller the fill factor will be because the space not used for quantum absorption remains independent of the pixel pitch. Indirect conversion therefore currently includes an intrinsic technological limit when it comes to approaching a pixel pitch smaller than around 0.1 mm. The use of a vertical pixel structure with a continuous photodiode above the TFT readout array may enable one to overcome this limit in the future [12.80].

Direct conversion flat panel detector

The direct conversion approach enables one to convert X-ray quanta directly into an electric signal and thereby avoid the additional noise caused by an intermediate stage. A typical detector [12.81, 12.82] of this kind has an amorphous selenium layer of 0.250 mm thickness and a pixel size of 0.07 mm. While the detector layer under the a-Se conversion layer is comprised of the a-Si pixel array (as in the case of the indirect approach), the pixel structure is simpler because there is no need for a photodiode. The pixel consists simply of the pixel electrode and the TFT readout switch. The effective fill factor can be close to one if the pixel electrodes are manufactured in a mushroom design overlapping the TFT [12.83]. The electric field is thereby shaped to attract nearly all of the charges. This permits one to make the pixel size smaller than what is currently possible with the indirect conversion type of flat panel detector.

The absorption of a-Se is considerably higher in the mammographic energy range than that of CsI at comparable thickness. This and the smaller pixel design lead to the conclusion that the a-Se detector is currently the concept of choice for FFDM. The measured results for the *DQE* shown in fig. 12.120 support this conclusion.

Charged coupled devices (CCD)

One advantage of working with an amorphous material (a-Si technology) is that it allows one to manufacture large area detectors. In contrast, CCD chips are manufactured from single-crystal silicon. CCD chips consist of an array of metal-oxide silicon capacitors that store the light-generated charges in the photosensitive silicon. It is necessary to create the light in a scintillation layer that is optically coupled to the CCD chip (as in the case of the indirect flat panel detector). The charge package in one pixel is transported during the readout process by switching voltages from pixel to pixel in one line (section 12.3.3).

High manufacturing costs per CCD detector area and limited silicon wafer size restrict CCD deployment to relatively small areas. For instance, they are well-suited for digital spot imaging [12.85].

New approaches were required to meet the challenge of covering the full area needed in diagnostic radiography. One initial approach involving the use of a lens system to optically minify the image from the phosphor screen onto the small area of the CCD had to be abandoned because it leads to a secondary quantum sink as too many photons get lost [12.86]. One more realistic concept involves the use of a linear (line) detector and the scanning of the object (see below).

Another approach pursued in the 90s involved the use of one CCD chip optically coupled (1:1) to the scintillator and scanned across a large area. The image was then constructed from the single images. This step-and-stitch procedure was abandoned, however, due to poor coupling efficiency, difficulties faced when stitching the images together, mechanical complexity and long acquisition and breast compression times.

A further concept involved the tiling of a large area detector with many (i.e. 3 by 4) CCD chips coupled via fiber optics to the CsI scintillator. While this solution was abandoned on account of its expense, a detector of this type was used at the beginning (2001) of the ACRIN-DMIST screening trial [12.87] involving 49,500 patients.

Whether the newly developed active pixel sensors based on complementary metal-oxide silicon (CMOS) technology are appropriate for medical imaging, remains to be investigated. These detectors continue to replace CCD cameras in the area of consumer imaging.

Slot-scanning systems

The motivation for slot-scanning systems is twofold. First, the area detector is smaller. This enables one to cut costs as the price of expensive digital detectors scales with area. All existing slot-scanning systems employ detectors not available in large area. Second, with the use of a slot defined by slit collimators, one can expect an efficient suppression of scattered radiation.

Nevertheless, slot-scanning systems have many drawbacks. Given that a fan beam does not exploit X-ray power like a cone beam, high tube load and reduced tube lifetime can be expected. The dose advantage due to reduced scatter might be smaller than suggested on account of scatter in the slot direction. The dose advantage depends on the width of the slot and on the precise adjustment of the slit collimators (i.e. to avoid overradiation due to the penumbra effect). This requires high mechanical precision synchronized to the detector readout.

One commercially available example of a slot-scanning system uses four CCD chips butted linearly to cover an area of 1 cm by 22 cm. This detector is scanned linearly together with the X-ray fan beam over the patient [12.88].

Photon counting detectors

In contrast to all of the detection technology discussed so far (i.e. involving the integration of energy or charge into pixels), a new imaging detector principle developed in high-energy physics is based on the detection and counting of single X-ray quanta.

Beneath their conversion material, counting detectors involve counting electronics for each pixel. The conversion material must be fast enough to secure high count rates without dead time. Typical count rates for medical imaging range from 10^5 to 10^6 photons/second/pixel. While gas and crystalline semiconductors would be capable of fulfilling these requirements, these materials do not permit the manufacture of large area detectors [12.89]. All of the existing devices thus use the slot-scanning principle.

One potential advantage of this technology centers on the fact that counting detectors would be virtually free of electronic detection noise, leaving only the quantum nature of radiation as a source of noise. For the standard mode of operation in mammography, however, a well designed radiation detector operates in the quantum noise limited range where electronic noise can be neglected in order to secure the soft tissue contrast resolution needed for a reliable diagnosis. Nevertheless, one can still expect the DQE of counting detectors to be somewhat higher than that of integrating detectors.

A further possible advantage centers on the potential for establishing a means of measuring the energy of the quanta or at least for including one or more energy thresholds in the counting process at the cost of more complex electronics. This could enable energy-selective methods (e.g. dual energy subtraction) with one X-ray acquisition. However, such future applications will depend on the capacity to produce large areas in counting technology.

12.6.2.3 Advanced applications

The introduction of digital mammography offers opportunities for developing new applications based on new technologies.

First, there is the benefit of soft-copy reading on digital viewing workstations, which also makes images from other modalities available and opens the door to telemammography and the reading skills of expert radiologists at remote locations. Workstations, display systems and networking technologies will have to be deployed in a manner that facilitates the quick and convenient handling of the images required for a reading session and that is otherwise appropriate for the mammographic workflow.

Computer-aided detection algorithms (CAD) were first developed for mammography so as to provide the radiologist with a second opinion. These methods can be expected to evolve in the direction of computer-assisted diagnosis (CAD) and computer-supported decision tools.

The digitization of image acquisition will enable the clinical implementation of further advanced applications. These new procedures may include digital tomosynthesis [12.90] for the rendering of 3D information to increase sensitivity and specificity. Dual-energy subtraction [12.91] is also a subject of current investigation, i.e. with an eye to facilitating the detection and diagnosis of lesions.

12.6.3 Other and new modalities

Although X-ray mammography is the only accepted screening modality for breast imaging today, there are other modalities in use [12.92]. Sonography [12.93] is routinely applied for the diagnosis and workup of suspicious lesions, particularly cysts found using mammography. Ultrasound imaging is also used for biopsy guidance.

Magnetic resonance imaging continues to improve and already excels in terms of versatility and high sensitivity. Its specificity, however, is still too low. It is therefore used today mainly as a diagnostic tool, for instance, to assess the extent of disease before surgery and to monitor response to therapy [12.94].

Nuclear medicine methods are well-suited for staging and finding malignant lymph nodes and metastatic disease. Dedicated breast devices (scintillation cameras, SPECT and PET systems) are currently being investigated in research projects.

Completely new methods are also in development [12.95]. Interesting examples include electrical impedance scanning [12.96] and optical imaging [12.97], in particular in the context of molecular imaging such as near-infrared fluorescence imaging (NIR). It can also be expected that non-imaging methods such as genetic profiling will establish themselves in the field as prognostic and diagnostic tools [12.99].

12.7 References

[12.1] N. Ashcroft, D. Mermin
Solid State Physics,
Saunders College Publishing, 1975

[12.2] Electron Emission and Gas Discharges
Encyclopedia of Physics, Volume 11 – I, edited by S. Flügge
Springer-Verlag, 1956

[12.3] K. Simonyi
Physikalische Elektronik,
Teubner Verlag, 1972

[12.4] O.W. Richardson
Emission of electricity from hot bodies
London, 1921

[12.5] S. Dushman
Thermionic Emission
Rev. Mod. Physics 2 (1930), 381

[12.6] E. Hell, D. Mattern, P. Schardt
Direct-heated flat emitter for emitting an electron beam
US 6115453 Patent, Siemens (05.09.2000)

[12.7] W. Espe
Werkstoffe der Hochvakuumtechnik
VEB Deutscher Verlag der Wissenschaften, Berlin 1959

[12.8] Dr. O. Goetze (Frankfurt a.M.)
Verfahren und Glühkathodenröntgenröhre zur Erzeugung scharfer Röntgenbilder (Strichfokus).
DP 370 022 (2. Feb. 1918)

[12.9] Standard für Brennfleckbezeichnung und Toleranzen der Brennfleckgrößen
DIN/IEC 60 336/1981

[12.10] W.D. Coolidge
X-Ray Apparatus
US 1215116 Patent, GE (1917)

[12.11] H. Bittdorf, H. Bittl, W. Dörfler
Gebrauchsmuster BRD, Rollennummer G8713042.4, Siemens (28.09.87)

[12.12] P. Schardt, E. Hell
Rotating X-ray tube
US 5883936 Patent, Siemens (16.3.1999)

[12.13] E. Hell, P.Schardt
X-ray Radiator
US 6272205 Patent, Siemens (07.08.2001)

[12.14] E. Hell, P. Schardt, D. Mattern
X-ray tube with flying focus
US 6292538 Patent, Siemens (18.09.2001)

[12.15] E. Hell, D. Mattern, P. Schardt
X-ray source with selectable focal spot size
US 6181771 Patent, Siemens (30.01.2001)

[12.16] M. Levy
Röntgenröhre mit aus verschiedenen Stoffen zusammengesetzter Antikathode
DRP 114 455, Fabrik Elektr. App. Berlin (9. Nov. 1899)

[12.17] Röntgenröhre mit Wolfram-Elektroden
DRP 165 138, Siemens & Halske (8. Nov. 1904)

[12.18] W. Föhre
Röhre mit justierbarem Vakuum
Röntgenröhre mit durch Wasser gekühlter Antikathode
DRP 113 430, C.H.F. Müller (21. Mai, 1899)

[12.19] E. Pohl
Über Relativbewegungen von Kathode und Antikathode
DRP 376 359 (11. Feb. 1914)

[12.20] J.C. Brown
DC Braking for Rotating Anode X-ray Tube
US 2 242 182 Patent, GE (24. Nov. 1939)

[12.21] K. Silbermann
Drehanodenteller für eine Drehanoden-Röntgenröhre (2 Winkel auf Anodenteller)
DP 956 708, SRW (1. Okt. 1954)

[12.22] R. Friedel, W. Wiche
Röntgenröhren-Drehanode mit einem Verbundkörper aus einem Schwermetallteil und wenigstens einem Graphitteil und Verfahren zu ihrer Herstellung
DP 1951 383, Siemens (11. Okt. 1969)

[12.23] K. Silbermann
Drehanoden-Verbundteller für Röntgenröhren (Rhenium).
DP 1 270 192, Siemens AG (30. Juli 1960)

[12.24] A. Elsaß, Th. Zimmer
Höhere Belastung von Drehanodenröhren durch Verwendung von legierten Anoden.
Fortschr.Röntgenstr.97 (1962)

[12.25] High emissive coatings on X-ray tube components
US 6,456,692 B1 Patent, (2002)

[12.26] A. Bouwers
Über den Temperaturverlauf an der Anode einer Röntgenröhre.
Z.f. techn. Phys. 8 (1927)

[12.27] W.J. Oosterkamp
The heat dissipation on the anode of an X-ray tube.
Philips Res.Rep. 3 (1948)

[12.28] M. Wutz, H. Adam, W. Walcher
Theorie und Praxis der Vakuumtechnik,
Friedr. Vieweg & Sohn, Braunschweig/Wiesbaden 1988

[12.29] Kerspe et al.
Vakuumtechnik in der industriellen Praxis
Expert Verlag, Ehningen 1987

[12.30] J. Bretting
Technische Röhren
Hüthig, Heidelberg 1991

[12.31] F.P. Incropera, D.P. Dewitt
Fundamentals of Heat and Mass Transfer
John Wiley, New York 2002

[12.32] E.A. Hoxter, A. Schenz
Röntgenaufnahmetechnik
Siemens AG, Berlin, München 1991

[12.33] IEC-Publication 60601-2-7 (1998)
Medical electrical equipment – Part 2-7: Particular requirements for the safety of high-voltage generators of diagnostic X-ray generators
IEC/TR 60788 (2004)
Medical electrical equipment – Glossary of defined terms

[12.34] J. Meiler
Die in der Röntgendiagnostik verwendeten Spannungskurvenformen und ihr Einfluss auf Bildqualität und Röhrenbelastung
Fortschr. auf dem Geb. der Röntgenstrahlen (vereinigt mit Röntgenpraxis) 72 (1949), 222

[12.35] H. Aichinger, J. Dierker, S. Joite-Barfuß, M. Säbel
Radiation Exposure and Image Quality in X-Ray Diagnostic Radiology
Springer-Verlag, Berlin Heidelberg New York 2004

[12.36] A. Berger
Zum Problem der Bewegungsunschärfe im Röntgenbild der Lunge und des Herzens
Röntgenblätter 14 (1961), 369

[12.37] DIN EN 61223: Bewertung und routinemäßige Prüfung in Abteilungen für medizinische Bildgebung;
Teil 2-6 (1997): Konstanzprüfungen – Röntgeneinrichtungen für Computertomographie
Teil 3-1 (2001): Abnahmeprüfungen – Bildgebungsleistung der Röntgeneinrichtung bei radiographischen und Durchleuchtungssystemen
Teil 3-2 (2001): Abnahmeprüfungen – Abbildungsqualität von Röntgen-Einrichtungen für die Mammographie
Teil 3-3 (2000): Abnahmeprüfungen – Leistungsmerkmale zur Bildgebung von Röntgeneinrichtungen für digitale Subtraktionsangiographie

[12.38] W. Kühnel
Der Schwingkreiswechselrichter mit Gegenspannungslast zur Versorgung von Verbrauchern mit gepulstem Gleichstrom
Dissertation, Technische Fakultät der Universität Erlangen-Nürnberg (1986)

[12.39] I. Takahashi
SiC power technology in future
International Electric Machines & Drives Conference, Madison WI 2003

[12.40] J.W. Coltmann
Fluoroscopic image brightening by electronic means
Radiology 51, 359 (1948)

[12.41] T. Jing, et al.
IEEE Transactions on Nuclear Science 39, 1195 (1992)

[12.42] W. Greschat, H. Heinrich, P. Römer
Quantum yield of Cs_3Sb photocathodes as a function of thickness and angle of incidence
Advances in Electron. and electron. Phys. 40A, 397 (1976)

[12.43] CEI IEC 1262-6 (1994)
Medical electrical equipment – characteristics of electro optical X-ray intensifiers, part 6: determination of the contrast ratio and veiling glare index

[12.44] H.J. Zwieg
Detective quantum efficiency of photodetectors with some amplifying mechanism
J. Opt. Soc. Am. 55 (1965) 525

[12.45] L. Strüder, C. von Zantier
Elektronische Bildwandlung – Fortschritte bei Charge Coupled Devices (CCD) und Active Pixel Sensors (APS)
Phys. Bl. 54 (1998), 519

[12.46] CCD Image Sensor Noise Sources
Application Note MTD/PS-0233 (2001)
Eastman Kodak Company – Image Sensor Solutions, Rochester, NY

[12.47] L.E. Antonuk
Thin-film, flat-panel imagers – a coming revolution in megavoltage and diagnostic imaging?
Phys. Med. 9 (1993), 63-68

[12.48] R.L. Weisfield, M. Hartney, R. Schneider, K. Alfatooni, R. Lujan
High performance amorphous silicon image sensor for X-ray diagnostic medical imaging applications
SPIE 3659 (1999), 307-317

[12.49] C. Chaussat, J. Chabbal, T. Ducourant, V. Spinnler, G. Vieux, R. Neyret
New CsI / a-Si 17"× 17" X-ray flat panel detector provides superior detectivity and immediate direct digital output for General Radiography systems
SPIE 3336 (1998), 45-56

[12.50] M. Spahn, M. Strotzer, M. Völk, S. Böhm, B. Geiger, G. Hahm, S. Feuerbach
Digital Radiography with a large-area, amorphous-silicon, flat-panel X-ray detector system
Invest Radiol 35 (2000), 260-266

[12.51] M. Völk, M. Strotzer, N. Holzknecht, C. Manke, M. Lenhart, J. Gmeinwieser, J. Link, M. Reiser, S. Feuerbach
Digital radiography of the skeleton using a large-area detector based on amorphous silicon technology: image quality and potential for dose reduction in comparison with screen-film radiography
Clinical Radiology 55 (2000), 615-621

[12.52] J.C. Dainty, R. Shaw
Image Science
Academic Press, London 1974

[12.53] K. Stierstorfer, M. Spahn
Self-normalizing method to measure the detective quantum efficiency of a wide range of X-ray detectors
Med Phys 26 (1999), 1312-1319

[12.54] P. Hertrich
Practical Radiography
Publicis Corporate Publishing, Erlangen 2005
German edition: Röntgenaufnahmetechnik, 2004

[12.55] M. Völk, O.W. Hammer, S. Feuerbach, M. Strotzer
Dose reduction in skeletal and chest radiography using a large area flat-panel detector based on amorphous silicon and thallium-doped cesium iodide: technical background, basic image quality parameters, and review of the literature.
Eur. Radiol. 14 (2004), 827-834

[12.56] M. Völk, P. Angele, O.W. Hammer, S. Feuerbach, M. Strotzer
Digital image composition in long-leg radiography with a flat-panel detector: first clinical experiences.
Invest. Radiol. 38 (2003), 189-192

[12.57] H. Zhao, S.C.B. Lo, M.T. Freedman, Y.J. Wang
Enhanced lung cancer detection in temporal subtraction chest radiography using directional edge filtering techniques.
Proceedings of SPIE 4684 (2002), 698-703

[12.58] R.A. Robb, E.A. Hoffman, L.J. Sinak, L.D. Harris, E.L. Ritman
High-speed three-dimensional X-ray computed tomography: The dynamic spatial reconstructor
Proceedings of the IEEE 71 (1983), 308-319

[12.59] D. Saint-Felix, Y. Trousset, C. Picard, C. Ponchut, R. Romeas, A. Rougee
In vivo evaluation of a new system for 3D computerized angiography
Phys. Med. Biol. 39 (1994) 583-595

[12.60] R. Baba, K. Ueda, H. Ueki, K. Umetani
Ellipsoid scan: chest cone-beam CT with a large ellipsoidal view field using a 16-inch X-ray image intensifier
Proceedings of the SPIE 3032 (1997), 349-357

[12.61] L.A. Feldkamp, L.C. Davis, J.W. Kress
Practical cone-beam algorithm
J. Opt. Soc. Am. A1 (1984), 612-619

[12.62] R. Fahrig, A.J. Fox, S. Lownie, D.W. Holdsworth
Use of a C-arm system to generate true three-dimensional computed rotational angiograms: preliminary in vitro and in vivo results
Am. J. Neuroradiol. 18 (1997), 1507-1514

[12.63] M. El-Sheik, J.T. Heverhagen, H. Alfke, J.J. Froelich, J. Hornegger, T. Brunner, K.J. Klose, H.-J. Wagner
Multiplanar reconstructions and three-dimensional imaging (computed rotational osteography) of complex fractures by using a C-arm system: initial results
Radiology 221 (2001), 843-849

[12.64] U. Linsenmaier, C. Rock, E. Euler, S. Wirth, R. Brandl, D. Kotsianos, W. Mutschler, K.J. Pfeifer
Three-dimensional CT with a modified C-arm image intensifier: feasibility
Radiology 224 (2002), 286-292

[12.65] J.D. Foley, A. van Dam, S.K. Feiner, J.F. Hughe
Computer graphics: principles and practice (2nd ed.)
Addison-Wesley Longman Publishing Co., Inc. (1990)

[12.66] D.L. Parker
Optimal short scan convolution reconstruction for fan-beam CT
Med. Phys. 9 (1982), 254-257

[12.67] K. Wiesent, K. Barth, N. Navab, P. Durlak, T. Brunner, O. Schuetz, W. Seissler
Enhanced 3-D-reconstruction algorithm for C-arm systems suitable for interventional procedures
IEEE Transactions on Medical Imaging 19 (2000), 391-403

[12.68] National Cancer Institute: http://www.cancer.gov/

[12.69] The breast health resource: http://www.imaginis.com/

[12.70] American Cancer Society: http://www.cancer.org/

[12.71] R.H. Gold, L.W. Bassett, B.E. Widoff
Highlights from the history of mammography
RadioGraphics 10 (1990), 1111-1131

[12.72] P.C. Johns, M.J. Yaffe
Characterization of normal and neoplastic breast tissues
Phys. Med. Biol. 32 (1987), 675-695

[12.73] J.M. Boone
X-ray production, interaction, and detection in diagnostic imaging
in J. Beutel, H.L. Kundel, R.L. Van Metter (eds), Handbook of Medical Imaging
SPIE Press, Bellingham, Washington USA, 2000

[12.74] J.M. Boone, T.R. Fewell, R.J. Jennings
Molybdenum, rhodium, and tungsten anode spectral models using interpolating polynomials with application to mammography
Med. Phys. 24 (1997), 1863-1874

[12.75] M. Flynn, C. Dodge, D. Peck, A. Swinford
Optimal radiographic technique for digital mammograms obtained with an amorphous selenium detector
Proc. SPIE 5030 (2003), 147-156

[12.76] J.M. Lewin, C.J. D'Orsi, R.E. Hendrick, L.J. Moss, P.K. Isaacs, A. Karellas, G.R. Cutter
Clinical comparison of full-field digital mammography and screen-film mammography for detection of breast cancer
Am. J. Rad. 179 (1992), 671-677

[12.77] R. Schaetzing
Computed Radiography Technology
in E. Samei, M.J. Flynn (eds), Syllabus: Advances in digital radiography – categorial course in radiology physics
Oak Brook, Illinois: Radiological Society of North America, 2003

[12.78] K.A. Fetterly, B.A. Schueler
Performance evaluation of a "dual-side read" dedicated mammography computed radiography system
Med. Phys. 30 (2003), 1843-1854

[12.79] S. Vedantham, A. Karellas, S. Suryanarayanan, I. Levis, M. Sayag, R. Kleehammer, R. Heidsieck, C.J. D'Orsi
Full breast digital mammography with an amorphous silicon-based flat panel detector: physical characterization of a clinical prototype
Med. Phys. 27 (2000), 558-567

[12.80] L.E. Antonuk, K.W. Jee, Y. El-Mohri, M. Maolinbay, S. Nassif, X. Rong, Q. Zhao, J.H. Siewerdsen
Strategies to improve the signal and noise performance of active matrix, flat-panel imagers for diagnostic X-ray applications
Med. Phys. 27 (2000), 289-306

[12.81] J.G. Yorker, L.S. Jeromin, D.L.Y. Lee, E.F. Palecki, K.P. Golden, Z. Jing
Characterization of a full field mammography detector based on direct X-ray conversion in selenium.
Proc. SPIE 4682 (2002), 21-29

[12.82] R.S. Saunders Jr., E. Samei, J.L. Jesneck, J.Y. Lo
Physical characterization of a prototype selenium-based full-field digital mammography detector
Med. Phys. 32 (2005), 588-599

[12.83] J.A. Rowlands, J. Yorkston
Flat panel detectors for digital radiography
in J. Beutel, H.L. Kundel, R.L. Van Metter (eds), Handbook of Medical Imaging
SPIE Press, Bellingham, Washington USA, 2000

[12.84] P.C. Bunch
Advances in high-speed mammographic image quality
Proc. SPIE 3659 (1999), 120-130

[12.85] S. Thunberg, H. Sklebitz, B. Ekdahl, L. Bätz, A. Lundin, H. Möller, F. Fleischmann, G. Kreider, T. Weidner
OPDIMA: Large-area CCD-based X-ray image sensor for spot imaging and biopsy control in mammography
Proc. SPIE 3659 (1999) 150-158

[12.86] S. Hejazi, D.P. Trauernicht
System considerations in CCD-based X-ray imaging for digital chest radiography and digital mammography
Med. Phys. 24 (1997), 1-11

[12.87] B. Galen, E. Staab, D.C. Sullivan, E.D. Pisano
American College of Radiology Imaging Network: The Digital Mammographic Imaging Screening Trial – An Update
Acad. Radiol. 9 (2002), 374 –37

[12.88] M.M. Tesic, M.F. Picarro, B. Munier
Full field digital mammography scanner
Eur. J. Rad. 31 (1997), 2-17

[12.89] K.F.G. Pfeiffer, J. Giersch, G. Anton, L. Bätz, M. Hoheisel
Large scale images taken with the Medipix-1 chip
Nuclear Instruments and Methods in Physics Research A 509 (2003), 340

[12.90] T. Wu, A. Stewart, M. Stanton, T. McCauley, W. Phillips, D.B. Kopans, R.H. Moore, J.E. Eberhard, B. Opsahl-Ong, L. Niklason, M.B. Williams
Tomographic mammography using a limited number of low-dose cone-beam projection images
Med. Phys. 30 (2003), 365-380

[12.91] J.M. Lewin, P.K. Isaacs, V. Vance, F.J. Larke
Dual-energy contrast-enhanced digital subtraction mammography: feasibility
Radiology 229 (2003), 261-268

[12.92] S. Heywang-Koebrunner, I. Schreer
Bildgebende Mammadiagnostik, 2. Auflage
Thieme, Stuttgart, 2003

[12.93] E.B. Mendelson
Current Status of Breast US.
in A.G. Haus, M.J. Yaffe (eds), Syllabus: Categorial Course in Diagnostic Radiology Physics: Physical Aspects of Breast Imaging – Current and Future Considerations
Oak Brook, Illinois: Radiological Society of North America, 1999

[12.94] R. Dakins
Clamor for breast MRI could be boon or boondoggle
Diagnostic Imaging, September 2003, 35-43

[12.95] S.J. Nass, C. Henderson, J.C. Lashof (eds)
Mammography and beyond: Developing technologies for the early detection of breast cancer
National Academic Press, Washington, DC, USA, 2001

[12.96] B. Scholz
Towards Virtual Electrical Breast Biopsy: Space-Frequency MUSIC for Trans-Admittance Data.
IEEE Trans. Med. Imaging 21 (2002), 588-595

[12.97] S. Fantini, O. Schütz, J. Edler, S. Heywang-Köbrunner, L. Götz, M.A. Franceschini,

[12.98] H. Siebold
Clinical applications of frequency-domain optical mammography
Proc. SPIE 3566 (1999), 194-199

[12.99] M.J. Van de Vijver, Y.D. He, L.J. van't Veer, H. Dai, A.A.M. Hart, D.W. Voskuil, G.J. Schreiber, J.L. Peterse, C. Roberts, M.J. Marton, M. Parrish, D. Atsma, A. Witteveen, A. Glas, L. Delahaye, T. van der Velde, H. Bartelink, S. Rodenhuis, E.T. Rutgers, S.H. Friend, R. Bernards
A gene-expression signature as a predictor of survival in breast cancer
N. Engl. J. Med. 347 (2002), 1999-2009

13 Computed X-ray tomography

13.1 Principles

Computed tomography (CT) was the first technology to combine a computer with a medical imaging system, the first to display X-ray images in cross section, and the first to herald a new era of digital imaging. Methods of image reconstruction were pursued in other disciplines such as radio astronomy as early as the 1950s [13.1, 13.2]. Several independent investigations involving methods of image reconstruction in the context of medical applications were carried out in the early 1960s [13.3-13.5]. The first clinically useful X-ray CT scanner, developed by Sir Godfrey Hounsfield [13.6], was introduced in the early 1970s by EMI, a company that had previously been known for electronic components and records. The monopoly on this technology ended around two years later when Siemens became the first medical X-ray system manufacturer to introduce a CT head scanner (Siemens Siretom) (fig. 13.1).

13.1.1 Measurement principle

The measurement process of X-ray computed tomography is based on the rectilinear propagation and attenuation of X-rays that pass through an object. In general, objects are inhomogeneous, i.e. they exhibit varying local compositions and densities. The linear attenuation coefficient is accordingly a function of the spatial coordinates. The task of computed tomography in the context of object imaging is to represent the spa-

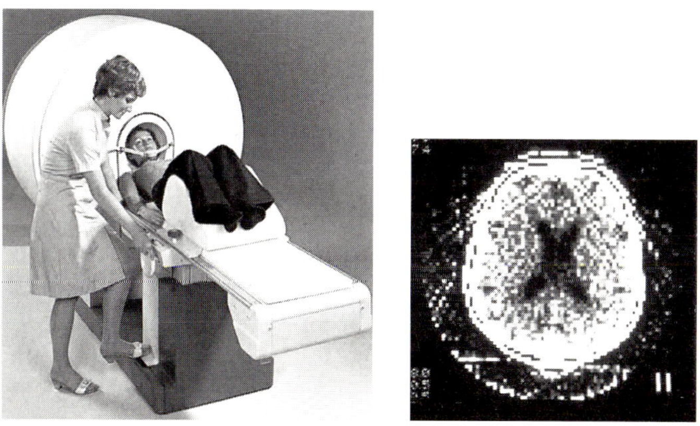

Figure 13.1
CT head scanner: **(left)** the Siretom introduced by Siemens in 1974 and **(right)** a head scan obtained using the Siretom

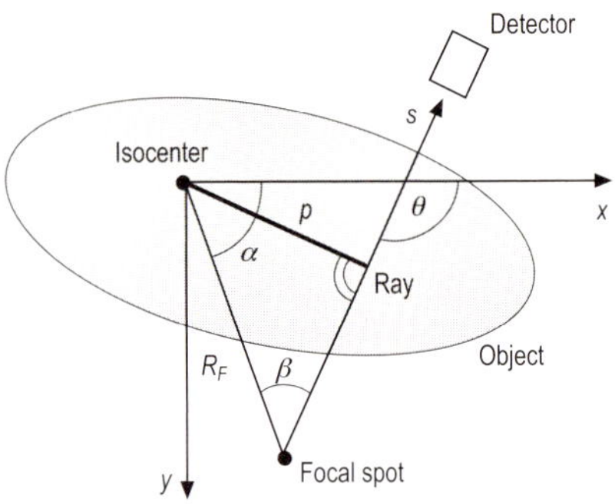

Figure 13.2
CT measurement geometry: Fan-beam coordinates α, β and parallel-beam coordinates θ, p. (A left handed x, y coordinate system has been chosen to stay in accordance with the system image matrix).

tial variability of the attenuation coefficient μ without superimposing structures. Two-dimensional tomography is thus required to supply the values $\mu(x,y)$ as a function of the spatial coordinates x and y.

To this end, the degrees of attenuation for all of an object's parts are measured in a large plurality of directions, with each measurement value being characterized by a projection angle and a channel coordinate. Fan-beam coordinates are appropriate for scanners of the so-called third generation: the projection angle α and the fan-beam angle β. For the sake of simplicity, however, we frequently use equivalent parallel-beam coordinates in this context to characterize the ray path, i.e. the projection angle θ and the distance p to the isocenter (fig. 13.2). Using the focus-isocenter distance R_F, the relation between both sets can be expressed by the following coordinate transformation:

$$p = R_F \sin\beta \qquad \theta = \alpha + \beta \tag{13.1}$$

The result of the measurement is a plurality of intensity ratios $I(p,\theta)/J_0$. The set of all measurement values for any given angle θ is referred to as a projection. Given the inhomogeneity of the object, the attenuation of the X-ray beam is not simply given by the product of μ and the object diameter. Instead, one is required to sum up all of the contributions $\mu(x, y)$ds over the length elements ds along the path defined by θ and p, a calculation that yields a line integral. The integration over s, the coordinate along the ray path (perpendicular to p), is performed over the whole object range. In order to see the dependence of the line integral on θ and p more clearly, the coordinates x, y are expressed by p, s and vice versa:

$$\begin{aligned} x(p,s) &= p\cos\theta + s\sin\theta \\ y(p,s) &= p\sin\theta - s\cos\theta \end{aligned} \tag{13.2}$$

The resulting line integral of the linear attenuation coefficient can thus be expressed as follows:

$$L(p,\theta) = \int_{-\infty}^{\infty} \mu(x(p,s), y(p,s))\,\mathrm{d}s = -\ln\left(\frac{I(p,\theta)}{I_0}\right) \tag{13.3}$$

For instance, in practice one might have $N_p = 600$ projections for θ in the range from 0 to π, where each projection typically contains values for $N = 800$ channels.

13.1.2 Basic image reconstruction

The reconstruction formula

The reconstruction of the attenuation coefficient from projections has already been outlined in chapter 10. The linear attenuation coefficient for pixel x,y is calculated in two steps. The first step is the convolution step according to which all line integrals L are convolved with the function G (see eq. 10.11). The second step is the backprojection step according to which the convolved line integrals are summed up for all projection angles between 0 and π (see eq. 10.10). This leads to the following reconstruction formula:

$$\mu(x,y) = \int_0^{\pi}\int_{-\infty}^{\infty} L(p',\theta)G(x\cos\theta + y\sin\theta - p')\mathrm{d}p'\mathrm{d}\theta \tag{13.4}$$

The function $G(p)$ is the convolution kernel for an exact reconstruction of the object from its line integrals: one obtains the true image by using $G(p)$.

Convolution kernels

As discussed in chapter 10, the one-dimensional Fourier transform of $G(p)$ is the ramp function $|v|$. $G(p)$ exhibits a singularity at $p = 0$. Only a finite number of θ and p samples for the line integrals is available in any practical realization of CT. It will be necessary to replace the integrals in eq. (13.4) by sums and apply an interpolation function after the convolution before performing the backprojection. Instead of the distribution $G(p)$, the coefficients K_n of the kernel $K(p)$ will have to be considered.

If we assume that the line integrals (or projections) are collected by N detectors with spacing a, then the signal detected at position na is obtained as an average over the detector width, which can be considered a convolution of the line integral with a rectangle of width a. If one convolves the filter function G in the same way, the singularity at $p = 0$ is removed and the Shepp-Logan convolution kernel is obtained

$$K^{SL}(p) = -\frac{2}{(\pi a)^2}\frac{1 - 2\frac{p}{a}\sin\pi\frac{p}{a}}{4\left(\frac{p}{a}\right)^2 - 1}, \quad K^{SL}(\pm 0.5a) = \frac{1}{(\pi a)^2}, \tag{13.5a}$$

which then reduces at the detector positions na to

$$K_n^{SL} = -\frac{2}{(\pi a)^2}\frac{1}{4n^2 - 1}, \quad 0 \le n \le N \tag{13.5b}$$

Since a convolution is equivalent to a multiplication in the Fourier domain, the Shepp-Logan kernel corresponds to the ramp filter multiplied by the Fourier transform of a rectangle (i.e. sinc($\pi a v$)), see fig. 10.7. In the limit of an infinite number of p-samples of distance a, the Fourier-transform of the Shepp-Logan kernel approaches $|\sin(\pi a v)|$, a function in frequency space which is periodic with $1/a$.

Convolution kernels used in clinical scan protocols are realized as modifications of the periodic ramp function or of $|\sin(\pi a v)|$; in particular, the high frequency contents in the filter is reduced. This is feasible because the object spectrum only contains frequencies up to a certain limit, due to the fact that the measuring process involves detector elements and a focus of finite size. Note that the reduction of the high frequency components occurs in addition to the broadening of the line integrals by the finite detector width.

Image data

The spatial distribution of the linear attenuation coefficient is displayed in a matrix of pixel values measured in Hounsfield units (HU):

$$I_{ij} = 1000\left(\frac{\mu(x_i, y_i)}{\mu_w} - 1\right) \text{HU} \tag{13.6}$$

The matrix dimension corresponding to a field of view ranging from 50 to 500 mm is usually 512. The quantity μ_w is adjusted so as to give water a pixel value of zero independent of the X-ray spectrum. This value is typically $\mu_w \approx 0.192$/cm.

The CT values of human tissue depend on the spectrum involved. In general, lung and fat have negative CT values, muscle has positive I_{ij} and bone has rather large values of up to 2000 HU (fig. 13.3).

The normal CT scale is characterized by a range of −1024 HU to 3071 HU. An extended CT scale is available for metallic implants.

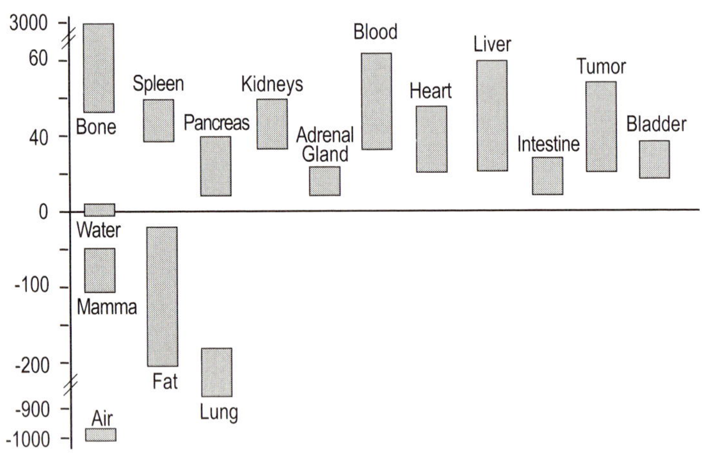

Figure 13.3 CT values of human tissue in Hounsfield Units (HU)

13.1.3 Single-slice axial CT and spiral CT

A complete and consistent data set is an important prerequisite for successful image reconstruction: at least one data value must be available for each coordinate pair of the channel coordinate p and the projection angle θ (completeness); and the scan geometry must be planar (consistency).

Standard scans

Both conditions are fulfilled in the case of standard scans. A complete set of data is acquired during a full 360° rotation and all measurement values belong to the same plane (i.e. as long as the patient does not move).

Incomplete scans

Situations arise in which the data are incomplete or over-complete. The partial fan detectors, which are characterized by an asymmetric fan that does not completely cover the whole object field, represent one example. The so-called quick-scan or partial-scan measurement mode in which data are only acquired for a fraction of the full rotation (usually around 240°) represents a further example.

In these two and in similar cases, the measurement values have to be weighted appropriately prior to reconstruction in order to avoid artifacts. The in-plane resolution and the slice sensitivity profile at the isocenter are not influenced by the weighting procedure. However, the noise amplitude is increased compared to a standard scan because a smaller number of quanta contributes to the image.

Single-slice spiral scans

CT scanners with continuous gantry rotation based on slip-ring technology and the continuous transport of the patient during data acquisition were introduced in 1990. This so-called spiral or helical method of data acquisition [13.7, 13.8] introduced clinical possibilities that went beyond those offered by axial step-and-shoot scanning. Spiral CT enables one to avoid the misregistration of anatomical details and it allows for overlapping in image reconstruction at arbitrary z-positions. However, given that the

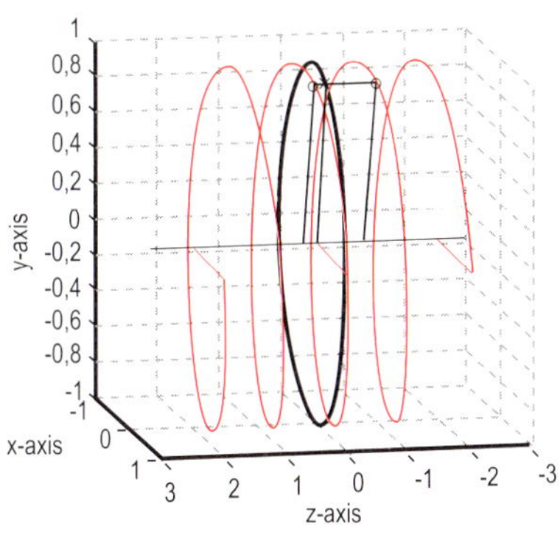

Figure 13.4
Helical path of the focal spot during scanning with table-feed and interpolation to the plane of the black circle using algorithm 360-LI

scan geometry is nonplanar (the X-ray tube does not move on a circular path, but on a helical path as shown in fig. 13.4) it is necessary to process the measurement values prior to reconstruction in order to create consistent data for a plane.

The wide or 360-LI single-slice spiral algorithm

The helical path of the focal spot in fig. 13.4 is displayed in a 3D view. The black circle represents the focal spot positions needed for a proper reconstruction of that plane. Measured data are available only at the intersection of the helical path and the black circle. It is necessary to obtain the missing data for image reconstruction by interpolation (figs. 13.4 and 13.5).

The use of fan-beam coordinates offers a convenient way of explaining the interpolation formula. In this case, the line integrals $L(\beta, \alpha, z)$ measured during spiral scanning depend on the fan angle β as channel coordinate, on the projection angle α, and on the axial position z. As long as the table travels at a constant speed, the relation between projection angle and axial position is linear:

$$z = \frac{z_{rot}}{2\pi}\alpha \tag{13.7}$$

Here, z_{rot} is the table-feed per rotation, and $\alpha = 0$ is characterized by $z = 0$. Accordingly, it suffices to use the shorthand notation $L(\beta, \alpha)$.

Let us denote the projection angle of the line integral lying exactly in the image plane at z_{ima} by α_{ima}. It follows that the angle $\alpha' = \alpha - \alpha_{ima}$ can be interpreted as the (angular) distance of the left focal spot position to the image plane and $2\pi - \alpha'$ of the right focal spot position. The interpolation formula for the line integrals through the plane z_{ima} for $0 \leq \alpha' < 2\pi$ is

$$\begin{aligned} L'(\beta,\alpha') &= w_1 L(\beta,\alpha'+\alpha_{ima}) + w_2 L(\beta,\alpha'+\alpha_{ima}-2\pi) \\ w_1 &= 1 - w_2 \qquad w_2 = \frac{\alpha'}{2\pi} \end{aligned} \tag{13.8}$$

This is known as the 360-LI (LI stands for linear interpolation) or wide algorithm.

While it may seem remarkable that the table-feed z_{rot} does not enter into the interpolation formula eq. (13.8), this can be explained by the fact that the distance between

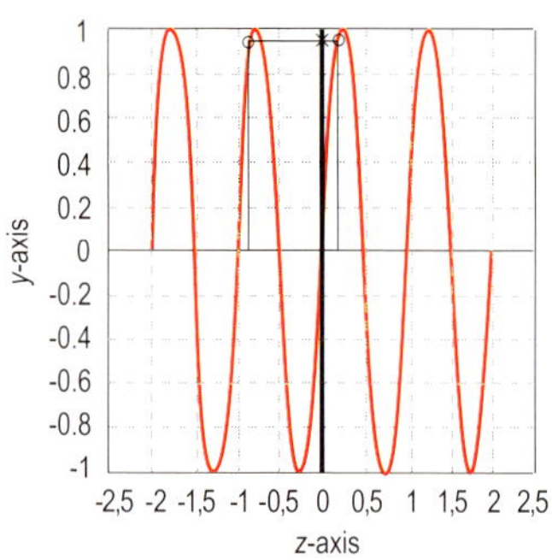

Figure 13.5
Projection of fig. 13.4 into the y, z-plane

the measured samples (i.e. in terms of angles) is always 2π. In terms of distances, it is z_{rot}.

It is convenient in spiral CT to characterize the motion of the patient bed by a dimensionless figure. The so-called pitch factor p_f is defined as the ratio of table-feed z_{rot} to z-collimation S

$$p_f = \frac{z_{rot}}{S}. \tag{13.9}$$

Given that the interpolation partners of the 360-LI algorithm lie 360° apart, data are needed from a point 360° before the reference plane to a point 360° behind the reference plane. This comprises a total angular data range of 720°. The interpolation leads to a broadening of the spiral slice sensitivity profile (SSP). Taking $p_f = 1$ as an example, the full width at half maximum (*FWHM*) of the SSP in the isocenter is 27% larger than that of a corresponding axial slice. Moreover, the noise in an image reconstructed with the wide algorithm is 18% less than that of a corresponding axial slice. The wide algorithm is thus recommended whenever low contrast detectability and dose (noise) reduction are an issue.

The slim or 180-LI single-slice spiral algorithm

While the wide algorithm is computationally simple and numerically stable, it has a number of drawbacks. In particular, image quality will be degraded for higher pitch values due to the large z-distance between the interpolation partners. In order to reduce this distance, it will be necessary to identify interpolation partners closer to the reference plane. An interpolation partner is indeed available for each ray after approximately half a rotation [13.9], i.e. when the X-ray tube and detector have interchanged their positions. This is the so-called complementary ray $f(\hat{\alpha}, \hat{\beta})$.

The interpolation partners are exactly 180° apart only for the central detector channel $\beta = 0$. In general, the following relations hold:

$$\begin{aligned} \hat{\alpha}(\beta) &= \alpha + 2\beta + \pi \\ \hat{\beta} &= -\beta \end{aligned} \tag{13.10}$$

Fig. 13.6a offers an example.

This redundancy permits one to calculate a set of auxiliary measurement values for z-positions between the turns of the measured spiral that can be used as interpolation partners, thus giving a distance between the interpolation partners that is smaller than in the case of 360-LI (see fig. 13.6b).

Two interpolation situations may occur. If the direct focus path is to the left of the image plane and the complementary path is to the right, then the following interpolated line integral will result ($-\pi - 2\beta \le \alpha' \le 0$):

$$\begin{aligned} L'(\beta, \alpha') &= w_1 L(\beta, \alpha' + \alpha_{ima}) + w_2 L(-\beta, \alpha' + \alpha_{ima} + 2\beta + \pi) \\ w_1 &= 1 + \frac{\alpha'}{\pi + 2\beta} = 1 - w_2 \qquad w_2 = \frac{-\alpha'}{\pi + 2\beta} \end{aligned} \tag{13.11a}$$

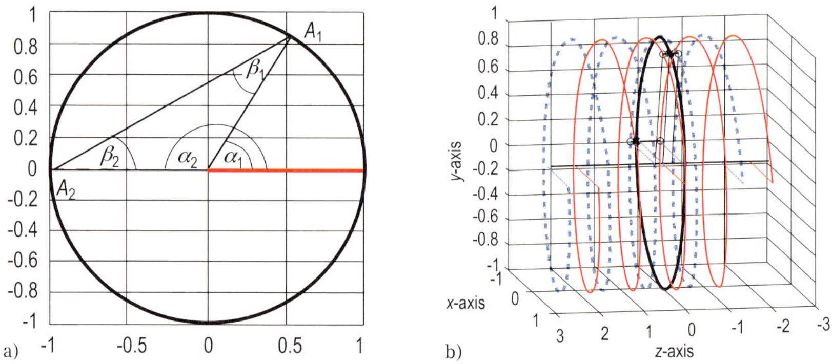

Figure 13.6
(a) Complementary interpolation (projection into the x,y plane). The black circle represents the path of the focal spot in the x,y plane. The attenuation measured for projection angle α_1 and fan angle β_1 (focus position A_1) is the same as the attenuation measured for projection angle $\alpha_2 = \alpha_1 + 2\beta_1 + \pi$ and fan angle $\beta_2 = -\beta_1$ (focus position A_2). **(b)** Interpolation to the plane of the black circle with algorithm 180-LI.

If the reverse is true (i.e. the direct focus path is to the right of the image plane and the complementary path is to the left), then the following interpolated line integral will result ($0 \leq \alpha' \leq \pi - 2\beta$):

$$L'(\beta,\alpha') = w_1 L(-\beta,\alpha'+\alpha_{ima}+2\beta-\pi) + w_2 L(\beta,\alpha'+\alpha_{ima})$$
$$w_1 = \frac{\alpha'}{\pi-2\beta} = 1 - w_2 \qquad w_2 = \frac{\pi-\alpha'-2\beta}{\pi-2\beta} \tag{13.11b}$$

This typical form of the linear spiral interpolation over approximately 180° for an estimation of line integrals in the image plane at z_{ima} is known as the 180-LI or slim algorithm.

Given that the interpolation partners in the 180-LI algorithm are approximately 180° apart, the data range extends across projection angles of at least 180° before the image plane and 180° behind the image plane in addition to two times the fan angle (i.e. about 2 × 50°) due to the fan-beam geometry. This comprises a total angular data range of approximately 460°. One consequence of the reduced data range (compared to 360-LI) is a reduced broadening of the slice-sensitivity profile (SSP). Taking $p_f = 1$ as an example, the SSP at the isocenter has about the same full width at half maximum (*FWHM*) as that of a corresponding axial slice. Moreover, the noise in an image reconstructed with the 180-LI algorithm is 15% more than that of a corresponding axial slice. This is because, due to the weighting procedure, the image is reconstructed with a reduced number of X-ray quanta.

Common properties of 360-LI and 180-LI

Longitudinal (z-axis) resolution in spiral CT is not only determined by the collimated beam width as in axial scanning, but also by the effective slice width, which is established during the spiral interpolation process. The effective slice width S_{eff} is usually

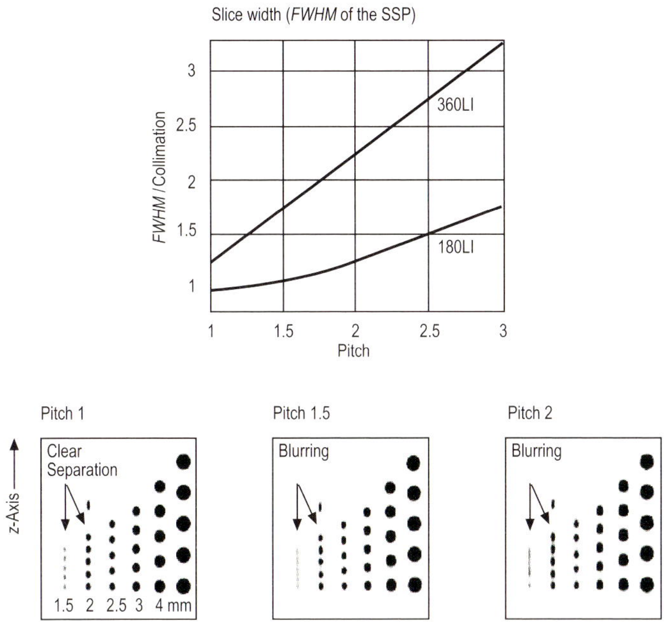

Figure 13.7
Top: the FWHM of the SSP as a function of the pitch for the two most commonly used single-slice spiral interpolation approaches (180-LI and 360-LI). The slice significantly widens along with increasing pitch in both cases. **Bottom:** MPRs of a spiral z-resolution phantom scanned with a collimation of 2 mm (180-LI) show increased blurring of the 1.5 mm and 2 mm cylinders with increasing pitch as a consequence of the increasing effective slice width.

defined as the FWHM of the spiral SSP. Some well-known common features of 180-LI and 360-LI single-slice spiral algorithms include:

- The FWHM of the SSP increases monotonically and the longitudinal resolution degrades along with increasing pitch p_f (fig. 13.7). This is a consequence of the increasing longitudinal distance of the projections used for spiral interpolation.
- The width of the spiral SSP is always smaller for 180-LI than it is for 360-LI at equal pitch p_f. This is a consequence of the smaller z-distance of the interpolation partners. While S_{eff} equals the collimated slice width S at a pitch of 1 in the case of 180-LI, $S_{eff} = 1.27\ S$ at a pitch of 2: a collimated slice of 5 mm is actually a slice of 6.4 mm at a pitch of 2. The degradation of the SSP is significantly worse in the case of 360-LI: at a pitch of 2, $S_{eff} = 2.25\ S$ and a collimated slice of 5 mm is in fact a slice of 11.25 mm.
- Two interpolation partners are used for every projection angle independent of the pitch. Therefore, if the tube current (mA) is left unchanged, the image noise will be independent of the pitch and the patient dose will decrease along with increasing pitch.

Due to its narrower SSP, 180-LI is used almost exclusively for single-slice spiral scanning, despite its increased susceptibility to artifacts and its increased image noise. Spiral artifacts gradually increase with increasing pitch. Typical spiral artifacts appear as hyper- or hypo-dense structures that surround z-inhomogeneous high-contrast objects.

The option of scanning at a higher pitch in single-slice CT is often selected so as to reduce patient dose, although it comes at the expense of slice broadening (i.e. if the collimation is kept constant) and increased spiral artifacts. It is more advantageous, particularly in the case of angiographic (CTA) applications, to scan a given volume for a given period of time using narrow collimation at high pitch than to use a wider collimation at low pitch. The motivation for increasing pitch and reducing collimation is to improve the longitudinal resolution by narrowing the spiral slice profile [13.10].

13.1.4 Image quality

Image quality is a matter of the degree to which a system is capable of accurately imaging an object. This implies that a good image is free of structures that are not present in the object and that its noise level is low. Here, streaks, rings, large-scale inhomogeneities, etc. qualify as artifacts while the structures and effects due to the finite number of X-ray quanta are subsumed under the term noise. Moreover, a good image is expected to exhibit the correct size and contrast of the object's details, i.e. the system is required to supply appropriate spatial and contrast resolution both within the scanning plane and perpendicular to it.

13.1.4.1 Modulation transfer function

The relation between the object and its image in an ideal image that is free of artifacts and noise is completely determined by the modulation transfer function or *MTF* (see chapter 9). The image function $B(\underline{x})$ for a two dimensional system can be represented on the basis of the object function $O(\underline{x})$ via convolution with the point spread function $PSF(\underline{x})$:

$$B(\underline{x}) = \iint O(\underline{x}')PSF(\underline{x}-\underline{x}')\mathrm{d}^2x' \qquad (13.12a)$$

Alternatively (i.e. in the frequency domain), this function can be expressed as:

$$B(\underline{x}) = \iint O(\underline{v})MTF(\underline{v})\exp(-\mathrm{i}2\pi\underline{v}\cdot\underline{x})\mathrm{d}^2v \qquad (13.12b)$$

The functions *MTF* and *PSF* are related to one another by a 2D Fourier transform. Polar coordinates can be used in the case of radial symmetry where the functions *PSF* and *MTF* depend only on the lengths r and v of the vectors $\underline{x}$ and $\underline{v}$. This enables one to perform angular integration with the following results:

$$MTF(\underline{v}) \rightarrow M(v) = 2\pi\int P_S(r)J_0(2\pi vr)r\mathrm{d}r \qquad (13.13a)$$

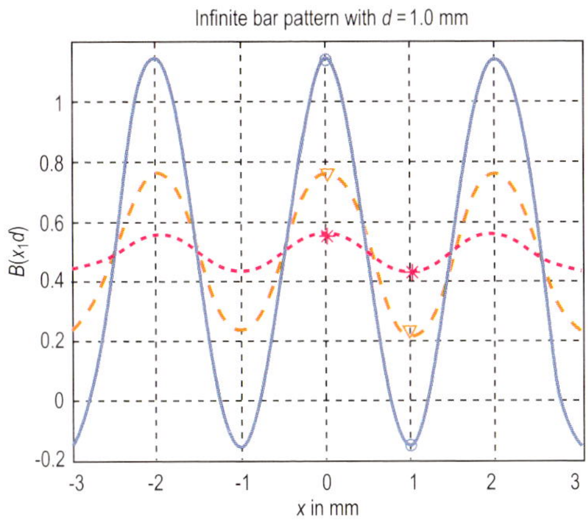

Figure 13.8
Infinite bar pattern for $d = 1$ mm ($\nu_d = 5$/cm) and images with 3 body kernels (soft, medium, and sharp)

$$PSF(\underline{x}) \rightarrow P_S(r) = 2\pi \int M(\nu) J_0(2\pi\nu r)\,\nu \mathrm{d}\nu \tag{13.13b}$$

J_0 denotes the 0-order Bessel function and $P_S(r)$ and $M(\nu)$ are one-dimensional Hankel transforms of one another. The normalization $M(0) = 1$ is chosen.

As has been outlined in chapter 9, the *MTF* can be measured via contrasting bar patterns (fig. 13.8). The use of bar patterns with different periodicities yields the *MTF* curves shown in fig. 13.9.

The *MTF* of a CT system can be broken down into two factors that reflect the influence of the reconstruction algorithm and the measuring system:

$$M(\nu) = M_A(\nu) M_M(\nu) \tag{13.14}$$

The algorithmic contribution $M_A(\nu)$ is determined by the Fourier transforms of the convolution kernel and of the interpolation applied during backprojection. The Shepp-Logan kernel (raster a) with linear interpolation represents a simple example:

$$M_A^{SL}(\nu) = |\mathrm{sinc}(\pi a \nu)|^3 \tag{13.15}$$

(For the sinc-function the definition $\mathrm{sinc}(x) = \sin(x)/x$ is used, with $\mathrm{sinc}(0) = 1$).

The contribution made by the measuring system, $M_M(\nu)$, contains the blurring due to the finite size of the detector aperture and the effective width of the focus. The $M_M(\nu)$ function for a rectangular aperture b_D and focus width b_F (both projected to the system axis) can be simply expressed as:

$$M_M(\nu) = \mathrm{sinc}(\pi b_D \nu)\,\mathrm{sinc}(\pi b_F \nu) \tag{13.16}$$

with zeros at $\nu_D = 1/b_D$ and $\nu_F = 1/b_F$ and with the lower of these two spatial frequencies limiting the image sharpness. Typical values are $b_D = 0.6$ mm and $b_F = 0.5$ mm, i.e. $\nu_D = 16.67$ /cm, $\nu_F = 20$ /cm.

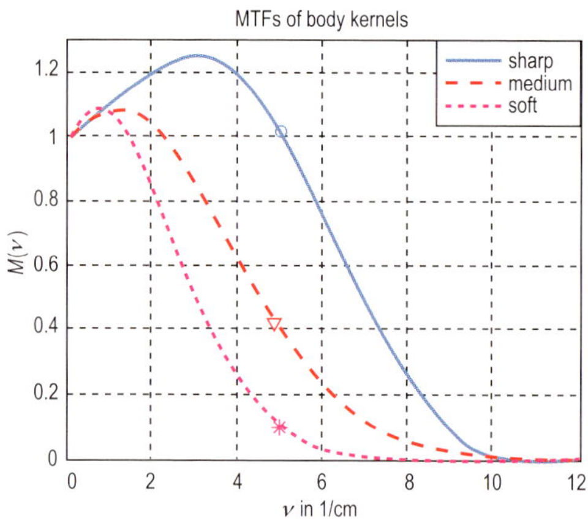

Figure 13.9
MTF of 3 body kernels (soft, medium and sharp)

The image sampling procedure represents a practical limitation on sharpness. If a square image of length D_B (the field of view) is displayed as an m_B by m_B matrix, the pixel size is $l_B = D_B/m_B$. Consequently, only frequencies below the Nyquist frequency $\nu_B = 1/2l_B$ are represented correctly in the image. A reconstruction kernel with a cut-off frequency larger than ν_B would be too sharp for such an image, given that it could result in Moiré-like artifacts. While such artifacts can be avoided by multiplying the kernel by an l_B-dependent factor (the Moiré filter) in frequency space, thereby suppressing frequencies above ν_B, doing so may reduce the sharpness compared to that of the pure kernel. For instance, the critical frequency for a 512 by 512 matrix with a field of view $D_B = 400$ mm is $\nu_B = 6.4$ /cm. While the Moiré filter has no effect on images with soft kernels, it reduces higher frequencies with medium and sharp kernels. On the other hand, no effect is observed with the kernels discussed so far where $D_B \leq 250$ mm and $\nu_B \geq 10.24$/cm.

13.1.4.2 Noise

Fluctuations in the number of X-ray quanta absorbed in the detector represent the origin of uncertainties in the signal, in the line integral and, ultimately, in the reconstructed values $\mu(x,y)$ of the image. In the present section, we address systems in which quantum noise is the predominant source of uncertainty in the measuring process. That being said, it warrants pointing that the electronic noise generated by the data acquisition system also plays a role in the case of low-dose scans where it can lead to artifacts (dark streaks) in directions of high attenuation.

The probability of counting n X-ray quanta with a detector when the average value is $\bar{n}$ can be expressed by the Poisson distribution:

$$P(n) = \frac{\bar{n}^n}{n!} e^{-\bar{n}} \tag{13.17}$$

The variance is identical to the mean value $\bar{n}$, with the standard deviation being $\sqrt{\bar{n}}$.

The illumination of an object with a quantum flux density of j_n for a time τ will yield an average number of quanta that can be expressed as

$$\bar{n} = b_D S j_n \tau \tag{13.18}$$

b_D: Detector aperture, S: Slice thickness

The average number of quanta per unit length (along scan direction) detected behind an object with an X-ray attenuation of

$$A_S = e^{\int \mu ds} \tag{13.19}$$

after N_R readings (summed over all projection measurements) is

$$neq = \eta_D \frac{\bar{n}}{A_S a_D} N_R \tag{13.20a}$$

where η_D ($0 < \eta_D \leq 1$) is the detector efficiency, and a_D is the detector pitch. The value of the noise equivalent quanta neq determines the signal-to-noise ratio in the image (see also chapter 9).

According to eqs. (13.18) and (13.20a), the relation

$$neq = \frac{1}{A_S} \eta_D \frac{b_D}{a_D} S T_S j_n \propto \frac{1}{A_S} \eta_D \eta_G S Q \tag{13.20b}$$

holds, i.e. neq is proportional to the detector efficiency η_D, the geometric efficiency $\eta_G = b_D / a_D$, to the slice thickness S and to the mAs-product Q. $T_s = N_R \tau$ is the rotation time, and j_n is proportional to the tube current.

Owing to the radial data acquisition in CT, decreases in the density of noise equivalent quanta in frequency space $NEQ(\nu)$ are inversely proportional to frequency

$$NEQ(\nu) = \frac{neq}{\pi |\nu|} \tag{13.21}$$

It therefore follows from eq. (9.33) that the noise power spectrum (measured in Hounsfield units times cm^2) can be expressed as (eq.(9.33))

$$NPS(\nu) = \left(\frac{1000}{\mu_W} HU\right)^2 \frac{\pi |\nu|}{neq} M_A^2(\nu) \tag{13.22}$$

The easiest way of measuring the noise generated by a CT system is to take the standard deviation σ of the CT values in the image of a homogeneous object (e.g. a water phantom with a diameter of 20 cm). The variance (standard deviation squared) is related to the noise power spectrum by:

$$\sigma^2 = 2\pi \int NPS(\nu) \nu \, d\nu \tag{13.23}$$

This can be rewritten as:

$$\sigma = \frac{500\, HU}{\mu_W} \frac{f_A}{\sqrt{a^3 neq}} \tag{13.24}$$

a: Kernel raster

The factor f_A depends on the reconstruction algorithm and can be expressed as:

$$f_A^2 = 8\pi^2 a^3 \int M_A^2(\nu)\nu^2 \mathrm{d}\nu \tag{13.25}$$

The Shepp-Logan kernel with linear interpolation for backprojection yields $f_A = 1$. Diagnostic kernels can vary in the range $0.2 < f_A < 3$ from soft to sharp. Noise increases along with increasing sharpness. Typical σ values for the kernels in fig. 13.9 include 3 HU (soft), 5.9 HU (medium) and 13.2 HU (sharp).

The selections $a = a_D$ and $a = a_D/2$ are frequently made for the kernel raster a. When comparing noise for Shepp-Logan kernels with rasters $a/2$ and a, the standard deviation (for fixed NEQ) increases by a factor of $2^{3/2} \approx 2.83$.

If the slice thickness S and the mAs product Q are varied, the noise amplitude will change according to:

$$\sigma \propto \frac{f_A}{\sqrt{SQ}} \tag{13.26}$$

To gain an impression of the magnitudes of the quantities involved, one can treat a numerical example with plausible parameters for σ in the center of the 20 cm water phantom, i.e. $A_S = e^{20\mu_W} \approx 47$:

$$j_n = 6 \cdot 10^{10}/(\mathrm{s\,cm}^2),\ \tau = 0.5\ \mathrm{ms},\ S = 10\ \mathrm{mm},\ b_D = 0.6\ \mathrm{mm}$$
$$\rightarrow \bar{n} = 1.8 \cdot 10^6,$$

$$N_R = 2000\ (T_S = 1\ \mathrm{s}),\ a_D = 0.8\ \mathrm{mm}\ (\eta_G = 0.75),\ \eta_D = 1$$
$$\rightarrow neq = 9.57 \cdot 10^8/\mathrm{cm},$$

$$a = 0.4\ \mathrm{mm},\ f_A = 1,\ \mu_W = 0.192/\mathrm{cm}$$
$$\rightarrow \sigma = 10.52\ \mathrm{HU}.$$

The neq can be estimated (*vice versa*) from the values for σ, f_A and a.

In characterizing quantum noise, we have thus far only considered its amplitude σ. However, in the case of objects with low contrast, it is also important to assess the noise structure, i.e. the spatial appearance of the noise *grains*. Kernels with a large number of high frequencies in the Fourier transform exhibit a fine-grained image noise. If the high frequencies are cut off, then the noisy image will be coarse-grained. Moreover, small noise pixels will improve the visual sharpness. Fine-grained kernels sometimes yield better images than coarse-grained kernels, even if their σ is higher.

Noise in images from non-standard scans

The considerations that have been presented so far are valid for complete and consistent scans in the sense outlined in section 13.1.3. However, as indicated in section 13.1.3, it is necessary in the case of nonstandard scans (i.e. spiral scans) to apply an appropriate weighting factor in order to obtain images that are free of artifacts. This weighting factor also influences noise. It is assumed that the measurement values in the different channels and projections are statistically independent. The variances can then be added. If all measurements exhibit the same measurement noise, then the procedure for calculating the image noise of a nonstandard scan reduces to a summation of the squared weights. By way of illustration, one can consider the result for spiral weighting. If the weighting function exhibits a triangular shape with width W at the bottom, one obtains

$$\frac{\sigma_{\text{tri}}^2}{\sigma^2} = \frac{4z_{\text{rot}}}{3N_S W} \tag{13.27}$$

for a detector with N_s slices. Here, the image noise σ_{tri} of a weighted scan is compared with the image noise σ of a standard scan with the same noise equivalent quanta (*neq*) and the same kernel. In the case of single-slice spiral CT scanners, the algorithm slim has the width $W = z_{\text{rot}}$, leading to $\sigma_{\text{tri}} = \sqrt{4/3}\,\sigma$ for $N_s = 1$. The algorithm wide has the width $W = 2z_{\text{rot}}$, leading to $\sigma_{\text{tri}} = \sqrt{2/3}\,\sigma$. In the case of multi-slice spiral CT scanners, the width of the weighting function can be set to values $W \geq 2S$, independent of the table-feed. Hence, the image noise will increase along with z_{rot} if no additional actions are taken. If weighting functions other than triangles are used for multi-slice spiral CT scanners, then the corresponding relations can be derived.

13.1.4.3 Low-contrast detectability

The properties of images with high contrast objects are essentially determined by high-contrast resolution, i.e. by the *MTF* of a proper kernel. Noise does not play a major role. However, a low noise level is of central importance for the observation of details exhibiting small contrast, i.e. for low-contrast resolution. Given that small image details of low contrast will deteriorate as a result of the high noise, it will be necessary to raise the dose to an appropriate level to guarantee reasonable detectability within noisy surroundings. Special phantoms (e.g. the low-contrast module of the CATPHAN) are currently used to obtain a well-defined arrangement for specification. Such phantoms are typically comprised of several sections, with each section containing a series of holes of diameter d and a given contrast ΔCT. The task of specifying low-contrast detectability will involve confronting the following problem:

- We want to detect a small object (of diameter d)
- with a certain contrast (ΔCT)
- in a particular phantom (e.g. CATPHAN with a diameter of 16 or 20 cm)
- with a certain slice thickness (S)
- at a particular mAs product (Q)
- at a particular dose (in mGy).

The statistical nature of noise generally prevents one from obtaining identical results for detectability when scans are performed repeatedly. For the sake of specification, one usually gives values of d (at a certain ΔCT), which can be *seen* in the majority of scans (i.e. in around 5 of 9 scans). Fig. 13.10 shows two images of the 20 cm CATPHAN that were measured with an Emotion at 130 kV, 10 mm, Q = 73 mAs and Q = 225 mAs respectively. All 4 sections with ΔCT = 10, 5, 3, 1 HU can be seen (e.g.

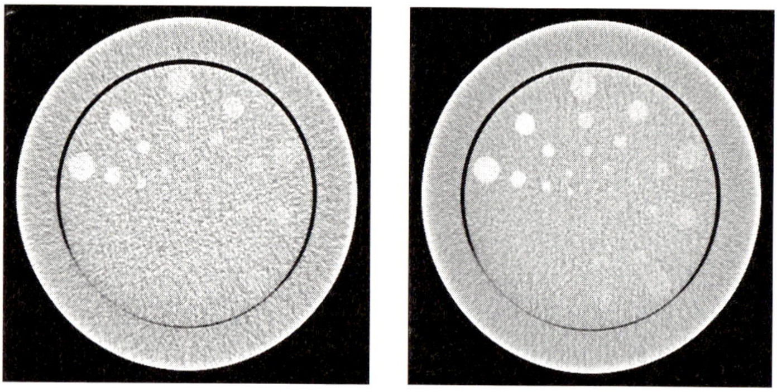

Figure 13.10
Image of a low-contrast phantom (20 cm CATPHAN) **(left)** generated by the Somatom Emotion at Q = 73 mAs (130 kV, 10 mm) and **(right)** the same image taken at Q = 225 mAs (130 kV, 10 mm)

even the 3 mm holes in the 3 HU block) in the high-dose image shown in fig. 13.10 (right). The detectability in the low-dose image (fig. 13.10, left) is much worse, with the 1 HU block being *drowned* in noise.

As outlined in chapter 2, the minimum recognizable contrast in an image depends on the object size and on the noise level. As a simple rule of thumb applicable to the range 2 mm ≤ d ≤ 5 mm, this dependency can sometimes be approximated as follows:

$$\Delta CT \propto \frac{\sigma}{d^{3/2}} \tag{13.28}$$

The dose that is sufficient for seeing the 5 mm/3 HU is thus too low for the detection of 3 mm/5 HU holes and will have to be raised by a factor 5/3 (e.g. from 90 mAs to 150 mAs). Actually, the situation is a little more complicated due to the fact that both the noise amplitude and the noise structure play a role: kernels with fine-grained noise perform better than coarse-grained kernels, even if σ is higher. Consequently, the approximate relation should only be used for kernels of the same type.

13.1.4.4 Artifacts

The simplest type of artifact appears as a streak or a ring in the image. If the measuring value of one channel in a single reading is disturbed, a single streak occurs. If one channel drops out over a full rotation, a ring is produced (fig. 13.11). Rings will also show up if differences in the sensitivities of neighboring detector channels are not adequately corrected.

Patient movement (e.g. related to peristalsis, breathing, heart beat, etc.) represents another source of artifacts. Such motion artifacts result in local contour blurring, double contours and streaks or shadowing throughout the entire image (fig. 13.12). Motion leads to inconsistencies in the start angle region and these inconsistencies then lead to motion artifacts. Such inconsistencies can be reduced using sophisticated algorithms designed to correct motion artifacts. An even better way of reducing the

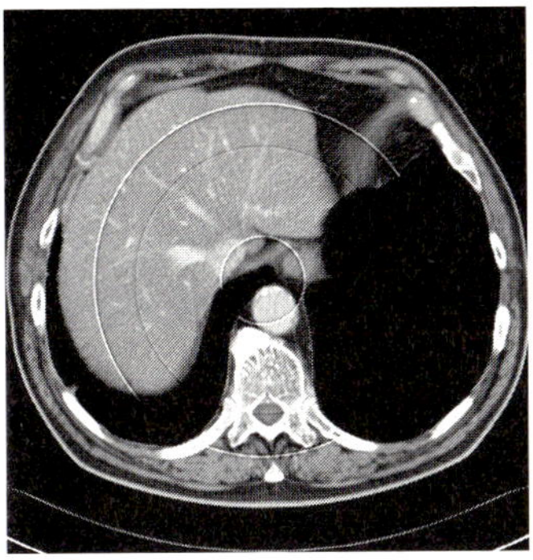

Figure 13.11
Ring artifacts in a body scan

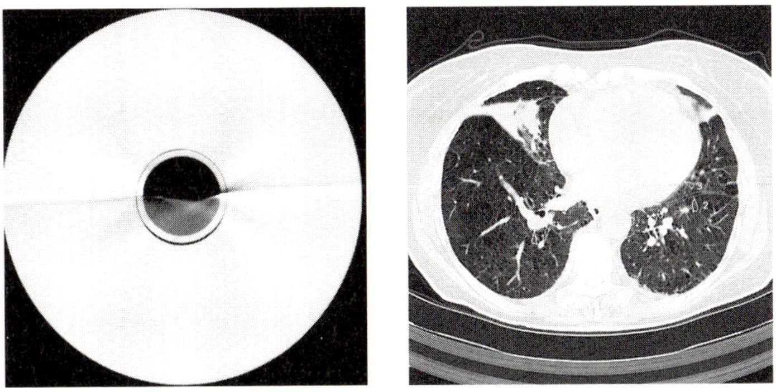

Figure 13.12
Images showing motion artifacts. The first image is produced with the help of a phantom **(left)** where the inner water surface was agitated during the sequence scan. The second image is that of a lung that shows **(right)** blurring at the marked positions 1 and 2 and double contours at position 3.

probability and intensity of motion artifacts is to use short acquisition times and appropriate start angles.

In cases where high contrast steps in the scan plane are present in an object, sampling artifacts can show up (e.g. as fine streaks originating from these discontinuities). Here, it is advisable to use a finer detector pitch or a doubling of the sampling rate (e.g. via a flying focal spot focus) as a remedy. Such effects are also known as lateral partial volume artifacts.

Longitudinal partial volume artifacts (in z-direction perpendicular to the scan plane) occur whenever high-contrast structures extend only partly into the slice. These may appear as relatively broad streaks and as dark or light zones in the image. The source here is actually a nonlinear effect originating from an averaging (by the detector elements) of signals over the slice. Fig. 13.13 shows an image of two cylinders extending halfway into the slice. This is the result of data simulated with monoenergetic X-rays. The use of thin slices is the only reasonable measure against partial volume artifacts.

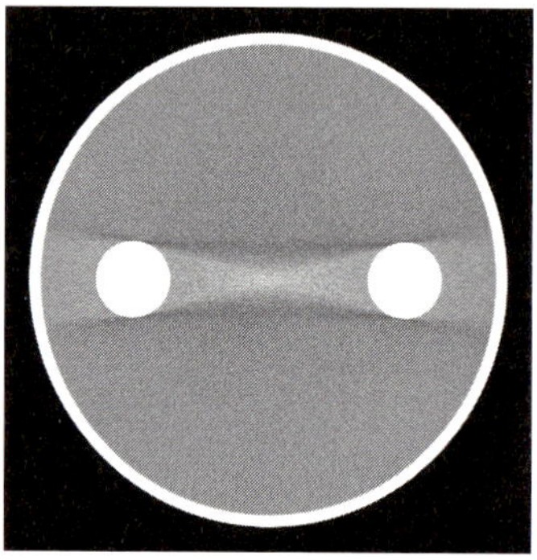

Figure 13.13
Images showing longitudinal partial-volume artifacts in a simulated phantom

If the images of several thin slices are summed up, the noise can be reduced to a level comparable to that of a thick slice image, but essentially without the partial-volume effects.

Beam hardening leads to artifacts that resemble those stemming from partial-volume effects. The X-ray beam used in CT is characterized by a broad polychromatic spectrum. Given that the linear attenuation coefficients depend on X-ray energy, the spectrum of measured line integrals depends on the size and composition of the object and on the viewing direction. As the attenuation of X-ray energy decreases, the spectrum behind an object will contain relatively more high-energetic quanta than it originally contained, i.e. it will have become harder. In the case of a homogeneous object, the central beam with the longest path corresponds to the hardest spectrum, mimicking a lower effective μ than would result from a peripheral beam. This leads to the appearance of a bowl in the image, i.e. to lowered HU values in the center. Water phantom images can be flattened by applying a global beam-hardening correction. Despite this correction, however, pronounced beam-hardening artifacts will appear in images of objects that contain materials exhibiting quite different attenuation properties (e.g. bone and soft tissue).

This is demonstrated in fig. 13.14 using a simulated image and an image showing the base of a patient's skull. The dark zone between the petrous bones is typically referred to as the Hounsfield bar. While such effects can be slightly reduced by using a harder original spectrum, much greater effort is required for a good image. Excellent results can be obtained by deploying an iterative beam-hardening correction that starts from a first rough image in order to locate soft tissue and bone, and then uses this knowledge to apply a selective spectral algorithm, usually for two components (e.g. water and bone). This is the procedure used to obtain the images in fig. 13.15.

The artifacts due to metallic implants can be reduced in many cases by modifying the iterative beam-hardening algorithm. However, if the attenuation is so large that the signal is dominated in some directions and channels by electronic noise, the image will show overall deterioration (i.e. not only in the vicinity of the metal). The only possible remedy in this case is to increase the signal by using larger slice-thickness, tube-current and voltage values.

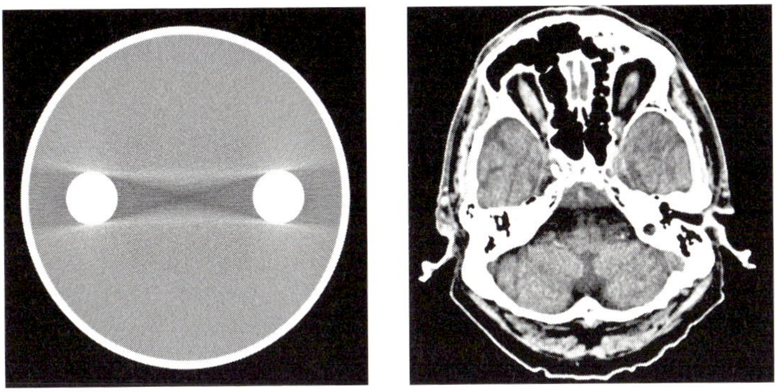

Figure 13.14
Images showing beam-hardening artifacts in a simulated phantom and in the head

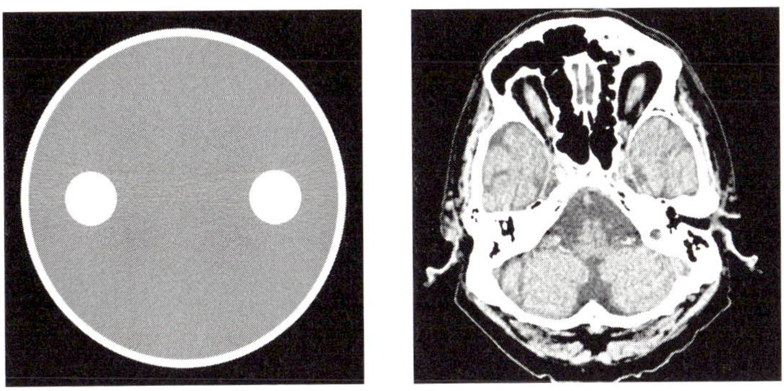

Figure 13.15 Result of the iterative beam-hardening correction of the images from fig. 13.14

Objects of extreme elliptical shape (e.g. the shoulder) show peculiar image artifacts, i.e. heavy noise streaks in directions of high attenuation. This streak pattern can be leveled out using particular algorithmic procedures such as local smoothing controlled by the attenuation value or, better still, dose modulation, which involves the use of a hardware device that varies the tube current during the rotation according to the expected attenuation, i.e. by applying high dose and low dose in directions of high and low attenuation respectively.

The main contribution to the signal stems from the attenuation in the direct ray connecting the focus with a detector element. An additional signal contribution arises from radiation that scatters upon contact with the object and then strikes the detector element from a plurality of directions. Scattered radiation increases the signal, and thus mimics reduced attenuation. This leads to smaller CT values and a deterioration of spatial and contrast resolution. Collimators can be used to suppress scattering in the case of single-slice (and even multi-slice) scanners.

In summary, the main sources of error in quantitative CT are beam hardening and scattered radiation.

13.1.4.5 Dose profiles and slice sensitivity profiles

One can infer from the term tomography that the definition of the part of the object that is to be scanned is an important issue. The volume that is irradiated by X-rays is referred to as a slice. Slice definition is controlled by several parameters: the emission profile of the focal spot, the opening of the pre-patient (tube-side) collimator, the opening of the post-patient (detector-side) collimator and the structure of the detector slice (if applicable). In general, a slice profile is calculated via the convolution of the emission profile with the respective apertures. It will be necessary to apply different geometric relationships depending on whether a dose profile or a sensitivity profile is to be calculated.

Calculation of the dose profile

The dose profile (DP) can be defined as the spatial distribution of the primary radiation dose delivered to the object as a function of the z-coordinate. Any post-patient collimation will accordingly not influence this quantity. Fig. 13.16 offers a quantitative explanation of the shape of an ideal dose profile.

In general, the dose profile is calculated as a convolution of the focal spot's emission profile $P_F(z)$ and the effective aperture $P_{FB}(z)$ of the pre-patient collimator:

$$P_{DP}(z) = \frac{\int P_F(z')P_{FB}(z-z')dz'}{\int P_F(z')dz'} = \frac{P_F(z) \otimes P_{FB}(z)}{\int P_F(z')dz'} \qquad (13.29)$$

If rectangular profiles are used (as before), the convolution will result in a trapezoidal dose profile as shown in fig. 13.17. The effective slice thickness or *FWHM* of the dose

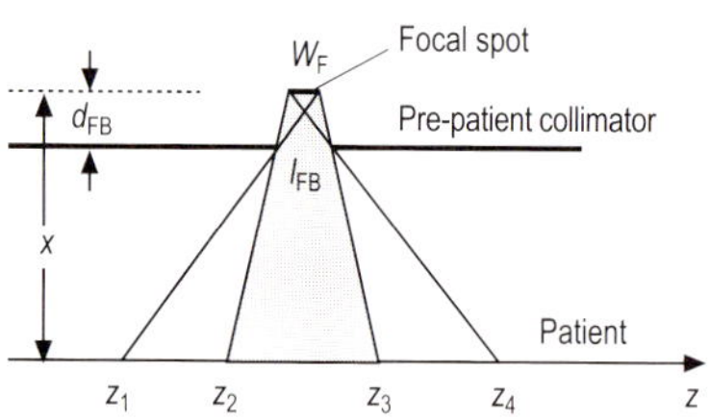

Figure 13.16
Formation of a dose profile at a distance x from the focal spot. Given that point z_1 and all points left of z_1 receive no energy flux from the focal spot, the dose profile is set to zero. The entire focal spot can be seen from any point between z_2 and z_3. The energy flux is at its maximum. The (normalized) dose profile is set to one and exhibits a plateau. The following is true for all points z between z_1 to z_2: an increasing part of the focal spot comes into view, the energy flux increases and the dose profile rises linearly from zero to one. The energy flux decreases from z_3 and z_4 and the dose profile falls linearly from one to zero. Both the energy flux and the dose profile remain at zero for all points to the right of z_4.

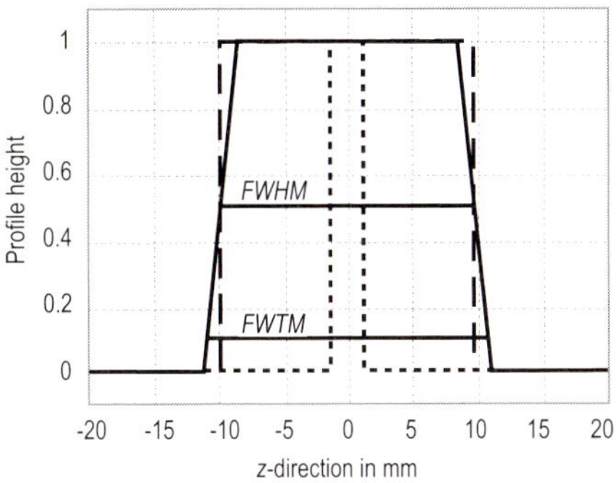

Figure 13.17
Trapezoidal profile (line) resulting from the convolution of two rectangular profiles (dotted and slash-dotted)

profile is equal to the width of the wider of the two rectangular profiles being convolved.

These considerations are valid if the opening l_{FB} of the tube-side collimator is wide enough that the focal spot is seen in full length by at least one point on the isocenter. If the opening l_{FB} of the pre-patient collimator l_{FB} is too small, so that the focal spot is no longer seen in its full length at the isocenter, then the use of the X-ray quanta from the tube will not be optimally efficient. The maximum value of the profile will be reduced from 1 to $(l_{FB}\,x)/(w_F(x - d_{FB}))$ and the slice thickness at the isocenter will be independent of the collimator opening and will show a value of $S_{eff} = w_F(x - d_{FB})/x$.

Calculation of the slice-sensitivity profile

The slice-sensitivity profile (SSP) can be defined as the response of the entire measurement system (including the detector) to a δ-shaped object detail. Accordingly, the convolution introduced in eq. (13.29) is also required to include the effective widths $P_{DB}(z)$ of the post-patient collimator and the effective aperture $P_{D,q}(z)$ of the respective detector slice q:

$$P_{SSP,q} = \frac{P_F(z) \otimes P_{FB}(z) \otimes P_{D,q}(z) \otimes P_{DB}(z)}{\int P_F(z')\mathrm{d}z'} \tag{13.30}$$

In the case of an axial scan (slice by slice), all measurement values are acquired at the same z-position and the superimposition of the SSPs from the individual projections has the same functional form as the SSP of an individual projection.

- DP and SSP are equal in the case of single-slice scanners without post-patient collimators.
- DP and SSP are not equal in the case of single-slice scanners with post-patient collimators. While the SSP is a trapezoid, the boundaries of its profile are sharper.
- DP and SSP are not equal in the case of multi-slice scanners where the SSP of a single slice is determined by the aperture w_D of a single detector row.

In the case of spiral (helical) scans, the projections are acquired at different z-positions and the (weighted) superimposition of the SSPs differs from the SSP of an individual

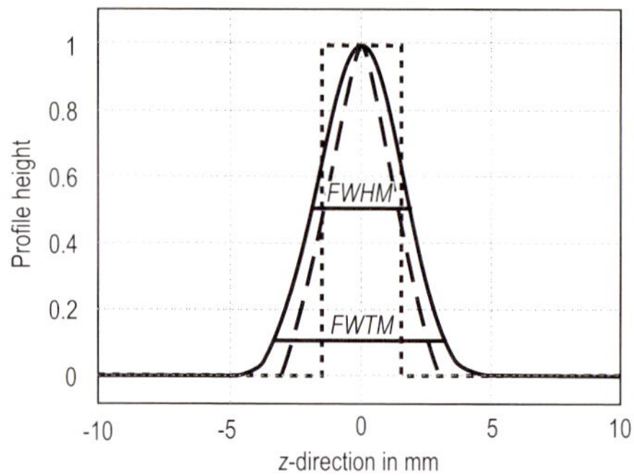

Figure 13.18
Piecewise parabolic profile (lined) resulting from the convolution of a rectangular collimation profile and a triangular spiral weighting function

projection. If we assume, for instance, that the SSP of an individual projection is rectangular and the spiral weighting function shows a triangular shape, then the resulting spiral SSP will be a piecewise parabolic function of the sort demonstrated in fig. 13.18. The broadening of the foot of the slice profile entails that it will not be sufficient to characterize its width on the basis of the FWHM alone. Additional quality parameters such as the full width at tenth maximum (FWTM) will also have to be provided.

The rectangular profile of width S in fig. 13.18 represents the sensitivity of the collimator. The triangular profile represents a spiral weighting function (linear interpolation) of width W. The resulting slice sensitivity profile is bell-shaped and its width can be characterized as follows:

$$FWHM = \begin{cases} S & W \leq S \\ S + W - \sqrt{2WS - S^2} \quad \text{for} & S \leq W \leq 2.5\,S \\ \dfrac{W}{2} + \dfrac{S}{4} & 2.5\,S \leq W \end{cases} \tag{13.31}$$

Notes: In the case of single-slice spiral CT scanners, the slim algorithm (see section 13.1.3) shows an interpolation width of $W = z_{\mathrm{rot}}$ and the wide algorithm shows an interpolation width of $W = 2z_{\mathrm{rot}}$. The effective slice width in these cases increases along with the table-feed (fig. 13.7). More versatile weighting functions can be used for multi-slice spiral CT scanners (see section 13.3).

13.2 From single-slice to multi-slice CT

The introduction of spiral CT in the early nineties represented a major advance in the development and ongoing refinement of CT imaging. The technique enabled one for the first time to acquire volume data and to avoid the misregistration of anatomical details. Volume data became the very basis for applications such as CT angiography [13.11], which has revolutionized noninvasive approaches to assessing vascular disease. The ability to acquire volume data also paved the way for the development of three-dimensional image processing techniques such as multiplanar reformation

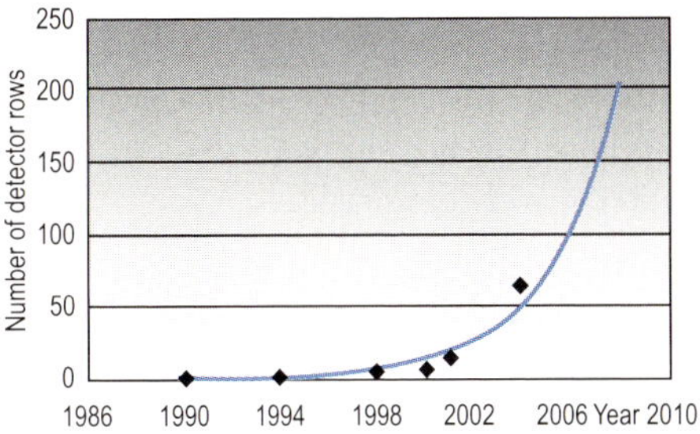

Figure 13.19
The number of slices offered by new CT scanners at the time of their market introduction

(MPR), maximum intensity projection (MIP), surface-shaded display (SSP) and various volume rendering techniques (VRT) [13.12] that have come to play an important role in medical imaging today.

Volume data that are isotropic in nature (i.e. each data element or voxel is of equal dimensions in all three spatial axes) and exhibit high spatial resolution offer an ideal basis for image display in arbitrarily oriented imaging planes. When applied in most clinical scenarios, single-slice spiral CT with a gantry rotation time of 1 s does not offer these properties. Spiral CT body examinations need to be completed within a certain time frame (usually one patient breath-hold or 25 to 30 s) in order to avoid motion artifacts and to optimally utilize the contrast bolus. If one is required to cover a large scanning range such as the entire thorax or abdomen (30 cm) within a single breath-hold, one will have to use a thick collimation of 5 to 8 mm. While the in-plane resolution of a CT image depends on the system geometry and on the reconstruction kernel selected by the user, the longitudinal (z-)resolution along the patient axis is determined by the collimated slice width and the spiral interpolation algorithm. Using a thick collimation of 5 to 8 mm results in a considerable mismatch between the longitudinal resolution and the usual in-plane resolution of 0.5 to 0.7 mm (i.e. depending on the reconstruction kernel). Single-slice spiral CT therefore permits one to achieve ideal isotropic resolution only when one is working with very limited scanning ranges [13.13].

The strategies that have been developed to achieve greater volume coverage and improved longitudinal resolution center on the simultaneous acquisition of more than one slice and reductions in the gantry rotation time. It is interesting to note in this context that the very first medical CT scanners (the EMI head scanner introduced in 1972 and the Siemens SIRETOM introduced in 1974) were 2-slice systems. However, 2-slice acquisition was abandoned following the introduction of whole-body fan-beam CT systems for general radiology. Apart from a dedicated 2-slice system for cardiac applications (the IMATRON C-100 introduced in 1984), the first step towards multi-slice acquisition in general radiology was a 2-slice CT scanner introduced in 1993 (Elscint TWIN). All of the major CT manufacturers introduced multi-slice CT (MSCT) systems in 1998. These typically enabled one to acquire 4 slices simultaneously at a rotation time of 0.5 s, thus introducing considerable improvements in terms of scanning speed, longitudinal resolution and the efficient utilization of available X-ray power [13.14-13.17]. The revolutionary potential in these developments for enabling real isotropic 3D imaging was soon recognized and the vendors pushed towards more and more slices, effectively elevating number of slices to the most important CT scanner performance characteristic. Fig. 13.19 shows the number of slices specified by new CT systems at the time of their market introduction. In analogy to Moore's law, the development is exponential, approximately doubling every two years.

The simultaneous acquisition of M slices results in an M-fold increase in speed so long as all of the other parameters (e.g. slice thickness) remain unchanged. This increased MSCT performance over single-slice CT allowed for the optimization of a variety of clinical protocols. For instance, the significant reductions in examination time for standard protocols proved to be of immediate clinical benefit for the quick and comprehensive assessment of trauma victims and of non-cooperative patients. Furthermore, the scanning range that one was able to cover within a certain scanning time was extended by a factor of M, which is relevant for oncological staging or for CT angiography with extended coverage (e.g. of the lower extremities). The most important clinical benefit, however, was the capacity to scan a given anatomic volume within a given scanning time with substantially reduced slice width at M times increased longitudinal resolution. This placed the goal of isotropic resolution within reach for many clinical applications. Examinations of the entire thorax and abdomen were now routinely performed using a collimated slice width of 1 mm or 1.25 mm. Despite these promising advances, however, clinical challenges and limitations remained for 4-slice CT systems. True isotropic resolution for routine applications had not yet been achieved, since the longitudinal resolution of about 1 mm does not fully match the in-plane resolution of around 0.5 to 0.7 mm in a routine scan of the chest or abdomen. It was necessary to select thicker collimated slices (2.5 mm) in order to complete the scan within a reasonable time frame for large volumes (e.g. in CT angiography of the

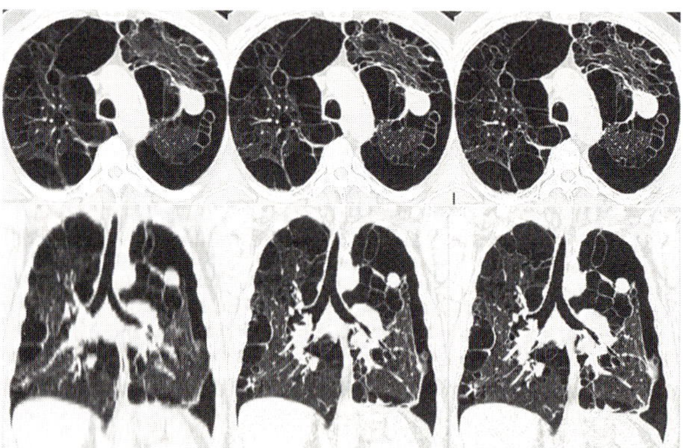

Figure 13.20
Case study (axial slices and coronal MPRs) of a thorax examination illustrating the clinical performance of single-slice CT (8 mm slices, left), 4-slice CT (1.25 mm slices, center) and 16-slice CT (0.75 mm slices, right). The difference in diagnostic image quality is most obvious in the MPRs. The single-slice and 4-slice images were synthesized from the 16-slice CT data. (Source: Dr. U.J. Schoepf, MUSC, Charleston, USA)

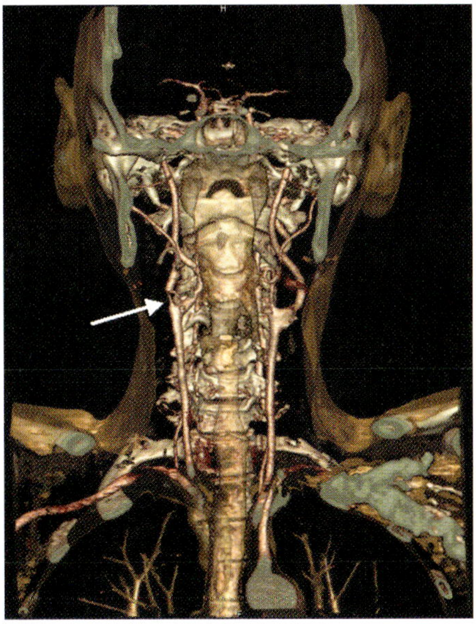

Figure 13.21
Clinical case illustrating the performance of 64-slice CT with a z-flying focal spot: CTA of the carotid arteries and the circle of Willis. Scanning parameters: 120 kV, an effective mAs of 150, a collimation of 64 × 0.6 mm, a gantry rotation time of 0.375 s, a pitch of 1.4 and a 6 s scanning time for 350 mm. The arrow indicates a severe stenosis. (Source: Dr. Lell, Dr. Anders, University Erlangen, Germany)

lower extremity run-off). Scanning times were often too long to permit image acquisition during the pure arterial phase. For instance, a CTA of the circle of Willis required one to cover a scanning range of around 100 mm. This volume can be covered in around 9 s of scanning time (not fast enough to avoid venous overlay if one assumes a cerebral circulation time of less than 5 s) using a 4-slice CT at a collimated slice width of 1 mm, a pitch of 1.5 and a gantry rotation time of 0.5 s.

While the introduction of an 8-slice CT system in 2000 enabled shorter scanning times, it did not yet provide improved longitudinal resolution (thinnest collimation: 8 × 1.25 mm). This was achieved with the introduction of 16-slice CT [13.18], which enabled one to routinely acquire substantial anatomic volumes with isotropic submillimeter spatial resolution and scanning times of less than 10 seconds for 300 mm of coverage (fig. 13.20), although the in-plane spatial resolution was not substantially improved. The two major advantages offered by fast MSCT acquisition include true isotropic through-plane resolution and short acquisition times that enable high-quality examinations in severely debilitated and severely dyspneic patients.

Traditional CT applications have been enhanced by the remarkable, albeit incremental, improvements in scanner performance stemming from the deployment of additional detector rows. MSCT technology has also made dramatic inroads in areas previ-

Table 13.1
Scanning protocols for thorax scans using different generations of CT scanners: older single-slice CT scanners forced users to compromise longitudinal resolution in favor of scanning speed.

	Collimation	**Rot. time**	**Typical scan time for 35 cm range**
1992 Single Slice SOMATOM Plus 4	e.g. 1 mm	e.g. 0.75 s	175 s
	e.g. 10 mm	e.g. 0.75 s	17.5 s
1998 Four Slice SOMATOM Volume Zoom	e.g. 4 × 1 mm	e.g. 0.5 s	29 s
2001 16-Slice SOMATOM Sensation 16	e.g. 16 × 0.75 mm	e.g. 0.5 s	10 s
2003 64 Slice SOMATOM Sensation 64	e.g. 64 × 0.6 mm sampled at 0.3 mm	e.g. 0.5 s	6 s

ously considered beyond the scope of 3rd generation CT scanners that are based on the mechanical rotation of X-ray tubes and detectors. One such application is cardiac imaging with the addition of an ECG-gating capability.

The race for more slices continues. In 2004, all of the major CT manufacturers introduced next generation MSCT systems featuring the capacity to acquire 32, 40 or even 64 slices simultaneously. This has brought a further leap in volume coverage speed. Some of these scanners use refined z-sampling techniques enabled by periodic focal spot motion in the z-direction (z-flying focal spot) so as to further improve longitudinal resolution and image quality in routine clinical procedures. These systems enable CT angiographic examinations with sub-mm resolution in the pure arterial phase even for extended anatomical ranges. A CTA of the carotid arteries and the circle of Willis with a collimation of 64 × 0.6 mm, a rotation time of 0.375 s and a pitch of 1.5 requires only 5 s for a scanning range of 350 mm (see fig. 13.21). A whole-body submillimeter CTA with a scanning range of 1,500 mm, a collimation of 64 × 0.6 mm, a rotation time of 0.375 s and a pitch of 1.2 to 1.4 can be completed in around 22 to 25 s.

Table 13.1 shows scanning protocols for different generations of CT scanners. Very useful up-to-date information regarding multidetector row CT is also readily available on the Internet (e.g. www.medical-devices.gov.uk, www.ctisus.org).

13.3 Multi-slice CT (MSCT)

The fundamental demands on a modern volume scanner can be summed up by the following two requirements:

1. Continuous data acquisition (the capacity to reconstruct images at any z position)
2. The capacity to scan a long range in a short time without compromising longitudinal (z) resolution

The first requirement calls for spiral acquisition. The second requirement calls for a defining of the maximum z-resolution via the detector pixellation alone rather than via a combination of spiral pitch and detector collimation, i.e. as is the case in single-slice spiral. This second requirement has been fulfilled since the introduction of multi-slice spiral CT in 1998. Moreover, multi-slice spiral scanners provide the new feature of allowing one to specify the z-resolution during the post-scanning reconstruction phase.

The technical challenges presented by MSCT are manifold: one is required to (1) design a detector capable of measuring several thousand channels simultaneously, (2) provide for the transfer of the data to the image reconstruction system and (3) devise a suitable reconstruction algorithm.

13.3.1 System design

The design of modern MSCT scanners is required to cover the full range of diagnostic techniques, ranging from standard tomographic scanning to trauma applications, radiation therapy planning and special applications such as ECG gating and respiratory gating. An MSCT scanner (fig. 13.22) comprises the following subsystems:

- Patient handling system (PHS)
- Gantry
- Computer systems
- Control unit in the operator room
- Line connection and network connections
- Cooling system

The patient table (patient handling system PHS) is required to enable exact positioning both in the vertical and horizontal direction while providing all of the necessary tools for comfortably fixing the patient to the table board. The table-feed in the horizontal direction covers a wide range (from 1 mm/s to more than 100 mm/s) and offers a positioning exactness of less than 0.5 mm. The vast majority of patient examinations today are performed in spiral (helical) mode, requiring continuous gantry rotation

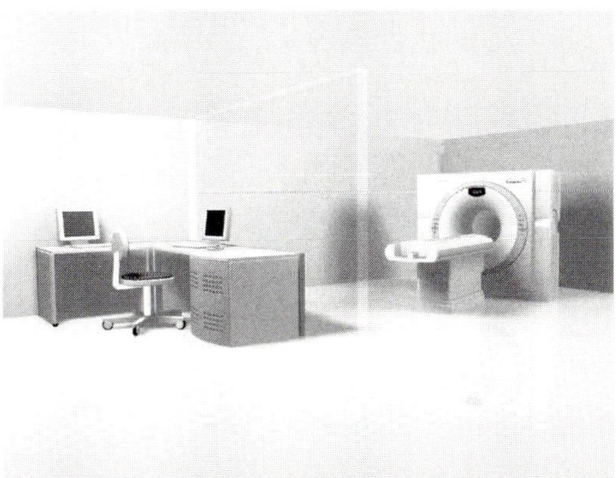

Figure 13.22
Major CT system components

and table movement during scan acquisition. While standard MSCT systems have a bore diameter of 70 to 73 cm, a trend towards widening the bore is in evidence, in particular, for radiation therapy planning and the examination of severely obese (bariatric) patients. Large-bore MSCT scanners are characterized by bore diameters of larger than 80 cm. The SOMATOM Sensation Open, for instance, has an 82 cm bore. The gantry is required to provide all of the necessary interfaces for performing examinations with external equipment (injector, ECG monitor, respiration control, etc.). The gantry and patient table are located in a lead-shielded examination room and the computer terminals and the control components (e.g. to start the examination and release X-rays) are located in the operator room. An optional X-ray release (e.g. a foot switch) and an additional image monitor can be installed in the examination room to offer support for interventional examinations. A lead window or a camera system provides the necessary visual contact to the patient. Communication with the patient is established via a two-way communication system. The cooling components and the line connection components may be located in the examination room or in a separate utility room. Air cooling is a feasible option for low-power systems. Cooling is then achieved by blowing the warm air from the gantry into the examination room and using the examination room's air-conditioning system to remove the heat.

In the remainder of the present section, we describe a number of the MSCT scanner's subsystems and components in greater detail. We begin with the gantry and the components on the rotating part of the gantry before moving on to the stationary components.

Gantry

The gantry is the subsystem used to acquire raw CT data with the necessary degree of precision and reproducibility (fig. 13.23).

An adequate combination of both mechanical and electrical components on the gantry provides a basis for a state-of-the-art MSCT acquisition system: X-rays are generated by an X-ray tube and precisely collimated by a tube collimator (pre-patient collimator). The attenuation of the X-ray beam is measured by a solid-state detector. The signals

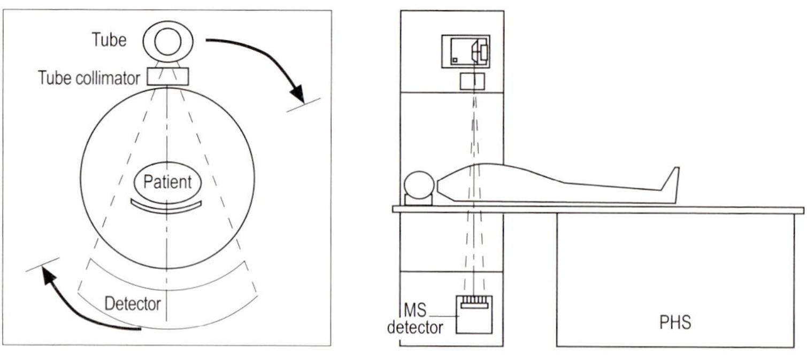

Figure 13.23 Drawing of a CT gantry enabling the acquisition of raw CT data

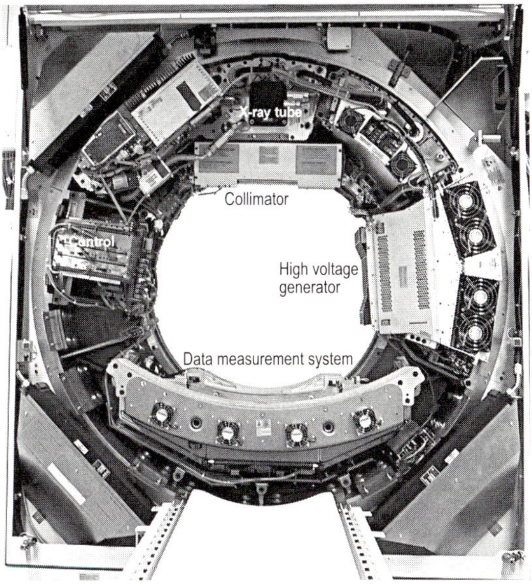

Figure 13.24
Somatom Sensation 64 gantry

are amplified and digitized by the data acquisition electronics. Both the X-ray tube and the detector in 3rd generation CT systems rotate around the patient. The measurement data are transferred from the rotating part of the gantry to the stationary part before being sent to the image reconstruction computer.

The rotating part of the gantry (fig. 13.24) is comprised of the following items:

- X-ray generation components: the X-ray tube, the high voltage generator, the control system for the electromagnetic deflection of the focal spot (if applicable) and the tube collimator
- Data generation components: the detector, the detector electronics and the data transmission system
- Various control and power supply components

The control components must be capable of rapid interaction during the examination in order to stabilize the X-ray beam with respect to gravitational and thermal influences, to acquire the data at the proper angular and longitudinal positions and to prevent X-ray exposure in cases of system malfunctioning. The control of the gantry's rotation must exhibit narrow tolerances and all negative influences caused by environmental factors such as temperature, vibration, etc., must be eliminated.

The following components are located on the stationary part of the gantry:

- Gantry tilt control
- Cooling control
- Bearing and drive system

- Power and data transmission link between the gantry's rotating and stationary parts
- Operator interface to control the patient handling system, gantry tilt and additional functions such as the positioning lasers

A key requirement for the mechanical design of the gantry is the stability of both focal spot and detector position during rotation, in particular with regard to the rapidly increasing rotational speeds of modern CT systems (0.75 s in 1994 and 0.33 s in 2003). The design of the mechanical support for the X-ray tube, the tube collimator and the data measurement system (DMS) is therefore required to account for the high gravitational forces associated with fast gantry rotation. The importance of proper weight distribution within the rotating part of the gantry increases as the rotation speed increases. It is essential that the gantry be precisely balanced to prevent any movement or vibration. Today's gantries are dynamically balanced in all three axes to minimize any negative influence on image quality. Fig. 13.25 offers an illustration of the radial force on gantry components at radial distances of 0.4 m, 0.6 m and 0.8 m from the isocenter. The static weight of components at a distance of 0.6 m from the isocenter will increase ten-fold at a gantry rotation speed of 0.5 s.

The electrical system is required to link all of the gantry's necessary functions. Two control system options are available for state-of-the-art MSCT systems. The first is a centralized control system comprised of a powerful controller and a multitask operating system. All sensors and power drivers are then linked to this central controller (fig. 13.26).

The second possibility is a de-centralized control system (fig. 13.27). A communication link (e.g. a controller area network) is used to connect the different function controllers for the generator, the tube collimator, the gantry drive, etc. The required control parameters are sent during the scan-preparation phase. Each function is then independently controlled during the scan by the small function controller.

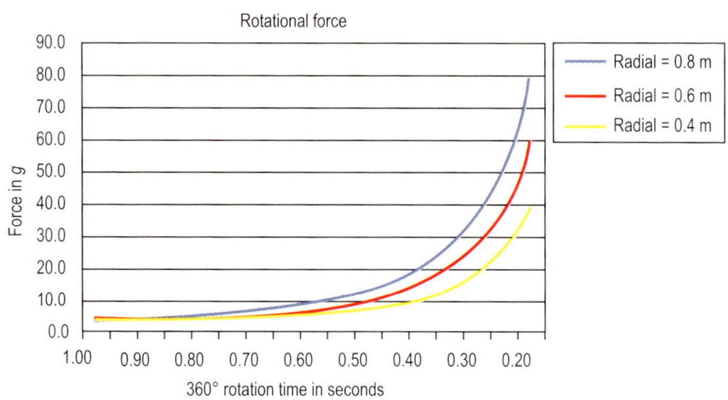

Figure 13.25
Gravitational force on gantry components at distances of 0.4 m, 0.6 m and 0.8 m from the isocenter as a function of the gantry rotation time

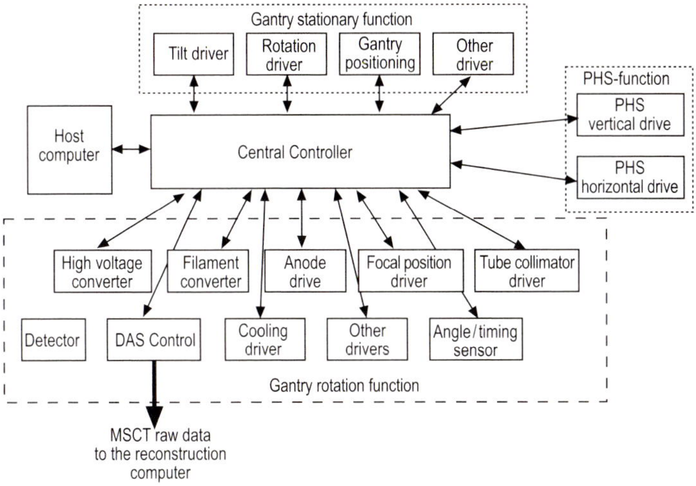

Figure 13.26 Centralized control system for an MSCT scanner

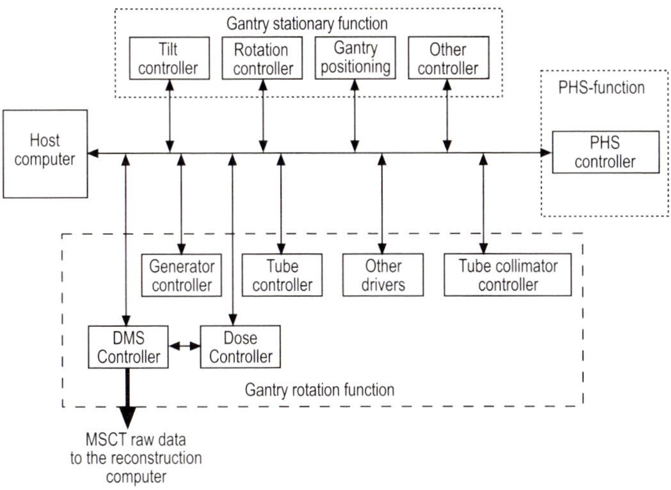

Figure 13.27 De-centralized control system for an MSCT scanner

High voltage generator

Depending on the system geometry and on the intended application spectrum, the necessary generator power will range from 40 kW to 100 kW for MSCT systems, i.e. usually at various user-selectable voltages (e.g. 80 kV, 100 kV, 120 kV and 140 kV). Different clinical applications require different X-ray spectra and hence different kV settings for optimal image quality and/or signal-to-noise ratio at the lowest dose. CT angiographic examinations, for instance, generally benefit from lower tube voltage. State-of-the-art CT generators make use of high-frequency converters that enable the scanner to start scanning at a high and stable voltage. The significance of a stable dose output has increased in light of the increasingly shorter examination times, which have now dropped to only a few seconds. One important feature of fast switching generators is the capacity to rapidly and effectively modulate the dose output according to the patient attenuation using an on-line anatomical dose-modulation approach such as CARE Dose 4D. This technique has been introduced to reduce the overall patient dose.

X-ray tube

MSCT tube design has been governed over the past few years by the high power demands for faster gantry rotation speeds and increased spatial resolution. Conventional tube design includes an anode plate with a typical diameter of 160 to 220 mm that rotates in a vacuum housing (see section 12.1). The heat storage capacity of the anode plate and the tube housing determines the performance level. Design efforts aim at increasing both the heat storage capacity and the heat dissipation rate, for instance, by increasing the anode diameter, by using circular grooves in the anode support to increase the contact area for improved cooling, or by employing special liquid-metal vacuum bearings that allow for faster anode rotation. The rotating envelope tube (e.g. STRATON) represents an alternative design (figs. 12.18 and 12.19). Thanks to their fast anode cooling rotating envelope tubes are capable of performing high-power scans in rapid succession. The performance of both conventional and rotating envelope tubes is ultimately limited by the maximum heat dissipation of the CT system itself. The absence of moving parts and bearings in the vacuum permits a compact tube design (anode diameter of 12 cm) and greater resistance to the high gravitational forces associated with gantry rotation times of < 0.4 s. However, the weight of the anode plates in conventional X-ray tubes has become more problematic as a result of the increasing rotational speeds.

The capacity to ensure the stability of both the size and the position of the focal spot relative to the detector represents an important requirement for CT tubes. The position of the focal spot in modern MSCT systems is controlled by an electromagnetic deflection system with a high-precision driver. The concept of an in-plane flying focal spot was introduced along with conventional X-ray tubes. The focus periodically moves between two slightly shifted positions in the fan-angle direction (β-direction), with the aim of improving sampling to increase in-plane resolution and reduce sampling artifacts. The STRATON tube has an even more versatile electromagnetic deflection system. Its central rotating cathode requires the permanent electromagnetic deflection of the electron beam for the sake of positioning and shaping the focal spot on the anode. The STRATON tube enables one to use an additional flying focal spot in the z-direction, which is a prerequisite for the double z-sampling technology used in the recently introduced SOMATOM Sensation 64 (a 64-slice CT system).

Tube collimator (pre-patient collimator)

The tube collimator (pre-patient collimator) is used to shape the X-ray fan beam before it penetrates the patient. A set of collimator blades made of highly absorbing materials such as tungsten or molybdenum is positioned behind the tube entrance window. The opening of these blades is adjusted according to the selected slice width and the size and position of the focal spot. Various additional pre-filters (e.g. bowtie filters) can usually be moved into the X-ray beam to modify both its spectrum and intensity distribution. The stability of the collimator opening throughout the entire examination (i.e. its imperviousness to rotational forces) is essential for excellent image quality. It is necessary to perform the tasks of positioning the collimator blades and changing the collimator opening sufficiently quickly so as to avoid influencing the detector signal.

Data measurement system (DMS)

The data measurement system (DMS) is comprised of the detector, the electronics to convert the small analog detector signal into a digital signal, and the detector controller, which combines the measurement data with the necessary system data.

Gantry drive

While belt drives were commonly used in previous generations of CT gantries and CT systems with low rotation speeds, state-of-the-art CT gantries make use of direct drives because they are more precise and stable and because they permit higher rotation speeds. Direct drives are comprised of a multipole stator and a rotor with permanent magnets.

Various techniques can be used to measure the actual angular position of the gantry's rotating part. The actual angular position in position-triggered systems is measured by an encoder that is directly connected to the rotating drum. In the case of time-triggered systems, a fixed time slot is defined for the sake of collecting data for each view. A reference position for each rotation is required in both systems so as to prevent any over or underrunning of the counting pulses.

Gantry bearing

The main bearing is required to enable a firm, uniform rotation with as little torque as possible. Given the increasing speed of today's MSCT systems, the bearing has become a major source of the noise produced during rotation. It is necessary to keep the rotation speed of the bearing balls as low as possible within the tight spatial confines of the bearing itself in order to effectively minimize noise. Modern MSCT scanners reach rotation speeds of 3 rotations per second or 180 rpm.

Power and data transmission

The link between the stationary and rotating parts of the gantry becomes a bit of a technical challenge as the rotation speeds increase. The generator supply requires a current of more than 100 A. A large brush contact area is necessary to transfer this current via carbon brushes and slip-rings. The fast rotation means that these brushes will be subject to heavy wear and carbon dust. This makes it necessary to clean the gantries periodically. The electronic noise generated by the brushes should be kept at a sufficiently low level to prevent any distortion in the signal path for data transfer.

Given the increasing number of detector rows and decreasing gantry rotation times, the data transmission systems used by the MSCT scanners must be capable of handling high transmission rates: a 4-slice CT system with a rotation time of 0.5 s generates roughly 1,000 × 700 × 4 × 2 bytes (5.6 MB) of data per rotation (i.e. 11.2 MB/s), a 16-slice CT scanner with the same rotation time generates 45 MB/s and a 64-slice CT system can produce up to 180 to 200 MB/s. This stream of data represents a challenge for data transmission off the gantry and for real-time data processing in the downstream image reconstruction systems. Contactless transmission technology is generally used in modern CT systems to handle data transfer that is either based on laser transmission or electromagnetic transmission. Laser transmission systems involve the sending of data from the rotating part of the gantry to the stationary part via a laser diode, with the stationary part being outfitted with several equidistant receivers to ensure that the laser always strikes one receiver. A stack of laser diodes can be used in combination with appropriate multiplexing/de-multiplexing methods to increase the data transmission rate. An electromagnetic transmission system uses the coupling between a rotating transmission ring antenna and a stationary receiving antenna. This technology is currently used in the SOMATOM MSCT family.

Gantry cooling

Cooling is a major requirement when it comes to modern MSCT systems that are designed to accommodate up to 100 kW of tube power and very high patient throughput. Low cost CT systems use fans to dissipate the expended thermal power into the air-conditioned examination room. The drawbacks associated with air cooling include the noise generated by the fans and the potential contamination of the examination room via the dust and dirt that comes with the heavy airflow (up to 4,000 m^3 air/h is required). Air-cooled systems thus qualify as problematic in the case of interventional applications. High-end CT systems such as those in the SOMATOM Sensation family use water cooling. A closed gantry distributes the expended thermal power to a heat exchanger inside the gantry where it is transported via water to a cooling device outside of the examination room.

Gantry control elements

All of the necessary control elements for patient positioning and for preparing ECG-controlled examinations are located on the gantry covers. Some of the positioning functions can be executed both from the front and from the back of the gantry, i.e. to give the clinic staff maximum workflow flexibility. Some MSCT systems that are equipped for cardiac scanning include the display of the ECG signal on the gantry screen.

Patient handling system (PHS)

Key requirements for the PHS include positioning accuracy and the capacity to transport the patient at constant speeds during spiral scanning. The table position measurements are added to the raw CT data for the sake of image reconstruction. The PHS can be moved vertically to enable one to position the patient at the isocenter. Positioning lasers in the gantry support the operator when it comes to the vertical and horizontal positioning of the patient on the table. Table stability is a major requirement for radiotherapy planning. While it is important to avoid overlaying the location of the tumor due to table instability and bending, it is also essential that the board on which the patient is positioned in the gantry does not produce any image artifacts. This places limits on the thickness of the board itself and the materials used.

13.3.2 Detector design for MSCT

Various detector technologies have been used since the introduction of CT. Gas detectors, frequently used in previous generations of single-slice CT systems, essentially consist of a wire chamber filled with xenon at high pressure (20 to 25 bar). Gas detectors have meanwhile become obsolete due to their limited detection efficiency. Furthermore, they cannot be extended to multi-slice systems.

Modern CT systems generally use solid-state detectors. Each detector element consists of a radiation-sensitive solid-state material (such as cadmium tungstate, gadolinium oxide and gadolinium oxisulfide) combined with suitable doping agents to convert the

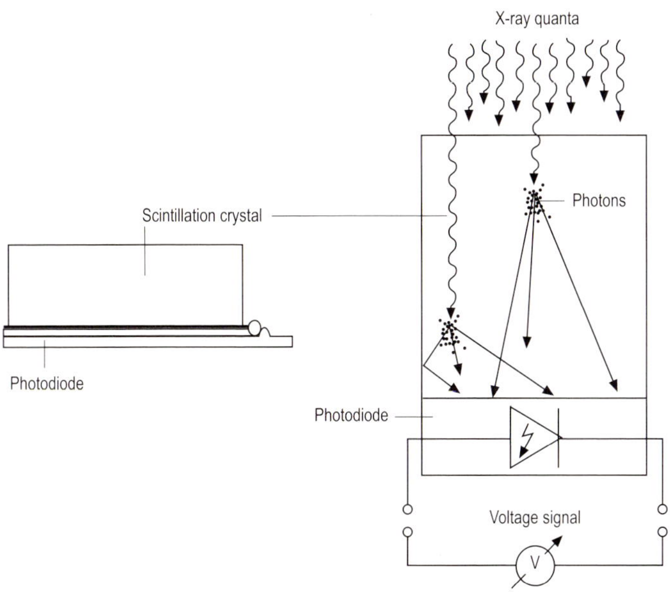

Figure 13.28 Detection principle of a solid-state CT detector

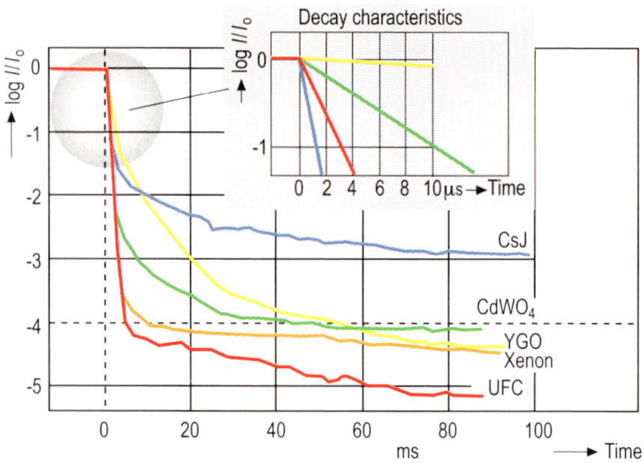

Figure 13.29 UFC afterglow characteristics compared to those of other detector materials

absorbed X-rays into visible light. The light is then detected by a Si photodiode. The resulting electrical current is amplified and converted into a digital signal. The detection principle is illustrated in fig. 13.28.

The key specifications for a suitable detector material include high detection efficiency (i.e. high atomic number) and very short afterglow times to enable the fast gantry rotation speeds that are essential for ECG-gated cardiac imaging. The detector itself is to be constructed in a way that ensures both a geometric efficiency of better than 80% and anti-scatter collimation. The typical sample rate for a modern CT detector is 5 kHz (i.e. one view is acquired every 200 µs). The UFC (ultra fast ceramics) material used in Siemens detectors is optimized to ensure extremely short afterglow times (fig. 13.29). Once the radiation has been switched off, the signal drops by two orders of magnitude in less than 500 µs and by four orders of magnitude in 3.5 ms.

Further requirements for a suitable CT detector include high dynamic range (> 16 bit), good linearity, minimal radiation drift and low-noise measurement electronics (< 6 ppm full scale electronic noise). The purpose of the latter requirement is to ensure that data noise is dominated by quantum noise and not by electronic noise.

The CT detector must allow for different slice widths to enable one to adjust the optimum scanning speed, z-resolution and image noise for each application. When using a single-slice CT detector, different collimated slice widths are obtained via a pre-patient collimation of the X-ray beam. When using a very elementary model of a 2-slice CT detector consisting of $M = 2$ detector rows, different slice widths can be obtained by pre-patient collimation if the detector is separated midway along the z-extent of the X-ray beam.

Whenever $M > 2$, it will be necessary to replace this simple design principle with more flexible concepts requiring more than M detector rows to simultaneously acquire M slices. The various manufacturers of MSCT scanners have introduced various detector designs. All of these scanners combine several detector rows electronically to a smaller number of slices according to the selected beam collimation and the desired slice width in order to permit one to select different slice widths.

Two detector types are commonly used in the 4-slice CT systems introduced in 1998. The first is the fixed-array detector that consists of detector elements of equal size in the longitudinal direction. An example of this scanner type is the Lightspeed scanner manufactured by General Electric (GE). This scanner has 16 detector rows. Each row defines a collimated slice width of 1.25 mm in the center of rotation [13.15, 13.17, 13.19]. The total coverage in the longitudinal direction is 20 mm at isocenter, with the actual detector being about twice as wide due to geometrical magnification. The following slice widths (measured at the isocenter) are realized via pre-patient collimation and by combining the signals of the individual detector rows: 4 × 1.25 mm, 4 × 2.5 mm, 4 × 3.75 mm, 4 × 5 mm (fig. 13.30, top left). The same detector design is used for the 8-slice version of this system, which provides collimated slice widths of 8 × 1.25 mm and 8 × 2.5 mm.

The second type of detector involves the use of an adaptive-array design that is comprised of detector rows of different sizes in the longitudinal direction. Scanners of this type (e.g. the Philips Mx8000 4-slice scanner and the Siemens SOMATOM Sensation 4 scanner) have 8 detector rows [13.14]. Their widths in the longitudinal direction range from 1 mm to 5 mm (at the isocenter) and allow for the following collimated slice widths: 2 × 0.5 mm, 4 × 1 mm, 4 × 2.5 mm, 4 × 5 mm, 2 × 8 mm and 2 × 10 mm (see fig. 13.30, center left).

The selection of the collimated slice width determines the intrinsic longitudinal resolution of a scan. Any multiple of one detector slice's collimated width can be obtained in step-and-shoot axial mode by adding the detector signals during image reconstruction. The effective slice width in spiral mode, which is usually defined as the full width at half maximum (*FWHM*) of the spiral slice sensitivity profile (SSP), is adjusted separately in the spiral interpolation process during image reconstruction. Both narrow slices for high-resolution detail or for 3D post-processing and wide slices for better low contrast resolution or quick review and filming can thus be derived from the same data set.

The available 16-slice CT systems are generally equipped with adaptive-array detectors. An example of this scanner type is the Siemens SOMATOM Sensation 16 scanner, which uses 24 detector rows [13.20]. The 16 central rows define a collimated slice width of 0.75 mm at the isocenter, the 4 outer rows on both sides define a collimated slice width of 1.5 mm (fig. 13.30, bottom left). The total coverage in the longitudinal direction is 24 mm at the isocenter. One can acquire either 12 or 16 slices (with collimated slice widths of 0.75 mm or 1.5 mm) simultaneously by appropriately combining the signals in the individual detector rows. The GE Lightspeed 16 scanner makes use of a similar design that provides 16 slices with a collimated slice width of either 0.625 mm or 1.25 mm. The total coverage in the longitudinal direction is 20 mm at the isocenter. The Toshiba Aquilion scanner implements yet another design that permits the use of 16 slices with a collimated slice width of 0.5 mm, 1 mm or 2 mm and with a total coverage of 32 mm at the isocenter.

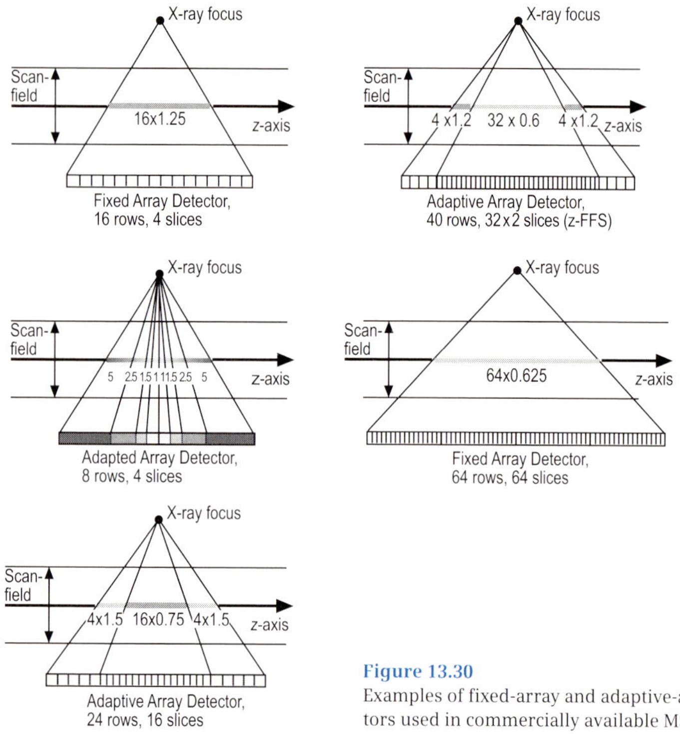

Figure 13.30
Examples of fixed-array and adaptive-array detectors used in commercially available MSCT systems

The latest generation of MSCT systems providing more than 16 slices was introduced in 2004. The Siemens SOMATOM Sensation 64 scanner is equipped with an adaptive-array detector that has 40 detector rows. The 32 central rows define a collimated slice width at the isocenter of 0.6 mm, the 4 outer rows on both sides define a collimated slice width of 1.2 mm (fig. 13.30, upper right). The total coverage in the longitudinal direction is 28.8 mm. The deployment of periodic focal spot motion in the z-direction (z-flying focal spot) enables one to shift two subsequent 32-slice readings with a collimated slice width of 0.6 mm slightly in the z-direction and combine them into one 64-slice projection with a sampling distance of 0.3 mm at the isocenter, and thereby acquire 64 overlapping 0.6 mm slices per rotation. Alternatively, one can acquire 24 slices with 1.2 mm slice width. The Toshiba, Philips and GE systems are equipped with fixed array detectors. The Toshiba Aquilion scanner has 64 detector rows with a collimated slice width of 0.5 mm. Appropriate combining of the signals of the individual detectors enables one to acquire either 64 slices with 0.5 mm slice width or 32 slices with 1 mm slice width. The total z-coverage at the iso-center is 32 mm. Both the GE VCT scanner and the Philips Brilliance 64 have 64 detector rows with a collimated slice width of 0.625 mm, thus enabling the simultaneous read-out of 64 slices (see fig. 13.30, center right) with a total coverage of 40 mm in the longitudinal direction.

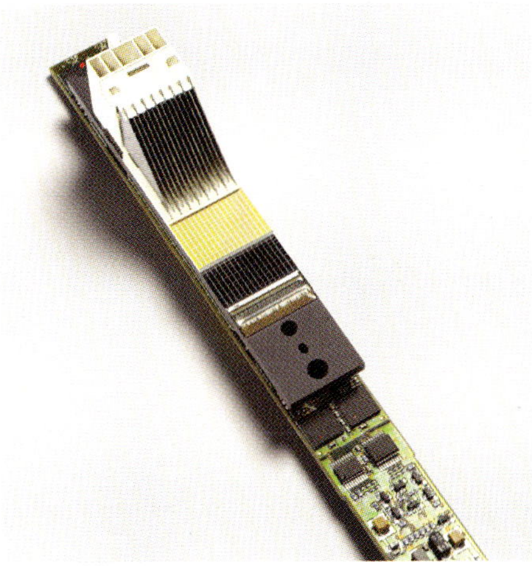

Figure 13.31
Detector module (SOMATOM Sensation 64). Each module consists of 40 × 16 detector pixels with the corresponding electronics. The anti-scatter collimators are cut diagonally so as to open the view onto the detector ceramics (yellow).

Fig. 13.31 shows a picture of one of the SOMATOM Sensation 64's detector modules. Each module consists of 40 × 16 detector pixels and the corresponding electronics. The anti-scatter collimators are cut diagonally so as to open the view onto the detector ceramics.

13.3.3 The cone-angle problem

The methods of two-dimensional image reconstruction that are used in commercially available single-slice CT scanners (e.g. convolution-backprojection reconstruction) require that all of the measurement rays that contribute to an image run in a plane perpendicular to the patient's longitudinal axis. This requirement is violated in MSCT systems. Fig. 13.32 shows the geometry of a 4-slice scanner: the measurement rays are tilted with respect to the center plane by the so-called cone angle. The cone angle is largest for the slices at the outer edges of the detector and it increases as the number of detector rows increases so long as their width remains constant.

The cone angle τ for detector row m in an M-slice scanner can be expressed as:

$$\tan(\tau) = \left(\frac{M-1}{2} - m\right)\frac{S}{R_F} \qquad (13.32)$$

where m counts from 0 to $M-1$, S is the collimated slice width of a detector row at the isocenter and R_F is the focus-isocenter distance. As a first approximation, the cone angle is neglected in MSCT reconstruction approaches: the measurement rays are treated as if they traveled perpendicular to the z-axis and modified two-dimensional image reconstruction algorithms are used. The resulting data, however, are inconsistent, and this inconsistency leads to the creation of cone-beam artifacts in high-contrast objects such as bones. While interchanging the positions of the X-ray tube and the detector will lead to the acquisition of identical measurement values in single-slice CT systems, this is not the case with MSCT systems, owing to the cone angle of the measure-

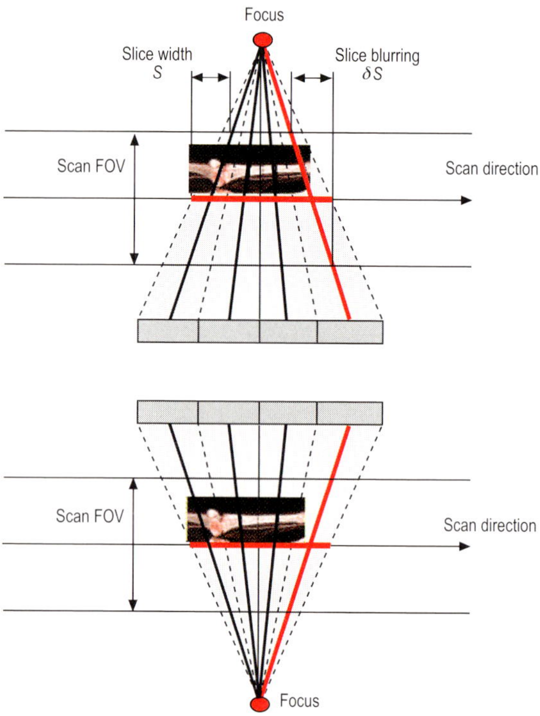

Figure 13.32
Geometry of a 4-slice CT scanner demonstrating the cone-angle problem: the measurement rays are tilted with respect to the center plane by the so-called cone angle. **Top** and **bottom**: illustration of two different axial-scan viewing angles that are shifted by 180° so that the positions of the X-ray tube and the detector are interchanged. Single-slice CT systems yield identical measurement values. MSCT systems yield different measurement values and their acquired data are inconsistent.

ment rays. Furthermore, the slices of nominal slice width S suffer from widening and SSP degradation (fig. 13.32). The slice broadening δs is a good indicator of whether one may justifiably neglect the cone angle of the measurement rays for a given scanner geometry. δs can be expressed as follows for a multi-slice CT scanner's outermost detector row:

$$\frac{\delta s}{S} = (M-1)\frac{R_{FOV}}{R_F} \tag{13.33}$$

R_{FOV} is the diameter of the scan field of view.

It has been demonstrated [13.21] that the ratio of $\delta s/S$ should not be allowed to exceed 1 if the user is interested in keeping cone-beam artifacts to a tolerable level in CT procedures that make use of reconstruction approaches that neglect the cone-beam geometry. The typical geometry of a medical CT system ($R_{FOV} = 250$ mm and $R_F \approx 600$ mm) leads to a maximum number of simultaneously acquired slices of $M \leq 4$.

As a consequence, the methods of image reconstruction used in all commercially available CT systems with 4 slices (and in some systems with even more slices) neglect the cone angle of the measurement rays, and either extend 180° or 360° single-slice spiral interpolation techniques to multi-slice spiral scanning (180-MLI or 360-MLI) or they introduce generalized z-filter approaches [13.23, 13.25]. While these approaches are fully adequate for 4 slices, they will lead to artifacts and image quality degradation if applied to spiral scanning with 16 or more slices.

13.3.4 MSCT spiral scan and reconstruction techniques

The advent of MSCT has lead to a reduction in the use of axial step-and-shoot scanning. The few clinical applications for which this technique is still used include head scanning, high-resolution lung scanning, perfusion CT and various interventional procedures. A detailed theoretical description of how to predict the performance of MSCT in sequential mode can be found in the literature [13.22]. Spiral/helical scanning is the method of choice for the vast majority of all MSCT examinations.

13.3.4.1 Definition of "pitch"

"Pitch" represents an important parameter by which to characterize a spiral/helical scan. According to IEC specifications (International Electrotechnical Commission 2002), the pitch p (eq.(13.9)) is given by the ratio of the table-feed per rotation to the total width of the collimated beam. This definition holds both for single-slice CT and MSCT. The definition shows whether data acquisition includes gaps ($p > 1$) or overlap ($p < 1$) in the longitudinal direction. The pitch for a 4-slice CT scanner with a collimation of 4×1 mm and a table-feed of 6 mm/rotation is $p = 6/(4{\times}1) = 6/4 = 1.5$. At a collimation of $16{\times}0.75$ mm and a table-feed of 18 mm/rotation, the pitch is also $p = 18/(16 \times 0.75) = 18/12 = 1.5$. The term "volume pitch" was also used in the early days of 4-slice CT. This term accounts for the width of a single slice in the denominator. In the case of a beam collimation of 4×1 mm, the beam consists of 4 sub-beams, each 1 mm wide at the center of rotation. Assuming a table-feed of 6 mm per rotation, the volume pitch is $p_{vol} = 6/1 = 6$. In the interest of clarity and avoiding ambiguity the term volume pitch should no longer be used.

13.3.4.2 180° and 360° multi-slice linear interpolation

The 360-LI and 180-LI single-slice spiral reconstruction can be extended to multi-slice spiral scanning in a straightforward way [13.19, 13.23, 13.24]. Both 360-MLI and 180-MLI are characterized by a projection-wise linear interpolation between two rays on either side of the image plane at z_{ima}. The cone angle of the measurement rays is not taken into account and the rays are treated as if they traveled perpendicular to the patient axis. In the interest of accounting for the multi-slice geometry, the interpolation is not restricted to data from the same detector slice. Instead, the interpolation may also be performed for two rays of different slices if these rays are closest to the image plane for the projection angle under consideration. Fig. 13.33 offers an illustration of 180-MLI and 360-MLI for a 4-slice spiral.

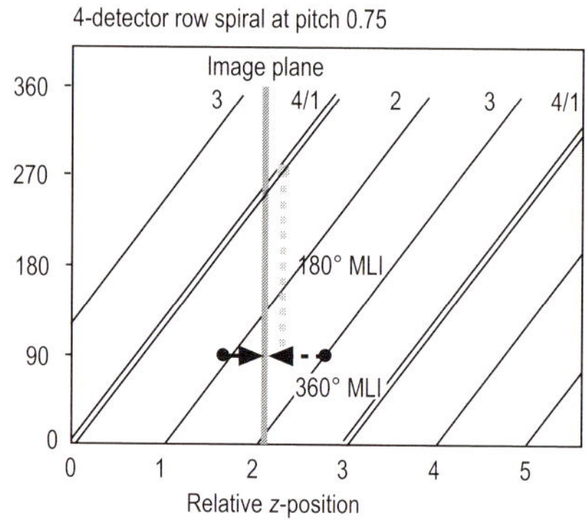

Figure 13.33
Illustration of 180-MLI and 360-MLI for a 4-slice CT system at pitch 0.75. The projection angle for the central channels of the 4 detector rows (in degrees) is indicated as a function of their relative z-positions (in multiples of the collimated slice width). The detector travels 3 collimated slice widths in a full rotation (360°) and the z-positions that were sampled by detector row 4 are resampled by detector row 1. Rays measured at the same projection angle are used in 360-MLI. These may either be taken from subsequent rotations or from different detector rows in the same rotation. Data from detector rows 2 and 3 are used for the projection angle indicated in this example (90°) and the sampling distance equals the collimated slice width (see the two dark arrows). Complementary rays from opposite directions are used in 180-MLI. These are shifted by 180° at the center of rotation. The direct interpolation partner from row 3 at 90° is replaced in this example by complementary partners from row 1 and row 4 at 270° (see the dashed light grey line). The sampling distance, which is now half the collimated slice width, yields the desired narrow SSP.

The result of the spiral interpolation is a complete set of one-dimensional fan-beam projections $L'(\beta, \alpha')$ at z_{ima} that are used as input for a conventional single-slice convolution-backprojection reconstruction. It is necessary to determine the contributing detector rows m_1 and m_2 and the index k for each projection angle α in such a way that the distances $\Delta z(\alpha, m_1) = z_{ima} - z(\alpha, m_1)$ and $\Delta z(\alpha + k2\pi, m_2) = z(\alpha + k2\pi, m_2) - z_{ima}$ of the corresponding projections $L(\beta, \alpha, m_1)$ and $L(\beta, \alpha + k2\pi, m_2)$ from the image plane at z_{ima} are minimized. The following equation represents the local sampling distance along the z-axis for 360-MLI:

$$\delta z_{360\text{-MLI}} = (Mkp - m_2 + m_1)S \tag{13.34}$$

M: Number of slices, k: Index of rotation, p: Pitch
m_1, m_2: Detector rows used at interpolation, S: Slice width

Two observations can be made from eq. (13.34):

- Up to a pitch of $p = 1$, there are always two rays, i.e. even from subsequent rotations ($k = 1$) with a distance that does not exceed the nominal slice width S. In other words: up to a pitch of 1, two 360-MLI interpolation partners can be found with a z-distance less than S for any image position z_{ima} and any projection angle α. The maximum distance S corresponds to a single slice 360-LI spiral at pitch 1.

- In contrast to single-slice spiral scanning, the sampling distance $\delta z_{360\text{-MLI}}$ is not constant, but depends on the projection angle and on the z-position under consideration (local sampling distance, nonequidistant sampling).

In the case of 360-MLI, some pitch values deserve special attention. Let us assume in the present discussion that $M = 4$. The following relation will then hold for a pitch of $p = 1/4$:

$$z(\alpha + m2\pi, m) = z(\alpha, m = 0), \quad m = 0, 1, 2, 3 \tag{13.35}$$

At a pitch of $p = 1/4$, the same z-position is sampled by all 4 slices in subsequent rotations. These measurement values may be added prior to spiral interpolation. The result is a 360-LI spiral at a pitch of 1 with 4-fold dose accumulation.

At pitch $p = 1/2$, we have a 360-LI spiral at pitch 1 with 2-fold dose accumulation. Finally, at pitch $p = 1$, the sampling scheme is again identical to that of a 360-LI spiral at pitch 1, without dose accumulation. While slightly narrower slice sensitivity profiles may be obtained for pitch values in between these special pitches, this will come at the cost of dispensing with dose accumulation.

In contrast to 180-LI single-slice spiral interpolation, which always involves the measuring of interpolation partners at opposite projection angles, the interpolation partners in 180-MLI multi-slice spiral interpolation may originate from opposite or corresponding projection angles. Again, it will be necessary to determine the contributing detector slices m_1 and m_2 for each projection angle α so as to bring about a minimization of the distances of the corresponding rays from the image plane at z_{ima}.

While the following argument resembles that used for the 360-MLI approach, it is only valid for 180-MLI at the center of rotation:

- Up to a pitch of $p = 2$, there are always two rays, i.e. even from subsequent rotations with a distance that does not exceed the nominal slice width S. In other words: up to a pitch of 2, two 180-MLI interpolation partners can be found with a z-distance of less than S at the isocenter for any image position z_{ima} and any projection angle α. The maximum distance S corresponds to a single slice 360-LI spiral at a pitch of 1 or a 180-LI spiral at a pitch of 2.

In contrast to single-slice spiral scanning there are pitch values that correspond to the falling of direct and complementary rays onto the same z-positions.

Owing to the complicated z-sampling schemes and in contrast to single-slice spiral scanning, the spiral slice sensitivity profiles for 180-MLI are not necessarily smaller than those for 360-MLI. Direct and complementary rays interleave in the z-direction at the isocenter only for selected pitch values. This leads to a significant reduction in the distance between measured samples to half of the collimated slice width S, which results in the desired narrow SSPs.

Scanners that rely on 180-MLI or 360-MLI techniques generally provide the user with selected discrete pitch values such as 0.75 and 1.5 for 4-slice scanning and 0.5625, 0.9375, 1.375 and 1.75 for 16-slice scanning. It is necessary that the user be aware of pitch-dependent effective slice widths s. For low-pitch scanning (at $p = 0.75$ using 4 slices and at $p = 0.5625$ or 0.9375 using 16 slices), $s \sim S$ and the resulting effective slice width remains at 1.25 mm for a collimated slice of 1.25 mm. The narrow SSP, however, is achieved via 180-MLI reconstruction using conjugate interpolation at the price of increased image noise. For high-pitch scanning (at $p = 1.5$ using 4 slices and at $p = 1.375$ or 1.75 using 16 slices), $s \sim 1.27\,S$ and a collimated slice width of 1.25 mm results in an effective slice width of 1.5 to 1.6 mm. It is necessary to take the widening of the SSP into account when comparing dose and image noise for different pitch values. In order to obtain the same image noise as in an axial scan of the same collimated slice width, it will be necessary to apply 0.73 to 1.68 times the dose (i.e. depending on the spiral pitch), with the lowest dose being applied at the highest pitch. Some manufacturers provide a semiautomatic adaptation of the mA value in order to keep the image noise constant when the pitch is changed. When selecting the scan protocol for a particular application, one should bear in mind that while scanning at low pitch optimizes image quality and longitudinal resolution at a given collimation, it does so at the expense of an increased patient dose. In order to reduce the patient dose, one should either reduce the mA settings at low pitch values or select high pitch values.

13.3.4.3 MSCT z-filter approaches

The spiral interpolation for each projection angle in a z-filter multidetector row spiral reconstruction [13.23, 13.25] is not restricted to the two rays in closest proximity to the image plane. All of the direct and complementary rays within a selectable distance $|z_{max}|$ from the image plane contribute to the image. The cone angle of the measurement rays, however, is still neglected. The weight of the contribution depends on the

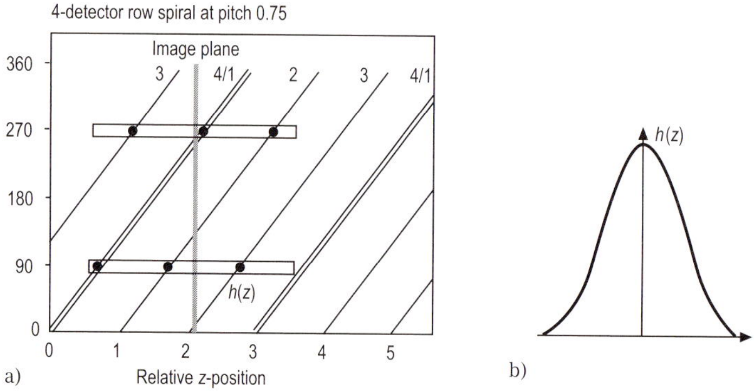

Figure 13.34
Illustration of z-filter reconstruction (adaptive axial interpolation) for a 4-slice CT system at a pitch of 0.75 (cf. fig. 13.33). The contributions from all of the projections at corresponding or opposite projection angles within a selectable distance from the image plane are used (as indicated by the two boxes at 90° and 270°). The weighting function $h(z)$ is selectable **(b)**.

distance of the respective measurement ray from the image plane. The weighting function $h(z)$ is selectable. This allows one to adjust both the functional form and the FWHM of the spiral SSP. The larger the $|z_{max}|$ is, the more the spiral SSP will widen. The MUSCOT algorithm used by Toshiba offers a good example of a z-filter approach. Another example is the adaptive axial interpolation implemented in Siemens CT scanners illustrated in fig. 13.34. The adaptive axial interpolation works on parallel projection data. The first step in the reconstruction pipeline is a partial rebinning from fan-beam multi-slice projections $L(\beta,\alpha,m)$ to non-equidistantly sampled parallel multi-slice projections $L(\beta,\theta,m)$ by resorting and interpolation in the azimuthal (i.e. projection angle direction). The second step is the actual spiral interpolation. The third and final step is the interpolation from the non-equidistant β-grid to an equidistant sampling in the p-direction for subsequent filtered backprojection.

The adaptive axial interpolation can be expressed as:

$$L'(\beta,\theta) = \sum_{v}\sum_{m} h(z_{ima} - z(\theta + v\pi, \delta_v\beta, m))L(\theta + v\pi, \delta_v\beta, m)$$
$$\delta_v = \begin{cases} 1 & \text{for even } v \\ -1 & \text{for odd } v \end{cases} \tag{13.36}$$

δ_v takes into account that $\beta' = -\beta$ for complementary projections. Given the irregular distribution of the samples along the z-axis, the sum of all weights does not necessarily add up to 1. This makes it necessary to normalize the applied weights by dividing through the weighting sum. If the weights for even and odd index v are normalized separately, the result of the adaptive axial interpolation will correspond to a 360°-type interpolation. If all v are normalized together, the result will correspond to a 180°-type interpolation.

z-filtering allows to trade off z-axis resolution (SSP) for image noise (which directly correlates to the required dose). Adaptive axial interpolation enables one to select the spiral pitch within a range of 0.5 to 2 and to generate the same effective slice width, which is defined as the *FWHM* of the spiral SSP, for all pitch values [13.14, 13.23, 13.26]. The longitudinal resolution is therefore independent of the pitch, in contrast to single-slice spiral CT and MSCT, which rely on 180-MLI and 360-MLI. The sampling scheme with multiple slices along the z-direction represents a major reason why it is possible to realize a pitch-independent SSP. Although both the sampling pattern and the sampling density vary along with the pitch, the sampling distance at the isocenter is never larger than the sub-beam collimation S for any pitch up to 2. A constant SSP is achieved by automatically adapting the functional forms and the widths of the spiral weighting functions to the pitch using edge-enhancing, linear, cosine and trapezoidal functions.

Fig. 13.35 shows the SSPs of the 2 mm slice (for a collimation of 4 × 1 mm) and multiple slice reformations (MPRs) of a spiral z-resolution phantom for selected pitch values. Given the pitch-independent spiral slice width, the image noise for a fixed mA (fixed tube current) decreases along with decreasing pitch due to the increasingly overlapping spiral acquisition. This is why the effective mAs-concept has been introduced.

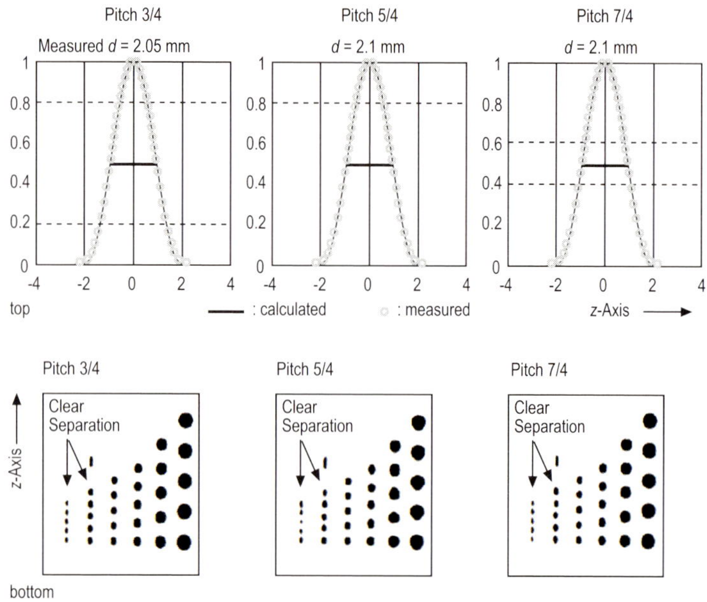

Figure 13.35
Adaptive axial interpolation for a 4-slice CT system. **Top:** SSPs of the 2 mm slice (for a collimation of 4 × 1 mm) at selected pitch values. The functional forms of the SSPs, and hence the slice widths, are independent of the pitch. **Bottom:** MPRs of a spiral *z*-resolution phantom scanned with a slice width of 2 mm show a clear separation of the 1.5 mm and 2 mm cylinders for all pitch values as a consequence of the pitch-independent SSPs.

The user selects an effective mAs value, and the tube current (mA) is automatically adapted to the pitch of the spiral scan to compensate for dose accumulation. The dose for fixed effective mAs is independent of the spiral pitch and equals the dose of an axial scan with the same mAs. In contrast to single-slice spiral CT, changing the pitch will not change the patient dose. Accordingly, the use of higher pitch will not result in dose saving, which is an important practical consideration in the case of CT systems that rely on adaptive axial interpolation.

The intrinsic resolution of a multidetector row spiral scan is determined by the choice of collimation (e.g. 4 × 1 mm or 4 × 2.5 mm). *z*-filtering enables one to reconstruct images retrospectively using different slice widths from the same raw CT data set. Only slice widths equal to or larger than the sub-beam collimation can be obtained. In many cases, both thick slices for initial viewing and filming and thin slices for detailed diagnosis or as an input for advanced 3D post-processing are routinely reconstructed.

The thinnest available slice $s = S$ (1 mm for a collimation of 4 × 1 mm) is created by using nonlinear spiral weighting functions at the cost of increased image noise and increased susceptibility to artifacts. The following equation represents a suitable weighting function:

$$h_{\text{enh}}(z) = \begin{cases} 1 + w - (0.5 + 0.75w)\dfrac{8|z|}{L} & \text{for} \quad |z| \le \dfrac{L}{4} \\ \left(\dfrac{2|z|}{L} - 1\right)w & \text{for} \quad \dfrac{L}{4} \le |z| \le \dfrac{L}{2} \\ 0 & \text{for} \quad |z| > \dfrac{L}{2} \end{cases} \tag{13.37}$$

This function is used for the high resolution modes of the SOMATOM Sensation 4 with enhancement parameter $w = 0.05$. The thinnest available slice should only be used in clinical routine for high-contrast applications such as high-resolution lung imaging. A slice width of 1.25 mm for a collimation of 4 × 1 mm (and 3 mm slice width for 4 × 2.5 mm collimation) is recommended for general purpose scanning as the most suitable trade-off among the factors longitudinal resolution, image noise and artifacts, in particular, when thin slices are reconstructed as input for 3D post-processing such as MPR, MIP and VRT. In the case of a spiral slice width of 1.25 mm that is reconstructed from a collimation of 4 × 1 mm, one is required to apply 0.61 to 0.69 times the dose (depending only slightly on the spiral pitch) in order to maintain the image noise of an axial scan at the same collimation. In contrast to 180-MLI and 360-MLI, image noise is therefore practically independent of the pitch at a constant dose.

Image quality can be optimized with regard to spiral artifacts for a given collimation (e.g. 4 × 2.5 mm) by lowering the pitch . Another means of reducing spiral artifacts is to use a narrow collimation: a given slice width (e.g. 3 mm) can be obtained with different collimations (in this case 4 × 1 mm and 4 × 2.5 mm). It is advisable to use a narrow collimation relative to the desired slice width in order to achieve optimal image quality and to bring about a more rectangular SSP. As with single-slice spiral CT, narrow collimation at high pitch is preferable to wide collimation at low pitch when it comes to artifact reduction.

With the exception of a minor dose increase due to the different relative contributions of the dose profile's penumbral zones, scanning at narrow collimation does not result in higher radiation dose to the patient as long as the effective mAs is kept constant.

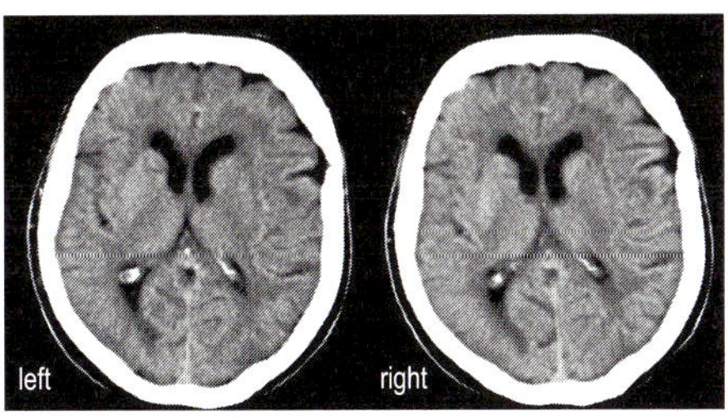

Figure 13.36
Head examination using a 4-slice CT system, offering a comparison of an axial scan (2 × 8 mm, **left**) and a spiral scan (8 mm slice width from 4 × 1 mm collimation, **right**) for the same patient. The image quality can be considered equivalent owing to the narrow-collimation z-filter reconstruction. (Source: Dr. R. Bruening, Klinikum Großhadern, Munich, Germany)

The protocol of choice for all applications that require 3D post-processing as a part of the clinical evaluation should therefore include narrow-collimation scanning. The use of wider collimation may be considered when it comes to the clinical management of uncooperative patients or trauma victims or for protocols involving routine oncological staging. The best suppression of spiral artifacts can be achieved by using both narrow collimation relative to the desired slice width and reducing the spiral pitch. In general, protocols that involve more challenging clinical examinations (e.g. of the spine and of the skull base) rely on a combination of narrow collimation and low pitch. When multidetector row spiral scanning of the head is performed with narrow collimation, low pitch and z-filter reconstruction of wider slices, the results are equivalent to traditional axial sequential CT scanning. Fig. 13.36 shows a head scan generated by a 4-slice CT system that offers a comparison of an axial scan (2 × 8 mm, left) and a spiral scan (8 mm slice width from 4x1 mm collimation, right) for the same patient.

Some manufacturers of systems that use z-filter approaches do not place spiral pitch entirely at the discretion of the user. Instead, these systems operate on the basis of a recommended selection of fixed pitch values that are determined in the interest of optimizing the z-sampling scheme and reducing spiral artifacts. These fixed values might include, for instance, pitches of 0.625, 0.75, 0.875, 1.125, 1.25, 1.375 and 1.5 for 4-slice scanning (MUSCOT algorithm).

13.3.4.4 MSCT reconstruction algorithms for the cone-beam problem

It is necessary to consider modified reconstruction approaches that account for the cone-beam geometry of the measurement rays in the case of CT scanners with 16 or more slices. Cone-beam reconstruction algorithms can be broken down into two classes: *exact algorithms* and *approximate algorithms*. Exact cone-beam reconstruction approaches [13.27, 13.28] rely on 3D radon inversion and offer a theoretically exact solution to the cone-beam reconstruction problem. 3D radon inversion is a generalization of the 2D case. A two-dimensional function – in the context of medical CT, this is the patient's X-ray attenuation coefficients in an axial slice – can be reconstructed when all of the function's line integrals are known. These line integrals are the measurement values in standard single-slice CT. A three-dimensional function – the patient's X-ray attenuation coefficients in the entire examination volume – can be reconstructed when all of the function's plane integrals are known. This, however, is a difficult task because the primary measurement values in cone-beam CT are also line integrals and plane integrals are not easy to obtain. As a consequence, exact image reconstruction approaches are computationally expensive and result in image reconstruction times that far exceed what would be acceptable in a clinical environment. An exact multi-slice spiral reconstruction algorithm that does not use 3D radon inversion has been proposed recently [13.29]. While this approach shows promise with respect to reduced computational complexity, it is still in the developmental stage.

Approximations are used in the field of approximate multi-slice spiral algorithms to handle the cone-beam geometry. Most approaches involve extending two-dimensional convolution-backprojection reconstruction algorithms to three dimensions. Although these algorithms are theoretically not exact, image artifacts may be controlled for a moderate cone angle and a moderate number of simultaneously acquired slices and kept at a level tolerable for medical CT. All of the commercially available MSCT systems that provide cone-beam reconstruction rely on approximate algorithms. Some manufacturers (Toshiba, Philips) extend the Feldkamp algorithm [13.30], an approximate 3D-filtered backprojection reconstruction that was originally introduced for axial scanning (see chapter 10), to multidetector row spiral scanning [13.31, 13.32]. Other manufacturers use variations and extensions of nutating slice algorithms [13.33, 13.34, 13.35] that split the 3D reconstruction task into a series of conventional 2D reconstructions on tilted intermediate image planes. Examples of such algorithms include the adaptive multiple plane reconstruction (AMPR) used by Siemens [13.36, 13.37] and the weighted hyperplane reconstruction (WHR) proposed by GE [13.38].

3D-filtered backprojection

An example of a 3D convolution-backprojection reconstruction is the true cone beam tomography algorithm (TCOT) implemented in the Toshiba 16-slice , 32-slice and 64-slice scanners. The algorithm involves subjecting the measurement rays to a filter operation (convolution) in the fan-angle direction β and then backprojecting them into a 3D volume along the lines of measurement, thereby accounting for their cone-beam geometry. In order to reconstruct a pixel i located at the coordinates (x_i, y_i) on the image plane of interest, the ray that passes from the X-ray source through the pixel to the detector array is selected for each viewing angle α. This backprojection ray falls on the detector at fan angle β and slice position d. The filtered detector values for all ray sums passing through the pixel for all views are summed up and normalized to create the final reconstructed image. 3D backprojection is computationally demanding and requires dedicated hardware to achieve acceptable image reconstruction times.

It has recently been shown that the choice of the proper direction along which the data are to be filtered is of critical importance for the degree of image quality achieved using 3D-filtered backprojection [13.39]. If the fan beam projections are filtered along the fan-angle direction β, as proposed in the original Wang algorithm [13.31], severe artifacts appear for larger cone angles (fig. 13.37, left). Filtering the data in the direc-

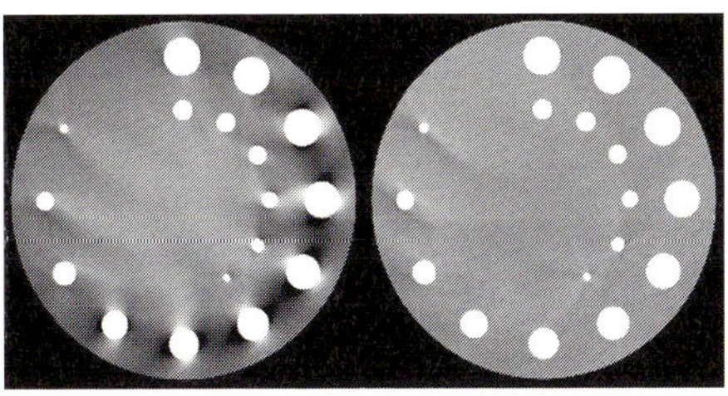

Figure 13.37
3D-filtered backprojection reconstruction of the Turbell clock phantom for scanning data with a collimation of 64×1 mm and a pitch of 1. The phantom's diameter is 480 mm. **Left:** filtering of the fan data along the detector-row direction causes severe artifacts. **Right:** filtering of the rebinned data in the direction of the spiral tangent considerably reduces artifacts.

tion of the spiral tangent can markedly improve image quality (fig. 13.37, right). Filtering the data in the p-direction after rebinning to parallel geometry represents a good approximation in this context.

Adaptive multiple plane reconstruction (AMPR)

The AMPR algorithm is an extension and generalization of the advanced single-slice rebinning (ASSR) algorithm [13.33, 13.35]. AMPR allows one to freely select the spiral pitch with optimized dose utilization, which is beneficial for medical applications.

The ASSR algorithm involves the use of a partial-scan data interval in fan-beam geometry ($\pi + \beta_{fan}$), which corresponds to a π-segment of data in parallel geometry after rebinning, for image reconstruction. The image planes are no longer perpendicular to the patient axis, but are tilted to match the spiral path of the focal spot. The focal spot is positioned in or near the image plane for every viewing angle in this partial scan interval, i. e. measurement rays running in or very close to the image plane are available. These conditions need to be fulfilled for a standard 2D reconstruction. The mean squared z-distances of all focus positions on the spiral segment to the image plane are minimized in order to determine the optimal tilt angle. The image plane in our geometry using reference angle $\theta_r = 0$ is tilted by an angle γ around the x-axis. The normal vector for this plane is:

$$\vec{n}_{\mathrm{ASSR}}(\gamma) = \begin{pmatrix} 0 \\ -\sin\gamma \\ \cos\gamma \end{pmatrix} \qquad (13.38)$$

The optimal tilt angle γ depends on the pitch p. The scan geometry, including a tilted image plane, is illustrated in fig. 13.38. The traditional axial images are calculated in a final z-reformation step via an interpolation involving the original tilted image planes.

ASSR encounters its limitations when the spiral pitch is reduced to make use of the overlapping spiral acquisition and the resulting dose accumulation. Using a range of projection angles much larger than π (in parallel geometry) for an image makes it impossible to optimally fit the image plane to the spiral path. The AMPR algorithm addresses this problem: instead of using all of the available data for a single image, the data are distributed to several partial images on double oblique image planes that are individually adapted to the spiral path. In order to ensure full dose utilization, the number of partial images as well as the length of the data interval per image are made to depend on the spiral pitch. Any given z-position z_{ima} at pitch p will be measured by a spiral segment of length $2\pi/p$ (in parallel geometry). This spiral segment is subdivided according to the AMPR into a number n_{ima} of overlapping subsegments, each exhibiting the length $\theta_{sub} \geq \pi$ and separated by a maximum of π. An individual image with an optimally adjusted image plane is calculated at z_{ima} for each of these subsegments. Any subsegment of length θ_{sub} and centered at reference angle θ_r will equivalently be used to calculate n_{ima} images at different z-positions with differently tilted image planes. Given that each of these n_{ima} partial images has the same reference projection angle, the images fan out like the pages of a book. Subsegments centered at $\theta_r = 0$ are handled by introducing a tilt angle around the y-axis in addition to

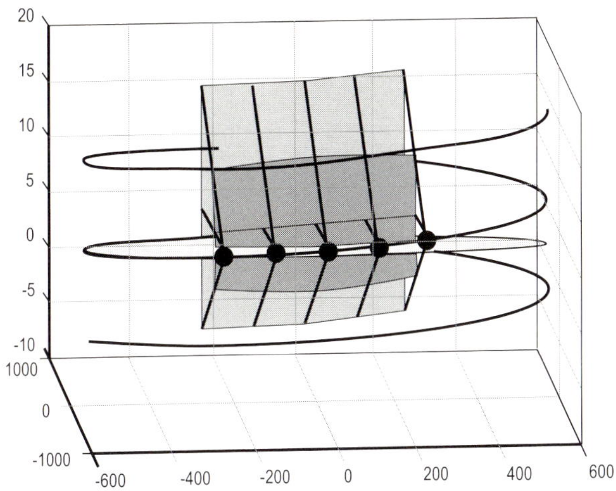

Figure 13.38
Illustration of the ASSR algorithm (data in mm). The image plane is attached to the focus at reference projection angle $\theta_r = 0$ (see left side of figure). It is tilted by an angle γ around the x-axis (with normal vector $\vec{n}_{ASSR}$). A parallel projection at projection angle $\theta = \pi/2$ is indicated. The dots represent the focus positions for selected rays within this parallel projection. Both the virtual detector D_c located in the center of rotation and the physical detector D_P that results from parallel rebinning are plotted. The reconstruction plane optimally fits the spiral path in a projection angle range $(-\pi/2, \pi/2)$.

the tilt angle around the x-axis. The normal vector of the respective image plane can then be expressed as:

$$\vec{n}(\gamma, \delta) = \begin{pmatrix} \sin\delta \\ -\cos\delta\sin\gamma \\ \cos\delta\cos\gamma \end{pmatrix} \tag{13.39}$$

The scan geometry is illustrated in fig. 13.39. γ and δ are again determined by an optimization process. First, γ is optimized for $\delta = 0$, i.e. in the same way as in the original ASSR approach. Using this optimized γ_0 we optimize δ. The optimization criterion for δ is two-fold. On the one hand, the intersection line of the image plane with a virtual detector in the center of rotation, which is obtained by projection from the actual detector, must be contained within the active detector area for any projection angle within the subsegment of length θ_{sub}. On the other hand, the intersection lines for all partial images should make use of as much of the detector area as possible for optimal dose utilization.

Using the optimal δ_{max}, the available range of tilt angles $-\delta_{max} \dots \delta_{max}$ is subdivided for the n_{ima} images that are to be calculated. Each image plane $0 \le i \le n_{ima} - 1$ is characterized by the tilt angles γ_0 (which are the same for all planes in our approach) and

$$\delta_i = \delta_{max} \frac{2i - (n_{ima} - 1)}{n_{ima} - 1} \tag{13.40}$$

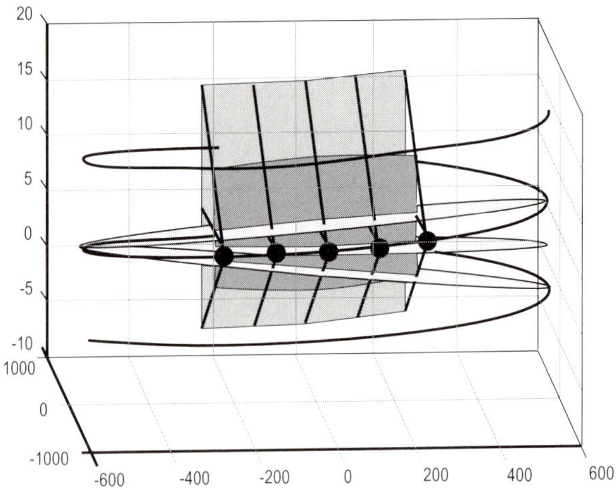

Figure 13.39
Illustration of the AMPR algorithm for a 16-slice detector at pitch $p = 0.75$ using the same perspective as in fig. 13.38. $n_{ima} = 3$ double oblique image planes are attached to the focus at reference projection angle $\theta_r = 0$ (see left side of figure). The three image planes fan out like the pages of a book. A parallel projection at projection angle $\theta = \pi/2$ is indicated. Both the virtual detector D_c located in the center of rotation and the physical detector D_p that results after parallel rebinning are plotted. The optimization of the double oblique image planes is such that the intersection lines of the image planes with the virtual detector D_c must be contained within the active detector area and make use of as much of the detector area as possible. The lowest image plane in the present case hits the lower boundary of the virtual detector.

The final axial (or arbitrarily oriented) images are calculated via z-interpolation between the tilted partial image planes. The shape and the width of the z-interpolation functions are selectable. Different SSPs and different slice widths can therefore be adjusted so that z-axis resolution (SSP) can be traded off for image noise. The spiral pitch is freely selectable and the slice width – and consequently z-axis resolution – are independent of the pitch. The concept of effective mAs and automatic adaptation of the tube current to the pitch also applies to AMPR. Excellent image quality can be obtained using the AMPR approach for all pitch values between 0.5 and 1.5. Fig. 13.40 shows an axial slice and an MPR of an anthropomorphic thorax phantom. Scanning data for a collimation of 16 × 0.75 mm at a pitch of 1 were reconstructed with a slice width of 1 mm using z-filtering (top), the AMPR algorithm (center) and 3D backprojection (bottom). Neglecting the cone angle leads to artifacts in high-contrast objects and geometric distortions, particularly in MPRs (top). AMPR (center) and 3D backprojection (bottom) restore the spatial integrity of the high-contrast objects, reduce cone-beam artifacts and are fully equivalent for 16-slice scanning. Recent studies have demonstrated the adequacy of extended versions of AMPR for medical CT systems with up to 64 rows [13.40].

The remaining artifacts in fig. 13.40 are spiral interpolation artifacts (windmill artifacts), as opposed to cone-beam artifacts. Unrelated to the cone-beam geometry, wind-

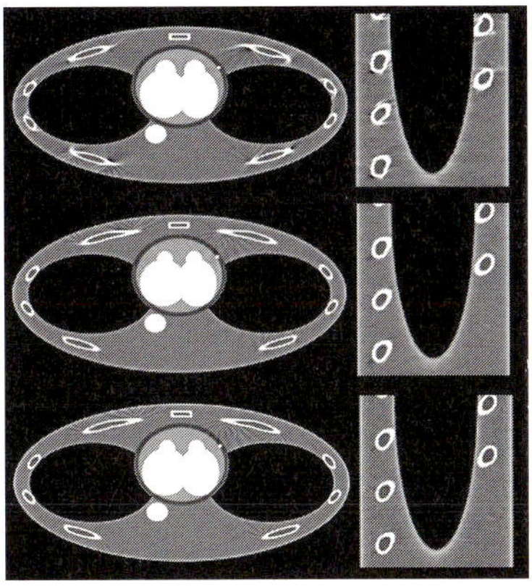

Figure 13.40
Axial slice and MPR of an anthropomorphic thorax phantom. Scan data for a collimation of 16 × 0.75 mm at a pitch of 1 were reconstructed using a slice width of 1 mm and z-filtering neglecting the cone angle of the measurement rays (top), the AMPR algorithm (center) and 3D backprojection with optimized filter direction (bottom). Neglecting the cone angle leads to artifacts in high-contrast objects, particularly in MPRs (top). AMPR (center) and 3D back-projection (bottom) reduce cone-beam artifacts and are fully equivalent for 16-slice scanning.

mill artifacts result from the finite width of the detector rows that require inter-row interpolation for image reconstruction. Their occurrence is thus independent of the reconstruction approach. They appear in exaggerated form in the mathematical phantom shown and can be reduced by either decreasing the pitch and/or increasing the reconstruction slice width relative to the collimation (fig. 13.41).

Multidetector row spiral scanning using AMPR is characterized by the same key properties as adaptive axial interpolation (as outlined in the above section on z-filter reconstruction). All of the recommendations that have been made so far regarding the selection of collimation and pitch thus also apply to AMPR. In particular, changing the pitch will not change the radiation exposure to the patient, and using higher pitch will not result in dose saving. Narrow-collimation scanning should be performed whenever possible. With a collimation of 16 × 0.75 mm, the thinnest available reconstruction slice width (0.75 mm) is created by using nonlinear weighting functions during the image z-reformation step at the expense of increased image noise and increased susceptibility to artifacts. Again, this slice should only be used for high-contrast applications such as high-resolution lung imaging. When reconstructing thin slices as input for 3D post-processing (e.g. MPR, MIP and VRT), a slice width of 1 mm is recommended as the most suitable means of balancing longitudinal resolution, image noise and artifacts.

Weighted-hyperplane reconstruction (WHR)

While weighted-hyperplane reconstruction (WHR) makes use of concepts that are related to AMPR, these concepts are derived in a different manner [13.38]. As in the case

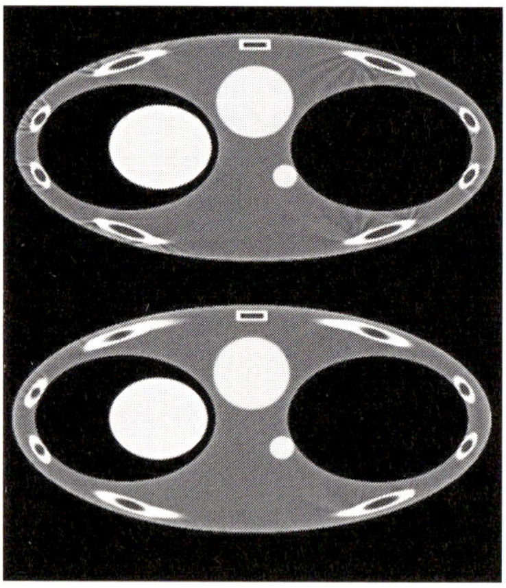

Figure 13.41
Axial slice of the anthropomorphic thorax phantom for a collimation of 16×0.75 mm at a pitch of 1, reconstructed using the AMPR approach with a slice width of 1 mm (top) and a slice width of 3 mm (bottom). Spiral interpolation artifacts are reduced when using a wider slice width relative to the collimation. Best image quality for a desired slice width can be obtained in clinical practice by acquiring narrow collimation data.

of AMPR, the 3D reconstruction is broken down into a series of 2D reconstructions. Instead of reconstructing traditional axial slices, convex hyperplanes, which are selected as sloped lines in the sinogram space, constitute the region of reconstruction. The fan angle of a measurement ray in the sinogram space is plotted as a function of its viewing angle (projection angle). Multiple convex hyperplanes with different slopes can be defined for each detector row to improve the smoothness of the interpolation. The increasing spiral overlap that occurs with decreasing pitch is handled by introducing subsets of detector rows, which offer a sufficient basis for reconstructing an image at a given pitch value. When using a 16-slice scanner at a pitch of $p = 0.5625$, the data collected by detector rows 1 to 9 form a complete projection data set. Similarly, projections from detector rows 2 to 10 can be used to reconstruct another image at the same z-position, projections from detector rows 3 to 11 yield a third image, and so on. In a way, these subimages are related to the book pages of AMPR. The final image is based on a weighted average of the subimages. Excellent image quality for a 16-slice CT system (GE Lightspeed 16) has been demonstrated using the WHR approach [13.84]. An optimal balance of various system performance parameters, including noise, artifacts and SSPs, can be achieved by performing parameter optimizations.

13.3.5 Double z-sampling

A new concept for multidetector row spiral scanning, which makes use of periodic focal spot motion in the longitudinal direction to improve data sampling along the z-axis, was introduced in 2004 [13.42]. The focal spot is wobbled between two different positions on the anode plate via the permanent electromagnetic deflection of the elec-

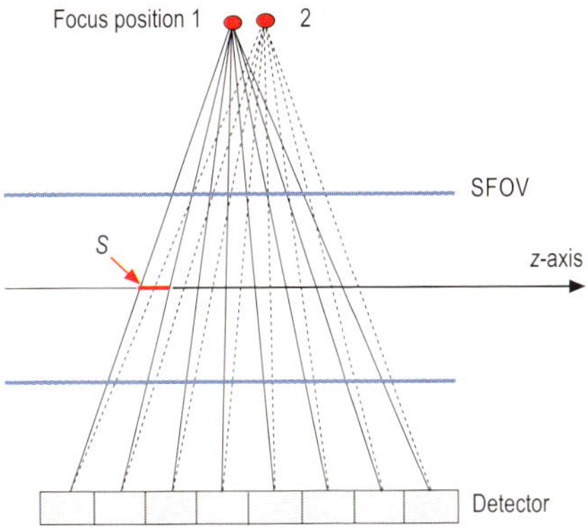

Figure 13.42
Principle of double z-sampling. Due to periodic focal spot motion in the z-direction, two subsequent *M*-slice readings are shifted by half a collimated slice width *S*/2 at isocenter and can be interleaved to one 2*M*-slice projection. To simplify the drawing, the radial motion of the focal spot is not shown.

tron beam in the X-ray tube. Given the typical anode angle of 7 to 9°, this translates into motion both in the radial direction and in the z-direction. The radial motion is a side effect that one will have to take care of in the image reconstruction, preferably during the so-called rebinning procedure, which is the interpolation of the measured fan-beam data to parallel geometry. The amplitude of the periodic z-motion is adjusted such that two subsequent readings are shifted by half a collimated slice width in the patient's longitudinal direction (fig. 13.42). The measurement rays of two subsequent readings with a collimated slice width of *S* therefore interleave in the z-direction and each pair of *M*-slice readings is combined into one 2*M*-slice projection with a sampling distance of *S*/2.

The SOMATOM Sensation 64, a multidetector CT system that relies on double z-sampling, has a detector that provides 32 collimated slices of 0.6 mm. Two subsequent 32-

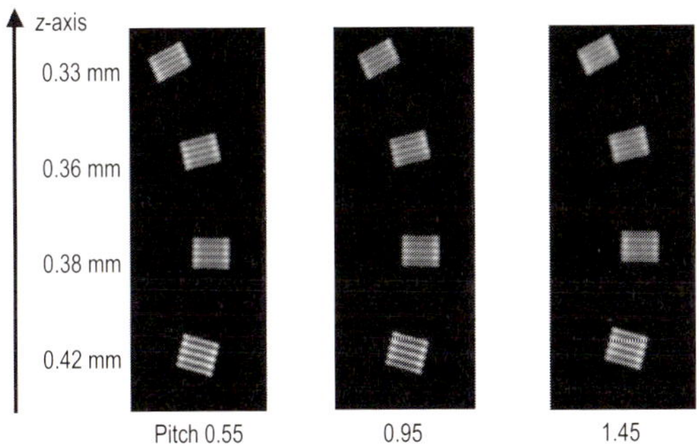

Figure 13.43
Demonstration of spatial resolution with double z-sampling. The grid pattern in the high resolution insert of the CATPHAN has been aligned in the longitudinal direction (at isocenter). The scan data have been acquired with the SOMATOM Sensation 64 with a collimation of 32 × 0.6 mm and double z-sampling using a sharp body kernel (B70). Independent of the pitch, the 0.36 mm grid is clearly visible.

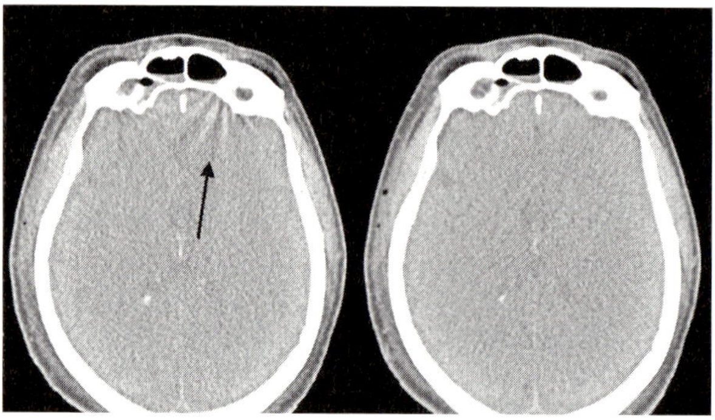

Figure 13.44
Reduction of spiral windmill artifacts via double z-sampling. **Left:** head specimen scanned using a conventional 32 × 0.6 mm scanner at a pitch of 1.4. **Right:** double z-sampling, 64 × 0.6* mm, pitch 1.4. The improved longitudinal sampling enables one to suppress spiral interpolation artifacts (the windmill structures indicated by the arrow) without causing any degradation to z-axis resolution.

slice readings are combined into a single 64-slice projection with a sampling distance of 0.3 mm at the isocenter. This technique involves the acquisition of 64 overlapping 0.6 mm slices per rotation. The sampling scheme is similar to that of a 64 × 0.3 mm detector, and the AMPR algorithm is used for image reconstruction. This enables one to increase spatial resolution in the logitudinal direction and routinely resolve objects with diameters of < 0.4 mm at any pitch (fig. 13.43). A further benefit of double z-sampling that is even more clinically relevant is the suppression of spiral windmill artifacts at any pitch (fig. 13.44). Double z-sampling provides a sampling distance of $S/2$ that is independent of the pitch. The improved sampling along the z-direction is not restricted to the isocenter, but is maintained for a large portion of the scanned field of view (SFOV). Longitudinal resolution is therefore not severely degraded for off-center objects. This represents a major difference to approaches that involve attempts to improve longitudinal resolution by specifying optimized small pitch values to ensure that data acquired in different rotations interleave in the z-direction. A sampling distance of $S/2$ in such cases is only achieved close to the isocenter.

13.3.6 Dose in MDCT

The average CT dose in the scanning plane can be best described by the weighted computerized tomographic dose index $CTDI_w$ [13.43]:

$$CTDI_w = \frac{1}{3} CTDI_{100}(\text{center}) + \frac{2}{3} CTDI_{100}(\text{periphery}) \tag{13.41}$$

The CT dose index $CTDI_{100}$ is measured using a 100 mm ionization chamber both in the center and on the periphery of a Lucite head or body phantom (with a diameter of 16 or 32 cm) for a single slice. $CTDI_w$ offers a good estimate of the average patient dose as long as the patient size is similar to the size of the respective phantoms.

$CTDI_w$, expressed in mGy, is always measured in an axial scanning mode. Its value depends on scanner geometry, slice collimation and beam prefiltration as well as on X-ray tube voltage, tube current I_{Tube} and gantry rotation time t_{rot}. The product of mA and t_{rot} is the mAs value of the scan. To obtain a parameter characteristic for the scanner, it is helpful to eliminate the mAs dependence and to introduce a normalized $(CTDI_w)_n$ expressed in mGy/mAs:

$$(CTDI_w)_n = \frac{CTDI_w}{I_{Tube}t_{rot}} \tag{13.42}$$

$CTDI_w$ is a measure of the dose in a single axial scan and depends on the X-ray tube voltage and filter (i.e. the X-ray spectrum) and on slice collimation. Both parameters are needed to fully characterize a $CTDI_w$ value. In the case of multidetector row CT systems, $CTDI_w$ tends to increase along with decreasing collimated slice widths on account of the increasing relative contribution of the penumbral zones of the dose profiles. In order to represent the dose in a spiral scan, it is essential to account for gaps and overlaps between the radiation dose profiles from consecutive rotations of the X-ray source. $CTDI_{vol}$, the volume $CTDI_w$, has been introduced for this purpose:

$$CTDI_{vol} = \frac{CTDI_w}{p} = \frac{I_{Tube}t_{rot}(CTDI_w)_n}{p} \tag{13.43}$$

The factor $1/p$ accounts for the increasing dose accumulation that is associated with decreasing spiral pitch due to the increasing spiral overlap. In general, eq. (13.43) holds for single-slice CT and for MSCT. A higher pitch is often used in single-slice CT to reduce patient radiation exposure at the expense of a wider SSP and a loss in longitudinal resolution. The image noise, however, is independent of the pitch. The situation is more complex in the case of MSCT. Many MSCT scanners use z-filter approaches for image reconstruction (see above). Owing to the increasing longitudinal sampling density (overlapping spiral sampling), z-filtering leads to decreases in image noise along with decreasing pitch so long as the tube current mA is left unchanged. It is necessary to use different mA settings (depending on the spiral pitch) in order to maintain constant image noise. Some manufacturers make provision for a semiautomatic adjustment of the mA settings upon a change in the pitch of a spiral scan. Others adapt the tube current to the pitch per default [13.14, 13.26, 13.37]. The user selects a desired image noise level (and thus a certain image quality) by choosing an effective mAs value that accounts for the pitch:

$$(mAs)_{eff} = \frac{I_{Tube}t_{rot}}{p} \tag{13.44}$$

The tube current is increased in direct proportion to the pitch in order to keep the $(mAs)_{eff}$ at a constant level. The dose of a multidetector row spiral scan can thus be expressed simply as:

$$CTDI_{vol} = (mAs)_{eff}(CTDI_w)_n \tag{13.45}$$

This procedure ensures that the spiral dose remains constant and equal to the dose of a sequential scan with the same mAs.

$CTDI_w$ is a measure of physical dose. It does not provide full information about the radiation risk associated with a CT examination. An interest in providing information about the risk of radiation was the impetus behind the introduction of the concept of effective dose by the ICRP (International Commission on Radiation Protection). The effective dose is expressed in mSv and constitutes a weighted sum of the dose applied to all organs in a CT examination, including both direct and scattered radiation. The weighting factors depend on the biological radiation sensitivities of the respective organs. The effective dose can be measured using whole-body phantoms (e.g. the Alderson phantom) or computer simulations based on Monte Carlo techniques to determine scattered radiation. Typical values for the effective patient dose that are specified in CT protocols include 1 to 2 mSv for a head examination, 5 to 7 mSv for a chest CT and 8 to 11 mSv for a CT of the abdomen and pelvis. These degrees of radiation exposure can be best understood in relation to the average annual background radiation, which is 2 to 5 mSv (3.6 mSv in the United States).

13.4 Multi-slice cardiac CT

13.4.1 Introduction

Cardiac imaging represents a demanding application for any noninvasive imaging modality. On the one hand, high temporal resolution is required in order to virtually freeze the cardiac motion and to avoid motion artifacts. On the other hand, sufficient spatial resolution – ideally submillimeter – is required to adequately visualize small and complex anatomical structures such as the coronary arteries. Moreover, it is necessary to examine the entire heart volume within one short breath-hold so as to avoid breathing artifacts and to limit the amount of contrast agent. Electron beam CT (EBCT) was introduced in 1984 as a noninvasive imaging modality for diagnosing coronary artery disease [13.44]. The temporal resolution of 100 ms enables motion-free imaging of cardiac anatomy in the diastolic heart phase even at higher heart rates. As a consequence of the restriction to non-spiral scanning in ECG-synchronized cardiac investigations, a single breath-hold scan of the heart requires slice widths that are no smaller than 3 mm. The resulting longitudinal resolution is limited and is not sufficient for the 3D visualization of the coronary arteries. While the introduction of subsecond rotation combined with prospective ECG triggering or retrospective ECG gating enabled one to use mechanical single-slice spiral CT (with its superior general image quality) for cardiac imaging [13.45, 13.46], the clinical results proved insufficient. Four-slice CT systems with the potential to overcome the drawbacks of single-slice CT were introduced in 1999 [13.47-13.49]. A gantry rotation time of 0.5 s and dedicated image reconstruction approaches enabled one to reduce the temporal resolution for the acquisition of a transaxial image to 250 ms or less [13.47, 13.50]. This proved to be sufficient for motion-free imaging of the heart during the mid to end-diastolic phase for slow to moderate heart rates (i.e. up to 65 bpm) [13.51]. The simultaneous acquisition of 4 slices made it feasible to cover the entire heart volume with thin slices (i.e. with a collimation of 4×1 mm or 4×1.25 mm) within a single breath-hold. The improved longitudinal resolution allowed for high-resolution CT imaging of the heart and the coronary arteries. Initial clinical studies have demonstrated multi-slice CT's capacity to differentiate and classify lipid, fibrous and calcified coronary types of plaque [13.52]. Since their introduction in 2001, MSCT systems capable of acquiring up to 16 submillimeter slices simultaneously and offering gantry rotation times as low as 0.37 s have led to further improvements in spatial and temporal resolution and considerable reductions in examination times: the entire heart volume can be covered with sub-mm slices in 15 to 20 s [13.20, 13.54]. Sixteen-slice systems have been used to establish ECG-triggered and ECG-gated multi-slice CT examinations of the heart and the coronary arteries in clinical practice [13.55, 13.56]. A further leap in clinical performance can be expected to result from the latest generation of MSCT systems that feature 64-slice simultaneous acquisition and gantry rotation times as low as 0.33 s.

13.4.2 ECG-triggered MSCT imaging

Prospective ECG triggering has long been used in conjunction with electron beam CT (EBCT) and single-slice spiral CT [13.57, 13.58]. A trigger signal is derived from the patient's ECG based on a prospective estimation of the present RR interval. The scan is started at a defined time point after a detected R-wave (usually during diastole). Multi-slice CT enables the simultaneous acquisition of several slices in one heartbeat with a cycle time that usually permits scanning during every second heartbeat (fig. 13.45a). This enables one to obtain shorter breath-hold times than those associated with single-slice scanners and to largely eliminate respiratory artifacts. In order to achieve the best possible temporal resolution, scanning data is only acquired during a partial scanner rotation (≈ 2/3 of a rotation with 240 to 260° projection data) covering the minimum amount of data required for image reconstruction. Conventional partial-scan reconstruction based on fan-beam projection data results in a temporal resolution that equals the acquisition time of the partial scan. Optimized temporal resolution can be achieved using parallel-beam-based half-scan reconstruction algorithms that provide a temporal resolution of half the rotation time in a center area of the scan field of view (250 ms for a 500 ms rotation time, 210 ms for a 420 ms rotation time, 188 ms for a 375 ms rotation time, etc.) [13.47, 13.60]. Prospective ECG triggering is therefore also the most dose-efficient method of ECG-synchronized scanning (i.e. given that only the very minimum of scanning data needed for image reconstruction is acquired). However, prospectively ECG-triggered techniques strongly depend on a regular heart rate and are bound to result in misregistration in the presence of arrhythmia.

13.4.3 ECG-gated MSCT imaging

Retrospective ECG gating overcomes the limitations of prospective ECG triggering with regard to scanning time and spatial resolution and can provide greater consistency with regard to image quality when it comes to examinations of patients whose heart rates may change during the scan. This approach requires multi-slice spiral scanning with slow table motion and simultaneous recording of the ECG trace that is used for the retrospective assignment of scanning data and heart motion [13.47]. Phase-consistent coverage of the heart requires a highly overlapping spiral scan with a spiral table-feed adapted to the heart rate in order to avoid gaps between image stacks that are reconstructed in consecutive heart cycles. These image stacks are reconstructed at the exact same phase of the cardiac cycle and cover the entire heart and adjacent anatomy in the considered scanning range (fig. 13.45b). Images are reconstructed in every heartbeat and faster scanning coverage is possible than that offered by prospective ECG triggering. Moreover, the continuous spiral acquisition enables the reconstruction of overlapping image slices and thus the achievement of a longitudinal spatial resolution of around 20% below the slice width (e.g. 2.5 mm for 3.0 mm slices, 1.0 mm for 1.25 mm slices, 0.8 mm for 1.0 mm slices and 0.6 mm for 0.75 mm slices). These advantages make retrospective ECG gating the preferred method for imaging small cardiac anatomy and the coronary arteries with thin slices and high spatial resolution in short single breath-hold times.

The data segments contributing to an image begin with a user-defined offset relative to the onset of the R-waves (i.e. similar to the method used in ECG-triggered axial scanning).

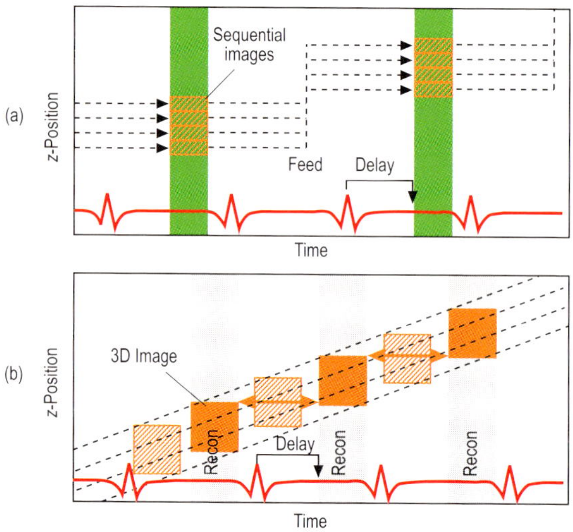

Figure 13.45
(a) Illustration of prospectively ECG-triggered MSCT scanning. Dashed lines indicate the z-positions of the detector slices relative to the patient as a function of time. The ECG signal is displayed at the bottom of the diagram. Multiple images (1 image per detector slice) are acquired at a time with a certain delay after a detected R-wave (hatched blocks). The temporal resolution equals half the rotation time. **(b)** A scan with continuous table-feed and continuous exposure is acquired for retrospectively ECG-gated MSCT spiral scanning. Stacks of overlapping images are calculated during every cardiac cycle. The temporal resolution for the basic single-segment approach equals half the rotation time. The selection of the data ranges that show certain phase relations to the R-waves enables the reconstruction of continuous 3D images during different phases of the cardiac cycle.

Image reconstruction generally consists of two parts: (1) multi-slice spiral interpolation to compensate for the continuous table movement and to obtain scanning data at the desired image z-position followed by (2) a partial scan reconstruction of the axial data segments. In the case of low heart rates, a single-segment reconstruction yields the best compromise between sufficient temporal resolution on the one hand and adequate volume coverage with thin slices on the other. Consecutive multi-slice spiral data from the same heart period are used in single-segment reconstruction to generate the single-slice partial-scan data segment for an image (fig. 13.45b). The temporal resolution of an image can be improved up to $t_{rot}/(2N)$ by using scanning data from N subsequent heart cycles for image formation in a so-called multisegment reconstruction [13.50, 13.61, 13.62, 13.63, 13.85, 13.86]. t_{rot} is the gantry rotation time of the CT scanner.

While increased N leads to superior temporal resolution, this is achieved at the expense of slower volume coverage: every z-position in the heart needs to be seen by a detector slice at every time during the N heart cycles. As a consequence, the larger N is and the lower the patient's heart-rate is, the more the spiral pitch will have to be reduced. As in the case of $N = 1$ (single-segment reconstruction, see above), a linear interpolation is performed between the data of those two detector slices that are in closest proximity to the desired image plane for each projection angle θ within subsegment l. This results in N single-slice partial-scan subsegments located at the given image z-position z_{ima}. It is necessary to properly desynchronize the patient's heart rate and the scanner's gantry rotation time when executing this technique in order to allow for improved temporal resolution. Two requirements apply. First, the start and end-projection angles of the subsegments will have to fit together to build up a full partial scan interval. This makes it necessary to shift the start projections of subsequent subsegments with respect to one another. Second, all of the subsegments will have to be acquired in the same relative phase of the patient's heart cycle in order to reduce the total time interval contributing to an image. In what follows, we derive the corresponding relations for a two-segment reconstruction. Let $T_s^l = T_R^{l+1} - T_{del}$ be the temporal position of the start angle of the projection data used in heart cycle l. T_R^{l+1} denotes the temporal position of the $(l+1)^{th}$ R-peak of the patient's ECG. The start angle of the data segment acquired in heart cycle l can then be expressed as:

$$\theta_s^l = \theta_{start} + 2\pi \frac{T_s^l}{t_{rot}} \tag{13.46}$$

In order to establish a proper fit for the start and end angles, the start angle of the segment acquired in heart cycle $l+1$ is expressed as:

$$\theta_s^{l+1} = \theta_s^l + \Delta\theta_l^l + n_l \cdot \pi \tag{13.47}$$

n_l is an integer and $\Delta\theta_l^l$ denotes the angular range of the data segment in heart cycle l. It is necessary to acquire the data segment in heart cycle $l+1$ at the exact same temporal distance from the corresponding R-peak. This yields the following equation:

$$\theta_s^{l+1} = \theta_s^l + 2\pi \frac{T_{RR}^l}{t_{rot}} \tag{13.48}$$

Using eq. (13.47) and eq. (13.48) we obtain:

$$\Delta\theta_1^l = 2\pi\frac{T_{RR}^l}{t_{rot}} - n_1 \cdot \pi \quad \text{with } n_1 = \left\lfloor 2\frac{T_{RR}^l}{t_{rot}} \right\rfloor \tag{13.49}$$

$T_{RR}^l = T_R^{l+1} - T_R^l$ is the duration of heart cycle l. It is obvious from eq. (13.49) that $\Delta\theta_1^l$ and hence the temporal resolution ΔT_{Recon} depend on the actual heart rate. The temporal resolution of the 2-segment reconstruction can be expressed as:

$$\Delta T_{Recon} = \frac{t_{rot}}{2}\frac{\max(\Delta\theta_1^l, \pi - \Delta\theta_1^l)}{\pi} \tag{13.50}$$

In the best case, i.e. when the gantry rotation and heart motion are properly de-synchronized, the temporal resolution reaches a quarter of the gantry rotation time $t_{rot}/4$. In the worst case, the achievable temporal resolution is no better than half the gantry rotation time. For instance, for a heart rate of 60 beats per minute (bpm) and a rotation time of 0.5 s, the same heart phase always corresponds to the same projection-angle segment and a partial scan interval cannot be divided into smaller subsegments acquired in successive heart periods. Depending on the relationship between the rotation time and the patient heart rate, the temporal resolution is generally not constant, but varies between one half and $1/(2N)$ times the gantry rotation time. One encounters sweet spots, heart rates with optimal temporal resolution and heart rates that prevent improvements in temporal resolution beyond half the gantry rotation time.

Multisegment approaches rely on complete heart-motion periodicity and they encounter limitations in the case of patients with arrhythmia and patients whose heart rates change during the examination. While these approaches may improve image quality in selected cases, their reliability when it comes to obtaining good quality images with N-segment reconstruction decreases as N increases. In general, clinical experience indicates the advisability of using one segment at lower heart rates and $N \geq 2$ segments at higher heart rates. The partial-scan data segment in Siemens CT scanners is automatically divided into 1 or 2 subsegments, depending on the patient's heart rate during examination. This proceeds according to the adaptive cardio-volume algorithm or ACV (fig. 13.46). Fig. 13.47 shows the temporal resolution that is achieved with the ACV algorithm at gantry rotation times of 0.42 s, 0.375 s and 0.33 s.

Some other CT scanners (e.g. GE) involve the prospective reconstruction of the single-segment partial-scan images as base-line images followed by a 2-segment retrospective reconstruction to bring about a potential gain of temporal resolution for higher heart rates. Another approach is to prospectively adjust the scanner's rotation time to the patient's heart rate to obtain the best possible temporal resolution for a multisegment reconstruction. Again, this approach requires stable and predictable heart rates during examination. Image reconstruction during different heart phases is made feasible by shifting the starting points of the data segments used for image reconstruction relative to the R-waves. Multi-slice data acquisition enables the reconstruction of a stack of images at different z-positions covering a small subvolume of the heart for a given start position.

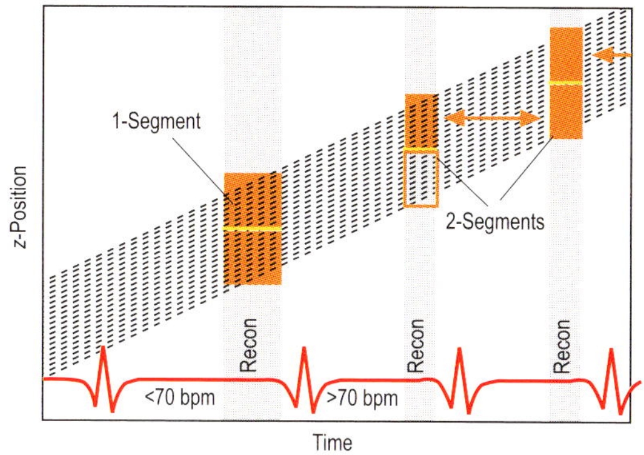

Figure 13.46
Illustration of the adaptive cardio-volume (ACV) approach for ECG-gated 16-slice spiral CT scanning at a gantry rotation time of 0.42 s. Dashed lines indicate the z-positions of the detector slices relative to the patient as a function of time. The ECG signal is recorded during scan acquisition and is displayed at the bottom of the diagram. One segment of consecutive multi-slice spiral data is used for image reconstruction involving heart rates below a certain threshold (70 bpm for a rotation time of 0.42 s). At higher heart rates, two subsegments from adjacent heart cycles contribute to the partial-scan data segment. A stack of images is reconstructed for each cardiac cycle at different z-positions covering a small subvolume of the heart, which is indicated as a box. The combination of subvolumes from all heart cycles during the scan provides a continuous 3D data set of the entire heart.

It has been demonstrated in recent publications [13.18, 13.36] that cone-beam reconstruction algorithms are mandatory for general purpose CT scanning with 8 and more slices in order to avoid substantial cone-beam artifacts. The severity of cone-beam artifacts depends on the number of simultaneously acquired slices, on the collimated slice width and on the distance of an object from the isocenter. Cone-beam artifacts are most pronounced in high-contrast structures. Typical sources of cone-beam artifacts are the ribs and the pelvic bones. Given that the heart is usually sufficiently centered and does not contain large high-contrast structures, the cone-beam artifacts that it generates are negligible for 16-slice CT scanners [13.20, 13.60]. Cardiac CT scanning with more than 16 collimated slices, however, requires advanced cardiac cone-beam algorithms [13.64]. One of these cone-beam algorithms is based on AMPR reconstruction [13.36, 13.37]. The basic idea is to reconstruct booklets containing double-oblique image pages similar to the AMPR booklets in selected phases of the cardiac cycle. It is necessary to reformat the double-oblique images to axial slices after reconstruction. Multisegment reconstruction approaches involve the calculation of segment pages that utilize projection data from a portion of a half turn only. It is then necessary to reformat each booklet separately to axial image segments after reconstruction. The pages of each segment booklet do not represent full CT images. A complete CT image is obtained only after all of the image segments have been combined at one slice location.

Prospective ECG triggering combined with the step-and-shoot acquisition of axial slices offers the benefit of a smaller patient dose than what is offered by ECG-gated spiral

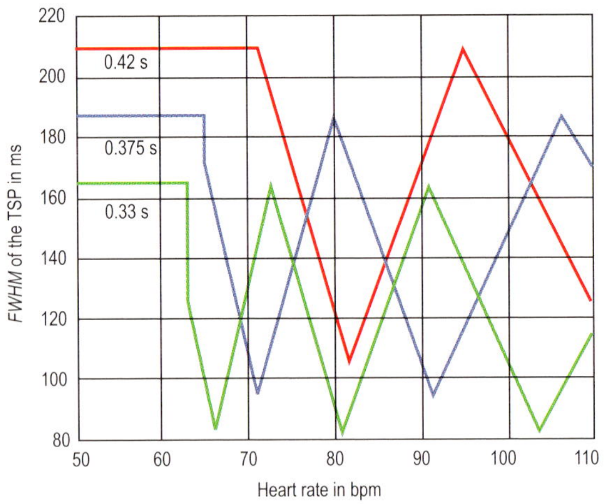

Figure 13.47
Temporal resolution as a function of the heart rate for the adaptive cardio-volume (ACV) approach with gantry rotation times of 0.42 s, 0.375 s and 0.33 s (TSP = temporal sensitivity profile). If data from 2 consecutive heart cycles are used for image reconstruction, the temporal resolution will depend on the heart rate. The temporal resolution for a rotation time of 0.42 s reaches its optimum of 105 ms at 82 bpm. Sweet spots exhibiting an optimal temporal resolution of 94 ms for a rotation time of 0.375 s include 71 bpm and 92 bpm. The optimal temporal resolution of 83 ms is achieved for a rotation time of 0.33 s at 66 bpm, 81 bpm and 104 bpm. Note that the rotation times of 0.42 s and 0.375 s and 0.375 s and 0.33 s are complementary.

scanning. This is owing to the fact that the scanning data are acquired during the previously selected heart phases only. However, the technique is more sensitive to arrhythmia than ECG-gated spiral scanning and it provides neither continuous-volume coverage with overlapping slices nor the reconstruction of images in different phases of the cardiac cycle for purposes of functional evaluation. ECG-controlled dose-modulation has been introduced to maintain the benefits of ECG-gated spiral CT while reducing patient dose [13.65]. The X-ray tube's output is modulated during the spiral scan according to the patient's ECG and is kept at its nominal value during user-defined phases of the cardiac cycle (in general, the mid to end-diastolic phase). The tube output is then reduced to 20% of its nominal value for the remainder of the cardiac cycle. Instead of being switched off, the tube current is kept at 20% of its nominal value to allow for image reconstruction throughout the entire cardiac cycle. Even though their signal-to-noise ratios are decreased, the low-dose images are sufficient for functional evaluation. Clinical studies involving 4-slice CT systems have demonstrated that one can achieve dose reductions of 30 to 50% (depending on the patient's heart rate) by using ECG-controlled dose modulation. Given that the modulation of the X-ray tube current depends on a reliable prediction of the patient's next RR interval – as in the case of ECG triggering – the method encounters limitations for patients with severe arrhythmia.

13.4.4 Performance evaluation

The evolution of MSCT from 4-slice to 16-slice and 64-slice systems has enabled significant improvements in both temporal and spatial resolution in the context of ECG-gated cardiac examinations while reducing the scan acquisition times. The progress in longitudinal spatial resolution can best be demonstrated using a z-resolution phantom consisting of a Lucite plate with rows of cylindrical holes of different diameters aligned in the z-direction. The 4-slice CT scanner with a collimation of 4 × 1 mm, a rotation time of 0.5 s and a table-feed of 3 mm/s (pitch 0.375) is capable of resolving 1.0 mm objects using a reconstructed slice width of 1.3 mm and an image increment of 0.7 mm. With a collimation of 16 x 0.75 mm, a rotation time of 0.42 s and a table-feed of 8 mm/s (pitch 0.31), 0.6 mm objects can be delineated using a reconstructed slice width of 0.8 mm and an image increment of 0.4 mm. The 64-slice CT scanner with double z-sampling, a rotation time of 0.33 s and a table-feed of 12 mm/s (pitch 0.20) can routinely resolve 0.4 mm objects (fig. 13.48).

A coronary artery phantom is used for a further evaluation of spatial and temporal resolution for ECG-gated cardiac scanning. This phantom is a contrast-filled Lucite tube with an inserted stent and a lumen of 4 mm. The tube is immersed in a water bath and can be moved periodically by a computer-controlled robot arm (both in the scan plane and perpendicular to it) to simulate heart motion.

Fig. 13.49 shows MPRs of the coronary artery phantom scanned with a 64-slice CT scanner using double z-sampling, a rotation time of 0.33 s and a table-feed of 12 mm/s (pitch 0.2), reconstructed with an artificial ECG signal of 82 bpm. The phantom was stationary during scan acquisition. The same scanning data were used to obtain both 0.6 mm slices and 1.0 mm slices to simulate the routine performance of a 16-slice CT scanner. The 0.6 mm slice width with z-flying focal spot allows for a considerably improved evaluation of the in-stent lumen (i.e. compared to what is available when using a 1.0 mm slice width). The vessel diameter of 4 mm is typical for the proximal, left anterior descending artery (LAD) and right coronary artery (RCA). The improved tempo-

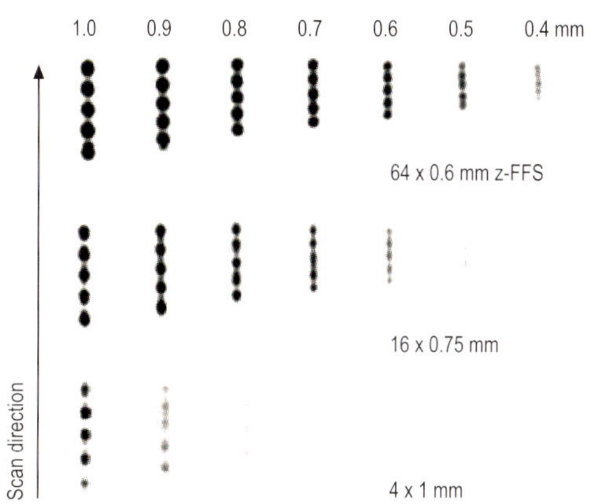

Figure 13.48
Demonstration of longitudinal resolution for ECG-gated spiral scanning with state-of-the-art 4-slice, 16-slice and 64-slice CT systems. The transition from 4-slice to 64-slice CT includes an improvement in longitudinal resolution from 1.0 mm to 0.4 mm.

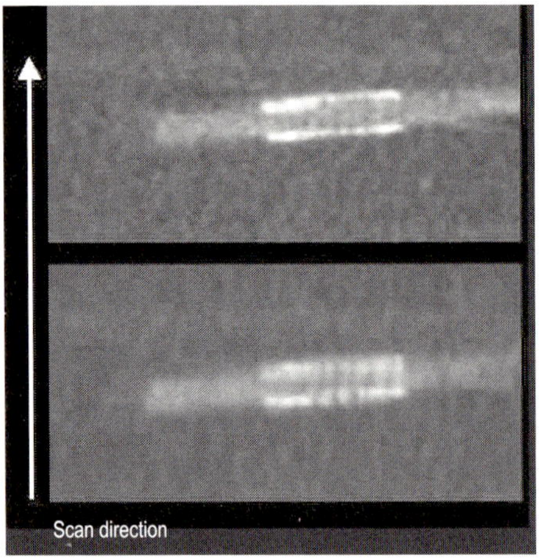

Figure 13.49
Coronary artery phantom with inserted stent at rest. The ECG-gated spiral scan data were acquired with a 64-slice CT scanner using double z-sampling, a rotation time of 0.33 s and a table-feed of 12 mm/s (pitch 0.2) and reconstructed with an artificial ECG signal of 82 bpm. The same scan data were used to obtain both 0.6 mm slices **(top)** and 1.0 mm slices **(bottom)**. The 0.6 mm slice width allows for a markedly improved evaluation of the in-stent lumen.

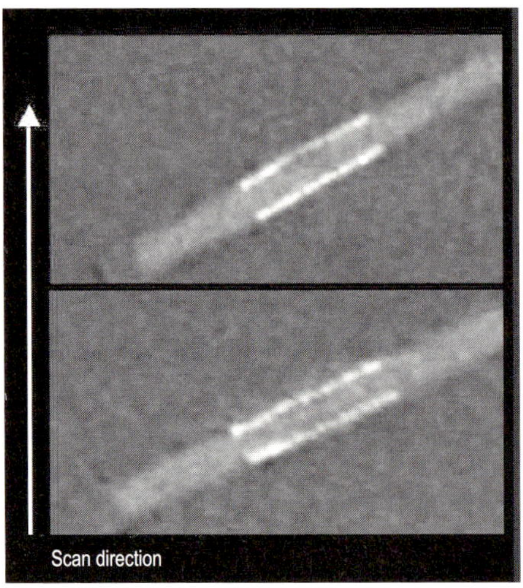

Figure 13.50
MPRs of the coronary artery phantom reconstructed using an artificial ECG signal of 82 bpm. **Top:** stationary phantom. **Bottom:** phantom moving at 82 bpm, rest phase 100 ms. Scan data were reconstructed using the ACV algorithm (2-segment reconstruction). The temporal resolution with a gantry rotation time of 0.33 s is around 85 ms at 82 bpm (see fig. 13.47).

ral resolution with a gantry rotation time of 0.33 s shows potential for enabling an increase in clinical robustness at higher heart rates, and thereby also reducing the number of patients requiring heart rate control. Fig. 13.50 shows MPRs of the coronary artery phantom (both stationary and with realistic motion corresponding to a heart rate of 82 bpm). The rest phase of the moving phantom was 100 ms. When using the ACV approach for image reconstruction, the temporal resolution at 82 bpm is approximately 85 ms with a gantry rotation time of 0.33 s (fig. 13.47). The depiction of the moving phantom is therefore nearly free of motion artifacts, thereby allowing for a reliable evaluation of the in-stent lumen even at this heart rate.

13.5 Clinical applications

13.5.1 Quantification of coronary calcification

Although their exact prognostic relevance is controversial, the presence of calcifications in the coronary arteries is an indicator of coronary artery disease. The use of electron beam CT scanning (EBCT) in combination with the Agatston scoring algorithm has proven to be an effective method of detecting and quantifying coronary calcium [13.58]. While single-slice [13.59] and dual-slice mechanical spiral CT [13.66] have also been used since the introduction of subsecond gantry rotation to evaluate coronary artery calcium, multi-slice CT can be expected to offer far greater quantification accuracy owing to its superior imaging performance in terms of temporal resolution and volume coverage [13.68]. Optimal acquisition techniques remain to be developed and Ca-scoring data acquired via MSCT will need careful clinical evaluation and comparison to EBCT.

Both ECG-triggered sequential and ECG-gated spiral scanning can be used as acquisition techniques. Scanning data are acquired without contrast enhancement in craniocaudal direction from the caudal part of the pulmonary artery trunk to the apex of the heart ($\approx$ 12 cm scan range). A slice width of 3 mm is routinely used for EBCT scanning as it represents the thinnest slice width that allows for a single breath-hold scan. Slice widths ranging from 2.5 to 3.0 mm are usually used with 4, 8, 16 and 64-slice CT scanners as the closest match to the standard EBCT protocols. A tube voltage of 120 kV is recommended because it provides the best balancing of contrast-to-noise ratio and radiation exposure.

ECG-triggered scanning allows one to cover the scanning volume in 20 to 25 s using 4-slice CT and in 10 to 15 s using 8 and 16-slice CT. Depending on the selected mA, the effective patient dose will vary between 0.5 and 0.7 mSv for male and between 0.6 and 0.9 mSv for female patients. Each scan covers a subvolume that consists of several adjacent slices, thus reducing the probability of interscan misregistration caused by heart movement in the z-direction and allowing one to expect greater detection accuracy compared to that offered by ECG-triggered single-slice acquisition. Comparative studies of EBCT and prospectively ECG-triggered multi-slice CT have demonstrated considerable agreement in measurements obtained in the context of phantom experiments as well as a high correlation in a clinical context [13.67]. However, a high average inter-examination variability of 22% to 32% (comparable to the inter-examination variability of 2 consecutive EBCT examinations) has been observed when using prospectively ECG-triggered multi-slice CT due to the presence of motion artifacts and misregistration between the sequential slices.

ECG-gated spiral scanning enables shorter breath-hold times when compared to ECG-triggered scanning as well as more consistent volume coverage based on overlapping slices. A 12 cm scanning range can be completed in 15 to 20 s using a 4-slice CT and in 6 to 10 s using 8 and 16-slice CT. The spiral interpolation algorithms generate a slice thickness of 3 mm (FWHM) based on a slice collimation of 1.25 to 1.5 mm for 16-slice CT scanners. Optimal detection accuracy in the case of small calcified lesions may be achieved with 16-slice scanners via the reconstruction of 3 mm slices acquired using submillimeter collimation. Retrospectively ECG-gated spiral scanning qualifies as the preferred scanning technique when it comes to minimized inter-examination variability. Independent studies have demonstrated an interscan variability of around 10% or even less for repeat 4-slice CT scanning [13.68, 13.69, 13.70]. This level may be accurate enough to enable one to reliably detect changes in the total atherosclerotic disease burden in patients with and without specific therapy. Interscan variability can be fur-

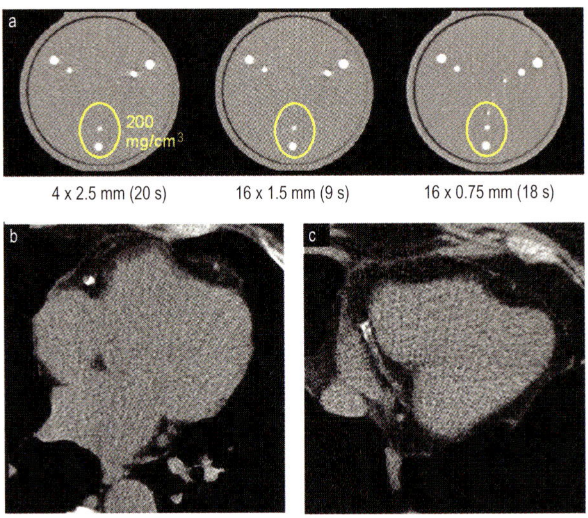

Figure 13.51
Various scanning protocols for 4 and 16-slice CT were compared in a phantom study to investigate detection sensitivity for small amounts of coronary calcification **(a)**. Slices of 3 mm were reconstructed based on scanning data acquired with an mAs of 133 and collimations of 4 × 2.5 mm, 16 × 1.5 mm and 16 × 0.75 mm. The smallest calcifications (1 mg mass) can only be detected with the 16 × 0.75 mm protocol. A case study performed with 16-slice CT and a collimation of 16 × 1.5 mm reveals small calcifications in the middle segment **(b)** and in the distal segment **(c)** of the right coronary artery. (Source: Department of Radiology, Klinikum Grosshadern, University of Munich, Germany)

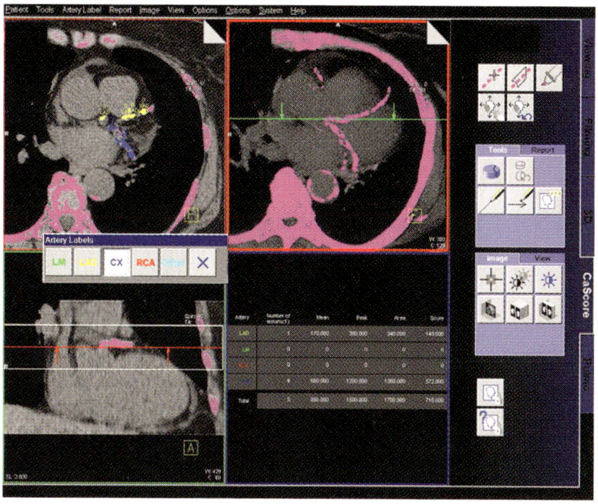

Figure 13.52
Platform used for the quantification of coronary calcification (*syngo* Calcium Scoring, Siemens, Forchheim, Germany). Lesions exceeding the calcium threshold of 130 HU are identified using 3D-based picking and viewing tools and are assigned to the various coronary arteries LM, LAD, CX and RCA. Coronary calcifications are quantified by means of Agatston scoring, calcium volume and calcium mass. Calibration factors that are pre-determined using phantom measurements and that depend on the scan protocol form the basis for calculating calcium mass. The quantitative measurements are displayed and reported in table format.

ther improved with the use of the latest 16-slice and 64-slice CT scanners, primarily on account of their faster rotation times and increased scanning speeds (fig. 13.51). When compared to the prospectively ECG-triggered technique, CT acquisition using retrospective ECG-gating shows higher levels of effective radiation exposure (1.9 mSv for males and 2.8 mSv for females). Healthy, asymptomatic individuals frequently undergo coronary calcium scoring in the context of primary prevention. In particular, with respect to this population, it is imperative to limit radiation dose to a minimum. This can be achieved by properly adapting scanning protocols and by using sophisticated technical developments such as ECG-based tube current modulation [13.65], which can decrease the effective radiation exposure to the patient by as much as 50%.

The most commonly used algorithm for the quantification of coronary artery calcium is the traditional semiquantitative score based on the slice-by-slice analysis of CT images described by Agatston [13.58]. Recent studies indicate better results for interscan and inter- and intra-observer variability with the use of quantitative measures as compared to the traditional Agatston scoring method [13.68, 13.69]. Advanced software platforms (fig. 13.52) enable one to assess equivalent volume and total calcified plaque burden in terms of absolute calcium mass based on scanner-specific calibration. This latter technique seems to show the greatest potential for increasing the accuracy, consistency and reproducibility of coronary calcium assessments [13.87] and could soon replace traditional scoring methods.

13.5.2 Cardiac and coronary CT angiography

Noninvasive cardiac and coronary CT angiography is required to meet demanding specifications with regard to spatial resolution, low-contrast detectability and temporal resolution. Image quality depends on various patient and scanner parameters. The optimization of examination protocols is critical to achieving the best balance of imaging parameters and the best examination results.

Cardiac and coronary CT imaging using MSCT requires ECG-gated thin-slice spiral scan protocols with a table speed adapted to the heart rate in order to ensure complete phase-consistent coverage of the heart with overlapping image slices. Most 16-slice CT scanners provide scanning protocols with a fixed overlapping spiral pitch (ranging from 0.22 to 0.3) that enables seamless volume coverage for heart rates higher than ≈ 40 bpm.

The established 16-slice CT scanners provide high-resolution cardiac scanning protocols with submillimeter slice collimation (0.75 mm) and in-plane spatial resolution of up to 0.5 × 0.5 mm. The image reconstruction protocols are adapted to clinical priorities. Slices that are not thinner than 1.0 mm are usually reconstructed with an in-plane resolution of 0.6 × 0.6 mm in order to achieve optimal contrast resolution for evaluations of coronary narrowing and coronary lesions (fig. 13.53). Rotation times as low as 0.375 s and an extended number of slices (up to 16) result in a reduced scanning time of 15 to 20 s. Thus, 16-slice CT is also capable of covering larger scanning ranges of 18 to 20 cm with ECG-gated thin-slice spiral scanning protocols in a reasonably short breath-hold of 25 to 30 s. This enables high-resolution imaging for most parts of the thoracic vasculature and for coronary bypass grafts.

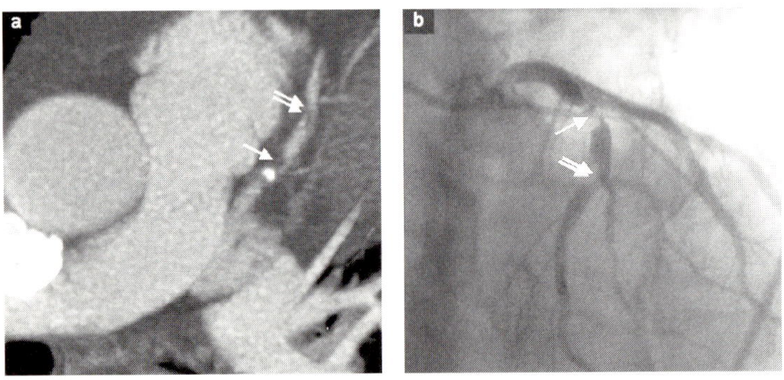

Figure 13.53
Coronary CT angiography examination of a patient with suspected coronary artery disease **(a)** using a 16-slice CT scanner with a detector collimation of 16 × 0.75 mm and a rotation speed of 420 ms and **(b)** using conventional coronary angiography. Coronary CT angiography reveals high-grade stenosis in the proximal left descending coronary artery near the bifurcation of the first diagonal branch (arrow, 90% stenosis) and in the middle segment of the left descending coronary artery next to the bifurcation of the second diagonal branch (double arrow, 70% stenosis). Both lesions are confirmed by coronary angiography. (Source: Dr. Soo, CS, HSC Medical Center, Kuala Lumpur, Malaysia)

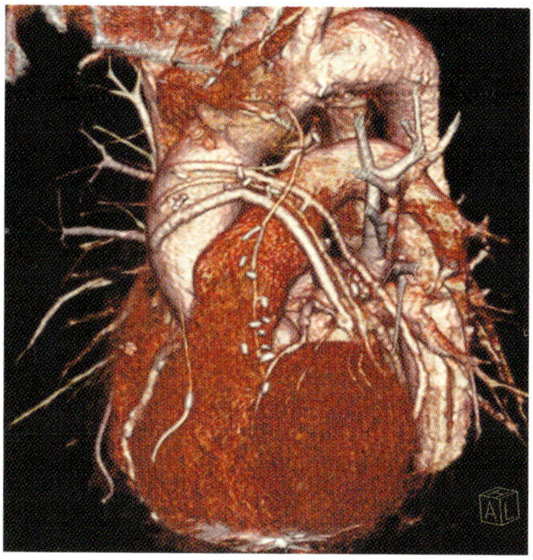

Figure 13.54
Clinical case illustrating the performance of ECG-gated 64-slice CT with z-flying focal spot: patient with 4 bypass grafts and a heart rate of 85 bpm. Scanning parameters: 120 kV, an effective mAs of 685, a collimation of 64 × 0.6 mm, a gantry rotation time of 0.33 s (pitch 0.2) and a scanning time of 21 s. The anastomoses of the bypass grafts can be clearly evaluated. (Source: Dr. Wintersperger and Dr. Becker, Klinikum Großhadern, Munich, Germany)

The most recent generation of 64-slice CT systems offers improved longitudinal resolution (as low as 0.4 mm with a slice width of 0.6 mm and double z-sampling), shorter examination times (8 to 10 s) and improved temporal resolution thanks to reduced gantry rotation times (0.33 s) for robust cardiac imaging at higher heart rates. Fig. 13.54 shows a VRT of a patient with 4 bypass grafts. The scanning parameters were 120 kV, an effective mAs of 685, a collimation of 64 × 0.6 mm with double z-sampling a gantry rotation time of 0.33 s (pitch 0.2) and a scanning time of 21 s. The average patient heart rate during the scan was 85 bpm. The anastomoses in the bypass grafts can be clearly evaluated. The fine vessel structures at the anastomoses demonstrate the good longitudinal resolution.

The optimization of scanning protocols by means of radiation exposure is particularly important for contrast-enhanced CT imaging of the coronary arteries. It is necessary to achieve sufficiently high spatial resolution and low-contrast resolution in normal-sized and larger patients at the lowest possible radiation exposure. A tube current of ≈ 350 to 400 mA is required in the case of a 16-slice CT with submillimeter slice collimation operating at a tube voltage of 120 kV and a rotation time of 420 ms. Retrospectively ECG-gated scan acquisition with a highly overlapping spiral pitch in a 10 cm scanning range requires radiation exposure of about 6 to 7 mSv for male and about 8 to 11 mSv for female patients using the above scan parameters. The radiation exposure increases along with a reduced spiral pitch and an extension of the scanning range. ECG-gated dose modulation enables one to reduce radiation exposure by 30 to 50% depending on the heart rate without compromising image quality in the fully exposed phase of the cardiac cycle. ECG-gated dose modulation reduces radiation exposure with 16-slice CT to around 3 to 5 mSv for male and to around 4 to 8 mSv for female patients and should be used for all patients who show reasonably stable heart rhythm during the scan.

The overall diagnostic quality of noninvasive cardiac and coronary CT angiography largely depends on the selection of an appropriate reconstruction time point within the cardiac cycle, on patient heart rate during the examination and on contrast enhancement. While the motion patterns of the left heart and the left anterior descending (LAD) and circumflex (CRX) coronary arteries follow the left-ventricular contraction, the right coronary artery (RCA) moves synchronously to the right heart (i.e. the right atrium). These different motion patterns mean that different reconstruction time points in the cardiac cycle may result in the optimal display of different parts in the cardiac anatomy and different coronary arteries. Most studies indicate that patient heart rate is inversely related to image quality in cardiac and coronary CT angiography on account of motion artifacts. It has been shown that multi-slice CT offers the best diagnostic accuracy and reliability in patients with slow heart rates. While the technique allows one to obtain adequate image quality in many cases involving higher heart rates, the overall results are less consistent and reproducible. The robustness of image quality despite motion is remarkably increased in the case of scanners offering faster rotation times (e.g. between 0.375 s and 0.33 s). In general, it appears advisable to slow down the heart rate of individuals undergoing CT coronary angiography pharmacologically via the oral administration of beta-blockers so long as one is able to rule out contraindications. The reliable evaluation of larger cardiac morphology (e.g. the cardiac chambers and the large vessels) is also possible in patients who present with higher heart rates during the scan although some image artifacts may be present.

While the reliability of multi-slice cardiac and coronary CT angiography in patients with arrhythmia is limited, misinterpretations of the ECG signal can be partially compensated for by the retrospective editing of the ECG trace.

The presence of severe calcification represents a limitation in CT coronary imaging because beam hardening and partial-volume effects can completely obscure the coronary lumen and thus prevent an assessment of the integrity of the coronary lumen.

The optimization of contrast-media injection protocols for cardiac and coronary CT angiography is aimed at providing homogenous enhancement within the entire course of the coronary arteries in order to facilitate density-threshold-dependent 2D and 3D visualization. The optimal contrast attenuation within the vessel is high enough to allow for lesion detection, but not so high as to obscure calcified lesions in the coronary-artery wall with a higher Hounsfield unit (HU) attenuation (i.e. > 350 HU). The amount of contrast media in the case of 16-slice CT (≈ 20 s scan time) may range from 80 to 100 ml (delivered at an injection rate of 3 to 4 ml/s).

13.5.3 Evaluation of cardiac function

Besides the diagnosis of cardiac and coronary morphology, the evaluation and quantification of cardiac function also plays an important role in the development of sound assessments of cardiac and coronary diseases. In addition to image reconstruction in

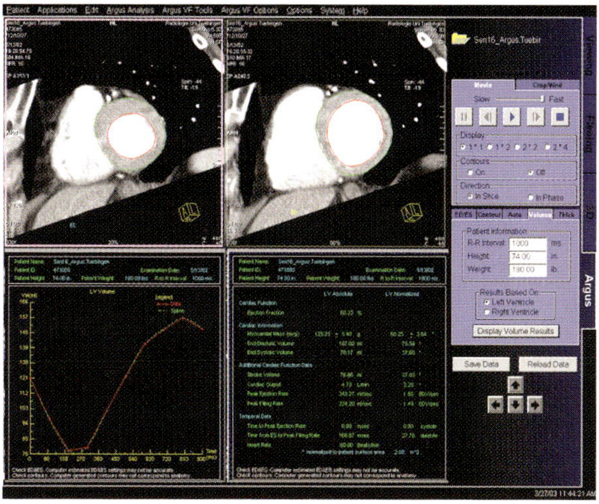

Figure 13.55
CT angiographic examination of a patient with an occlusion of the left descending coronary artery using a 16-slice CT scanner with a detector collimation of 16×0.75 mm and a rotation speed of 420 ms. In addition to reconstruction of the coronary artery tree, ECG-gated spiral image reconstruction was performed at 10 different time points during the cardiac cycle with a distance of 10% of the RR interval to provide input data for an evaluation of cardiac function. The end-diastolic volume and end-systolic volume of the left ventricle as well as the ejection fraction can be readily assessed based on short axis and long axis multiplanar reformations with a thickness of 5 mm that are processed by dedicated evaluation software (*syngo* Argus, Siemens, Germany). (Source: Department of Radiology, Tübingen University, Germany)

the diastolic phase of the cardiac cycle in order to support morphological assessments, ECG-gated multi-slice spiral CT can provide additional 3D reconstructions in various heart phases that are based on the same scanning data. The diagnosis of cardiac and coronary morphology as well as of basic parameters of cardiac function (e.g. left and right ventricular ejection fraction and end-diastolic and end-systolic volume) can be derived from a single contrast-enhanced ECG-gated spiral examination using thin-section acquisition.

Initial study results [13.71] show that the basic parameters of cardiac functioning that are derived using 4-slice CT correlate well with the gold-standard techniques of MRI and coronary angiography based on a standardized heart-phase selection for end-diastolic and end-systolic CT reconstruction and semiautomated evaluation tools (fig. 13.55).

Although dose is significantly reduced during end diastole and systole in the case of ECG-controlled tube-current modulation, sufficient contrast resolution can still be obtained for purposes of functional evaluation. The use of multiplanar reformation along the short and long axis of the heart with a thickness of 5 to 8 mm enables one to achieve an appropriate delineation of the ventricle wall in both end-diastolic and end-systolic reconstruction. The automated direct 3D reconstruction of oblique planes in pre-defined views such as the short and long axes of the heart and in multiple phases of the cardiac cycle will enable one to establish a more efficient workflow for the analysis of cardiac function.

13.5.4 Preventive care: CT of the lung and colon

Preventive care involves the examination of patients who are at high risk of developing a certain disease before the disease becomes manifest. Methods conceived to enable the detection of lung cancer at an early stage and CT colonography represent promising applications in the field of preventive care.

Initial studies of the use of CT to detect lung cancer at an early stage in a screening population were published in 1999 [13.72]. The basic system requirements center on the capacity to cover the entire lung in a single breath-hold at a resolution that is sufficient to detect small, suspicious nodules while keeping the dose to an acceptable level. While single-slice CT is essentially capable of meeting these requirements, one can enhance the clinical workflow substantially by using MSCT. In the Early Lung Cancer Action Project (ELCAP) study [13.72], which was performed using single-slice CT, suspicious nodules were found in about 25% of the screened population. These individuals received further workup involving the careful monitoring of the small nodules or their surgical removal, depending on various factors. Given that an accurate volume assessment of small nodules requires high spatial resolution, which was not available during the initial screening examination on account of limited volume coverage, the respective patients had to be rescheduled. In contrast, MSCT allows one to perform the screening examination at high resolution, thereby making such rescheduling unnecessary. The entire thorax (350 mm) can be covered in 25 to 30 s using a collimation of 4×1 mm and a gantry rotation time of 0.5 s. Using a collimation of 16×0.75 mm enables one to reduce the scanning time to around 10 s. The use of CT as a screening tool in a healthy population at risk for lung cancer requires a reduction in the patient dose to the lowest clinically acceptable level. Using 120 kV and an effective mAs of 20, one can reduce the effective patient dose to a range below 1 mSv, which is less than the average exposure to natural background radiation over a period of six months.

The ELCAP study demonstrates that CT screening is capable of detecting lung cancer far earlier than what can be achieved using chest X-rays. While it has not been proven that CT screening for lung cancer is capable of reducing mortality rates, earlier detection of lung cancer is commonly considered to have a favorable impact on the effectiveness of therapy.

Application packages are available to improve clinical workflow. These enable the characterization and follow-up of suspicious nodules, for instance, by providing 3D evaluation tools (e.g. spinning MPRs to facilitate the differentiation of lesions and vessels) and volume measurement tools to reliably monitor the growth of nodules (LungCare, Siemens Medical Solutions, fig. 13.56). New software tools have also been developed for the automatic detection of suspicious nodules. These can be used as second readers to support the radiologist (nodule enhanced visualization or NEV).

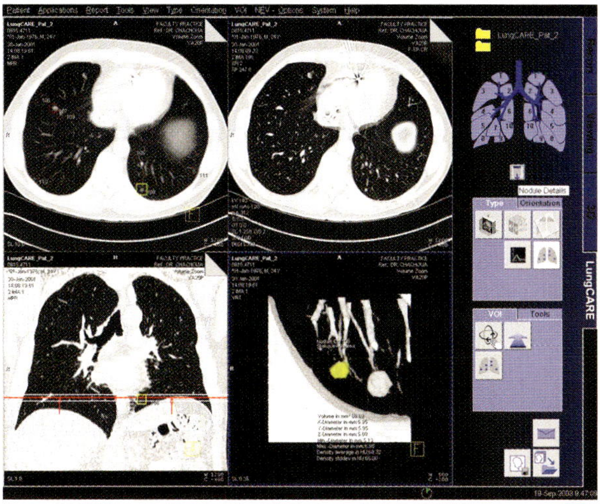

Figure 13.56
Thorax examination of a patient with lung nodules. Thin slice images are processed by dedicated evaluation software (*syngo* LungCare, Siemens, Germany) that represents an effective tool for the characterization and follow-up of suspicious lung lesions.

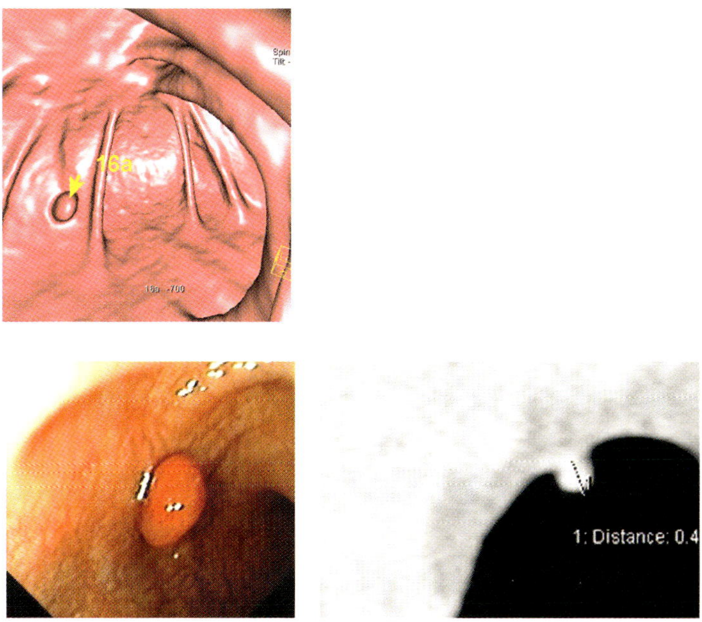

Figure 13.57
Virtual CT colonography **(upper left and bottom right)** versus conventional optical colonoscopy **(bottom right)** for a polyp with a diameter of 4 mm.
(Source: Klinikum Großhadern, Munich, Germany)

CT colonography (fig. 13.57) is used to detect suspicious polyps in the colon. Although the technique remains controversial, a recent study has shown that the method compares favorably to conventional colonoscopy when it comes to detecting polyps with a diameter of at least 10 mm [13.73]. The study involved the application of CT colonography in 68 asymptomatic men with an average risk, followed by the application of optical colonoscopy on the same day. A per-patient specificity of 89.7% was obtained for CT colonography. A similar study in 1,233 asymptomatic adults resulted in sensitivity levels of 93.8%, 93.9% and 88.7% for the detection of adenomatous polyps with diameters of at least 10 mm, 8 mm and 6 mm respectively. The specificity was 96.0%, 92.2% and 79.6% for the three sizes of polyps respectively. Two polyps in the screening population were malignant, with both of them being detected by virtual colonography and one being missed by optical colonoscopy [13.74].

Narrow-collimation scanning (4 × 1 mm/4 × 1.25 mm, 16 × 0.625 mm/16 × 0.75 mm) is the method of choice for CT colonography. While no difference in sensitivity was observed for thick-section reconstructions, specificity markedly improved for thin sections [13.76]. Again, the radiation dose should be kept as low as possible (e.g. by using 120 kV and 120 mAs_{eff}/40 mAs_{eff} for the supine/prone scans). As with the early detection of lung cancer, new software tools are being developed that automatically detect suspicious polyps. These can also be used as second readers to support the radiologist (polyp-enhanced viewing or PEV, Siemens Medical Solutions).

13.6 The future of CT

13.6.1 From multi-slice to area-detector CT

What we are currently witnessing in the area of MSCT is a further increase in the number of simultaneously acquired slices, which is perceived as the most important performance characteristic of a CT scanner. This new generation of CT systems offering 32, 40 and 64 simultaneously acquired slices – some of them using refined z-sampling techniques – was introduced in 2004. However, in contrast to the transition from single-slice to 4-slice and 16-slice CT, clinical performance can only be expected to improve incrementally along with a further increase in the number of detector rows. The resulting clinical benefits will have to be carefully considered in the light of the necessary technical efforts and cost. It is more likely that clinical progress will come from further improvements in spatial and temporal resolution than from an increase in the volume coverage speed. Clinical reality suggests that the latter is only rarely a limiting factor (i.e. ever since the introduction of 16-slice CT). Once the point has been reached where all relevant examinations can be performed in a comfortable breath-hold of not more than 10 s, a further increase in the slice number will not provide any significant clinical benefits. Future trends towards a larger number of slices will therefore not be driven by the need to increase scanning speed in spiral acquisition modes, but rather by the desire to increase volume coverage in non-spiral dynamic acquisitions, for instance, via the introduction of area detectors large enough to cover entire organs such as the heart, the kidneys and the brain in a single axial scan (~ 120 mm scan range).

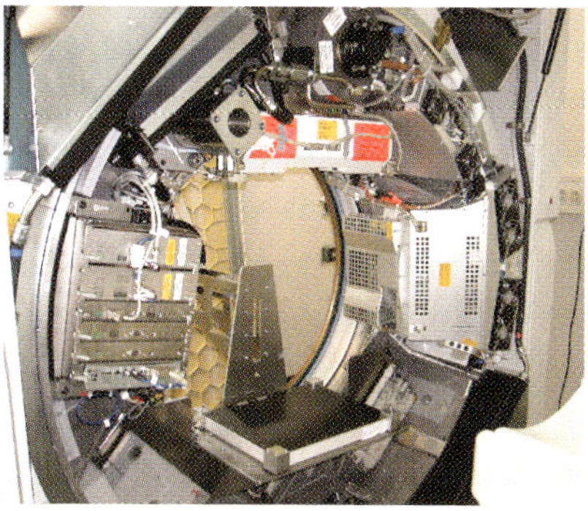

Figure 13.58
Prototype of an area detector CT scanner based on a SOMATOM Sensation gantry with modified Akron tube (anode angle 16°) and an a-Si detector with CsI scintillator plate

Such systems would make dynamic volume scanning feasible, and thereby open up a whole spectrum of new applications such as functional and volume perfusion studies. Area-detector technology is currently in development (cf. cone-beam CT in section 12.5). Prototype systems use CsI-a-Si flat-panel detector technology originally intended for conventional catheter angiography (fig. 13.58), e.g. a Varian Paxscan 4030A flat-panel detector with a pixel pitch of 191 µm. A frame rate of 30 fps can be achieved in a 2×2 binning mode. This results in acquisition times of 20 s for the acquisition of 600 projections. Both the high intrinsic signal lag as well as limitations in the acquisition electronics limit the frame rates to values at least one order of magnitude smaller than what is typically required for CT. However, the spatial resolution of such systems is excellent on account of the small detector pixel size. The prototype provides isotropic spatial resolution of approximately $(0.25\ \text{mm})^3$ in a field of measurement with a diameter of 25 cm and a length along the z-axis of 18 cm. Excessive dose requirements, however, have so far precluded the examination of larger objects. The initial experimental results are thus limited to small high-contrast objects such as joints, the inner ear and contrast-filled vessel specimens [13.77, 13.78].

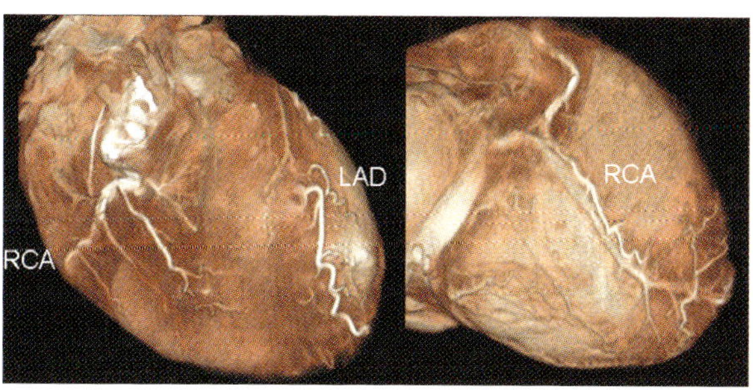

Figure 13.59
Volume-rendered display of a stationary heart specimen scanned with the flat-panel CT prototype with the CsI-a-Si detector shown in fig. 13.58. The isotropic resolution of $0.25\ \text{mm}^3$ enables an exquisite delineation of small side branches in the contrast-filled coronary artery tree. (Source: Dr. U.J. Schoepf, MUSC, Charleston, USA)

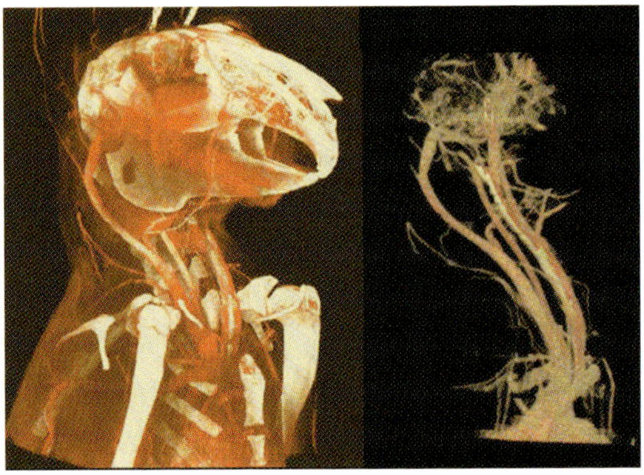

Figure 13.60
CTA of the head and neck of a rabbit, scanned with the flat-panel CT prototype with the CsI-a-Si detector shown in fig. 13.58. (Source: Dr. Rajiv Gupta, MGH, Boston, USA)

Fig. 13.59 shows VRTs of a contrast-filled heart specimen (scan parameters: 80 kV, 20 mA, 20 s gantry rotation time) demonstrating excellent spatial resolution, which enables the visualization of even very small side branches of the coronary artery tree. The combination of area detectors that provide sufficient image quality and high gantry-rotation speeds represents a promising technical concept for medical CT systems. Other interesting applications beyond cardiac scanning include dynamic CTA examinations (e.g. of the carotids and the circle of Willis). Fig. 13.60 shows a CTA of the head and neck of a rabbit. While the vast spectrum of potential applications may bring about another quantum leap in the evolution of medical CT imaging, such systems will probably not be available in the near future.

13.6.2 Combined systems

While CT is primarily directed to the provision of morphological information, its use in combination with other modalities allows one to obtain functional and metabolic information [13.79]. The significance of combined systems for obtaining comprehensive structural and functional diagnoses can therefore be expected to increase in the near future (cf. section 17.2). The advantages of combining PET and SPECT with CT are twofold. First, CT provides fast and accurate imaging of morphology and thus provides reference landmarks when very specific tracers are used that image pathology, but provide no hints about the surrounding anatomy. Second, CT provides a fast attenuation map for the attenuation correction of emission measurements. Both PET and SPECT measure the spatial distribution of a radioactive tracer that emits positrons (PET) or gamma quanta (SPECT). The measurements carried out according to both techniques are impaired by the reduction in the number of detected quanta as a result of the attenuation caused by tissue situated between the place of emission and the detectors.

An attenuation map can be used to correct for the attenuation. In PET scanners, this attenuation map is usually based on line-integral measurements of the attenuation coefficients using a radioactive source outside the body. The drawbacks to this method include long measurement times and low image quality. Moreover, the radioactive

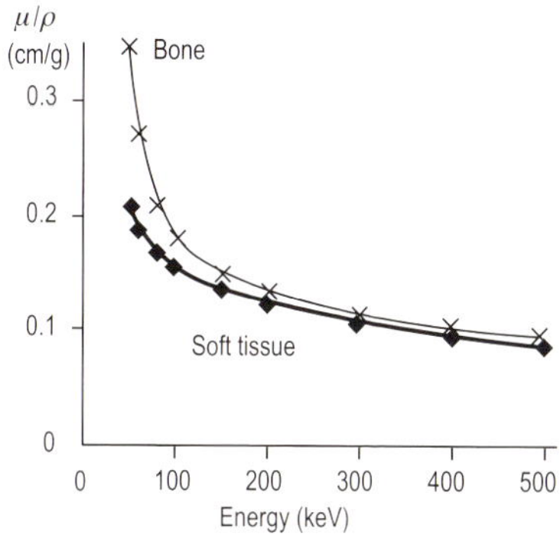

Figure 13.61
Attenuation depends strongly on photon energy and this dependence varies according to tissue type.

sources need to be replaced regularly and lead to increased maintenance costs. In the case of PET/CT, the attenuation map can be conveniently obtained using the CT scanner. One difficulty, however, is that the attenuation of tissue in the 50 to 100 keV range that is typical for CT is very different from its attenuation at 511 keV, i.e. the energy of gamma quanta resulting from positron annihilation (fig. 13.61). In response to this difficulty, methods have been devised to segment the CT images into the different types of tissue and to perform separate energy scaling for each type of tissue.

The capacity to reconstruct the CT images in a sufficient field of view (FOV) without the truncation of anatomical structures (e.g. arms) represents a prerequisite for ade-

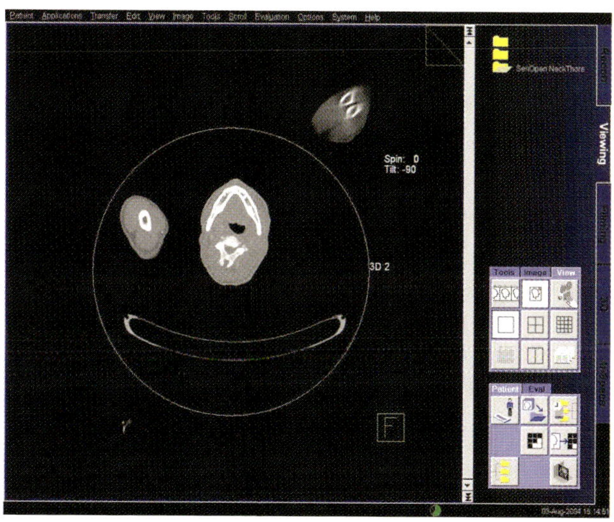

Figure 13.62
CT scan with enlarged FOV achieved by extrapolating from the original CT data. The original SFOV with a diameter of 50 cm is indicated by the circle.

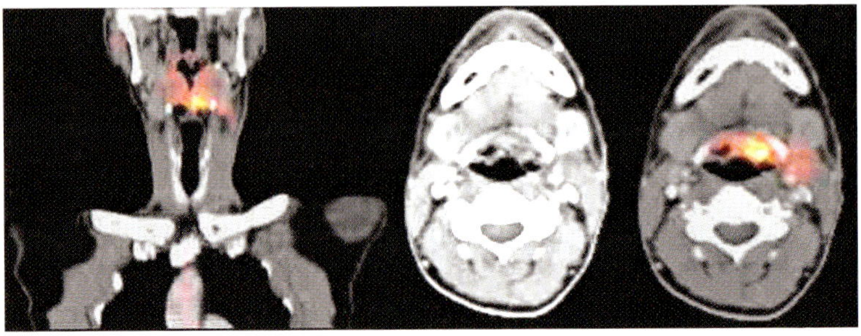

Figure 13.63
Case study illustrating the clinical performance of PET/CT. MPR and axial slices with superimposed PET images of a patient after excision of a malignant left-neck lymph node. The primary tumor can be localized via increased focal uptake of the FDG tracer in the left tongue base. (Source: University of Pittsburg Medical Center, Pittsburg, USA)

quate PET-image attenuation correction. An enlarged FOV of up to 70 cm can be realized by extrapolating from the measured CT data. Readers may wish to refer to the literature for pertinent algorithms [13.80] (fig. 13.62).

The combination of state-of-the-art MDCT and PET scanners opens a wide spectrum of applications, ranging from oncological staging to comprehensive cardiac examinations. The clinical potential of these scanners is currently being evaluated [13.81]. Fig. 13.63 shows CT images (MPRs and axial slices) with superimposed PET images of a 48-year-old patient following the excision of a malignant left-neck lymph node. While the clinical workup failed to reveal the primary tumor, it was identified in the PET/CT examination via the increased focal uptake of the FDG tracer in the left base of the tongue. This supports the notion that PET scanning adds a new contrast agent to CT.

Combined SPECT/CT systems are another promising modality. Potential applications are currently being investigated and range from the localization of parathyroid lesions and heterotopic splenic tissue to the detection of recurrent nasopharyngeal carcinomas and the imaging of aortic prosthesis infection.

Virtual CT simulation has gained in importance along with the more widespread adoption of three-dimensional conformal and intensity-modulated radiation therapy. Some patients (e.g. women with breast cancer) cannot always be scanned in the treatment position using general-purpose CT systems whose gantry openings typically have diameters of 70 cm. These applications, along with interventional procedures and trauma protocols, will be facilitated by CT systems with larger bores [13.82]. Concepts involving 4-slice, 16-slice and 20-slice CT scanners with bore diameters of up to 85 cm and reconstruction fields of up to 82 cm have been recently introduced in connection with image reconstruction based on data extrapolation. The significance of these systems is likely to grow in the near future in the areas of radiation therapy (cf. section 17.1) and emergency care as well as with regard to the dramatically increasing number of severely obese patients in western societies.

13.6.3 Alternative system concepts

Although sufficient diagnostic image quality can be achieved in most cases by administering beta-blockers, motion artifacts in patients with higher heart rates remain the most important challenge for multi-slice coronary CTA. Improved temporal resolution will be desirable in the future to avoid the need for heart-rate control. Increased gantry rotation speeds seem preferable to multisegment reconstruction approaches when it comes to robust clinical performance. The most recent generation of MSCT systems provides gantry rotation times as low as 0.33 s. Obviously, significant development efforts will be needed to account for the substantial increase in mechanical force (~ 17 G for a rotation time of 0.42 s and ~ 28 G for a rotation time of 0.33 s) and increased data transmission rates. The rotation times of less than 0.2 s (mechanical force of > 75 G) that would be required to provide a temporal resolution of less than 100 ms independent of the heart rate appear for the time being to be beyond mechanical limits. One alternative to further increased rotation speed involves a reconsideration of an earlier CT scanner concept based on two tubes and two corresponding detectors [13.83]. The two acquisition systems are mounted onto a rotating gantry with an angular offset of 90°. The half-scan sinogram, required for image recon-

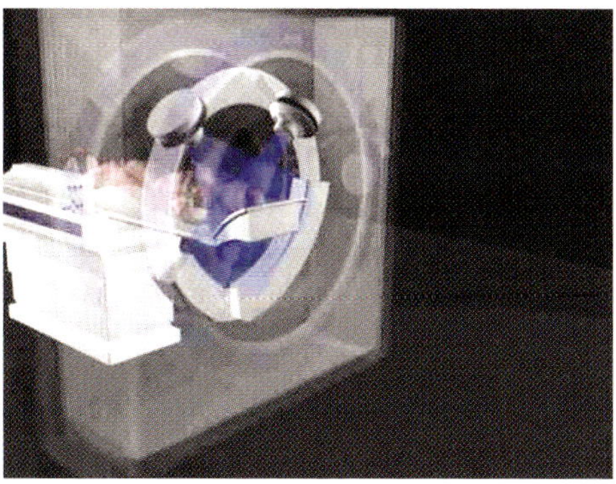

Figure 13.64
Illustration of a CT scanner concept based on two measurement systems (two tubes and two detectors) offset by 90°

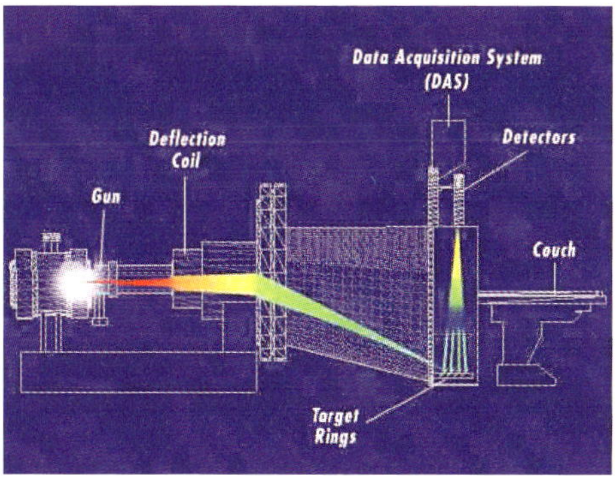

Figure 13.65
Illustration of the electron beam CT principle

struction, is composed of two quarter rotations acquired simultaneously by the two systems (fig. 13.64).

A scanner of this type provides temporal resolution roughly equivalent to a quarter of the rotation time (i.e. independent of the heart rate).

Electron beam CT (EBCT) represents an alternative scanner concept that enables one to avoid mechanically moving parts (fig. 13.65). This technology involves the emission of an electron beam from a powerful electron gun and the beam's magnetic deflection towards a circular anode surrounding the patient. The magnetic deflection sweeps the electron beam over the target, thus generating an X-ray source that virtually rotates around the patient. Given the absence of mechanically moving parts, a sweep can be accomplished in as little as 50 ms.

The EBCT principle is currently not regarded as an alternative to general purpose high-end CT scanners owing to inherent disadvantages in the measurement principle, including a large amount of scattered radiation, problematic geometric efficiency and insufficient X-ray peak power for a good signal-to-noise ratio.

13.6.4 Maximum data volumes and theoretical CT limitations

While early single-slice CT scanners required several seconds for a single rotation (generating roughly 1 MB of data), today's scanners (e.g. the SOMATOM Sensation 64) generate measurement data at a rate of up to 400 MB/s. This stream of data represents a challenge when it comes to data transmission off the gantry and real-time data processing in downstream image-reconstruction systems. Today, images are reconstructed at a rate of up to 40 images/s. Typical scanning protocols generate several thousands of images. Given that visualization and evaluation workstations need to cope with such volumes of data, it is important to try to estimate future developments with regard to data volumes. Here, it warrants bearing in mind that an image made up of N by N pixels of size a can only contain information up to spatial frequencies of $1/(2a)$. Typical scanners are capable of resolving details up to spatial frequencies of 20 lp/cm in the scan plane, corresponding to an object size of 0.25 mm. Consider, for instance, a CT scanner with a resolution of 0.25 mm in all three dimensions. The scanning range is limited to a diameter of 50 cm and a length of 200 cm. It follows that the maximum number of voxels required to adequately represent the data volume will be roughly $2{,}000 \times 2{,}000 \times 8{,}000$, or 64 GB worth of data. This volume can be regarded as an upper limit so long as only one point in time is to be represented.

We have shown in section 1 that the variance of the pixel noise is proportional to the 4th power of the resolution in 3D space. The variance of the pixel noise increases linearly along with an increase in longitudinal resolution and along with the third power of the in-plane resolution. Fig. 13.66 shows the increase in noise when the in-plane resolution is increased. Consequently, the maintenance of a given signal-to-noise ratio will require one to increase the applied dose by the power of 4 if the resolution is to be increased in all three dimensions. In order to double the resolution without increasing the pixel noise, the dose will need to be increased 16-fold! On the other hand,

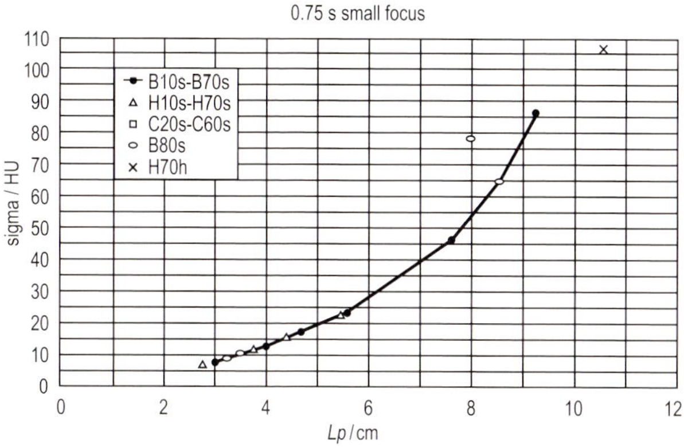

Figure 13.66
Noise levels for scans of a 20 cm water phantom on the SOMATOM Sensation 16 using a rotation time of 0.75 s, a collimation of 16 × 0.75 mm and various reconstruction kernels [13.88]

one cannot expect to be able to increase the patient dose significantly. Reference values and restrictions are currently being introduced in many countries. Ultra-high resolution imaging will therefore be limited to special applications in which high noise levels can be tolerated on account of high object contrast (e.g. in lung and bone imaging).

13.7 References

[13.1] R.N. Bracewell
Strip integration in radioastronomy
Aust. J. Phys. 9 (1956), 198

[13.2] R.N. Bracewell, A.C. Riddle
Inversion of fan-beam scans in radioastronomy
Astrophys. J. 150 (1967), 427

[13.3] W.H. Oldendorf
Isolated flying spot detection of radio-density discontinuities displaying the internal structural pattern of a complex object
IRE Trans. Biomed. Elect. BME 8 (1961), 68-72

[13.4] D.E. Kuhl, R.Q. Edwards
Rapid brain scanner with self contained computer and CRT display for both rectilinear and transverse section viewing
J. Nucl. Med. 9 (1968), 332

[13.5] A.M. Cormack
Representation of a function by its line integrals, with some radiological applications
J. Appl. Phys. 34 (1963), 2722-2727

[13.6] G.N. Hounsfield
Computerized transverse axial scanning (tomography), Part I. Description of system
Br. J. Radiol. 46 (1973), 1016

[13.7] C.R. Crawford, K.F. King
Computed tomography scanning with simultaneous patient translation
Med. Phys. 17 (1990), 967-982

[13.8] W. Kalender, W. Seissler, E. Klotz, P. Vock
Spiral volumetric CT with single-breath-hold technique, continuous transport and continuous scanner rotation
Radiology 176 (1990), 181-183

[13.9] A. Polacin, W.A. Kalender, G. Marchal
Evaluation of section sensitivity profiles and image noise in spiral CT
Radiology 185 (1992), 29-35

[13.10] G.D. Rubin, S. Napel
Increased scan pitch for vascular and thoracic spiral CT
Radiology 197 (1995), 316-317

[13.11] G.D. Rubin, M.D. Dake, C.P. Semba
Current status of three-dimensional spiral CT scanning for imaging the vasculature
Radiol. Clin. North Am. 33 (1995), 51-70

[13.12] S. Napel, G.D. Rubin, R.B. Jeffrey
STS-MIP: a new reconstruction technique for CT of the chest
JCAT 17 (1993), 832-838

[13.13] W. Kalender
Thin-section three-dimensional spiral CT: is isotropic imaging possible?
Radiology 197 (1995), 578-580

[13.14] K. Klingenbeck-Regn, S. Schaller, T. Flohr, B. Ohnesorge, A.F. Kopp, U. Baum
Subsecond multi-slice computed tomography: basics and applications
EJR 31 (1999), 110-124

[13.15] C.H. McCollough, F.E. Zink
Performance evaluation of a multi-slice CT system
Med. Phys. 26 (1999), 2223-2230

[13.16] B. Ohnesorge, T. Flohr, S. Schaller, K. Klingenbeck-Regn, C. Becker, U.J. Schöpf, R. Brüning, M.F. Reiser
Technische Grundlagen und Anwendungen der Mehrschicht-CT
Radiologe 39 (1999), 923-931

[13.17] H. Hu, H.D. He, W.D. Foley, S.H. Fox
Four multidetector-row helical CT: image quality and volume coverage speed
Radiology 215 (2000), 55-62

[13.18] T. Flohr, K. Stierstorfer, H. Bruder, J. Simon, S. Schaller
New technical developments in multislice CT, part 1: approaching isotropic resolution with sub-mm 16-slice scanning
Röfo 174 (2002), 839-845

[13.19] H. Hu
Multi-slice helical CT: scan and reconstruction
Med. Phys. 26 (1999), 5-18

[13.20] T. Flohr, H. Bruder, K. Stierstorfer, J. Simon, S. Schaller, B. Ohnesorge
New technical developments in multislice CT, part 2: sub-millimeter 16-slice scanning and increased gantry rotation speed for cardiac imaging
Röfo 174 (2002), 1022-1027

[13.21] Y. Saito, T. Suzuki
Evaluation of the performance of multi-slice CT system in non-helical scanning
Radiology 209(P) (2000), 578

[13.22] J. Hsieh
Investigation of the slice sensitivity profile for step-and-shoot mode multi-slice computed tomography
Med. Phys. 28 (2001), 491-500

[13.23] S. Schaller, T. Flohr, K. Klingenbeck, J. Krause, T. Fuchs, W.A. Kalender
Spiral interpolation algorithm for multi-slice spiral CT – part 1: theory
IEEE Trans. Med. Imag.19 (2000), 822-834

[13.24] J. Hsieh
Analytical models for multi-slice helical CT performance parameters
Med. Phys 30 (2003), 169-178

[13.25] T. Taguchi, H. Aradate
Algorithm for image reconstruction in multi-slice helical CT
Med. Phys. 25 (1998), 550-561

[13.26] T. Fuchs, J. Krause, S. Schaller, T. Flohr, W.A. Kalender
Spiral interpolation algorithms for multislice spiral CT – part 2: measurement and evaluation of slice sensitivity profiles and noise at a clinical multislice system
IEEE Trans. Med. Imag. 19 (2000), 835-847

[13.27] M. Defrise, R. Clack
A cone-beam reconstruction algorithm using shift variant filtering and cone-beam backprojection
IEEE Trans. Med. Imag. 13 (1994), 186-195

[13.28] S. Schaller, F. Noo, F. Sauer, K.C. Tam, G. Lauritsch, T. Flohr
Exact Radon rebinning algorithm for the long object problem in helical cone-beam CT
IEEE Trans. Med. Imag. 19 (2000), 361-375

[13.29] A. Katsevich
Theoretically exact filtered backprojection-type inversion algorithm for spiral CT
SIAM Journal of Applied Mathematics 62 (2002), 2012-2026

[13.30] L.A. Feldkamp, L.C. Davis, J.W. Kress
Practical cone-beam algorithm
J. Opt. Soc. Am. A 1 (1984), 612-619

[13.31] G. Wang, T. Lin, P. Cheng
A general cone-beam reconstruction algorithm
IEEE Trans. Med. Imag. 12 (1993), 486-496

[13.32] I. Hein, K. Taguchi, M.D. Silver, M. Kazarna, I. Mori
Feldkamp-based cone-beam reconstruction for gantry-tilted helical multislice CT
Med. Phys. 30 (2003), 3233-3242

[13.33] G. Larson, C. Ruth, C. Crawford
Nutating slice CT image reconstruction
Patent Application WO 98/44847, filed 8 April, 1998

[13.34] H. Turbell, P.E. Danielsson
An improved PI-method for reconstruction from helical cone beam projections
IEEE Medical Imaging Conference, Seattle, 1999

[13.35] M. Kachelrieß, S. Schaller, W.A. Kalender
Advanced single-slice rebinning in cone-beam spiral CT
Med. Phys. 27 (2000), 754-772

[13.36] S. Schaller, K. Stierstorfer, H. Bruder, M. Kachelrieß, T. Flohr
Novel approximate approach for high-quality image reconstruction in helical cone beam CT at arbitrary pitch
Proc. SPIE Int. Symp. Med. Imag. 4322 (2001), 113-127

[13.37] T. Flohr, K. Stierstorfer, H. Bruder, J. Simon, A. Polacin, S. Schaller
Image reconstruction and image quality evaluation for a 16-slice CT scanner
Med. Phys. 30 (2003), 832-845

[13.38] J. Hsieh, T.L. Toth, P. Simoni, B. Grekowicz, C.C. Slack, G.E. Seidenschnur
A generalized helical reconstruction algorithm for multi-slice CT
Radiology 221(P) (2001), 271

[13.39] K. Stierstorfer, R. Rauscher, J. Boese, H. Bruder, S. Schaller, T. Flohr
Weighted FBP- a simple approximate 3D FBP algorithm for multislice spiral CT with good dose usage for arbitrary pitch
Phys. Med. Biol. 49 (2004), 2209-2218

[13.40] K. Stierstorfer, T. Flohr, H. Bruder
Segmented Multiple Plane Reconstruction – a novel approximate reconstruction scheme for multislice spiral CT
Phys. Med. Biol. 47 (2002), 2571-2581

[13.41] T.L. Toth, P. Simoni
A quantitative measure of CT helical artifact
Radiology 221(P) (2001), 218

[13.42] T. Flohr, K. Stierstorfer, R. Raupach, S. Ulzheimer, H. Bruder
Performance evaluation of a 64-slice CT-system with z-flying focal spot
Röfo 176 (2004), 1803-1810

[13.43] R. Morin, T. Gerber, C. McCollough
Radiation dose in computed tomography of the heart
Circulation 107 (2003), 917-922

[13.44] M. Budoff, D. Georgiou, A. Brody, A.S. Agatston, J. Kennedy, C. Wolfkiel, W. Stanford, P. Shields, R.J. Lewis, W.R. Janowitz, S. Rich, B.H. Brundage
Ultrafast computed tomography as a diagnostic modality in the detection of coronary artery disease: a multicenter study
Circulation 93 (1996), 898-904

[13.45] M. Kachelriess, W. Kalender
Electrocardiogram-correlated image reconstruction from subsecond spiral

computed tomography scans of the heart
Med. Phys. 25 (1998), 2417-2431

[13.46] M. Bahner, J. Boese, A. Lutz, et al.
Retrospectively ECG-gated spiral CT of the heart and lung
Eur. Radiol. 9 (1999), 106-109

[13.47] B. Ohnesorge, T. Flohr, C. Becker, A. Kopp, U. Schoepf, U. Baum, A. Knez, K. Klingenbeck-Regn, M. Reiser
Cardiac imaging by means of electro-cardiographically gated multisection spiral CT
– initial experience
Radiology 217 (2000), 564-571

[13.48] A. Knez, C. Becker, A. Leber, B. Ohnesorge, M. Reiser, R. Haberl
Non-invasive assessment of coronary artery stenoses with multidetector helical computed tomography
Circulation 101 (2000), e221-e222

[13.49] K. Nieman, M. Oudkerk, B. Rensing, P. van Oijen, A. Munne, R. van Geuns, P. de Feyter
Coronary angiography with multi-slice coputed tomography
The Lancet 357 (2001), 599-603

[13.50] M. Kachelriess, S. Ulzheimer, W. Kalender
ECG-correlated image reconstruction from subsecond multi-slice spiral CT scans of the heart
Med. Phys. 27 (2000), 1881-1902

[13.51] C. Hong, C.R. Becker, A. Huber, U.J. Schoepf, B. Ohnesorge, A. Knez, R. Brüning, M.F. Reiser
ECG-gated reconstructed multi-detector row CT coronary angiography: effect of varying trigger delay on image quality
Radiology 220 (2001), 712-717

[13.52] S. Schroeder, A. Kopp, A. Baumbach, C. Meisner, A. Kuettner, C. Georg, B. Ohnesorge, C. Herdeg, C. Claussen, K. Karsch
Noninvasive detection and evaluation of atherosclerotic coronary plaques with multi-slice computed tomography
JACC 37 (2001), 1430-1435

[13.53] S. Schroeder, T. Flohr, A.F. Kopp, C. Meisner, A. Kuettner, C. Herdeg, A. Baumbach, B. Ohnesorge
Accuracy of density measurements within plaques located in artificial coronary arteries by X-ray multislice CT: results of a phantom study
JCAT 25 (2001), 900-906

[13.54] T. Flohr, U.J. Schoepf, A. Kuettner, S. Halliburton, H. Bruder, C. Suess, B. Schmidt, L. Hofmann, E.K. Yucel, S. Schaller, B. Ohnesorge
Advances in cardiac imaging with 16-section CT-Systems
Acad. Radiol.10 (2003), 386-401

[13.55] K. Nieman, F. Cademartiri, P.A. Lemos, R. Raaijmakers, P.M.T. Pattynama, P.J. de Feyter
Reliable noninvasive coronary angiography with fast submillimeter multislice spiral computed tomography
Circulation 106 (2002), 2051-2054

[13.56] D. Ropers, U. Baum, K. Pohle, K. Anders, S. Ulzheimer, B. Ohnesorge, C. Schlundt, W. Bautz, W.G. Daniel, S. Achenbach
Detection of coronary artery stenoses with thin-slice multi-detector row spiral computed tomography and multiplanar reconstruction
Circulation 107 (2003), 664-666

[13.57] D.P. Boyd, M.J. Lipton
Cardiac computed tomography
Proceedings of the IEEE 71 (1982), 298-307

[13.58] A.S. Agatston, W.R. Janowitz, F.J. Hildner, N.R. Zusmer, M. Viamonte, R. Detrano
Quantification of coronary artery calcium using ultrafast computed tomography
JACC 15 (1990), 827-832

[13.59] C.R. Becker, T.F. Jakobs, S. Aydemir, A. Becker, A. Knez, U.J. Schöpf, R. Brüning, R. Haberl, M.F. Reiser
Helical and single-slice conventional CT versus electron beam CT for the quantification of coronary artery calcification
AJR 174 (2000),543-547.

[13.60] T. Flohr, B. Ohnesorge, H. Bruder, K. Stierstorfer, J. Simon, C. Suess, S. Schaller
Image reconstruction and performance evaluation for ECG-gated spiral scanning with a 16-slice CT system
Med. Phys. 30 (2003), 2650-2662

[13.61] H. Bruder, S. Schaller, B. Ohnesorge, T. Mertelmeier
High temporal resolution volume heart imaging with multirow computed tomography
Proc. SPIE Int. Symp. Med. Imag. 3661 (1999), 420-432.

[13.62] T. Pan, Y. Shen
New multi-sector reconstruction for cardiac CT
Nuclear Science Symposium Conference Record, 2000 IEEE

[13.63] K. Taguchi, H. Anno
High temporal resolution for multi-slice helical computed tomography
Med. Phys. 27 (2000), 861-872

[13.64] H. Bruder, K. Stierstofer, B. Ohnesorge, S. Schaller, T. Flohr
A novel reconstruction scheme for cardiac volume imaging with MSCT providing cone-correction
Proc. SPIE Medical Imaging Conf. 4684 (2002), 60-71

[13.65] T.F. Jakobs, C.R. Becker, B. Ohnesorge, T. Flohr, C. Suess, U.J. Schoepf, M.F. Reiser
Multislice helical CT of the heart with retrospective ECG gating: reduction of radiation exposure by ECG-controlled tube current modulation
Eur. Radiol. 12 (2002), 1081-1086

[13.66] J. Shemesh, S. Apter, C.I. Stroh, Y. Itzchak, M. Motro
Tracking coronary calcification by using dual-section spiral CT: a 3-year follow-up
Radiology 217 (2000), 461-465

[13.67] C.R. Becker, T. Kleffel, A. Crispin, A. Knez, Y. Young, U.J. Schöpf, R. Haberl, M.F. Reiser
Coronary artery calcium measurement: agreement of multirow detector and

electron beam CT
AJR 176 (2001), 1295-1298

[13.68] A.F. Kopp, B. Ohnesorge, C. Becker, S. Schröder, M. Heuschmid, A. Küttner, R. Kuzo, C.D. Claussen
Reproducibility and accuracy of coronary calcium measurement with multi-detector-row versus electron beam CT
Radiology 225 (2002), 113-119

[13.69] B. Ohnesorge, A.F. Kopp, R. Fischbach, A. Knez, S. Schröder, U.J. Schöpf, A. Crispin, E. Klotz, T. Flohr, M.F. Reiser, C.R. Becker
Reproducibility of coronary calcium quantification in repeat examinations with retrospectively ECG-gated multislice spiral CT
Eur. Radiol. 12 (2002), 1532-1540

[13.70] K. Moser, T. Bateman, J. Case, et al.
The influence of acquisition mode on the reproducibility of coronary artery calcium scores using multi-detector computed tomography (abstract)
Circulation 106 (Suppl. II) (2002), 479

[13.71] K.U. Juergens, M. Grude, E.M. Fallenberg, W. Heindel, R. Fischbach
Using ECG-gated multidetector CT to evaluate global left ventricular myocardial function in patients with coronary artery disease
AJR 179 (2002), 1545-1550

[13.72] C.I. Henschke, D.I. McCauley, D.F. Yankelevitz, D.P. Naidich, G. McGuinness, O.S. Miettinnen, D.M. Libby, M.W. Pasmantier, J. Koizumi, A.K. Altorki, J.P. Smith
Early lung cancer action project, overall design and findings from baseline screening
Lancet 354 (1999), 99-105

[13.73] M. Macari, E.J. Bini, S.L. Jacobs, S. Naik, Y.W. Lui, A. Milano, R. Rajapaksa, A.J. Megibow, J. Babb
Colorectal polyps and cancers in asymptomatic average-risk patents: evaluation with CT colonography
Radiology 230 (2004), 629-636

[13.74] P.J. Pickhardt, J.R. Choi, I. Hwang, J.A. Butler, M.L. Puckett, H.A. Hildebrandt, R.K. Wong, P.A. Nugent, P.A. Mysliwiec, W.R. Schindler
Computed tomographic virtual colonoscopy to screen for colorectal neoplasia in asymptomatic adults
N. Engl. J. Med. 349 (2003), 2191-2200

[13.75] J. Weßling, R. Fischbach, N. Meier, T. Allkemper, J. Klusmeier, K. Ludwig, W. Heindel
CT colonography: protocol optimization with multi-detector row CT – study in an anthropomorphic colon phantom
Radiology 228 (2003), 753-759

[13.76] Y.W. Lui, M. Macari, G. Israel, E.J. Bini, H. Wang, J. Babb
CT colonography data interpretation: effect of different section thicknesses – preliminary observations
Radiology 229 (2003), 791-797

[13.77] C. Enzweiler, P. Chan, U. Hoffmann, et al.
In vitro coronary stent imaging: novel flat-panel volume CT versus multidetector

CT
Eur. Radiol. 13(S) (2003), 195

[13.78] K. Nikolaou, T. Flohr, K. Stierstorfer, C.R. Becker, M.F. Reiser
Flat panel computed tomography of human ex vivo heart and bone specimens: initial experience
Eur. Radiol. 15 (2005),329-333

[13.79] D.W. Townsend, S.R. Cherry
Combining anatomy and function: the path of true image fusion
Eur. Radiol. 11 (2001), 1968-1974

[13.80] B. Ohnesorge, T. Flohr, K. Schwarz, J.P. Heiken, K.T. Bae
Efficient correction for CT image artifacts caused by objects extending outside the scan field of view
Med. Phys. 27 (2000), 39-46

[13.81] M. Namdar, P. Kaufmann, T. Hany, G. von Schulthess
Combined CT-angiogram and PET perfusion imaging for assessment of CAD in a novel PET/CT: A pilot feasibility study
Eur. Radiol. 13(S) (2003), 165

[13.82] I.J. Garcia-Ramirez, S. Mutic, J.F. Dempsey, D.A. Low, J.A. Purdy
Performance evaluation of an 85 cm bore X-ray computed tomography scanner designed for radiation oncology and comparison with current diagnostic CT scanners
Int. J. Radiat. Oncol. Biol. Phys. 52 (2002), 1123-1131

[13.83] R. Robb, E. Ritman
High speed synchronous volume computed tomography of the heart
Radiology 133 (1979), 655-661

[13.84] J. Hsieh, B. Grekowicz, P. Simoni, J.B. Thibault, M.C. Joshi, S. Dutta, E.C. Williams, C. Shaughnessy, P. Sainath
Convolution reconstruction algorithm for multi-slice helical CT
Proc. SPIE Int. Symp. Med. Imag. 2003

[13.85] T. Flohr, B. Ohnesorge
Heart rate adaptive optimization of spatial and temporal resolution for ECG-gated multi-slice spiral CT of the heart
JCAT 25 (2001), 907-923

[13.86] E. Cesmeli, M. Edic, M. Iatrou, A. Pfoh
A Novel Reconstruction Algorithm for Multiphasic Cardiac Imaging Using Multislice CT
Proc. SPIE Int. Symp. Med. Imag. 4320 (2001), 645-654

[13.87] S. Ulzheimer, W.A. Kalender
Assessment of calcium scoring performance in cardiac computed tomography
Eur. Radiol. 13 (2003), 484-497

[13.88] T. Fuchs, W.A. Kalender
On the correlation of pixel noise, spatial resolution and dose in computed tomography: Theoretical prediction and verification by simulation and measurement
Physica Medica XIX (2003), 153-164

14 Nuclear medicine

14.1 Introduction

Nuclear medicine imaging involves image formation through the detection of high energy photons. Many of the steps in this process resemble those in diagnostic radiology. A fundamental difference, however, is that nuclear medicine involves the emission of radiation from the organ or tissue under examination, whereas radiology involves the transmission of radiation through the tissue.

Clinical applications in nuclear medicine involve injecting patients with a radioactively labeled pharmaceutical (i.e. a radiopharmaceutical) that accumulates in target organs or pathologic tissue. The decay of the radioactive atoms supplies the photons used to produce the nuclear medicine image. The temporal course of the radioactivity measured within the organ often permits diagnosis of functional abnormalities. Kidney filtration and excretion rates, for example, can be measured during a 30-minute dynamic scan, dynamic in the sense that many time points are measured during the 30-minute acquisition. The ability to gather information about biochemical, metabolic, and functional processes in vivo with no pharmacologic effect (via the tracer principle) is a unique feature of nuclear medicine imaging. Two broad areas in nuclear medicine imaging can be distinguished according to the type of radioactive decay exhibited by the nuclide attached to the pharmaceutical:

a) Imaging with single photon emitters

A nuclear medicine image can be formed by counting the individual photons emitted by a radionuclide. The energy and the location of each detected photon are recorded and the image is formed via the accumulation of many thousands of individual photons. When deployed in conjunction with parallel hole collimation, single photon imaging back-projects the detected locations of the photons onto a life-sized image of the distribution of radioactivity within the patient. Single photon images are referred to as planar scintigraphy or projections, analogous to projection radiography. Three-dimensional images are produced by single photon emission computed tomography or SPECT when cross sectional images are reconstructed from multiple projections in a manner analogous to X-ray computed tomography.

b) Imaging with positron emitters

Positron emission imaging involves the use of nuclides that have an excess positive charge in their nuclei, and thereby exhibit a tendency to emit a positively charged positron. The positron is the antiparticle of the negatively charged electron. Positron decay results in an annihilation of the positron and a neighboring electron and the emission of oppositely-directed gamma-ray photons, each exhibiting an energy level of 511 keV. Three-dimensional digital imaging of the original decay sites results from the coincidence detection of these gamma-rays via detectors located on opposite sides of the patient's body.

The practice of nuclear medicine pioneered the use of digital imaging techniques years before X-ray CT came into clinical use [14.1]. The close cooperation between physicians, physicists, engineers, radiochemists and biochemists in clinical research and industrial environments has been crucial in the establishment of the technology and its applications.

14.2 Imaging with single photon emitters – measurement principles and devices

Despite considerable progress in the area of semiconductor detectors [14.2, 14.3], the clinical imaging devices currently in use are based on the scintillation detector. We therefore preface our discussion with a review of some basic considerations relating scintillation detectors.

14.2.1 The scintillation detector

Fig. 14.1 offers an illustration of basic scintillation detector design [14.4]. The primary element of detection is an optically transparent scintillation crystal with a high atomic number. This crystal absorbs γ-ray photons and converts each photon's energy into a multitude of visible light photons (N_{ph}). A good scintillator is distinguished by high detection efficiency, high light yield and rapid signal decay. Sodium iodide doped with thallium (NaI(Tl)) meets the requirements for SPECT imaging and lutetium orthosilicate (LSO) meets the requirements for PET imaging.

Each photon generated in the scintillation crystal has a probability p of producing a photoelectron at the cathode of the photomultiplier (PM). For each gamma ray detected, the signal from the photoelectrons undergoes low-noise amplification in the PM's dynode system and further amplification and shaping in the preamplifier (PA). The integrator (I) (fig. 14.1) smoothes the signal while the pulse height analyzer (PHA) performs a rough pre-selection of signal amplitude. The signal then undergoes analog-to-digital (A/D) conversion and is passed on to a multichannel analyzer (MCA) in which individual signals are binned according to their pulse amplitudes. Given that this pulse height is proportional to the energy of the absorbed gamma-ray photon, the accumulated spectrum of pulse heights will represent the energy spectrum of the gamma-radiation incident on the detector.

The spectrum shown in fig. 14.1 features a peak at energy level E_0 that corresponds to the incident gamma-ray energy. This peak exhibits a finite width ΔE that reflects an important scintillation detector property: energy resolution. Even in the case of monoenergetic radiation (i.e. all incident photons have the same energy), the system produces a peak exhibiting a finite width centered on the original energy E_0. This broadening is

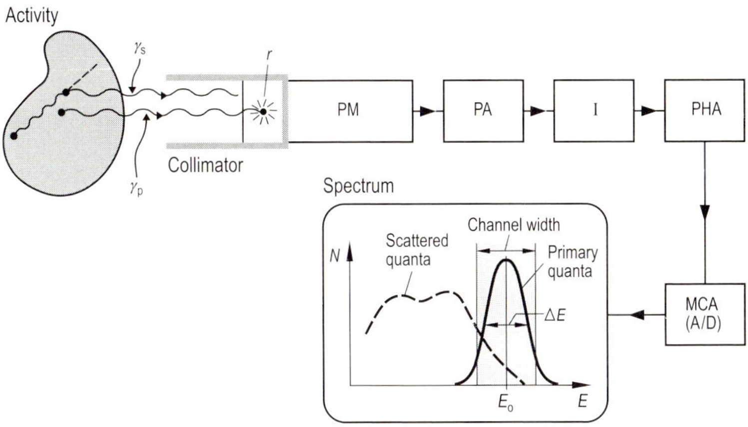

Figure 14.1
Diagram of a scintillation detector's components (PM: photomultiplier; PA: preamplifier; I: integrator; PHA: pulse height analyzer; MCA: multichannel analyzer; *N*: number of pulses; γ_p: primary quanta; γ_s: scattered quanta; *E*: energy, ΔE: pulse width)

due to statistical fluctuations associated with the various energy conversion processes within the scintillation detector and electronic amplification system. The relative value of the full width at half maximum $\Delta E/E_0$ (usually expressed as a percentage) represents a quantitative measure of the detector's energy resolution.

The mean number N_{Ph} of visible light photons generated by a detected gamma ray can be described to a good approximation by a Poisson distribution [14.5]. Given the probability *p* that a single photon will produce a single photoelectron at the cathode of the photomultiplier (PM), the mean number of photoelectrons can be expressed by pN_{Ph} and the statistical fluctuation by $\sqrt{pN_{Ph}}$.

Considering other sources of noise to be negligible compared to that associated with the number of visible light photons, the energy resolution can be expressed as

$$\frac{\Delta E}{E_0} = \frac{1}{\sqrt{pN_{Ph}}} \tag{14.1}$$

A scintillation detector will exhibit good energy resolution if the following criteria are met: high light yield, efficient light transmission to the photomultiplier cathodes and high quantum efficiency in the conversion of visible light photons to photoelectrons. Practical values of about 10% for $\Delta E/E_0$ can be achieved with clinical gamma cameras (at E_0 = 140 keV, i.e. the γ-ray energy resulting from the decay of ^{99m}Tc).

Given the fact that the detected photons may have undergone significant scatter inside the patient's body, good scintillation detector energy resolution is very important for clinical applications. In contrast to the primary photons, the scattered photons do not contribute directly to the image's information content (as indicated in fig. 14.1). The underlying reason for this is that the location of the detected photon does not correspond to the position of its original emission inside the patient. The scattered radiation may exceed the useful primary radiation for many clinical applications.

The corresponding pulse heights recorded for scatter in the energy spectrum shown in fig. 14.1 are less than the primary energy E_0 because the photons lose energy during the scattering process (via Compton-effect collisions with outer-shell electrons in patient tissue).

A large fraction of the scattered quanta can be eliminated by adjusting the pulse height analyzer to accept only primary events. Doing so enables one to avoid the image quality degradation associated with improperly placed events.

14.2.2 The gamma camera (Anger camera)

When nuclear imaging was first introduced in the early 1950's, objects were scanned using collimated single detectors [14.6, 14.7] to obtain two-dimensional images of the activity distribution inside the body. Various designs were investigated throughout the same decade with the aim of developing a large area detector with good spatial resolution and shortened acquisition times [14.8]. The gamma camera, also known as the Anger camera after its inventor H.O. Anger [14.9], emerged as the standard device for single photon nuclear imaging. Decades of technological improvements have since led to the availability of gamma cameras that perform near the physical limits.

14.2.2.1 Image generation

Fig. 14.2 offers an example of a γ-camera design and illustrates the basic principles of γ-camera imaging. The key element is a large NaI(Tl) single crystal that absorbs the γ-rays emitted from the patient. A mechanical collimator (e.g. parallel hole collimator) is placed in front of the crystal. This collimator defines the direction of the projection imaging. Due to collimation, only those γ-rays that impinge nearly perpendicularly to the crystal surface are recorded, while obliquely incident γ-rays are absorbed in the collimator walls (also known as septa). A series of PMs is optically coupled to the rear face of the crystal. The electrical output signals from these PMs are used for localization (i.e. to determine the position (x,y) absorbed within the crystal) and for pulse height analysis following summation. The sum of the PM signals forms the event energy used for pulse height analysis.

The gamma camera's active area is divided into a generally square matrix of image elements (pixels) to set up the nuclear emission image. Each pixel (i, j) contains the events that have been recorded during the time of measurement, i.e. the number $n_{ij}(t)$ of quanta absorbed at the location (x_i,y_j).

The gamma camera's output provides at least three signals for each event: the X-signal and the Y-signal, representing the spatial coordinates x and y, and the Z-signal (sum of all individual PM signals), representing the energy of the absorbed quantum.

Each event is added to a bin of events (one bin per pixel) following analog-to-digital conversion. The matrix of pixel bins is formatted and displayed on a computer monitor. These elements are shown in a simplified graphical form in fig. 14.3.

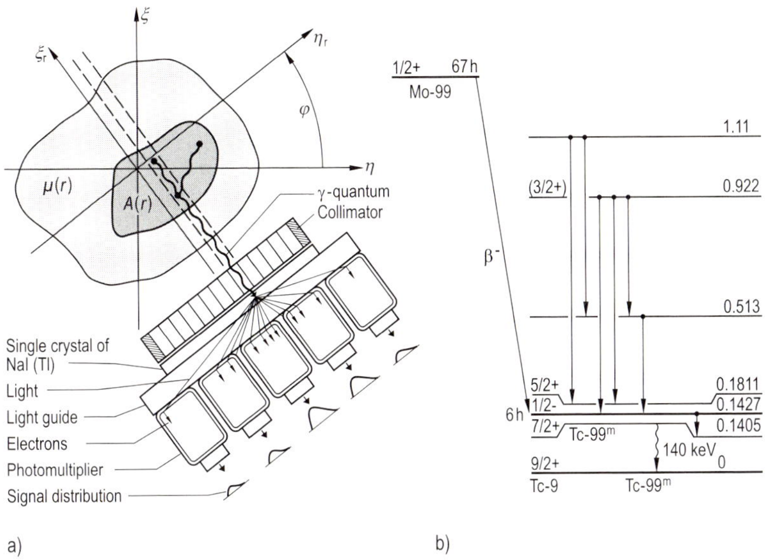

Figure 14.2
Representation of image generation with a gamma camera **(a)** and decay of the nuclides ^{99}Mo and ^{99m}Tc **(b)**. Energy levels are indicated in MeV.

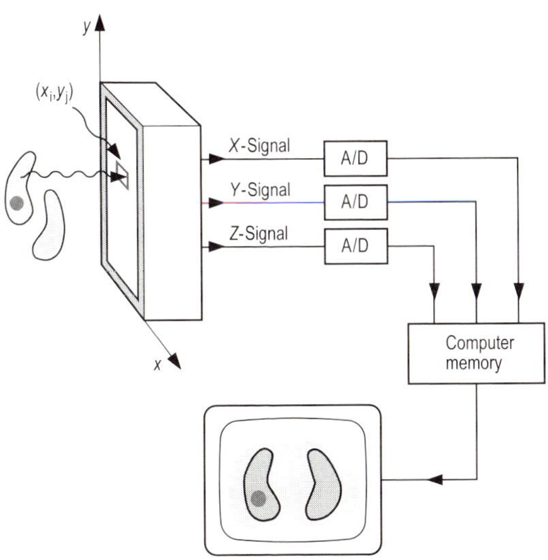

Figure 14.3
Imaging with a gamma camera

The total number N_γ of quanta per image and the number n_{ij} per pixel represent important features in nuclear emission images. Given that the emission of γ-quanta during nuclear decay is a statistical process, the numbers N and n_{ij} are subject to statistical fluctuation. The corresponding standard deviations for a Poisson distribution for nuclear decay can be expressed as

$$\frac{\Delta N_\gamma}{N_\gamma} = \frac{1}{\sqrt{N_\gamma}}. \tag{14.2}$$

For n_{ij} holds an analogous equation. It follows that the statistical accuracy of the measured activity distribution increases along with an increase in the numbers of events per image and per pixel.

Fig. 14.2b shows the decay diagram for the nuclide ^{99m}Tc (the most-often-used nuclide in single-photon clinical applications). γ-ray photons with energy of 140 keV are generated by transitions from an excited, metastable state to the ground state. The metastable state has a half-life of 6:02 h and is populated by the γ-decay of the mother nucleus ^{99}Mo.

14.2.2.2 Collimators

As mentioned above, the collimator defines the direction of projection for the emission image. Photons emitted from the patient that assume the appropriate angle of incidence can traverse the collimator via one of the narrow holes in the array of narrow holes. These photons can then enter the scintillation crystal for detection and localization. The geometric characteristics of a collimator therefore strongly influence the spatial resolution and sensitivity of a nuclear camera. Given that both of these parameters are of great importance to the quality of the nuclear emission images, we discuss them in greater detail in the following paragraphs.

Spatial resolution

To gain a basic understanding of the parameters, it will suffice to consider a single collimator hole. Fig. 14.4 offers an illustration of the relevant geometrical relationships for a round collimator hole. The figure can be regarded as rotationally symmetric with respect to the hole's axis.

The radius R_G defines the circular field of view from which photons can propagate through the collimator hole. R_G can be expressed as follows:

$$R_G = \frac{D}{L}\left(z + \frac{L}{2}\right) \tag{14.3}$$

If a point source of radioactivity is scanned along a line at a constant distance z from the collimator surface, the point spread function (PSF) (fig. 14.4) is represented by the response of the detector to photons passing through the collimator hole. The full width at half maximum (*FWHM*) of the PSF defines the collimator's spatial resolution Δr_{coll}. Given the geometrical relationships shown in fig. 14.4, the collimator resolution can be derived as follows:

$$\Delta r_{\text{coll}} = \frac{D}{L}(L + z) \qquad (14.4)$$

Applying these simple geometric relationships to a real collimator with a plurality of closely spaced holes is complicated by the distance dependence of the point spread function response. As a consequence, the PSF is not shift-invariant.

The solution derived by H.O. Anger [14.10] is based on the concept of an averaged PSF. A rigorous mathematical derivation based on the sampling theorem can be found in [14.5].

The calculation of the collimator's spatial resolution in the case of parallel, round holes [14.5] is as follows:

$$\Delta r_{\text{coll}} = 0.808\, D\left(1 + \frac{z}{L} + \frac{A}{L}\right) \qquad (14.5)$$

A denotes the distance from the collimator to the scintillation crystal's center plane.

It follows from eq. (14.5) that the following criteria are important for optimal spatial resolution: the shortest possible distance from the collimator to the scintillation crystal (A), deep holes (L) and a small hole diameter (D) (i.e. a maximized grid ratio L/D). The magnitude of the grid ratio L/D is limited by the requirement that the collimator's sensitivity (eq. (14.7)) be clinically acceptable.

As can be seen in fig. 14.4, the collimator's spatial resolution depends linearly on the object distance z. This dependence plays a dominant role in actual imaging situations. When it comes to actual clinical applications involving an object distance of several centimeters, this part of the collimator resolution dominates the camera system's overall resolution.

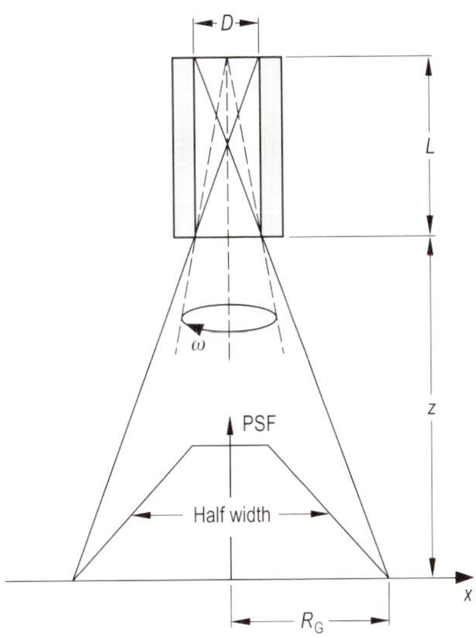

Figure 14.4
Geometry of a single collimator hole. PSF denotes the point spread function response to a point source scanned along the x-axis at a distance z above the collimator.

Sensitivity

Collimator sensitivity (i.e. the fraction of all incident gamma-ray photons that pass through the collimator holes and enter the detector crystal) represents a second important parameter.

To analyze collimator sensitivity, we again consider the case of a single collimator channel (fig. 14.4). For a point source directly in front of the collimator hole ($z = 0$) this fraction is determined by the solid angle ω, which is subtended by the collimator hole:

$$\omega = \frac{\pi D^2}{4L^2} \tag{14.6}$$

The geometrical sensitivity ε can thus be expressed by the ratio of ω to the total solid angle of 4π:

$$\varepsilon = \frac{D^2}{16L^2} \tag{14.7}$$

The collimator's overall geometrical sensitivity can be expressed to a good approximation by:

$$\varepsilon = \alpha \frac{D^2}{16L^2} \tag{14.8}$$

where α denotes the packing density of the collimator (i.e. accounts for the fact that lead septa cover a fraction of the detector surface). A comparison of the sensitivity of eq. (14.8) and the spatial resolution of eq. (14.5) shows that these collimator features impose competing requirements on geometrical design, particularly with respect to the grid ratio D/L. It is therefore important to consider specific clinical applications when seeking to optimize collimator design.

A variety of collimator designs are in use. These range from the LEAP (low energy, all purpose) to the UHRES (ultra-high resolution) collimator.

Finally, it should be pointed out that the relationships discussed are valid for the case of round collimator holes. Readers may wish to refer to [14.11 and 14.12] for a discussion of other hole shapes and a derivation of the corresponding modulation transfer functions. In addition to the parallel hole collimator discussed here, other collimator designs (e.g. cone and fan beam collimators) are used for specific applications.

14.2.2.3 Localization

The most important feature of the Anger camera is its ability to localize detected γ-rays, i.e. to determine the (x,y) coordinates (fig. 14.3) of the location within the crystal where the γ-rays have been absorbed.

The intrinsic spatial resolution r_{int} of the camera does not depend on the collimator. One method of measuring intrinsic spatial resolution is to use a sharply collimated point source (i.e. a pencil beam) directed perpendicularly to the surface of the uncollimated detector.

The spatial resolution of the imaging system can be expressed by the following combination of collimator and intrinsic spatial resolution contributions:

$$\Delta r = \sqrt{\Delta r_{\text{coll}}^2 + \Delta r_{\text{int}}^2} \tag{14.9}$$

Basic principles

Fig. 14.2a offers an illustration of the basic design of an Anger camera's measuring head. Fig. 14.5 shows a two-dimensional array of PMs in a densely packed hexagonal arrangement on a round NaI crystal. The crystals for large field-of-view cameras may exhibit diameters of up to 55 cm and PM numbers greater than 100. Rectangular crystals are deployed in the cameras used in modern multihead systems. These cameras retain an adapted hexagonal arrangement of PMs.

Fig. 14.6 shows a typical profile of the distribution of light $L(x)$ around the absorption site x_A. If the event is sufficiently distant from the crystal edge, this light distribution can be described to a good approximation as rotationally symmetric. The detailed shape of the light distribution and its FWHM strongly depend on the camera's optical elements (e.g. crystal thickness, surface preparation and reflection properties, and the presence and optical properties of a light guide between the crystal and the PM array).

A pattern of electronic output signals $(S_1(x_A), \ldots S_N(x_A))$ that is unique to the absorption site x_A is generated by the array of PMs for any individual event at x_A. As shown in the lower portion of fig. 14.6, the relative PM signal heights comprise the pattern that is characteristic of the absorption position. In other words, the optical elements of the camera effectively encode the absorption position into a vector $(S_1 \ldots S_N)$ of electrical

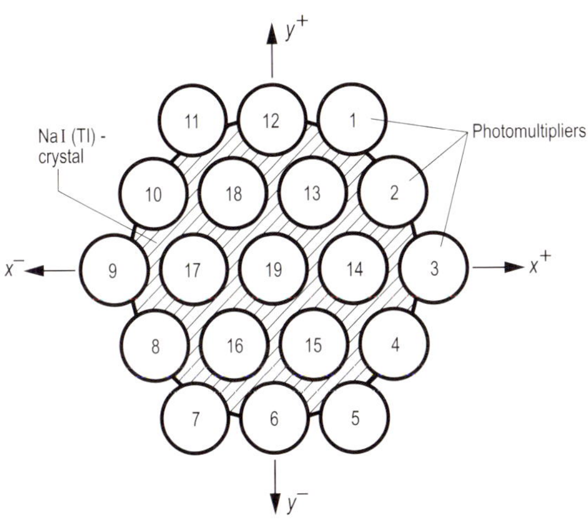

Figure 14.5
Hexagonal arrangement of photomultipliers coupled optically to the crystal surface. The example shows 19 photomultipliers.

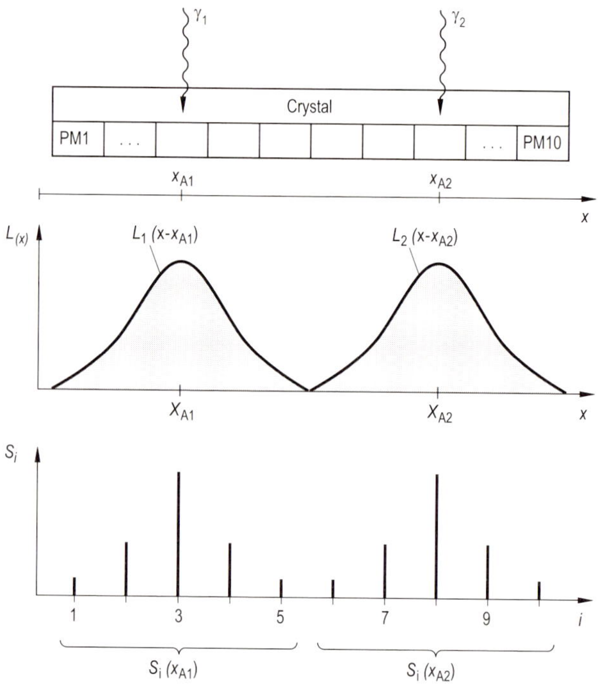

Figure 14.6
Distribution of light $L(x)$ (continuous) and photomultiplier signals $S_i(x_A)$ (discrete, $i = 1..10$) for absorption at two different positions x_{A1} and x_{A2}

output signals. Consequently, the general task of localization is to perform a decoding operation on the ensemble of PM signals.

Center of gravity algorithm

The center of gravity algorithm (also known as Anger localization or Anger logic) represents the standard approach to event localization using the signal vector (S_1 ... S_N). This algorithm is formally analogous to the determination of the center of gravity of a spatial distribution of discrete masses. Here, the spatial center of gravity of an event's discrete signal vector is evaluated and identified with the position of absorption. Using the coordinate system defined in fig. 14.5, the coordinates of the center of gravity can be expressed as:

$$\bar{x} \propto \frac{1}{S}\sum_i x_i S_i \tag{14.10a}$$

Given that the x- and y-direction localization algorithms are independent, it will suffice to consider the one-dimensional case (i.e. y_A is determined analogously to x_A). In eq. (14.10a), $S = \sum S_i$ denotes the sum or the energy signal and x_i denotes the distance of the PM number i to the center of the crystal (fig. 14.6).

The center of gravity algorithm offers the clear advantage of convenient implementation for real-time applications. While alternatives for localization based on statistical estimates (e.g. the maximum likelihood estimator [14.13]) have been proposed and evaluated in the literature, they involve greater computational challenges.

The statistical fluctuations of the S_i signals discussed in section 14.2.1 imply a corresponding uncertainty in the location of the absorption site calculated according to eq. (14.10a). Given that the S_i signals are proportional to the number N_i of photoelectrons at the PM numbered i (apart from a constant gain factor) and the signals of different PMs are statistically independent, the localization error at eq. (14.10a) can be expressed as:

$$\langle \Delta x \rangle^2 = \sum_i \left(\frac{\partial \bar{x}}{\partial S_i} \right)^2 \langle \Delta S \rangle_i^2 \qquad (14.11)$$

Differentiating eq. (14.10a) yields

$$\frac{\partial \bar{x}}{\partial S_i} = \frac{x_i - \bar{x}}{\sum_i S_i} \qquad (14.10b)$$

and therefore

$$\sqrt{\langle \Delta x \rangle^2} = \frac{\rho}{\sqrt{\sum S_i}} \qquad (14.12)$$

where

$$\rho^2 = \frac{\sum (x_i - \bar{x})^2 S_i}{\sum S_i} \qquad (14.13)$$

In eq. (14.13), ρ is the radius of inertia for the signal distribution in fig. 14.6. As such, ρ is a measure of the width of the light distribution within the scintillation crystal. Consequently, the intrinsic resolution of the gamma camera is essentially determined by the width of the light distribution, by the diameter of the PMs used and by the amplitude of the summed PM signals. The PM signals are proportional to the number of photoelectrons released, which in turn is determined by the number of light photons produced by each gamma-ray photon detected.

The intrinsic resolution of a gamma camera is commonly defined as the *FWHH* of a Gaussian point spread function. The corresponding relation between the *FWHH* and the mean standard deviation of eq. (14.12) is:

$$FWHH = 2\sqrt{2\ln 2}\,\sigma = 2.35\,\sigma \qquad (14.14)$$

The intrinsic resolution of large field of view gamma cameras is on the order of a few mm. A visual evaluation of the inherent resolution can be performed using lead slit patterns. A quantitative evaluation of typical imaging geometries, particularly for organs at some depth, shows that the collimator usually dominates the achievable spatial resolution (eqs. (14.5, 14.9, 14.14)).

14.2.2.4 Corrections

In order to achieve optimal image homogeneity and linearity, certain corrections need to be applied to the (X,Y,Z) signals at the camera output. Inhomogeneous light yield across the crystal can cause inhomogeneities in a uniform image. While eq. (14.12) implies that narrowing the light distribution will result in improved spatial resolution, doing so will create a greater dependence on the light yield as a function of the absorption position. As a consequence, the amplitude of the energy signal varies as a function of the absorption position. Variations in the energy signal at different locations will result in inhomogeneities in a camera image of a uniform source of radiation when a fixed energy window is applied to the spectrum.

Image distortions and count-rate fluctuations may also be caused by deviations from spatial linearity. Edge packing generated by distortions in the light distribution as a result of crystal edge reflections constitutes a familiar example. Given that the center-of-gravity localization expressed in eq. (14.10) is a strictly linear algorithm, such non-linear effects result in the misplacement of an event's calculated (x,y) position.

Several methods have been introduced to overcome deterioration of image quality. One involves a sophisticated optical coupling of the photomultipliers to the crystal. Other methods rely on electronic and/or digital corrections of the energy signal Z and the position signals (x,y). As these corrections can be carried out in real time for each event, other camera properties (e.g. counting rate) remain unaffected.

The counting rates of a gamma camera are physically limited by the so-called pile-up effect [14.14]. Pile-up occurs when the temporal interval between the begins of two events is too short, and thus results in the superimposition of the corresponding signals during signal processing. Extensive investigations [14.15, 14.16] of the underlying causes of pile-up have led to the design of effective correction schemes. Recent advances in electronic performance and fast digital algorithms have made it possible to fulfill the most demanding requirements with respect to dynamic, high-count-rate data acquisition in nuclear medicine.

14.3 SPECT systems

14.3.1 General SPECT principle

Single photon emission computed tomography (SPECT) enables one to visualize the distribution of radiotracers in the human body in 3D (x,y,z) or even 4D (x,y,z,t) [14.17]. The availability of radiotracers with various decay energies enables one to apply this imaging capacity to specific organs and body parts. Having provided a review in the previous section of the basic principles behind obtaining projections with Anger systems, we now turn to a discussion of SPECT:

- The γ-camera acquires a 2D projection of the radiotracer distribution within a patient's body at a projection angle θ. Outfitted with large field of view (FOV) detector heads, modern cameras are capable of covering a large part of the human body (fig. 14.7).

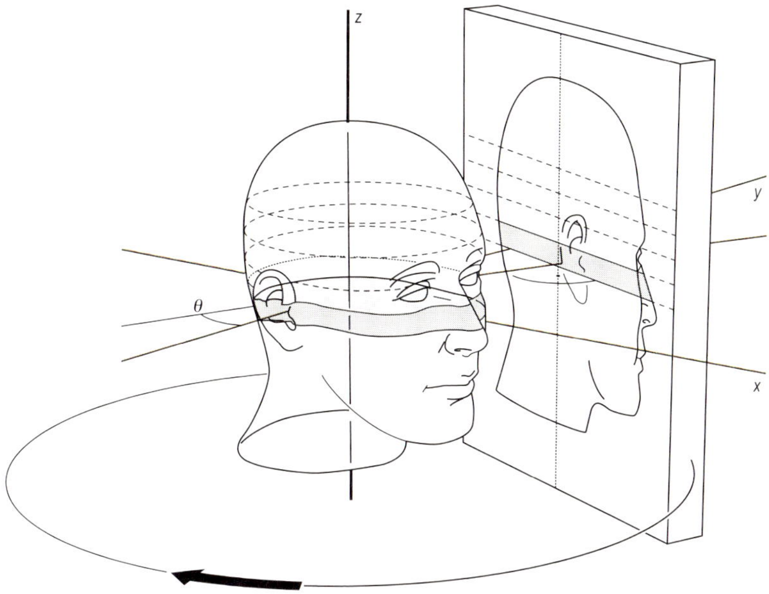

Figure 14.7
SPECT acquisition. The 2D projection of the radiopharmaceutical distribution within the patient's body is imaged at various angles θ. A 3D (x,y,z) or even a 4D (x,y,z,t) view of the functioning of individual organs can be obtained by moving the camera head all the way around the patient.

- The camera head revolves at a certain angular step $\Delta\theta$ around the patient's body to scan the entire region of interest (ROI).
- This movement either describes a circular or non-circular orbit (NCO). The system's spatial resolution varies according to the orbit type used.
- The patient can also be moved along the axis of the camera system's center of rotation (COR) so as to enable one to image larger parts of the body than are covered by the FOV itself.
- The acquired patient body projections are used to compute the volume distribution (non-quantitatively and/or quantitatively) of the radioactively marked tracers according to a mathematical reconstruction procedure that is carried out on modern workstations.
- The reconstructed images are then read by physicians for the sake of diagnosing disease or determining the function of a specific organ.

A camera system will need to meet several requirements in order to yield high quality images: (i) high sensitivity coupled with high spatial resolution and the capacity to image across a wide energy range (70 to 511 keV), (ii) precise camera head movement around the patient's entire body and (iii) reduced or corrected γ-quanta scatter effects.

The patient handling system, in particular, is to be designed for a low γ-attenuation. Finally, fast data acquisition and processing electronics in the camera head are a prerequisite for image reconstruction that yields optimal image quality for downstream workstations.

A variety of γ-cameras is currently available for handling various applications in nuclear medicine. In what follows, we discuss a number of these systems.

14.3.2 Overview of current systems

Two types of γ-cameras are currently in use: (i) general purpose cameras covering all nuclear medicine applications and (ii) cameras dedicated to cardiac SPECT imaging. These camera types can be broken down further according to their head design: single head, dual head and triple head. General purpose cameras are usually outfitted with two large FOV detectors capable of moving relative to one another into a 90° orientation for cardiac applications and a 180° orientation for other applications. Dedicated cardiac cameras are outfitted with smaller detectors that are fixed in 90° orientation. The dual detector camera has turned out to provide the best combination of clinical flexibility, patient throughput and cost efficiency.

While solid-state detector technology remains a subject of investigation (see section 14.3.4), most currently available γ-camera detectors still make use of NaI crystals in two degrees of thickness (3/8" or 5/8"). Owing to their higher γ-absorption, thicker crystals provide better system sensitivity (especially when it comes to imaging medium and high-energy isotopes) but offer lower resolution. Some dual detector γ-cameras are also available with coincidence imaging capacity for positron emission tomography (PET). Segmented 1" crystals are deployed here (fig. 14.8) to bring about improvements in absorption and count rate when it comes to the high energy of the 511 keV positron annihilation radiation.

The importance of nuclear cardiology studies in the noninvasive diagnosis of coronary artery disease, the assessment of heart function and cardiac patient outcome pre-

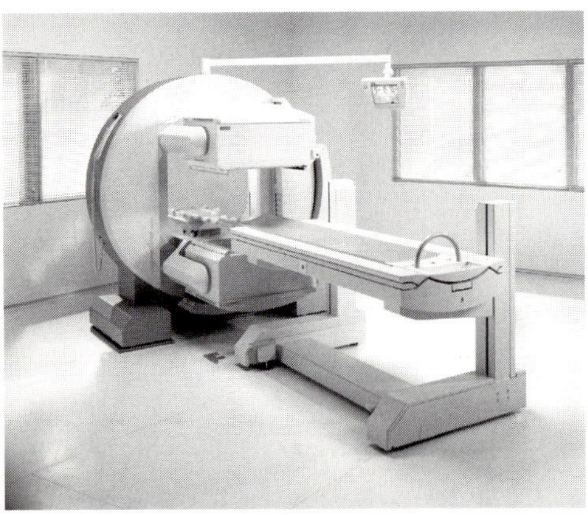

Figure 14.8
SPECT/coincidence camera system with 1" segmented NaI crystal technology (Siemens e.cam^{duet})

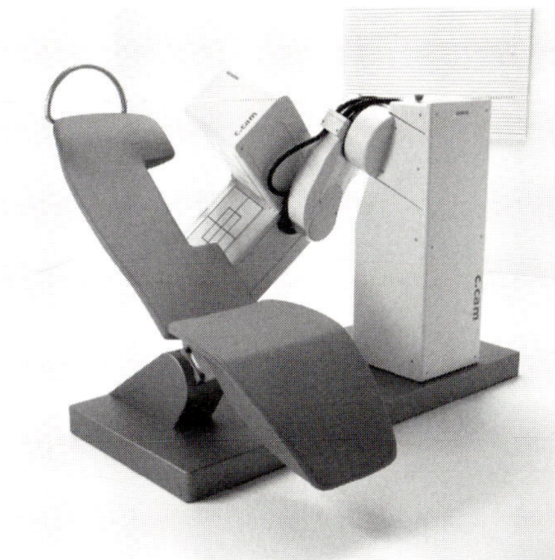

Figure 14.9
Dedicated cardiac camera with a reclining chair (Siemens c.cam)

dictions continues to increase. Around 85% of myocardial procedures are currently performed with SPECT. Fig. 14.9 offers an illustration of a dedicated cardiac camera.

Interest in the development of small dedicated detectors for use in nuclear medicine (e.g. for the diagnosis and localization of breast cancer and for intraoperative imaging) has increased in recent years. Owing to their small size, these new detectors can be placed closer to the objects of investigation and can be used for specialized applications and for areas where space constraints prevent the use of full-sized γ-cameras. Such a system may be referred to as a small FOV gamma imager.

14.3.2.1 Data acquisition and quality control

Data acquisition

Nuclear medicine includes five basic acquisition types: static (planar), dynamic, whole-body, gated and SPECT. In the case of static acquisition, neither the patient nor the camera moves while a time-integrated image of an organ (e.g. a thyroid) is obtained. Dynamic acquisition involves the same fixed orientation and the taking of several images over a pre-defined period of time. Such investigations are performed, for instance, to assess renal function.

In the case of whole-body investigations, the patient bed is moved with respect to the camera head to permit, for instance, the scanning of the entire skeleton. ECG-triggered data acquisitions are generally referred to as gated. These enable one to obtain images of the individual contraction phases (usually 16) of the cardiac cycle. As mentioned above, SPECT involves the revolving of the individual camera heads around the patient's body. This rotation is typically performed in step-and-shoot mode, which amounts to an angular sampling at determined positions while also permitting continuous rotation.

In order to achieve high count rates and high spatial resolution the distance between the region of interest and the position of the detector should be kept as small as possible. This can be achieved by deploying patient body contouring systems that ensure that the camera head describes a noncircular orbit around the patient's body. Light barriers attached to the detector heads prevent the detectors from moving too close to the patient. The actual radius of rotation is registered for each viewing angle θ for the subsequent image reconstruction.

Reconstructed SPECT image data are stored as a matrix in a workstation's memory. Typical matrix sizes include 64×64, 128×128 and occasionally 256×256 picture elements (pixels). Matrix size is usually selected according to the spatial resolution of the acquired image, as determined by the collimator. Final image quality is limited by quantum noise, i.e. the number of counts per pixel [14.18].

Image reconstruction relies on the accuracy and stability of the entire γ-camera system during data acquisition. Reproducible functioning and image quality can strongly influence a physician's diagnosis. This has led lawmakers to introduce strict regulations to govern γ-camera performance and quality controls.

Quality control

As with X-ray CT, SPECT images are reconstructed numerically from the acquired data. The reconstruction algorithm is required to account for several experimental parameters relating to the sensitivity of the SPECT system (e.g. setting of electronics, crystal contamination) and the movement of the system as a whole (e.g. gantry rotation, collimator alignment). If not maintained, parameter values may change over time, leading to image artifacts or even erroneous diagnoses. Lawmakers have therefore seen fit to define quality control procedures that are to be performed on a daily, weekly or monthly basis to ensure the clinical quality of the SPECT system.

Radioactive contamination close to the camera system represents a danger that can seriously corrupt a SPECT acquisition. The user is therefore obliged to make daily checks of the background count level with the camera. Any source of background contamination that is detected (i.e. count rates greater than 500 counts per second (cps)) will have to be identified and eliminated prior to image acquisition.

The setting of the window acquisition photo-peak is also to be checked to ensure that it has not shifted beyond a certain limit (typically 5%). This test is usually performed using ^{99m}Tc. If the peak shift exceeds manufacturer's recommendations, the γ-camera will have to be retuned. The retuning procedure involves adjusting the gain response of the camera's photomultiplier tubes (PMTs) so that they are uniform and fixed for a known radiation source. A total spectrum may also be acquired at this point to enable one to check for a clean photo-peak response.

Precise information about the detector's response to a uniform flux of radiation is necessary for correcting unavoidable local detector variations. A monthly calibration procedure involving the flooding of the detector with a known radiation flux is usually required. The resulting image is used to establish a correction matrix that is applied to the clinical images. In addition to the monthly calibration flood, the SPECT system user can test camera head quality at any time using phantoms. Either a single point

Figure 14.10
Flood quality control test. The acquisition on the left indicates a defective PMT. The image on the right shows a homogenous flood.

source at a fixed position is imaged with the uncollimated system in order to check the homogeneity of the crystal (intrinsic flood) or an image of a homogenously radioactive planar phantom is taken with the collimator deployed to control system homogeneity (extrinsic flood). Subtle variations in phantom uniformity indicate a need to correct the calibration matrix. More serious variations such as the one shown in fig. 14.10 indicate hardware failure and the need for camera servicing.

The reconstruction algorithm requires a precise indication of the actual head position with respect to the center of rotation (COR). A calibration procedure is applied using point sources at defined positions to correct for mechanical variations in the gantry over time. The actual COR is determined on the basis of an analysis of the sinograms produced by these point sources.

It is also necessary to check linearity and resolution on a regular basis. Linearity refers to the system's capacity to image lines as straight and resolution refers to the system's capacity to resolve closely spaced lines. Both can be monitored using a four-quadrant bar pattern to cover the uncollimated detector's entire FOV.

Readers may wish to refer to [14.19] for a discussion of a comprehensive set of tests that accounts for the entire complexity of SPECT acquisition. These tests can be carried out to quantify specific aspects of system performance (e.g. quality control and conformity with system specifications).

14.3.2.2 Reconstruction methods

As in CT and MR, image reconstruction in nuclear medicine is based on projections of the object to be reconstructed. Filtered back projection (FBP) remains the most commonly used method for SPECT [14.20].

Filtered backprojection (FBP)

The projection data obtained during a SPECT acquisition are comprised of photon numbers generated by the local activity of radioactive tracers along the projection path and attenuated by absorption and scatter. The 2D projection profile of the 3D activity distribution that is generated can be regarded as a stack of 1D slice projections. Each slice can be reconstructed via filtered backprojection and the methods described in section 10 (it is not necessary to take the logarithm of the data). Filtering is performed by (Fourier) transforming the single projections and multiplying them by a ramp function. High frequency noise can be reduced by multiplication with a Hanning or a Butterworth function whose cut-off frequency determines the grade of image smoothing. The filtered data are then transformed in reverse and backprojected.

In order to obtain a quantitative estimate of local activity, the backprojection of the filtered profiles must take account of absorption and scatter. Chang's method [14.21] is often applied in this context. The method involves multiplying each reconstructed pixel (x,y) activity by a correction factor

$$C(x,y) = \frac{M}{\sum_{i=1}^{M} e^{-\mu(x,y)l_i}} \qquad (14.15)$$

M: Number of projections
l_i: Distance from the pixel to the object edge along projection direction

This correction depends on a precise indication of the shape of the slice and the local absorption coefficients $\mu(x,y)$. An elliptic contour and a constant μ may be sufficient for a rough estimate. More sophisticated methods improve the correction iteratively, minimizing the difference between the measured projection and the projections calculated on the basis of the reconstructed activity distribution.

Iterative reconstruction (IR)

Iterative image improvement techniques are not restricted to absorption correction, but can also be applied to the entire image reconstruction process. Such IR algorithms model the imagining physics to various degrees of sophistication in order to predict the image [14.22]. This enables one to account for the distance dependant resolution produced by the collimator (fig. 14.11) and to better assemble the attenuation distribution (e.g. from CT images).

The stochastic process of quantum noise prevents an exact quantification of the model parameters from the measured projections. It is therefore necessary to estimate the

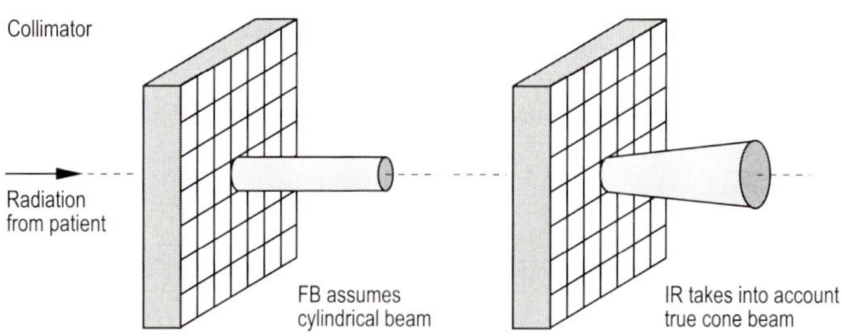

Figure 14.11
Comparison of beam models reaching the detector behind the collimator. While a narrow, pencil-like beam is assumed for FBP, the geometry is much closer to reality for a 3D IR because this latter takes account of the depth-related degradation of the collimator's geometric resolution.

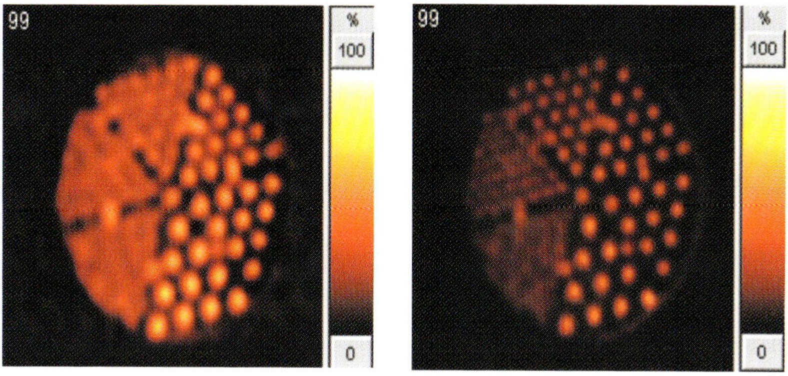

Figure 14.12
Comparison of FBP and 3D OSEM plus CT attenuation correction in an identical phantom study. The fine structures are obviously more clearly visible when reconstruction is performed with 3D OSEM plus CT AC **(right)** than with FBP **(left)**.

most likely parameter combination. The maximum likelihood expectation maximization (MLEM) algorithm involves the establishment of a model that is the most likely to give the same projection set as measured from the object. The deviations between modeled and measured projections are used to improve the model parameters (i.e. activity and absorption) in an iterative process. The determination when to stop iterating warrants special care given the fact that the system tends to also model image variations that are related to stochastic changes, a tendency that results in increasingly noisy images.

Ordered subset expectation minimization (OSEM)

OSEM is a derivative of MLEM that enables one to accelerate image reconstruction through the use of a single subset (e.g. 8 instead of 64) of projections when comparing the estimated and the measured projections during iteration [14.23]. The other projection sets are used progressively for subsequent iterations. It is necessary to carefully determine the order of projections so as to maximize image improvement upon each iterative step. Fig. 14.12 shows an example of a phantom study involving one reconstruction with basic FBP and one with a 3D OSEM algorithm that applies attenuation correction from CT data.

14.3.3 Clinical applications

Nuclear medicine enables one to perform functional imaging of the human body. The perfusion and metabolism of various organs can be visualized by administering various radiopharmaceuticals, typically based on ^{99m}Tc, ^{131}I, ^{123}I, ^{111}In, ^{201}Tl and ^{67}Ga. In order to guide these radioisotopes to the organ of interest, it is necessary to attach them to nonradioactive tracer substances (fig. 14.13) [14.24]. Given that no more than submicromolecular substance concentrations are required, the imaging procedure has

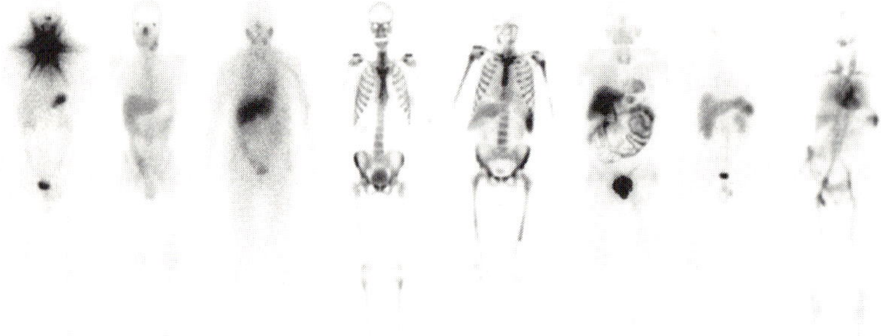

(1) (2) (3) (4) (5) (6) (7) (8)

Figure 14.13
Comparison of various radiopharmaceuticals. ^{131}I **(1)** shows high tracer accumulation in the thyroid (with septal penetration via the deployed high energy collimator) as well as less intense uptake in the stomach and bladder. ^{67}Ga-Citrate **(2)** behaves like iron molecules in the human body and binds to iron receptors, for example, in patients with lymphoma (in this case the left neck). The ^{123}I-MIBG study **(3)** shows the distribution in the so-called sympathetic nerve system, including tumors of this origin. ^{99m}Tc DPD **(4)** visualizes the activity of bone cells to permit the detection of bone metabolism abnormalities (e.g. metastases and fractures). The ^{99m}Tc-labeled antibodies against white blood cells **(5)** reflect the distribution of the bone marrow and permit the diagnosis of infections. ^{99m}Tc -MIBI **(6)** is used as a clinical perfusion marker mainly for cardiac perfusion studies and parathyroid imaging. The physiological distribution for ^{111}In SMS **(7)** includes the spleen, liver, kidneys and bladder. It is used for the diagnosis of hormone producing tumors. The last image **(8)** shows ^{99m}Tc-labeled red blood cells, reflecting distribution to the blood vessels in the human body. This tracer is routinely used to evaluate cardiac function and to depict the origin of bleeding in the bowel.

no effect on biological processes. Patient radiation exposure ranges from 1 to 5 mSv, values that can be further decreased (e.g. by hydrating the patient). The majority of nuclear medicine examinations thus do not exceed twice the natural annual radiation exposure of 2 to 5 mSv.

The most frequently used nuclear medicine procedures include bone, thyroid, heart, lung and renal scanning. In bone scanning, the tracer bonds chemically to the active bone cells. Bone scans are useful for diagnosing pathologies such as metastases, bone tumors, infections and occult fractures. In combination with ultrasound, thyroid scintigraphy enables one to evaluate hormone production in the thyroid gland and to determine the risk of malignancy in thyroid nodules. Myocardial perfusion and viability studies are important clinical tools when it comes to assessing the severity of coronary artery disease and arriving prognoses for patients suffering from it. Lung perfusion scans are routinely used to rule out pulmonary embolism, an occlusion of one of the pulmonary vessels. Renal scintigraphy enables one to easily evaluate kidney perfusion, function and urinary excretion.

New tracers for oncology imaging have been developed in recent years. Given that cell function in a tumor changes before the tumor starts to grow, nuclear medicine allows one to detect diseases at an early stage. Nuclear medicine has come to represent an important tool for treatment planning and monitoring in the field of oncology when combined with CT and MR for anatomical information. New techniques such as image fusion and the availability of hybrid devices such as SPECT/CT and PET/CT are gaining in importance.

14.3.4 New detector technologies

The Anger camera has proven over the years to be a reliable and indispensable work horse in the field of nuclear medicine. New detector principles, however, promise a number of practical advantages. The removal of the photo multiplier tubes (PMTs) from the gamma camera would entail a dramatic reduction in size and would have a cascading impact on overall system design. For instance, making the detector an order of magnitude thinner (e.g. a reduction from 25 cm down to 2.5 cm) would significantly reduce the need for lead shielding and with it the weight of the camera head. This would make the head easier to configure, simplify gantry construction, increase flexibility with respect to bringing the detector closer to the patient and thereby lead to improvements in image quality.

Two new detector designs are currently being investigated: (i) scintillation crystals in new configurations with light detectors and (ii) direct conversion semiconductor detectors.

The new scintillator-based detectors can be broken down into three main designs: (i) an array of crystals (typically 2.5 mm × 2.5 mm single crystals of 6.0 mm thickness) coupled to a position-sensitive PMT (PSPMT), (ii) an array of crystals coupled to a corresponding array of photodiodes and (iii) a single crystal coupled to an array of silicon-drift photodiodes. The probabilistic localization algorithm used in the Anger camera is replaced in these designs by a direct spatial sensing of the scintillation event.

The use of an array of detector crystals and position-sensitive PMTs [14.25] enables one to enlarge the FOV and the intrinsic spatial resolution of the detector. Replacing the PSPMT with photodiodes reduces the size of the detector [14.26]. The deployment of an array of very low noise photodiodes (silicon-drift photodiodes) [14.27] coupled to the camera's single scintillation crystal instead of photomultipliers enables one to enhance the spatial resolution of the scintillation event. Silicon-drift detectors (SDDs) consist of a silicon substrate with a structure of p^+ junctions on both sides and a small n^+ contact that acts as an anode. This composition leads to the generation of an electric field with a strong lateral gradient that guides all photon-generated charges to the anode. The size of the SDD can be enlarged without significantly increasing detector capacity, thereby enabling one to maintain low noise levels.

Owing to their high γ-absorption, monolithic cadmium telluride (CdTe) and cadmium zinc telluride (CdZnTe) substrates represent suitable materials for semiconductor γ-detectors [14.28, 14.29]. A slab with a solid-state thickness of several mm is equipped with a continuous electrode on one side and with an array of pixel electrodes on the other. Each absorbed γ-photon generates many thousands of electron-hole pairs that are then separated by an electric field applied across the detector and driven to the electrodes. The accumulated charges are amplified and then digitized at each pixel. Proper pixel electrode size and spacing and an adequately fine collimator allow one to achieve a spatial resolution of 1 to 2 mm. In addition to improved spatial resolution, semiconductor detectors may also provide an increased energy resolution that can be used for reducing the signals from scattered radiation. To date, γ-cameras with semiconductor detectors have only been built in sizes that permit the imaging of small animals such as mice.

It warrants mention that any improvements in intrinsic spatial resolution that result from the deployment of the new detector designs will not result in any noticeable improvements in image quality in the case of parallel hole collimators. A detector head offering significantly higher intrinsic spatial resolution will require novel collimator designs. The pinhole collimator may be an alternative. This collimator operates on the same principle as a pinhole camera, with the pinhole acting as an aperture through which a photon is required to pass in order to be seen by the detector. Spatial resolution is given by the pin hole diameter and the magnification factor, i.e. the ratio of the distances of the detector and the object to the pinhole. Field of view is then limited by the size of the detector. In the SPECT reconstruction, it will also be necessary to account for the fact that a thick object contains areas that will be imaged at different magnifications. Multiple pinhole configurations improve the count rate by providing simultaneous views from several angles. Special encoding strategies have to be applied in order to account for the overlap of the projections by the single pinholes [14.30]. This technique, therefore, is often referred to as coded aperture imaging.

The prospect of helping to achieve significant improvements in both practical design and image quality provides ample motivation in the quest to develop these new detectors into tomorrow's clinical nuclear imaging devices.

14.4 PET systems

Positron emission tomography (PET) uses tracers labeled with positron emitters to characterize the biochemical function of cells, organs and body structures in vivo. The special features of the positron emitters and their decay characteristics permit an absolute quantification of tracer distribution and metabolic activity at a molecular level. This enables diagnostic examinations of high sensitivity and specificity.

14.4.1 Principles of PET

Positron emitters

Positron emitters are nuclides whose nuclei contain a high number of protons compared to neutrons, a composition that leaves the nuclides unstable. As the nuclides decay, they emit a positron. One of the protons p in the nucleus converts into a neutron n (which stays within the nucleus), an emitted positron β^+ (or e^+) and a neutrino ν.

$$p \rightarrow \beta^+ + n + \nu \tag{14.16}$$

Due to its negligible mass, the neutrino does not interact with matter and therefore cannot be detected. The positron, on the other hand, is scattered by the atoms surrounding the positron emitter and loses its kinetic energy. When it comes to a stand still, it unites with an electron e^- and forms a two-particle object known as a positronium. Given that the electron and the positron are identical particles (with the only difference being their charge), the half-life of the positronium is very short and the electron and positron annihilate into two γ-quanta:

$$\beta^+ + e^- \rightarrow 2\gamma \tag{14.17}$$

Due to the conservation of energy and momentum, the energy E_γ of each of the two γ-quanta is 511 keV ($E_\gamma = m_e c^2$ with m_e being the mass of the electron and positron, respectively, and c the speed of light). These two γ-quanta will fly in exactly opposite directions. While this is true for most of the positron/electron annihilation, there is a small possibility that not just two but three quanta will be created. In this case, the sum of the energy of all gammas created will also equal 1,022 keV. Given that the probability that one of the quanta will have an energy level of 511 keV is very small, this effect does not have a significant impact on PET imaging.

If the momentum of the electron and the positron is not exactly zero at the moment of annihilation, a deviation from the co-linearity of the two gamma rays might occur.

Positron emitters can be found for a large number of nuclides. Some common positron emitters are listed in table 14.1.

Table 14.1 Common positron emitters

Positron emitter	**Half-life**	**Daughter**	**Maximum positron energy**	**Mean linear range in tissue**
^{11}C	20.4 min	^{11}B	0.96 MeV	0.3 mm
^{13}N	9.9 min	^{13}C	1.19 MeV	0.4 mm
^{15}O	2.9 min	^{15}N	1.72 MeV	1.5 mm
^{18}F	110 min	^{18}O	0.64 MeV	0.2 mm
^{68}Ga	68 min	^{68}Zn	1.89 MeV	1.9 mm
^{82}Rb	1.3 min	^{82}Kr	3.35 MeV	2.6 mm

The half-life of positron emitters is relatively short. While ^{68}Ga and ^{82}Rb represent generator-produced positron emitters (daughters of isotopes with a longer half-life, e.g. ^{68}Ge and ^{82}Sr, respectively), the other positron emitters need to be produced in close proximity to the PET center. Only ^{18}F, with its half-life of 110 minutes, is capable of being distributed a certain distance.

Most positron emitters are produced by cyclotrons. Today's clinical cyclotrons are optimized to produce high amounts of the clinically relevant positron emitters (in particular, ^{18}F). Such negative-ion, deep-valley cyclotrons are compact and self-shielded, to allow for their integration into clinical environments.

Positron emitters are produced in cyclotrons by means of a high energy beam of protons p (typical 10 to 20 MeV) that is directed, for instance, to an $H_2{}^{18}O$ target. This leads to the production of ^{18}F:

$$^{18}O(p,n)^{18}F \tag{14.18}$$

The emitted neutron n will be shielded by the cyclotron shield or vault.

PET tracers

PET tracers are labeled with positron emitters. A variety of tracers is available. Automatic chemistry boxes have been designed to synthesize the most common PET tracers and to label them with the positron emitter. Used in more than 90% of all PET studies, FDG (2-[^{18}F]fluoro-2-deoxy-D-glucose) is the current tracer of choice.

Coincidence detection

Once the positron and an electron are annihilated, the two emitted gamma quanta can be detected by opposing detectors (fig. 14.14) as a coincidence event.

Such coincidence events based on the detection of two gamma quanta by two detectors are used to reconstruct the local distribution of the tracer in the patient. In the case of fast detectors, the coincidence window within which two events are defined as being in coincidence is on the order of 4.5 to 6 ns.

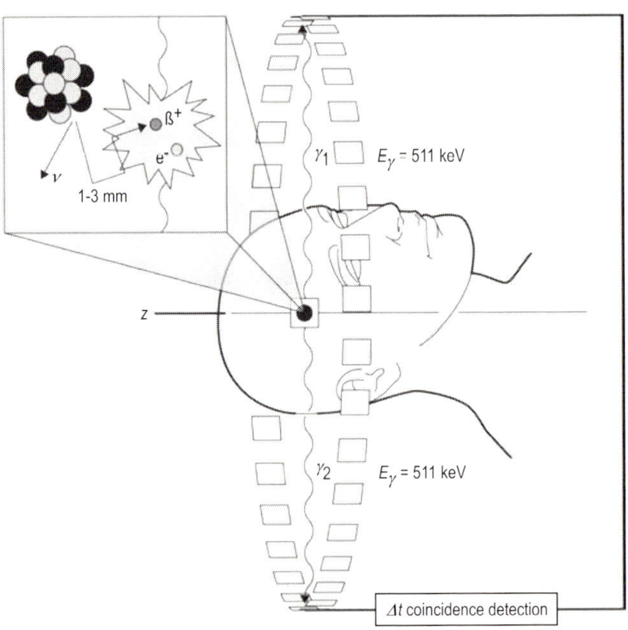

Figure 14.14 Coincidence detection

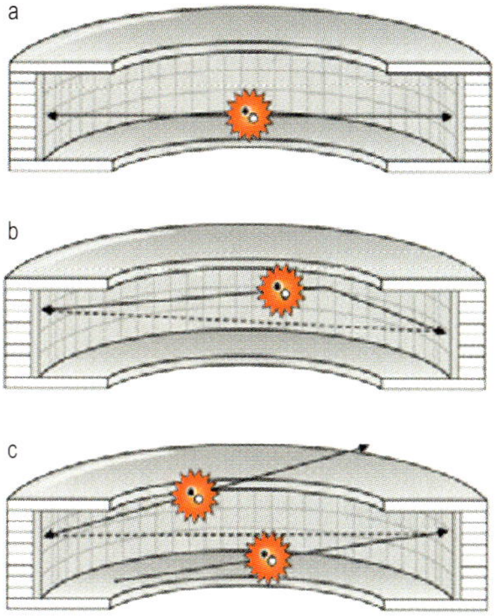

Figure 14.15
a) True coincidence, **b)** scattered coincidence, **c)** random coincidence

Two distinct events (singles) detected by opposing detectors are measured as a coincidence only if the two events are detected within the coincidence window $\tau = \Delta t$. If these two events stem from the same annihilation and the two quanta have not been scattered, the occurrence is referred to as a case of true coincidence (fig. 14.15a). If one or both quanta have been scattered, the result of the measurement is referred to as a case of scattered coincidence (fig. 14.15b). Scattered events are measured if the energy of each of the quanta falls into the energy window ΔE (e.g. typically 425 to 650 keV).

Owing to the finite width of the coincidence window τ, two events stemming from two different annihilations may be recorded. The rate r of these random coincidences (fig. 14.15c) is related to the single rates r_{si} ascertained by each individual detector element i and the length of the coincidence window. The random rate r is thus proportional to the squared activity A^2 in the patient and the length of the coincidence window τ.

PET detectors

The capacity of PET detectors to efficiently detect annihilations depends on their exhibiting a high absorption coefficient for 511 keV photons and high spatial, temporal and energy resolution. Table 14.2 offers a list of the scintillation crystals currently available.

While BGO (bismuth germanate) was the detector of choice for many years owing to its short mean free path length (i.e. high attenuation coefficient for 511 keV photons), its long decay time limits the count rate performance of PET scanners. Furthermore, its low relative light output limits design options. Other detector materials such as cerium-doped lutetium oxyorthosilicate (LSO) and gadolinium oxyorthosilicate (GSO) offer more favorable properties. While LSO, in particular, offers nearly the same short mean free path length as BGO, it exhibits a much shorter decay time and very high light output. Given this combination of characteristics, LSO outperforms all other cur-

Table 14.2 Characteristics of PET scintillators at photon energy 511keV [14.31, 14.32]

	LSO	BGO	GSO	NaI
Density	7.4 g/cm^3	7.1 g/cm^3	6.8 g/cm^3	3.7 g/cm^3
Effective atomic number	66	75	59	51
Mean free path	1.16 cm	1.05	1.43	2.88
Hygroscopic?	No	No	No	Yes
Rugged?	Yes	Yes	No	No
Decay time	40 ns	300 ns	60,600 ns	230 ns
Relative light output	75	15	25	100
Energy resolution	10%	10.1%	9.5%	7.8%

rently available PET scintillators and makes it the preferred detector material for many of today's high performance PET scanners.

As soon as the 511 keV photon is detected in the scintillator, the scintillation light is converted by photomultipliers (PMTs) into an electric signal that is then analyzed and processed with the help of dedicated electronics. Several individual scintillators are typically combined into a block (usually 8 × 8 or 13 × 13) of crystals to increase efficiency, reliability and affordability. The location of the scintillation can be determined using a center of gravity algorithm similar to that used with the Anger camera and four PMTs replete with a light guide for coded light distribution (fig. 14.16).

Real-time electronic systems enable one to analyze the output of the four PMTs, and thus to determine scintillation time and energy. Such systems also enable one to determine whether two events have been detected within the coincidence window.

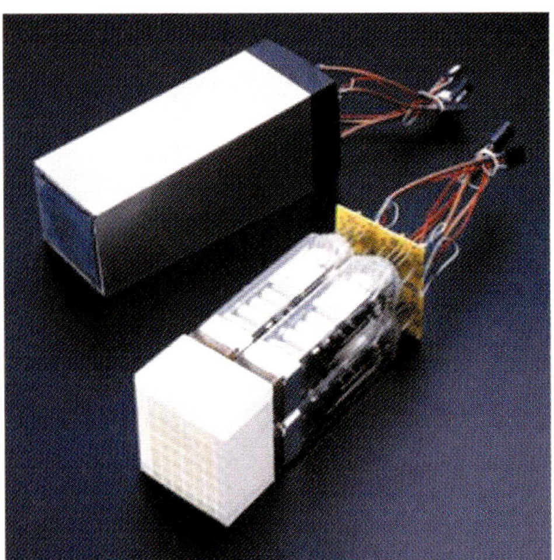

Figure 14.16
PET block detector

Gantry design

The PET detectors are positioned in rings surrounding the patient so as to cover a large solid angle. Today's systems feature up to 24,000 individual crystals or more in 13 × 13 blocks to cover an axial field of view (FOV) of 16.2 cm. The compact gantry has a wide patient aperture to ensure the highest degree of patient comfort (fig. 14.17). The gantry electronics allow for full 3D acquisition to ensure optimal sensitivity and clinical flexibility (fig. 14.18).

Reconstruction and corrections

Once they have been detected for each line of response, the coincidence events need to be reconstructed. 3D acquisitions require either direct 3D reconstruction or 2D re-binning. The most common approach is to use Fourier re-binning (FORE) to re-sort the 3D datasets into 2D projections, which are then iteratively reconstructed by AW-OSEM (attenuation weighted ordered subset expectation maximization algorithm) [14.33]. The data are normalized and the decay and dead-time effects are corrected during the reconstruction process.

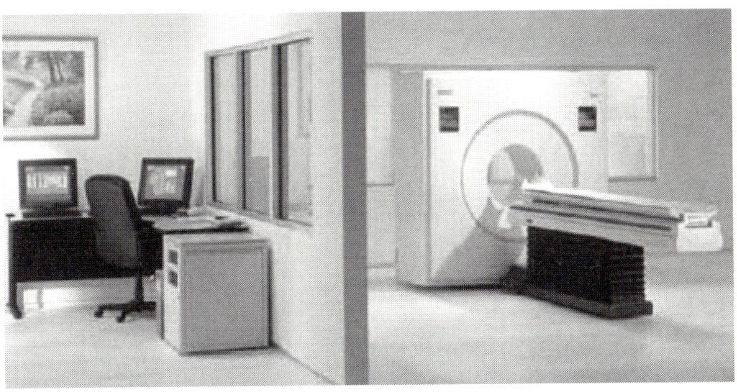

Figure 14.17 3D PET scanner (ECAT ACCEL, Siemens Medical Solutions)

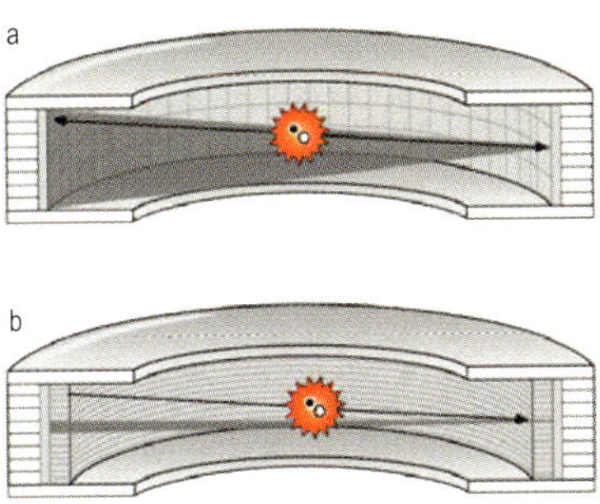

Figure 14.18
3D PET imaging **(a)** with high sensitivity compared to the limited acceptance angle of 2D imaging **(b)**

The projection $p(l,\theta)$ is a product of the activity distribution $f(x,y)$ and the local attenuation integral along the line of response (LOR) for each line of response.

$$p(l,\theta) = \int f(x,y)\,\delta(l - x\cos\theta - y\sin\theta)\,dx\,dy\; e^{-\int \mu(x,y)\,\delta(l - x\cos\theta - y\sin\theta)\,dx\,dy} \tag{14.19}$$

Attenuation can therefore be corrected by means of external sources. $^{68}Ge/^{68}Ga$ sources represent the most commonly used sources for this task. A transmission scan measures the local distribution of the attenuation coefficient $\mu(x,y)$ in the patient. A correction factor can be calculated for each line of response.

The distribution of the attenuation coefficient also describes the patient scatter characteristics. The residual scatter component in the reconstructed data can be minimized by applying an inverse Monte Carlo simulation of the patient [14.34].

Random coincidences for each LOR can either be corrected for by calculating the random rate from the single rate of each detector and the length of the coincidence window or by using a second delayed coincidence window of the same length. Random coincidences can be corrected in real time using the delayed coincidence window.

14.4.2 Characterization of PET scanners

Various parameters can be used to characterize a PET scanner. National and international standardization organizations such as the National Electric Manufacturers Association (NEMA) [14.35] and the International Electrotechnical Commission (IEC) [14.36] have established performance tests that can be used to characterize PET scanners.

The most important performance criteria that apply to PET systems designed for clinical use include spatial resolution, noise equivalent count-rate performance and patient throughput.

Resolution

The size of the individual detector defines the system's intrinsic spatial resolution. The resolution of the reconstructed image is also dependent on detector sharing and reconstruction parameters. The 4 mm by 4 mm LSO crystals in a 13 × 13 block (fig. 14.19) provide a reconstructed resolution of 4.2 mm (fig. 14.20).

The system is required to provide high effective sensitivity (e.g. a noise equivalent count-rate performance that is optimized for the clinical range of activity concentrations in the patient) in order to achieve such high resolution in clinical studies.

Noise equivalent count-rate performance

The noise equivalent count rate (*NEC*) has been defined to characterize the effective sensitivity of PET scanners for purposes of clinical imaging. The *NEC* compares the statistical quality of a PET scanner (measuring a true coincidence rate t) and an ideal system that is resistant to random coincidences (random coincidence rate r) and scat-

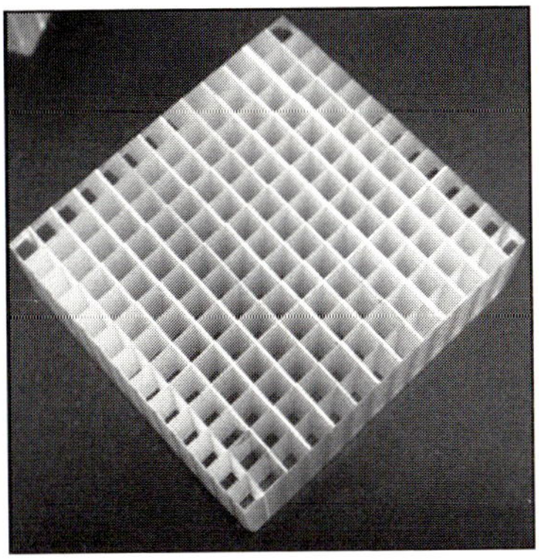

Figure 14.19
LSO block detector with 13 × 13 individual elements providing a reconstructed resolution of 4.2 mm

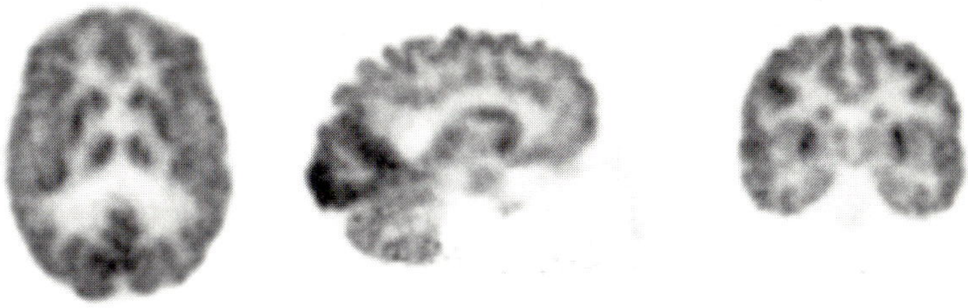

Figure 14.20 High resolution FDG uptake in the brain

tered radiation (rate of scattered coincidences s), i.e. the two most important sources of statistical noise in a PET study. Depending on the method of random correction the constant k is either 1 or 2.

$$NEC = \frac{t^2}{t + s + kr} \tag{14.20}$$

The *NEC* can be optimized by using a fast detector, short coincidence window to reduce the random coincidences (e.g. $\tau = 4.5$ ns), high energy resolution (e.g. 14%), tight energy windows (e.g. 425 to 650 keV), optimized electronics and high intrinsic sensitivity by implementing fully 3D acquisitions (fig. 14.21).

Patient throughput

While the PET system's sensitivity and count-rate performance have a direct impact on patient throughput, the system's user interface and workflow integration also play an important role. High patient throughput (e.g. scanning times of less than 10 minutes for a whole body study) relies on the integration of all steps (fig. 14.22).

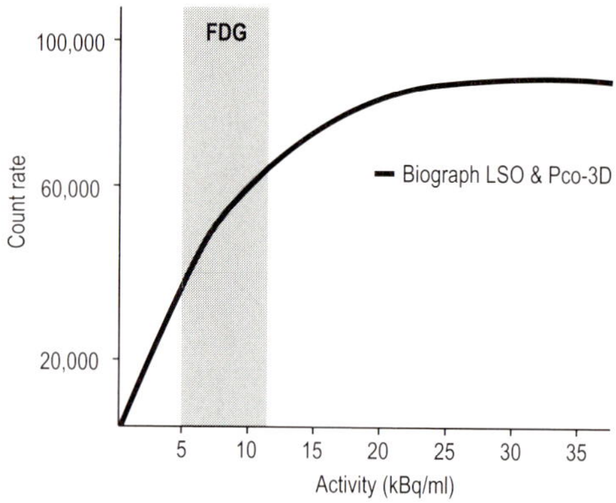

Figure 14.21
Typical noise equivalent count-rate performance (Biograph, Siemens Medical Solutions)

14.4.3 Clinical applications

PET has demonstrated great potential as a diagnostic tool since the 1990s. The results of several studies verify the sensitivity and specificity of PET [14.37]. In most countries PET is an accepted procedure for a variety of oncology applications. Applications in the fields of cardiology and neurology have also become a matter of diagnostic routine.

Oncology

The high glucose metabolism of most tumors makes FDG a perfect tracer for oncology. Although its uptake is relatively unspecific, PET provides diagnostic results of high sensitivity and specificity (fig. 14.23).

The following oncology applications with FDG are accepted in the United States [14.38]:

- Lung cancer – diagnosis, initial staging and restaging of single pulmonary nodules in non-small cell lung cancer
- Colorectal cancer – diagnosis, staging and restaging
- Melanoma – diagnosis, initial staging and restaging
- Esophageal cancer – diagnosis, initial staging and restaging
- Head and neck cancers – diagnosis, initial staging and restaging
- Lymphoma – diagnosis, initial staging and restaging
- Breast cancer – initial staging, restaging and therapy response
- Hodgkin's and non-Hodgkin's disease – initial staging and restaging
- Thyroid cancer – in patients for whom the usually accurate ^{131}I whole body scan proves unhelpful at localizing the disease.

Other tracers and applications include ovarian cancer, testicular tumors, pancreatic cancer, brain tumors, musculoskeletal tumors, prostate cancer, bladder cancer, kidney cancer, liver cancer, gastrointestinal stromal tumors (GIST) and others.

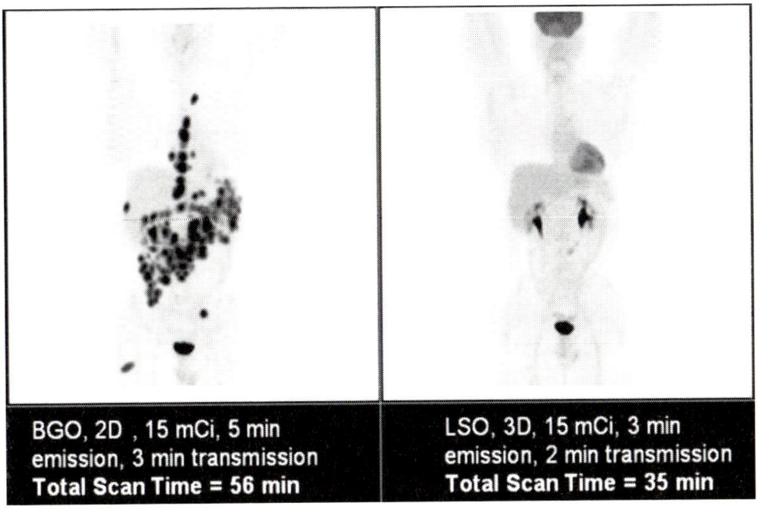

Figure 14.22
Short acquisition time with the LSO detectors of the ECAT ACCEL compared to a BGO PET scanner (same patient before and after chemotherapy and stem cell transplantation, data courtesy of NCPIC, Sacramento, CA, USA)

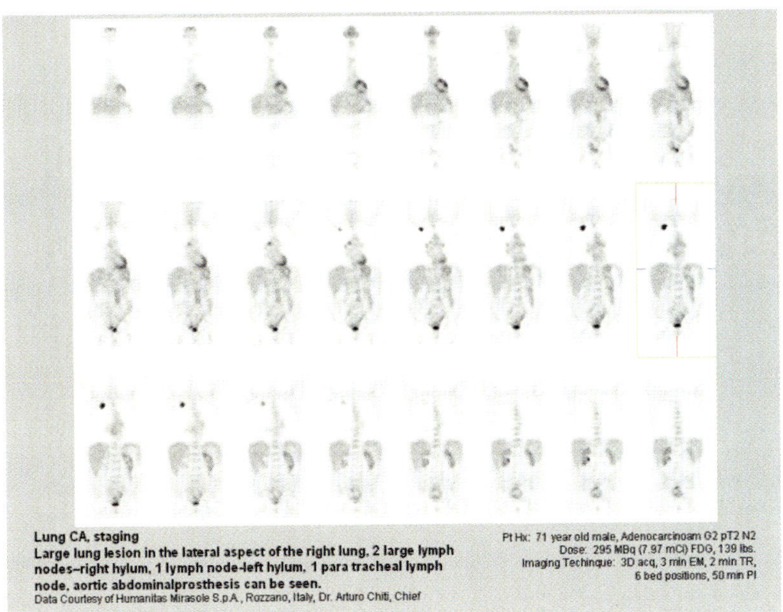

Figure 14.23 Lung cancer staging (Source: Humanitas Mirasole S.p.A., Rozzano, Italy)

Cardiology

PET applications in cardiology center on myocardial viability (fig. 14.24).

The following applications are typically reimbursed in the United States:

- Myocardial viability with FDG – following inconclusive SPECT scan
- Myocardial perfusion with $^{13}NH_3$ – under rest and/or pharmacologic stress conditions to evaluate myocardial perfusion in patients with suspected or existing coronary disease
- Cardiac perfusion – with ^{82}Rb

Other tracers and applications include diagnosis of hibernating myocardium, hibernation and congestive heart failure, receptors and others.

Neurology

Around 20% of the injected FDG accumulates in the brain. Deviations from the normal uptake lead to diagnostic results (fig. 14.25).

The following FDG indications are reimbursed in the United States:

- Seizures – pre-surgical evaluation of patients with refractory seizures
- Alzheimer's disease – patients with documented cognitive decline of at least six months and a recently established diagnosis of dementia.

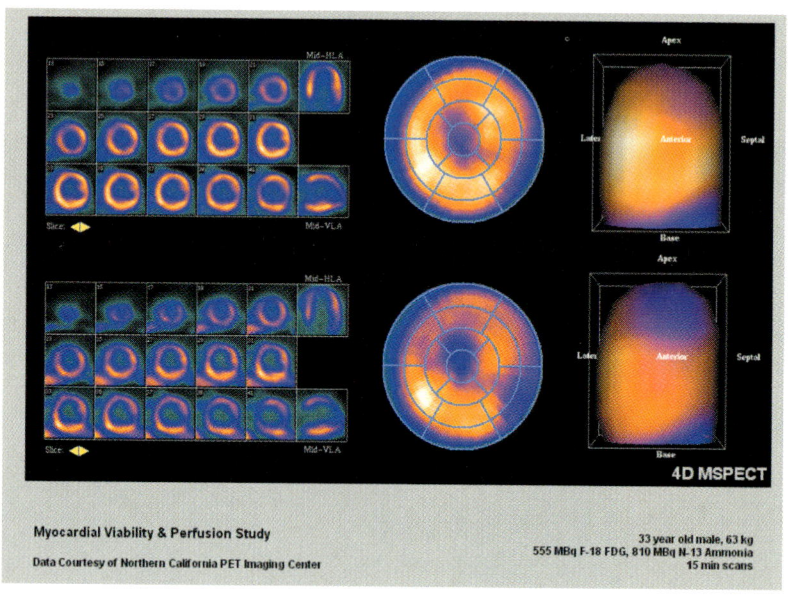

Figure 14.24
FDG and NH_3 cardiology study with the ECAT ACCEL (Source: NCPIC, Sacramento, CA, USA)

Other tracers and applications include differential diagnosis of dementia, detection of Morbus Huntington, Parkinson's disease, schizophrenia, depression, substance abuse and several others.

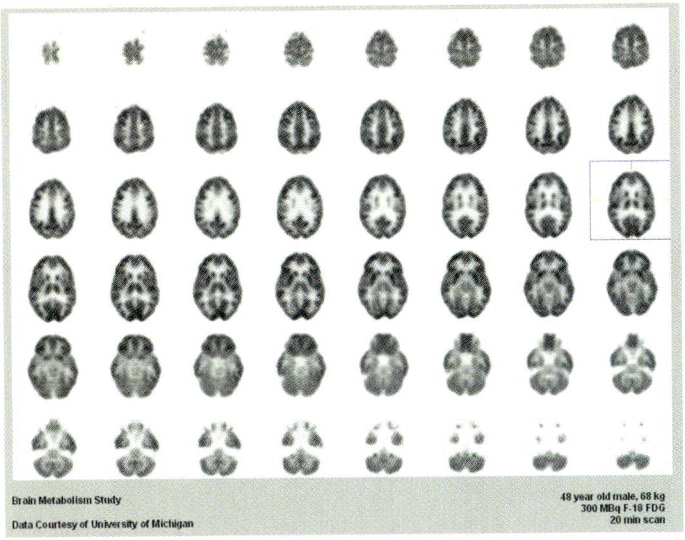

Figure 14.25 FDG uptake in the brain (Source: University Michigan, USA)

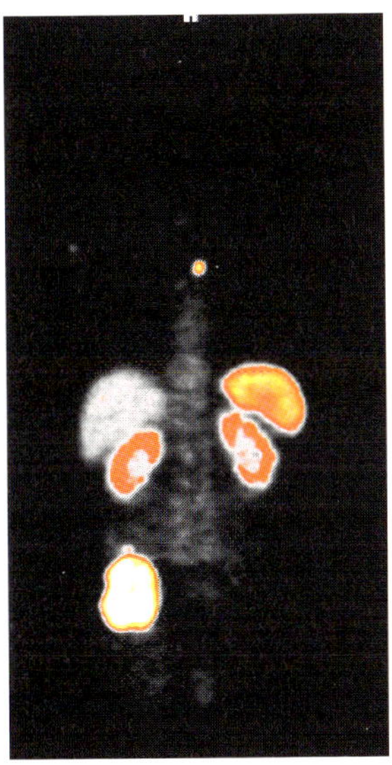

Figure 14.26
Specific uptake of ^{68}Ga-DOTATOC
(Source: MHH Hannover, Germany)

Molecular Imaging

High sensitivity, high resolution and a large variety of physiological tracers make PET an ideal tool for imaging metabolism at a molecular level. The use of dedicated tracers enables one to visualize and characterize nearly all biochemical pathways. Highly specific tracers such as ^{68}Ga-DOTATOC highlight specific tumors or receptors in the body (fig. 14.26).

The tracer principle permits the administration of minimal quantities of labeled substances and thus the avoidance of physiological effects. Newly developed pharmaceuticals and therapeutic regimes can be tested and their biochemical pathways can be quantified in vivo without significant side effects.

14.5 References

[14.1] D.E. Kuhl, R.Q. Edwards
Reorganizing data from transverse section scans of the brain using digital processing
Radiology 101(1968), 1075

[14.2] L. Kaufman, J. Ewins, W. Rowan, et al.
Semiconductor gamma cameras in nuclear medicine
IEEE Trans. Nucl. Sci. NS-27 (1980), 1073-1079

[14.3] H.B. Barber, H.H. Barrett, T.S. Hickernell, D.P. Kwo, J.M. Woolfenden, G. Entine, C. Ortale Baccash
Comparison of NaI(Tl), CdTe, and HgI_2 surgical probes: physical characterization
Med. Phys. 18 (1991), 373-381

[14.4] G.F. Knoll
Radiation detection and measurement
John Wiley, N.Y. (1979)

[14.5] H.H. Barrett, W. Swindell
Radiological imaging, Vol. 1 and 2
Academic Press (1981)

[14.6] B. Cassen, L. Curtis, C. Reed, et al.
Instrumentation for I^{131} use in medical studies
Nucleonics 9 (1951), 46-50

[14.7] W.V. Mayneord, R.C. Turner, S.P. Newbery, H.J. Hodt
A method for making visible the distribution of activity in a source of ionizing radiation
Nature 168 (1951), 762-765

[14.8] J.G. Kareiakes
The history and development of medical physics instrumentation – nuclear medicine
Med. Phys. 14 (1987), 146

[14.9] H.O. Anger
Scintillation camera
Rev. Sci. Instrum. 29 (1958), 27

[14.10] H.O. Anger
Scintillation camera with multichannel collimators
J. Nucl. Med. 5 (1964), 515

[14.11] C.E. Metz, F.B. Atkins, R.N. Beck
The geometric transfer function component for scintillation camera collimators with straight parallel holes
Phys. Med. Biol. 25 (1980), 1059-1070

[14.12] B.M.W. Tsui, G.T. Gullberg
The geometric transfer function for cone and fan beam collimators
Phys. Med. Biol., Vol. 35 (1990) pp. 81-93

[14.13] T.D. Milster, J.N. Aarsvold, H.H. Barrett, A.L. Landesman, L.S. Mar, D.D. Patton, T.J. Roney, R.K. Rowe, R.H.3rd. Seacat
A full-field modular gamma camera
The Journal of Nuclear Medicine 31 (1990), 632

[14.14] S.L. Blatt
Characteristics of random-sum peaks in nuclear radiation spectra
Nucl. Instr. and Meth. 128 (1975), 277

[14.15] R. Adams, C. Jansen, G.M. Grames, C.D. Zimmerman
Dead time of scintillation camera systems – definitions, measurements and applications
Medical Physics 1 (1974), 1908

[14.16] I.A. Sorenson
Methods of correcting Anger-camera deadtime losses
J. Nucl. Med., Instrumentation and Physics 17 (1975), 412-416

[14.17] H. Wagner, Z. Szabo, J. Buchanan (eds.)
Principles of Nuclear Medicine
W B Saunders, Philadelphia 1995

[14.18] G. Saha
Physics and Radiobiology of Nuclear Medicine
Springer Verlag, New York 1993

[14.19] Performance Measurements of Scintillation Cameras
NEMA Standards Publication NU 1-2001
National Electrical Manufacturers Association, Rosslyn 2001

[14.20] I.P.C. Murray, P.J. Ell (eds.)
Nuclear Medicine in Clinical Diagnosis and Treatment
Churchill Livingston, New York 1994

[14.21] L.T. Chang
A method for attenuation correction in radionuclide computed tomography
IEEE Trans Nucl Sci 26 (1979), 2780

[14.22] T.R. Miller, J.W. Wallis
Fast maximum-likelihood reconstruction
J Nucl Med 33 (1992), 1710

[14.23] A.H. Vija, E.G. Hawman, J.C. Engdahl,
Analysis of SPECT OSEM reconstruction method with 3D beam modeling and optional attenuation correction: Phantom studies
Conference Record, IEEE MIC 03

[14.24] H. Schicha, O. Schober
Nuklearmedizin
Schattauer, New York 2003

[14.25] Hamamatsu Corporation
314-5, Shimokanzo, Toyooka-village,
Japan

[14.26] S. Kumita, K. Tanaka, K. Cho, N. Sato, H. Nakajo, M. Toba, Y. Fukushima, S. Mizumura, T. Takano, T. Kumazaki
Assessment of left ventricular function using solid-state gamma camera equipped with a highly-sensitive collimator
Annals of Nuclear Medicine 17 (2003) 517

[14.27] R. Farrell, F. Olschner et al.
Advances in semiconductor photodetectors for scintillators
Nucl. Instr. and Meth. A387 (1997), 194

[14.28] C. Scheiber, G.C. Giakos
Medical applications of CdTe and CdZnTe detectors
Nucl. Instrum. Methods Phys. Res. A458 (2001), 12

[14.29] K.B. Parnham, J. Grosholz, R.K. Davis, S. Vydrin, C.A. Cupe
Development of a CdZnTe-based small field of view gamma camera
IEEE/NSS Symposium Conference record (2000), 21

[14.30] D.W. Wilson, H.H. Barrett, and E.W. Clarkson
Reconstruction of two and three-dimensional images from synthetic collimator data
IEEE Transactions On Medical Imaging 19 (2000), 412

[14.31] R. Nutt
For: Is LSO the future of PET?
Eur. J. Nucl. Med. 29 (2002), 1523-1525

[14.32] J.S. Karp
Against: Is LSO the future of PET?
Eur. J. Nucl. Med. 29 (2002), 1525-1528

[14.33] T.J. Hebert, R. Leahy
Fast methods for including attenuation in the EM algorithm
IEEE Trans. Nucl. Sci. 45 (1990), 754-758

[14.34] C.C. Watson
New, Faster, Image-Based Scatter Correction for 3D PET
IEEE Trans. Nucl. Sci. 47 (2000), 1587-1594

[14.35] Performance Measurements of Positron Emission Tomographs
NEMA Standards Publication NU 2-2001 (2001)

[14.36] Radionuclide imaging devices – Characteristics and test conditions – Part 1: Positron emission tomographs
IEC 61675-1 (1998)

[14.37] S.S. Gambhir, J. Czernin, J. Schwimmer, D.H. Silverman, R.E. Coleman, M.E. Phelps
A tabulated summary of the FDG PET literature
J. Nucl. Med. 42 (2001), 1S-93S

[14.38] Centers for Medicare & Medicaid Services (CMS) 2005
http://www.cms.hhs.gov

15 Magnetic resonance imaging

15.1 MR systems and components

15.1.1 System overview

A magnetic resonance imaging (MRI) system is quite similar to a computer-controlled nuclear magnetic resonance (NMR) spectrometer of the sort that has been used for years in analytical chemistry for the purpose of determining molecular structures. The additional components that are needed to make an MR imager out of an NMR spectrometer include: three field coils (driven by power amplifiers) to create pulsed linear magnetic gradient fields in three orientations for the spatial encoding of the magnetic resonance (MR) signal and an image display unit. The size of the system is adapted to accommodate an adult human body and the control and image processing software is designed to meet the requirements of medical diagnosis.

Fig. 15.1 illustrates the basic arrangement and interactions of an MRI system's various components. In what follows, we discuss the important features of these components

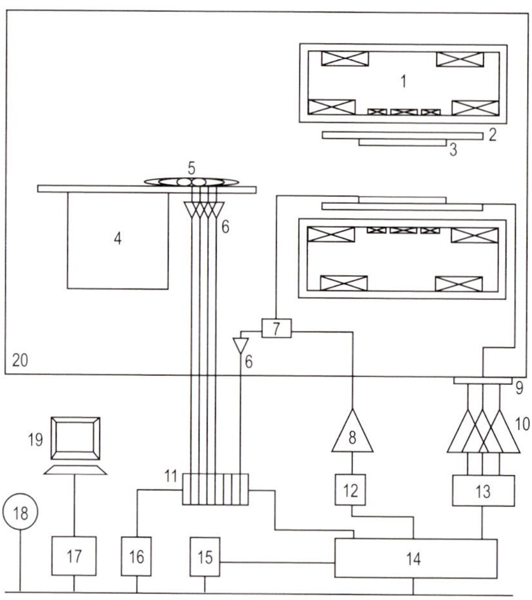

1 Magnet
2 Gradient coil (with shim)
3 RF transmit coil (and whole body receive coil)
4 Patient table
5 Multichannel local receive coils
6 RF preamplifiers
7 Transmit-receive switch
8 RF power amplifier
9 RF penetration filters
10 Gradient amplifiers
11 Multichannel receiver/digital demodulators
12 Digital RF transmitter modulator
13 Gradient waveform generators
14 Pulse sequence control
15 Synthesizer and master clock
16 Image processor
17 Host computer
18 Mass storage
19 Display and control keybord
20 RF cabin

Figure 15.1 Wiring diagram for an MRI system

(i.e. the magnet and its shim system, the gradient system, the radio frequency (RF) equipment and the system controls).

The main magnet generates a strong and constant magnetic field in order to polarize the nuclei of the atoms in the patient's body. Ferromagnetic shims (e.g. sheets of iron) are placed inside the magnet's bore to obtain the necessary spatial homogeneity within the measurement volume. While a set of shim coils (i.e. coils creating spatial gradients of a higher order than linear gradients) is optional, it may be necessary for applications that are sensitive to the residual field inhomogeneity caused by the human body itself. These applications include spectral saturation, spectroscopic techniques and echo planar imaging (EPI) (see section 15.2). The gradient coil consists of three sets of windings, each causing a linear magnetic gradient field in the x (horizontally across the patient), the y (vertically across the patient) or the z (along the patient) axis when a current is driven through it. The gradient coil contains a radio frequency (RF) coil or resonator. The purpose of this component is to convert pulsed RF current from a power amplifier into a magnetic RF field to excite nuclear spins in the tissue that is the focus of the examination. The same coil or resonator may be used to detect the tiny RF field created by the precessing nuclear spins (i.e. the NMR signal) that contain the information needed to create a cross-sectional image. However, special local pick-up coils (antennas) are often used to receive the MR signal because the signal-to-noise ratio (S/N) they generate is much better than that of a whole-body receiver coil. The signal is forwarded to a preamplifier and then to the RF small signal processing unit where it is converted into a digital form that can be processed by the image reconstruction computer.

Given that the MR signal is very weak compared to the virtually ubiquitous electromagnetic interferences caused by broadcasting stations, computers and other electric devices, it will be necessary to enclose all of the MRI system's field-generating and receiving components in an RF-tight metal housing and to route all of the relevant cables through appropriate RF filters.

The image-creating MR process is guided entirely by the pulse sequence control unit. Once the unit has been appropriately programmed it runs the measurement largely independently of the main computer (the so-called host). The pulse sequence controller's main task is to create the data for the RF and gradient pulses (which are forwarded to the RF power transmitter and the gradient power drivers after digital-to-analogue conversion) and to trigger data acquisition. This procedure is referred to as the pulse sequence. In order to obtain clear and artifact-free MR images, it is necessary to run the pulse sequence according to a precisely timed schedule that is synchronized to the main system clock.

The host computer runs the system start-up, status, and watch-dog processes, the system's user interface (i.e. controls and image monitor), the measurement recording database, the patient database (including the image data archives) and various film and image post-processing applications.

15.1.2 The main magnet

15.1.2.1 Main magnet properties

The magnets that are used in medical MR systems are characterized by their field strength, their field homogeneity (i.e. within the usable measurement volume), their field stability (including the influence of fluctuations caused by external sources) and their fringe field.

The primary property of any magnet is its field strength. The task of selecting a field strength is of vital importance and will be discussed in greater detail in the next section.

It warrants emphasizing that the magnet characteristics mentioned above are not mutually independent and that they also depend to a significant degree on the type of technology used. In what follows, we present the two design schemes that are most frequently used in modern MR imagers, i.e. axial superconducting air-core magnets and iron-yoke magnets driven by permanently magnetic material.

Magnetic field homogeneity

As shown in chapter 7, the spatial encoding of the MR signal emerging from the measurement object (i.e. the patient's body) is performed by selectively exciting certain spins (i.e. applying a band-limited RF pulse while a slice selection gradient is superimposed on the main field so that, in first approximation, only those spins in a plane are excited where the resonance condition is met), deploying a phase-encoding gradient pulse of a well-defined strength and duration prior to the acquisition of the signal and then reading the MR signal after switching on the third gradient (the read-out or frequency-encoding gradient).

While the phase encoding of nuclear magnetization is independent of the actual local field, the position of the excited spins will be determined by the frequency of the RF pulse, the selection-gradient field and the main field $B(x,y,z)$. The same is true for fre-

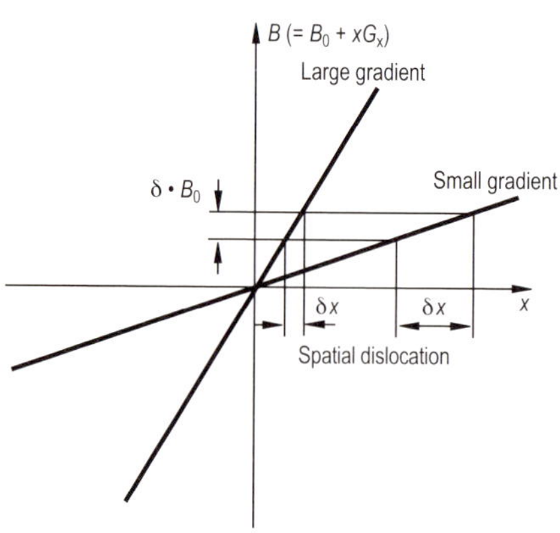

Figure 15.2
Spatial shift between fat and water as a function of gradient strength.

quency encoding: the actual precession frequency of the nuclear magnetization at a location x, y, z is not only a function of the read-out gradient (assumed in this case to be perfectly linear), but also of the actual local field. This can be seen in fig. 15.2. The amount of misregistration δr in slice-select and read-out direction will be:

$$\delta r = \delta B / G, \quad (15.1)$$

where δB is the deviation from the ideal homogeneous field and G is the (slice-select or read-out) gradient. While one could naturally select a larger gradient strength to reduce the influence of the field inhomogeneity, this remedy includes the drawback of a higher bandwidth for the selective RF pulse, which in turn entails a shorter duration and hence the need for increased RF amplitude or power. A higher read-out gradient results in a larger read-out bandwidth, which means more noise and, as a result, a lower S/N.

It may be helpful to take a different approach (namely, from the point of view of image distortion) when seeking to arrive at an estimate of the homogeneity requirement: The local field deviation δB translates into a frequency shift via the fundamental Larmor equation $\delta\omega = \gamma\delta B$. This frequency shift may be compared to the bandwidth of the selective RF pulse (typically 1 to 2 kHz) and the bandwidth per pixel (typically anything between 50 and 200 Hz for spin-echo sequences) of the deployed pulse sequence. The field inhomogeneity of a magnet is usually expressed in relative units $\delta B/B$ (ppm). For instance, the 5 ppm inhomogeneity of a 1 T magnet would result in a slice bending of approximately 20% of the slice thickness (assuming a selective pulse bandwidth of 1 kHz) and an in-plane dislocation of 4 pixels (assuming a pixel bandwidth of 50 Hz).

A more straightforward and stringent requirement for field homogeneity can be derived by considering spectroscopic (imaging) applications. The most important of these involves separating the hydrogen bound in water (intra- and intercellular fluids such as muscle tissue and blood, respectively) from that bound in aliphatic compounds (fatty tissue). This separation is possible because the NMR frequency of water-bound hydrogen spins is approximately 3.5 ppm lower than that of fat-bound hydrogen spins. However, such spectroscopic applications will only succeed if the (relative) homogeneity of the main magnetic field is sufficiently better than 3.5 ppm within the volume of interest.

Field stability

The Fourier MRI procedure requires an extremely stable main magnetic field in order to generate images free of artifacts. The reason for this is that the spatial information of at least one dimension is encoded in the phase of the NMR signal. It can be shown by computer simulation that phase errors of only a few degrees can generate visible artifacts. The phase error due to a time-varying field $\Delta B(t)$ will accumulate for a simple gradient echo pulse sequence during the period between the occurrence of the excitation pulse and the read-out time t:

$$\Delta\varphi(t) = \gamma \int_0^t \Delta B(t')\,\mathrm{d}t' \quad (15.2)$$

If $\Delta B(t)$ shows sinusoidal modulation with a ripple frequency ω_r and a ripple phase φ_r such that

$$\Delta B(t) = \Delta B \sin(\omega_r t + \varphi_r), \tag{15.3}$$

then the phase error can be calculated by inserting equation 15.3 into 15.2:

$$\Delta\varphi = -\frac{1}{\omega_r}\gamma\Delta B[\cos(\omega_r t + \varphi_r) - \cos\varphi_r] \tag{15.4}$$

At a very low ripple frequency ($\omega_r << \pi/t$) and an unfavorable ripple phase $\varphi_r = \pi/2$, eq. (15.4) can be approximated by:

$$\Delta\varphi = \gamma\Delta B t \tag{15.5}$$

The worst possible phase error diminishes with increasing frequency at high ripple frequencies:

$$\Delta\varphi \le \frac{1}{\omega_r}\gamma\Delta B \tag{15.6}$$

Assuming that artifacts may become visible at a phase error of 3° (i.e. assuming also that the image is of low noise), a slow field variation may not exceed 40 nT_{pp} if the echo time of a gradient echo sequence is only 5 ms. This is a challenging requirement because it forces one to consider not only the inherent stability, which is in principle very good for permanent magnets and superconducting magnets operated in a closed loop without an external power supply, but also the time-varying magnetic field caused by external sources. The most common of these sources include ferrous objects magnetized either by the earth field or the fringe field of the MR magnet moving in the vicinity, as well as power lines, transformers and large electric motors. The most critical sources include electric street cars and trains because these are ferromagnetic and generate large and rather unpredictable magnetic fringe fields.

The following example suggests that this problem is by no means a trivial one: Let's assume a single power line. Its fringe field can be calculated by:

$$B = \frac{\mu_0 I}{2\pi r} \tag{15.7}$$

If this line is as close as $r = 3$ m and carries a time-varying current I of 10 A_{pp}, the value for B will be 10 times more than the allowed value.

It is thus important to carefully consider the sensitivity of MR systems to minute time-varying magnetic fields (of any source) during the planning process and prior to making any siting decisions.

The selection of specific magnet properties and the implementation of additional remedies can help to resolve siting difficulties. For instance, the highly conductive cryoshields in superconducting magnets are quite effective at dampening the 50 or 60 Hz power line and transformer fringe fields (depending on the openness of the magnet). The same is true for permanent magnets, especially if they have two yokes. Superconducting magnets can make use of the Meissner-Ochsenfeld effect, even if they are actively shielded. For this purpose, one will need a few windings of superconducting wire outside the screen coil to effectively ward off any uniform external interference. Active interference suppression systems are available for use (mostly) in combination with permanent magnets. Such systems make use of highly sensitive probes to measure external time-varying fields. The signals sent by the probes are then processed to control an auxiliary coil (or the system's RF reference generator).

Fringe field and screening

The main magnet's fringe field is another factor when it comes to the siting of MR systems. Nearness to the fringe field (essentially its gradient) during operation and maintenance represents a major risk management issue due to the considerable hazardous forces it exerts on ferromagnetic objects of even moderate size such as screwdrivers and wrenches. Similarly, it is also important to consider devices that are sensitive to small magnetic fields (in particular, life-supporting devices such as heart pacemakers) as these may malfunction when exposed to the magnet's fringe field (table 15.1). In light of these considerations, it is generally accepted that static fringe fields may not exceed 0.5 mT outside the controlled area of the MR suite. Given the importance of space, magnets that have a low fringe field are at an advantage. High field superconducting magnets are actively shielded so that the 0.5 mT line does not extend beyond a few meters from the isocenter (mostly 3 to 5 m). The cost and weight (tens of tons) of the once popular passive iron screens has made them obsolete and their deployment is largely restricted to special measures. Given that their fringe field does not extend more than a few meters (2 to 3 m) beyond the isocenter, low field yoke type magnets are usually not in need of additional screening.

15.1.2.2 Field strength selection criteria

As shown in chapter 7, the signal to noise ratio (*S/N*) of an MR signal emerging from a lossy object generally increases in proportion to the field strength B_0. While this may lead one to conclude that the higher B_0 values will lead to better image quality (either expressed in *S/N* or traded in for better spatial resolution and/or acquisition speed), the conclusion is only partially true owing to the fact that several inevitable physical problems arise when one aims for higher B_0 values, i.e. higher MR frequency [15.1]. It

Magnetic disks or tapes	3 mT
Video monitors with shielding or correction	3 mT
CRT video monitors (monochromatic)	1 mT
Cardiac pacemakers	0.5 mT
X-ray units	0.2 mT
Image intensifiers	50 µT
Photomultipliers	50 µT
Earth's magnetic field for comparison	50 µT

Table 15.1
Sensitivity of various instruments to static magnetic fields (approximate values)

also warrants mention that higher B_0 values are associated with higher system investment and life cycle costs.

In what follows, we offer a summary of the relevant physical constraints (in the order of their importance).

RF losses heating the patient (*SAR*) and required peak RF power

According to Maxwell's equations, an electric field E is always connected to a time-varying magnetic field:

$$\oint \vec{E}\,\mathrm{d}r = -\int_F \frac{\partial \vec{B}}{\partial t}\,\mathrm{d}\vec{F} \tag{15.8a}$$

This yields the following for a homogeneous magnetic field B_1 varying harmonically in time:

$$2\pi r_\perp E = -\pi r_\perp^2 \omega \hat{B}_1 \tag{15.8b}$$

The electric field $\vec{E}$ causes eddy currents of density $\vec{j}$ inside conductive objects (conductivity σ), such as the human body, that increase linearly along with the distance $r_\perp$ from the object's center:

$$\vec{j} = \sigma \vec{E} \tag{15.9}$$

The electric power losses thus amount to

$$P = \int_V \vec{j}\,\vec{E}\,\mathrm{d}V = \int_V \sigma E \mathrm{d}V = \frac{\sigma}{4} B_1^2 \omega^2 \int r_\perp^2 \mathrm{d}V. \tag{15.10}$$

The RF transmitter will be required to compensate for these losses. RF losses in the patient are proportional to MR frequency squared and can create heat.

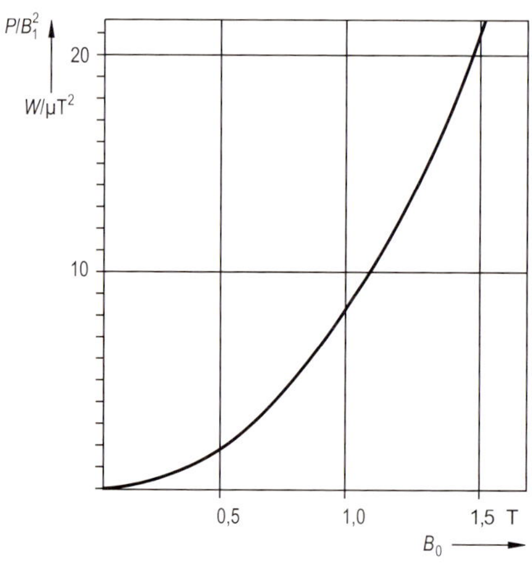

Figure 15.3
Absorbed RF power per B_1^2 by an average person weighing 70 kg as function of the main magnetic field B_0 when imaged with proton MR applying a circular polarized RF field B_1.

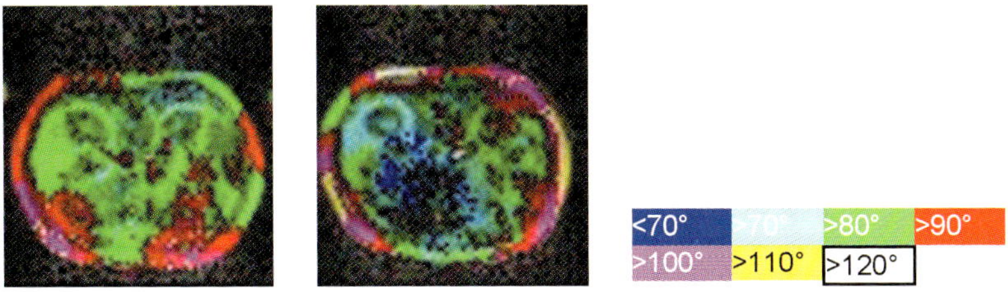

Figure 15.4
Flip angle distribution due to an inhomogeneous B_1 field in a human object at 63 MHz **(left)** and 126 MHz **(right).**

National and international standards have been introduced to restrict the exposure of humans to RF heating (see fig. 15.3). For instance, the IEC standard 60601-2-33 which has been adopted by most national regulatory authorities requires that the whole-body specific absorption rate (*SAR*) may not exceed 2 W/kg (or 4W/kg under special supervision of the patient). The lower limit can cause limitations in the repetition rate of short high peak power 180° pulses at 1.5 T or 63 MHz. Here, it warrants bearing in mind that the required RF transmitter's peak power capacity also increases. While 15 kW might be considered sufficient to support 180° pulses of 0.5 ms at 1.5 T, one would need approximately 60 kW to perform the same sequence at 3 T. This high power would introduce considerable challenges, not only for RF transmitter design, but also for transmitter resonator design (seeing as how the latter would be required to withstand the high RF voltage of several kV).

RF object penetration, dielectric resonance effects

Conductive material such as human body tissue also prevents the penetration of the electromagnetic RF field. This is referred to as the skin effect. Penetration depth decreases along with increasing frequency. The explanation for this phenomenon is the same as that for the power losses discussed above: eddy currents weaken the effect of the RF field by shielding the inner portions of the body. The effect referred to as dielectric resonance plays a similar role. The human body consists mostly of water with a relative dielectric constant of $\varepsilon_r \approx 81$. The wavelength inside the body is therefore shortened by a factor of 9 compared to that in free space. While the wavelength in free space is around 2.4 m at 126 MHz (B_0 = 3 T), it is only 26 cm inside a watery object, thereby clearing the way for the occurrence of standing waves that undermine the homogeneity of the RF field. This is shown in fig. 15.4, which offers a comparison of the flip angle distribution at 63 MHz (1.5 T) and at 126 MHz (3 T).

Size, weight, fringe field and cost

A magnet's size, weight, fringe field (i.e. if a high field magnet is scaled from a medium field magnet) and cost (for the system as well as for its infrastructure requirements) are likely to increase along with its field strength. While a degree of juggling is permitted when combining these variables, it is impossible to gain anything without paying a penalty. For instance, if one would like to keep the weight, size and cost of a 3 T magnet comparable to that of a 1.5 T magnet, then one will have to sacrifice homogeneity volume and a significant portion of fringe field shielding capacity.

Relative field homogeneity and chemical shift

Field homogeneity (as a property of design and inevitable manufacturing tolerances) and MR chemical shift are expressed in relative units (ppm) because they are proportional to B_0. As a consequence, image distortion and chemical shift (i.e. in the frequency encoding and slice-select direction) will increase along with the magnetic field unless one refrains from increasing the pixel bandwidth and the selective pulse bandwidth. The drawbacks here include lower *S/N* and increased peak and average power requirements for RF pulses. The latter is especially unfavorable because it can make the *SAR* and power requirement issue even more problematic.

T_1 frequency dependence

Given that T_1 relaxation times increase along with MR frequency [15.2], it is necessary to increase the repetition time of the pulse sequences accordingly when going to higher B_0 values so as to maintain image contrast. The associated increase in total acquisition time represents no more than a minor drawback that is usually outweighed by the *S/N* gain.

Concluding remarks

There is as yet nothing conclusive to add to the optimal field strength debate of recent years. No one solution has been revealed to be clearly better than the rest. If one looks at the issue with the eye of a physicist and engineer, one will see dramatic gains in image quality and performance in the transition from 0.1 T (the first systems capable of scanning human beings) to (let's say) 1.5 T, which is the most popular field strength used for clinical purposes today. That being said, it warrants pointing out that the transition from 1.0 T to 1.5 T includes a number of drawbacks, largely centering on system costs and *SAR*, but also on issues of RF field inhomogeneity. These drawbacks have to some extent been mitigated by (continuing) price decreases, optimized transmission antennas and greater flexibility on the part of standardization and regulatory authorities (i.e. with respect to *SAR* limits). The introduction of fast, low-flip, angle-pulse sequences has also been helpful. However, it will be important to continue to consider drawbacks and general clinical usefulness as developers seek to move beyond 1.5 T. While manufacturers and research institutions are aiming for 3 T (and even higher), clinicians should make sure to carefully assess their needs and all system advantages and disadvantages when making purchasing decisions.

15.1.2.3 Superconducting magnet construction

Superconducting magnets form the basis of the majority of medical MR imaging systems and are likely to continue to do so in light of the trend in the direction of ever higher field strengths (an area where iron-based permanent magnet and resistive-coil magnets cannot compete).

Coil design

A typical cylindrical superconducting magnet consists of several coils (usually six or seven) run in series to form a solenoid which provides a cylindrically symmetric field. The size and position of the coils are designed to minimize the field fluctuations, which are described in terms of spherical harmonics – mathematical solutions to the Laplace equation which describe magnetic fields in free space:

$$B_Z(r,\vartheta,\varphi) = \sum_{n=0}^{N}\sum_{m=0}^{M\le N}\left(\frac{r}{R}\right)^n P_n^m(\cos\vartheta)[A_n^m\cos m\varphi + B_n^m\sin m\varphi] \qquad (15.11)$$

The equation is akin to Fourier synthesis where a square wave is constructed from many sine waves; the many harmonics combine to make a uniform field. Fig. 15.5 shows how each coil influences the design harmonics of a magnet, revealing the characteristic twelve fingered (12th-order) harmonic of any 6-coil system. The final homogeneity for a typical system over a 50 cm diameter spherical volume (DSV) is 1 to 3 ppm V_{rms} and 20 to 40 ppm (peak to peak) when plotted with a degree of accuracy sufficient for measuring the 12th and higher orders. The degree to which these harmonics are to be controlled will have a major impact on the external dimensions of the system. Control of these harmonics is a major influence on the external dimensions of the system. Short and open magnets are fighting physics and pose challenging problems to magnet designers.

A typical magnet contains 20 to 40 km of superconducting wire composed of superconducting filaments embedded in a copper matrix for added strength. This strength is required because the magnetic field near the coils is greater than the central field, which means they generate large forces between themselves. These forces range from

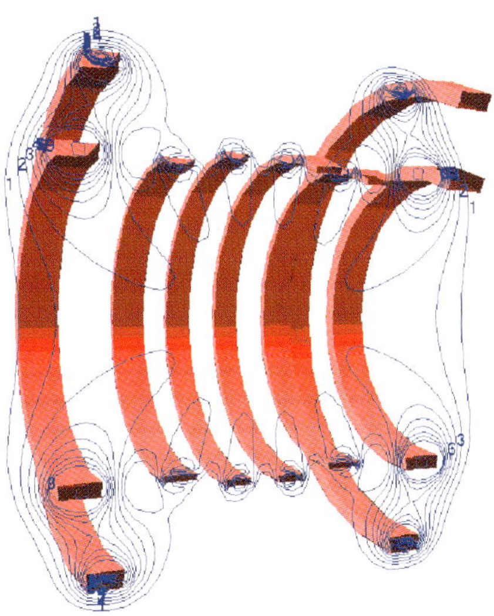

Figure 15.5
Magnetic field distributions for the single coils in a 6-coil MR magnet.

just a few tons to several hundred tons in the case of high field systems. Such forces place limits on the achievable absolute field and on the use of the superconductor since superconductivity is lost above a certain magnetic field. The forces are borne by the coils themselves and the supporting magnet former on which the coils are wound. For a 1.5 T magnet, there are regions of 4 T or more, but these are carefully controlled within the volume of the outer vessel.

Shielding

Early systems had very large stray fields requiring large and costly magnet or room steel shields to contain them. Today, active shielding is employed, where counter-running coils surround the main field coils, constricting the magnetic field (figs. 15.5 and 15.6). Whilst this requires a small increase in the magnet dimensions and cost (it reduces the magnet efficiency), the savings in external shielding cost and weight are far greater. Concomitantly, the magnet becomes easier to site and is safer for personnel near the system.

Cryostat

Conventional superconductors (e.g. Nb-Ti) function at only a few degrees (~4 K) above absolute. High temperature superconductors do exist, but these are still very much in the development phase. In order to maintain very low temperatures necessary, the magnet former is placed inside a strong non-magnetic steel cryo-vessel and bathed in liquid helium. This in turn is encased in a very efficiently insulated, outer vacuum housing made of non-magnetic steel or aluminium (fig. 15.6). The helium vessel is

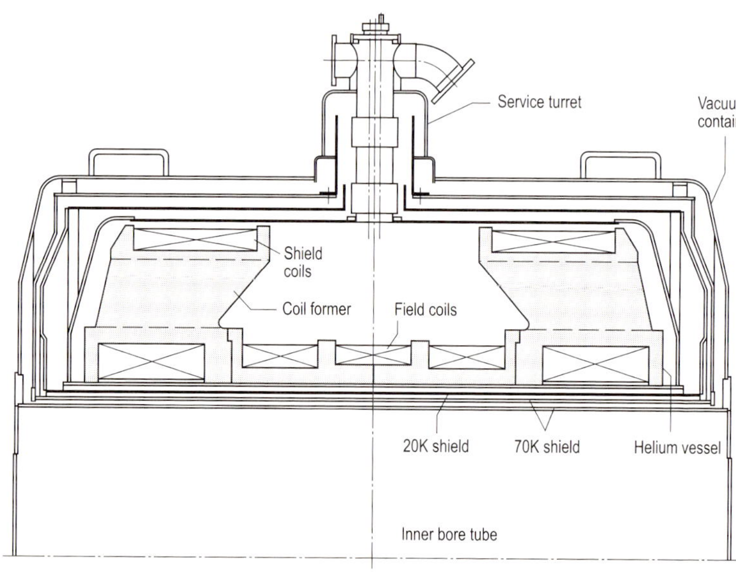

Figure 15.6 Cross section of an actively screened superconducting magnet.

suspended from thermally insulating rods in a system of concentric aluminum cylinders or heat shields, each insulated using layers of high-tech super insulation. There are generally two intermediate layers that are kept at 20 K and 70 K by the cryo cooler or fridge. The use of state-of-the-art technology recondenses the helium internally, thus allowing zero-boil-off systems to be built.

The fridge turret connects the cooler to the various cryoshields and the service turret (sometimes combined with the fridge) and allows access to the magnet for the sake of attaching power cables (i.e. for ramping), refilling the helium and routing system diagnostics.

Ramping

Superconducting systems are energized by an external power supply that is temporarily plugged into the magnet. This ramping procedure takes time (typically 30 minutes) due to the inductance of the coils opposing the change in current. Once the correct current has been introduced, a superconducting switch is activated that effectively shorts out the current leads so that they can be removed whilst the magnet current remains. Once a superconducting magnet has been ramped up, the current decay is so slow that it seldom needs adjusting (normally once every two to three years, depending on the field strength and the bandwidth of the associated measurement electronics).

Quenching

A quench occurs when there is a sudden loss of superconductivity. This may occur as a result of a fault or due to the activation of the emergency run-down button. As soon as one small part of a coil becomes resistive, it rapidly dissipates heat, spreading the quench zone and causing the current and field to drop rapidly to zero. The magnet's inductance opposes this change, with large voltages (several kV) being generated in the process. If not properly controlled, this can be very destructive to the coil, even if the quench is deliberate. Passive circuits are therefore deployed to limit damage. Activated by the start of a quench, these circuits spread the quench to all of the coils so that the potentially destructive energy (several MJ) is distributed throughout the magnet and the voltages are lowered to safe levels.

An emergency quench activated by the operator represents a very quick way of switching off the field in the event of an emergency. The mechanism involved deliberately heats the coils to cause a loss of superconductivity, thus switching off of the field in a matter of seconds. The procedure is carefully controlled so as to ensure that no damage is done to the system. This still results in a large loss of helium, which must be safely vented outside the MR facility. The magnet must be subsequently checked, refilled with helium and ramped back to field.

Stability

One major advantage of superconducting systems is their inherent stability: better than 0.1 ppm change per hour for the central field and no rapid changes. A group of superconducting coils also effectively screens external magnetic effects such as those generated by passing vehicles. A secondary superconducting screening circuit is usually included to augment this screening effect.

15.1.2.4 Iron yoke magnets

Resistive systems

Resistive magnets are limited by their electrical power requirements to around 0.3 T and are therefore used for low field, low-cost installations. These magnets are generally sold as open systems, with a C-yoke providing some degree of access to the patient during scanning as well as reducing the claustrophobic effects. Due to their openness, these systems are deployed for various applications in the area of real-time MRI, a technique used for guiding invasive surgical procedures.

In general, a pair of coils is used to generate a vertical field between the poles of an iron yoke. The large mass of iron is needed to guide the magnetic flux to boost the field strength and reduce the stray field to some extent. The poles are specially shaped to improve the homogeneity, but typically the imaging volumes are smaller and less homogeneous than those of superconducting systems. However, this degree of homogeneity is sufficient for many applications and the advantages of size, openness and cost make such systems a viable alternative to superconducting systems.

One of the critical factors for a resistive magnet is the stability of the power supply. This must be able to produce a very constant current, otherwise the central frequency fluctuations will be too great. Because such systems are generally ramped down overnight to conserve energy, they require some time (about one hour) to achieve equilibrium after being re-energized. However, the stability of superconducting systems easily exceeds that of state-of-the-art resistive systems.

Permanent magnets

Permanent magnet materials offer an alternative to resistive coils for low field applications of around 0.3 T. One obvious advantage to such materials is that they do not require a stable power supply. However, given that the magnetic remanence of permanent magnetic materials (e.g. the popular NdFeB) is sensitive to temperature changes, the system in question will need to be subject to tight thermal control to achieve the required stability.

Permanent systems do not need ramping, therefore they do not suffer from the switch on and stabilisation time delay of a resistive system: one obvious drawback is the concomitant inability to switch off the field should it be desired. In particular, transportation and installations of such systems must be strictly controlled, since they leave the factory energized.

Open systems

Many systems are marketed as 'open': the current superconducting systems available are shorter than before and 'openness' is used to describe the clear reduction in patient claustrophobia, but a true open system allows patient access too. While C-shaped magnets achieve this to some extent, it remains a Holy Grail of magnet design to provide a system of around 1 T that offers good access to the patient. The systems that have been developed so far (from 0.5 T up to 1 T) are too costly and complex for general use.

Such systems represent a major challenge for designers: the gap for patient access is exactly where the magnetic materials are placed for greatest control of the final homogeneity.

15.1.2.5 Shimming

All types of MR magnets require passive shimming to achieve optimal homogeneity. Passive shimming corrects for minor imperfections in the build of the system and for the effects of any magnetic materials present on site. This is particularly important for mobile applications where the amount of steel necessary for the tight magnetic shielding requirement leads to large distortions.

Shimming is also required to compensate for the paramagnetic effects exhibited by the human body (commonly referred to as susceptibility). Such effects vary from patient to patient, usually ranging from 0.5 to 1 ppm at a field strength of 1.5 T. The highest quality images are achieved when these patient-induced variations are compensated for by an active shim.

Passive shims

There are two main techniques for passive shimming to compensate for field inhomogeneities. The first and more common technique involves the use of small iron shims that are placed in the pockets of long thin trays within the magnet bore. The second technique involves the use of electric shims consisting of many variously shaped coils. These are either resistive ones that are placed in the bore or superconducting coils mounted inside the magnet vessel.

Field corrections

Field imperfections are also described in terms of spherical harmonics. In order to compensate for these imperfections, the shim engineer (guided by sophisticated software) places thin pieces of iron to generate distortions that oppose (i.e. cancel out) existing distortions. The same technique applies to electrical shims where each coil is designed to cancel out one particular spherical harmonic; however, it is physically impossible to fit a magnet with all of the coils that would be required to cancel out every distortion. Iron shims allow far more degrees of freedom and give the engineer more flexibility when it comes to effectively shimming the magnet.

Field measurements

It is important to measure distortions correctly when shimming a magnet. What applies to imaging also applies to shimming, namely, the smaller the pixel, the greater the resolution (i.e. the more planes used to measure the field, the better the information). It is important to ensure that the shimming procedure uses enough planes to map all the dominant harmonics, such as the 12th-order harmonic shown in the coil diagram above. If only 12 planes are used in the measurement, then the true distortion will remain concealed and the magnet will appear to be better than it really is.

The use of spherical harmonics is an elegant mathematical solution. Physics tells us that if the field on the surface of a volume is well known, then the field within that volume is uniquely defined. Thus, if the spherical harmonics describe the surface variation, they also describe the complete volume. This principle can be reliably used in the volume *RMS* definition to achieve greater accuracy than that made available by a set of measurements throughout the volume.

Measurement techniques with for example 24-planes concentrate on measuring the surface of the imaging volume very accurately, where the field distortions are greatest. The V_{rms}-algorithm subsequently fits the harmonics to this surface data and then integrates the route mean square (rms) deviation over the whole volume to give a true representation of the magnetic field homogeneity throughout the entire usable imaging volume.

Active shims

The insertion of a patient into the magnet bore causes further field distortions. These must be corrected for if one wishes to achieve the highest image quality. First order correction is possible by subtly adjusting the gradients, but for off-centre imaging, the best solution is to also have second order shims, which can be set before each new clinical study to optimize the field. A quick MR sequence maps out the field and applies the required corrections to the coils before the main image is acquired. This is particularly helpful in the case of off-axis imaging (e.g. shoulder investigations).

15.1.3 The gradient system

15.1.3.1 The relevant properties of the gradient system

The MR scanner's gradient system can be characterized by maximum achievable gradient field strength (mT/m), minimum possible switching time or slew rate (i.e. the time needed to switch the gradient from 0 to G_{max} given in mT/m/ms), spatial nonlinearity over the specified usable volume (usually expressed as % deviation of the actual vs. the ideal field), gradient pulse stability and reproducibility and eddy-current-induced dynamic distortions. Derived properties that are important in the case of high performance gradient systems include the field change rate dB/dt at a given slew rate, which can cause peripheral nerve stimulation and patient discomfort, and acoustic noise, which can cause hearing impairment.

One should be aware that not all of these characteristics are mutually independent. For instance, a gradient system capable of delivering a high gradient strength at a high slew rate with low nonlinearity over a large usable volume will cause stimulation significantly below its power limits. Such a design would be unnecessarily expensive.

Maximum gradient strength and slew rate

When attempting to determine the optimal maximum gradient and slew rates for an MR imager, it can be instructive to have another look at the reason why gradient pulses are necessary. Gradient pulses are used in an imaging sequence to select a slice (in 3D sequences: a slab) together with a band-limited RF pulse, then to carry out phase encoding (one in 2D and two in 3D imaging) and finally to carry out frequency encoding (i.e. reading the MR signal while a gradient is on). The three types of gradients are mutually orthogonal and are switched on at the beginning and off at the end of the select, phase-encode and read-out periods.

The fact that it is necessary to switch the gradients several times during an imaging pulse sequence makes the slew rate issue quite important: the switching periods are parasitic (i.e. they take time and are good for nothing). Therefore, the slew rate should as high as possible.

Other gradient functions include spatial saturation (which is similar to the slice selection process), flow encoding and diffusion weighted imaging. Smaller pixels and/or shorter acquisition times require stronger gradients.

It thus appears at first glance that a system with the highest gradients (and slew rates) will offer the greatest flexibility when it comes to selecting imaging protocols (especially in terms of speed and spatial resolution). However, it is likely that a number of practical, physiological and physical difficulties will restrict the growth of gradient system power as the technology develops.

The practical concerns include power supply requirements, cooling capacity and cost. The patient-related constraints associated with switched gradients include peripheral nerve stimulation (PNS) and acoustic noise. The first patient-related concern is of a fundamental nature and has been limited by regulatory standards. The latter concern can be resolved to some extent by deploying dampening material between coil and patient bore. This solution is limited by spatial constraints within the magnet.

The Maxwell gradients, also referred to as concomitant gradients, represent a physical problem. The static Maxwell equations for magnetic fields in homogeneous media $\nabla\vec{B} = 0$ and $\nabla\times\vec{B} = 0$ indicate that a gradient field (e.g. $G_x = \partial B_z/\partial x$) will inevitably cause field components to point in a perpendicular direction to the main field (assumed to be parallel to z). These concomitant fields increase along with the square of the desired gradient (for G_x: $\frac{G_x^2 z^2}{2B_0}$) with the result that bipolar gradient pulses, for instance, do not properly rephase the nuclear magnetization, and thereby cause image quality problems in certain pulse sequence types [15.3]. While this can be compensated for by additional gradient pulses in many cases, it will entail a penalty in the form of lost speed. Maxwell gradients are negligible if the gradient coil field is small compared to B_0.

Spatial linearity

Spatially nonlinear gradients will cause spatial image distortions. The mechanism involved is analogous to the effect of an inhomogeneous B_0 field. However, in the case of the nonlinear gradient, the deviation δB (in eq. (15.1)) results from the imperfection in the gradient coil's field distribution:

$$B_{\mathrm{Gr}}(r) = G_r r + \delta B_{\mathrm{Gr}}(r) \tag{15.12}$$

The relative gradient nonlinearity $\delta B_{\mathrm{Gr}}/B_{\mathrm{Gr}}$ increases as the distance from the gradient center increases, as does the spatial distortion resulting from it. However, this kind of distortion is independent as well of gradient strength and whether it is employed for slice selection, phase encoding or readout. It is necessary to accept a few percentage points of nonlinearity at the edge of the imaging volume in order to keep the ($\mathrm{d}B/\mathrm{d}t$)-stimulation level, the gradient amplifier power and the size of the gradient coil within reasonable limits.

Stability and reproducibility

The requirements that apply to the gradient fields are as high as those that apply to the stability of the main magnetic. This is the case because the phase of the MR signal carrying the spatial information is determined by all of the acting magnetic fields.

We can make this obvious by replacing $\Delta B(t)$ in eq. (15.2) with $r\Delta G(t)$:

$$\Delta\varphi(r,t) = \gamma r \int_0^t \Delta G(t')\mathrm{d}t' \tag{15.13}$$

Again, one can run quantitative calculations (e.g. for periodic gradient instabilities caused by the current ripple of the gradient amplifier) and one will again find that the effect of high frequency ripple is smoothed out by the integration in equation 15.13.

Given that the gradient coils generate fields that are approximately 2 to 3 orders of magnitude less than the main field, the relative instability (and reproducibility of the gradient pulse time integrals) may be less demanding. Nonetheless, they are still on the order of 10^{-5} (i.e. depending on the overall properties of the gradient system). This is still a very challenging specification for the gradient current amplifier.

Eddy current effects

The fact that the gradient coil is surrounded by conductive parts in the main magnet (e.g. the cryostat and cold shields of a superconductive magnet) means that the coil's switched fringe field will generate eddy currents in these structures that will in turn cause a time-dependent weakening of the gradient field. As shown in fig. 15.7a, a rectangular current pulse through the coil will result in a gradient field that is distorted (as if it had been filtered by a simple low pass). One can compensate for this effect by applying a high pass pre-emphasis to the current pulse shape (fig. 15.7b). However, this sort of eddy-current compensation only works locally because the eddy currents flow along a different path than the currents in the coil. A time-dependent gradient field (mainly of the 3rd order) will therefore remain. This turns out to be detrimental

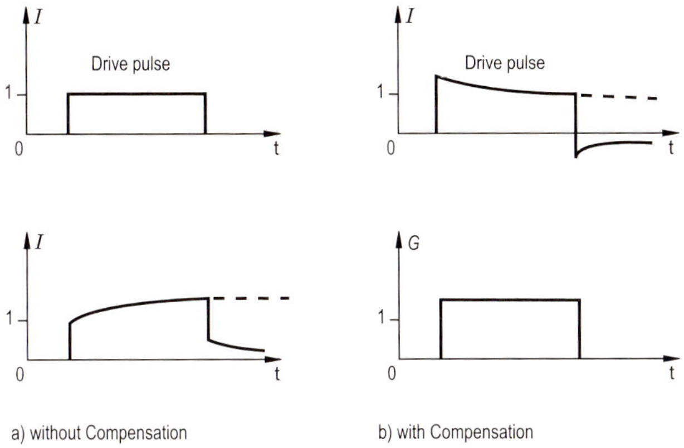

Figure 15.7
Gradient pulse shape caused by eddy currents in the surroundings **(a)** and its compensation via the pre-deformation of the current drive pulse **(b)**

to the imaging quality of sophisticated pulse sequences such as turbo spin echo. To avoid such difficulties, modern MRI systems deploy so-called actively shielded gradient coils [15.4] that need almost no eddy-current compensation.

Concluding remarks

The issue of maximum gradient power appears to be somewhat more complex than that of field strength. Unlimited gradient strength together with the highest slew rate appears at first glance to be desirable. However, going beyond peripheral nerve stimulation (PNS) and acoustic noise levels does not make sense because such overpowered gradient systems cannot be applied in patients without creating unacceptable risks. The upper limit of gradient performance depends on the size of the imaging volume. The same is true if the ratio of concomitant gradient to main field is large enough to cause image quality degradation.

15.1.3.2 Gradient coils

Given the fact that magnetic field gradients are used in MRI to perform 3D mapping from the object into image space, the role of gradient coils in MRI can be compared to some extent to that of lens systems in optical instruments. For example, deviations from the ideally desired gradient fields are directly related to geometrical image distortions.

Furthermore, gradient coils need to be designed to enable almost perfect control of their magnetic field dynamics via driving electric current pulses.

The fact that one can focus exclusively on the field component parallel to the main magnetic field (i.e. perpendicular components can be neglected to a large extent) is helpful when it comes to the practical gradient coil layout because the static B_0 field is 2 orders of magnitude larger.

Gradient coils are required to cope with strong Lorentz forces because they are driven by large pulsed electrical currents in the environment of a strong static magnetic B_0 field. This exposure means that the coils are a source of mechanical vibration and acoustic noise.

Fundamental winding structure (cylindrical gradient coils)

Each of the three subsystems G_x, G_y, G_z is usually set up as a separate layer within a single solid isolating coil structure.

Cylindrical coils (with current flowing in opposite directions) are used to generate a z-gradient (fig. 15.8a). A *y*-gradient can be generated by deploying four current arcs (all carrying currents of the same direction) located at opposite *y* positions. Given that the paths of the arcs need to be closed after their technical realization, the windings are comprised of four saddles, each extending over one quarter of the coil (fig. 15.8b).

An *x*-gradient coil shows the same structure as a *y*-gradient coil except that it is rotated by 90°. Saddle coils are less efficient with respect to the ratio of the gradient strength to the current than longitudinal coils because their only their central arcs are positively contributing to the desired gradient field.

Fundamental gradient-coil properties

Gradient nonlinearity

Given that it is essentially impossible to generate a perfect gradient $G = \text{const}$, gradient coils are designed with a specified maximum deviation (nonlinearity) from ideal field linearity within a defined volume of interest. The fact that these deviations are determined via calculations enables one to correct geometrical distortion in MR images offline. Typical actual nonlinearities amount to around 5% for a spherical volume of interest with a diameter of 45 cm.

Shielding performance

Gradient coils can cause eddy currents in their electrically conductive surroundings (e.g. in the magnets that house them). These eddy currents generate unwanted addi-

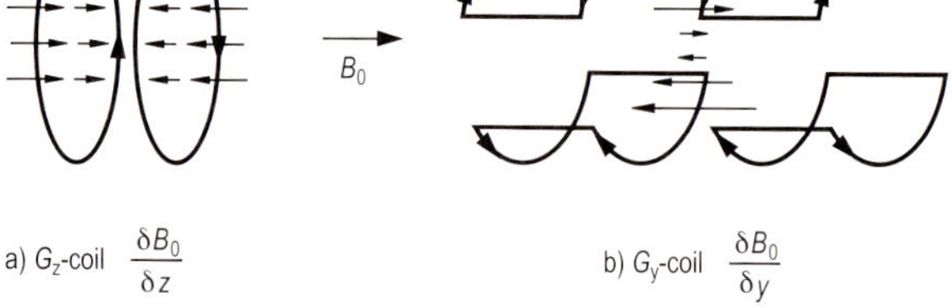

Figure 15.8
Fundamental winding arrangement in a cylindrical longitudinal (z) gradient coil **(a)** and in a cylindrical transversal (here: *y*) gradient coil **(b)**.

tional magnetic fields that cause severe imaging artifacts. The use of shielded gradient coils enables one to minimize the stray field in the conductive environment and thereby suppress the eddy currents.

A shielded gradient coil is comprised of two layers. The inner or primary layer generates the gradient field in the volume of interest. The outer layer (with its reversed currents) acts as a shield that essentially nullifies the magnetic stray field at the coil's outer surface.

Gradient strength and slew rate

Gradient performance increased between 1988 and 2000 from 6 mT/m to 30-40 mT/m, with the electrical driving power scaling with the square of the gradient strength. The rate of gradient change (slew rate) increased during the same period to 125-200 Ts/m. Peripheral nerve stimulation may prevent further performance increases. It is necessary to match the electrical properties of gradient coils and gradient power supplies. Today's MRI gradient systems use currents of around 500 A and voltages of around 2,000 V.

Gradient coil technologies

Design calculation methods

Coil design can be optimized by applying mathematical methods that generate winding patterns according to input specifications such as:

- Geometrical limitations (like coil length)
- Gradient strength, nonlinearity, volume of interest
- Shielding performance
- Inductance
- Resistive power losses and current density limitations
- Lorentz forces and torque

These specifications are used as boundary conditions in the optimization procedure. An entire gradient axis, including primary and shielding layers, is usually calculated within a single optimization procedure.

Fingerprint design

As a result of numerical optimization, the wire paths of actual transversal coils differ from that shown in fig. 15.8. The rectangular frames are replaced by saddles comprised of wire paths that look like finger prints (fig. 15.9).

3D-design

In the case of shielded transversal coils, some of the loop-closing wires (which don't contribute positively to the desired field) can be avoided if the current paths are allowed to change radially between the primary and shielding layers. These short-cuts enable both more efficient and shorter gradient coil designs.

Mechanical assembly and electrical insulation

Vacuum potting with a special epoxy resin is performed to achieve proper fixation of the gradient wires and to make sure that the coils can be operated at voltages of up to 2,000 V without coronary discharge or flashovers.

Cooling

The high density of the electrical power losses due to the actual gradient performance data requires the use of water cooling for the gradient coils.

Additional functions

The space between the primary and the shielding layers in shielded gradient coils can be put to use, for instance, to provide pockets for the housing of passive shim iron or to enable the integration of active shim coils (fig. 15.10).

The inner surface of the gradient coil can be used for the integration of an RF screen that is electrically connected to the RF resonator system.

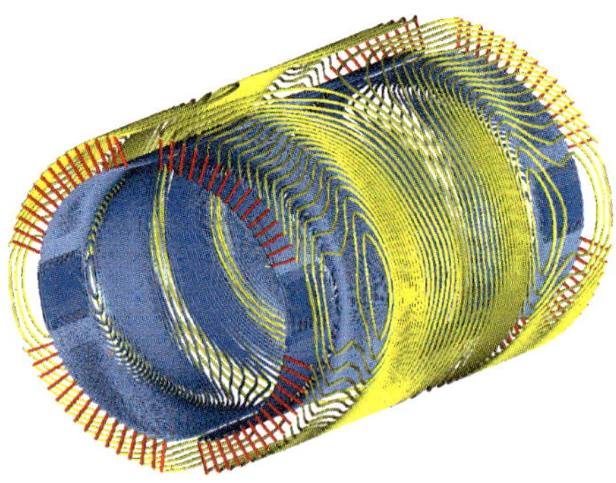

Figure 15.9
Example of a transversal 3D fingerprint design using wire paths that partially change between primary and shielding layer.

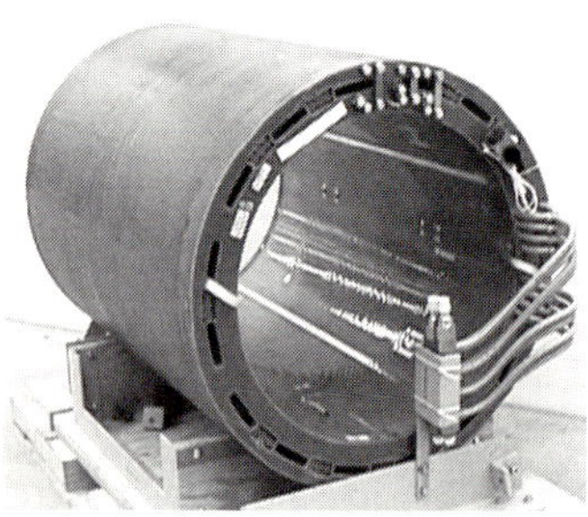

Figure 15.10
A cylindrical gradient coil potted in filled resin, with attached manifolds for cooling water, pockets for passive shim iron and an integrated RF screen

Alternative gradient coil layouts

Flat gradient coils

Open MRI scanners exhibit a different gradient coil winding structure. Here, the gradient coils are arranged as flat plates with their surfaces perpendicular to the B_0 field.

Head-only gradient coils

Special engineering solutions are necessary in the case of head-only gradient coils with an inner bore diameter of approx. 36 cm. Asymmetric transversal coils offer a positioning advantage in that the volume of interest is close to their frontal edges, thus enabling proper access for the patient to the imaging volume. Nonaxial-symmetric longitudinal coil designs allow for shoulder cutouts. Head-only coils (fig. 15.11) offer the advantages of higher thresholds for peripheral nerve stimulation and greater feasibility when it comes to their integration in dedicated magnets with reduced inner bore diameters.

15.1.3.3 Gradient power supply

The basic function of a gradient power supply or amplifier is to drive currents of correct amplitude and duration into the gradient coils. A pulse sequence controller calculates the required current pulses, including the eddy current compensation and shim-offset currents.

Modern high power gradient amplifiers generate currents of more than 600 A with maximum output voltages of around 2,000 V. Current rise times in the gradient coil of about 3,200 kA/s are possible.

The instantaneous output power of each axis in a three-axis amplifier reaches more than 1 MW. The stored energy is returned to the amplifier during the period when the magnetic field in the gradient coil is driven to zero. The integrated power supply is therefore only required to provide the power for the gradient system's resistive and switching losses. Optimal efficiency is achieved by using switch-mode amplifiers exhibiting an efficiency of better than 99%.

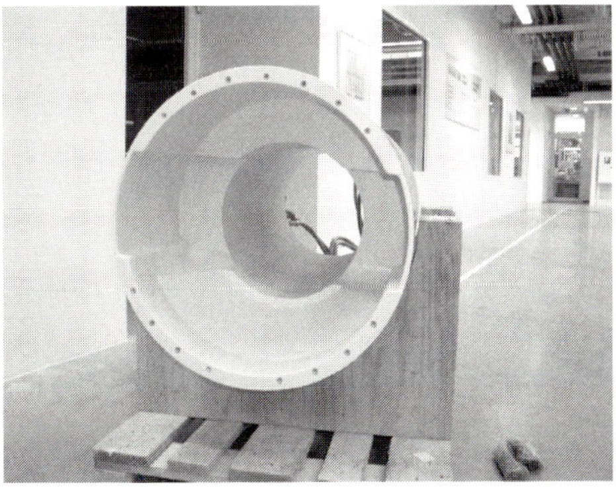

Figure 15.11
Dedicated head-only gradient coil with shoulder cutouts using transversal windings with an asymmetric design

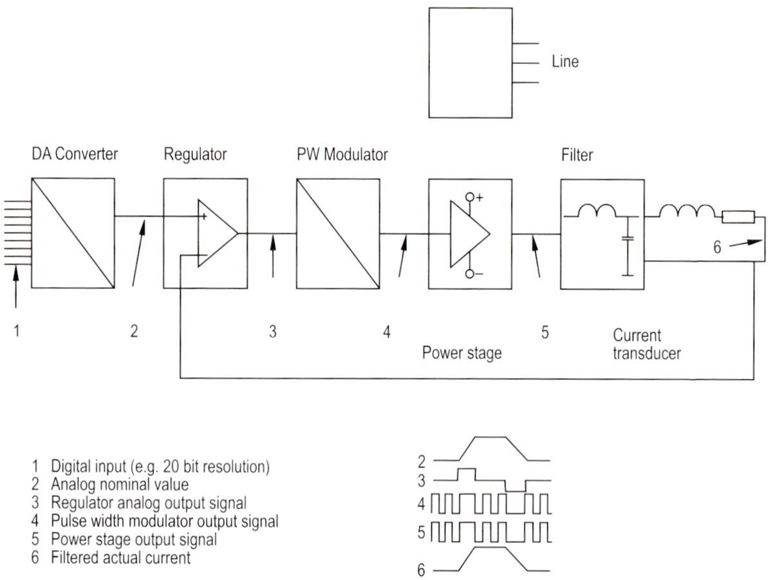

Figure 15.12 Block circuit diagram of a single gradient amplifier axis

The gradient system is comprised of the amplifier, cable, filter and gradient coil (fig. 15.12).

The digital gradient pulse signal is converted by a digital-analog converter (DAC) into an appropriate analog voltage pulse and then supplied to the regulator. The resolution of the DAC is about 1 mA/bit. The regulator output signal is transformed in the modulator to a digital switching signal for the final stage power transistors and is often referred to as the pulse width modulation signal. The switch-on time can vary between 0% to decrease the current and 100% to increase the current. The switching frequency is fixed to several 100 kHz. Output current flows through a low pass filter to the gradient coil. High precision current transducers measure the current and provide the regulator with actual current values. All of the components in the regulator circuitry and the amplifier chain need to comply with the highest precision standards in order to meet performance requirements.

Linear amplifiers are not a practical alternative to the described switching design. They are poor in efficiency due to high final stage power losses. Hybrid designs that use booster stages to get around this limitation are sometimes used. While this design increases the output voltage during the ramping procedure in order to achieve high current slew rates, it has some critical limitations. The output voltage (and therefore the slew rate) is only variable within tightly defined limits. This introduces severe restrictions for sequence programming. Furthermore, the cross-over characteristic of these amplifiers (i.e. as they switch from normal to booster stage) is not linear. This can cause artifacts.

15.1.4 The RF system

15.1.4.1 The relevant properties of the RF system

As discussed in chapter 7, the task of the RF system is twofold. First, it is necessary to expose the nuclear magnetization caused by the static magnetic field B_0 to a magnetic RF field B_1 perpendicular to B_0 and rotating at the Larmor frequency in order to turn the magnetization away from the B_0 axis at an angle determined by the strength and (pulse) duration of the RF field. As soon as the RF pulse ceases, the nuclear magnetization begins to precess around the B_0 axis at the Larmor frequency, causing a tiny rotating RF field. The second task of the RF system will thus be to pick up this signal.

The first task is performed by the RF transmitter (Tx) and the second task is performed by the receiver (Rx) system. As will be shown later, it might be advantageous to have a multi-channel Rx system.

The transmitter and receiver are comprised of signal processing electronics, amplifiers and coils or resonators that transform electrical currents into magnetic fields and vice versa. The coil or resonator used to create the B_1 field may also be deployed to receive the MR signal. The transmit and receive functions are controlled and synchronized to a master clock by the MR system's control unit.

In what follows, we first outline the main requirements for the RF system components before moving on to describe the components in greater detail.

Tx RF field strength B_1

The required B_1 field depends on the flip angle and (effective) pulse duration. In the case of MR imaging pulse sequences, almost every RF pulse is selective (i.e. it has a limited bandwidth). Starting with a slice selection gradient of 20 mT/m, a slice thickness of 1 mm will result in a pulse bandwidth of $\Delta\omega_z/2\pi = 852$ Hz. The main peak of such a pulse will have a duration (the effective pulse length) of $2\pi/\Delta\omega_z \approx 1.2$ ms.

Some degree of flexibility in pulse sequence design can be achieved if one has the capacity to generate a 180° pulse in 0.5 ms. This means that the Tx system (Tx coil and RF power amplifier) should be able to generate a rotating (circularly polarized) B_1 field of 23.6 μT.

The question arises in this context as to how much RF power is necessary to achieve this B_1 amplitude. While an answer could be obtained by modeling the RF losses in a human body, it would be easier to simply conduct experiments on prototype coils or resonators. A range of 10 to 15 kW would represent a reasonable quantification for a 63 MHz whole-body Tx resonator. It warrants bearing in mind that the RF losses go with the square of the Larmor frequency. It follows that 3 T systems would essentially need 4 times more RF power than 1.5 T systems, with the precise amount of power necessary depending on patient size, position and fat-to-muscle ratio. An adjustment procedure is thus needed to determine the RF power per B_1^2.

Another issue is the heating of the patient by the applied RF power. While it might be desirable to increase imaging speed via shorter RF pulses requiring stronger B_1 fields, the limits that have been established for RF deposition are reached rapidly.

In summary, it does not make much sense to require shorter RF pulses than can be delivered by a 10 to 20 kW transmitter. Doing so would only result in higher costs (not only because of the RF power amplifier, but also because the whole Tx system would have to be high voltage proof) without leading to any practicable performance gains.

B_1 uniformity

The RF field generated should naturally be as homogeneous as possible over the MR system's applicable volume to enable uniform excitation and a uniform signal response from the measured object (i.e. the patient). Although it is possible to design resonators with a vacuum space RF homogeneity of better than 20%, the object (patient) itself will, as mentioned above, distort the RF field at high MR frequencies (≥ 40 MHz). Fig. 15.4 above shows this effect on the basis of an MR pulse sequence that displays the flip angle as a color scale a) for 1.5 T (63 MHz) and b) for 3 T (123 MHz). As one can see, the flip angle varies at 3 T by more than 100% across the object despite the fact that the resonator itself exhibits a homogeneity of approx. 20%. It is difficult to compensate for this physical effect.

Coil Q and coil filling factor

As has been discussed in chapter 7, Rx coils and Tx coils and resonators should exhibit a high unloaded Q factor in order to ensure a minimization of the coil losses that contribute to noise in the received MR signal and additional RF power dissipation during excitation. However, optimization will be required only to the extent that the coil losses are significantly lower than the patient losses.

For the same reason, the filling factor should be as high as possible for Rx coils. This requirement has led to the availability of a variety of special local coils that have been optimized for the various specific regions of the patient's body.

Dynamics and noise figure

MR scanners should ideally be outfitted with receivers (multiple receivers to support array coils) that exhibit a very low overall noise figure so as not to contribute to the image noise (which is then predominated by patient-generated noise).

The receiver's required dynamic range may well exceed 100 dB, especially in the case of high field 3D scanning where large object volumes are excited. If the Rx system is not capable of handling this, artifacts may occur due to signal compression or clipping and signal-to-noise degradation may result as the noise becomes predominated by preamp noise or ADC digitization.

RF system stability and reproducibility

Short-term phase stability (i.e. statistical variation over the acquisition time of one image) is of utmost importance. It will be necessary to adhere to even higher specifications than those described in section 15.1.2.1 to avoid phase-encoding artifacts. The overall phase instability for the complete RF system must remain below 0.5°.

With respect to amplitude (amplifier gain) stability, an overall short-term reproducibility of 2% appears to be sufficient to avoid the same kind of phase-encoding artifacts. However, higher demands apply to more sophisticated MR imaging applications, e.g. fMRI (functional MRI) and DTI (diffusion tensor imaging). Here, long-term reproducibility of better than 0.5 to 1% is required.

15.1.4.2 Overview of the radio frequency (RF) system

An MR system's RF system is comprised of three major blocks: the transmit path, the antennas and the receive path. Fig. 15.13 offers an overview of the components. The synthesizer, generating the local oscillator frequencies, and the transmit/receive (T/R) switches represent the internal interfaces of the three major RF blocks.

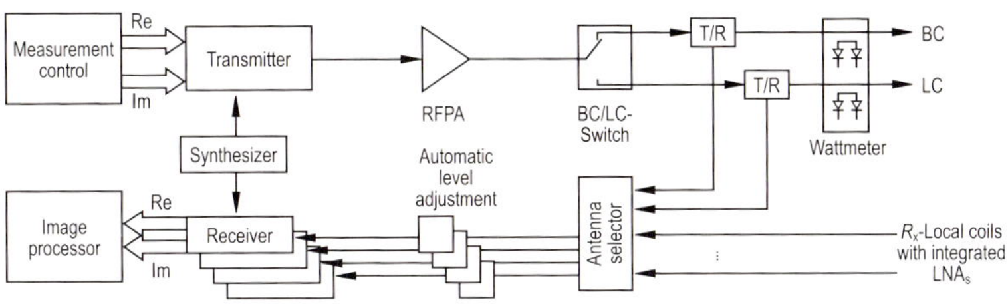

Figure 15.13 Block diagram of the RF system of an MR system

15.1.4.3 Transmit path

Overview and tasks

The RF transmit (Tx) path delivers amplitude and phase-controlled RF pulses to one or more transmit antennas. Its major components, the small signal transmitter and the RF power amplifier (RFPA), are described below. As can be seen in fig. 15.13, a body-coil/local-coil switch distributes the output power to the antenna and an RF power level meter (watt meter) monitors the delivered RF power.

Transmitter

The RF small-signal transmitter provides full amplitude and phase control for the applied RF pulses. The measurement control system (MC) usually describes the complex rotating baseband signal $F(t)$ via its in-phase $A(t)$ and quadrature $B(t)$ components as two digital series with a certain time step T. A single sideband modulation with an in-phase and quadrature phase local oscillator (LO) of frequency ω_0 yields the desired RF transmitter signal:

$$u(t) = A(t)\cos\omega_0 t + B(t)\sin\omega_0 t \tag{15.14}$$

The imaging slice may be shifted by either varying the LO or the baseband frequency.

This modulation is technically implemented in the form of a multi-stage processing consisting of digital and analog components. The details of the processing stages are similar to those of the RF receiver described below.

Dynamic range

In-pulse dynamic range (*DR*) is limited by the digital-to-analog converter (DAC) dynamic, which can be expressed as

$$DR_{\mathrm{dB}}^{\mathrm{DAC}} = (6n + 1.8)\mathrm{dB} \tag{15.15}$$

where n is the number of effective bits. Additional gain control elements are used to expand the pulse-to-pulse dynamic. These gain elements are adjusted automatically by the MC.

Radio frequency power amplifier (RFPA)

The maximum power required in an MR imaging experiment scales as

$$\hat{P} \propto \frac{\alpha^2 \omega_{\mathrm{r}}^2}{t_\alpha^2} \tag{15.16}$$

α: Flip angle, t_α: Pulse duration, ω_{L}: Larmor frequency

while the average power can be derived from the pulse-pause ratio. In the case of a gradient echo sequence

$$\bar{P} = \hat{P}\frac{t_\alpha}{T_{\mathrm{R}}} \approx (0.05\ldots0.1)\hat{P} \tag{15.17}$$

T_{R}: Pulse repetition time

RF pulses generated by the modulator must be amplified to kW power levels. This is performed by the RFPA, which consists of one or more RF driver stages, a power amplifier (PA) stage, a source of high voltage (power supply and capacitor bank) and a directional coupler for output power monitoring (fig. 15.14). The amplifier is required to provide additional range to also account for the following factors:

- The attenuation of transmit cables and T/R switches typically ranging from 0.5 to 1 dB
- *VSWR* (voltage standing wave ratio) derating of the RFPA. Due to the PA stage's maximum permissible voltage/current swing, the delivered peak power P_{d} is restricted to

$$P_{\mathrm{d}} = P_{\mathrm{forward}} - P_{\mathrm{reflected}} = \frac{\hat{P}}{VSWR} \tag{15.18}$$

Essentially, one will have to accommodate a *VSWR* of 1.5 (equivalent to a reflection coefficient of 20%).

Typical peak power values are given in table 15.2.

It is worth noting that the RFPA design does not need to account for continuous wave (CW) operation at these power levels. The design can take advantage of the fact that

Table 15.2 The RF power amplifier's peak power for protons at different main magnetic fields.

System field strength	0.2 T	1 T	1.5 T	3 T
RFPA peak power	2 kW	10 kW	15 kW	35 kW

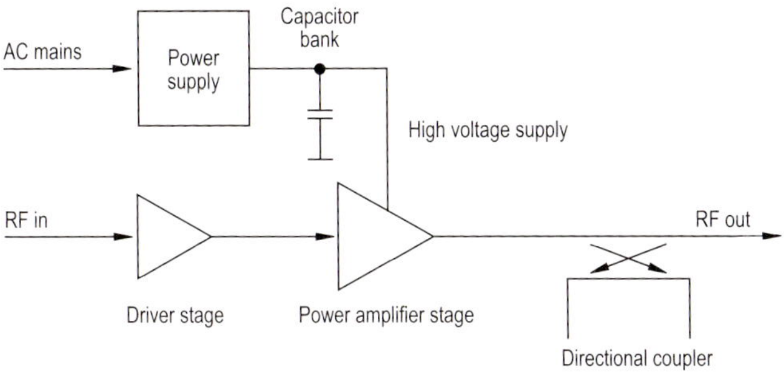

Figure 15.14 Block diagram of an MR's RF power amplifier (RFPA).

the required average power is considerably smaller. The energy for the RF pulses is delivered by a capacitor bank (fig. 15.14) that is recharged by the power supply during the pauses between pulses.

What follows is a list of the most important remaining requirements that the RFPA designer will have to consider:

- *Maximum pulse length and pulse droop*
  Both values are mainly controlled by the size of the capacitor bank.
- *Linearity*
  The implementation of cost and efficiency considerations will entail power amplifier stages that are characterized by poor linearity and that thus lead to RF pulse-shape distortion. The following measures are employed to overcome this problem: software predistortion within the MC, hardware predistortion within the RFPA driver and various feed-forward and feedback techniques borrowed from the field of telecommunications electronics.
- *Pulse reproducibility*
  Excellent pulse reproducibility is a prerequisite, especially for functional MR imaging. Pulse reproducibility can be degraded by various effects, including transistor and tube-parameter thermal drifting, microphony and interference. Microphony and interference can be avoided via an optimized mechanical design and an internal electromagnetic interference (EMI) concept. Thermal drift, which causes slow amplifier-gain variation, must be controlled via temperature sensing and compensation mechanisms.
- *Noise*
  The MR image's signal-to-noise ratio (*SNR*) should not be compromised by the noise of the blanked RFPA. This noise should thus remain at least 20 dB below thermal noise (–174 dBm/Hz). Since the isolation of the T/R switch is 30 dB, $P_N^{blanked} < -164$ dBm/Hz.
- *Spurious signals*
  It is important to make sure that coherent spurious signals do not cause artifacts in the MR image. Note that a Fourier transform of *N* samples will amplify the spectral

power of a coherent spur by a factor of N compared to incoherent noise. A 256×256 MR image with $B = 10$ kHz receive bandwidth will thus require spurious levels of less than $kTB/256^2$ or approx. −182 dBm.

The state-of-the-art RFPAs that are currently deployed in MR systems are either based on tube or solid-state technology, with a clear trend favoring solid-state technology on account of space and serviceability considerations. Both water and air cooling is possible. Most RFPAs operate in class AB, which combines the benefits of class A (linearity) and class B (efficiency) [15.5].

15.1.4.4 Receive path

Overview and tasks

The receive (Rx) path usually consists of signal conditioning electronics including low noise amplifiers (LNAs), antenna selectors and automatic level adjustment and several RF receivers. The MR signals received by a set of antennas are processed and delivered to the image processor as digital series of the in-phase and quadrature components $u_1(t)$ and $u_2(t)$ of the complex rotating frame signals. LNAs are mounted close to the T/R switches of the Tx/Rx coils or directly to the Rx coils in order to minimize the impact of cable losses on the overall noise figure. Automatic level adjustment may be used to further amplify the MR signals so as to adapt them to the receiver level range. Modern matrix coils may have considerably more Rx elements than RF receivers within the MR system. It is therefore necessary to use an antenna selector to connect subsets of Rx-coils to the available number of receivers. These subsets are defined by the patient table position and sequence requirements (e.g. parallel acquisition techniques).

Receiver

The receiver performs a quadrature demodulation by multiplying the MR signal $u(t) = A(t)\cos\omega_L t + B(t)\sin\omega_L t = \sqrt{A^2 + B^2}\cos\left(\omega_L t - \arctan\frac{B}{A}\right)$ by an in-phase LO signal $\cos\omega_0 t$ and a quadrature LO signal $\sin\omega_0 t$. This yields

$$\begin{aligned} u_1(t) &= u(t)\cos\omega_0 t \\ &= \frac{A(t)}{2}(\cos((\omega_L - \omega_0)t) + \cos((\omega_L + \omega_0)t)) \\ &+ \frac{B(t)}{2}(\sin((\omega_L - \omega_0)t) + \sin((\omega_L + \omega_0)t)) \end{aligned} \tag{15.19a}$$

and

$$\begin{aligned} u_2(t) &= u(t)\sin\omega_0 t \\ &= \frac{B(t)}{2}(\cos((\omega_L - \omega_0)t) - \cos((\omega_L + \omega_0)t)) \\ &+ \frac{A(t)}{2}(-\sin((\omega_L - \omega_0)t) + \sin((\omega_L - \omega_0)t)) \end{aligned} \tag{15.19b}$$

One can suppress the terms with $\omega_L + \omega_0$ using low pass filters (LPFs) so that $u_1(t)$ and $u_2(t)$ directly represent the in-phase and quadrature components of the nuclear mag-

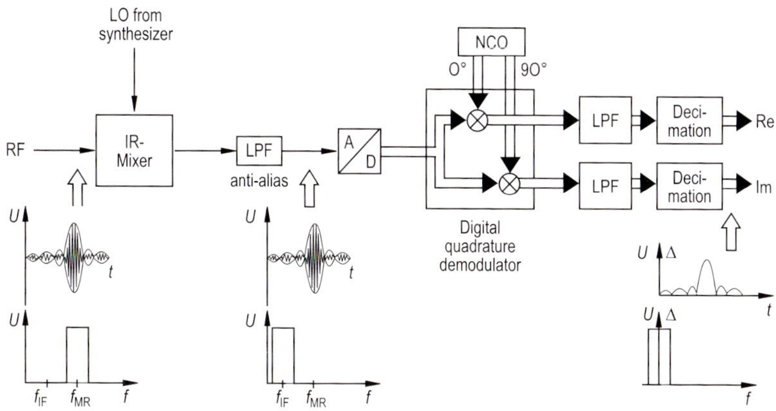

Figure 15.15 Block diagram of a state-of-the-art MRI receiver

netization precessing in a frame rotating with ω_0. These are fed as a digital time series into the image processor for image reconstruction.

Like the transmitter, modern receivers make use of a fully digital demodulator (fig. 15.15). The digitized signal $u(t)$ is simultaneously digitally multiplied by $\cos \omega_0 t$ and $\sin \omega_0 t$ series that are realized by a numerically controlled oscillator (NCO). This fully digital demodulator overcomes a number of problems associated with the previously used analog demodulator and baseband analog-to-digital converter such as ADC offset, low frequency noise and the balancing of the in-phase and quadrature output signals $A(t)$ and $B(t)$. The following digital LPF eliminates the $\omega_L + \omega_0$ components and avoids the aliasing of the noise in the decimation to the final sampling rate of the MR raw data used for image reconstruction.

Given that the clock rates of commercially available ADCs do not yet permit the direct conversion of the RF signals of high-field MR scanners, they are first mixed down from the Larmor frequency to an intermediate frequency (IF) ω_{IF} via analog image rejection (IR) mixer stages (fig. 15.15). The IF signal is then fed into the digital quadrature demodulator.

State-of-the-art MR scanners apply a large number of independent receiver channels (> 8) for imaging based on array coils. Array coils provide a superior signal-to-noise ratio and allow for parallel acquisition techniques (PAT) that shorten image acquisition time.

Dynamic range

The dynamic range (DR) of a signal is defined as the ratio of the maximum signal peak power P_S and the thermal noise kTB:

$$DR = \frac{P_S}{kTB} \tag{15.20a}$$

This ratio is often expressed on a logarithmic scale in decibels (dB):

$$DR_{\mathrm{dB}} = \left(10\lg\frac{P_s}{\mathrm{mW}} + 174 - 10\lg\frac{B}{\mathrm{mW}}\right)\mathrm{dB} \qquad (15.20b)$$

Given that thermal noise depends on bandwidth B and temperature T, it is necessary to specify these values whenever DR values are given. For instance, in the case of a local coil at 1.5 T, $P_S \triangleq -24$ dBm and $kTB \triangleq -174$ dBm where $B = 1$ Hz at $T = 300$ K (1 dBm $\triangleq$ 1 mW). This yields $DR_{\mathrm{dB}} = 150$ dB. However, a smaller dynamic range of 110 dB would be required at a bandwidth of $B = 10$ kHz.

The DR^{ADC} of the ADC is generally the limiting factor on the receive path. If one applies digital bandpass filtering [15.6], an n-bit ADC with sample rate f_s will cover a dynamic range of

$$DR_{\mathrm{dB}}^{\mathrm{ADC}} = \left(6n + 1.8 + 10\lg\left(\frac{f_s}{2B}\right)\right)\mathrm{dB} \qquad (15.21)$$

A modern 14-bit ADC with a sample rate of 10 MHz will thus allow for a dynamic range of 153 dB at a bandwidth of 1 Hz and 113 dB at a bandwidth of 10 kHz. Further DR expansion will require automatic level adjustment. The present MR signal level is matched to the maximum level of the ADC via additional switchable gain elements (attenuators). The SNR of small MR signals will thus not be affected by the limited dynamic range of the ADC. Modern MR systems will automatically adjust the MR signal level in accordance with one or more of the following three methods:

1. Gain is fixed for the entire image acquisition time. A forecast of the maximum signal level is made on the basis of the deployed coils, sequence, slice thickness and number of slices.
2. Gain is reduced for certain raw data lines. Usually, only a few k-space lines (within the center of k-space) have maximum level. All other lines can be collected with a higher gain level.
3. Gain is dynamically adjusted depending on the present MR signal level. This exploits the fact that only the center portion of the acquired k-space lines have the maximum level. Thus, only a very small percentage of the k-space values are affected by the limited ADC dynamic range. The dynamic switching may be based on a forecast or on a level-detection circuit.

15.1.4.5 Resonators and coils

Early MR systems made use of the same RF coil for receive and transmit operation. Today, the majority of MR applications involve the use of a volume transmit (body) coil to generate the exciting B_1 field and dedicated receive antennas to pick up the MR signals from the patient's body. Detune circuits in the individual coils suppress coupling to neighboring coils.

A homogeneous RF magnetic field transverse to the direction of the static magnetic field is necessary for the excitation of the spins [15.7-15.10]. The standard structure for the generation of this RF magnetic field in solenoid magnets is the birdcage antenna (fig. 15.16).

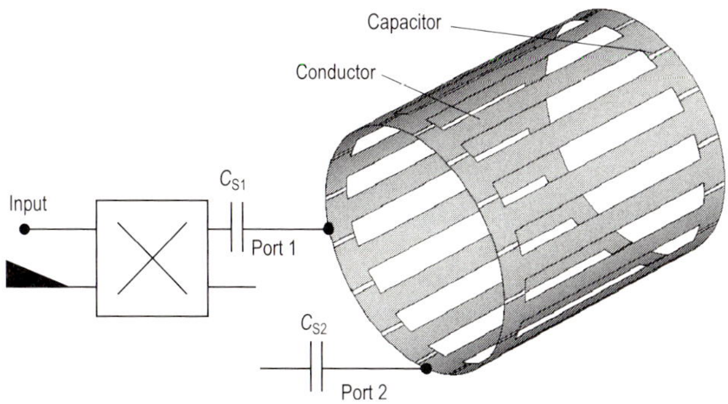

Figure 15.16 The birdcage antenna and a typical feed circuit

The birdcage antenna typically consists of $N = 16$ rods or rungs, connected by end rings. Capacitors in the end rings and/or in the rungs tune the antenna to the operating frequency. PIN diodes in the rungs or end rings acting as DC-controlled RF switches are used as detune elements (not shown in fig. 15.16).

The birdcage is the discrete approximation of an ideal current density distribution that yields a homogeneous transverse magnetic field (fig. 15.17). One-port excitation will yield a sinusoidal rod current distribution and a linear polarized magnetic field. Two signals with a 90° phase difference fed to two orthogonal antenna feed ports will deliver a homogeneous amplitude and a phase increment of $2\pi/N$ for the rod currents, resulting in a circular polarized RF magnetic field.

The transverse dimensions of the body resonator are mainly dictated by the space required for the patient, the safety distance between the patient and the electrical parts of the body coil and the necessary room for the magnetic field reflux. The length of the

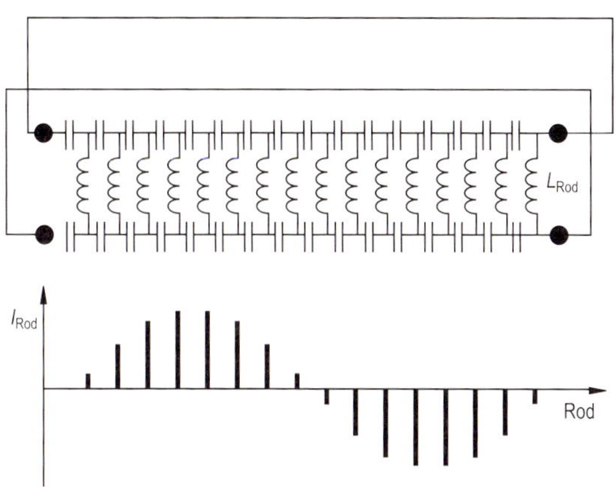

Figure 15.17 Equivalent electrical circuit and current distribution in the birdcage antenna

body coil amounts to a compromise between minimum exposed patient volume and sufficient homogeneity for the exciting magnetic field.

The different sizes, weights and positions of the patients inside the body coil result in varying impedances at the feed ports. In the past, the body coil was matched and tuned to every change in coil loading. The current state of the art is a so-called no-tune system. The matching capacitors C_{s1} and C_{s2} at the body coil feed ports are adjusted once to deliver an optimal match for the maximum patient load and are not changed in response to different load conditions. In the case of light coil loads, a non-negligible fraction of the RF power is reflected and absorbed in a dummy load via the hybrid. This sort of power loss can be tolerated in practice because light loads do not require full RF power and can even be used as a power-limiting safety mechanism.

An essential part of the body coil's RF function is handled by the so-called RF screen. This screen is glued or molded to the inner surface of the gradient coil. Typically formed by two slotted copper foils isolated by a thin low-loss dielectric layer, the screen performs a number of tasks:

- It prevents the coupling of the RF magnetic fields to the gradient coil windings and thus minimizes RF power losses.
- It suppresses residual RF noise emanating from the gradient coil.
- It establishes a well-defined RF environment for the body coil in order to ensure a homogeneous transmit field.

Given the space constraints in the magnet bore, the body coil is required to permit the integration of additional tasks, such as acting as a casing in the patient bore, carrying the patient table and dampening the noise generated by the vibrating gradient coil. Gradient-induced eddy currents in the metallic parts of the body coil can lead to imaging artifacts (ghosting) and generate additional noise. It is also indispensable that the whole-body coil (as is the case for all parts inside the gradient coil) is designed to minimize eddy currents.

A local transmit-receive coil represents the optimal choice for special applications such as head and extremity imaging and spectroscopy. Depending on the individual

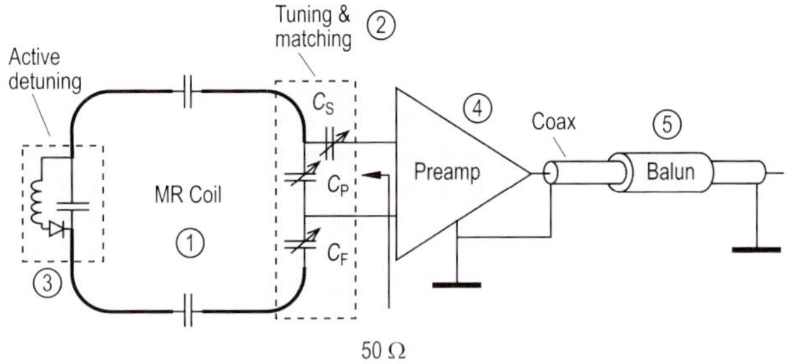

Figure 15.18 Typical components for a receive (RX)-only MRI coil

requirements involved, these coils may include components such as T/R switches, hybrids and preamplifiers. The transmit-receive coils also offer the advantages of reduced whole-body *SAR* values, increased excitation magnetic fields and the capacity for multi-nuclei spectroscopy.

While the main focus of design in the case of transmit antennas is homogeneity, receive antennas (also referred to as local coils) are optimized for high signal-to-noise ratio (*SNR*) within a certain region of interest (ROI) and typically do not offer homogeneous sensitivity.

A receive-only MR coil consists of the following components (fig. 15.18):

1. Antenna structure (size-optimized to extract maximum *SNR* from the ROI)
2. Tuning and matching network to minimize noise contributions from the preamplifier
3. Active detuning circuit to prohibit the flow of RF currents on the antenna during the transmit cycle
4. Low noise preamplifier
5. Shielded cable with one or more balun structures that minimize the flow of shield currents and thus prohibit the cable itself from acting as an antenna.

The achievable *SNR* is a function of receive coil geometry and the distance between the receive coil and the region of interest [15.11-15.15]. Under quasi-magnetostatic conditions, the signal from a pixel at position y on the main axis of a circular loop coil with radius r can be expressed as

$$s(y) \propto \frac{r^2}{(r^2 + y^2)^{3/2}}. \tag{15.22}$$

The average noise voltage picked up by the loop is also a function of the coil radius:

$$\bar{n} \propto r^{3/2} \tag{15.23}$$

For a given distance y_0 between the coil and the point of interest, the signal-to-noise ratio can be maximized by optimizing the coil radius to

$$r_{\text{opt}} = \frac{y_0}{\sqrt{5}}. \tag{15.24}$$

The signal received by a local coil is inherently weak on account of the nature of the MRI experiment. It is therefore important to minimize signal loss in the receive path. A very effective method of doing so involves the use of low-noise preamplifiers in immediate proximity to the coil terminals.

For optimum performance, it is necessary to transform the coil impedance Z_{Coil} to 50 Ω by means of a low loss matching network (i.e. to offer noise match at the input to the amplifier). With the same network, the amplifier input impedance Z_{Amp} is transformed to a quasi open circuit at the terminals of the antenna. This method, which reduces coil currents and unwanted coupling effects between neighboring antennas, is

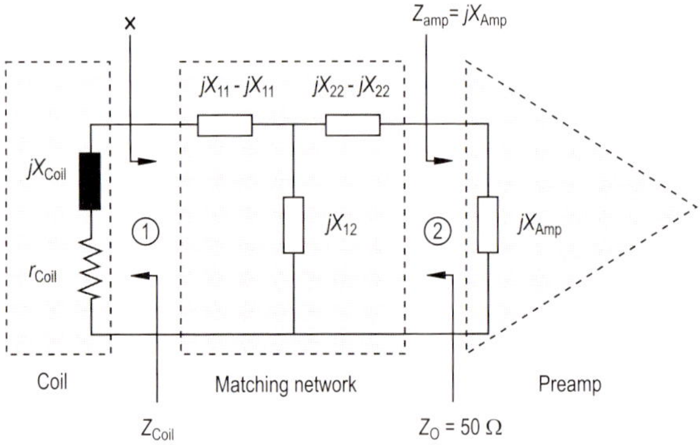

Figure 15.19 Matching network for receive (RX) coils

referred to as preamp decoupling or isolating preamp (fig. 15.19). The reactance values for the network are given by the following equations:

$$\begin{aligned} X_{11} &= -X_{\text{Amp}} \\ X_{22} &= -X_{\text{Amp}} \cdot \frac{r_{\text{Coil}}}{Z_0} - X_{\text{Coil}} \\ X_{12} &= \mp\sqrt{Z_0 \cdot r_{\text{Coil}} \cdot \left[1 + \left(\frac{X_{\text{Amp}}}{Z_0}\right)^2\right]} \end{aligned} \tag{15.25}$$

High Q capacitors represent a good choice for the components of the matching network. A well-matched, low-noise preamp has a typical noise figure of less than 0.5 dB, which is equivalent to 5% of additional noise added to the receive signal.

While the signal produced by the precessing spin sample amounts to a circular polarized (CP) high frequency magnetic field, a single antenna loop will pick up only one of this field's linear polarized (LP) components. The *SNR* of an ROI can be improved by up to a factor of $\sqrt{2}$ by detecting both of the field's LP components and combining them with an appropriate 90° phase shift.

The birdcage antenna has established itself as the CP antenna of choice for volume coils such as the whole-body resonator. A loop-antenna and butterfly combination is often used in the case of local coils to retrieve the full CP signal from an ROI. As shown in fig. 15.20, the loop picks up the B_1 field's vertical LP component and the butterfly detects the corresponding horizontal LP component. Both signals are independently matched to their own preamplifiers and then united using a 90° combiner.

Although they offer high *SNR*, surface coils are limited when it comes to their FOVs. However, this limitation can be overcome by deploying an array of several surface coil elements. The signals detected by the individual elements are not combined in the way that LP signals are combined to form CP signals. Instead, the signal detected by each coil element in the array is independently fed into a separate receiver channel and the final signal combination is performed on a pixel-by-pixel basis in the image

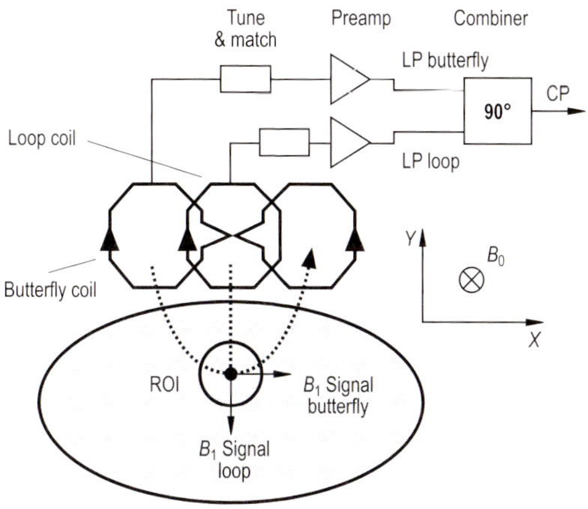

Figure 15.20 Loop/butterfly coil combination for circular polarized (CP) signal reception

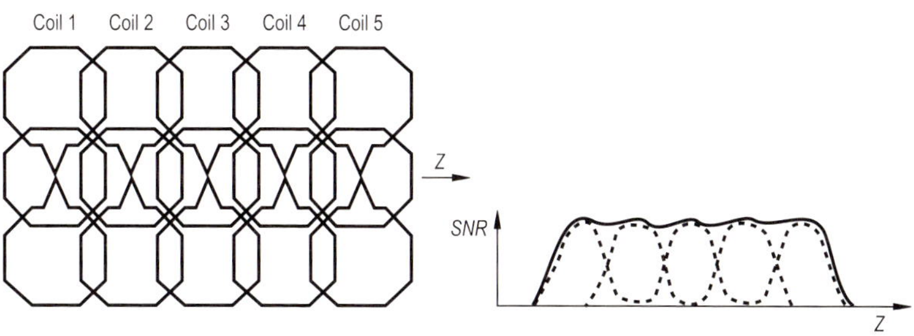

Figure 15.21 Enlarging the field of view (FOV) using array technology

domain. This approach ensures that the high *SNR* of each array element is preserved while exploiting the advantage that the array offers a much larger FOV (fig. 15.21).

Array imaging depends on a minimization of coupling and thus of the signal and noise correlation among the elements in the array. Array elements that are direct neighbors can be inductively decoupled by selecting the element overlap so as to ensure that the mutual inductance is cancelled and the total flux generated by coil 1 and induced into coil 2 is zero (fig. 15.22).

The mutual inductance of elements that are not direct neighbors (e.g. coil 1 and coil 3 in fig. 15.22) is usually fairly low and it is sufficient to reduce the coupling effect by

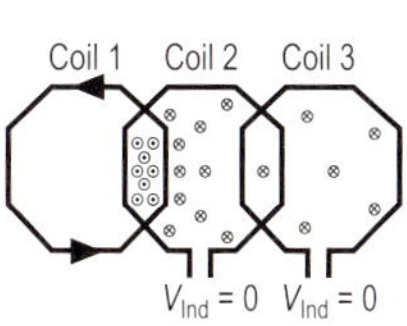

Figure 15.22 Decoupling of neighboring coils through overlap

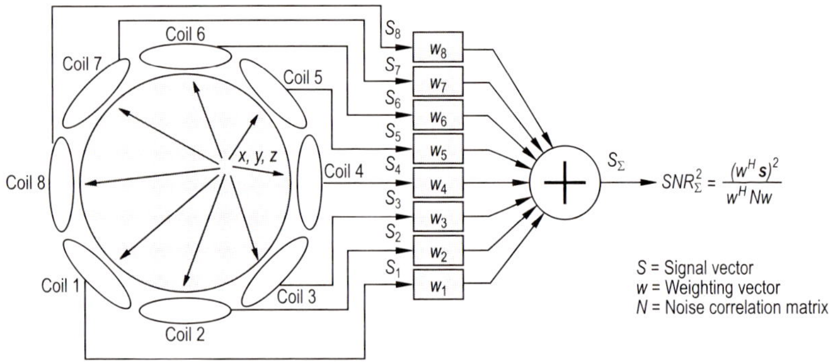

Figure 15.23 Weighted signal combination in a coil array for a pixel *x,y,z*

minimizing the current in the first coil via the isolating preamplifier method described above.

After simultaneously extracting the signals from all elements in the array, a combined image is formed by weighting and combining the individual images on a pixel-by-pixel basis (i.e. after individual image reconstructions). Fig. 15.23 shows the signal flow chart for the signal from a selected pixel *x,y,z* within an object surrounded by an 8-element coil array.

The pixel signals $s_i(x,y,z)$ from each single coil are weighted using a complex weighting factor $w_i(x,y,y)$ and then added up to form a combined signal

$$s_\Sigma(x,y,z) = \sum_i w_i(x,y,z)s_i(x,y,z) = \boldsymbol{w}^H\boldsymbol{s}, \tag{15.26}$$

where $\boldsymbol{w}^H$ is the conjugate transpose of the column vector $\boldsymbol{w}$ with values w_i and $\boldsymbol{s}$ is the vector of s_i. The weighting factors may be normalized to $\sum w_i = 1$. The noise power of coil *i* can be expressed as $\sum_j n_{ij}$ where n_{ii} is the noise power from coil *i* (in the absence of all others) and n_{ij} is the noise power added by coil *j*.

Having included n_{ij} in the noise correlation matrix N, one can express the squared combined signal-to-noise ratio $SNR_\Sigma^2\,(x,y,z)$ as

$$SNR_\Sigma^2(x,y,z) = \frac{(\boldsymbol{w}^H\boldsymbol{s})^2}{\boldsymbol{w}^H N\boldsymbol{w}} \tag{15.27a}$$

Differentiating the above equation with respect to the weighting factors and nullifying the result yields

$$\boldsymbol{w}^{\text{opt}} = cN^{-1}\boldsymbol{s}, \tag{15.28}$$

with c being a normalization factor.

It follows that the best possible $SNR_\Sigma^{\text{opt}}\,(x,y,z)$ is

$$SNR_{\Sigma\text{opt}}^2(x,y,z) = \boldsymbol{s}^H N^{-1}\boldsymbol{s}. \tag{15.27b}$$

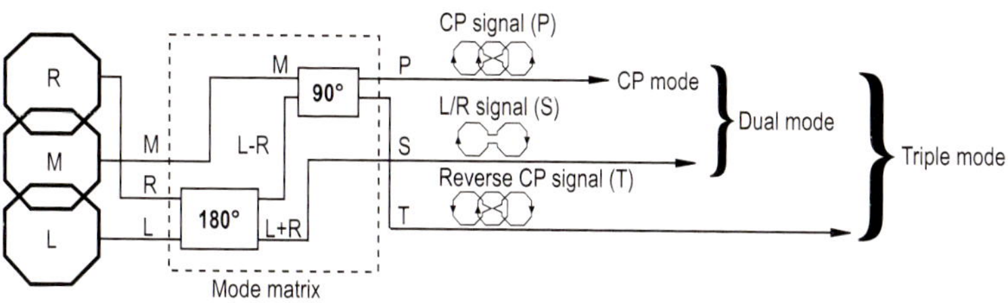

Figure 15.24 Mode matrix for a three-element coil cluster

The method described above requires information about the pixel signals $s_i(x,y,z)$. If one assumes sufficient *SNR* (≥ 10) in the uncombined images, the uncombined images themselves will represent a good estimate. Furthermore, if the noise correlation in the uncombined images is low (≤ 40%), the noise correlation matrix can be reduced to a matrix with zero non-diagonal elements, i.e. $n_{ij} = 0$. The *SNR* of the combined pixel signal can thus be expressed as follows:

$$SNR^2_{\Sigma opt}(x,y,z) = \sum_i \frac{s_i^2(x,y,z)}{n_{ii}} = \sum_i SNR_i^2(x,y,z) \tag{15.27c}$$

Thus, the sum-of-squares combination of the pixel signals from all coils yields an *SNR* that is larger or equal than that for each individual coil.

While array coils used to be designed using LP or CP coil elements, the most recent developments involve matrix coil arrays consisting of clusters of LP coil elements that are pre-combined to a set of mode signals. Fig. 15.24 shows an example of a cluster with three elements. The original signals *R*, *M*, *L* are fed into a so-called mode matrix and combined into three new signals *P*, *S*, *T*. Eq. (15.29) shows the corresponding mode matrix.

$$\begin{bmatrix} P \\ S \\ T \end{bmatrix} = \underbrace{\begin{bmatrix} \frac{1}{2} & -\frac{i}{\sqrt{2}} & -\frac{1}{2} \\ \frac{1}{\sqrt{2}} & 0 & \frac{1}{\sqrt{2}} \\ \frac{1}{2} & \frac{i}{\sqrt{2}} & -\frac{1}{2} \end{bmatrix}}_{\text{Mode Matrix}} \cdot \begin{bmatrix} R \\ M \\ L \end{bmatrix} \tag{15.29}$$

The primary signal *P* is equivalent to the CP signal of a loop-butterfly combination as shown in fig. 15.20. The two other signals contain array signal information from those imaging regions where the CP combination is not equal to the optimum array weighting.

The CP mode contains sufficient *SNR* to achieve high image quality in the case of non-parallel imaging applications. However, if parallel imaging techniques like SENSE, SMASH or GRAPPA are used (see section 15.2.2), the additional signals from dual or triple mode deliver the spatial information needed for this type of image reconstruc-

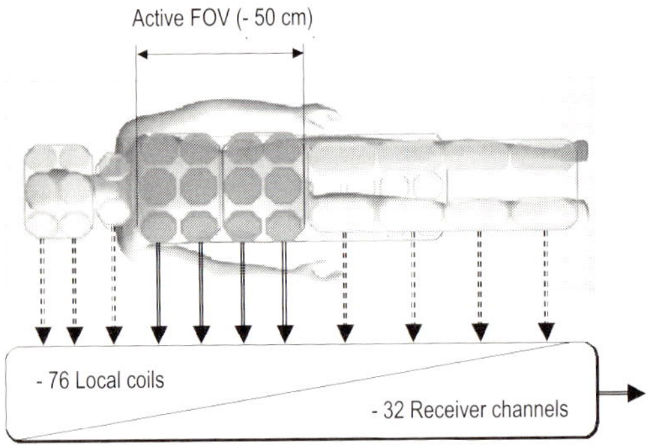

Figure 15.25 Total imaging matrix for whole-body scans

tion. Dual and triple mode signals can also be used for nonparallel imaging in order to improve *SNR* on the periphery of the images.

While the *SNR* for the combined array is the same when using all three mode signals *P, S, T,* as when using the original signals *R, M, L,* the new signals *P, S, T* offer the user greater flexibility given that each of the original signals covers only a part of the FOV while the mode signals cover the entire FOV. It is thus possible in the case of mode signals to scale the number of receiver channels between one and three, depending on the application.

Fig. 15.25 shows how matrix coils can be combined to form a total imaging matrix (Tim) for whole-body coverage. Up to 76 local coil elements can be connected to the

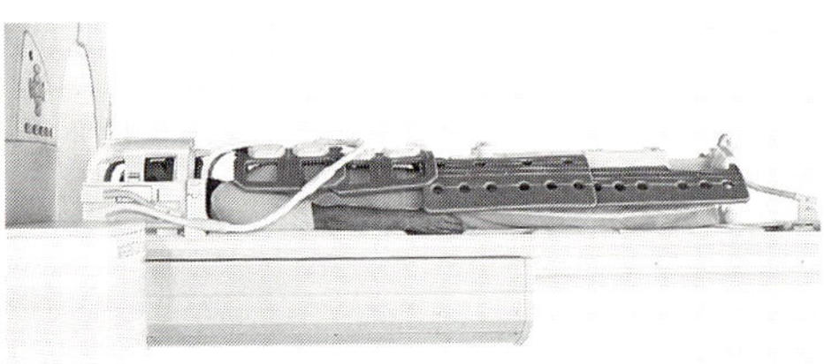

Figure 15.26 Patient setup for whole-body scan using matrix coils

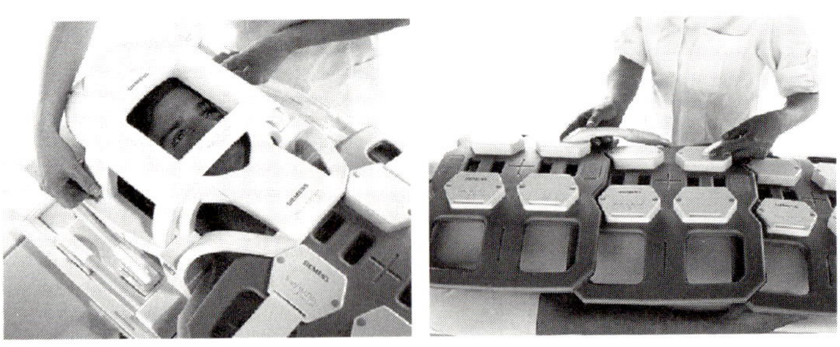

Figure 15.27 Details of patient setup for whole-body scan using matrix coils

system in this specific example. Of these 76 elements, a subgroup of up to 32 elements in the current FOV can be selected for image acquisition.

Figs. 15.26 and 15.27 show patient setups for whole-body imaging using a combination of matrix coils for the head, neck, torso, spine and extremities.

15.1.5 System control

Several processors are usually deployed to control the MR scanner and permit one to run the various system functions independently of one another. A common high speed data bus allows for the exchange of data and programs among the processors. Extensive software is needed to program these for their specific tasks.

Siemens Magnetom MR systems use a host computer with a basic Windows operating system and a basic *syngo* imaging platform. All of the other processors are provided with data (control parameters) and executables from the host computer. The host computer, with its display, keyboard and mouse, also serves as a user interface that allows the operator to administer patient data and image files.

Further processors control the measurement (i.e. the sequence of RF and gradient pulses and the analog-to-digital conversion of the MR signal) and the image reconstruction from the acquired data. The measurement requires high precision real-time operation (i.e. in the ns range). The image reconstruction (2D and 3D Fourier transform of a previous measurement) should proceed simultaneously to speed up the patient workflow. Given that measurements may last up to a few minutes, provision should also be made for the handling of parallel activities such as image viewing, post processing and archiving.

One can thus expect the requirements for computer speed and storage capacity to be relatively high. For example, the acquisition of a 3D FLASH sequence data set with a 256^2 pixel matrix and 128 partitions, a T_R of 5 ms and a 4-channel array receiver coil will result in a 134-Mbyte raw data file (4 bytes per complex data sample) that is to be handled in less than 3 minutes. The resulting image data add up to 16.7 Mbytes (after combination). The average data stream is approx. 1 Mbyte/s and the peak value may come above 10 Mbyte/s.

Clinical MR exams frequently result in more than 500 images per patient. Busy sites handle more than 30 patients per day. This means that several Gbyte of data (depending on the image resolution) may have to be handled, stored, and archived on a daily basis.

15.1.6 Image quality

15.1.6.1 System calibration

Although MR scanners are tuned and calibrated when they are installed and at regular servicing intervals, there is nevertheless a need for continuous fine adjustment on a patient-by-patient basis. This is due to the fact that each patient represents a unique imaging subject whose individual anatomy variously affects the radio frequency (RF) transmit and receive circuits as well as the homogeneity of the magnetic field. Once the scan table has been moved into the magnet, a number of preparatory steps (often referred to as prescan, adjustment or calibration) are carried out to determine and compensate for any patient-specific factors that would otherwise have an adverse effect on image quality. Depending on the scheduled examination and prescribed imaging techniques, this calibration procedure will comprise some or all of the following steps:

- Load matching for the RF transmit/receive coils
- RF transmit power calibration to achieve the desired flip (nutation) angles
- Restoring the magnetic field homogeneity via extra field gradient (shim) setting
- Matching the RF center frequency to the MR resonant frequency
- Adjusting the RF receive gain for optimum dynamic range performance
- Miscellaneous, i.e. application dependent (e.g. identifying local coils for parallel imaging)

Attention should be paid to the validation of the calibration results. While this may involve a whole-body examination, the specialized prescans are often related to the body region of interest, the patient table position, and the particular selection of local RF coils. This specificity can be taken into account whenever necessary by acquiring unique calibration data for each clinical series (i.e. rather more than once per examination). Given that previous adjustment results are identified and updated each time the scanner prepares for a new series, the prescan time may vary from one series to the next.

It is common practice to implement two alternative control modes: automatic and manual. Automatic mode corresponds to routine operating procedure and does not call for any user interaction. Manual mode typically features step-by-step processing and a comprehensive user interface that provides intermediate results and allows for a number of interventions on the part of the operator. Manual mode is sometimes used to optimize field homogeneity (shim) within delicate areas of the body that exhibit large local variations in magnetic susceptibility (e.g. the base of the brain and the heart).

Coil tuning

Although RF coils come in various designs, their circuit diagrams are always comprised of an effective resistance R, inductance L, and capacitance C (the damped resonant circuit) as well as a matching network connecting the coil to the transmission line. Transmit and receive efficiency depend on coil positions close to the patient's body. A human being represents a conductive and lossy medium in radio-technological terms. As a result of coil-patient interaction, the coil parameters R, L, and C undergo individual changes. The task of coil tuning is to compensate for these patient-related influences via the appropriate control of trim components integrated into the coil circuit. The objective here is to restore the resonance condition and to match the coil impedance to the impedance of the transmission line.

Recent developments include so-called no-tune coils that utilize a dedicated matching network and a fixed setting adapted to the average patient load. Such coils do not require individual tuning. They thus serve to reduce complexity and accelerate the overall calibration process.

Transmit-gain calibration

RF excitation pulses are deployed to generate the correct RF magnetic field B_1 and thereby bring about the desired flip angles. Although they pass identical unit currents through the coil, B_1 fields may differ significantly depending on the specific patient load and transmit coil arrangement. In order to ensure consistent flip angles, it is therefore necessary to subject the RF transmitter output level to individual calibration.

One widely accepted method that is fast, accurate and insensitive to patient motion involves the application of a sequence of three RF pulses of as yet unknown flip angles α, β, and γ. These RF pulses generate several (Hahn and stimulated) echoes, with each exhibiting a specific signal intensity dependence $I \sim f(\alpha,\beta,\gamma)$ on the flip angles. Expressions for the flip angles can be established by evaluating various combinations of these echo responses. In particular, certain echo intensity ratios are independent of the relaxation times T_1 and T_2 as well as the sequence timing parameters. This ensures clean results and the capacity to repeat the sequence quickly. This RF sequence is typically accompanied by field gradient pulses that limit the adjustment to a localized plane or volume of interest, thus taking care of the inhomogeneous B_1 field distribution in the transmit coil. The Fourier transform of the echo signal represents the spatial excitation profile whose central part alone is used for further evaluation. The beneficial side effect of this procedure is the elimination of disturbing signal contributions resulting from the decreasing flip angles towards the edges of the slice profile.

One particular version of the method involves confining the three RF pulses to the flip angle scheme $\alpha/2 - \alpha - \alpha/2$ and evaluating only two echoes as a sufficient condition for determining the single unknown α. Eligible candidates include the first Hahn echo of intensity $I_H \sim \sin^3(\alpha/2)$ and the stimulated echo of intensity $I_S \sim (1/2)\sin(\alpha)\sin^2(\alpha/2)$. The resulting simple expression for the flip angle $\alpha = 2\arccos(I_S/I_H)$ will provide unambiguous figures across the 0° to 360° range. The sequence may be repeated several times if the initial a varies significantly from the desired value (e.g. 180°). In any case, the calibration procedure will take only a few seconds.

Shimming procedure

Placing a subject in the magnet will affect the homogeneity of the magnetic field on account of the differing magnetic susceptibilities of air, water, tissue, bone, etc. The MR scanner is equipped with adjustable extra field gradients (shims) with field shapes that nominally form an orthogonal basis set of spherical harmonics for the sake of restoring some degree of the initial high homogeneity. First-order terms x, y, z are generated via static offset currents in the pulsing gradient system. Optional high-order shims typically include the second-order terms xy, xz, yz, x^2-y^2, z^2 and require additional resistive field coils and controllable current supplies. The objective of shimming is to adjust the strength of the shims (i.e. currents through the shim coils) to optimize the field homogeneity within the body region of interest.

The type of measurement that is required for shimming is similar in terms of spatial encoding to common imaging measurements. The necessary information about the local magnetic field is taken from the phase evolution φ of gradient-recalled echoes. To eliminate phase interferences originating from other sources, two consecutive echoes with different echo times TE_1 and TE_2 are acquired and the phase difference $\Delta\varphi = \gamma B_0(x,y,z)(TE_2 - TE_1)$ alone is used to determine the spatial field distribution $B(x,y,z)$. The phenomenon of *phase wrapping* demands careful attention and, depending on the extent of the field inhomogeneity, may impose restrictions on sequence timing parameters, spatial resolution and data interpretation. A further constraint emerges in connection with simultaneous fat and water signal contributions that exhibit slightly different resonant frequencies (chemical shift $\delta \sim 3.4$ ppm). A proven remedy for this constraint involves confining the echo times TE_n to the *fat-water-in-phase* condition $\gamma\delta B_0 TE_n = 2\pi n$, resulting, for instance, in $TE_1 = 4.6$ ms and $TE_2 = 9.2$ ms at $B_0 = 1.5$ T. Once the field map data are available, one can arrive at a best fit for the field shapes that are to be shimmed, for instance, by deploying a least-squares metric. This yields the specific correction amount that is to be added to the present shim setting. The objective is to converge on a stable optimum in a single iteration. Volume-selective shimming confines the evaluated field map data accordingly. This permits one to accept a suboptimal shim at all locations except in the volume of interest and gives one an opportunity to improve quality within the volume.

Depending on the prescribed MR techniques, shimming may have little impact, or it may improve image quality significantly. Beneficial effects have been particularly evident in cases involving ambitious applications such as fat suppression, echo-planar imaging and spectroscopy.

Center frequency setting

Both the patient's magnetic susceptibility and the fine tuning of the shim setting change the effective field strength and hence the MR resonant frequency. The necessary matching of the RF center frequency is based on the Fourier analysis of MR signals acquired without simultaneous gradient pulsing and is required to reach an accuracy of a few Hertz. The resulting spectrum is typically dominated by the fat and water lines. An automated peak-fitting routine is used to identify the reference (e.g. water) resonance. This calibration will clearly determine the quality of any subsequent spectral saturation/excitation technique. The obligatory localization may be incorporated into the MR signal excitation procedure, consisting, for instance, of three selective RF pulses (i.e. one in each of the three spatial orientations). The resulting stimulated echo emerges from the intersection of the three planes, the volume of interest. A single excitation is sufficient and takes less than a second.

Receive-gain calibration

It is necessary to take two concomitant factors into account: the receive gain should be set as high as possible to optimize signal-to-noise performance without causing the as yet unknown maximum MR signal to exceed the distortion limit of any receiver component. The optimal gain setting has traditionally been determined by prescanning each clinical series and identifying the maximum recording level. This time consuming procedure has been made unnecessary by today's state-of-the-art scanners that are equipped with digital receiver systems whose dynamic ranges (in excess of 130 dB) allow for default gain setting that is free of adverse effects.

Miscellaneous

Further calibration procedures tend to be associated with very specific MR techniques. Their lack of generality places them beyond the scope of this chapter. For instance, in the case of parallel imaging, the different sensitivity profiles of the local receive coils are used to supplement the gradient encoding steps in order to reduce scan time. The required sensitivity maps may be derived from rapidly acquired low-resolution prescan images that also provide information about the spatial coil positions, and thereby offer assistance when it comes to the task of configuring the parallel imaging application. If the prescan is extended in a manner that leads to the acquisition of both local-coil and body-coil images, the pixel-intensity ratios will provide further helpful information that can be used to filter (brightness smoothing) the local coil images.

15.1.6.2 Image quality properties

The quality of an imaging system can be very generally described in terms of the following properties:

1. Spatial resolution (i.e. the ability to display two tiny individual objects separately in an image)
2. Contrast resolution (i.e. the ability to make an object visible despite the fact that there is only a minimal signal difference between the object and its background)
3. Image fidelity (i.e. the ability to display an object without spatial distortion and with uniform intensity when it is homogeneous)
4. Absence of artifacts (i.e. the absence of objects in an image that do not exist in reality)

Spatial resolution

As discussed in section 7.3.2, spatial resolution is determined by the pixel size

$$\Delta x = \frac{\pi}{\gamma G_x T_x} \tag{15.30}$$

as long as the read-out time T_x is shorter than any signal decay due to T_2 (or T_2^*) or diffusion in the read-out gradient G_x. The signal decay acts as a weighting factor on the MR signal in the time domain, which corresponds to the image's spatial frequency spectrum. In the case of more sophisticated sequences such as turbo-spin-echo and EPI, it is necessary to extend this consideration to the phase encoding process as well (i.e. one is required to compare the signal decay time constants to the total read-out

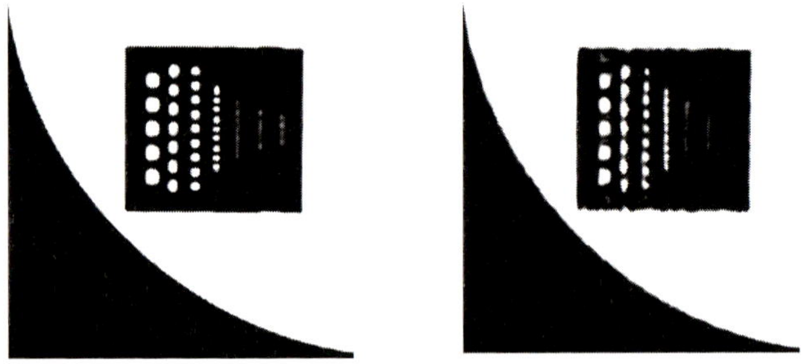

Figure 15.28
Degradation of spatial resolution due to poor eddy current compensation (resolution test object measured using a turbo-spin-echo sequence). **a)** Perfectly adjusted eddy current compensation, **b)** Maladjusted (3%) eddy current compensation (time constant 12.4 ms).

duration after each excitation pulse). This corresponds to the total acquisition time in single shot sequences like EPI or HASTE.

Theoretically, one can deliberately reduce the pixel size by extending T_x or increasing G_x. The physically feasible limit of resolution is reached when the T_2 of the object becomes comparable to T_x or (supposing one keeps T_x short enough and increases G_x) when the signal decay due to diffusion in G_x becomes significant. T_2 and diffusion are properties of the object that is to be imaged and show a positive correlation (i.e. a long T_2 normally goes together with a high diffusion coefficient). The physical resolution limit of MRI can thus be estimated to be a few μm. However, this does not appear to be significant in clinical practice because even an immobilized patient will move by a larger order of magnitude during data acquisition.

Technical deficiencies may also have an impact on the spatial resolution of an MR system. For instance, inadequate compensation for eddy current fields can cause a loss of spatial resolution (image blurring), especially when the time constants are comparable to the read-out time T_x (fig. 15.28).

Contrast resolution

The ability of an MR imager to resolve (i.e. make visible) objects despite the fact that there is only a slight signal difference (i.e. contrast) between the objects and their backgrounds is directly related to the signal-to-noise ratio. It is safe to assume that it will be difficult to discern an object if its contrast is close to the image noise level. However, the detectability of a low-contrast object also depends on its size (see chapter 2). The larger the object is, the easier it will be to detect it, even if the contrast to its surrounding is below the pixel noise level. The reason for this is that the human visual sensing system performs a degree of averaging over the area of the object's image. Given that MR permits one to adjust the size of the object in the image and the image intensity with the gradient, it will be important to determine the best parameters for imaging an object of diameter A and nuclear magnetization M_0:

If we assume

$$S_{\min} D_{\min} \propto S_{\text{Noise}} \,, \tag{15.31}$$

then the minimum recognizable signal intensity $S_{\min}$ can be expressed as

$$S_{\min} \propto M_0 \Delta x \Delta y N_y \tag{15.32}$$

N_y: Number of acquisitions (e.g. phase encoding steps)

and the minimum recognizable diameter $D_{\min}$ (measured in pixels) can be expressed as

$$D_{\min} = \frac{A_{\min}}{\Delta x} \,. \tag{15.33}$$

If we assume that $\Delta x = \Delta y$ and also take into account that the noise in the image can be expressed as

$$S_{\text{Noise}} \propto \sqrt{\frac{N_y}{T_x}} \,, \tag{15.34}$$

then the minimum recognizable physical diameter (e.g. measured in mm) of a low contrast detail $A_{\min}$ will amount to

$$A_{\min} \propto \frac{1}{M_0} \frac{1}{\sqrt{N_y T_x}} \frac{1}{\Delta x} \tag{15.35a}$$

or

$$A_{\min} \propto \frac{1}{M_0} \sqrt{\frac{T_x}{N_y}} G \,. \tag{15.35b}$$

This leads to the astonishing conclusion that increasing the spatial resolution in MRI (increased gradient, decreased pixel size) will make it necessary to introduce a larger diameter $A_{\min}$ for the sake of discerning low contrast details (fig. 15.29).

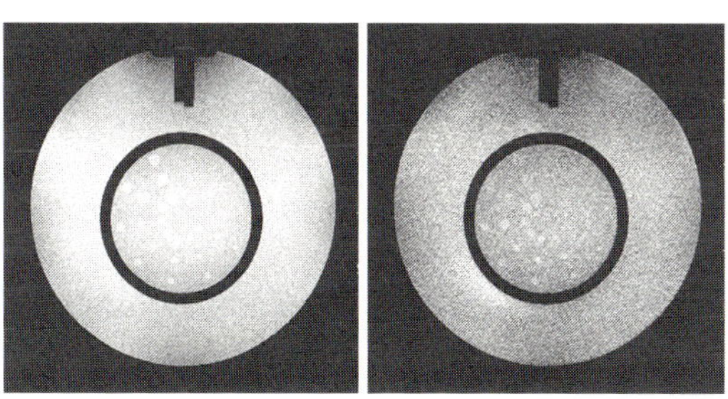

Figure 15.29
The low contrast test object containing various spokes of low contrast spots demonstrates that the MRI contrast resolution declines as the spatial resolution increases (provided all other sequence parameters remain unchanged). **a)** Pixel size 1×1 mm^2; **b)** Pixel size 0.5×0.5 mm^2 (fewer spokes are visible).

Spatial distortion

Spatial distortion can be defined as the deviation between the location of an object detail as shown in the image and in reality. Distortions are generally not restricted to the 2D image plane, but can also occur perpendicular to the selected slice (potato chip distortion). Distortion can thus be described as a 3D vector that is itself a function of the three spatial coordinates. A Cartesian and a polar coordinate system would both be appropriate for quantifying distortion.

As outlined in the previous sections, the location of an MRI pixel is encoded by the magnetic field (main magnet and gradients) present during excitation, phase-encoding and signal acquisition. Spatial distortions are inevitable in MR imaging because it is not possible to make the homogeneity of the main magnet field and the linearity of the gradients ideal. Unless the main field remains unchanged locally on account of the magnetic properties (susceptibility) of the measured object itself, the spatial distortions will be negligible close to the center of the imaging volume and increase to a few % in proportion to the distance from the center depending on the design of the gradient coil and the ratio of the local pixel bandwidth to the field deviation. As shown in fig. 15.30, such design data can be used to conveniently correct in-plane distortions.

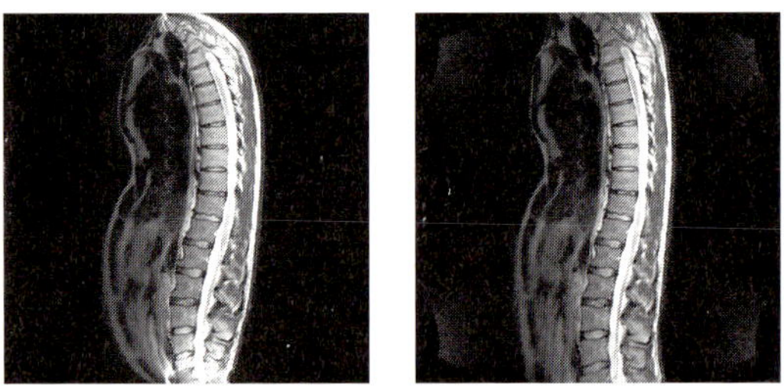

Figure 15.30
Image of a volunteer demonstrating the effect of correcting spatial distortions due to gradient nonlinearity in a field of view of 5000 mm × 5000 mm: **a)** Without correction; **b)** With distortion correction based on the gradient design specification.

Image uniformity

One might expect all of the pixels in an image of a uniform object (e.g. a cylinder filled with water) to show the same signal, as long as the following prerequisites for a uniform MR image are fulfilled: the RF transmit field B_1 that excites the nuclear magnetization is homogeneous within the object and the sensitivity of the receiving coil that picks up the MR signal is spatially uniform. However, as already mentioned, this can hardly be achieved. Nonuniformity can be removed to a certain extent. Given that the B_1 field map of the RF coils is not sufficient because the measured object itself distorts the RF field, correction algorithms are frequently based on data from the imaged objects. This is clearly no remedy for nonuniformity in the MR relaxation contrast that arises on account of the nonlinearity of the Bloch equations describing the MR excitation.

15.1.6.3 Objective methods of determining MR image quality

While at least one objective method is available for measuring each of the image quality characteristics described in the previous section, it is less clear which of the numerous pulse sequence types and parameters (that come with state-of-the-art MR systems) should be selected for the sake of measuring image quality. A degree of standardization would be desirable in this area, but is difficult to achieve because of the many options and their associated advantages and disadvantages. Although the IEC established a task force to find a solution in February of 2002, it is doubtful that any standards will have been finalized [15.16] by the date of this book's publication. This is a good indication of the complexity of the issue.

The question as to exactly what the objective of image quality measurement is supposed to be also warrants consideration. If it is meant to assess the systems of different manufacturers, it will be necessary to maintain commensurability by ensuring that all measurement details are comprehensively defined and uniformly applicable. This should not only include obvious parameters such as sequence type and timing, phantom properties, etc., but also potentially hidden parameters such as bandwidth per pixel and image processing (e.g. nonlinear filtering). The person or institution doing the assessing may have difficulties gaining full control of all of the necessary test conditions. The task would be easier if the purpose were to demonstrate the fulfillment of specifications as defined by the manufacturer (and sometimes explicitly required by the customer). Such acceptance testing may represent a baseline for periodic quality assurance (QA) tests to make sure that the system continues to perform as specified. In order to increase efficiency, such QA testing could be made fully automatic (except for the placing of a test object in the bore) and could be restricted to properties that are not inherent to the system's design (such as spatial resolution and spatial distortion), but might deteriorate slowly and less obviously (e.g. signal-to-noise ratio). In what follows, we offer a number of examples of how to measure image quality parameters.

Measurement of spatial resolution

The most comprehensive and quantitative method of assessing spatial resolution would be to calculate the modulation transfer function (*MTF*) from the point spread function (*PSF*) or the edge response function, which is the spatial integral of the *PSF*. The *MTF* is the Fourier transform of the *PSF*. It is difficult in MRI to record a reasonable image of a needle-like object because contrast is poor in the case of objects that are much thinner than a single pixel. The *MTF* is therefore derived from an edge phantom image (fig. 15.31). Another difficulty associated with this method involves the flipping of the negative lobes of the Gibbs ringing in the signal void area of the edge image to positive values because MRI images are modulus images. This may generate artifacts in the *MTF* diagram.

Other popular methods are semiquantitative and require the visual inspection of object images, which contain regular patterns of various spatial frequencies such as a set of pinholes or bars of various sizes (gap and thickness, e.g. 3.0, 2.5, 2.0, 1.5, 1.0, 0.8,

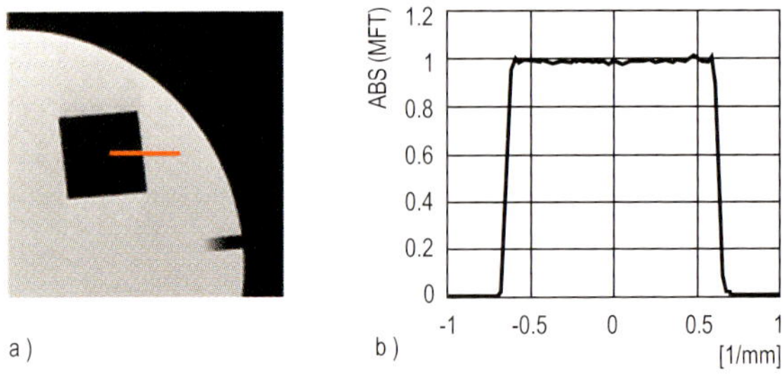

Figure 15.31
a) Image of an edge phantom; **b)** Modulation transfer function (*MTF*) derived from the edge image

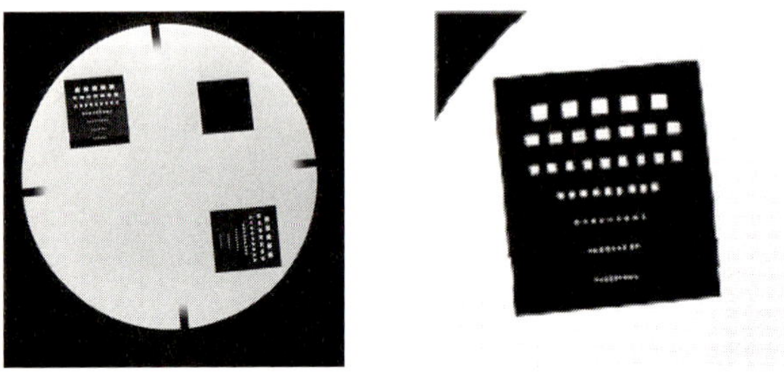

Figure 15.32
MR image of a resolution test object containing rows of pinholes (opening of gap between holes: 2.5, 2.0, 1.5, 1.0, 0.7, 0.5, 0.4 mm). The pixel size was 0.39 mm. As expected, the row with the 0.4 mm holes is still resolved.

0.5 mm). Fig. 15.32 offers an example. Spatial resolution is defined as the smallest detail that can be visually discerned. However, such methods are not suitable for automatic QA evaluation.

Measurement of signal-to-noise ratio

Measuring signal-to-noise ratio may appear to be a trivial matter. One needs only to acquire an image of a uniform object such as a sphere or a cylinder filled with water and then take the mean value (for the signal) and the standard deviation (for the noise) over a region (ROI) within the image of the phantom. However, it will be necessary to take into account that an MR image of such an object will never be perfectly uniform, and if it is corrected for uniform appearance, then the noise will vary along with the location. One approach to getting rid of this difficulty [15.17] involves acquiring two consecutive images under identical conditions, and then taking the mean value from the ROI of one image and the standard deviation of the difference of both images divided by $\sqrt{2}$.

Another option is to take the standard deviation of the MRI background. However, the background noise has a Rayleigh and not a Gaussian distribution because a negative pixel signal is flipped to positive. It is therefore necessary to divide the S/N result by $\sqrt{2-\pi/2}$ to obtain the same value obtained using the method described above.

Irrespective of the particular method used, it is important to be careful about the measurement conditions, including the phantom's properties (e.g. T_1 and T_2), the sequence type and timing, the absence of artifacts in the evaluation ROI and/or the signal de-rating at the image margins due to analogue filters in the receive path.

Measurement of spatial distortion

One will need to image a regular object to measure spatial distortion. A sphere or cylinder will suffice if no more than radial distortions are of interest. Given that the distortions increase or decrease in proportion to the distance from the magnet's center, the phantom will have to be of a reasonable size to obtain meaningful results. 2D and 3D measurements require regular 2D and 3D grids or pinhole phantoms as shown in fig. 15.33a. An evaluation SW recognizes the pinholes (or grid crossings) and compares their positions to those of a perfectly regular grid as shown in fig. 15.33b. The deviation is often given in distance units (mm) in x, y direction of the image plane or in % relative to the distance of the grid point to the image center.

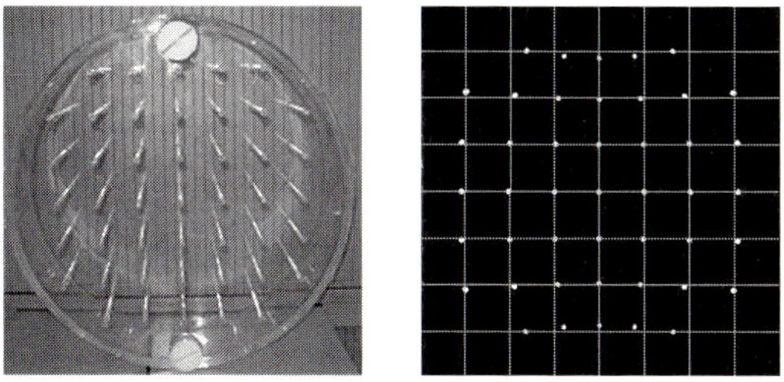

Figure 15.33
Determination of spatial distortion: A regular grid is overlaid by an image of the test object with a regular pattern of pinholes. The distance between the grid lines is derived from a central set of pinholes that are hardly distorted. The distance between the crossings of the gridlines and the corresponding pinhole is a measure of distortion at that location.

Measurement of image uniformity

One may dispute the importance of image uniformity because it is not determined by the characteristics of the RF coils alone, but is also a matter of the imaging object. Indeed, many applications involve the use of local receive coils that trade uniformity for contrast resolution. Nevertheless, audits and acceptance testing still require a uniformity measurement. The most popular method [15.18] is to image a homogeneous object such as a cylinder or sphere filled with doped water (less suitable for very high field strength) or oil, search the image for the minimum (S_{min}) and maximum (S_{max}) signal and then run the following calculation: $(S_{max} - S_{min})/(S_{max} + S_{min})$. One can avoid mistaking noise spikes for the S_{max} or S_{min} in this context by selecting appropriate measurement parameters or applying a strong low pass filter to the image to achieve a sufficiently high *S/N*.

15.1.6.4 Artifacts

Given the many artifact types and the many reasons for their occurrence in MRI, a comprehensive treatment of this issue would go beyond the scope the present handbook [15.19]. We will therefore restrict our discussion to a description of the most important artifacts. The causes of artifacts include imperfections or defects in the imaging system, improper pulse sequence design, improper selection of measurement parameters and the (natural) inability of patients to keep their body (organs) sufficiently motionless during the data acquisition procedures.

Ghosting

The most frequently observed artifact is ghosting, i.e. more or less faint multiple overlaid images of the object extended in the phase encode direction. An example is shown in fig. 15.34a. This can occur with any kind of imaging sequence. Unfortunately, the ghosting phenomenon has many causes. The major cause involves the encoding of the 2nd (and 3rd) dimension in 2D (and 3D) Fourier imaging into the phase of the MR signal. It follows that even very tiny deviations in phase (a few degrees) and amplitude (a few %) will lead to inconsistencies in the acquired raw data and thus to ghosting as well. While instability in signal amplitude usually reveals a deficiency in the RF transmit or receive system, the root cause of phase deviations is field (main B_0, shim, or gradients) instability. The RF system is seldom the culprit. The movement of the measurement object in the imaging gradients is equivalent to field variation.

The first step in the procedure for identifying the reasons for ghosting is to rule out patient movement. This can be done by scanning a test object. If the ghosting vanishes, then the problem is the patient's inability to hold still and the remedy will center on the selection of suitable measurement protocols that, for instance, run faster or synchronize the scan to periodic physiological functions such as heart beat and breathing.

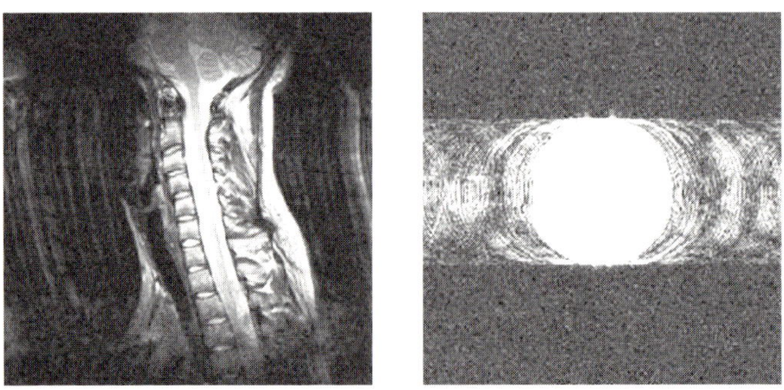

a) b)

Figure 15.34
a) MRI ghosts in a patient. Faint multiple duplicates of the spinal cord can be seen that result from the physiological pulsatile flow of the CSF inside the spinal canal. **b)** To exclude system instability as a cause of such artifacts one scans a uniform phantom. If ghost images appear as in the example, it will be necessary to inspect the system (or its environment) for sources of interference.

If ghosting appears in the phantom images (fig. 15.34b), then it will be necessary to examine the system components for malfunctioning. Various test procedures are available for this purpose. These procedures allow the service engineer to identify those system parts that have become defective. However, if one ascertains that the main field B_0 is unstable (after ruling out all other system components including the main RF system's synthesizer), it will be necessary to search the environment for sources of field variations such as moving ferromagnetic objects (e.g. clinic beds, cars, elevators, etc.) or for field-generating items such as electric power lines, transformers, electric trains, etc. Floor vibrations can also cause field instability. If the pre-installation site survey revealed no such problems, then one might begin by considering post-installation environmental changes.

So-called Nyquist ghosts represent a special case. This kind of artifact is shifted by exactly half of the image size due to a slight variation in the signal strength and phase of every other Fourier projection – an artifact that is very typical for EPI where every other line in *k*-space is acquired in the opposed direction. Any tiny off-resonance effect, asymmetry in the gradient power unit for positive and negative pulse lobes, etc. will cause this problem.

Wavelike patterns (spikes in raw data)

Wavelike patterns in images occur when the acquired raw data (the time domain signal) contain a few individual spikes. Such signal peaks normally result from electric discharges inside the RF cabin that are picked up by the receiver coil while data acquisition is in progress. While discharges may be caused by a person moving in plastic shoes on a non-conducting floor, they are usually caused by loose parts in the scanner (e.g. covers and electric connectors) that are shaken by gradient coil vibrations. The Fourier transform will spread out every single spike as a wave pattern across the entire MR image. The wavelength, amplitude, and direction depend on the distance of the spike from the *k*-space center ($k = 0$), its amplitude and its location in the raw data matrix. While many low amplitude spikes will lead to a noisy image, a few high amplitude spikes will make an image nondiagnostic (fig. 15.35).

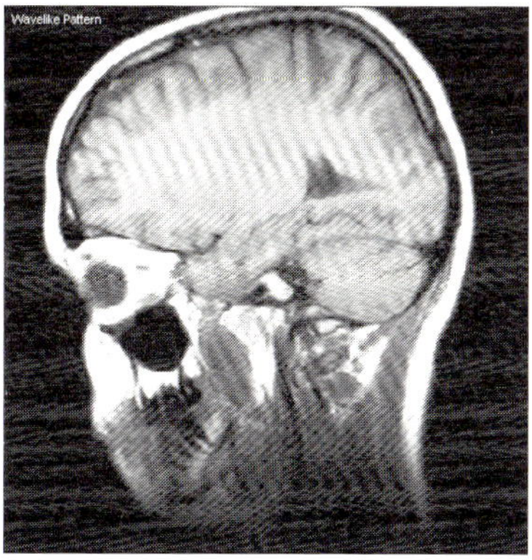

Figure 15.35
Patient MR image with a wave-pattern artifact. An analysis of the measured raw data would reveal a single spike. The most probable cause: electric discharges inside the RF cabin picked up during data acquisition.

Dots and stripes (spikes in image data)

Image dots and stripes caused by periodic signals in the acquired raw data represent quite a reversed type of artifact. Single dots occur if the interfering signal is perfectly synchronous to the system clock controlling the data acquisition. If the periodic signal is not synchronized (i.e. shows an arbitrary phase with respect to each Fourier projection), the dots will smear out in phase encode direction and appear as stripes (fig. 15.36). The causes of such artifacts often involve components inside the RF cabin such as patient monitoring systems that transmit RF energy in the deployed receive band. Virtually ubiquitous RF energy emerging from broadcasting stations, computer clocks, switched power supply sources, etc. may penetrate the RF cabin if its door is left open, if cables are routed through holes without appropriate RF filtering or if the cabin lacks tightness at certain locations due to improper assembly. Single dots usually reflect interference resulting from a deficiency inside the system (e.g. improper grounding or imperfect shielding of RF components in the scanner).

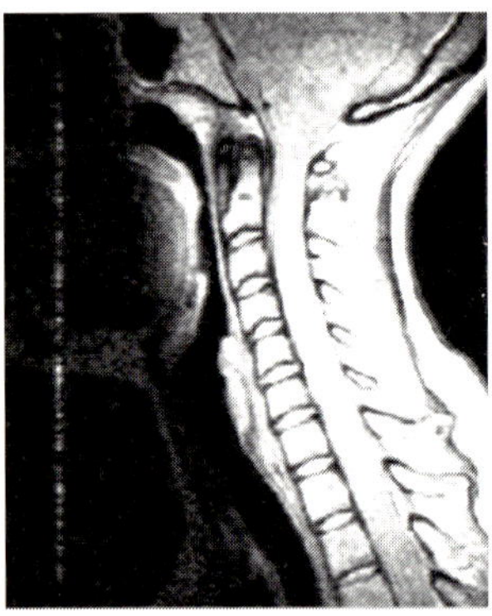

Figure 15.36
Patient MR image with a prominently visible stripe due to RF interference in the RF cabin

15.1.7 MR safety

The MR system comprises three different types of fields (i.e. static magnetic field, pulsed gradient field and RF field) that may be hazardous for both patients and staff.

Static magnetic field

The considerable gradient in the static magnetic field (fringe field) outside the magnet tunnel is the reason for the attractive force on magnetizable (in particular ferromagnetic) objects. Given that the force arises suddenly and magnetizable objects can be accelerated like projectiles, their use is strictly prohibited in the examination room. Special attention should be given to devices (e.g. transport trolleys and objects such as scissors) that are brought into the examination room. It is essential to proper conduct during an emergency that the staff be aware of the availability of nonmagnetic rescue tools (e.g. fire extinguishers and oxygen tanks). Only MR-safe or MR-compatible equipment can be allowed in the MR examination room.

Given that magnetizable objects on the patient (e.g. hair slide) can lead to significant image artifacts and hinder proper diagnosis, these are to be removed from the patient's body prior to the examination.

The introduction of higher static magnetic fields (e.g. 3 T) can lead to physiological effects such as giddiness and nausea that may trigger a startle reflex in patients. These minor effects themselves, however, are reversible.

When using superconducting magnets, coolant (e.g. liquid helium) is applied to cool the wire coils through which the currents flow. In the event of an uncontrolled quench, it will be necessary to respond in accordance with the characteristics of the coolant used.

Pulsed gradient field

Quickly switching on and off the magnetic gradient fields will induce an electric field in the patient's tissue. Eddy currents can be generated that may lead to stimulation effects in the peripheral muscles and nerves (e.g. chest, shoulder, posterior or nose) of the patient. Certain MR systems may be equipped with safety devices that control the switching speed and the strength of the gradients so as to prevent peripheral nerve stimulation [15.20].

The combination of the pulsed gradient field and the static magnetic field causes considerable acoustic noise during MR examinations. The noise level of certain MR systems may require patients to wear protective devices over their ears (table 15.3).

Table 15.3 Excerpt from safety standard (EN/IEC 60601-2-33, [15.20])

		Normal operating mode	**First level controlled operating mode**	**Second level controlled operating mode*)**
Static magnetic field	B_0	≤ 2 T	≤ 4 T	> 4 T
Pulsed gradient field	$\frac{dB}{dt}$, 200 µs risetime	≤ 45 T/s	≤ 56 T/s	> 56 T/s
	$\frac{dB}{dt}$, 400 ms risetime	≤ 30 T/s	≤ 38 T/s	> 38 T/s
RF field**)	Whole body SAR, Body region: Whole body	≤ 2 W/kg	≤ 4 W/kg	> 4 W/kg
	Head SAR, Body region: Head	≤ 3.2 W/kg	≤ 3.2 W/kg	> 3.2 W/kg
	Local SAR, Body region: Head/trunk	≤ 10 W/kg	≤ 10 W/kg	> 10 W/kg
	Local SAR, Body region: Extremities	≤ 20 W/kg	≤ 20 W/kg	> 20 W/kg
Acoustic Noise	No ear protection required for	≤ 99 dB(A)		
	Noise shall be	< 140 dB peak		

*) Not allowed for clinical routine, research only.
**) All values given imply an averaging time of 6 min.

RF fields

The radio frequency (RF) fields that are applied to stimulate the magnetic resonance are absorbed by the body and result in a slight warming up of the body tissue. Given that the decisive parameter is the specific absorption rate *SAR*, an SAR monitor is integrated into all Siemens MR systems to prevent the energy absorbed by the body from exceeding the predetermined limits (table 15.3). These limits are specified in international safety standards [15.20] and may differ from country to country.

The occurrence of large surface current loops may result in patient burns at points of contact if parts of the patient's body (e.g. both feet) are touching one another. It is thus important to position the patient with the use of positioning aids that prevent extremities from touching one another.

Software

Software design also represents a key safety issue. For instance, it is essential to reduce to a minimum those cases in which artifacts are mistaken for pathological structures. Furthermore, special attention should also be given to image orientation and slice positioning in order to avoid misdiagnoses and incorrect treatment (e.g. amputation, skull surgery on the wrong side).

Additional information about contraindications

MR examinations are contraindicated in patients with electronic implants or metal-containing (in particular ferromagnetic) foreign bodies. Implant malfunctioning or total failure may occur in patients with electronic implants and ferromagnetic inclusions may be subject to dislocation. Given that implants may be comprised of various components and alloys, it is essential to have precise information about any implant prior to the examination. Information has been assembled relating to over 1,100 implants and devices and MR safety and MR compatibility [15.21]. In general, pacemakers (i.e. electronic implants) are not allowed in the 0.5 mT control area including the examination room.

Risk management processes are required for medical devices so as to ensure that potential risks are reduced to an acceptable level [15.22]. Safety manuals offer information on how to perform MR examinations ([15.23] and [15.24]) to eliminate hazards for patients and system operators.

15.1.7.1 Safety issues relating to the static magnetic field

The well-known actions of magnetic fields on matter may also cause biological effects in the human body. Readers may wish to refer to the relevant texts (e.g. [15.25]) for a more detailed discussion of the subject. The related factors discussed in the literature include:

- *Magnetic forces*
  Tissue is indeed susceptible to magnetic forces. Frogs, for instance, have been levered (although without sustaining injury) by very large inhomogeneous fields [15.26]. While the magnetic fields applied in magnetic resonance imaging are much

weaker and their magnetic forces have no significant impact on tissue, a great deal of attention has to be given to magnetic implants and objects introduced as a result of accidents (e.g. magnetic splinters). Such objects may move inside the body when exposed to magnetic fields and cause serious injuries.

- *Motion induced voltages*
  Given that objects moving in a magnetic field are exposed to an electric field $\vec{v} \times \vec{B}$, the motion of biological tissue in a strong magnetic field can produce physiological effects. Patients have reported experiencing nausea or strange tastes when being moved in or out of the static magnetic field of an MR system. No lasting adverse effects are known. Voltages induced by the blood flow have been identified as the cause of the altered ECG waveforms observed in persons located in MR scanners. Such changes can thus be regarded as artifacts. The induced voltages are far below levels that would cause nerve or muscle stimulation.
- *Influence on chemical reactions*
  Chemical reactions can indeed be influenced by static magnetic fields. This is due to interactions with electron orbits and spins. One can therefore not rule out the possibility of biomolecular effects stemming from static magnetic fields. However, no sound evidence has yet been presented demonstrating the existence of static-magnetic-field effects on metabolic processes in living beings.

No increased mortality or increased incidence of cancer has been observed in men who were exposed for more than one year to magnetic fields of about 10 mT while working in factories where chlorine is produced by electrolysis [15.27]. More than 1 million people worldwide have been exposed to the strong magnetic fields of MRI scanners since their introduction 25 years ago. No permanent physiological changes have been observed. It is thus more than likely that the magnetic fields used in MRI are totally harmless in physiological terms. That being said, it warrants pointing out that the forces these fields exert on ferromagnetic parts in the vicinity of an MRI magnet represent a very high risk. Fatalities have occurred as a result of such parts striking patients after being accelerated into the magnet.

The force on a magnetic object is proportional to its magnetization and to the gradient of the magnetic field. Actual self-screened magnets can be regarded in a far-field approximation as octupoles with a fringe field decaying as $1/r^5$. The force on a saturated ferromagnetic object, therefore, increases by $1/r^6$ when approaching the magnet. If the magnetization is not yet saturated and still proportional to the magnetic field, the force will even increase by $1/r^{11}$! This means that the magnetic force can change from being scarcely discernable to being destructive in the space of a couple of cm.

15.1.7.2 Stimulation induced by fast gradient switching

Peripheral nerve stimulation

The switching of whole-body gradient coils with amplitudes of more than 20 mT/m at a slew rate of about 100 mT/m/ms may cause the patient to experience peripheral nerve stimulation (PNS). The change in the magnetic flux generated by the gradient coil and expressed as dB/dt induces an electric field E within the patient's body according to the Maxwell equations. If the electric field exceeds a physiologically given threshold (which may vary considerably from subject to subject), stimulation of the peripheral nerve system is induced. While the sensation the patient feels is very weak when the stimulation threshold is reached (tingling sensations or muscular twitching experienced in the lower chest, upper abdomen and upper arm), the PNS can become uncomfortable and even intolerable if the initial threshold is exceeded.

The PNS threshold for a given gradient system depends on a number of gradient pulse parameters. The most important of these is the pulse duration τ, i.e. the stimulus duration within which the electric field is applied to the patient as a result of gradient pulse switching. The threshold value of the electric field E_{Th} at which stimulation starts can be expressed as

$$E_{\mathrm{Th}}(\tau) = E_{\mathrm{Rheo}}\left(1 + \frac{t_{\mathrm{Chron}}}{\tau}\right) \tag{15.36}$$

where the rheobase E_{Rheo} is the limit of the threshold stimulus for $\tau \to \infty$ and t_{Chron} denotes the so-called chronaxie. Taking into account that the electric field E applied to the patient is proportional to $\mathrm{d}B/\mathrm{d}t$, the hyperbolic dependence of Eq. (15.36) can be transformed into a linear dependence on τ to express the stimulation threshold B_{Th} in terms of magnetic flux change [15.28]:

$$B_{\mathrm{Th}} = B_{\mathrm{Min}}\left(1 + \frac{\tau}{t_{\mathrm{Chron}}}\right) \tag{15.37}$$

The B values here are directly proportional to the gradient amplitudes and B_{Min} denotes the minimum change of magnetic flux needed to cause stimulation.

Regulations such as the IEC standard 60601-2-33 [15.29] have been established to define limits for gradient systems according to eq. (15.36) to minimize the occurrence of intolerable PNS in patients. While the default values printed in [15.29] were ascertained on the basis of the published results of several stimulation studies, the IEC standard makes explicit provision for an alternative procedure to directly determine the limits for any given type of gradient system. The limits will thus have to be defined as the mean threshold PNS directly determined from an experimental study involving human volunteers. These limits will then have to be controlled in the MR system by means of an appropriate supervisory method.

Stimulation monitor

Fig. 15.37 shows an experimentally determined stimulation threshold for a typical y-gradient. Here, the thresholds have been specified in terms of the pulse duration (i.e. for bipolar pulses twice the rise time) for trapezoidal and sinusoidal gradient pulses, respectively. According to eq. (15.37), the data sets can be described by a linear fit.

Furthermore, the stimulation thresholds shown in fig. 15.37 can be described using the SAFE model (stimulation approximation by filtering and evaluation), which is an empirical model inspired by the physiological behavior of nerve cells [15.30]. One proceeds according to the model by first differentiating the gradient signal, which is then split into three low pass (exponential) filters. Two of the signals are rectified as

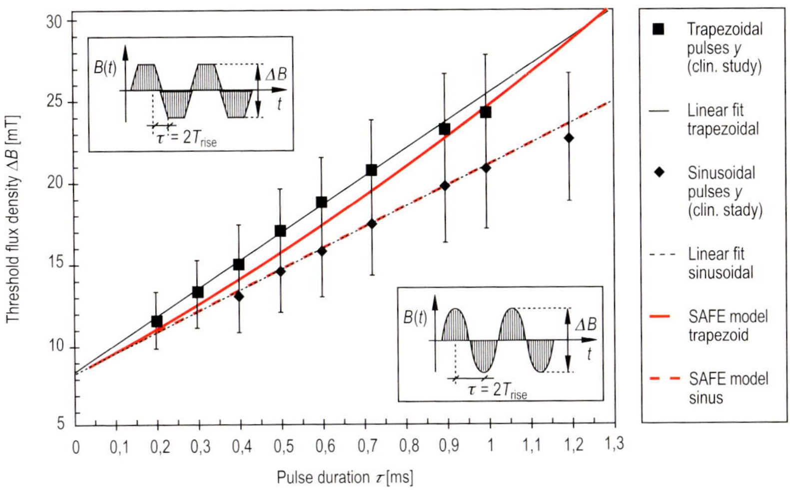

Figure 15.37 Stimulus threshold for sinusoidal and trapezoidal gradient pulses

soon as they have been filtered with a time constant (typically 100 to 700 μs), the 3rd signal is rectified first and then filtered on a time scale of 5 to 15 ms. The final step in the procedure involves recombining the filtered signals into a single value that can be compared to a given limit defining the 100% level. The SAFE model's set of parameters is characteristic of a given gradient system and needs to be determined carefully using a fit process so that the experimentally ascertained stimulation thresholds can be represented when applying the model. Given that the SAFE model generates certain predictions of the stimulation thresholds without incorporating explicit knowledge of the gradient waveforms and rise times, it is highly suitable for implementation as a gradient watchdog within the MR system.

The actual implementation of gradient supervision using the SAFE model is referred to as stimulation monitoring and typically works in two steps. Before the start of a measurement, a part of the corresponding sequence is analyzed by calculating the stimulation level of the deployed gradient pulses on the *x*-, *y*- and *z*-axes. The sequence will start if the stimulation level is below 100%. The real currents flowing through the gradient coil are sampled and evaluated online with the SAFE algorithm during the measurement run. If the defined limits are exceeded for any reason during the system run (e.g. the sequence uses more gradient power than expected or the gradient power amplifier is not working properly), the measurement is stopped immediately by directly switching off the gradient power amplifier.

15.1.7.3 RF heating

An inevitable side effect of the application of time-varying electromagnetic fields with frequencies in the MHz range is the generation of heat within the exposed tissue. As heating is the major effect of RF exposure, temperature increases are a focus of safety

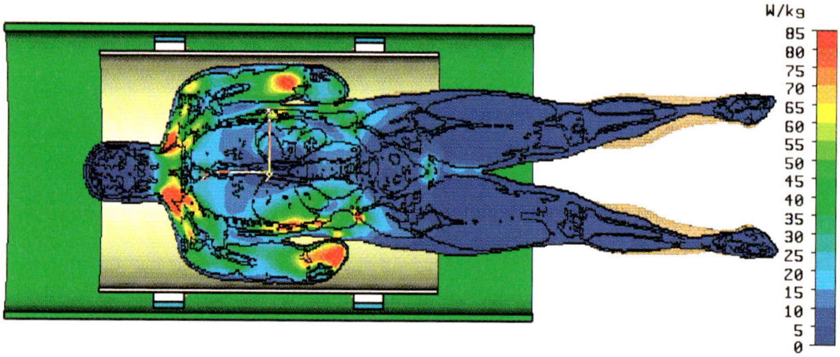

Figure 15.38
SAR distribution within the human voxel model positioned in the center of the body coil (bronze colored area) of the 1.5 T Siemens Symphony system (green colored area indicates the inner magnet bore) during the application of a 180° RF pulse (rectangle-shaped, 1 ms duration, ^{1}H frequency)

considerations. Energy dissipation within the tissue occurs due to the energy losses associated with the stimulated oscillations of permanent and induced electric dipoles and to the limited mobility of free charge carrier. Both mechanisms can be summarized via the generalized, frequency-dependent conductivity $\sigma(\omega)$ of the tissue [15.31]. Given that body/tissue temperatures are generally not accessible during routine clinical examinations, the RF power absorbed per kilogram of tissue – the specific absorption rate (SAR) – is used as a measure of patient load due to the RF. The *SAR* within the exposed tissue can be expressed as

$$SAR = \frac{jE}{\rho} = \frac{\sigma E^2}{\rho} \tag{15.38}$$

j: Current density, E: Electric field, ρ: Tissue density, σ: Electric conductivity

Taking account of eq. (15.8), it follows that

$$SAR \propto \omega_0^2 B_1^2 \propto B_0^2 \alpha^2 \tag{15.39}$$

According to eq. (15.39), the *SAR* scales both with the square of the main magnetic field and with the square of the flip angle α (assuming constant pulse duration). Doubling the main magnetic field strength/pulse flip angle will quadruple the *SAR*!

The finite difference time domain (FDTD) calculation using realistic voxel models of the human body enables one to determine the complex *SAR* distribution within the exposed part of the body (fig. 15.38).

The consequence of the energy absorption is an increase in tissue temperature. The resulting temperature increase depends on the local *SAR* and the duration of exposure (i.e. the energy deposition of the RF pulses in a sequence), the tissue heat conductance and perfusion, and the effect of the body's thermoregulation reaction. The most important physiological thermoregulation mechanisms include: vascular dilatation, sweating, increased heart rate and reduced basal metabolic rate [15.32].

SAR guideline limits are aligned to physiological temperature limits. A two-step limit concept is provided because the thermoregulatory capacity of the patient might be compromised. Experimental data indicate that exposure of up to 4 W/kg (averaged over total body mass) will not increase core body temperature above 1 °C in subjects with an unimpaired thermoregulatory capacity. No adverse health effects have been observed in humans in the case of exposure (head and torso) leading to body temperature increases that do not exceed 1 °C.

However, tissue exhibiting reduced blood circulation (e.g. the lens of the eye and the testicles) is especially sensitive to RF absorption and warrants special attention. While FDTD calculations do not show an increased risk for the eye lens when the RF is transmitted via a typical head coil, the application of RF coils with significantly inhomogeneous B_1 fields may pose a risk for the mentioned tissue regions.

15.2 Methods and clinical applications

15.2.1 Sequences and contrast

The MR pulse sequence is a unique feature in medical imaging that enables one to easily adjust image contrast via the timing and progression of RF and gradient pulses. The two basic sequence concepts in MR imaging, gradient-echo (GRE) and spin-echo (SE) imaging, have already been discussed in chapter 7. These two sequence types have been variously combined and otherwise modified to expand the range of available clinical applications. We are concerned in the present section to trace the development of these applications.

The main difference between spin-echo imaging and gradient-echo imaging centers on the influence that local field inhomogeneities have on image contrast. Inhomogeneities of the magnetic field cause the transverse nuclear magnetization to dephase rapidly. That dephasing is refocused in SE imaging. The field inhomogeneities that influence GRE contrast are mainly caused by local susceptibility gradients in the measured object. The excitation pulse applied in steady-state GRE techniques may also act as a refocusing pulse, causing spin-echo components to contribute to the image contrast.

The contrast in the SE and GRE groups can be manipulated further by preparing the longitudinal magnetization prior to starting the imaging sequence or prior to the measurement of a Fourier line.

The rephasing of the transverse magnetization after a Fourier line has been acquired and the acquisition of another induced echo is referred to as multi-echo imaging. Multi-echo imaging is possible within both the SE group and the GRE group. The use of only one excitation and multiple phase-encoded echoes to acquire all of the required Fourier- or *k*-space lines without a further excitation is referred to as a single-shot technique. All previously described acquisition schemes can be augmented by a preparation of the magnetization.

Table 15.4 Sequence classification scheme (Siemens acronyms)

	Spin-echo sequences (SE)	Gradient-echo sequences (GRE)
Single-echo techniques	SE	FLASH (fast low angle shot) FISP (fast imaging steady precession) PSIF (reversed FISP) trueFISP CISS (constructive interference steady state)
Multi-echo techniques	TSE (turbo spin echo)	DESS (double-echo steady state) MEDIC (multi-echo data image combination) SINOP (simultaneous in-phase opposed phase)
	TGSE (turbo gradient and spin-echo)	
Single-shot techniques	HASTE (half-Fourier acquired single-shot turbo spin echo)	EPI (echo-planar imaging)
Magnetization-prepared single-echo techniques	IR (inversion recovery) IRM (inversion recovery magnitude) STIR (short tau inversion recovery) FLAIR (fluid attenuated inversion recovery)	turboFLASH SR FLASH (saturation recovery FLASH) MP RAGE (magnetization prepared rapid gradient echo)
Magnetization-prepared multi-echo techniques	TIR (turbo inversion recovery) TIRM (turbo inversion recovery magnitude) turboSTIR, turboFLAIR	
Magnetization-prepared single-shot techniques	HASTIRM (HASTE inversion recovery magnitude)	Diffusion weighted spin echo echo planar imaging (DW-SE-EPI)

Table 15.5 Vendor-specific cross reference to sequence acronyms

Siemens	General Electric	Philips
FLASH (fast low angle shot)	SPGR (spoiled GRASS)	T1-FFE (T1 fast field echo)
FISP (fast imaging steady precession)	GRASS (gradient-recalled acquisition in the steady state)	FFE (fast field echo)
PSIF (reversed FISP)	SSFP (Steady-state free precession)	CE-T2-FFE (contrast enhanced T2 fast field echo)
trueFISP	FIESTA (fast imaging employing steady state acquisition)	balanced FFE
turboFLASH	FSPGR (fast spoiled GRASS)	TFE (turbo field echo)
TSE (turbo spin echo) TIR (turbo inversion recovery) RESTORE	FSE (fast spin echo) IR FSE (inversion recovery fast spin echo) DEFT FSE (driven equilibrium Fourier transform fast spin echo)	TSE (turbo spin echo) IR TSE (inversion recovery turbo spin echo) DRIVE
TGSE (turbo gradient and spin-echo)	GRASE (gradient and spin-echo)	GRASE (gradient and spin-echo)
HASTE (half-Fourier acquired single-shot turbo spin echo)	SSFSE (single shot fast spin echo)	SS-TSE (single shot turbo spin echo)

A sequence classification scheme is provided in table 15.4. New sequence acronyms have been introduced as researchers have devised new imaging strategies. These acronyms have sometimes been adapted by the major vendors. Table 15.5 represents a cross reference of the terms used by the three major vendors to describe identical underlying imaging mechanisms. All imaging strategies seem to be tailored to a specific application or seem to provide a specific contrast in a requested measurement time. Table 15.6 offers a short list that correlates sequence acronyms to typical applications.

Table 15.6 Primary sequence utilization (application and contrast)

Sequence acronym	Application
FLASH (fast angle low shot)	T_1-weighted imaging within a breath-hold (abdominal imaging) Time of flight MR angiography (MRA) and contrast-enhanced MRA
SINOP (simultaneous in-phase/opposed-phase)	In-phase/opposed-phase imaging to characterize lesion malignancy Joint studies (morphology)
FISP (fast imaging steady precession)	Low angle applications identical to FLASH T_2* weighted imaging
PSIF	Fast real-time T_2-sensitive technique Imaging of the internal auditory canal (IAC)
MEDIC (multi-echo data image combination)	T_2*-weighted imaging (e.g. transverse spine studies)
CISS (constructive interference steady state)	Imaging of the IAC (fluid-filled cavities)
DESS (double-echo steady state)	Imaging of degenerative joint disease (strong T_2 waiting)
trueFISP	Fast real-time sequence with strong T_2 contrast (e.g. cine cardiac studies, fetal imaging)
turboFLASH	Myocardial perfusion studies
MPRAGE (magnetization prepared rapid gradient echo)	T_1-weighted gapless imaging of the central nervous system (CNS)
TSE (turbo spin echo)	T_2-weighted imaging – whole body.
TIR (turbo inversion recovery)	T_1-weighted imaging – mostly CNS
TIRM (TIR magnitude)	TurboFLAIR: CSF-suppressed T_2-weighted imaging of the CNS Fat-suppressed imaging – whole body
RESTORE	T_2-weighted imaging – mostly CNS
TGSE (turbo gradient spin echo)	High resolution T_2-weighted imaging Increased sensitivity for hemorrhagic lesions as compared to TSE
HASTE (half-Fourier acquired single-shot turbo spin echo)	T_2-weighted imaging in uncooperative patients T_2-weighted abdominal imaging Fetal T_2-weighted imaging
HASTIRM (HASTE inversion recovery magnitude)	Fat-suppressed T_2-weighted abdominal imaging Fast T_1-weighted imaging

15.2.1.1 Spin-echo imaging

Contrast in single-echo imaging

The basic SE imaging sequence (fig. 7.24) was discussed in section 7.3.4. Image contrast can be altered by varying repetition time T_R and echo time T_E. Using the tissue specific relaxation times T_1 and T_2 and the maximum possible longitudinal magnetization M_0 (often referred to as proton density or *PD*) eq. (7.85) can be applied to optimize T_R and T_E for maximum contrast between two different types of tissue. For instance, at 1.5 T maximum, image contrast between gray (GM) and white matter (WM) is achieved by applying an echo time of 15 ms at a repetition time of 430 ms.

T_1-weighted protocols utilize short T_Rs and provide excellent morphologic information in short acquisition times. Tumorous tissue usually shows up slightly hypo- to isointense or causes displacement of normal anatomy (fig. 15.39). T_1-weighted imaging is also performed in conjunction with paramagnetic contrast agents. Given that relaxation times are shortened in the presence of paramagnetic contrast agents, active lesions appear hyperintense on T_1-weighted images (fig. 15.40).

In order to establish contrast based on differences in T_2 relaxation, it will be necessary to select a long T_E and a T_R that is long enough to suppress the influence of T_1 relaxation. T_2-weighted imaging is often used for lesion characterization. Given that the majority of pathologies involve an accumulation of fluid, lesions show up as hyperintense on T_2-weighted images (fig. 15.41).

Most anatomic areas and pathologic conditions can be best investigated using either T_1-weighted imaging or T_2-weighted imaging. A few areas and conditions are best in-

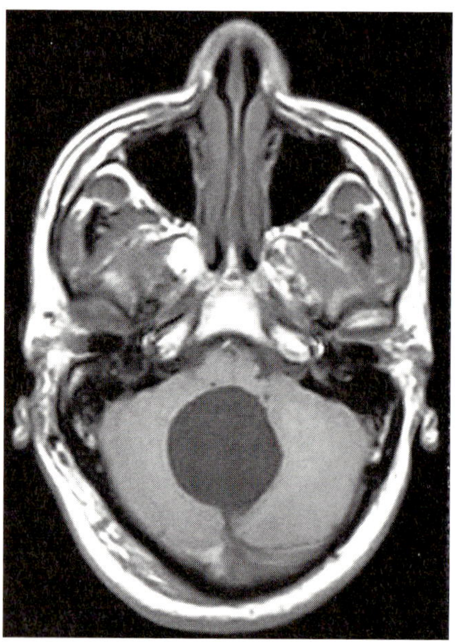

Figure 15.39
Spin-echo T_1-weighted image: fluid-filled cavities (cystic lesions or empty spaces) appear hyperintense due to the long T_1-relaxation times.

vestigated using so-called *PD*-weighted (i.e. proton-density-weighted) imaging. The protocol for *PD*-weighted imaging consists of a long T_R and a short T_E. This enables one to avoid contrast contamination by T_1 or T_2 relaxation.

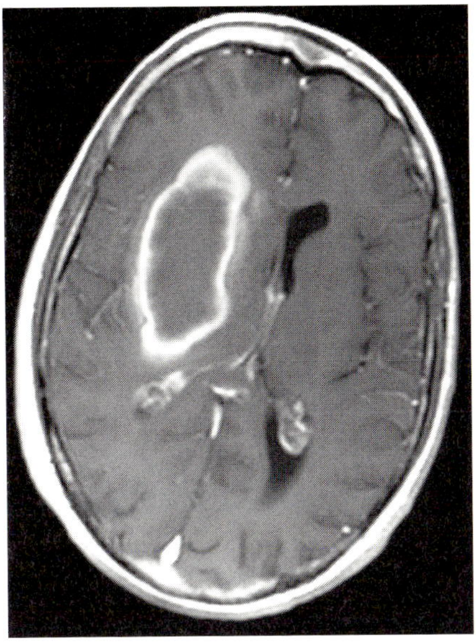

Figure 15.40
Spin-echo post-contrast T_1-weighted image: most contrast agents lead to shorter T_1-relaxation times. Active lesions appear hyperintense on T_1-weighted images.

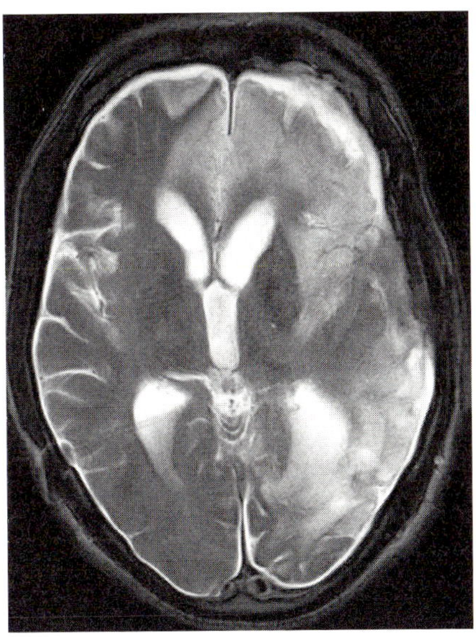

Figure 15.41
Spin-echo T_2-weighted image: long repetition times allow for a complete recovery of the longitudinal magnetization. Longer echo times T_E enhance tissue contrast based on the difference in T_2-relaxation times.

Multi-spin-echo imaging

The idea of using variously encoded subsequent spin echoes to rapidly fill the k-space surfaced as early as 1986 with the introduction of rapid acquisition with relaxation enhancement or RARE [15.33], also known as turbo spin echo (TSE). This sequence has replaced conventional spin-echo imaging in a majority of clinical applications (fig. 15.42). The decrease in the spin-echo amplitudes that results from transversal relaxation leads to the various weighting of the spatial frequencies along the encoding direction. Dedicated phase-encoding schemes are applied to soften the effect of T_2-decay during data acquisition, to reduce correlated image artifacts. The echo train length (ETL) or turbo factor is identical to the number of echoes used and describes the acquisition acceleration with respect to a normal SE sequence.

One can create a PD-weighted and a T_2-weighted image (similar to those created in conventional dual-echo spin-echo imaging) by using a different phase-encoding scheme. Early echoes are used for the PD-weighted image and late echoes are used for the T_2-weighted image. However, it turns out that this is only required for small k-values. For higher k-values echoes with intermediate echo times can be used for the reconstruction of both images. This procedure is therefore referred to using the term shared echo.

TSE imaging with T_1-weighting (short T_R) represents an option for some applications, although additional echoes will increase (unwanted) T_2-weighting. This technique is sometimes applied to investigate the central nervous system. In the case of the genitourinary system (uterus, cervix, bladder, etc.), around three echoes are used to improve the signal-to-noise ratio (SNR) or to reduce measurement time. In areas where the amount of T_2 weighting is less relevant (e.g. T_1-weighted imaging to detect degenerative disease in the cervical and lumbar spine), TSE is usually used with a turbo factor of 5. The same protocol is applied for contrast-agent-enhanced and non-enhanced studies of suspected vertebral metastases. T_1-weighted TSE imaging is rarely applied to abdominal studies because measurement time may be limited to a single breath-hold, a factor that underscores the advantages of T_1-weighted GRE imaging.

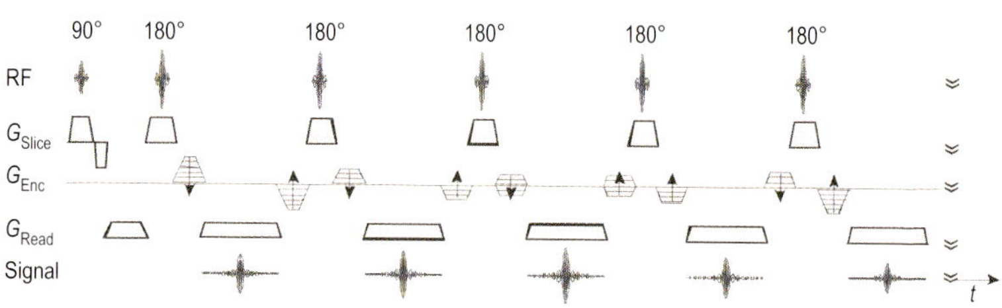

Figure 15.42
Turbo spin echo (TSE) acquisition scheme. After the acquisition of a Fourier line, the transverse magnetization that was de-phased with the phase-encoding gradient for the purpose of spatial encoding is re-phased. Another RF refocusing pulse is applied and the generated spin echo is again phase-encoded using a different phase-encoding amplitude that addresses another Fourier line.

Reduced sensitivity to susceptibility artifacts represents a remaining point of concern when comparing TSE imaging to conventional SE imaging. Hemorrhagic lesions appear less suspicious in TSE imaging than in conventional SE imaging [15.34].

Single-shot spin-echo imaging

Single-shot refers to a single excitation pulse and the use of multiple phase-encoded echoes to fill the required Fourier lines. The original RARE was introduced as a single-shot spin-echo technique. Combining RARE with a half-Fourier technique enables one to reduce measurement time even further. This technique is referred to as half-Fourier-acquired single-shot turbo spin echo or HASTE [15.35].

An image can essentially be constructed from data that fill only half of complex Fourier space (i.e. the part with positive k_ys). While the real part of the transformed data represents the distribution of the transverse magnetization, the imaginary part represents a dispersion image that displays the transverse magnetization folded with one over *y*. However, if a phase shift of transverse magnetization is present over the object of the investigation, the real part of the 2D Fourier transform will also contain dispersion parts that cause image blurring. Such phase shifts can arise from local field inhomogeneities and from gradient and sampling imperfections. Therefore, the full Fourier space is usually covered with data to prevent dispersion. Possible phase shifts are unimportant when the magnitude of the real and imaginary part of the reconstructed data is displayed.

Given the fact that limiting the measurement to half-Fourier space offers significant reductions in acquisition time, strategies have been developed to correct for possible phase shifts. It turns out that acquiring some Fourier lines beyond the center of *k*-space is sufficient [15.36]. For instance, in the case of a 128 by 256 matrix, a single-shot spin-echo technique using the half-Fourier approach would use 128/2 + 8 = 72 phase-encoded echoes to fill the *k*-space. The measurement time using this acquisition method is about one second per slice. The high number of echoes suggests that this technique will only be useful for T_2-weighted imaging and that the blurring effect due to the signal variation in *k*-space as a result of T_2-decay will prohibit the technique's use in high resolution studies.

Nevertheless, the technique remains an alternative to fast T_2-weighted studies (even for investigations of the brain) when clinicians are faced with patients who are either not willing or not able to cooperate. Given that it is an ideal technique for visualizing fluid-filled cavities, HASTE is used for magnetic resonance cholangiopancreatography (MRCP). The use of HASTE for obstetric imaging is increasing. Although sonography remains the imaging technique of choice for prenatal assessment, the complementary role of MR imaging is becoming more and more important as a tool enabling the early evaluation of prenatal brain development [15.37] and even the early detection of complications in the fetal circulatory system.

15.2.1.2 Gradient-echo imaging

The notion of gaining sensitivity via smaller excitation angles was introduced in 1970 [15.38] and proposed for application in MR imaging in 1979 [7.21]. Gradient-echo

(GRE) formation has been used in MR imaging since 1980 [15.39]. The combination of both ideas to achieve faster imaging was introduced in 1985 [15.40]. Signal encoding and readout occur during an FID that follows immediately after the excitation pulse. These techniques are referred to using the term gradient echoes (GRE) because they involve the formation of an echo in connection with the use of a bipolar read-out gradient pulse (also referred to as frequency encoding gradient). The duration of the FID is considerably shorter than the transversal relaxation time T_2 on account of magnetic field inhomogeneities (T_2^* relaxation, see section 7.2.5). Local magnetic field variations are present even in very homogeneous main magnetic fields on account of the differences in tissue-specific magnetic susceptibilities.

A short echo time is required in order to permit signal detection despite the rapid dephasing of the transverse magnetization. Shorter repetition times introduce the feasibility of extending phase-encoding from in-plane encoding to the direction of slice or slab selection leading to 3D imaging (fig. 7.23a). As discussed in section 7.2.7, the establishment of steady-state magnetization at short repetition times T_R depends strongly on the amplitude of the excitation pulses (fig. 15.43). Applying RF pulses of less then 90° results in a significantly larger MR signal.

Spoiled techniques

Following the acquisition of a Fourier line there will be residual transverse magnetization. It will be necessary to spoil this residue in order to avoid image artifacts. Spoiling can be accomplished by applying a gradient pulse to distribute the transverse magnetization evenly, and thereby prevent the next excitation pulse from generating

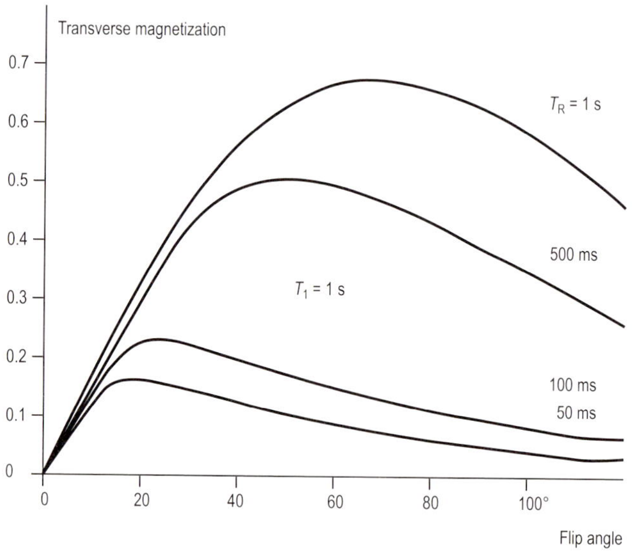

Figure 15.43 Signal strength in FLASH (fast low angle shot) as a function of the excitation angle

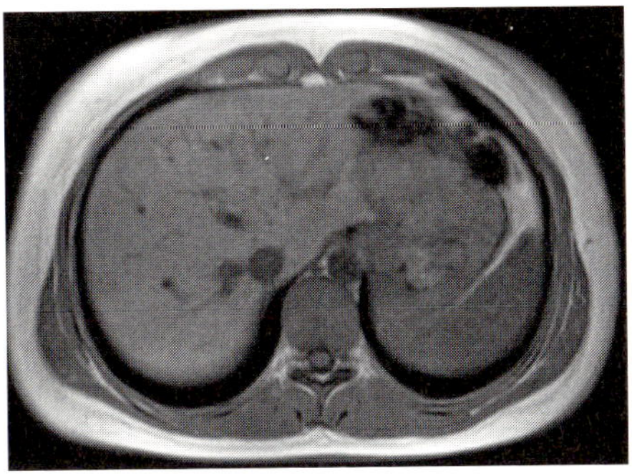

Figure 15.44
Abdominal imaging with FLASH during a breath-hold

a stimulated echo. Alternatively, the phases of the excitation pulses can be randomized to prevent the establishment of a steady state (RF spoiling). Spoiled, low-angle gradient-echo imaging was introduced as fast low angle shot (FLASH). This imaging technique enables one to achieve multi-slice imaging in measurement times short enough to permit single breath-hold acquisitions (fig. 15.44). FLASH images are usually referred to as T_1-weighted because the contrast mainly depends on the T_1-relaxation time.

The Larmor frequency is a function of the chemical environment. Given that frequency encoding is used to retrieve spatial information, images of adipose tissue are slightly shifted in relation to water images, thus leading to the fat-water chemical-shift artifact. This is true for SE as well as GRE imaging. In GRE imaging this phenomenon also affects the phase position of the transverse magnetization. With an appropriate selection of the echo time one can align the transverse magnetization of fat antiparallel to the transverse magnetization of water. The result is referred to using the term opposed phase. As a consequence voxels whose transverse-magnetization components are both about equal in amplitude will show no signal. The in-phase and the opposed-phase images can be acquired simultaneously via the deployment of a dual-echo gradient-echo technique. This technique is referred to as simultaneous in-phase/opposed-phase acquisition or SINOP (fig. 15.45).

SINOP is used, for instance, in the characterization of fat-containing adenomas and when screening for vertebral metastases.

Refocused techniques

Instead of spoiling the residual transverse magnetization after the Fourier line has been acquired, one can re-phase it in order to enhance the signal contribution for tissue with long T_2-relaxation times. This approach leads to a steady state not only for the longitudinal magnetization, but also for the transverse magnetization.

The RF pulse in a steady-state free precession (SSFP) sequence not only converts longitudinal magnetization to transverse magnetization, it also refocuses transverse magnetization. The signal directly after an RF pulse can therefore be regarded as an FID and the signal directly before an RF pulse as an echo [7.25].

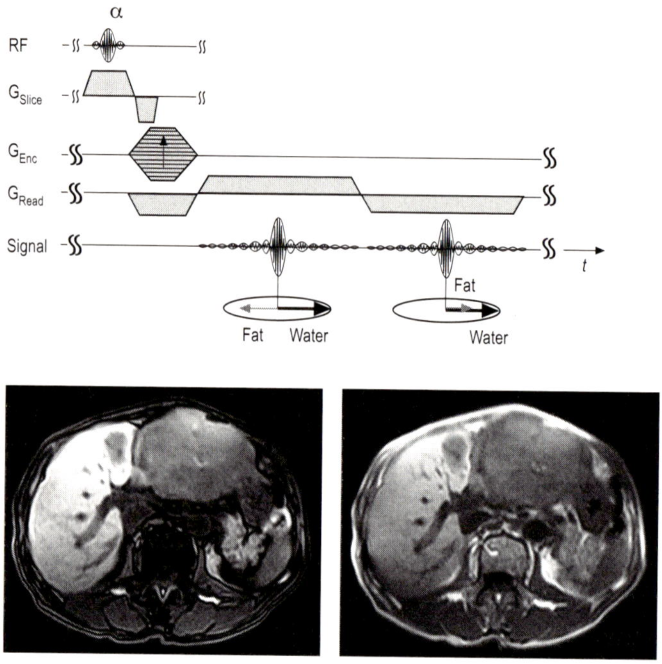

Figure 15.45
SINOP (simultaneous in-phase/opposed-phase) imaging. Depending on the echo time, transverse magnetization originating from fat and water may be in-phase or opposed phase. In the latter case, voxels containing approximately the same amount of water and fat appear hypointense. The two echoes can be acquired following a single RF excitation.

Fig. 15.46 shows an imaging sequence that reads out both the FID and the echo. One can superimpose the two separate images to obtain a single image of more intensity and some degree of T_2 contrast. This method is referred to as double-echo steady state (DESS [15.41]). Given the increased contrast between fat and fluid, DESS is a valuable imaging method in musculoskeletal applications.

Using a clever sequence design, one can encode the FID and the echo signal in a way that generates a single image with both components. This type of sequence, involving the application of phase-alternating RF pulses and a fully symmetric gradient scheme (fig. 7.23b), is referred to as trueFISP (the true having been added to the acronym retrospectively [7.14]).The trueFISP technique is primarily used in fast cardiac imaging (for cine snapshots of the beating heart), abdominal imaging, and even fetal imaging (fig. 15.47).

TrueFISP requires a very homogeneous main magnetic field and/or a short repetition time in order to prevent phase shifts between the FID and the echo. If the field homogeneity is not sufficient, signal canceling (banding) is observed in regions where the magnetization of the FID and the echo are opposed (fig. 15.48).

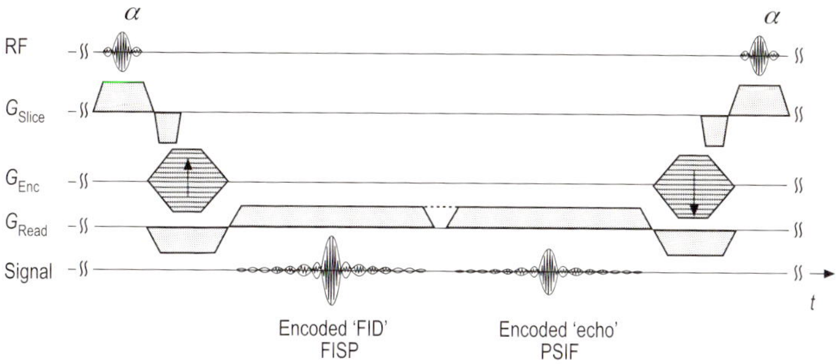

Figure 15.46
DESS (double-echo steady-state) sequence. A steady-state FID and a spin echo are simultaneously encoded to display two gradient echoes. The two images are superimposed to generate one image with T_2 contrast and improved signal-to-noise ratio.

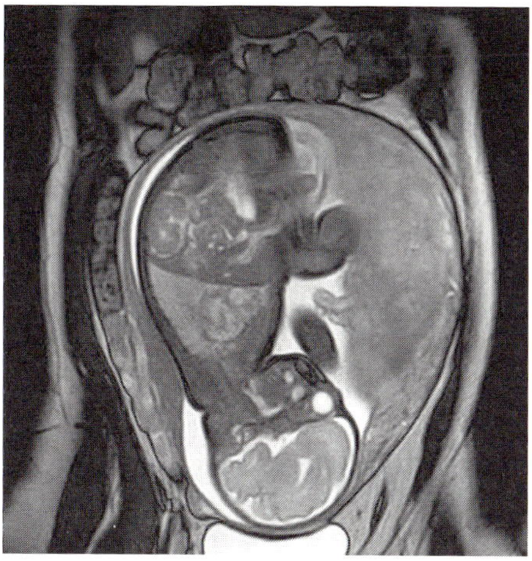

Figure 15.47
Fetal imaging using trueFISP. Contrast is governed by the ratio of T_1/T_2. T_2-weighted imaging in less than a second enables imaging of the unborn child – whereas slower sequences would fail on account of fetal motion.

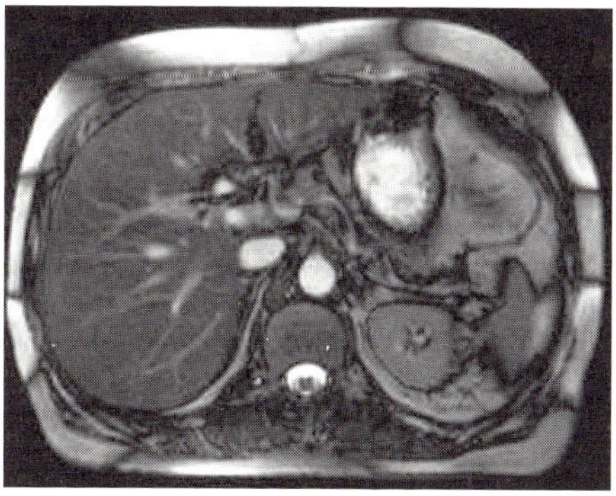

Figure 15.48
Interference artifacts in trueFISP related to poor magnetic field homogeneity

One can avoid this banding by abandoning the idea of a fully balanced sequence and rewinding the phase-encoding gradient only. Such sequences are referred to as FISP (without the true). However, in contrast to FLASH applications, differences in contrast will only be visible for short repetition times and large excitation angles and will only enhance signals within tissue that exhibits long T_2 relaxation times.

One can also avoid banding in a fully balanced GRE sequence by applying the constructive interference steady-state technique (CISS) [15.42]. This technique makes use of two data sets with a trueFISP sequence of alternating and non-alternating RF-pulses. The position of the dark bands is shifted in the second data set to the position of high intensity in the first data set. The complex adding of these two separate acquisitions results in a single image with a contrast that is similar to that of a trueFISP image without field inhomogeneity artifacts. CISS is even useful in regions with significant susceptibility gradients (e.g. imaging at the base of the skull). Given that this technique is a fast technique with the hyperintense appearance of fluid-filled cavities, it is primarily applied to study abnormalities in the internal auditory canal (IAC).

Instead of reading out only the FID part of a steady-state sequence as in FISP (without true), one also has the option of acquiring only the echo part. This leads to a backwards FISP scheme that is accordingly referred to using the acronym PSIF. Given that PSIF is a fast T_2-weighted sequence, it is deployed in the real-time imaging of T_2-enhanced lesions during interventional procedures. PSIF is very sensitive to flow and motion, and is therefore sometimes applied as an adjunct to demonstrate abnormal cerebral spinal fluid (CSF) flow patterns.

15.2.1.3 *k*-space acquisition schemes

As has already been mentioned above (see TSE imaging), one can achieve an additional degree of freedom for manipulating contrast via the raw data sorting scheme. The Fourier lines are usually sorted (from bottom to top) in the same manner as frequency encoding (from left to right). The high spatial frequencies are collected first, followed by the center of *k*-space and then the high spatial frequencies towards the last Fourier lines. This order is referred to as conventional. Timing is often critical in contrast-enhanced MR angiography. The goal is to catch the core of the passing contrast bolus while acquiring the low spatial frequencies (center of *k*-space). Centrally re-ordered *k*-space filling is sometimes desirable in such cases. The measurement starts with the filling of the center of *k*-space using low-phase encoding-gradient amplitudes. The high spatial frequencies containing Fourier lines are acquired later.

Another interesting acquisition scheme involves substituting projections similar to those used in computer tomography for phase encoding. Instead of proceeding through phase-encoding steps, the magnetic field gradient responsible for the frequency encoding is rotated around the isocenter with a different projection for each acquisition. This acquisition scheme is referred to as radial acquisition (see sections 7.3.1 and chapter 10). It will be necessary to re-grid the data so that they fit on a rectangular grid, and thereby allow the use of fast Fourier transformation for image reconstruction. The advantage of radial scanning is that the center of *k*-space is mea-

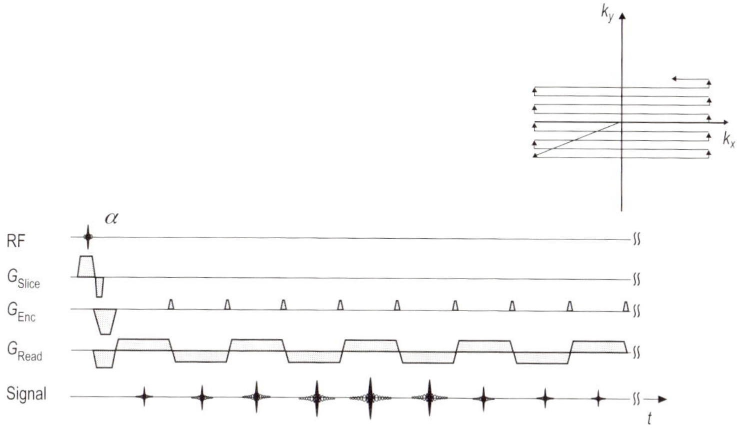

Figure 15.49
EPI (echo-planar imaging) acquisition scheme. The basic concept involves the filling of k-space (upper part of figure) with multiple phase-encoded gradient echoes following a single excitation. This version is referred to as blipped EPI.

sured with each acquisition, thus allowing real-time imaging of dynamic events with a subjectively higher temporal resolution than is afforded using Cartesian sampling.

The use of gradient echoes for multiple phase encoding was suggested by Sir Peter Mansfield as early as 1977. His proposal offered subsecond imaging at a time when conventional imaging took several minutes. The technique was referred to as echo-planar imaging (EPI [15.43]) and made provision for various methods of data acquisition. The original concept involved the deployment of a single excitation followed by multiple gradient echoes that were phase-encoded with a small constant gradient. k-space was thus traversed using a zigzag pattern that made the task of image reconstruction more elaborate. For the sake of simplicity, phase encoding is now usually performed using a gradient blip during the frequency-encoding gradient's ramping time (fig. 15.49). Another method of k-space sampling involves permitting both the frequency-encoding gradient and the phase-encoding gradient to oscillate, thereby creating a spiral trajectory through k-space. This method is referred to as spiral EPI.

The high sensitivity of EPI to local field inhomogeneities is utilized in brain perfusion imaging [15.44] and oxygen-level monitoring to identify cortical activation in BOLD (blood-oxygenation level-dependent) imaging [15.45]. As a single-shot technique, EPI covers the entire k-space during a single FID. Given less stringent acquisition time requirements, the k-space can be segmented using multiple gradient-echo trains to provide greater flexibility with respect to image quality and contrast.

Multiple echoes can also be used to improve the *SNR* rather than to speed up the measurement time. This type of multiple GRE imaging with low angle excitation is sometimes utilized in spine investigations to generate T_2^*-weighted images. The technique is referred to as multi-echo data-image combination (MEDIC).

Fourier or volume interpolation

The image of a small hyperintense structure (e.g. a small vessel in time-of-flight (ToF) MRA) will strongly depend on the position of the vessel relative to the voxel grid. If the vessel is contained in a single voxel, the hyperintensity of the representative pixel will likely be greater than if it is shared by adjacent voxels. One solution here is to shift the voxel grid and combine the generated images.

Interpolation via the zero-filling of *k*-space lines is equivalent to voxel-shifted interpolation [15.46]. The zero-filled interpolation is also referred to as Fourier interpolation and is routinely used in 2D imaging where, for instance, a 256 by 256 acquired raw data matrix is embedded in the center of a zero filled 512 by 512 matrix and the image is reconstructed into a 512 by 512 (interpolated) image matrix.

This concept can be extended to 3D imaging. Using the same Fourier interpolation in the direction of slice or slab selection allows one to calculate additional partitions in a 3D slab, similar to the manner in which one calculates additional pixel values in an expanded 2D image matrix. Unfortunately, the reduced partition thickness is often referred to as the spatial resolution after interpolation. This can lead to the false impression that the spatial resolution is improved, when it is really a matter of the partial volume effects being reduced due to a voxel-shifted interpolation.

Nevertheless, the appearance of the interpolated partitions is improved when compared to a thicker partition. Furthermore, more partitions can be calculated using the data of a measurement that may have been short enough to be acquired within a breath-hold. This technique is referred to as volume-interpolated breath-hold examination or VIBE [15.47]) and is also applicable during free breathing.

15.2.1.4 Imaging with magnetization preparation

Altering repetition time, echo time and/or excitation angle represent ways of influencing image contrast. A very powerful additional approach to modifying image contrast involves altering the available longitudinal magnetization prior to RF excitation. Doing so enables one to optimize imaging sequences with respect to specific tasks such as enhancing T_1 contrast, or suppressing the signal from fat or fluid.

Spectral saturation

The fact that protons in fat have a lower resonance frequency than those in water can be exploited in connection with the application of a spectral RF saturation pulse. A 90° RF pulse that covers the frequency range of the Larmor frequencies of the protons in the lipid compounds is applied in the absence of an activated magnetic field gradient. The resulting transverse magnetization is subsequently spoiled using large gradient pulses. No signal will be generated for the adipose tissue in the immediately following imaging sequence. This imaging method is used when investigating suspected pathologies: to distinguish between malign and benign conditions, to avoid the signal masking of pathologies (e.g. hyperintense tumors after contrast uptake in MR mammography), to reduce motion artifacts originating in subcutaneous fat and to simply

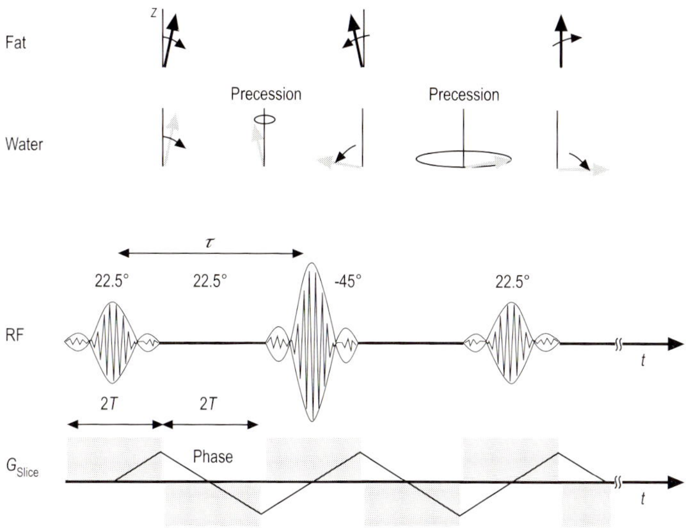

Figure 15.50
Spatially selective binomial 90° RF pulse (1-2-1 pulse) that excites water spins and no fat spins. The RF frequency is required to be identical to the Larmor frequency of fat.

increase the dynamic range for image windowing given that fat is usually very hyperintense due to it's short T_1 and relatively long T_2 relaxation times.

Binomial excitation

The quality of spectral fat saturation depends on the overall magnetic field homogeneity. If the homogeneity is poor, the water signal might be partially saturated, causing a loss in overall *SNR*. Instead of saturating the unwanted component in order to obtain a pure water or fat image, one might simply excite either fat or water. This can be achieved using a so-called binomial excitation pulse [15.48] that can be executed either selectively or non-selectively. Fig. 15.50 shows the mechanism of a 1-2-1 RF pulse for water excitation. An initial RF pulse tilts both the fat and the water magnetization by 22.5°. The transversal component of the water magnetization precesses by 180° with respect to the fat component during the ensuing waiting period τ:

$$\gamma_{H_2O}\delta B_0 \tau = \pi \tag{15.40}$$

A −45° excitation angle will then tilt the water magnetization to a −67.5° position with respect to the longitudinal direction while the fat magnetization is flipped back to the −22.5° position. After τ, another 22.5° excitation pulse will accomplish the −90° excitation for water while the fat magnetization is restored to the longitudinal position. The frequency range in which no excitation occurs can be broadened with longer binomial pulse trains as e.g. a 1-3-3-1 sequence (the underscore designating a negative pulse). Fat saturation is a technique that is commonly applied in orthopedics (fig. 15.51).

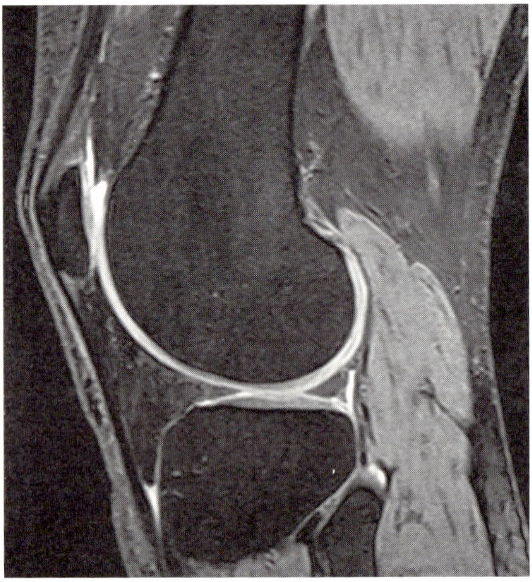

Figure 15.51
Fat-suppressed image of the knee acquired using DESS and applying spatially selective 1$\underline{2}$1 RF pulses

Inversion recovery SE

Placing an RF inversion pulse prior to the excitation pulse followed by the acquisition of a Fourier line will cause the signal not only to be a function of the repetition time and the echo time, but also of the inversion time – the time between the center of the inversion pulse and the center of the excitation pulse of the imaging sequence (see section 7.2.6).

The inversion pulse can be used to provide better contrast between tissues whose T_1-relaxation time differences are relatively small. If no more than the magnitude of the longitudinal magnetization is considered for the image contrast, the technique is referred to using the term inversion recovery magnitude or IRM. In the case of a phase-sensitive inversion-recovery technique, the parallel or antiparallel position of the longitudinal magnetization is considered by analyzing the phase of the generated transverse magnetization. In contrast to a positive longitudinal magnetization, a negative longitudinal magnetization will be converted to a transverse magnetization of the opposite phase. This (phase-sensitive) IR technique turns out to be very valuable in the documentation and evaluation of brain maturation in neonates (fig. 15.52).

Magnetization inversion prior to Fourier line acquisition can also be used to null the signal of tissue exhibiting a specific T_1-relaxation time. The RF excitation of the imaging sequence is applied at that point in time when the longitudinal magnetization passes zero. Given that fat has a relatively short T_1-relaxation value, the inversion time will also have to be short. An inversion-recovery technique that is used to suppress the fat signal is referred to using the term short tau inversion recovery or STIR. This technique is preferred in situations where local field inhomogeneities prohibit the spectral saturation of fatty tissue.

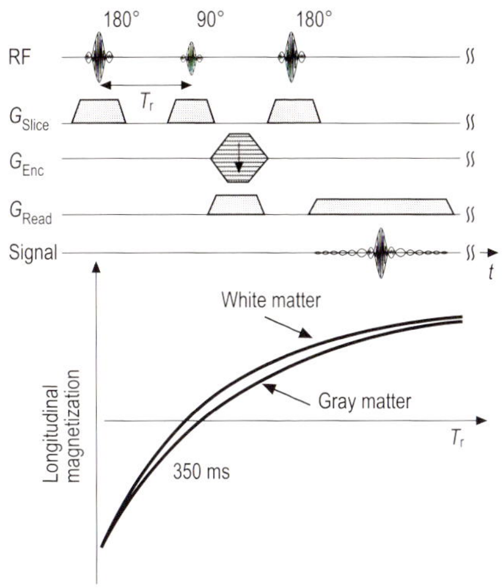

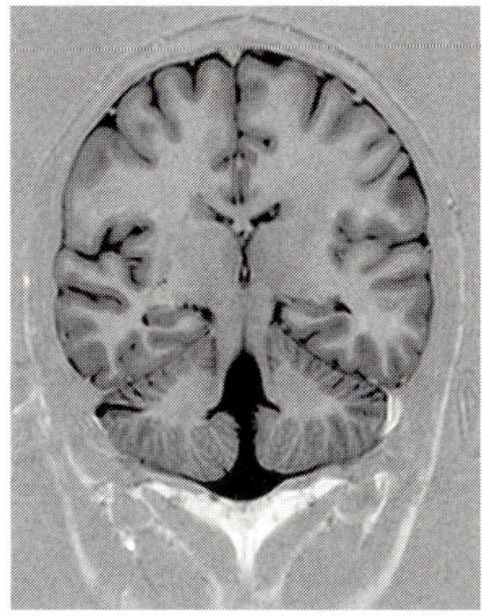

Figure 15.52
True inversion recovery imaging. Assuming that the inversion time has been properly selected, the inversion pulse prior to the excitation pulse will provide an optimal differentiation between gray and white matter. The parallel alignment of the longitudinal magnetization at the time of the excitation pulse of the imaging sequence is represented as a hyperintense signal. An antiparallel alignment is represented by a hypointense signal.

Inversion recovery multi-spin echo

Magnetization preparation in multi-echo imaging enables one to alter image contrast in a manner similar to that used in SE acquisition schemes. In general, the inversion time will need to be adapted to take account of the ETL. The use of multi-echo imaging has replaced single-echo protocols in most IR applications.

The application of an inversion pulse to bring about fat suppression with TSE represents a routine method of demonstrating bone infarctions and bone marrow abnormalities (e.g. bone marrow edema in sickle cell anemia). This fat suppression scheme is also used in genitourinary applications where the high signal intensity of fat may obscure contrast-enhanced tumor spread.

An inversion time of 1.9 s will suppress the CSF signal, which is referred to using the term fluid-attenuated inversion-recovery (FLAIR), a technique that was originally presented in conjunction with single-echo SE imaging. When combined with TSE imaging, the technique is referred to as turboFLAIR or TIRM (turbo inversion recovery utilizing the magnitude of the generated signal). The attenuated CSF signal allows for enhanced differentiation in the case of periventricular lesions and has demonstrated superior sensitivity for focal white matter changes in the supratentorial brain (although lesions located in the posterior fossa may be missed). The turboFLAIR method apparently allows for the identification of hyperacute subarachnoid hemorrhaging with MR, thereby precluding the need for an additional CT [15.49].

An inversion time of approximately 220 ms allows for an enhanced delineation of small differences in T_1-relaxation times (e.g. when it comes to documenting pediatric brain development). The improved tissue characterization between gray-matter and white-matter tracts allows one, for instance, to demonstrate mesial temporal sclerosis and to visualize hippocampal atrophy and temporal-horn dilation.

HASTE in conjunction with an inversion pulse is sometimes referred to as HASTIRM or HIR. This combination is designed to suppress the fat signal.

Dark-blood preparation

When augmented by ECG triggering, multi-echo spin-echo imaging enables one to achieve T_1 and/or T_2-weighted spin-echo imaging of the beating heart within a breath-hold. This capacity had been out of reach on account of the significant flow artifacts caused by the flowing blood until the introduction of the dark-blood preparation scheme revolutionized cardiac MR imaging [15.50].

The magnetization of the entire imaging volume is inverted non-selectively, followed by a selective re-inversion of the slice. This is done at end-diastole upon detection of the onset of the QRS complex. Most of the re-inverted blood is washed out of the slice (being replaced by the inverted blood) during the ensuing waiting period and the spin

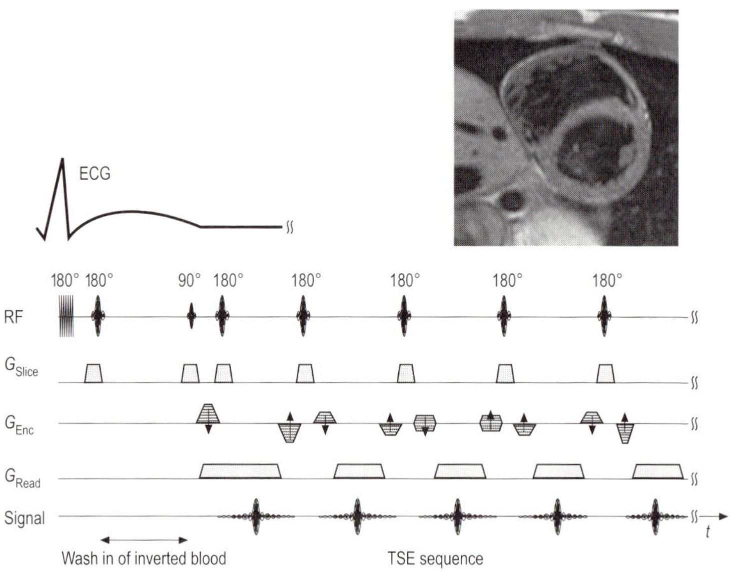

Figure 15.53
Dark-blood preparation used in cardiovascular imaging. A non-selective inversion pulse is applied at the time of the ECG's R wave and is immediately followed by a selective inversion pulse. Imaging begins close to the end of the diastole so that the inverted blood spins have already been washed in, causing the ventricles to appear hypointense. Tissue appears bright because the stationary tissue spins have been re-inverted.

echo train that is re-acquired towards end-diastole will show black blood (fig. 15.53). In addition to the black blood preparation, a double-inversion pulse will even permit the suppression of the fat signal. This capacity is helpful when it comes to characterizing fatty infiltration of the myocardium in arrhythmogenic right ventricular dysplasia (ARD).

Driven equilibrium

The transverse magnetization that remains after the measurement of a single Fourier line (i.e. after the measurement of the package of Fourier lines in the case of multi-echo imaging) is usually spoiled. By deploying the driven equilibrium method introduced by Becker et al. [15.51], one can also refocus the transverse magnetization at the end of the echo train and use an RF pulse to restore the residual transverse magnetization to the longitudinal direction [15.52]. This method enables one to accelerate the recovery of the longitudinal magnetization, and thereby allows for a further shortening of the repetition time without a loss of contrast. Driven equilibrium can also be applied with a magnetization prepared sequence.

Inversion recovery GRE

All of the magnetization preparation schemes described above can essentially be used for both SE and GRE sequences. It warrants bearing in mind, however, that GRE sequences usually make use of shorter T_E and shorter T_R than SE imaging and that some preparation schemes will therefore have to be altered slightly. The fat saturation scheme can be used as an example: the time necessary for a spectral saturation pulse followed by a gradient spoiler will add up to the slice-loop time for an otherwise short T_R GRE sequence. Skipping the fat saturation for a few slices (a technique referred to as quick fat sat) represents a feasible modification. Although this will introduce a slice-dependent recovery of the fat signal, the compromise is generally acceptable because the fat signal remains low and more slices can be measured per T_R.

As mentioned, T_1 contrast can be improved in SE imaging by placing an inversion pulse prior to the acquisition of the Fourier line. This approach is not feasible in GRE imaging because the inversion time would be much larger than the repetition time. Instead, the inversion pulse is used prior to the entire imaging sequence, a technique introduced as turboFLASH (TFL) [15.53]. The minor drawback here is that the longitudinal magnetization (available prior to the acquisition of a Fourier line) will change throughout the measurement. This violation of *k*-space symmetry will cause an under or overrepresentation of some spatial frequencies, and will thereby result in a slight image blurring.

The application of a saturation (i.e. 90°) instead of an inversion pulse has proven useful in studies of the first pass of a contrast bolus passing through the cardiac chamber, showing a hypointense signal in perfusion-restricted ischemic myocardial tissue [15.54]. In the early phase, normal myocardial tissue will be perfused with the T_1-shortening contrast agent and the perfusion-restricted ischemic myocardial tissue will remain hypointense.

This method of tissue-signal nulling can also be applied with trueFISP to demonstrate the late enhancement of the infarcted myocardium [15.55]. The advantage of trueFISP over turboFLASH is that the additional signal contributions due to refocusing and balancing (spin-echo components) allow for faster image acquisition (~450 ms for a total image). Moreover, trueFISP exhibits significantly lower sensitivity to flow and motion artifacts compared to turboFLASH, thus enabling virtually artifact-free images.

The introduction of short T_R gradient-echo acquisition schemes made 3D imaging feasible. Applying an inversion pulse prior to a 3D acquisition scheme would not represent a promising approach because the preparation of the longitudinal magnetization would rapidly diminish during the relatively long measurement time and on account of the significant number of low angle excitation pulses. A feasible alternative is to repeat the preparation of the longitudinal magnetization either in the partition-encoding loop or in the phase-encoding loop. Placing the preparation scheme in the partition-encoding loop eliminates the above-mentioned TFL artifact associated with the over and under representation of *k*-space lines. For a selected phase-encoding gradient amplitude the inversion pulse is applied followed by the rapid execution of the partition-encoding loop – during which the amount of longitudinal magnetization will change according to the course of the T_1 relaxation, with recovery being influenced by the low angle excitation pulses. This procedure is repeated for the next phase-encoding line. The amount of signal within each partition is identical for all phase-encoding steps and the *k*-space (in-plane) is again symmetric – resulting in artifact-free images. This technique has been introduced as magnetization prepared rapid gradient echo (MP RAGE) [15.56].

The MP RAGE sequence allows for seamless coverage of the entire brain in less than 6 minutes. However, susceptibility gradients (especially at the base of the skull) cause a geometrically distorted representation of the anatomy or even signal voids. Furthermore, MP RAGE does not always permit the reproduction of the commonly observed increase in signal intensity in the case of tumors upon the uptake of a paramagnetic contrast agent [15.57]. It thus follows that this sequence cannot yet replace standard T_1-weighted SE sequences despite its fast image acquisition time.

Diffusion-weighted EPI

As has been discussed in section 7.2.8, spin diffusion is one further parameter that can be used to characterize biological tissue. Diffusion-weighted and diffusion-tensor imaging represent additional forms of magnetization preparation. These will be discussed in greater detail in a later section. Magnetization is prepared prior to an EPI sequence using a 90° and a 180° pulse (or three 90° pulses) with diffusion gradients before and after the refocusing pulse. The echo is read out using an EPI gradient switching scheme. Diffusion-weighted imaging enables one to evaluate the extent of cerebral ischemia due to infarction (see section 15.2.5.2, fig. 15.96).

15.2.1.5 Hybride methods

Following the success of fast spin echo imaging, a variant of the technique was introduced so as to enable the acquisition of multiple phase-encoded gradient echoes in a spin-echo envelope. This technique is referred to the term gradient and spin-echo imaging (GRASE [15.58]) or turbo gradient and spin-echo imaging (TGSE). The potential reduction in measurement time scales with the number of gradient echoes used per spin-echo envelope, although the echo train length increases due to the additional read-out modules, and thus prolongs the slice-loop time or the minimum T_R. The spacing of the RF refocusing pulses is usually adjusted such that the echoes of fat oscillating due to homonuclear coupling (J-coupling) appear at intensities similar to a SE sequence. The introduction of gradient echoes has led one to anticipate an increase in sensitivity to susceptibility gradients and thus to an increase in sensitivity to hemorrhagic lesions [15.59].

15.2.2 Parallel imaging techniques (PAT)

Parallel imaging techniques (PAT) emerged as a method of parallelizing the sequential character of conventional MR image acquisition schemes in order to shorten imaging times. Despite the introduction of high performance gradients, RF electronics and sophisticated pulse sequences for many applications, scan time has remained limited by the time consuming sequential (line-by-line) acquisition of individual Fourier lines. The PAT concept involves the partial parallelization of the phase encoding process in order to substantially shorten conventional pulse sequences.

In addition to shorter scan times, the benefits of PAT include the ability to significantly increase image quality for certain applications. For instance, PAT may be applied to shorten the echo train length of EPI protocols, resulting in a reduction in susceptibility-induced distortions. This example also demonstrates the significance of the technique in general: it is hard to imagine that a similar improvement could be achieved by deploying more powerful gradients. Apart from the technical constraints (a factor of two in readout speed would require twice the gradient amplitude and a fourfold gradient slew rate!), patient peripheral nerve stimulation imposes a physiological limit on the applied gradient power.

PAT is not restricted to special sequence types. In general, it can be applied to any imaging protocol, a property whose significance should not be underestimated when it comes to clinical application given the fact that the contrast behavior of established protocols is preserved.

15.2.2.1 Basics of parallel imaging

Although the principles of PAT were first outlined in the 1980s [15.60-15.65], the technology was not implemented for clinical imaging until the late 90s. The basic idea behind PAT is to make use of the spatial information contained in the sensitivity profiles of local receiver coils. Array coils were originally introduced as dedicated signal reception devices designed to improve *SNR* in MRI [15.7]. In the case of PAT, they are incorporated into the spatial encoding process, which is conventionally based solely on RF excitation and gradient pulse schemes.

It is an intrinsic property of local coils that their sensitivity profiles vary in space, both in magnitude and phase. Hence, the detected signal is modulated with a spatially vary-

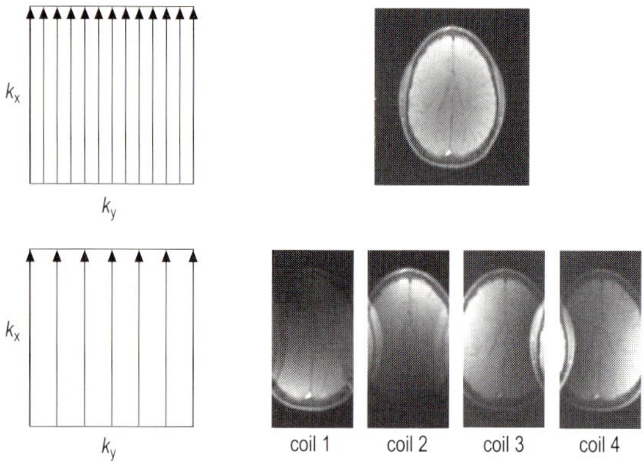

Figure 15.54
Typical parallel acquisition scheme. **Upper row:** non-accelerated, fully sampled k-space **(left)** and reconstructed image **(right)**. **Lower row:** accelerated acquisition via reduced phase encoding **(left)** leads to folded raw images **(right)**, in this example received by four individual coil elements.

ing function determined by the coil geometry. If a sample is covered by multiple, independently receiving coils, the spatial information contained in each receiver channel can provide part of the spatial encoding required for image reconstruction.

A typical parallel imaging scan will periodically leave out phase encoding steps, for instance, by skipping every other phase encoding line in k-space (fig. 15.54). These missing lines are calculated during image reconstruction with the use of the information contained in the scanned Fourier lines of the individual receiver channels.

Despite their sheer number, most of the parallel acquisition and reconstruction techniques that have been proposed [15.66-15.72] can be broken down into k-space-related methods and image-domain-related methods. These techniques are commonly referred to by the acronyms SMASH and SENSE that were coined by the authors of the first publications showing clinical results. In what follows, we offer a brief description of the techniques.

15.2.2.2 The SMASH technique

Introduced in 1997, the SMASH technique (simultaneous acquisition of spatial harmonics) was the first to incorporate processes of parallel acquisition into clinical MR imaging.

SMASH incorporates the coil sensitivity patterns $\sigma_l(x,y)$ into the spatial encoding function. As has been shown (section 7.3.1), the signal intensity in k-space $s_l(k_x,k_y)$ from the coil element l can be written as

$$s_l(k_x,k_y) = \iint \rho(x,y) \cdot \sigma_l(x,y) \cdot e^{i(k_x x + k_y y)} \mathrm{d}x\mathrm{d}y \tag{15.41}$$

$\rho(x,y)$: Spin density, $\sigma_l(x,y)$: Sensitivity profile for coil l

These signals are taken in linear combinations with weighting factors c_{lm} selected so as to yield the simulation of a magnetization pattern generated by phase encoding gradients (fig. 15.55). This requires combining the sensitivity profiles of the coils to form spatially varying harmonics:

$$\sum_l c_{lm}(x,y)\sigma_l = e^{i \cdot m \cdot \Delta k_y \cdot y} \tag{15.42}$$

Consequently, the signal combination

$$s_m(k_x,k_y) = \sum_l c_{lm} s_l(k_x,k_y) = \iint \rho(x,y) \cdot e^{i(k_x x + (k_y + m \cdot \Delta k_y)y)} dx dy \tag{15.43}$$

produces a new Fourier line at $k_y + m \cdot \Delta k_y$ in addition to the line at k_y that is generated by the gradient G_y. The gaps in k-space between acquired Fourier lines can thus be filled with n synthetic lines. In terms of image acquisition speed, this feature can be converted into an n-fold acceleration of image acquisition time compared to the conventional, purely gradient-based acquisition scheme. The theoretical maximum acceleration factor n is determined by the number of receive coils.

The original SMASH technique faces two major problems. The first is the dependence on the coil profiles. If spatial harmonics cannot be properly assembled in phase encoding direction, image reconstruction will result in residual fold-in artifacts. Furthermore, while the coil profiles should ideally remain invariant in the readout direction (i.e. orthogonal to the phase direction) experience shows that they do vary, a problem that may be solved by deploying a segmentation of the reconstruction process along readout direction, using different sets of coefficients for each segment. A second disadvantage of SMASH is found in its inferior signal-to-noise (*SNR*) performance [15.73]. It has been shown that a linear combination of signals from a coil array

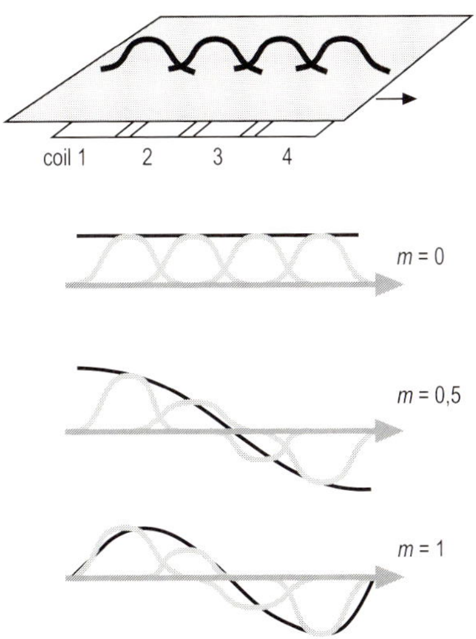

Figure 15.55
Generation of coil sensitivity patterns in SMASH. Different coil profile weightings are used to approximate different spatial harmonics.

(as is applied in SMASH) compares unfavorably in terms of *SNR* to the quadratic combination routinely used in standard imaging.

Methods related to the original SMASH approach have also been presented [15.67-15.69]. The aim of these methods is to refine the algorithms deployed so as to achieve robust, artifact-free and *SNR*-optimized reconstructions.

15.2.2.3 The SENSE technique

While the SENSE (sensitivity encoding) technique resembles SMASH in that it uses the sensitivity patterns of local coils as a substitute for gradient phase encoding steps, its mathematical approach to image reconstruction is rather different. Instead of generating phase encoding lines directly in *k*-space, reconstruction is performed in the image domain (i.e. after the Fourier transform).

For instance, if every other gradient phase encoding step in *k*-space is skipped for an acceleration factor of two, the result is equivalent to an image with half the field of view (FOV) in phase encoding direction. Those regions of the scanned object that are located outside the reduced FOV will fold over (aliase) as shown in fig. 15.54 (see also section 7.3.2). In other words, the PAT accelerated acquisition scheme (i.e. periodically skipping lines in *k*-space) translates into an unfolding problem in the image domain.

SENSE image reconstruction is a matter of restoring the full FOV by using each coil channel's tendency to display pixel intensities differently due to its sensitivity profile.

The concept of unfolding can be demonstrated using the following example (fig. 15.56): We assume that spin densities $\rho(P_1)$ and $\rho(P_2)$ at two locations P_1 and P_2 superimpose in the aliased images reconstructed from the signals of two coils that have different sensitivity profiles σ_A and σ_B. The aliased pixel intensity for the two coils can thus be expressed as

$$\begin{aligned} I_A &= \sigma_A(P_1)\rho(P_1) + \sigma_A(P_2)\rho(P_2) \\ I_B &= \sigma_B(P_1)\rho(P_1) + \sigma_B(P_2)\rho(P_2) \end{aligned} \tag{15.44}$$

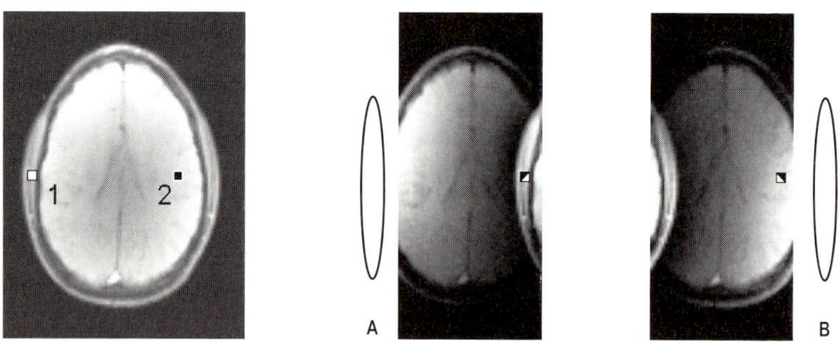

Figure 15.56
Unfolding aliased pixels with SENSE. **Left:** fully sampled, unfolded image. **Middle/right:** folded SENSE images prior to reconstruction, as received by coil A and coil B; folded image points 1 and 2 are no longer separate, but appear with different intensity values in both coil channels A and B.

Obviously, this set of equations can be solved for $\rho(P_1)$ and $\rho(P_2)$ if the sensitivities $\sigma_A(P_1)$ and $\sigma_A(P_2)$ are known. The noise characteristics of the receiving coil channels have to be taken into account for an *SNR*-optimized reconstruction. A detailed treatment of the SENSE reconstruction is given in [15.70]. Due to its pixel-by-pixel reconstruction, the SENSE technique is less demanding than the SMASH technique in terms of dedicated coil sensitivity profiles.

However, SENSE is subject to a tedious limitation in that the unfolding will fail whenever the image is pre-aliased, i.e. whenever the object extends beyond the chosen FOV in phase encoding direction [15.74] (fig. 15.57). In this case a two-fold ambiguity occurs: pixels beyond the borders of the FOV are folded back onto other parts of the image and, if phase encoding is reduced by PAT, these parts of the image fold in a second

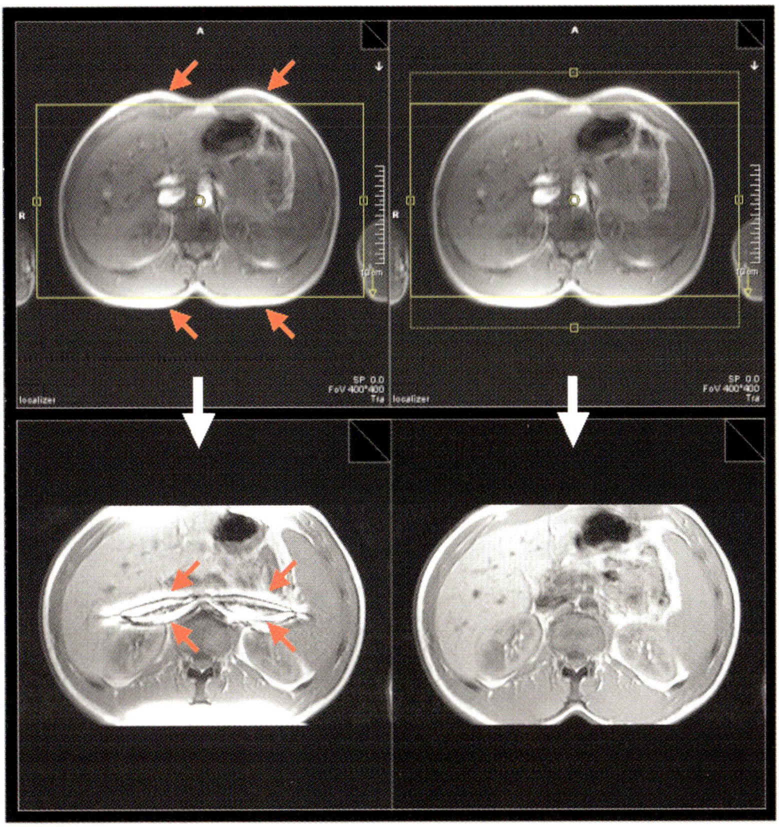

Figure 15.57
SENSE reconstruction of aliased images. **Left:** the selected FOV in phase encoding direction is smaller than the subject size (**upper row:** scout image with planned slice); the resulting aliasing cannot be handled by SENSE reconstruction (**lower row**), leading to severe artifacts. **Right:** folding is avoided by a few percent of phase over-sampling; the SENSE image is free of artifacts. Note that the additional time required for phase over-sampling reduces the net acceleration.

time. This problem does not occur in SMASH because the signal combination from the individual receiver channels takes place before the Fourier transform.

15.2.2.4 General technical aspects

The fact that PAT links the phase encoding process to the receiver coil geometry implies some noteworthy peculiarities. The most significant restriction is that PAT cannot be applied with the same flexibility as conventional, purely gradient-based imaging. The quality of the reconstructed image is strongly dependent on the encoding ability of the coil array. This implies a dependence on the selected phase encoding direction. Even coil arrays designed specifically for PAT allow only limited acceleration factors in certain phase encoding directions.

An inherent *SNR* reduction in parallel imaging is related to the applied coil array. Apart from the loss caused by the reduced number of Fourier line acquisitions, which leads to a relative *SNR* reduction by the square root of the acceleration factor, the data combination process may add a considerable amount of noise to the final image. Insufficient sensitivity variation or inappropriately located coils can result in excessive noise amplification. The so-called *g*-factor, which was originally introduced along with the SENSE technique [15.70], describes the amount of additional local *SNR* degradation (eq. 15.45):

$$SNR_{\text{accel.}}(x,y) = \frac{SNR_{\text{non-accel.}}(x,y)}{g(x,y)\cdot\sqrt{F}} \tag{15.45}$$

g: *g*-factor describing local *SNR* degradation, *F*: Acceleration factor

Note that the *g*-factor is not a constant in space. This leads to the phenomenon of intra-image *SNR* variation (sometimes even with sharp edges) commonly observed in parallel imaging. Simulated or measured *g*-factor maps are a common tool for investigating the parallel encoding capacity of coil arrays.

The relationship between coil setup and geometric scan parameters (phase encoding direction, size and position of the field of view) on the one hand and the resulting image quality on the other is confusing for most users because it is neither intuitive nor commonplace in conventional imaging. Moreover, even small changes in slice orientation (and hence the phase encoding direction) and FOV size can have a considerably adverse effect on image quality.

15.2.2.5 Coil calibration

The fact that PAT is based on the local sensitivity profiles of the receiving coils makes sensitivity calibration a crucial part of image reconstruction. PAT reconstruction requires precise information about the sensitivity vector (magnitude and phase) of each coil for each pixel. This causes substantial practical problems.

It warrants mention that it is not sufficient in most practical settings to work with a time-invariant set of coil maps that have been calibrated once. This simple approach does not work for the following reasons:

- Coils that are used routinely may be bent and moved to fit the patient.
- Coils always show a certain degree of mutual coupling, which varies with different settings.
- The actual sensitivity profile of a coil array will vary depending on its electrical environment (including the dielectric properties of the human body).

A method is therefore required that includes coil profile calibration upon each individual examination. In what follows, we discuss two basic approaches. The first involves acquiring a volume scan immediately prior to examination to serve as a basis for coil profile extraction (prescan method). The second approach involves incorporating the acquisition of calibration data into each examination scan (auto calibration method).

One would normally assume that sensitivity profiles change rather smoothly in space and that coil maps would thus not need to be measured at high resolution. However, this assumption is not valid if the location of a coil is too close to the body: both magnitude and phase are subject to strong local variations near the coil wires. This makes it necessary in practice to find a reasonable tradeoff between resolution and scan time for the prescan.

The prescan method

A calibration prescan is ideally performed only once per examination. However, any displacement of the patient or the coil after the calibration scan will lead to a mismatch when the image is reconstructed.

A 3D-scan is typically performed to cover the full imaging volume. Such a calibration scan still consists of a superimposition of the coil sensitivity profiles and the anatomically-induced signal variations. A common method of canceling the anatomical caused signal variation is to acquire the coil map twice: for one scan the local coil array is used for signal reception, for the second scan the large whole-body coil with its homogenous receive profile is used. Dividing each local coil image by the homogeneous body coil image results in a pure sensitivity map of the coil array.

Further processing may be necessary (e.g. interpolation to handle anatomical structures exhibiting very low signal strength such as lungs and bones.

The auto calibration method

The auto calibration method incorporates a few additional phase encoding lines into the acquisition process for each image. These lines are typically placed around the center of *k*-space, which would otherwise be generated by the PAT scheme (dotted lines in fig. 15.58). One thereby obtains a fully sampled region in the *k*-space center, which represents a low resolution image that is free of aliasing for each coil. The required individual coil sensitivity maps can be obtained by normalizing to the sum of the single images.

The effective image acceleration factor is reduced in proportion to the number of added calibration lines. In the case of high resolution scans (e.g. full 256-matrix size or

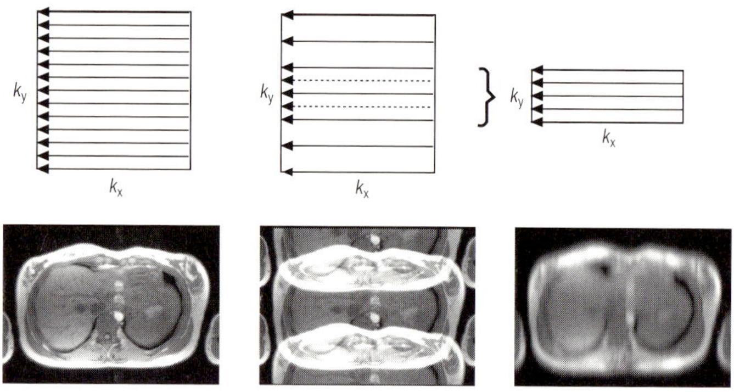

Figure 15.58
Coil map auto calibration. **Left:** non-accelerated acquisition. **Middle:** accelerated acquisition with a few lines added for auto calibration (dotted lines). **Right:** fully sampled central region of the accelerated scan provides a low resolution, but unfolded image that can be used to extract the coil sensitivity information.

higher), 12 additional lines are typically well tolerated while this number of additional lines might counteract the scan-time benefit of fast low-resolution scans. Given that each slice carries its own calibration data, the autocalibration method is hardly affected by potential changes in local coil profiles (e.g. due to patient movement).

PAT schemes based on k-space, in particular, benefit from the autocalibration approach. The explicit extraction of sensitivity calibration maps for each receiving coil can be skipped. As has been shown in the case of AUTOSMASH [15.67, 15.68] and as elaborated upon in further investigations, a procedure involving the direct fitting of the calibration lines to other measured lines provides the weighting coefficients for the signal combinations in advance. Interpolation problems within regions of low or vanishing signal strength do not occur.

Some *k*-space acquisition techniques even provide inherent calibration information. Radial scanning, where the *k*-space center is sampled much more densely than required by the sampling theorem, represents an example. As with AUTOSMASH, information can be generated from these samples to fill in for the missing values in the case of high *k*-values. Protocols for dynamic studies involving the continuous scanning of the same region represent another example [15.75]. For instance, each of the scans may be accelerated by a factor of two. If scans 1, 3, 5, ... skip every even line in *k*-space, and scans 2, 4, 6, ... skip the odd lines, then each set of two successive measurements will provide a fully sampled image that can be used to extract the PAT weighting factors. The assumption that the coil sensitivity variation between two successive measurements can be neglected is valid.

15.2.2.6 Applications-related aspects

PAT was originally introduced with a focus on imaging speed. Indeed, applications such as cardiac imaging and breath-hold abdominal imaging (including angiography) benefit from either shorter scan times or increased resolution. However, PAT provides a still wider range of applications. The two main areas center on improvements in image quality and reductions in RF power.

Reducing unwanted relaxation effects

Shorter acquisition times following the excitation pulse reduce signal loss due to T_2 and T_2^* decay, the most obvious example being single-shot imaging [15.76]. Single-shot, turbo-spin echo imaging is restricted in terms of resolution (T_2 signal decay along the echo train). Echo planar imaging (EPI) suffers from susceptibility-induced distortions due to T_2^* dephasing, leaving this method impractical for many applications. In both cases, image quality can be greatly improved by applying PAT for a reduction in the echo train length.

Furthermore, the contrast properties of certain sequences can be improved by shortening the readout period following magnetization preparation (e.g. after inversion or saturation pulses).

SAR reduction

The application of many RF pulses within a short time may lead to an unwanted heating of the subject within the scanner. For high field strengths, in particular 3 T and above, this effect becomes a limiting factor for many clinical imaging protocols. This is because the RF power per RF pulse is proportional to the square of the field strength. Given that it reduces the number of RF pulses, PAT can be deployed to keep imaging protocols within specific absorption rate (SAR) limits.

Drawbacks

Despite all of the benefits mentioned, PAT is also associated with a number of drawbacks:

- Gain in imaging speed and/or image quality is counteracted by a loss in *SNR*.
- Specific requirements related to the coil setup complicate application.
  This represents a potential source of image degradation.
- Coil calibration adds to total scan time.

PAT significantly increases the complexity of both software and hardware in clinical environments. A robust and flexible PAT implementation requires scanners that are equipped with a large number of independent receiver channels and appropriate coil arrays (PAT has introduced a completely new paradigm for RF-coil design). A large number of simultaneously receiving channels alone represents a demanding task in terms of data rate, storage space and image reconstruction speed. User dependence on the data acquisition scheme and local coil setup introduces questions such as: what is the maximum acceleration factor for a given phase encoding direction? Dedicated user interfaces (UI) must provide convenient support to facilitate the avoidance of unfavorable settings.

15.2.2.7 Conclusion

Parallel imaging has opened new horizons for MR imaging in terms of scan speed and improved applications. In turn, it has added a new level of complexity to MRI concerning all system components, ranging from RF electronics, data acquisition and image reconstruction to pulse sequence design and (last but not least) user interfaces.

15.2.3 Whole-body imaging

Some MRI examination types (e.g. spine imaging) require a field of view (FOV) along the magnet bore (z-direction) that is larger than the magnetic field's region of homogeneity (i.e. the intrinsic FOV). The natural approach to extended FOV imaging is to break up the desired z-range into smaller parts (stations). This then requires one to shift the patient position between the stations relative to the system's homogeneous region (isocenter) and to provide adequate coverage of local RF receiver coils for the extended FOV. The individual images can then be used separately or they can be combined into a composite image via a process called composing.

The development of extended FOV imaging was facilitated by the introduction of advanced scanner hardware such as patient tables capable of automatic movement and local RF coil arrays covering larger sections of the body. Fig. 15.59 shows an integrated patient table and local-coil concept that provide for automatic translation over a z-range of more than 2 m and table-mounted connections for up to 76 coil elements. Also shown is a composite multi-station image acquired in one contiguous exam on a 1.5 T MRI system with simultaneous reception by up to 32 individual RF receiver channels.

While extended FOV and whole-body imaging were developed from special applications involving standard scanners with intrinsic FOVs of approximately 0.5 m, the concept was a prerequisite for the development of imaging using ultra-short bore systems with much shorter intrinsic FOVs.

There are two groups of applications in which the scope of extended FOV imaging may encompass the whole body: examinations of the vascular system to determine the presence of malformations and atherosclerotic disease (see also section 15.2.4.3 on MR angiography) and metastasis imaging for the detection, characterization and staging of tumors. MRI competes in both of these areas with other imaging modalities, including X-ray imaging, CT, scintigraphy and PET. In many cases, MRI delivers at least equivalent diagnostic value, and may even provide additional diagnostic information thanks to its unique contrast mechanisms.

Angiography relies primarily on fast gradient-echo imaging and paramagnetic contrast agents. While peripheral angiography from the aorta to the foot has achieved the status of an accepted technique, whole-body applications have only been demonstrated recently [15.77, 15.78]. Efforts are being made to include cardiac imaging so as to provide comprehensive cardiovascular protocols. The resulting long examination times can be substantially shortened using parallel imaging techniques [15.79, 15.80].

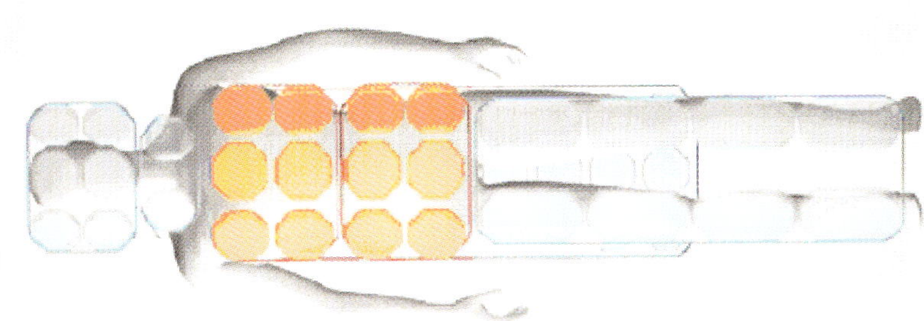

a)

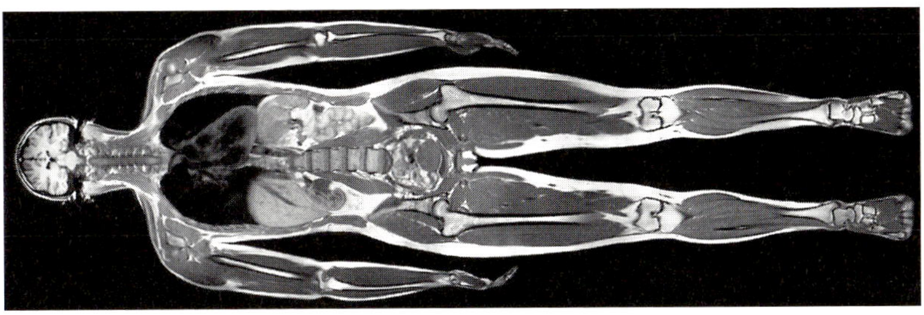

b)

Figure 15.59
Comprehensive coil setup **(a)** and composite multi-station whole-body MR image **(b)**

MRI is already the modality of choice in many areas of tumor diagnosis. Various MR imaging sequences have been deployed for metastasis screening, in particular short tau inversion recovery or STIR. Extensions to whole-body screening have recently been introduced [15.81].

The quality of extended FOV images is highly dependent on the accurate removal of geometric distortions induced by gradient nonlinearities in the MRI system. These cause a three-dimensional deformation that can be corrected via interpolation techniques. Given that the warping characteristics are time-invariant, each MRI system can be calibrated accordingly. The composing software uses the corrected images and their known positions to derive a single extended FOV image. A degree of station overlap is necessary to match images with remaining distortions.

Move during scan

One recent development involves the acquisition of data while the patient table is deliberately moved, a procedure referred to as move during scan (MDS) or continuously moving table MRI [15.82-15.84]. MDS removes the need to interrupt data acquisition between stations and is thus especially advantageous when the number of stations is high. Image deformations are minimized in that the data are mainly acquired from the isocenter. The remaining system-related spatial nonlinearities are distributed among the image data and therefore do not cause discontinuities between stations.

The movement of the object under investigation normally leads to unacceptable MR image artifacts. It is therefore necessary when using MDS to correct for the movement of the object during image acquisition and reconstruction. Two different approaches can be distinguished in this regard: one can place the readout gradient direction along the z-direction (direction of motion) or perpendicular to it. In the case of the latter approach (i.e. axial imaging), one can shift the excited slice along with the patient table by continually adjusting the system's center frequency (frequency sweeping). Doing so will entail that the image reconstruction process is the same as that in stationary cases. Frequency sweeping is of special importance in spin-echo imaging because the refocused slice is required to match the excited slice.

Coronal and sagittal slices are measured with a read-out gradient along the z-direction. It is necessary to correct the measured k_z-lines in Fourier space prior to image reconstruction in light of their acquisition at different object positions. Making use of the Fourier shift theorem, the known spatial shift of the object can be compensated for by multiplying the k_z-lines by a phase factor that takes the table speed into account.

Encouraging results have been presented based on various hardware setups, ranging from manually moved patient tables to shielded system table drives and from the RF body coil to integrated local coil arrays. Modern systems are already designed for MDS compatibility. One point of inquiry that has just recently appeared in the literature is that of system adjustments (e.g. the RF transmit level, which is dependent on the changing coil load). The resulting problems here include varying signal intensities along the z-direction and difficulties remaining within the limits of RF power deposition. Significant gradient nonlinearities are generally harder to correct for in MDS imaging owing to the fact that every *k*-space line is affected differently.

The targeted applications for MDS are the same as those for multi-station approaches: angiography [15.85] using coronal slices and metastasis screening [15.86] based on axial slices.

Discussion and conclusion

The advantages of multi-station whole-body imaging over MDS center on the fact that it can be performed with any desired orientation, FOV, resolution and station order. Furthermore, any contrast mechanism can be used without additional requirements relating to experimental design and image reconstruction. Only composing, if desired, will require sufficient overlap in the spatial coverage.

MDS has not yet reached the stage of product implementation. Data acquisition and image reconstruction are much more interdependent, making it difficult to vary imaging parameters over the course of an acquisition. Nevertheless, MDS would seem to be a promising complement to multi-station approaches, especially in settings where scanning time is crucial and where the intrinsic z-FOV is short.

Whole-body imaging as a diagnostic concept has made its way into clinical practice. It is on the verge of replacing examinations based on ionizing radiation and can be expected to lead to in a variety of new diagnostic possibilities. Future applications are likely to consist of flexible combinations of whole-body and locally focused MR imaging.

15.2.4 MRI and macroscopic motion

15.2.4.1 Real-time imaging

Real-time MRI involves the acquisition of data on a time scale comparable to the motion that occurs during the investigation of a patient. Real-time (RT) imaging is comprised of two major aspects:

- RT acquisition, i.e. acquiring images fast enough to freeze the process under investigation (e.g. the motion of an object)
- RT display to enable RT control, i.e. presenting images fast enough after completing the measurement to allow the observer to control the process

RT acquisition is used to either measure a static snapshot image only or to record the motion in time for the sake of a detailed study later.

Typical uses for RT acquisition include the imaging of cardiac-wall motion, contrast angiography and functional imaging. The periodicity of heart motion during a breath-hold enables one to stretch out the acquisition of data over several heartbeats. However, RT imaging is used for scouting, for cases of severe arrhythmia and whenever ECG data are unavailable (see section 15.2.6.2).

Further applications in which RT display figures prominently include interventional MRI fluoroscopy to control the insertion of a device and bolus timing where one monitors the arrival of a bolus of contrast agent into the field of view (FOV) before starting an angiography measurement.

RT acquisition

The timescale for the real-time condition depends on the application:

Given the necessity in cardiac imaging of freezing cardiac-wall motion, a time resolution of better than 150 ms is required. Functional imaging, on the other hand, requires the distinguishing of activation states with switching times of around one full second.

Achieving the real-time condition is a matter of minimizing the measurement time for an image while maintaining sufficient image quality. The measurement process for an image must fulfill two basic requirements. First, it must create enough signal intensity to achieve a sufficient signal-to-noise ratio in the image. Second, it must cover enough of the *k*-space to achieve sufficient image quality (i.e. spatial resolution and low intensity undersampling artifacts). These two requirements are directly linked. While the time needed to traverse *k*-space can be reduced by increasing the bandwidth of the acquired signal, doing so will also increase the signal's noise level. It will thus be necessary to arrive at an acceptable trade-off within the limitations posed by the scanner's gradient and RF systems and within the physiological limits of permissible RF power deposition and gradient-induced nerve stimulation.

The high signal amplitudes created by the trueFISP sequence make it especially suitable for most RT imaging applications. It can be combined with magnetization preparation pulses (e.g. dark-blood pulses to null the inflowing blood signal) in order to achieve contrasts other than its inherent T_2/T_1 contrast. Given that maintaining the transverse steady state of trueFISP places high demands on the deployed system, it is sometimes replaced by FLASH for robust applications (despite FLASH's lower signal strength).

The time required for a single trueFISP readout line typically ranges from 2.2 to 3.5 ms. Measurement times for a fully sampled 128-by-128 point image thus range from 282 to 448 ms.

The duration of the slice-selective RF excitation is not negligible compared to the read-out time. It is therefore useful to maximize the amount of *k*-space data measured after an RF excitation. While the length of a read-out train is ultimately limited by T_2, flow-related, off-resonance and susceptibility artifacts dictate much tighter limits in most applications. With their extremely long readouts, EPI techniques are limited to functional imaging where the brain structure is stationary and the contrast only changes on a timescale that is long compared to the read-out length. Readouts are typically limited in most other applications to less than 6 ms. TrueFISP is especially sensitive to the pulse separation time, and is therefore typically run with a read-out duration of less than 2 ms.

The following methods are used to further reduce image acquisition time:

1. *Fractional k-space sampling*
   As has already been discussed in section 15.2.1, image acquisition time can be shortened when the image is reconstructed from signal data covering half of the *k*-space. However, additional lines in the *k*-space center are needed for phase correction. In practical applications, sufficient image quality can be achieved with partial *k*-space filling factors ranging down to 5/8. While iterative reconstruction techniques such as projection onto convex sets (POCS) [15.87] may increase image quality for low filling factors or permit a further reduction in the number of additional lines, they will increase the reconstruction time.
2. *PAT*
   The application of receiver coil arrays allows one to reduce imaging time by making use of the spatial sensitivity distribution of the individual coils (see section 15.2.2). The possible acceleration factor follows from the number of coils covering the FOV and the tolerable signal-to-noise ratio.
3. *Echo sharing*
   Data sharing between successive images represents a further method of increasing the image update rate. The simplest case is twofold line sharing, i.e. the splitting of the *k*-space into two interleaved segments (e.g. one containing the odd and one containing the even Fourier lines). These segments are acquired in an alternating fashion. An image is reconstructed after the acquisition of each segment using data from this segment and the previously acquired one. Each image is therefore based on a complete *k*-space data set. Manifold line sharing corresponds to sliding window reconstruction. Note that echo sharing does not increase the temporal resolution of a single image, but provides interpolation between successive images.

4. *Keyhole methods*
   Increases in the size of a (structureless) object in an image go hand in hand with a greater concentration of corresponding signals near the center of k-space. Given that imaging parameters are normally adjusted to ensure that an image's important features always cover several pixels, the signals of these important features are well-concentrated around the center of k-space. These features can therefore be imaged with sufficient quality without measuring the outer portions of k-space. The image that results from this central portion of k-space is low pass filtered in phase encoding direction. To enhance this low-pass-filtered image, the data are combined with a sliding window data set of the outer portion of k-space. Only a fraction of the missing outer k-space lines is recorded for each image, so that the outer portion is fully updated only after several images. Skipping parts of the outer k-space lines for each image reduces image acquisition time. The keyhole method thus combines a low-pass-filtered image of high temporal resolution with a high-pass-filtered image of low temporal resolution. Many variations of this scheme exist. The success of this method depends on the shape and motion of the imaged object. The method is especially well-suited to monitoring needle advancement for biopsies and to placing ablation probes [15.88].
5. *Reduced FOV*
   This approach assumes that the moving object covers only a fraction of the FOV, while the rest of the image remains static. If the distance between k-space lines is increased (e.g. by omitting every second line), the object is aliased in the FOV, resulting in a discrete ambiguity as to where the object is really located. If the missing k-space lines are measured over several images, it will be possible to determine the true position of the object assuming that it has not moved from one aliased position to another [15.89].
6. *Non-Cartesian sampling*
   Cartesian sampling is the most common method of covering k-space. Here, the data is collected in parallel equidistant lines. Non-Cartesian sampling schemes can also be used. The most prominent of these include spiral and radial sampling schemes. In the case of Cartesian sampling, signals from objects outside the FOV result in the display of these objects inside the FOV (fold-in artifact). While spiral and radial sampling schemes do not suffer from fold-in artifacts, they do lead to stripes starting at some distance from object edges. A certain amount of these artifacts can be tolerated in many applications, thus allowing one to reduce the number of acquired radial lines from the theoretically required number. Another advantage that radial and segmented spiral sampling schemes offer over Cartesian sampling schemes is that each line passes the centre of k-space and is thus of similar importance, making both schemes ideally suited to manifold-echo sharing. Furthermore, the fact that radial schemes oversample the centre of k-space means that they can automatically provide a keyhole mechanism.
7. *Roadmap*
   A further technique that is deployed to provide real-time MRI information involves the display of dynamic information (e.g. in a small FOV) or fast visualizations of in-

strument positions on a previously acquired high resolution roadmap. Here, the roadmap might be a slice that is automatically selected from a 3D data set to contain the instrument position.

RT display and control

The real-time display of images is necessary only if the observer needs to react to them to either influence the imaging process or the situation displayed in the image. This places limits on the permissible lag time between the measurement and the real-time display. The bolus timing sequence that the observer uses to ascertain the arrival of the bolus in the FOV and thus to ascertain the optimal starting time for the angiographic measurement represents an example.

A further example is interventional imaging where the operator is required to observe tools such as needles, catheters and guide wires that are inserted into the patient. The particular tool can be made visible either by passive or active features. While susceptibility differences to surrounding tissue create a signal void and attached markers exhibiting a short T_2 appear bright, it is also possible to furnish the tool with a tiny receiver. The operator may use the RT image to reposition the device. Given that only a thin slice is measured in most applications – a slice that the device might leave when repositioned – it is useful to be able to adjust the slice position on the fly. In light of the fact that the operator will need to access the patient inside the magnet during intervention, the relevant visualization and control devices will need to be situated inside the RF cabin next to the patient table and will also need to be compatible with the MR data acquisition. Fig. 15.60 shows an MRI console with a track ball as an input device.

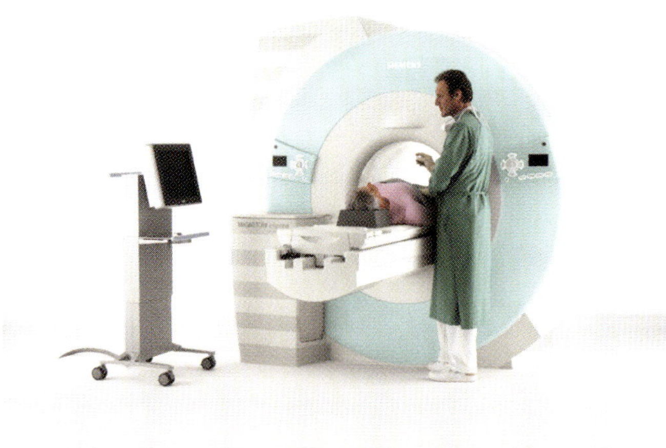

Figure 15.60 MRI-guided needle biopsy

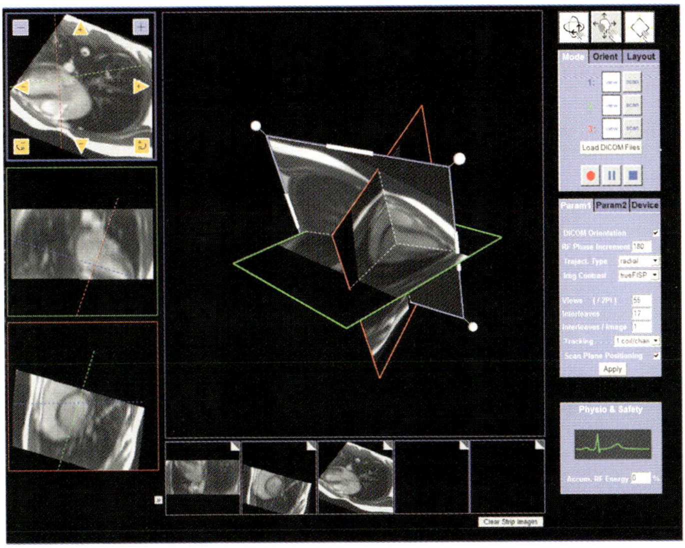

Figure 15.61 User interface (UI) for interactive scanning

Letting the scanner follow the device automatically represents an alternative to interactive positioning whenever the device is equipped with an active signal source, e.g. a tiny receive coil (tip tracking [15.90]). The position of the signal source and thus the position of the device can be automatically determined by recording a few non-slice selective projections between images. The image plane for the next image is then adjusted to contain the signal source. If the device is equipped with more than one signal source, one will be able to track both the position and the orientation of the device.

Presently available computing power and image-reconstruction algorithms enable one to deploy all of the described methods of accelerated image acquisition in conjunction with RT image display.

Fig. 15.61 shows a prototype of an interactive user interface (UI) for an MRI scanner. The real-time images are displayed and can be manipulated in three-dimensional space. Diverse imaging parameters such as scan-plane orientation, image contrast and time resolution can be adjusted interactively. The scan-plane center can be tracked if the device is equipped with a micro coil.

15.2.4.2 Motion correction

In various MR applications motion can detrimentally influence results and image quality. Various strategies of avoiding and dealing with motion artifacts have been invented in the ongoing development of MR imaging.

The use of methods such as triggering and gating to control image acquisition and reconstruction in response to periodic motion (e.g. motion associated with breathing and heart beat) is widespread. The emerging capabilities built into modern MRI systems allow to process data and even adapt pulse-sequences in real-time. Due to the enormously increased computational power, advanced methods for dealing with motions have been developed.

In general one can differentiate between retrospective and prospective approaches. In case of the retrospective methods after acquisition data is suitably processed and reconstructed taking information about the motion into account. In contrast using prospective methods, the motion information is evaluated in real-time and used for motion compensation by feeding back to the measurement system.

Triggering and gating

Triggering (also referred to as prospective gating) may offer a solution for periodic motion whose intervals match or are quicker than the acquisition time. One major area of application involves imaging of the heart or abdomen where motion due to breathing and/or the cardiac cycle occurs. Input for triggering includes physiological signals acquired via external devices (e.g. breathing belt, pulse oxymeter, ECG). MR signals such as navigators can also be used to supplement the necessary information.

In case of triggering, the input signal is used to monitor the motion and perform all steps required within the acquisition in a similar state of the motion. All other states are thus masked out. The trigger signal is generated when a striking feature appears in the physiological signal (e.g. R-wave in ECG). A certain pause may be required after the triggering event in order to start the acquisition during a desirable or advantageous phase (e.g. diastole). A certain amount of time can be used to acquire data depending on the state of the motion involved, the speed of the motion and the imaging technique used. For example, the standard time-frame used in cardiac MRI for imaging during systole is less than 50 ms while it may range from 200 to 300 ms during diastole. Further *k*-space lines or, for instance, data from other slices are acquired in subsequent trigger intervals.

Retrospective gating is performed vice versa to triggering. Data are acquired continuously and assigned to different states of motion on the basis of the physiological data. To a certain extent this permits successful imaging in cases of arrhythmia, given that the individual intervals can be adapted to one another retrospectively. This requires assumptions to be made about the progression of the motion within a motion cycle, which represents a challenging problem – in particular in cardiac imaging there this can be demanding, as the heart moves rapidly during systole and comparatively slowly during diastole.

Navigators

Additional MR experiments, which are not necessary for image formation, but provide information about the state of motion of an organ or a part of the body, are referred to as navigators or navigator scans.

The fastest navigator technique is the acquisition of a one-dimensional projection of an excited slice or volume. 1D information from a pencil-shaped region can also be collected. This region can be excited by a spin-echo technique where excitation and re-

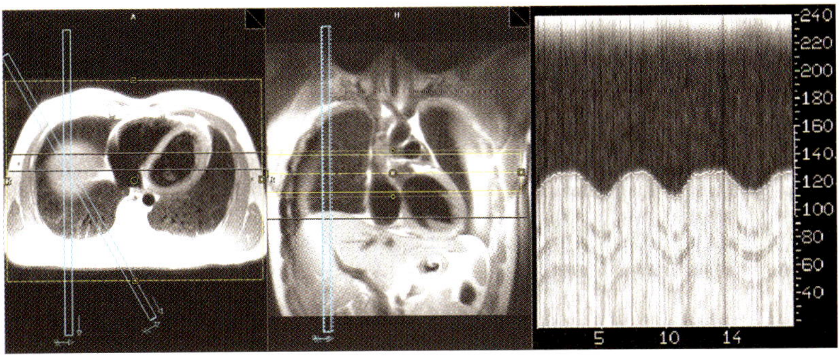

Figure 15.62
Creation of a navigator pencil through the diaphragm. Signal from the pencil-shaped region is evoked by angulating an excitation and a refocusing slice.

focusing pulses address differently angulated slices. Thus the spin-echo signal results from the intersection area. Care has to be taken to make sure that the additional navigator excitations do not adversely affect the imaging experiment (fig. 15.62). Alternatively, a navigator pencil or any other arbitrarily shaped volume can be defined by using 2D or 3D excitation pulses. The MR signal of the excited volume is read out using a 1D spatial-encoding method. The acquisition of a navigator usually takes less than 30 ms and can thus be smoothly incorporated into most MRI techniques.

Fig. 15.62 shows a navigator measurement providing information about the position of the diaphragm, i.e. the possibility of acquiring the actual state of breathing. This information can be used in combination with ECG data to enable MR imaging of the heart by triggering as well as gating. Furthermore, one can also use position information to adapt the position of the imaging slice. This tracking can be used to remain within the acceptance window of the trigger as long as possible even if breathing characteristics change.

The navigator methods described can be extended arbitrarily. Longer navigation scans can be performed depending of the speed of the motion that is to be detected. This may also include complete 2D imaging experiments. One example involves examinations of the liver using transversal slices. Patients are often not able to hold their breath long enough to permit the complete acquisition of all of the desired slices at once. The examination is therefore divided into multiple breath-holds. A coronal GRE image is acquired at the beginning of each breath-hold (fig. 15.63). The use of a low flip angle ensures that no noticeable saturation of the magnetization occurs and the subsequent imaging remains unaffected. By evaluating the GRE image one can detect and compensate for differences in the breath-hold positions. Shifts along a predefined vector or even a 2D shift vector including image rotation can be detected from such data by applying the methods described in the next section. Alternatively the breathing pattern can be observed by subsequent application of the navigator scan. Whenever a comparable position occurs, the imaging process is started.

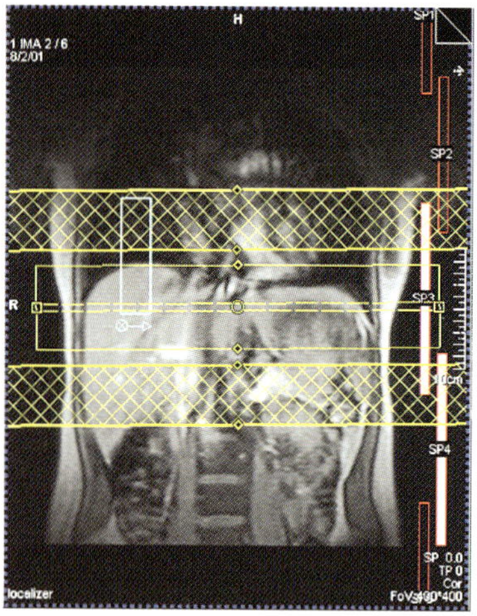

Figure 15.63
Coronal navigator scan for planning a liver examination in multiple breath-holds. A coronal image is acquired as a 2D navigator. The information contained in the turquoise rectangle is used to estimate the breathing phase.

If 3D motion or position information is necessary, usually a full spatially encoded acquisition of a volume cannot be performed due to temporal constraints. In some cases the desired information can be obtained by running several 1D navigation scans. Likewise, subsets of the full k-space may already contain all of the relevant information. A technique referred to as the orbital navigator or spherical navigator technique may be promising if the object that is to be imaged is completely contained within the measurement volume and does not deform. A rotation in the frequency domain results in the same rotation in the temporal domain. In contrast a translation only affects the phase of the Fourier-transformed data, while the rotation changes both the phase and the magnitude. This allows to separate the problem of object shifts and rotations into two separate problems in k-space. First an annulus in k-space is acquired using a navigator scan. Then the rotation is determined (e.g. by applying a cross-correlation method to the magnitude of data acquired at two different object positions). Finally, after correcting the data for the rotation effect, the phase difference of the annulus data can be used to detect shifts.

The extension of this method to 3D is possible. The information on a sphere in k-space is acquired fully or partially after the excitation of the measurement volume [15.91, 15.92]. The magnitude of the k-space data is again analyzed in the first step to separate the translation from the rotation.

The method of orbital and spherical navigators is based on the properties of the Fourier-transform. Also the strongest restrictions of these techniques are based on these properties. If the object deforms or if parts of it leave the measurement volume, the k-space data will change completely, because the magnitude and phase of each point in k-space depend on the complete image information. The method presented thus presupposes that the object that is to be measured is a rigid body that is completely contained within the navigator's FOV and will remain within this FOV despite the occurrence of motion. It follows that this method would seem to be promising for implementing motion correction in the head. Still, it warrants bearing in mind that the neck will violate the FOV requirement. This results in limitations with respect to the size of the motions that are detectable and detection accuracy.

Image-based motion detection and correction

In the present section, we present several methods of image-based motion correction. In general, we assume that the acquired image data are free of motion artifacts. However, looking at the time course of data motion effects are evident. Examples include the multi-breath-hold technique discussed above and applications such as BOLD and first-pass perfusion imaging. In the latter cases the information is contained in temporal changes in contrast behavior. Thus motion will affect the analysis of time domain voxel vectors. Discussions of the methods presented in the following are often referenced using the term image registration [15.93].

To determine changes in the position of image information, a suitable measure for similarity of different datasets must be defined. One may simply use the center of gravity of an image, where the definition follows the one used in mechanics:

$$\vec{r}_S = \frac{\sum I_j \cdot \vec{r}}{\sum I_j} \tag{15.46}$$

Here, voxel j has the position vector r_j and the brightness I_j. The difference vector of the center of gravity of two images can be used to calculate a shift. The magnitude of the difference vector can thus be regarded as a kind of similarity. It should be noted here that this instructive example will usually not lead to good results in practice.

If there is no major change in contrast between the images that are to be aligned, a valuable method is the search for transformation parameters q (e.g. spatial shift and/or rotation), which minimize the magnitude of the difference image. An additional spatially independent linear scaling of the intensity values is usually incorporated. This yields:

$$|X - c \cdot Y(q)| = min \tag{15.47}$$

Here, X is the voxel vector of all intensity values in the reference image. Y is created in the same way from a second image, which one will want to align to the reference data using the transformation parameters q. One may conduct a search for the minimum in a certain region of the data or for the complete image data available. The best transformation may be found by brute force if the transformation does not involve too many variables q, the amount of motion is known a priori to be small and demands for accuracy are not too high. In general, searching the complete parameter space is not a realistic approach, especially if the requirement for accuracy is below voxel size.

As is the case for most minimization problems, efficient algorithms are available that enable one to robustly find optimal solutions for typical data, although these algorithms may fail in the case of degenerate data. The Gauss-Newton method presented below requires a certain amount of smoothness in the similarity criterion when changing the transformation parameters [15.94]. The first step is a linearization of the problem:

$$X = \underbrace{\begin{pmatrix} \frac{\partial Y_1}{\partial q_1} & \cdots & \frac{\partial Y_1}{\partial q_m} & Y_1 \\ \cdot & \cdots & \cdot & \cdot \\ \frac{\partial Y_n}{\partial q_1} & \cdots & \frac{\partial Y_n}{\partial q_m} & Y_n \end{pmatrix}}_{A} \cdot \underbrace{\begin{pmatrix} q_1 \\ \cdot \\ q_m \\ c \end{pmatrix}}_{q} + O(q^2) \tag{15.48}$$

Here, q_1 ... q_m and c are the transformation parameters. $\partial Y_n / \partial q_m$ gives the rate of change of voxel n when altering q_m. These local derivatives can for example be estimated by applying a small transformation to the data and calculating the differential quotient. The linear system given is usually heavily overestimated. E.g. when looking for rigid body motion in 3D, 7 transformation parameters are to be estimated (3 for shift, 3 for rotation, 1 for scaling). The number of voxels typically ranges from 10^4 to 10^7. The least squares solution of the linearized problem can be calculated by using a Moore-Penrose pseudoinverse, while the higher orders of (15.48) are neglected here:

$$\begin{aligned} \vec{X} &= A \cdot \vec{q} \\ \Rightarrow A^T \cdot \vec{X} &= A^T \cdot A \cdot \vec{q} \\ \Rightarrow (A^T \cdot A)^{-1} \cdot A^T \cdot \vec{X} &= \vec{q} \end{aligned} \tag{15.49}$$

If the linearization was a good idea and the higher orders do not dominate, the solution q can be calculated by using an iterative approach. In practice, it is useful to exchange the reference data X for the data Y that are to be aligned, as it is not necessary to recalculate matrix A. In fact, matrix A remains the same for all iterations and all alignments to the same reference image. Fig. 15.64 shows the progress of an optimization process when using the presented algorithm. It can be shown that the accuracy of the detection is not limited by voxel-size, but by noise, artifacts and the characteristics and imperfections of the sampling process used. When applied to BOLD imaging using a voxel-size of 3 by 3 by 3 mm^3, motion can be detected with an accuracy of 100 microns and 0.2 degrees within a few tenths of a second [15.95].

A further very robust method of motion estimation, often referred to as cross entropy, joint entropy and mutual information (see chapter 4), is based on the assumption that the joint or mutual information of two images is maximal if they have been aligned successfully. The amount of joint information is estimated using statistical methods borrowed from information theory. The Shannon entropy for a common distribution $p(i,j)$ is defined as:

$$H(A,B) = \sum_{i,j} p(a,b) \cdot log(p(a,b)) \tag{15.50}$$

The two-dimensional histogram of two datasets that are to be aligned is often used as a common distribution. The fraction of voxels at identical voxel-positions that have intensity value a in dataset A and value b in B is expressed as $p(a,b)$. The transformation that maximizes the mutual information $H(A,B)$ yields the registration of the datasets.

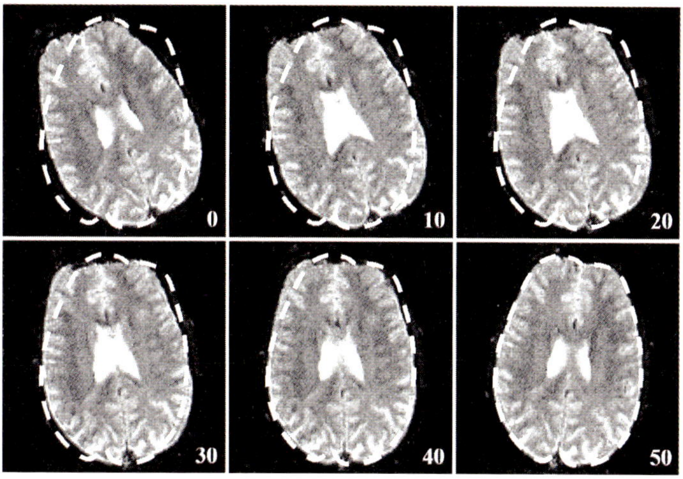

Figure 15.64
Iterative alignment of a 3D dataset to reference data (contour dotted) using a Gauss-Newton method. A transversal slice from a volume is shown after 0, 10, 20, 30, 40 and 50 iterations.

The search for the maximum can usually be conducted using the simplex algorithm. In the most cases H changes smoothly and for a not too large initial misregistration the danger of terminating in a local maximum is low. The proposed similarity measure is dependent on the overlap of image information. This problem can be reduced using the following normalized method [15.96]:

$$NMI = \frac{H(A) + H(B)}{H(A,B)} \tag{15.51}$$

Mutual information methods offer the advantage of enabling one to align datasets with very different contrast behavior. In particular, no prior knowledge of the contrast dependencies is required. This gives these methods a broad range of application, e.g. when it comes to the fusion of data generated by different imaging modalities (e.g. MR-CT, MR-PET). One major disadvantage is based on the statistical approach. A large number of independent voxels is required to achieve a reliable estimate of the entropy. The method is therefore not suitable for handling registration problems involving low resolution or local problems involving a focus on a small portion of the image.

Related to the mutual information methods are similar techniques for reducing motion artifact within single images or datasets [15.97]. After the repeated reconstruction of an image based on the MR raw data using different motion models, the entropy of the magnitude image is calculated. The motion artifacts can be reduced by maximizing the entropy. Such methods are demanding in computational terms because they involve a considerable number of reconstructions.

If the transformation for matching two datasets is known, a correction of the image data is required. In general this is performed via interpolation, as it is necessary to calculate intensity values for positions between the originally sampled voxels. Although still quite often used, simple linear interpolation is only acceptable in few cases because it involves considerable data degeneration. The most striking artifact is image blurring after linear interpolation.

Given that the full information of a band-limited continuous signal is contained in the finite number of samples, it is perfectly possible to reconstruct all values that lie between the known sample values. It can be inferred from digital signal processing theory that Whitakker reconstruction is the solution for this task. A convolution of the sampled data-points with a sinc function is performed. The sinc is placed where a value shall be interpolated. Given that the sinc-function decays only reciprocally, the influence of the convolution is assumed to be negligible for larger distances to the origin. Usually the sinc is apodized by multiplication with a Hanning window function. Typical window widths are 3 to 5 neighboring sample points to each side of the point that is to be interpolated. The values of 216 to 1,000 neighboring points have to be taken into consideration for the 3D case in order to reconstruct a single value. While this method is accurate, it is quite inefficient.

If the problem is not a general transformation but a rigid-body transformation (i.e. shifts and rotations), the so-called k-space methods are attractive. In contrast to general interpolation, the points that are to be resampled are placed in a systematic scheme. The simplest case is that of a translation in which all of the image-space points that are to be resampled have the same distance to the measured neighboring values. Given that a shift in image space is identical to an additional phase in k-space, the translation can be applied by the multiplication of a linear phase to the Fourier transformed data (Fourier shift theorem). One can extend Fourier interpolation to rotations by decomposing the rotation matrix to three shears (shown here for the 2D case [15.98]):

$$\begin{pmatrix} \cos\alpha & -\sin\alpha \\ \sin\alpha & \cos\alpha \end{pmatrix} = \begin{pmatrix} 1 & -\tan\frac{\alpha}{2} \\ 0 & 1 \end{pmatrix} \cdot \begin{pmatrix} 1 & 0 \\ \sin\alpha & 1 \end{pmatrix} \cdot \begin{pmatrix} 1 & -\tan\frac{\alpha}{2} \\ 0 & 1 \end{pmatrix} \quad (15.52)$$

α: Angle of rotation

A shear in column direction operates as a row-wise growing translation of the image columns. These translations can be accomplished by the column-wise use of the Fourier shift theorem. The method is easy to use in 3D and can also be extended to non-isotropic voxels [15.99] that are often used in MR imaging. In a nutshell, the k-space methods allow for a very efficient solution to the interpolation problem and enable one to achieve a high quality result.

Readers may wish to refer to the literature on so-called b-splines for more information on how to solve general interpolation problems efficiently and achieve high quality results [15.100]. Splines of degree n construct a polynomial representation of degree n of the data that is $(n - 1)$ times continuously differentiable. Efficient methods of constructing splines and resampling data are available. Degrees of 3 to 5 are often used to achieve good quality.

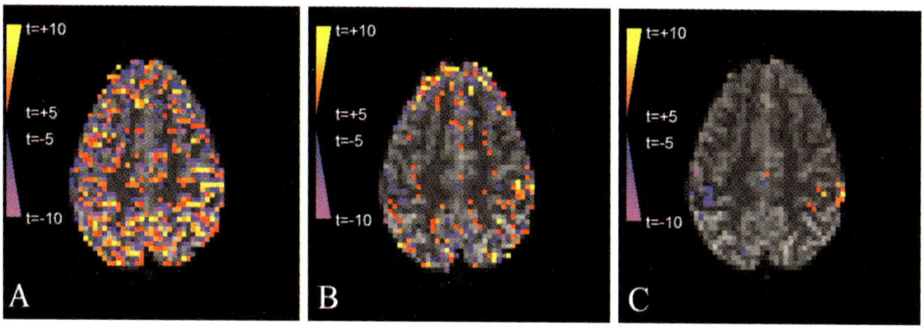

Figure 15.65
Results of a BOLD examination for identification of the motor areas. In this case, a strong stimulus-correlated motion of approx. 1.5 degrees was present. Voxels are colored if the statistical analysis of the BOLD data shows a significant relation between voxel time courses and stimulus. Image **C** shows the expected result, while artifacts dominate the other data. **A**: Result without any motion correction. **B**: Result when using retrospective correction. **C**: Result when using a prospective approach.

The results of image-based motion detection are suitable for more than retrospective correction via interpolation. With the use of modern computer systems, such methods have been run in real time for a number of years. In addition one can prospectively adjust the measurement coordinate system using image-based motion information [15.99]. This has been successfully implemented for BOLD imaging (fig. 15.65). Here, a new dataset of the brain is generated every 2 to 4 seconds. This data can be used to analyze the position of the brain and correct the measurement prospectively throughout the experiment. This enables one to suppress motion artifacts more efficiently as compared to retrospective methods.

15.2.4.3 MR angiography (MRA)

The clinical significance of MR angiography (MRA) has grown rapidly since its first implementation in the early/mid 1980s. MRA offers a number of advantages over conventional angiography. When applied without a contrast agent, it is noninvasive, using the intrinsic mechanisms of blood flow to depict flow. By going beyond the mere depiction of vascular anatomy to provide insight into underlying functions, MRA gives one access to important information that is not available via conventional angiography. The three components that form the basis of MRA include the time-of-flight technique (TOF), the phase effect, and the use of MR contrast agents to detect blood flow in a more indirect fashion [15.101, 15.102]. These components can be used to generate MR angiograms, evaluate vessel stenoses, detect flow direction and quantify blood flow. Although the use of contrast agents prevents MRA from achieving the attractive status of an entirely noninvasive procedure, it does qualify as a minimally invasive procedure, given that the contrast agents involved are delivered only intravenously and in small amounts.

15.2.4.3.1 The time-of-flight approach (TOF)

TOF is the most common angiographic technique [15.103]. The technique involves the excitation of slices or volumes via the application of an RF-pulse repetition time (T_R) that is shorter than the T_1 of the stationary tissue. Lacking sufficient time to regain their longitudinal magnetization, the spins produce no more than a dim signal.

Blood outside the imaging volume is not affected by the slice-selective RF pulses. As it flows into the imaging slice with full magnetization, it produces a bright signal and gives rise to inflow enhancement or flow-related enhancement (fig. 15.66). The vascu-

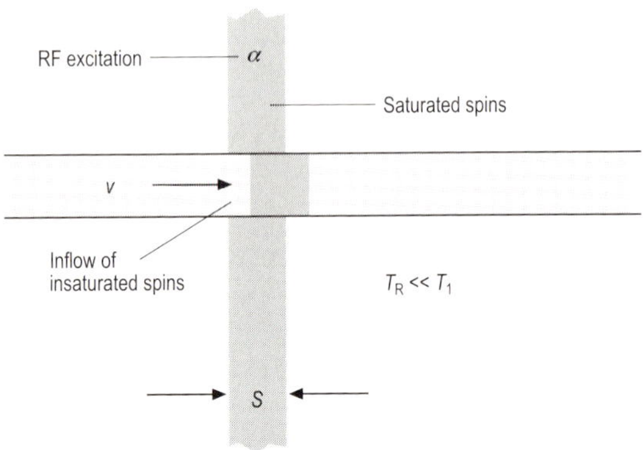

Figure 15.66
Principle of inflow enhancement. All tissues in the slice are partially saturated, and produce little signal, particularly when the T_R is much shorter than the T_1 of the tissue in the slice. Blood flow that is perpendicular to the slice replaces partially saturated spins with unsaturated spins of maximum magnetization.

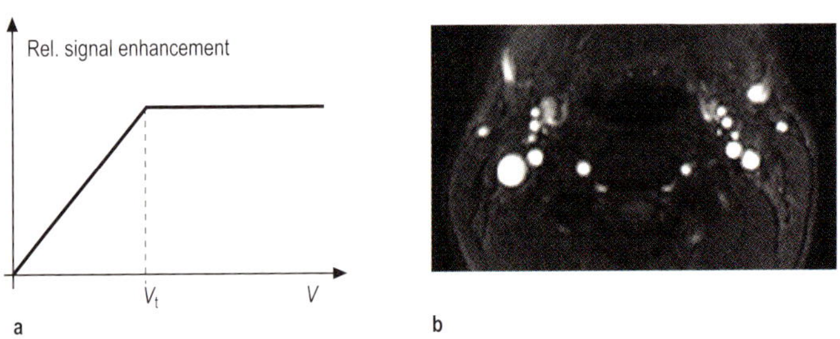

Figure 15.67
Signal enhancement as a function of blood flow **(a)**. The signal intensity of blood flowing at a constant velocity *v* perpendicular to the imaging slice increases in proportion with the flow velocity, given that more spins are replaced by unsaturated spins at higher velocities. Signal enhancement terminates at the transit velocity v_t, when all of the spins within the slice have been replaced during one T_R interval. This is demonstrated in an axial image through the neck **(b)**. The background tissues are partially saturated, and show only little signal intensity. All blood vessels are displayed with high contrast due to inflow enhancement.

lar signal in TOF increases linearly with the velocity of blood until it reaches a plateau at which all of the spins within the slice have been replaced by fully magnetized spins after each RF pulse (fig. 15.67). For flow orthogonal to the imaging slice, the transit velocity v_t at which the blood has been completely replaced can be expressed as

$$v_t = \frac{s}{T_R} \qquad (15.53)$$

where T_R is the repetition time and s is the slice thickness. The total replenishment of spins for a given T_R occurs at lower velocities for thin slices than for thick slices.

Dependence on sequence parameters

MRA offers considerable flexibility when it comes to the depiction of flow. Flow typically appears bright, but it can also be made to appear dark. Flow contrast in TOF varies in accordance with a number of image parameters, including T_R, echo time (T_E), flip angle (FA), size of the imaging volume, pixel size and slice orientation. Angiographic contrast also depends on flow conditions such as velocity, pulsatility and vessel tortuosity. A good understanding of how the sequence parameters affect vascular contrast enables one to tailor sequences to specific applications.

RF pulses are delivered at a T_R that is much shorter than the T_1 of the tissue to cause effective spin saturation and to suppress background signal. Typical T_R values range from 20 to 50 ms. A shorter T_R will also result in a shorter acquisition time. This offers further incentive to select short T_R values. However, one should avoid making the T_R values too short, as doing so may leave too little time for the inflow of fresh spins.

Effective saturation is also achieved by using large FA values. However, the same RF pulses that reduce the tissue signal can also affect the blood signal. This is particularly true in the case of slow-moving blood that spends a relatively long time within the imaging volume, thereby resulting in a diminished signal. A long T_R and a small FA should be used to minimize the blood's spin saturation and maximize its signal. Unfortunately, this leads to a relatively high background signal and low flow contrast (the difference in signal between flowing blood and stationary tissue). The selection of T_R and FA therefore represents a compromise between saturating background tissue and not saturating blood. The optimal values for T_R and FA depend on the blood velocity and the anatomic distances to be covered. Typical FA values range from 15° to 35° for three-dimensional (3D) TOF and from 30° to 60° for two-dimensional (2D) TOF.

Inflow can be maximized when performing 2D acquisition by positioning the imaging slice perpendicular to the direction of flow. This effectively replenishes the slice with fresh spins and permits one to use a large flip angle excitation for maximum flow contrast. A large FA is associated with an increase in ghost artifacts resulting from pulsatile flow. One should refrain from placing the imaging slice in the plane of the vessel because slow-moving spins become progressively saturated, an effect that worsens as the flip angle is increased. This is known as in-plane saturation. When performing 3D TOF, the vessel segment of interest should be near the entry point for flowing blood and not at the far end of a large slab, where the flowing blood will already have been saturated.

The spins within a voxel move at different velocities in various directions when flow is incoherent. This leads to phase cancellation and therefore a loss of signal. This signal loss can be reduced by using smaller voxels (i.e. higher spatial resolution). Small voxels are therefore often used to better visualize small vessels, given a sufficient signal-to-noise ratio. 3D sequences usually yield a better signal-to-noise ratio for small voxels than 2D sequences.

Unwanted loss of flow signal also occurs as a result of phase dispersion within a voxel caused by turbulent flow. The amount of phase dispersion can be reduced by using flow compensation. Flow compensation works by establishing the phase alignment of the stationary and moving spins at the time of the echo. The phase angle ϕ of an ensemble of spins moving at velocity v follows from

$$\phi = \gamma \int_0^t G(t) r(t) \mathrm{d}t \tag{15.54}$$

The actual position r of a spin at movement with velocity v and acceleration a can be expressed as

$$r(t) = r_0 + vt + \frac{a}{2} t^2 + \ldots \tag{15.55}$$

so that

$$\phi(t) = \gamma \left(r_0 \int_0^t G(t) \mathrm{d}t + v \int_0^t t G(t) \mathrm{d}t + \frac{a}{2} \int_0^t t^2 G(t) \mathrm{d}t + \ldots \right) \tag{15.56}$$

The phase of stationary spins is determined by the 0th moment $\int G(t)\mathrm{d}t$, the phase of spins with uniform flow by the 1st moment $\int tG(t)\mathrm{d}t$, and the phase of accelerated spins by the 2nd moment $\int t^2 G(t)\mathrm{d}t$ of the applied gradient sequence.

The phase of stationary spins will not have been changed after the application of a bipolar gradient pulse, while the phase of uniform flow is restored only after the application of two back-to-back bipolar gradient pulses (fig. 15.68). This means that at least three gradient lobes are needed for velocity compensation (also referred to as first-order flow compensation). Higher order forms of motion, such as acceleration, are not refocused by first-order flow compensation and are best dealt with by using a short T_E. The TOF method typically uses a gradient-echo sequence with a short T_E and velocity compensation. Fig. 15.69 shows a pulse sequence diagram of a 2D TOF sequence that is flow-compensated along the read and slice-select directions. One can reduce T_E by sampling the echo earlier in time with an asymmetric echo.

Additional methods for background tissue suppression

Saturation is a particularly insufficient method of suppressing the background signal when fat tissue is present. An unwanted bright fat signal can present a problem for MRA of the thoracic, abdominal and peripheral vasculature. MRA can be performed with a T_E to switch the protons in fat and water out of phase and thereby minimize the

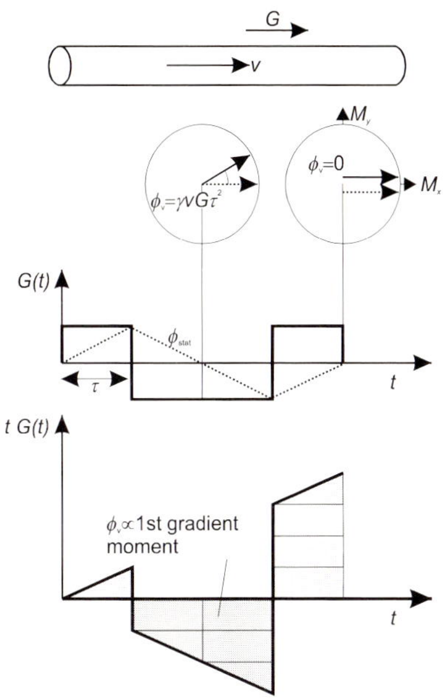

Figure 15.68
Development of the phase of stationary and moving spins during the application of gradient pulses. The phase of stationary spins is proportional to the area (0th order moment) under the gradient, the phase of uniformly flowing spins is proportional to the 1st order moment (the area under the function $tG(t)$). After a bipolar gradient stationary spins have no phase accumulated, while for the same effect at uniform flow two bipolar gradients are required.

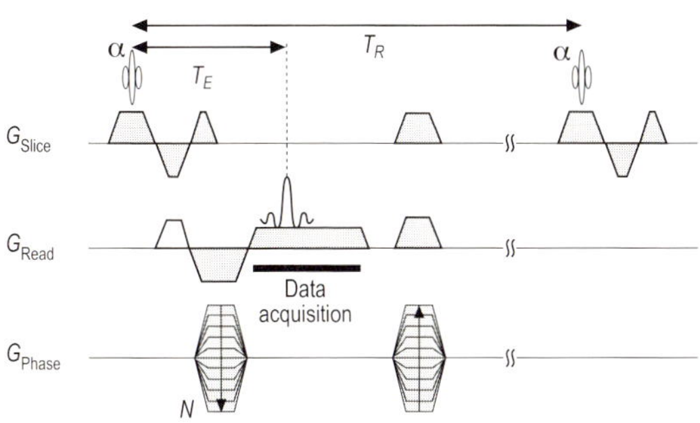

Figure 15.69
Pulse sequence for 2D time-of-flight MRA. First-order flow compensation is applied in the slice-select and read-out directions. Asymmetric sampling is applied during echo readout to keep the higher order moments of the readout gradients as small as possible.

fat signal. This occurs at approximately 7, 11.5, or 16 ms on a 1.5 T system. Given that the out-of-phase time is inversely proportional to the instrument's field strength, longer T_Es are recommended for lower field strengths. In general, the shortest possible echo time for out-of-phase fat and water is selected.

Selective saturation enables one to achieve a more complete suppression of the fat signal. This is particularly useful for MRA of the lower extremities. Effective fat suppression requires a homogeneous magnetic field. A selective water excitation that is less sensitive to field inhomogeneities and produces less inadvertent saturation of the arterial signal represents an alternative.

The background of stationary tissue can be further reduced by applying magnetization transfer (MT) pulses. The protons in bound water, which have a broad resonance peak compared to the sharp, narrow peak of protons in free water, are saturated with an off-resonance RF pulse. Water diffusion leads to an exchange between saturated bound protons and free water protons. This causes some of the free water protons to become saturated. MT tissue suppression is most effective when the ratio of bound to free water in a tissue is large. MT has been particularly effective in intracranial angiography where the large number of bound protons in brain parenchyma contrasts (grey and white matter) with the predominant free water in blood serum.

Selective presaturation

Given that arteries and veins are often companion structures, one will often be required to remove venous signal to gain an unobscured view of the arteries (and vice versa). This can be readily achieved by using a presaturation band to saturate the unwanted vessel, either upstream or downstream of the region of interest (fig. 15.70). In most applications, the presaturation band should be close to the acquired slice, and may partially overlap with it. A presaturation band that moves in tandem with the acquired slice in sequential 2D TOF is called a walking or a traveling saturation band.

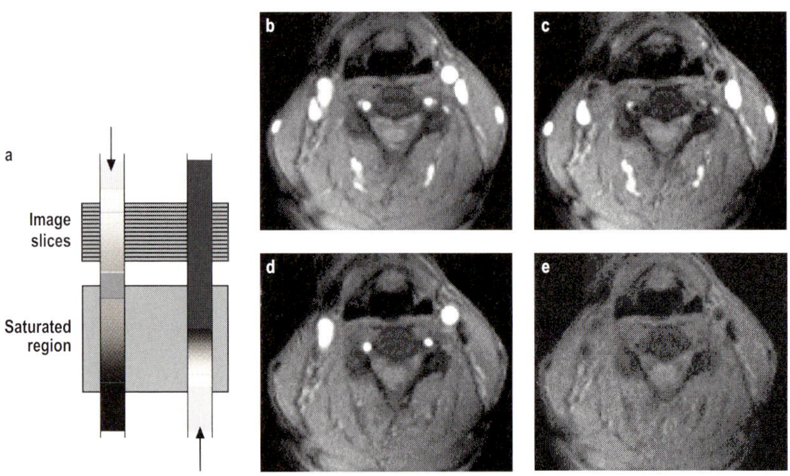

Figure 15.70
Spatial presaturation pulses are used to suppress venous or arterial flow depending on the flow direction. Similar strategies are applied for multi-slice 2D and 3D TOF techniques. The saturation band travels along with the imaging slice in the 2D technique to ensure that the distance between slice and saturation band remains constant irrespective of the slice's actual position. Saturation depends on the positioning of the saturation band relative to the slice and the flow direction **(a)**. The effect of the saturation band is demonstrated in the neck: **(b)** no saturation band, **(c)** arterial saturation, **(d)** venous saturation and **(e)** parallel saturation to remove all inflow effects.

Saturation bands may also be used to reduce flow artifacts or artifacts resulting from respiratory and/or cardiac motion. For example, a saturation band can be applied to the anterior chest wall to minimize ghost artifacts related to breathing. A clever use of saturation bands involves determining the feeding vessels of an arteriovenous malformation, the cervical vessels supplying a middle cerebral artery or the direction of flow. Placing a saturation band over the vessel causes all of the vessel's downstream branches to disappear from the angiogram.

Two and three-dimensional time of flight

TOF may be implemented either as a 2D or a 3D sequence. 2D TOF consists of individual thin slices that are acquired in a sequential fashion [15.101]. These slices are positioned perpendicular to the direction of the blood flow to maximize inflow effects. One proceeds by acquiring a first slice, and then acquiring a second slice adjacent to the first. The second slice is followed by a third, and so on. Note that this sequential method of slice acquisition is different from the familiar multi-slice 2D acquisition used in spin-echo imaging in which the slices are all acquired at once. Sequential 2D acquisition maximizes the inflow effect.

3D TOF offers substantially better spatial resolution than 2D TOF and has many useful clinical applications [15.104]. Here, rather thick slices (2 to 4 cm) are taken to subdivide the volume into smaller sections (< 1 mm) called partitions. The partitions exhibit no contiguity with interslice gaps. The increase in resolution, however, comes at a price. Blood is required to enter a larger volume and travel a longer distance within the imaging volume. The inflow effect persists for only a short distance into the volume before the signal from the blood is lost and the vessel intensity fades. The challenge is therefore to provide RF pulses that adequately suppress the background tissue without noticeably diminishing the blood signal. The selection of an optimal RF pulse is especially difficult in the case of imaging vessels with slow flow. Use of 3D TOF is therefore limited to vessels with moderately high rates of flow.

The progressive saturation of blood as it flows across a thick 3D TOF slab often results in high blood signal intensity at the entry side of the slab and lower signal intensity at

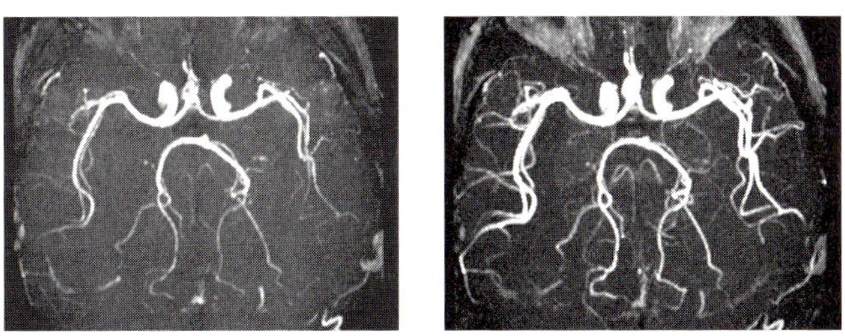

Figure 15.71
Signal intensity in a standard 3D TOF technique **(left)** drops towards the periphery of the intravascular system as a result of partial spin saturation effects as the spins travel through the imaging volume. The overall vessel contrast can be significantly increased by adding magnetization transfer contrast (MTC) and using a ramped RF pulse (TONE) **(right)**.

the exit side. This gradient in blood intensity may be partly corrected by gradually increasing the flip angle across the slab, a technique referred to as tilted optimized nonselective excitation (TONE). Lower flip angle values are applied at the entry side of the imaging volume to minimize saturation effects, and higher flip angle values are applied at the exit side to more distally maximize the blood signal. For instance, vascular structures at the inflow end of the slab (e.g. carotid siphons) can be made as bright as structures at the outflow end (e.g. small distal vessels) in a TONE 3D TOF axial acquisition of the circle of Willis. The effect of TONE and MT suppression is demonstrated in fig. 15.71. Although this technique is effective in improving the angiographic intensity across a 3D volume, it does not eliminate the tendency of vessels with slow flow to become saturated. It also presupposes that flow crosses the slab predominantly in one direction, which may not be the case in tortuous vessels such as renal arteries.

Some applications are best performed with 2D TOF, others with 3D TOF. These sequences are seldom interchangeable. The choice of 2D or 3D techniques is determined by several factors.

2D TOF is sensitive to slow blood flow. 3D TOF is often incapable of detecting vessels with slowly flowing blood (e.g. veins and peripheral arteries) because of spin saturation effects. This results from the difference in thickness between the volumes into which the blood is required to enter: a thin slice in the case of 2D and a thick slab in the case of 3D.

2D TOF can be acquired with breath-holding to minimize respiratory motion artifacts. This makes 2D a favorite sequence for abdominal venous studies, because the anatomy may be covered by a series of breath-holds. 3D TOF requires longer scan times and is typically not compatible with breath-holding.

3D TOF provides higher spatial resolution than 2D TOF. The partitions of 3D acquisition are usually less than 1 mm thick, which compares favorably with the 2-mm or thicker slices of 2D acquisition.

3D TOF is less susceptible to turbulent signal loss (e.g. within a stenotic segment) than 2D TOF. This results from a smaller voxel size. It thus makes sense to select a 3D TOF acquisition to grade the percent of stenosis within an internal carotid artery lesion and select a 2D TOF sequence to reliably visualize the slow flow beyond a stenosis.

The 3D multislab technique (also referred to as multiple overlapping thin-slab acquisition or MOTSA, represents an attempt to combine the advantages of 2D and 3D acquisition [15.105]. As the name suggests, the procedure centers on the generation of a series of thin-slab 3D acquisitions. Thin slabs are chosen to reduce blood saturation and to improve sensitivity to slow flow. The slabs are acquired with overlap because the slices at the end of a 3D slab often exhibit low signal intensity. The redundant slices are discarded. Otherwise, they would create a Venetian blind artifact in the projected image. MOTSA is currently the preferred technique when high-resolution images are required over a large anatomic area (e.g. in the case of the carotid and intracranial arteries).

In summary, 2D TOF techniques are used in peripheral MRA and in carotid MRA (when the slice orientation can be adjusted so that it is perpendicular to the arteries), but

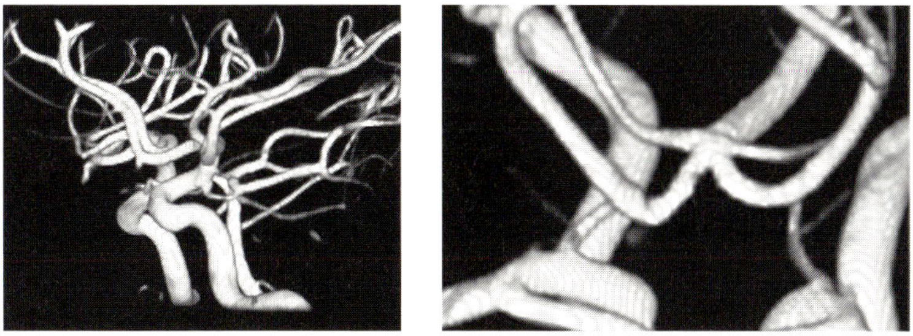

Figure 15.72
TOF MR angiography works better at 3 T due to the higher signal-to noise ratio (SNR) and longer T_1 times. Increased SNR can be used to improve the spatial resolution. In combination with parallel imaging techniques, the scan time is similar to that in 1.5 T systems. The result is a submillimeter resolution of 0.3 mm by 0.3 mm by 0.6 mm that offers exquisite vessel detail. **Left:** total imaging volume. **Right:** magnified view of the circle of Willis.

special care is required to ensure a correct interpretation of local signal losses and artifacts. The strengths of 3D TOF make it particularly useful for imaging the intracranial vasculature. Further improvements in 3D TOF MRA have arisen in connection with the higher field strengths that are becoming a more common element in clinical practice. Given the intrinsic increase in the signal-to-noise ratio that goes hand in hand with the higher field strengths, as well as the prolongation of T_1 times, 3D TOF techniques perform extremely well in the case of high fields (e.g. 3 T). The use of parallel imaging techniques enables one to noticeably reduce spatial resolution without increasing the scan time beyond a tolerable limit of several minutes (fig. 15.72).

Breath-hold acquisitions for thoracic and abdominal MRA

MRA of the thorax poses a greater challenge than intracranial MRA. This is due to motion artifacts caused by cardiac pulsation and respiration. The removal of such ghost artifacts requires fast acquisitions (e.g. high-speed cardiac-triggered MRA with a segmented *k*-space data acquisition scheme). Segmented *k*-space enables one to complete the entire cardiac-triggered acquisition within a single breath-hold, making the technique especially effective for thoracic studies.

A substantial reduction in scan time can be achieved by acquiring N phase-encode lines per *k*-space segment for each heartbeat (fig. 15.73). The reduction in scan time is determined by N. Faster acquisition is achieved at the expense of precise electrocardiographic triggering to a single time point within the cardiac cycle. When performing segmented acquisitions, the time interval over which the N echoes are acquired spans a portion of the cardiac cycle. For $T_R = 10$ ms, the acquisition window typically spans 160 ms for $N = 16$. This time interval increases along with N. Care should be taken to ascertain the optimal N when imaging moving objects because higher N values entail more time for blurring to occur. An acquisition window of up to 500 ms is acceptable for renal artery imaging, but not for coronary artery imaging, where cardiac motion is a problem.

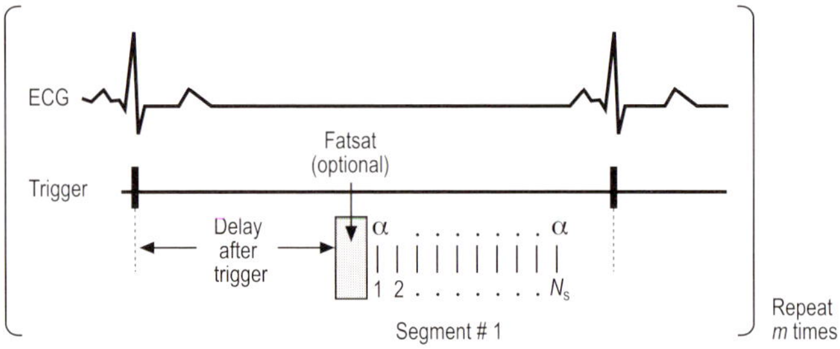

Figure 15.73
A segmented 2D FLASH technique is used for cardiac synchronization. *k*-space is segmented into *m* segments. Each segment contains *N* lines which are acquired during one heart beat. A trigger delay is used to push the data acquisition to a specific point in time during the cardiac cycle.

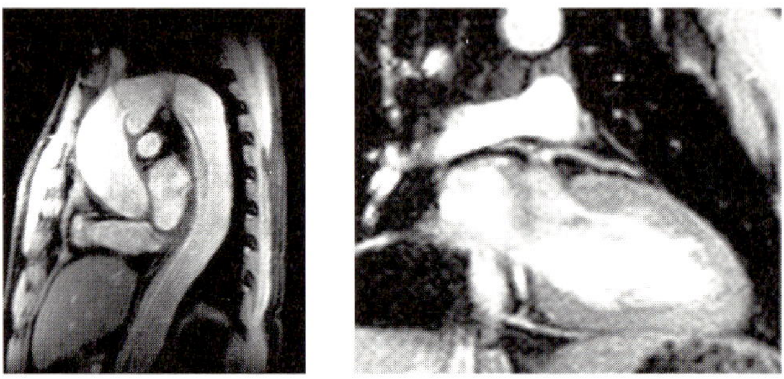

Figure 15.74
ECG-triggered 2D TOF techniques are useful for imaging vessels near the heart. **Left:** sagittal view of a coarctation. **Right:** double-oblique view of the heart showing the left ventricle and part of the left coronary artery. The images are acquired during a breath-hold of approximately 15 to 20 heartbeats.

The use of segmented acquisitions enables one complete cardiac-triggered acquisitions within 20 seconds. Before, these used to take 3 to 5 minutes. Both cardiac pulsations and respiratory motion are eliminated when segmented acquisition is combined with breath-holding. This has revolutionized thoracic imaging (i.e. segmented acquisitions have displaced the earlier spin-echo techniques in most cases). The segmented *k*-space technique has been applied to the acquisition of MR angiograms of the coronary artery and of larger arteries such as the aorta (fig. 15.74). The major advantages associated with segmented data acquisition include (1) speed, (2) elimination of physiological motion and (3) syncopated data acquisition for greater inflow (syncopation is discussed in the next paragraph).

Triggering and syncopation

Segmented *k*-space acquisition involves the syncopation of acquisitions, i.e. RF pulses are applied in clusters with a relatively long pause between clusters. For example, eight RF pulses are applied at a T_R of 4 to 8 ms when $N = 8$. The next set of RF pulses is then applied during the following heartbeat, which is approximately 1 second later. The pauses between the RF pulses allow fresh spins to flow into the imaging slice. The inflow for segmented data acquisition is thus larger than for standard TOF imaging. Pulmonary angiography, for example, has been achieved with a series of segments separated by a delay time to allow wash-in. This use of segmentation (i.e. triggered to the heartbeat or acquired at a constant interval that is independent of the heart rate) is referred to as syncopated acquisition.

Magnetization preparation

Magnetization preparation pulses are used in combination with segmented *k*-space sequences to tailor the desired image contrast. These preparation pulses are applied before each data segment acquisition to achieve certain purposes. For example, fat saturation pulses are used to suppress adipose tissue. Inversion pulses with an appropriate delay time can be used to suppress the background tissue.

Dark-blood imaging

While flow appears bright in standard TOF MRA images, a loss of flow signal may arise in the vicinity of a stenosis, as phase incoherence results from disrupted flow. One way to overcome this problem is to perform dark-blood imaging. This involves making the flow appear dark while maintaining a high signal intensity from the stationary tissue. Dark blood can be achieved in any of the following ways: (1) spin echo or fast spin echo with long T_E, a thin slice, and a dephasing gradient, (2) gradient echo with presaturation bands to suppress the flow signal and (3) segmented turboFLASH with magnetization preparation pulses to saturate the flow signal. The objective of dark blood imaging is to eliminate the flow signal completely while maximizing the signal from plaque and surrounding tissue (fig. 15.75).

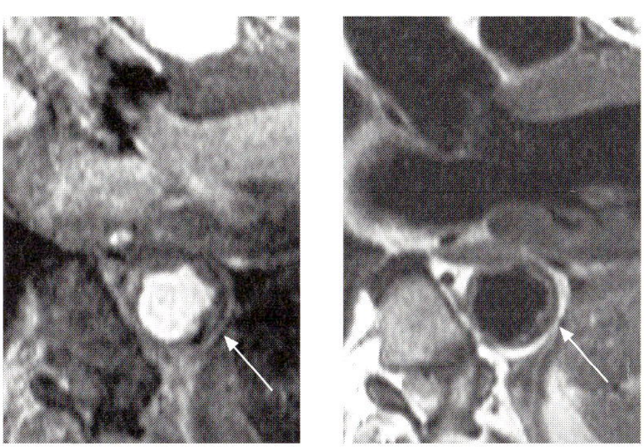

Figure 15.75
Standard 2D TOF techniques show blood with high signal intensity due to inflow enhancement **(left)**. A saturation pulse can be applied to suppress all inflowing blood **(right)**. This enhances the delineation of tissue in the vessel wall and the visualization of plaque (arrow).

Pulsatile flow and signal loss

Arterial flow is periodic in nature. The variation in the wash-in rate of spins between systole and diastole creates alterations in the amplitude of echoes acquired during the course of the acquisition. This variation results in ghost artifacts along the phase-encoding direction of TOF images. The use of large flip-angle values leads to increased ghosting. Such ghost artifacts can be selectively removed by using presaturation bands to eliminate the arterial signal when performing MR venography.

The variation in velocity over the cardiac cycle also causes phase modulations that cannot be eliminated by first-order flow compensation. This problem can, however, be addressed by using cardiac triggering to synchronize data collection to the cardiac cycle. If triggering is not used, the blood signal may vary and ghost artifacts may appear. Pulsatile artifacts can be quite complex in 3D imaging. 3D imaging involves two phase-encoding directions (in-plane and slice-select), with the ghost artifacts that result from respiration and pulsatile flow being capable of propagating in both directions. Artifacts in the slice-select direction may cause slice-to-slice variations in signal intensity.

Flow separation and recirculation

Flow saturation can be pronounced in vessel regions where the blood flow circles in one place (recirculation) or is stagnant. The most common example of this involves the carotid bulb, where blood moves forward in the anterior portion of the proximal internal carotid artery and in the reverse direction in the posterior portion. The laminar streamlines of flow depart from the vessel wall at that point, a phenomenon referred to as flow separation. The blood in the posterior bulb spends a long time in the acquired volume and appears dark, which might simulate the appearance of plaque. Flow separation may also occur beyond a stenosis or at the location of an ulcer or aneurysm, again with the result that these areas appear darker.

Flow misregistration

A blood signal often seems to arise from a point outside the vessel, as if the image of the blood and the image of the background were misregistered. This artifact occurs as a result of flow during the time delay between the phase-encoding and the frequency-encoding portions of the sequence. In other words, the position on the phase-encoding axis is determined at one point in time and the position along the frequency-encoding axis is determined at a slightly later point in time. Blood flowing at an angle to the phase-encoding axis appears displaced along the frequency-encoding axis. Displacement artifacts and signal pileup are often seen in tortuous vessels such as the carotid siphon. Misregistration can be detected by swapping the frequency and phase axes and repeating the MRA sequence. If the vessel takes on a new shape or position, then a displacement artifact is present.

The degree of misregistration depends on the blood velocity, the angle of the vessel with respect to the phase-encoding direction, and the time delay between phase encoding and frequency encoding. The displacement occurs in the same direction as the flow. This artifact differs from chemical-shift artifacts, which also occur along the frequency-encoding direction. Effectively reducing this artifact will require changes in the pulse-sequence design that bring about a minimization of the time between phase encoding and frequency encoding. The high performance gradients and short echo times offered by state-of-the-art imaging systems enable one to circumvent most of the above-mentioned problems.

15.2.4.3.2 Phase-contrast angiography

As has been shown, moving spins develop a phase shift with respect to stationary spins as they move in a pair of opposing magnetic field gradients, an effect that forms the basis of phase-contrast angiography (PCA). The shift involved can be exploited to indicate flow and calculate flow velocities, or it can be displayed as an angiogram [15.101, 15.106]. PCA is most commonly acquired in the context of thick-slice 2D PC MRA (used to generate scout views or rapid projections that can be viewed from one direction only), 3D PC MRA (used to generate higher resolution and rotatable angiograms) and cardiac-gated 2D PC flow velocity imaging (used for blood flow quantification).

The phase information is generated by applying an additional bipolar magnetic-field gradient pulse in the direction along which the flow is to be investigated (fig. 15.68). The phase shift in a voxel x,y,z can be measured by calculating

$$\phi(x,y,z) = \arctan\frac{\mathrm{Re}(I(x,y,z))}{\mathrm{Im}(I(x,y,z))} \qquad (15.57)$$

from the complex image intensity $I(x,y,z)$. The flow velocity v in that voxel will then follow from eq. (15.56).

Maximum encode velocity

It follows from the equivocality of eq. (15.57) that only flow velocities that cause phase shifts between ±180° can be unambiguously determined by applying a single bipolar gradient pulse. The maximum velocity at which a 180° phase shift occurs is referred to as the v_{enc}. Spins flowing forward are assigned the brightest signal intensity and those flowing backward at v_{enc} are assigned the darkest signal intensity. The v_{enc} of the pulse sequence can be adjusted by varying the gradient strength and duration. One can improve vessel visibility and the dynamic range of a quantitative flow study by matching the selected v_{enc} to the expected velocity.

However, one should always make sure to set the v_{enc} slightly higher than the maximum anticipated velocity in the vessel of interest. Velocity aliasing occurs and artifacts are produced within the vessel of interest whenever the peak velocity exceeds the v_{enc}. For example, if the v_{enc} is set to 20 cm/s and the blood is traveling at 21 cm/s, the image of the blood is not assigned to the brightest signal, but is wrapped around to display a low intensity (fig. 15.76). This yields the mistaken impression that the flow is going in the opposite direction. The presence of velocity aliasing can be readily detected in the image. While normal phase images show a gradual change of velocity within the vessel lumen, velocity aliasing tends to show an abrupt phase transition

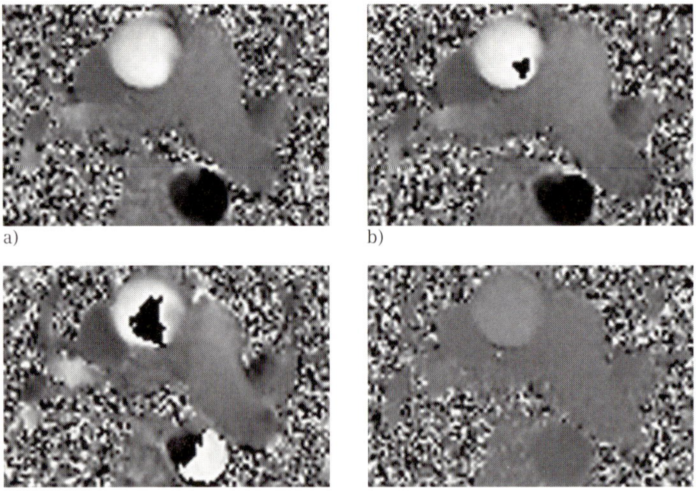

a) b) c) d)

Figure 15.76
The flow velocities in a flow quantification measurement are shown correctly when the selected v_{enc} is smaller than the maximum velocity range that occurs during the measurement **(a)**. If the v_{enc} is slightly lower than the maximum velocity, a small area of velocity aliasing will appear, as shown in the ascending aorta **(b)**. Lowering the v_{enc} further will result in larger areas of velocity aliasing that may affect both flow directions, as shown in the ascending and descending aorta **(c)**. If the v_{enc} is too high, the phase difference will be very small and the signal-to-noise ratio will also be very low **(d)**.

from positive to negative within a vessel. If this occurs, the study should be repeated with the correct v_{enc}.

Correction of phase errors

Magnetic field inhomogeneities and eddy currents are also capable of inducing local phase shifts in stationary spins. One can achieve background suppression in PCA by subtracting one phase image acquired with flow encoding and one phase image acquired with flow compensation (fig. 15.77). Alternatively, one can subtract one image acquired with a positive flow-induced phase shift and a second acquired with the polarity of the flow encoding reversed. This also produces a net phase shift for flow while subtracting out the background.

The measurement of the complete velocity vector requires repeated acquisitions with the gradient pulse pairs in three orthogonal axes , i.e. a total of 6 acquisitions. One can reduce the total number of acquisitions to 4 by using a single reference acquisition with flow compensation, and flow encoded images in three orthogonal directions.

Speed, complex-difference and phase-difference display

Once they have been acquired, the phase shifts resulting from flow encoding can be displayed in various ways.

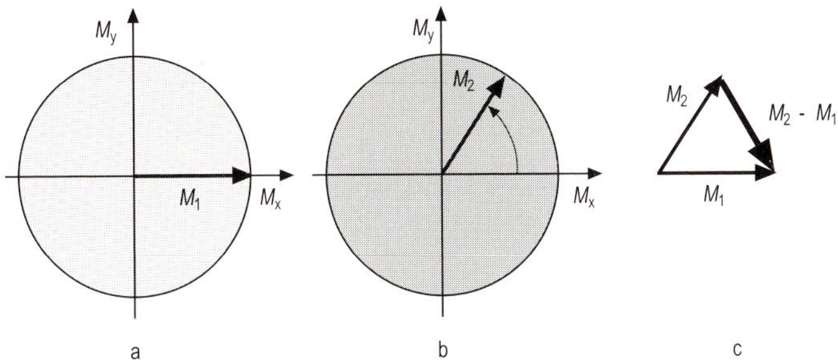

Figure 15.77
Phase contrast MRA is based on the acquisition of two data sets. In the first measurement, a flow compensation gradient is applied to rephase all spins, irrespective of their velocities **(a)**. In the second measurement, a flow-encoding gradient pulse pair is applied to add a phase shift that is proportional to the spin's velocity **(b)**. A final subtraction removes all other flow-independent phase shifts and creates a signal that depends only on the amount of flow-induced phase shifts **(c)**.

Net phase shift (phase difference) is used for flow quantification. The phase-difference image is computed from the phase difference between two acquisitions with different flow encodings (either 0 and v_{enc} or $+v_{enc}/2$ and $-v_{enc}/2$). The value of the phase difference is proportional to velocity. This image is thus also referred to as a velocity map and is used for velocity and flow volume calculations. In most cases, the measurement is cardiac-gated, with multiple measurements being acquired over each cardiac cycle. Flow encoding is usually performed in one direction only.

Complex difference is used mainly for 2D imaging. The complex-difference image is the vector difference (rather than the phase difference) between two acquisitions with different flow encodings. Rather than being simply a reflection of velocity, it is also proportional to the magnitude of the magnetization. The sequence's v_{enc} needs to be adjusted to the peak velocity to avoid signal cancellation effects. The complex difference obtained in these images, however, is no longer a matter of a simple linear relationship with velocity. While velocity quantification is therefore not so straightforward in the complex difference image, the information is very useful in the qualitative assessment of anatomical flow (fig. 15.78).

Magnetization vectors within pixels that exhibit little or no signal (e.g. those representing air and bone cortex) have random and meaningless phases. Air might therefore give the angiogram a speckled appearance and obscure the true vascular signal. This can be removed by setting pixels that correspond to small magnetic vectors to the value of the background signal. This is referred to as applying a mask.

Alternatively, one can use the signal intensity I as a weighting factor to generate the *SPEED* image. *SPEED* information is often used to generate an angiogram. *SPEED* is calculated at each pixel as follows:

$$SPEED = I\sqrt{v_x^2 + v_y^2 + v_z^2} \qquad (15.58)$$

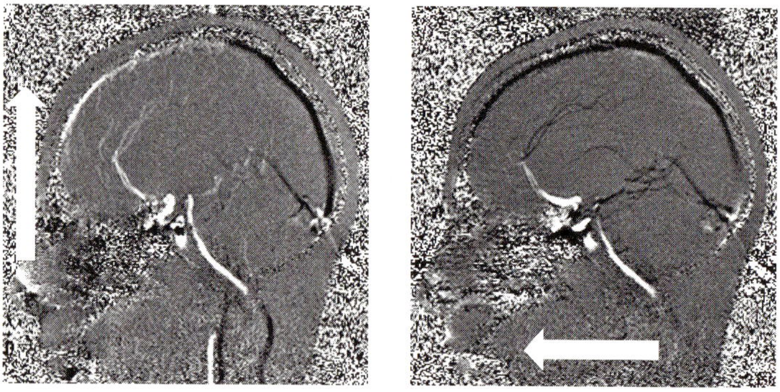

Figure 15.78
Phase-contrast techniques can be used to show magnitude and direction of flow. The images shown here are flow images in the S-I direction **(left)** and AP direction **(right)**. The flow component along S-I in the sagittal sinus is positive in the anterior part, but negative in the posterior part. However, the A-I component is always negative.

The *SPEED* image contains no information about the direction of flow. While velocity aliasing is less of a problem in the case of speed display, the proper setting of v_{enc} remains important. No sudden change from bright to dark occurs when the v_{enc} is exceeded. *SPEED* images are ideal for anatomic depictions of vascular anatomy.

Thick-slab 2D PCA

Thick-slab 2D PCA offers an assessment of flow within seconds and is often used to obtain a projective view of the vasculature. The slab thickness ranges from 2 to 10 cm. Partial voluming does occur because of the thicker slice, and the spatial resolution may sometimes be less than optimal. It is important to bear in mind that when two vessels cross within the slice, the acquired phase is the sum of the two. This means that various phase artifacts, whose degree worsens with increasing slice thickness, may be present. Multiple acquisitions are acquired when pulsatile flow is present in order to reduce respiratory and pulsatility artifacts. Alternatively, one may use electrocardiographic triggering.

3D PCA

3D PC MRA, like 3D TOF, generates a volumetric data set that can be reformatted and displayed in any chosen orientation by using the MIP (maximum intensity projection) algorithm. In addition to MR angiograms, flow-directional images can be generated to show flow along different axes. Repeated acquisitions are needed to encode flow along all three orthogonal directions. 3D streamline profiles can be generated from 3D PC data. Cardiac triggering is not used with 3D PC because of the prohibitive acquisition times. The flow velocity obtained is therefore averaged over the cardiac cycle. 3D PC is commonly applied in cerebral angiography, renal and other visceral angiography, and studies of distal extremities.

Flow velocity quantification and cine phase-contrast

Cine PCA allows one to measure pulsatile flow velocity [15.107]. This is done by acquiring data at multiple time points throughout the cardiac cycle (known as a cine measurement) using electrocardiographic triggering (fig. 15.79). The time resolution

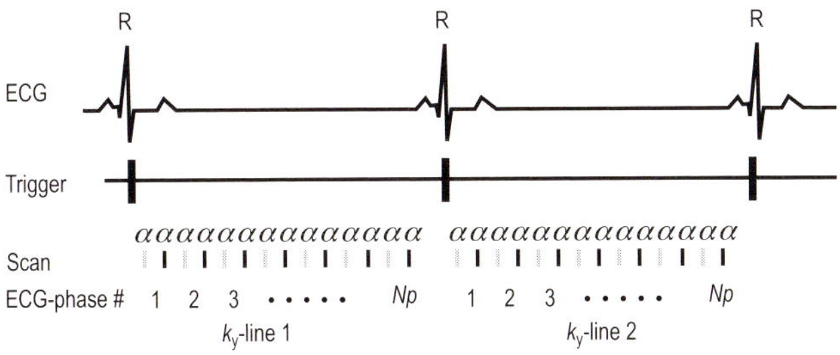

Figure 15.79
Flow quantification techniques are usually applied in a triggered mode to account for the pulsatile nature of blood flow in the body. The basic flow module consists of a flow-compensated (gray lines) and a flow-encoded (black lines) gradient echo sequence. This basic module is repeated N_p times with the same k_y encoding gradient during one ECG cycle. The different ECG phases are measured in the next cycle for a different k_y-line. The total time for this measurement is defined by the average R-R interval multiplied by the number of k_y-lines.

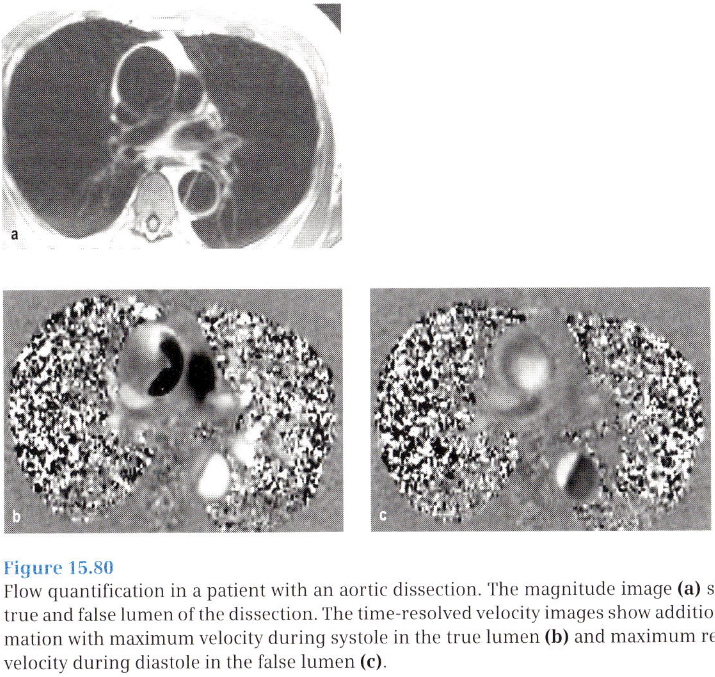

Figure 15.80
Flow quantification in a patient with an aortic dissection. The magnitude image **(a)** shows the true and false lumen of the dissection. The time-resolved velocity images show additional information with maximum velocity during systole in the true lumen **(b)** and maximum retrograde velocity during diastole in the false lumen **(c)**.

of the series is given by T_R, which is typically 30 to 40 ms. Multiple pairs of flow-sensitive and flow-compensated images are acquired in a triggered study. A time-velocity curve can be obtained by subtracting the images and determining the net phase shift at each time point. In addition, volumetric flow rates can be calculated by determining the product of the velocity and the cross-sectional area of the vessel lumen. Rapid flow quantification enables the completion of measurements within a single breath-hold (fig. 15.80).

Advantages and limitations of phase-contrast angiography

PCA offers the following advantages: First, it improves the detection of small vessels by virtue of its excellent background elimination. All stationary materials, even those with a short T_1 (such as fat and methemoglobin), are eliminated. As a result, hematomas are not mistaken for vascular structures, as may happen with TOF. PCA can often provide MIPs of a larger volume than TOF because of its superior background suppression. Second, PCA is well-suited for the imaging of slow flow, as in vein structures or large aneurysms. One can adjust the gradient strength and duration to create a pulse sequence that is sensitive even to exceptionally slow velocities such as those associated with cerebrospinal fluid motion. Third, cine PC can be used to perform flow quantification and to obtain the velocity-time curve in pulsatile flow.

PCA also has limitations: First, PC acquisitions, particularly in 3D PCA, take approximately two to three times longer than TOF acquisitions of comparable resolution. This is because the flow-encoded data along each of the three axes are acquired separately. Second, PC MRA is sensitive to instrument imperfections. The presence of eddy currents or field instabilities degrades the background suppression. The use of self-shielded gradient coils and careful eddy current compensation mitigate these problems. The need to partially dephase flowing spins to obtain flow sensitivity makes PC images more sensitive than TOF images to artifacts resulting from the complex flow that may occur distal to a stenosis or in some aneurysms.

15.2.4.3.3 Contrast-enhanced MR angiography

Certain limitations associated with conventional MRA techniques are revealed when the techniques are deployed to image large volumes of the vasculature. Very short T_Rs are used (5 ms or less) when imaging the thoracic or abdominal vasculature in order to keep the scan time short and allow for a breath-hold acquisition. However, this often leads to insufficient signal on account of spin saturation.

Several measures can be taken to mitigate this loss of signal. As described earlier in this chapter, one can acquire small volumes to ensure that spins are replaced quickly with unsaturated spins. One can select a small flip angle at the cost of tissue contrast and vessel conspicuity. Another option is to shorten the blood T_1 using contrast administration [15.102, 15.108].

The most common approach involves the use of chelates such as gadolinium diethylenetriaminepentaacetic acid (Gd-DTPA). The T_1 can be as short as 50 ms, depending on the actual concentration of gadolinium in the blood. Pulse repetition can thus be increased and more signal obtained by applying a larger Ernst angle (see section 15.2.1).

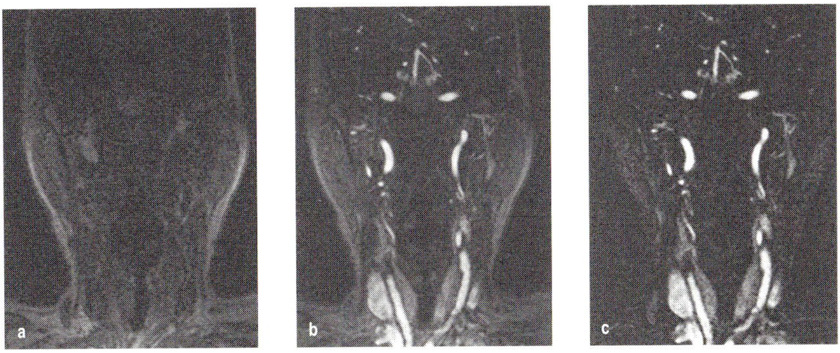

Figure 15.81
The blood is significantly saturated before contrast injection due to the long T_1 and the gradient-echo sequence's short repetition time **(a)**. Contrast injection shortens the T_1 of blood, resulting in strong signal in the blood vessels **(b)**. A subtraction removes a signal from stationary tissue and produces a subtraction angiogram **(c)**.

Despite the fact that stationary tissue remains unaffected by the contrast injection, it still produces a background signal that may obscure some vascular details in a projection image. Therefore, contrast-enhanced MRA is often applied as a subtraction technique that is similar to digital subtraction angiography (DSA). A mask image is applied before the contrast injection. This mask is later subtracted from the post-contrast acquisition of the same volume to remove all signal from stationary tissue and thereby leave signal only in those areas where the Gd-DTPA has been delivered (fig. 15.81).

Timing considerations in contrast-enhanced MRA

After its intravenous (IV) injection, the contrast agent is delivered to the vasculature of interest. The local blood signal is momentarily substantially enhanced. It is necessary to time the data collection (in particular for the center of *k*-space) to the arrival of the contrast agent at the vessels being imaged (fig. 15.82). The exact timing of the enhancement patterns will depend on many factors, particularly the patient's cardiac output, which pumps the contrast bolus through the vasculature. It is the center of *k*-space data acquisition that needs to be properly acquired when the contrast bolus passes through the arterial system.

Sequence considerations

The basis of contrast-enhanced MRA is a 3D gradient echo sequence with RF spoiling. The scan time T_S of this sequence can be expressed as

$$T_S = T_R N_P N_S \tag{15.59}$$

where N_p is the number of partition-encoding steps and N_s is the number of phase-encoding steps. T_R depends on the gradient strength and the spatial resolution that is to be achieved. The receiver bandwidth represents a further important factor. High receiver bandwidths are made possible by the high signal intensity of contrast-agent-

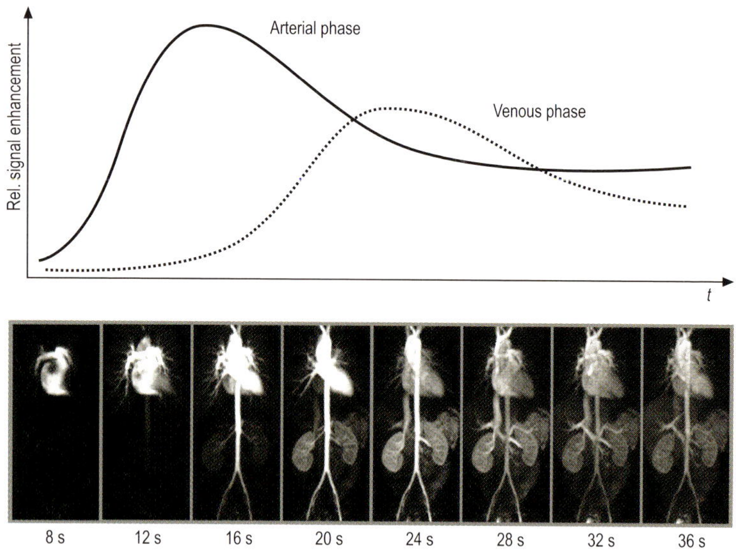

Figure 15.82
Timing of contrast-enhanced MR angiography. In this study, a series of ultra-fast 3D measurements with a scan time of only 4 s was acquired immediately after the bolus injection of a single-dose Gd-DTPA. Note, for instance, the rapid filling of the aorta and subsequent filling of the renal vein. This figure demonstrates the experimental result of a contrast injection study. The study was performed using an ultra-fast 3D gradient echo sequence with a T_R of 3 ms. 16 partitions were acquired with a reduced in-plane matrix of 80 by 256 to create one complete 3D data set in only 4 seconds. This measurement was repeated 10 times to ensure thorax scanning throughout the contrast injection. The images show the MIP projections from the central 8 measurements at the very moment the contrast arrives in the pulmonary artery, and then as it moves deeper into the vasculature (4-second measurements). A clear filling of the aorta can be seen at 16 seconds after contrast injection. Four seconds later, the kidneys begin to show enhancement. Filling of the renal veins and vena cava is then in evidence 24 seconds after injection.

enriched blood. These allow for rapid data sampling even at an increased noise level. State-of-the-art imaging systems enable one to easily achieve a T_R of 5 ms or less. More recent advancements in gradient technology (G_{max} ~ 40 mT/m, slew rates of up to 200 T/ms) enable the clinical use of repetition times of less than 2 ms. These ultra-fast gradient echo sequences permit one to realize scan times of 20 seconds or less while maintaining excellent spatial resolution. For instance, protocol scan times of 19.2 s can be achieved when $N_p = 200$, $N_s = 32$, and $T_R = 3.0$ ms. This time frame is short enough to permit most patients to hold their breath during the measurement. Contrast-enhanced MRA therefore also permits breath-hold investigations of the abdomen that are free of respiratory motion artifacts.

It is necessary to keep the scan time short not only because of the breath-hold length, but also because of the physiologic behavior of the contrast agent in the vascular system. It is only a matter of several seconds after arterial enhancement that venous enhancement begins to take place. The exact time depends on the vessel under consid-

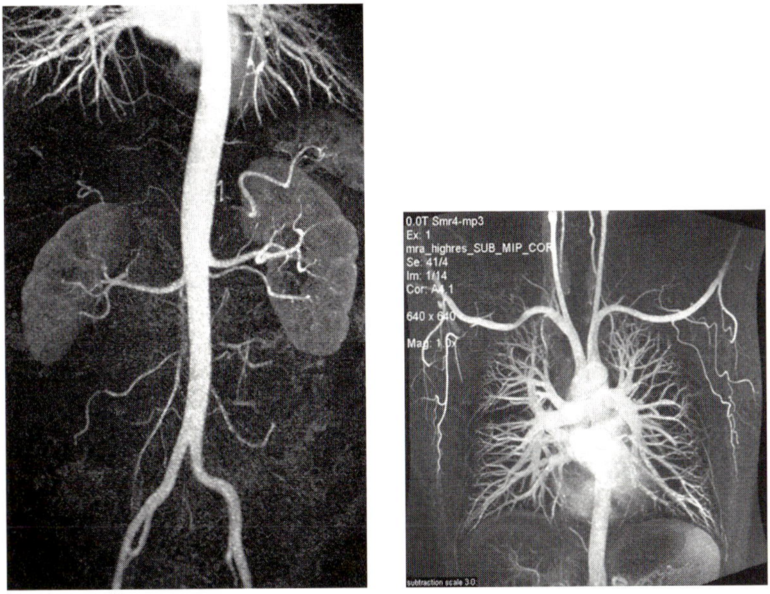

Figure 15.83
Application of contrast-enhanced MRA at 3 T. The higher field strength permits better spatial resolution. Shown here are two clinical examples of a submillimeter imaging protocol for imaging of the renal **(left)** and pulmonary arteries **(right)**. The imaging time is 22 s and the spatial resolution is 0.6 mm by 0.6 mm by 0.9 mm.

eration, as well as on the patient's condition. For example, while the arterial-venous delay in the carotid and renal arteries is only a few seconds (typically 5 to 8 seconds), the peripheral system is characterized by a slightly longer interval. Excellent spatial resolution is equally important when it comes to detecting and identifying vascular disease in the absence of conspicuity. In general, contrast-enhanced MRA techniques demand maximum spatial resolution with large vessel coverage in the shortest amount of time (fig. 15.83).

Timing considerations

Several techniques have been proposed to determine the optimal timing of contrast injection. Three major categories of contrast are applied in clinical settings:

- *Post-contrast-scan timing*
  Optimal results depend on a prior knowledge of the contrast arrival time. The contrast arrival time is best determined by administering a small test bolus and continuously monitoring for vascular signal enhancement in the region of interest. The full amount of contrast agent is administered following the test bolus measurement. A 3D scan is initiated to acquire data during the arterial enhancement. Breath-hold commands are added in the case of abdominal imaging to acquire the data during a breath-hold and thereby avoid any sort of respiratory motion arti-

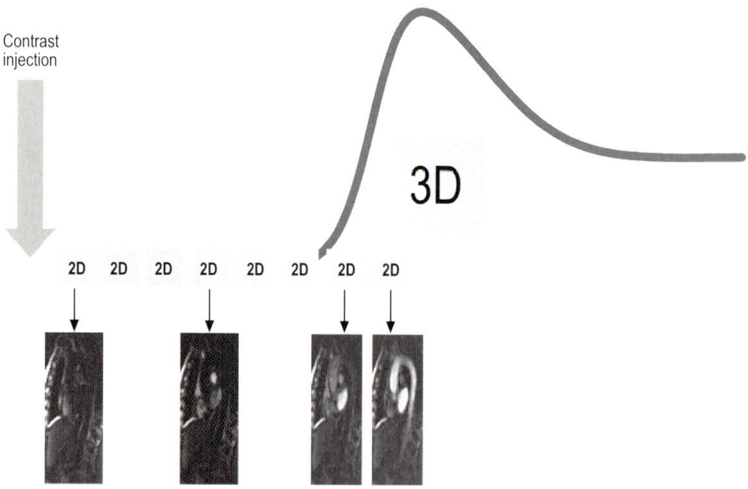

Figure 15.84
Fluoroscopic triggering of the ce-MRA sequence as soon as the contrast arrives in the vessel of interest. The contrast arrival is measured in real time using an ultra-fast 2D sequence at a rate of 1 image/s. A 3D sequence with a centric elliptical phase-encode order is initiated as soon as the contrast has arrived.

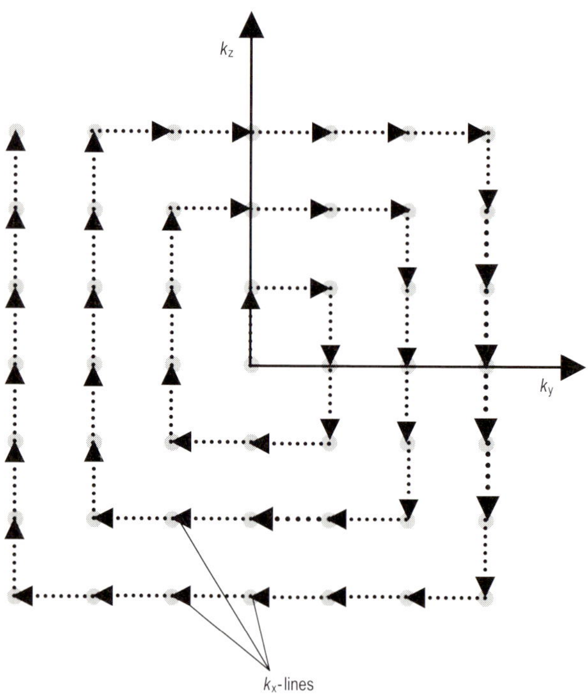

Figure 15.85
Centric elliptical phase-encode order

facts. After waiting briefly to allow for breathing, a second measurement can be added to scan the venous phase after contrast injection.

- *Fluoroscopic triggering*
  As shown in fig. 15.84, a series of ultra-fast 2D sequences provides a real-time view of the vessels of interest for the sake of triggering the 3D scan with a centric elliptical phase-encode order at the very moment of the contrast agent's inflow. The term elliptical centric refers to the filling of the center of *k*-space along two axes k_y, k_z (fig. 15.85). No test bolus is required, and venous overlay is minimal. However, the scan needs to be initiated as soon as the contrast shows up in the arteries so as to avoid venous contamination. This leaves little time for breath-hold commands.

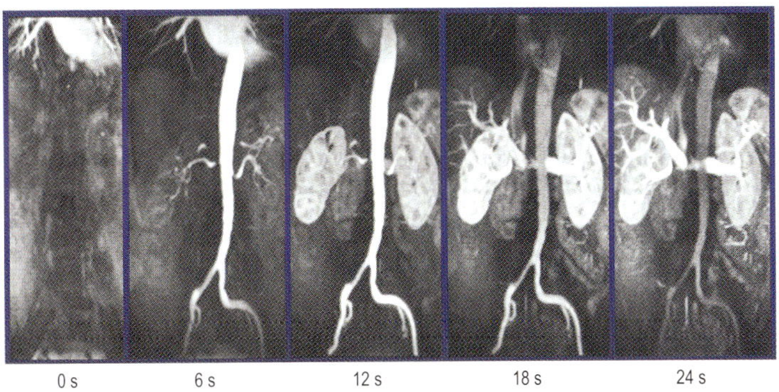

Figure 15.86
Dynamic contrast-enhanced MRA for imaging the renal arteries. A fast 3D sequence can be repeated every 3 seconds to show early arterial phase **(b)**, late arterial phase **(c)** and venous enhancement (**d** and **e**).

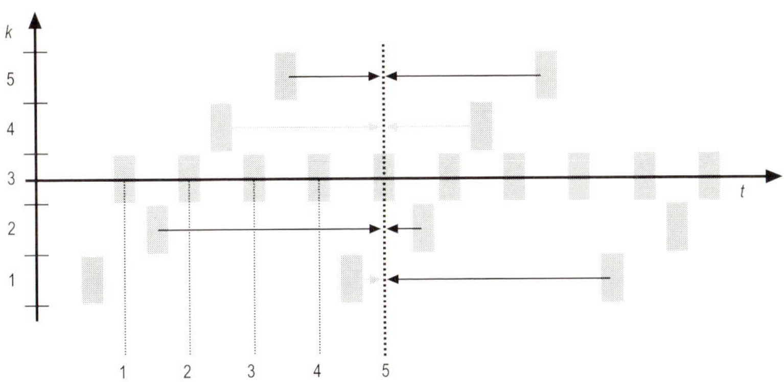

Figure 15.87
Time-resolved imaging of contrast kinetics: the temporal resolution of a contrast-enhanced sequence can be increased by scanning the center segment more frequently than the outer segments in *k*-space.

- *Dynamic image acquisition*
  Continuous rapid 3D image acquisition is initiated at the same time as the contrast injection. One set of images with good arterial enhancement will always be available for retrospective selection. Powerful gradients of up to 40 mT/m and slew rates of 200 mT/m/ms are necessary to avoid compromising spatial resolution during the short acquisition times required (around 3 s per 3D image) (fig. 15.86). Further improvements in temporal and spatial resolution can be obtained by using parallel acquisition techniques (see section 15.2.2) and *k*-space manipulation strategies. The outer parts of *k*-space are updated less often than the central part in time-resolved imaging of contrast kinetics (fig. 15.87) [15.109].

Large field of view MRA

The field of view in an imaging experiment is limited by the homogeneity and linearity volume of the MR instrument. A larger anatomy can be scanned by moving the patient to another position and repeating the measurement (fig. 15.88, see also section 15.2.3) [15.110]. Mask images are acquired at several positions before contrast injection in the case of whole-body contrast-enhanced MRA. The measurements are repeated with very rapid table movements after contrast injection to catch the contrast enhancement moving down to the legs. A whole-body MR angiogram is established by digital image subtraction and piecing together the single images (fig. 15.89).

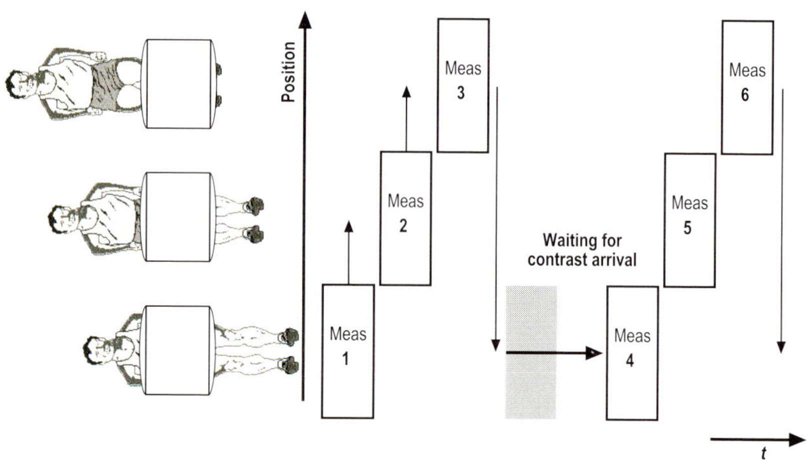

Figure 15.88
Whole-body ceMRA via patient movement. The field of view in an imaging experiment is limited by the homogeneity and linearity volume of the MR instrument. A larger anatomy can be scanned by moving the patient to another position and repeating the measurement. Several pre-contrast measurements are acquired before contrast injection in the case of contrast-enhanced MRA of the peripheral vessels. The measurements are repeated with very rapid table movements after contrast injection to catch the contrast enhancement moving into the legs.

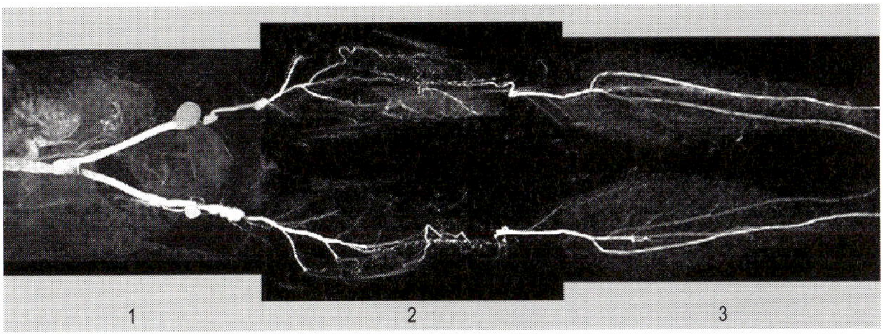

Figure 15.89
Contrast-enhanced peripheral MRA study. Three measurements were acquired at three different positions during constant contrast-agent infusion. Corresponding masks were acquired before contrast injection and subtracted from the post-contrast images.

15.2.4.5.4 MRA viewing: display and interpretation

The introduction of the MIP algorithm allowed for the calculation and display of realistic angiograms [15.111]. The algorithm permits one to combine individual slices of blood vessels that were acquired over a 3D volume and to render these slices in a 2D projection. Projection angiograms can be generated from a series of 2D images or from a 3D data set. The method has become so universal that it is nearly synonymous with MRA. Yet MIP is not always the best technique for vascular display. In what follows, we present a summary of the most important features of these methods.

Maximum intensity projection (MIP)

Blood vessels course across many slices in a typical angiographic acquisition. Displaying the entire vessel is a matter of combining the slices. An immediate problem arises if one simply sums the slice intensities: the background signal added from the many slices will exceed that of the vessels, thereby rendering the vessels invisible. The MIP algorithm was designed to overcome this problem. Rather than adding intensities, it uses only the largest single intensity at each position in the projection for the combined image.

First, the direction of projection is chosen. The computer algorithm then goes through the 3D data along that direction and automatically picks out and displays the highest signal intensity from the slices. Given that the program does not differentiate between blood and background tissue, the selection is based on signal intensity alone.

Although MIP is much better than simple pixel addition, weak vascular features may be lost in the projection because the vessel signal intensity is exceeded by the background signal intensity. Vessels may appear narrowed or may be absent on an MIP. When interpreting a study, one should therefore refer to the original images to determine the true vessel width.

Vessel depiction can be improved by targeted MIP, in which a selected volume of the 3D data is projected (fig. 15.90). Limiting the projection volume leads to the removal

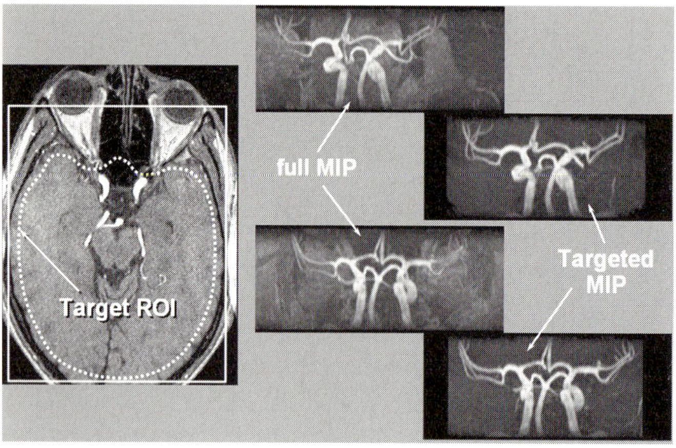

Figure 15.90
Targeted MIP: instead of projecting all data (marked as a rectangle in the left image) onto the projection plane to create the full MIP, only a subset of image data within the region of interest (dashed contour) is used to create the targeted MIP. The vessel conspicuity is significantly increased as shown by the maximum intensity projections on the right side.

of signals from other vessels and bright structures and reduces the chance that the vessel intensity will be exceeded by the background intensity. Another approach that can be helpful is to first perform multiplanar reconstructions of the 3D data and then obtain an MIP of these reconstructions.

Vessel tracking

Vessel tracking involves an attempt to identify the signal corresponding to blood vessels as a basis for removing all of the nonvascular voxels. This is done by picking out an object with contiguous voxels that exhibit a signal intensity above a certain threshold. The program is used to separate a volume into different contiguous objects, many of which are vessels. The nonvascular objects are then edited out by the operator.

The algorithm can be supported by seeding. Here, the operator selects a point in the vessel to serve as a seed. The computer then looks for bright voxels that are contiguous with that seed. These voxels in turn are used as seeds for the next iteration. The object grows outward until it reaches the vessel wall. The progression of the seed is based on signal comparison between neighboring voxels and is governed by criteria set by the user.

Surface rendering

Once the voxels corresponding to a vessel are identified, and assuming the angiogram is of adequate resolution, one may calculate the position of the lumen's outer margin. This can be rendered into a realistic surface using shading and perspective (i.e. as if a model had been made of the vessel). Although still uncommon, this method of presentation is effective for displaying complex anatomy.

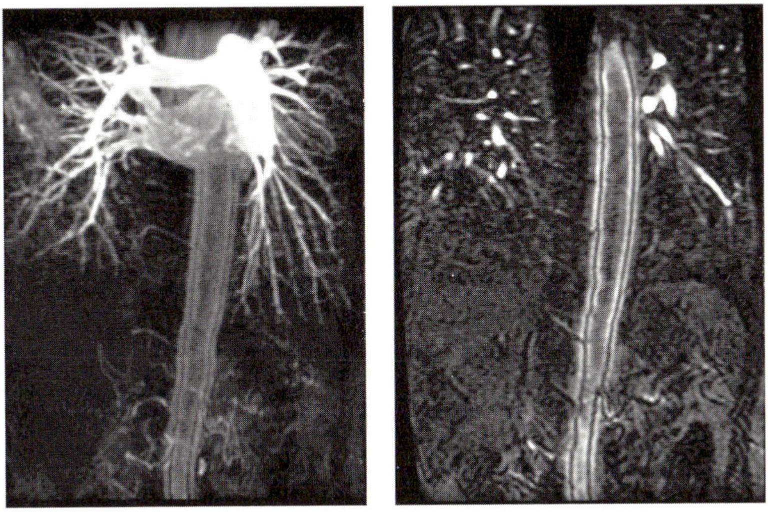

Figure 15.91
Pitfalls in contrast-enhanced MRA. Incorrect timing can mimic vessel disease such as in this MIP image of a 3D angiogram in the aorta (left). The source image on the right shows edge enhancement due to the high-pass filtering effects that occur when scanning is premature and the contrast only reaches the periphery of *k*-space data.

Source display

The original source images are important when it comes to determining the vessel widths and the degree of stenosis. The true lumen size is better evaluated in the cross-sectional views than in the projections. The introduction of whole-body MRA has made it possible to acquire more than 1,000 images within a short acquisition time. A rapid and time-efficient way of viewing the source images is required. Cine/movie display of images permits one to swim through the body and enables a quick overview of the vasculature. It is important to evaluate both the MIP and the selected source images when interpreting a study, as the source images are the key to making a diagnosis (fig. 15.91).

15.2.5 MRI and microscopic motion

15.2.5.1 Perfusion

The term perfusion is used to describe the amount of blood that flows into a tissue per unit of time and is typically expressed in ml/g/s [15.112]. It depends on the macroscopic blood flow of the afferent vessels and the microvascular structure of the tissue. The main motivation for its investigating is to obtain information on the functional state of an organ and its blood supply. Since the magnetic resonance signal is sensitive to changes in the microvascular structure and the signal contribution of blood, MR imaging lends itself very well as a tool for measuring perfusion. However, specific imaging techniques are required because dangerous blood supply deficits of an organ may otherwise not become visible, and because there is a need for quantification.

Various MR-based techniques for measuring perfusion have been developed. All of these techniques are based on changing the magnetization of the blood that flows to the organ and/or by modifying its relaxation times using contrast agents. The corresponding signal from the tissue of interest is then measured as a function of time or of the applied magnetization preparation of the blood.

Thus the available techniques for generating perfusion-specific signal changes can be separated 1) into techniques that depend on the intrinsic magnetic properties of blood only and 2) into techniques that utilize an additional tracer substance.

The first group includes techniques that utilize the specific oxygenation-level-dependent paramagnetic properties of blood (BOLD) [15.113]. Other techniques in this group employ various arterial-spin-labelling (ASL) techniques to prepare the magnetization of blood in order to modify the MR signal from the tissue [15.114]. Techniques that involve modifying the amount of blood flow to the tissue by selectively altering

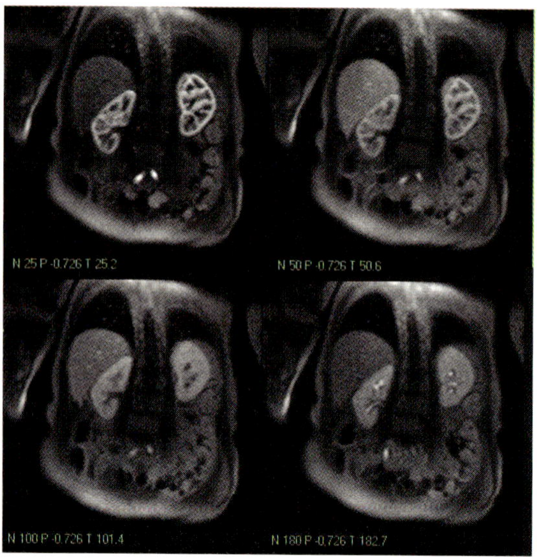

Figure 15.92
Examples of a 2D perfusion study of healthy kidneys taken with a 2D-FLASH sequence. The acquisition time for one image was 254 ms. Four parallel slices were scanned. The temporal resolution of the signal-time curve is 1 data point per second. The images were acquired during free breathing over 3 minutes. The **upper left** image shows the peak perfusion phase of the renal cortex. The medulla and the calyceal system remain relatively unenhanced. The **upper right image** and the **lower left image** represent the signal distribution 25 s and 75 s after the peak phase, when filtration of the paramagnetic tracer causes the contrast between cortex and medulla to vanish. The **lower right** image shows the bright appearance of the calyceal system during the excretion phase.

the local or global vascular resistance with medication or the application of mechanical restrictions should be mentioned here also.

The techniques included in the second group can be distinguished according to the kind of tracer substance used and the main effect they have on the magnetization properties of the tissue. The most common technique involves the injection of a paramagnetic contrast agent (e.g. Gd-DTPA) that decreases the T_1 and T_2 relaxation times of the water protons in the vicinity of the tracer molecules [15.115]. Considerable efforts have been made to further modify specific physiological and physical properties exhibited by the applicable agents. For instance, efforts have been made to enhance their relaxivity, to make them tissue specific and to bind them to other molecules and microspheres in order to restrict their distribution space [15.116]. Other techniques in this group make use of superparamagnetic substances (SPIO) [15.117] or hyperpolarized molecules (He, Xe, ^{13}C) that require specific modifications to conventional methods of image acquisition and methods of signal evaluation [15.118, 15.119].

Perfusion imaging is generally subject to small signal changes and is characterized by a low signal-to-noise ratio. Furthermore, in the event of a perfusion deficit, the signal change will also be relatively low. While the most endangered, ischemic or irreversibly damaged tissue exhibits the weakest available signal, sufficiently perfused tissue can be easily depicted (figs. 15.92, 15.93). Depending on the technique and the contrast agent used, it may be possible to repeat the acquisition multiple times and then average the signal. Doing so, however, will require the employment of motion compensation and correction, as unintentional movements and physiological motion can rarely be prevented.

All available techniques attempt to display the perfusion signal changes as accurate as possible. Much work has also been dedicated to the quantification of characteristic perfusion-dependent parameters and to the calculation of the amount of blood flow

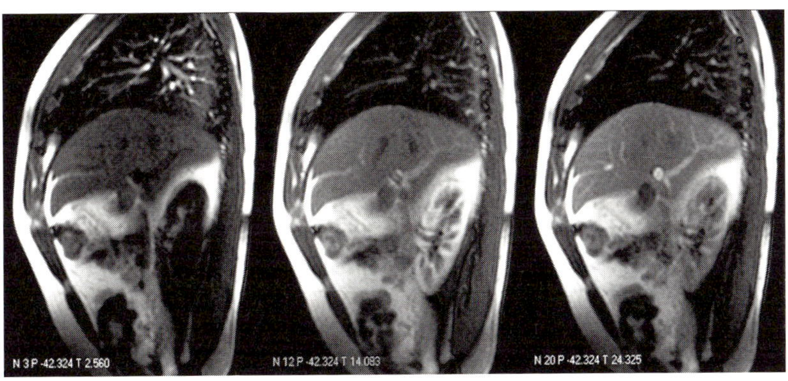

Figure 15.93
Examples from a 2D perfusion study using trueFISP. The maximum signal phase at lung **(left)**, kidney **(middle)** and liver **(right)** is depicted.

and blood volume in the tissue of interest [15.120, 15.121]. The difficulties encountered arise with the observation that the measured signal changes are not at all direct expressions of the blood flow and blood volume of the organ. Elaborate mathematical techniques for signal-time analysis are required in order to calculate the perfusion parameters as robustly and reproducibly as possible [15.122]. The quantification of the first pass perfusion is mainly based on the indicator dilution theory [15.123, 15.124] and the analytical description of the signal-time changes by a gamma variate function [15.125]. The calculation of tracer permeability and excretion is mainly based on the solution of multi-compartment models [15.126]. First-pass techniques take account of the arterial input signal in order to correct for the influence of the tracer administration and tracer distribution on the way to the tissue of interest [15.127]. The use of intravascular contrast agents promises significant improvements in the description of perfusion effects. These agents are characterized by a considerably reduced distribution to the interstitial space and therefore a considerably reduced distribution volume [15.128].

15.2.5.2 Diffusion imaging

Diffusion imaging in MR experiments enables one to indirectly observe the microstructures of soft tissue and the disease-related changes that these structures undergo (e.g. in the case of brain ischemia) [15.129].

Diffusion NMR schemes were first applied to in vivo human studies [15.130] shortly after the discovery of MRI. Researchers were able to ascertain in the early 1980s that subtle macroscopic motion (e.g. head movement, organ movement and even brain pulsation) had the effect of massively disturbing the conventional image-formation process. It was not until around 1990 that diffusion imaging became a useful tool in MRI. This development followed in the wake of two technological advancements. First, modern gradient hardware enabled the MR community to use the subsecond imaging technique known as EPI. Second, diffusion-weighted EPI (DW-EPI) offered a solution to the problem of motion-induced image artifacts by (1) separating diffusion-encoding and image-formation processes and (2) freezing motion via an intrinsically high data-acquisition speed of less than 0.1 seconds [15.131]. The application of such ultrafast imaging sequences to patients who had just experienced a stroke showed unprecedented degrees of contrast in areas of ongoing ischemic processes [15.132, 15.133].

Today, DW-EPI is used in hundreds of hospitals around the world to assist in the early diagnosis of stroke (see section 15.2.6.1). Diffusion imaging in acute brain ischemia is used to monitor changes in the fine architecture of neural tissue. The observed changes in diffusion behavior caused by the underlying pathological processes related to acute brain ischemia are isotropic in nature. This contrasts with the anisotropic water diffusion exhibited by many types of biological tissue (skeletal muscle, spine, tongue, eye lens, heart and cerebral white matter) [15.134].

Anisotropic diffusion behavior in MR imaging can be modeled by replacing a scalar diffusion constant with a diffusion tensor [15.135, 15.136]. Given that the diffusion tensor model is not sophisticated enough to handle (typical) situations in which the content of a voxel (as found in many sections of the human brain) is not given by a single homogeneous tissue component, other approaches are required (e.g. model-based and data-driven approaches) to more adequately display diffusion behavior in a voxel.

Various research groups are currently evaluating the viability of using anisotropic diffusion measurements to reconstruct (bundles of) nerve fibers in humans [15.137]. The complexity of the underlying (micro) anatomy (e.g. in sections of human white matter where some 10,000 nerve fibers run through a single voxel) may restrict this MR-based tractography to architecturally well-behaved portions of the human body.

Aspects of data acquisition

As an extension to the original Stejskal and Tanner experiment [15.138], one can apply predefined (large) diffusion-encoding gradient pulses to various kinds of pulse sequences to ascertain the diffusion properties of the investigated subject. It warrants pointing out, however, that all imaging gradients (even small ones) make a contribution (often negligible) to the diffusion encoding of an MR pulse sequence.

The introduction of diffusion encoding gradients represented one of the most demanding challenges to both the development of MR pulse sequences and the design of gradient systems: while the application of maximum gradient amplitudes of 20 to 80 mT/m for some tens of milliseconds brings about the desired diffusion encoding, it also produces unwanted side effects such as high sensitivity to subject motion. Two further problems also needed to be addressed. First, the maximum gradient amplitudes and minimum gradient rise times are limited by peripheral nerve stimulation. Second, the switching on and off of large magnetic field gradients introduces transient fields (e.g. eddy currents) even in well-designed modern MR systems. While such transient fields may disturb processes of image formation and image reconstruction, they can be largely compensated for by deploying corrective measures.

The application of diffusion-encoding radiance followed by single-shot EPI has been the most commonly used sequence for imaging diffusion in vivo for more than a decade (fig. 15.94). The diffusion-weighted signal obtained can be expressed as (see chapter 7):

$$\begin{aligned} M(\vec{q},\Delta) &= M_0 e^{-bD} \\ \vec{q} &= \gamma \vec{G}_D \delta \\ b &= q^2\left(\Delta - \frac{\delta}{3}\right) \end{aligned} \tag{15.60}$$

δ: Duration of the diffusion-encoding gradient G_D
Δ: Distance between the two diffusion-encoding gradient pulses

The image-formation part of the sequence is completely decoupled from the diffusion-encoding part. In diffusion-weighted EPI (DW-EPI), the imaging readout module typically takes less than 0.1 seconds, thereby freezing patient motion. As in photography, short exposure times are the key to obtaining sharp images from potentially moving objects.

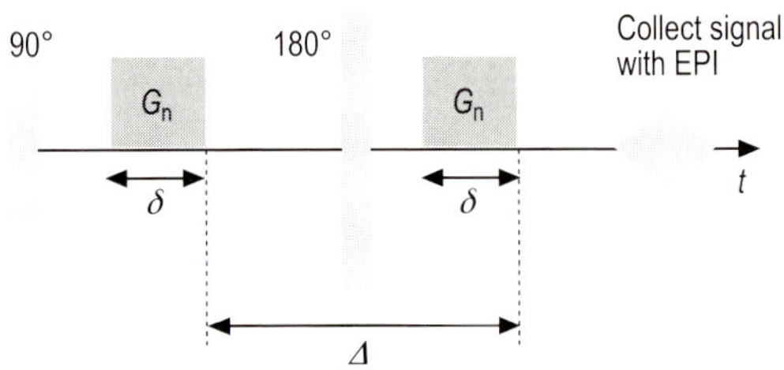

Figure 15.94
Basic diffusion-imaging sequence applying EPI for signal readout

The advent of feedback mechanisms in modern MR scanners has enabled one to acquire additional navigator information during all kinds of MR pulse sequences. Navigator technology has developed rapidly. Such navigators contain the necessary information about the state of motion in the object under investigation. Although it is obtained during the measurement, this information can be processed quickly enough to be used as feedback by the measurement-control system. The data acquisition can now be adjusted to eliminate (or at least greatly reduce) the effects of patient motion, even in sequences lasting for several minutes and in sequences where diffusion encoding runs parallel to image formation. These new developments have resulted in improved spatial resolution and improved image quality in MR diffusion imaging (at the cost of longer measurement times).

The speed of data acquisition is driven by the requirements of the specific application. For instance, the imaging of acute cerebral ischemia needs to be performed extremely quickly to obtain diagnostic information within a rapidly closing therapeutic window. MRI stroke centers thus prefer to use single-shot EPI-based measures of isotropic diffusion, which requires 3 multi-slice diffusion-weighted EPI scans and one reference ($b = 0$) scan covering the patient's whole brain within 1 minute. An EPI sequence is preceded in this scenario by diffusion-sensitizing blocks consisting of gradient pulses and RF pulses that encode the spin system subsequently along three perpendicular spatial directions. A fourth measurement without a diffusion-encoding block is used as a reference scan. This scan can also be used to make adjustments or for purposes of image registration.

The investigation of anisotropic diffusion (e.g. when imaging regions of brain white matter where bundles of fibers run parallel to one another) presupposes more than 3 gradient directions. Depending on the underlying assumptions, it will be necessary to measure between six (i.e. in the case of diffusion-tensor imaging or DTI, which assumes homogeneous Gaussian diffusion within each voxel) and several hundred (i.e. in the case of diffusion-spectral imaging or DSI, which is a 3-dimensional variant of the q-space method described in chapter 7.2.8) diffusion-encoding gradient directions to create diffusion images that display microscopic diffusion behavior on a voxel-to-voxel basis. Here, one is required to arrive at a proper balance of three factors: the spatial resolution of the underlying images, the intrinsic resolution of the voxel's diffusion-summary behavior and (from a practical point of view) the signal-to-noise ratio, which is governed by measurement time.

The use of EPI, preceded by a user-specified number of diffusion encoding directions ranging from 6 to around 1000 directions, still represents the method of choice for anisotropic diffusion imaging.

Variations of diffusion-weighted EPI involving the segmentation of *k*-space (along readout and phase-encode directions) and parallel-imaging techniques in combination with multichannel array coils have shown considerable potential as methods of eliminating imaging artifacts (e.g. the signal dropout and spatial distortion often seen in single-shot EPI). Other imaging techniques such as diffusion-weighted UFLARE, TSTEAM, PSIF, HASTE and trueFISP play a role in applications for regions other than the head and in applications involving systems that are not outfitted for diffusion-weighted EPI.

Image processing and data analysis

While diffusion-weighted images are usually stored in patient databases and can be inspected like other MR images (e.g. T_2-weighted or T_1-weighted images), the occurrence of anisotropic diffusion behavior means that the image contrast will often depend on the direction of the applied diffusion gradient, therefore making it difficult to interpret native diffusion-weighted images on the basis of simple visual inspection.

An elegant way of displaying diffusion information in MR images was introduced in 1994 when Basser proposed a diffusion-tensor model. Diffusive transport can be characterized in anisotropic media by a second-rank diffusion tensor that is assumed to be symmetric. The MR signal decay is given by the tensor product of the diffusion tensor D with a sensitivity tensor b, where b contains the experimental settings of the MR experiment, namely, the gradient timing and gradient amplitudes along the different spatial directions. The full determination of the diffusion tensor requires 7 measurements, i.e. in order to estimate the unattenuated ($b = 0$) signal as well as 6 b-tensor elements, represented by at least 6 different measured diffusion-encoding gradient directions.

The tensor can be decomposed into its eigensystem after the measurement and the principal diffusivities (eigenvalues) can be directly mapped pixel by pixel according to a color-coded scheme.

Various scalar invariants of D (which are independent of the laboratory reference frame) are often calculated in order to map the geometric properties of the tensor eigensystem: the trace (sum of the three principal diffusivities) of the diffusion tensor is commonly used when highlighting isotropic diffusion.

Dimensionless ratios of principal diffusivities such as the fractional anisotropy (FA) are used to highlight anisotropic diffusion. Other scalar measures and intuitive methods of visualizing tensor information are discussed in the literature.

Applications

Diffusion imaging has been routinely applied in clinical settings as a quick test of a third contrast (i.e. in addition to T_1-weighted and T_2-weighted routine brain imaging scans) since the beginning of the new century. Improvements in image quality that do

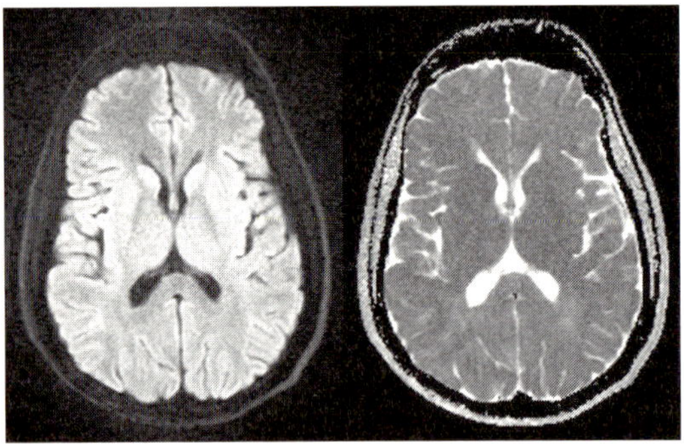

Figure 15.95
Segmented DW-EPI with the 2D navigator-based correction of motion [15.139]. **Left:** diffusion-weighted image, $b = 1{,}000\ s/mm^2$. **Right:** ADC map (in-plane spatial resolution 1 mm, 20 slices at 5 mm each, acquisition time 3 minutes).

not involve significantly prolonged measurement times have helped to increase diagnostic accuracy. Two major developments have supported this process:

1) Parallel imaging techniques in combination with multichannel array coils has enabled one to significantly reduce spatial distortion in EPI imaging.
2) Segmented EPI (controlled by navigator signals) has enabled one to generate high quality diffusion-weighted images at reasonable measurement times and in the absence of multichannel array coils. The combination of both developments may lead to high quality diffusion images and total acquisition times of less than a minute (fig. 15.95).

In what follows, we discuss a number of clinical applications for diffusion MR. One example is the immediate and robust visualization of pathological processes that change the behavior of isotropic diffusion in acute brain ischemia. A high signal in DW images indicates restricted diffusion, which is associated with cell swelling (cytotoxic edema). DW-EPI represents an important component in a comprehensive approach to diagnosing and treating acute stroke (fig. 15.96).

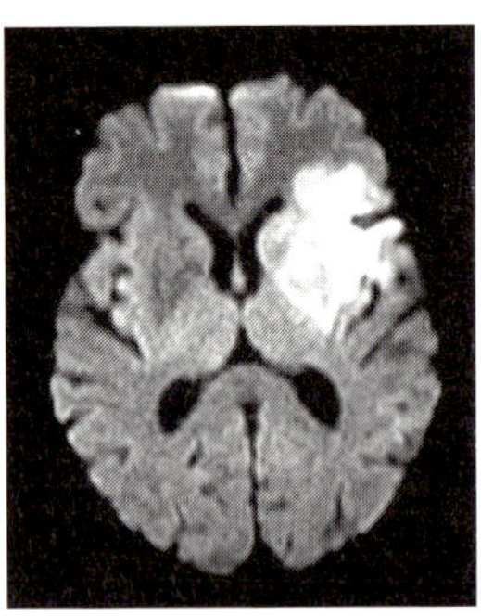

Figure 15.96
DW-EPI: transverse section of a patient's brain showing large regions of bright signal indicating acute brain ischemia (1.5 T Magnetom Avanto, multichannel array coil, parallel imaging, in-plane spatial resolution, in-plane 1.3 mm images) (Source: Professor Terwey, Dr. Lentschig, Bremen)

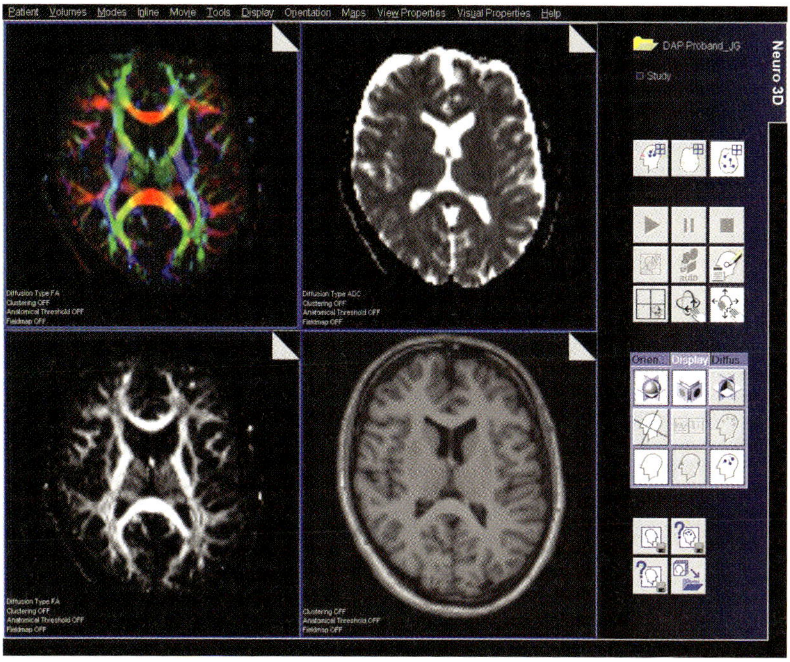

Figure 15.97
Comparison of a diffusion-tensor experiment with a T_1-weighted study of a healthy volunteer's brain. **Upper left:** colored anisotropy map, main diffusivity mediolateral: red, craniocaudal: blue, frontodorsal: green. **Upper right:** ADC map, bright signal means high diffusion constant. **Lower left:** fractional anisotropy map, scale from 0 (isotropic diffusion or zero anisotropy) to 1 (diffusion along one axis only). **Lower right:** corresponding T_1-weighted image from the same section of the brain.

Fig. 15.97 shows an example of a measurement of diffusion-tensor information featuring the side-by-side display of several images of a transverse section through the brain of a healthy volunteer.

Fig. 15.98 also shows a method of visualizing diffusion-tensor fields using a three-dimensional color-coded scheme. It is well known that nerve fibers show anisotropic diffusion behavior characterized by diffusivity levels that are significantly higher along the fiber axis than perpendicular to the fiber axis. On the other hand, it warrants bearing in mind that what is shown as fiber tracking is not a matter of fibers (which often have diameters on the order of tens of micrometers) but of some structural layer, consisting of bundles of nerve fibers running parallel to one another. The spatial resolution of the MR experiment is still restricted by measurement time and SNR. It is therefore necessary to arrive at an acceptable compromise between the spatial resolution of the underlying imaging experiment, as defined by a sampling of k-space (see chapter 7.3.2), and the number of diffusion encoding steps, as defined by a sampling of q-space.

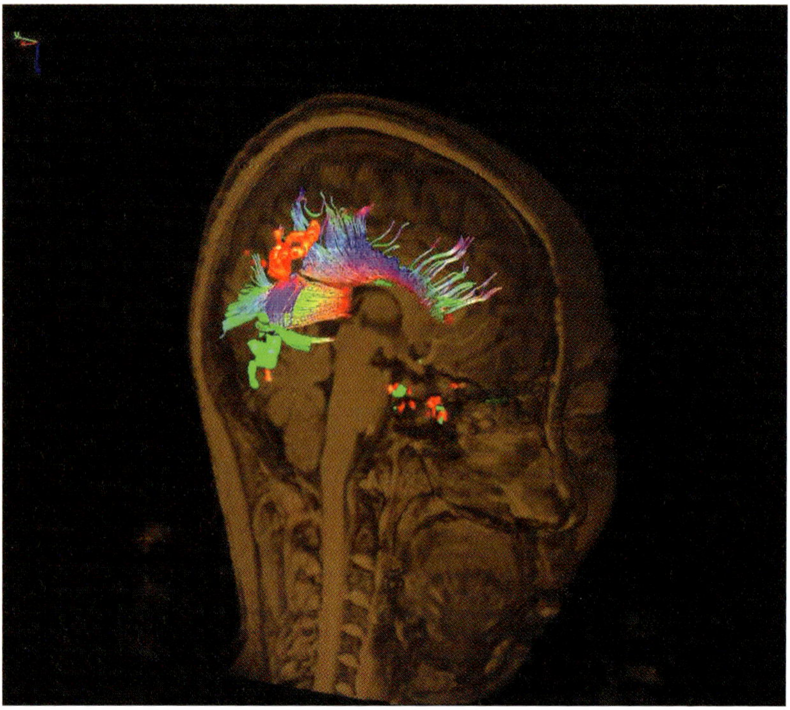

Figure 15.98
Visualization of measured diffusion-tensor field suggesting a colored tractography along regions of white matter in the human brain. The colored tractography (12 minute acquisition time, 2 by 2 by 5 mm resolution, DTI) is superimposed onto a 3D T_1-weighted representation of the brain (7 minute acquisition time, 1 mm isotropic resolution, MPRAGE).

15.2.5.3 Functional imaging

The BOLD effect

Prior to the late 1980s, T_2* relaxation caused by local magnetic field inhomogeneity was widely seen as a source of image artifacts. Around 1990, Ogawa [15.113] and Turner [15.140] showed in animal experiments that MR image contrast was altered by induced changes in local blood oxygenation. This observation was based on the fact (noted by Faraday and measured by Pauling [15.141] long ago) that deoxyhemoglobin is paramagnetic while oxyhemoglobin (as well as brain tissue) is diamagnetic.

One could thus regard deoxyhemoglobin as nature's own contrast agent, activated by any intervention creating an imbalance between oxygen uptake and local blood flow. The first human brain mapping experiment was successfully tested in the spring of 1991 at the MRI Center of the Massachusetts General Hospital in Boston where Kwong [15.142] showed that the change in deoxyhemoglobin in the human visual cortex that occurred while a subject viewed a bright light was sufficient to permit the detection of changes in T_2*-weighted MR images in a slice through the calcarine fissure. The technique was named blood oxygenation level-dependent contrast or BOLD.

Compared to other techniques using contrast agents or doses of radiation, this procedure was the first functional mapping of the human brain to be performed completely noninvasively. In identifying cortical areas active for a particular brain task, the experiment introduced a new investigational capacity that offered an unparalleled spatial resolution of 2 mm, temporal resolution of 1 second and the opportunity to rescan individual subjects as often as desired.

Within a decade, BOLD imaging (now mainly referred to as functional MRI or fMRI) became the preeminent tool for human brain mapping. This preeminence is echoed in the several thousands of scientific papers published each year that are devoted to its application in a variety of fields of brain research.

Indirect measurement of brain activation using BOLD imaging

Brain imaging techniques such as PET and fMRI are deployed in order to fill the gap between direct studies of brain function at the physiological level (e.g. EEG recordings, MEG (magneto-encephalogram)) and indirect studies of psychological processes at the cognitive level. Here, it warrants pointing out that fMRI studies, which rely on the BOLD effect, represent a rather indirect correlate of neural activity.

fMRI experiments involve exposing a subject to a sequence of stimuli (e.g. the visual presentation of objects or tasks, the application of sensory events, etc.) and observing the subject's responses by sampling T_2*-weighted images of the brain.

The presentation of stimuli causes a fraction of the human brain's 10^{12} neurons to communicate via electrical signals. This neural activation is followed by a change in local cerebral blood flow, a phenomenon postulated by Roy and Sherrington in 1890 [15.143] and measured by Fox and Raichle in PET experiments in 1986 [15.144]. Many experiments have since demonstrated that neural (electric) activity is indeed followed by transient increases in regional cerebral blood flow and regional cerebral blood volume as well as a slight increase in local oxygen consumption. A complete explanation of this transient hemodynamic response to neural activity has yet to be presented.

Studies have consistently shown that diamagnetic oxyhemoglobin flows into the active brain regions following stimulus presentation and a short deoxygenation period of around one second. This flow reaches a peak at around 6 to 8 seconds and then decreases in a matter of a few seconds.

BOLD images primarily show oxygenation changes in small venules overlying neurally active cortical tissue, i.e. given that these contain the majority of the blood that undergoes local changes in oxygenation [15.145, 15.146].

BOLD data acquisition

While the difference in the susceptibility of oxygenated and deoxygenated blood is small (about $2 \cdot 10^{-8}$ cgs units), it is sufficient to produce measurable signal intensity changes of a few percent in high field T_2*-weighted MR experiments.

Data acquisition in fMRI is mainly achieved via echo-planar imaging (EPI). While the intrinsic sensitivity of gradient-echo EPI to susceptibility effects is a clear factor, imaging speed is also important in enabling researchers to scan slices through the brain with a high signal-to-noise ratio in less than 100 ms and at a spatial resolution of about 2 mm. Today, fMRI imaging speed is no longer restricted by scanner hardware, but by patient safety considerations (avoiding potential peripheral nerve stimulation by fast switching imaging gradients) and the task of optimizing BOLD contrast imaging parameters, which requires a rather long echo time depending on the magnetic field strength of the fMRI scanner.

A typical fMRI experiment involves acquiring multi-slice volume data sets with an (isotropic) resolution of 2 to 3 mm from a subject's brain at equidistant spatial intervals every 2.4 seconds.

fMRI: experimental design

In a typical fMRI experiment, a subject lies on the patient table of an MRI scanner while viewing an LCD screen, listening to auditory input via head phones or performing cognitive tasks in response to specific instructions. During this time, a time series of MR images of the subject's brain is obtained (fig. 15.99). Some more advanced experiments include the simultaneous recording of physiological signals such as ECG and the electric conductivity of skin or eye movements for the sake of data analysis.

The majority of fMRI experiments involve the use of a block design: stimulus presentation is typically altered in temporal blocks of 20 to 60 seconds. The presentation of alternating checkerboards followed by the presentation of a fixation point (followed again by checkerboards, etc.) represents a simple example.

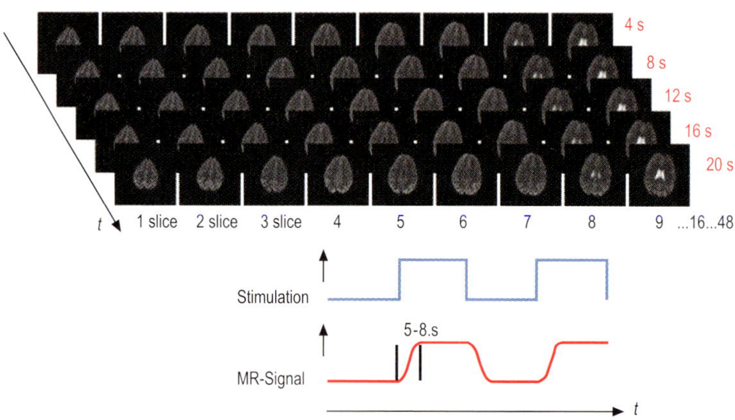

Figure 15.99
Typical fMRI experiment. The cognitive cortex is repeatedly stimulated while images are continuously acquired via EPI.

The experiment might last from a few minutes (e.g. 3 cycles with each cycle encompassing 30 seconds of stimulus-on conditions and 30 seconds of stimulus-off conditions) for common clinical applications to more than one hour for sophisticated experiments conducted at research centers.

The high spatial and relatively high temporal resolution involved makes it necessary to collect and process huge amounts of native images (see below).

Although the subject's head is fixed using passive means (e.g. foam pads and instructions given by the investigator), it is impossible to avoid some slight degree of head motion (e.g. 1 mm per minute) using passive means. This motion represents a major limiting factor when it comes to analyzing the data generated during fMRI time series.

Efforts to overcome this limiting factor have centered on the development of motion correction techniques (see section 15.2.4.2). Here, certain image-based techniques involving real-time prospective motion correction have been introduced [15.99] that enable a nearly complete removal of slow and tiny head motion effects during the fMRI experiment.

EPI sequences exhibit a high intrinsic sensitivity to the subtle magnetic-field changes that can arise in connection with the respiratory motion of the subject or external sources such as elevators that are located close to the MRI scanner. Modern MRI scanners are capable of correcting for these effects (which lead to small artificial image shifts in time series experiments) automatically via the use of navigators encoded into the EPI sequences [15.147].

Image processing and data analysis

Image time series are calculated after (or during) data acquisition. Such calculations may comprise the removal of artifacts from EPI images, navigator-based field correction, image-based motion correction and spatial and temporal smoothing.

The images undergo further analysis once this pre-processing work is complete. Such analysis may be model-based or data-driven. Model-based analysis was widely applied in the decade following the introduction of fMRI.

The aim of fMRI data analysis is to provide insight concerning statistically relevant relationships between a modeled signal-time course and the acquired data. A simple assumption is that signal-time course is directly reflected by (or identical to) the time course of the stimulus presentation used in the experiment. Given that observed changes in local blood oxygenation are delayed and dispersed compared to the primary (but not directly observed) neuronal activity of the brain, taking the hemodynamic response into account can improve the results of BOLD-type fMRI experiments. The time course of stimulus presentation is convolved with an assumed hemodynamic response function for purposes of data analysis.

Given that the BOLD signal is very weak, its analysis requires statistical methods [15.142, 15.148]. In the context of a simple *t*-test evaluation, the images are grouped into two parts: an *activated* (N_{active} images) and a *baseline* ($N_{passive}$ images) series of images. (It may be useful, however, to remove data acquired during or shortly after the transition of the stimulus to another state). In order to test whether the average MR signal <S> at location x, y of the two series is the same, the following equation is applied:

$$t = \frac{\langle S_{\text{active}} \rangle - \langle S_{\text{passive}} \rangle}{\sqrt{\frac{\text{var}(S_{\text{active}})}{N_{\text{active}}} + \frac{\text{var}(S_{\text{passive}})}{N_{\text{passive}}}}} \tag{15.61}$$

The significance of this value is evaluated on the basis of Student's t distribution $f(t, \nu)$, the number of degrees of freedom ν given by the number of samples and the variances [15.149]. If the value of the resulting significance is small, then the observed average signal difference is very pronounced.

Another evaluation method is to analyze the correlation of the BOLD signal $S(t_i)$ in one voxel with a model time course, which is in the most simple case the time course $s(t_i)$ of the applied stimulus or $s(t_i)$ convolved with a hemodynamic response function. From the correlation coefficient

$$r = \frac{\sum_{i=1}^{N} (S(t_i) - \langle S \rangle)(s(t_i) - \langle s \rangle)}{\sqrt{\sum_{i=1}^{N} (S(t_i) - \langle S \rangle)^2 \sum_{i=1}^{N} (s(t_i) - \langle s \rangle)^2}} \tag{15.62}$$

a test value

$$t = \sqrt{\frac{r^2}{1 - r^2}(N - 2)} \tag{15.63}$$

can be derived, which again allows one to derive the significance of the 0-hypothesis (i.e. the two functions are not correlated) from Student's t distribution. At typical $N = 60$ images a value of $t > 3.5$ means that the probability that the two functions are totally independent is less than 1/1,000. The map showing t values larger than the significance level can be superimposed onto the MR images to show regions of functional activity (fig. 15.100).

A more sophisticated and widely used analysis of BOLD experiments uses general linear model statistics (GLM) [15.150]. The BOLD signal $S(t_i)$ of each voxel is fitted to a model formed of several components, which could explain the observed data.

$$S(t_i) = \sum_j \beta_i M_i(t_i) + \varepsilon_i \tag{15.64}$$

The model may take into account various contributions M_j, e.g. the applied stimulus pattern convolved with the impulse response function describing the shape of the expected bold response, offsets, derivatives of the stimulation function, signal drifts etc. Minimizing the sum of the quadratic residual errors ε_i delivers parameters β_j describing the contribution of each model component M_j. Test statistics can be used to test for the significance of the model employing the Fischer F-test (i.e. comparing the vari-

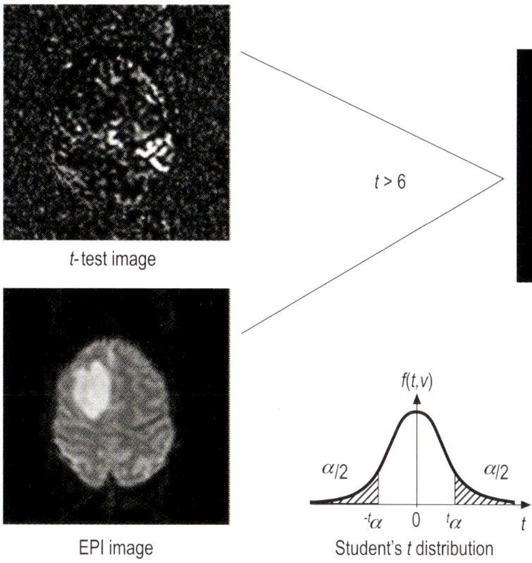

Figure 15.100
Evaluation of an fMRI experiment. A *t*-test image derived from the correlation of the MR signal with the stimulus function is superimposed on the MR image. The *t*-value allows one to determine the significance level for two events uncorrelated in Student's *t* distribution.

ances of model and BOLD signal) and the significance of single model parameters employing Student's *t*-test (i.e. comparing the means of model and the BOLD signal).

The multivariate data analysis of the GLM allows a better description of observed time courses of signal intensities in an fMRI experiment than simply comparing activated and not activated data or correlation with the stimulus. The model functions can describe covariates of interest as the stimulus presentation pattern convolved with a hemodynamic response function. Sophisticated patterns designed with components to stimulate different brain responses or areas can be analyzed. In addition covariates of no interest (like physiologically induced or hardware induced signal fluctuations, which are known and thus can be modeled, but which we are not interested in) can be added. By the use of multiple reference functions including covariates of no interest a better detection power of the statistics can be achieved. Prerequisite for a reasonable model design is a sufficient orthogonality of model time courses. As a result of the GLM analysis again a (pixelwise) *t*-map is obtained. For a detailed description of the GLM model applied to fMRI data sets we refer to [15.151].

The development of easy-to-use real-time fMRI products

Major advances in computer hardware and software have introduced a variety of applications. In less than a decade, the data processing times supported by commercially available MRI scanners have been accelerated by several orders of magnitude, thus enabling users to perform fMRI experiments (including data analysis and the 3D visualization of results) in real time.

While this increases the number of fMRI examinations that are possible in the context of established applications, it also opens the door to a wide array of new applications.

In addition to temporal performance, the quality of investigational results has significantly improved along with advances in computer vision and advances in the entire testing chain comprised of stimulus presentation, data acquisition and image analysis.

Image quality in fMRI experiments can be enhanced by properly registering the time series of volume data sets. Increases in computer power and algorithmic optimization have made it possible to accelerate the detection of tiny head movements to the level of real-time performance. Control processing units that make use of fast feedback loops between image calculation and measurement have led to prospective motion-correction techniques [15.99] involving the readjustment of measured slice positions and orientations during data acquisition in response to slight head movements. This has enabled the nearly complete removal of motion-based image artifacts.

Advances made at a variety of university research centers around the world have been optimized in terms of workflow, usability and temporal performance by large MR manufacturers and incorporated into commercially available products.

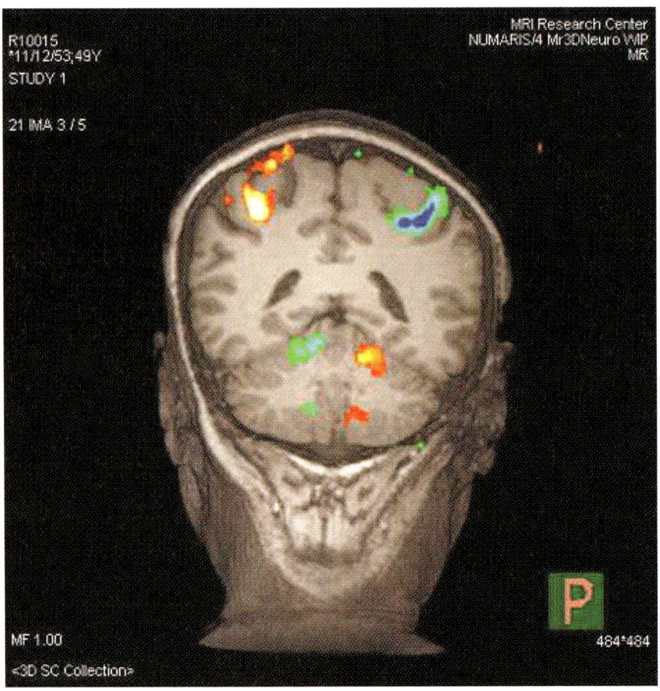

Figure 15.101
Color display of an fMRI experiment superimposed onto anatomical data. The bilateral finger tapping experiment shows contralateral cerebral activation of the corresponding primary motor areas and ipsilateral activation in the cerebellum of a normal subject.

Data acquisition has become more reliable thanks to the development of parallel imaging techniques that enable one to scan the whole brain with EPI and that are less susceptible to artifacts.

EPI image reconstruction (including ramp sampling and multichannel head array coils, spatial data filtering, rigid-body 3D motion correction, general linear model-based statistical analysis, and 3D color display of results superimposed onto high resolution anatomical data sets) can be performed on the fly, thereby allowing the user to watch the progress of the experiment in an interactive way while the subject performs the assigned tasks (fig. 15.101).

Data acquisition with multi-slice EPI covering the whole brain at an isotropic resolution of 3 mm has been performed with prospective motion correction. Image calculation, spatial filtering and statistical analysis are all performed on the fly. The user can navigate through the 3D data set during the experiment.

Applications

Since its introduction only 15 years ago, fMRI has led to the development of a broad spectrum of applications that have been reported in more than 10,000 publications. More than 2,000 MRI scanners around the world are capable of performing fMRI. Three major areas of fMRI investigation have emerged: 1) neurological imaging of functional mechanisms in the human and animal brain, 2) general presurgical mapping and various applications in psychiatry and, last but not least, 3) research at the point of convergence between psychology and economics (e.g. marketing research).

Research involving neurofeedback fMRI has even revealed a certain potential for transforming MR scanning from a purely diagnostic modality into a diagnostic and therapeutic modality: experiments have shown that patients learn to regulate their own brain activity during neurofeedback fMRI sessions. This may enable one to directly regulate and lower pain and phobias.

Applications in neuroscience

The imaging of functional mechanisms in the human brain can be carried out in an entirely noninvasive way. This permits one to perform longitudinal and group studies in all kinds of human subjects. Areas of investigation include sensation and perception, attention, cognition, learning and memory, motor function and language.

While the sensitivity of the EPI-based fMRI imaging technique to local field inhomogeneity has resulted in a more extensive investigation of the posterior division of the brain (the parietal, temporal and occipital cortices) than of the frontal lobes, recent advances in methods of data acquisition (e.g. parallel imaging using multichannel coils) have opened the entire brain to extensive investigation.

Presenting an overview of the fMRI-based advances in neuroscience would go beyond the scope of this book. Readers may therefore wish to refer to the literature for more information in this regard [15.151, 15.152].

Clinical applications

The clinical applications that have been reported include presurgical planning for tumor patients, mainly focused on somatosensory and primary motor function adjacent to lesions in the central region of the brain (fig. 15.102), lateralization of language and memory, detection of focal seizures in epilepsy, dementia, stroke (ascertaining risk and predicting the recovery of function) and chronic pain. New clinical applications are being rapidly introduced in the areas of psychiatry, mental illness and the study of human emotions (affective disorders). One of the most fascinating areas is pediatric fMRI, with applications centering on developmental disorders such as attention-deficit/hyperactivity disorder, obsessive-compulsive disorder, developmental dyslexia and childhood depression.

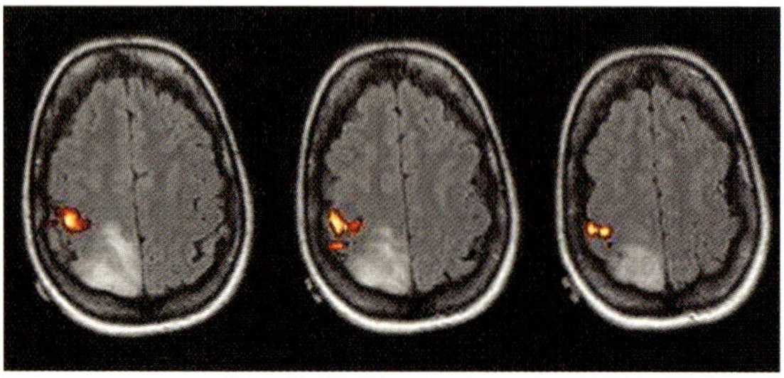

Figure 15.102
Presurgical planning in a patient with low grade glioma. Anatomy and function (color overlay) are obtained during a single session (display of three adjacent transverse slices, glioma hyperintense on T_1-weighted MPRAGE data). The fMRI experiment was based on multi-slice single-shot EPI. The result of the statistical analysis is superimposed onto the T_1-weighted study. The colored representation of the primary sensomotoric hand area can be used as safety-relevant information by a trained neurosurgeon. Markers outside the head were used in this case for neuronavigation during surgery. MR data are available online during surgery. (Source: German Cancer Research Center, Heidelberg).

fMRI is both convenient and safe for patients (in particular, when compared to invasive procedures such as WADA testing of language lateralization and EEG mapping during brain surgery) and it is cost-effective and fast. Furthermore, the availability of fMRI-capable MR scanners is high.

Readers may wish to refer to the literature for an overview fMRI's clinical applications [15.153].

15.2.6 Clinical examples

15.2.6.1 Comprehensive MRI stroke examination

Some facts about stroke

After myocardial infarction and cancer, stroke is the third leading cause of death in the industrialized countries of the world and is the leading cause of severe, long-term disability [15.154, 15.155].

The socioeconomic consequences that result from millions of disabled stroke patients, suffering from permanent deficits such as hemiparesis and aphasia are obvious. Average annual cost estimates for a patient who has survived a stroke range from USD 35,000 to USD 50,000. The incidence and prevalence of stroke are expected to continue to rise in the near future.

However, new therapeutic options (especially the use of recanalizing drugs) and new diagnostic capabilities (mainly involving CT and MRI) offer grounds for hope [15.152]. Dozens of stroke centers equipped with modern technology and trained personnel have shown that treatment can be very effective and can even offer a cure in many cases if patients exhibiting the symptoms of acute stroke make it to the 24-hour service centers on time!

On the other hand, clinicians in many countries have no access to CT and MRI and many stroke patients are still treated in departments of general internal medicine.

MRI as a multiparametric approach

MRI offers access to a variety of independent physical observables. Tissue can be characterized by relaxation times T_1, T_2 and by spin density. Other parameters that provide additional information include chemical shift (separation of fat and water, metabolic mapping by MR spectroscopy, measurement of tissue temperature), susceptibility (BOLD effect, brain function), diffusion (cytotoxic edema, highlighting of anisotropic diffusion structures) and spin velocity (TOF angiography, maps of blood flow velocity).

All of these multiple observables can be ascertained during a single measurement session that requires no patient repositioning and no patient transfer to other modalities.

A comprehensive MRI stroke examination generates all of the information that is necessary to make a sound diagnosis and to specify corresponding therapeutic measures.

An MRI stroke protocol

Patients who enter a stroke unit may exhibit severe neurological symptoms such as hemiparesis or aphasia. While cerebral ischemia is often the cause of the symptoms, it is necessary to first rule out other causes such as seizure, encephalitis and cerebral hemorrhaging.

A widely-accepted therapeutic procedure is available if the diagnostic evaluation indicates cerebral ischemia: apply fibrinolytic therapy within the first 3 hours of the onset of symptoms. Fibrinolytic therapy involves an attempt to recanalize an occluded brain artery and to prevent infarction in the tissue zone at risk [15.157]. Although the tissue in this zone may have been subject to inadequate perfusion, it can still be saved. The necessity of a rapid response means that any diagnostic procedures will have to be time-optimized. A typical MR-imaging protocol for acute stroke takes about 10 minutes to execute and comprises the following steps:

1) *TOF-MR angiography to show vessel occlusion*
   (approximately 50 slices of 1.2 to 1.6 mm, a 192×256 matrix at an FOV of 22 cm and an acquisition time of < 4 minutes)

2) *Diffusion-weighted imaging (DWI) to show the infarcted region, i.e. the region rapidly progressing towards a state of infarction*
   (20 slices of 6 mm, a 64 or 128 matrix at an FOV of 24 cm, $b = 1000$ s/mm^2, 3 directions and an acquisition time of < 2 min)
3) *Perfusion-weighted imaging (PWI) in combination with DWI to show the tissue at risk*
   (intravenous injection of 0.1 mmol/kg body weight contrast agent, 12 slices of 6 mm, a 64 or 128 matrix at an FOV of 24 cm, maximum $T_R = 1.5$ s and an acquisition time of 1.5 minutes)
4) *Fluid attenuated inversion recovery (FLAIR) to exclude subarachnoidal hemorrhaging*
   (20 slices of 6 mm, a 256 by 192 matrix at an FOV of 24 cm, flip angle = 90° and an acquisition time of < 2 min)

Axial and coronal MIPs of the MRA as well as diffusion maps (trace-weighted and ADC maps) and perfusion maps are available immediately after data acquisition. The data allow the physician to:

1) Exclude other sources of neurological symptoms, especially cerebral hemorrhaging
2) Localize areas affected by ongoing pathological processes
3) Detect a mismatch between abnormal regions in DWI and PWI images, and thus create a mental image of an ischemic penumbra that might help when it comes making a decision about how to proceed (e.g. whether fibrinolysis should be carried out)

A fast T_2-weighted imaging procedure may be added to the protocol to enable one to differentiate between new and old infarction zones. Diffusion-tensor imaging and proton spectroscopy are sometimes used for research purposes (i.e. to obtain additional and more specific information). However, in deference to the golden rule that admonishes clinicians in stroke situations that time is brain, these additional examinations are usually not carried out in most clinical settings.

Careful assessments of the feasibility, practicality and logistics of the multisequence MRI stroke protocols currently in use will continue to influence the design of MR scanners and will ultimately lead to more effective scanners and an enhanced capacity to carry out diagnoses in emergency care units.

Success in the diagnosis and treatment of acute cerebral ischemia continues to be limited by basic matters of infrastructure – the world is home to only a few hundred stroke centers – and deficient public awareness about stroke symptoms. Readers may wish to refer to the literature for an excellent overview of the use of MRI in diagnosing stroke [15.158].

15.2.6.2 Comprehensive cardiac exam

One of the driving forces behind the rapid development of cardiovascular MR (CMR) has been its comprehensive nature. Whereas typical evaluation of ischemic heart disease may include a variety of diagnostic tests such as echocardiography, ECG, nuclear stress imaging, cardiac CT, and coronary X-ray angiography, CMR has the potential to provide much of the diagnostic power of the individual tests in a single examination. A single examination for the patient has the potential to reduce the time to diagnosis and treatment, and also provides the managing physician with inherently registered imaging data of global ventricular function, regional wall motion, valve function, myocardial perfusion, myocardial viability, and proximal coronary anatomy.

In the past several years, advances in MR scanner hardware and software have made real-time and near real-time imaging possible for many CMR applications. These advances in speed have made it possible to combine multiple modes of CMR imaging in a single exam session. Concurrently, advances in image analysis software have made interpretation and presentation of quantitative results possible. As a result, CMR is moving steadily into diagnosis of ischemic heart disease in addition to some of its more traditional areas of anatomic evaluation of congenital heart disease, pericardial disease, and the aorta.

Ventricular function

Ventricular function has long been the mainstay of echocardiography, due to its wide availability, and real-time capability. Echocardiography has some disadvantages, however, including limited acoustic windows due to intervening structures, relatively poor ability to assess the right ventricle, and variability in blood-myocardial contrast. Due to these limitations, reproducibility of cardiac function parameters by echocardiography is less than that of CMR. CMR's advantages for ventricular function include no limitation on scan plane selection, ability to evaluate both the right and left ventricles simultaneously, and excellent blood-myocardial contrast even in patients with poor ventricular function. With fast imaging techniques, both high spatial and temporal resolution images can be acquired in a single breath-hold, or in real-time for resting heart-rates. Disadvantages however, include the need to bring the patient to the MR scanner (as opposed to being able to bring the echocardiography machine bedside, even in the operating room), and a limited number of imaging physicians who practice CMR.

Wall motion abnormalites can be assessed both qualitatively and quantitatively with CMR, and high resolution functional imaging can also be obtained during the high heart rates of dobutamine stress testing to elucidate ischemic areas of the myocardium. Fig. 15.103 shows an example of a trueFISP MR image in the short-axis plane.

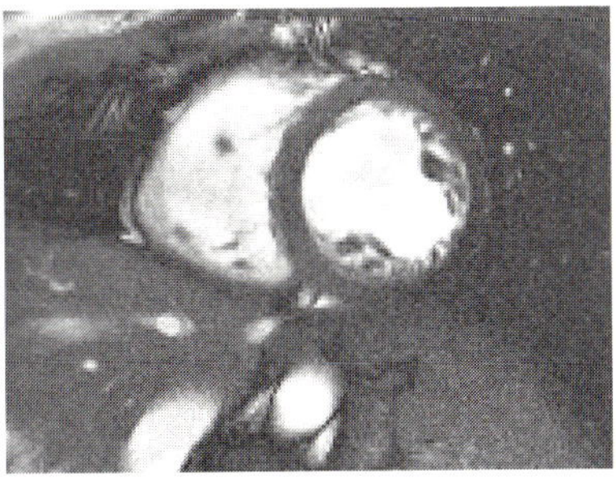

Figure 15.103
TrueFISP short axis image at end-diastole shows high blood-myocardial contrast.

Valvular function

As with ventricular function, echocardiography has been the main modality for assessment of valvular disease due to its real-time nature and ability to image both structure and flow. CMR has some advantages for pixel-by-pixel quantitation of flow dynamics as compared to echocardiography, but is not as flexible and easy to incorporate into an entire examination. Therefore, it has been used so far mainly for problem-solving in evaluation of valvular disease, or in research studies where high accuracy is required.

Myocardial perfusion imaging

SPECT and PET imaging have been the traditional modalities for evaluation of myocardial perfusion. SPECT is widely available and provides qualitative assessment of myocardial perfusion, but has relatively poor spatial resolution, masking small perfusion deficits, and exposing patients to ionizing radiation. PET provides quantitative myocardial blood flow measures, but is not as widely available as SPECT, and also suffers from relatively poor spatial resolution.

With CMR, using fast dynamic imaging one can track the passage of a contrast agent through the heart (T_1 shortening) in order to estimate parameters related to myocardial perfusion, or to visualize perfusion deficits qualitatively. Imaging approaches have included saturation-recovery TurboFLASH, trueFISP or segmented EPI. In general multiple slices are acquired, with an acquisition time of 100 to 200 ms, each heartbeat. Images are acquired pre-contrast arrival for baseline estimation, and for 60 to 90 s post contrast arrival. Nominal voxel size is on the order of 2 to 4 mm in plane and 5 mm through-plane, as compared to approximately 4 to 8 mm in plane and 10 mm through-plane for SPECT imaging. Further, since the images are each acquired in a short period at each cardiac cycle in CMR, blurring due to cardiac motion is minimized.

Quantitative analysis of the resulting time-intensity curves can be done to estimate parameters related to myocardial perfusion, such as upslope and area under the time-intensity curve. With additional analysis of the left ventricular input function, quantitative results in ml/min/100 g tissue can be derived, although to date, these measurements are still in evaluation in research studies. Fig. 15.104 shows sample images at various stages post-contrast administration. Due to the demonstrated ability of CMR to detect small perfusion defects and register perfusion images with those of function and infarction, there is intense interest in the cardiac imaging community to make perfusion CMR a robust clinical tool. Ongoing work in standardization of acquisition methods, and analysis methods will allow these methods to move from the research environment to clinical use in the next years.

Late enhancement imaging

Methods for distinguishing live from dead myocardium have long been sought after in the area of ischemic heart disease and also for evaluation of cardiomyopathies. The previous standard for detecting myocardial infarction with imaging was SPECT imaging (stress/delayed imaging). However, due to limitations in spatial resolution, SPECT is not ideal for detection of small subendocardial infarcts. Late enhancement CMR, due

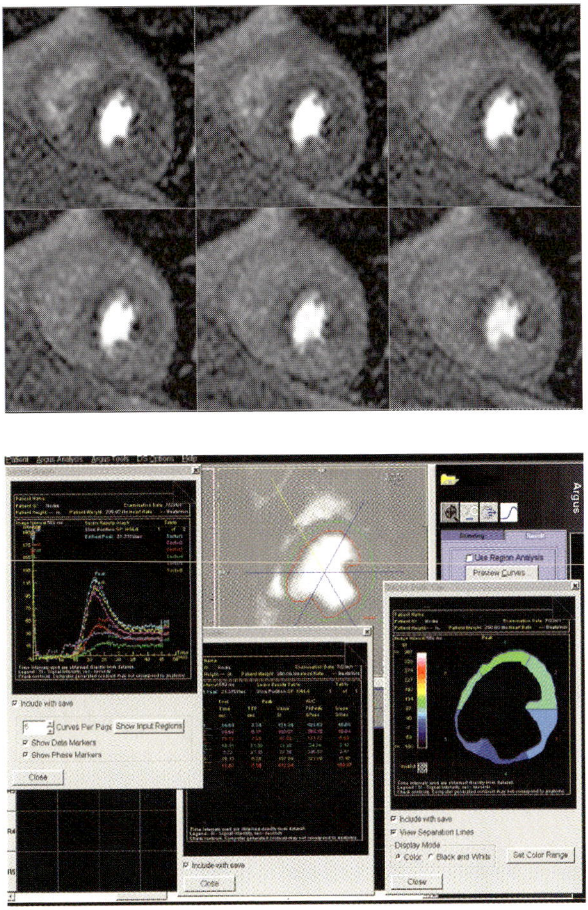

Figure 15.104
Myocardial perfusion images (TurboFLASH) showing a subendocardial perfusion defect in a patient with hypertension and exertional chest pain **(top)** (Source: Sir Run Run Shaw, Heart Center, Hong Kong) and time intensity curves and semiquantitative analysis of myocardial perfusion by CMR

to its high spatial resolution, is ideal for this application, and has become widely adopted for clinical evaluation of infarcts and cardiomyopathies in the past few years.

The basic principle involves use of an inversion-recovery imaging sequence and taking advantage of the kinetics of the contrast agent Gd-DTPA. Gd-DTPA is cleared from normal myocardium rapidly but accumulates in non-viable regions (infarcts, other areas of dead fibrotic tissue). The shortened T_1 of the non-viable tissue allows it to be separated easily from normal myocardium using an IR sequence between 10 and 30 minutes post-contrast administration. The inversion time is set to null for normal myocardium, which provides high contrast-to-noise for infarcts compared to background

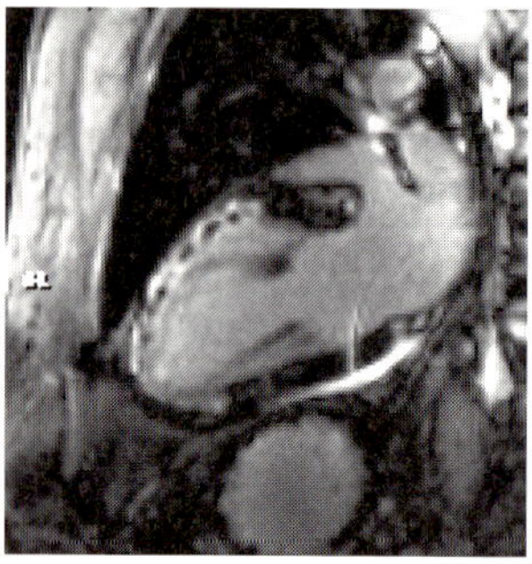

Figure 15.105
Late enhancement CMR image of myocardial infarction in the anterior wall of the left ventricle (Source: University of Erlangen)

tissue. Imaging can be performed in either 2D or 3D, during respiratory gating, in a breath-hold or during free-breathing in real-time. Fig. 15.105 shows an example of a myocardial infarction using this technique.

Coronary imaging

One of the most challenging areas, and potentially one of the most rewarding areas in CMR is imaging of the coronary arteries. Clinicians have long sought noninvasive methods for evaluation of the coronary arteries, and both CT and MR are candidates. This CMR application requires sub-millimeter spatial resolution, rapid imaging to freeze cardiac and respiratory motion, high signal-to-noise, and high contrast between the blood in the coronary artery and background fat or myocardial tissue. The general approach is to acquire several lines of *k*-space each cardiac cycle, during a portion of the heart cycle where motion is minimized. Respiratory motion is compensated for by either breath-holding (at the expense of spatial resolution), or by use of navigator echoes to track the respiratory motion and restrict acquisition to narrow acceptance windows (at the expense of scan efficiency). Although many improvements in coronary imaging have been made in the last years, the technique is still not widely used. CT is faster at the moment than MR, and has more robust image quality. However, research in evaluation of the coronaries by MR is also driven by MR's ability to image the coronary wall and potentially characterize plaque noninvasively. Ultimate ap-

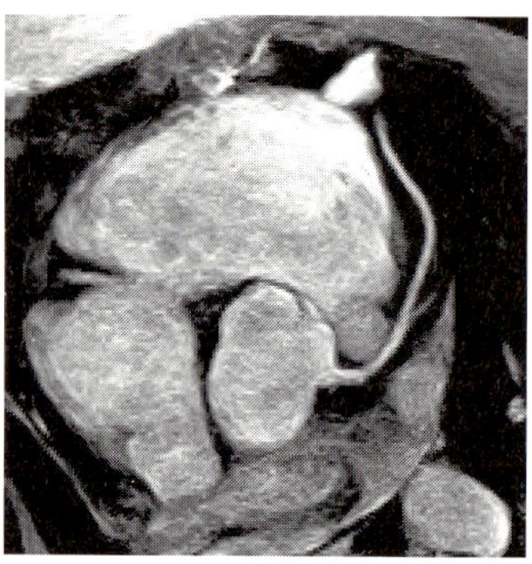

Figure 15.106
Coronary imaging with trueFISP
(Source: Northwestern University)

plication may be assisted by use of intravascular contrast media that are under development by several companies. The combination of high resolution coronary lumen imaging and vessel wall characterization is the ultimate goal. Fig. 15.106 shows an example of a high resolution MR coronary image obtained in a breath-hold.

Future directions

Though almost all the components of comprehensive cardiovascular MR are in place, and cardiologists as well as radiologists are using it, there is still work to be done to streamline the overall workflow and make CMR easy to perform in a routine clinical setting. Thus, continued work in real-time methods, interactive imaging, intelligent software parameter settings, and automated image analysis will be key to the dissemination of this technology. Also, as real-time interactive imaging becomes a reality, other applications such as interventional cardiovascular procedures are emerging. Readers are referred to any of the recent comprehensive textbooks in the area of CMR [15.159-15.162], for in depth description of CMR methods and clinical application.

15.2.6.3 Interventional MR

As the importance of minimally invasive procedures in medicine continues to grow, so too does the need for more advanced and accurate methods of guiding and controlling these procedures. MRI offers many advantages when it comes to guiding diagnostic and therapeutic procedures. These advantages include high soft-tissue contrast, unrestricted multiplanar imaging capabilities, absence of ionizing radiation, thermomonitoring capabilities and the capacity to provide functional information about blood flow, diffusion and perfusion. Interventional MRI has evolved during the last 10 years from a topic of research to a procedure offering a number of valuable clinical applications. The general technical advances that amongst others have helped to further establish interventional MRI include more open magnet designs, faster imaging techniques, interactive imaging, fast image reconstruction and improved MR angiography techniques.

Diagnostic intervention

The first MRI-guided clinical procedures involved diagnostic biopsies using closed-bore systems. As in the case of computed-tomography-guided (CT-guided) biopsies, puncture and needle advancement were performed outside of the magnet, with the patient being repeatedly placed into the magnet's isocenter for the sake of visualizing the needle position. Needle visualization was only possible using special MRI-visible compounds that produce small local-field distortions that show up as areas of signal loss on MR images. These needle artifacts are related to pulse-sequence type and parameters as well as to the orientation of the needle with respect to the main magnetic field and the readout gradient direction [15.163].

The continuous imaging of needle advancement became possible as more open MR systems were introduced. It is important to note that ultrasound (US) and CT guidance are still used for the vast majority of image-guided biopsies. Due to the higher associated costs and the lower availability of MR scanner time, MR-image guidance is mostly

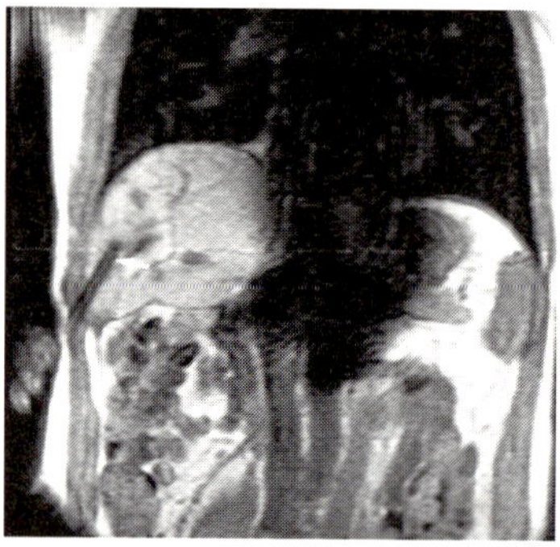

Figure 15.107
MR imaging guidance for liver biopsy with 16 G biopsy needle (arrow). Sagittal, virtually real-time imaging facilitates access to subphrenic lesions.

restricted to cases where it offers clear benefits. MRI guidance can be used in children in order to avoid the radiation exposure that is inherent to CT. MRI is also beneficial when it comes to investigating lesions that are difficult to reach using US and CT (e.g. subphrenic liver lesions). The multiplanar imaging capabilities of MR make such lesions easily accessible under MRI guidance (fig. 15.107). MRI guidance can also be used as a substitute for CT guidance in patients with known allergies to iodinated contrast agents. Furthermore, MRI guidance is required when pathologic lesions can only be seen via MR imaging. Typical examples here include bone marrow edema of unknown origin and suspicious breast lesions that require either biopsy or wire localization using MRI guidance.

Therapeutic intervention

Ablation therapy monitoring

Percutaneous, image-guided thermal ablation has received much recent attention as a promising method of treating primary and secondary focal malignant disease. Although US and CT are generally considered to be the most practical imaging modalities for ablation-probe placement, not all tumors can be properly visualized using these techniques. Another drawback associated with US is that heat-producing ablation procedures induce relatively strong artifacts within and around the treated tumor due to cavitation effects. This makes it difficult to provide immediate therapy control and probe repositioning for additional treatment. On the other hand, the use of CT guidance requires multiple contrast injections, first for tumor visualization prior to ablation and second for therapy monitoring after ablation. Furthermore, CT does not offer continuous monitoring of the thermal energy application. In light of these drawbacks that are inherent to US and CT guidance and even more importantly on account of MRI's unique, non-invasive thermo-monitoring capabilities, many investigators have proposed using MR imaging to monitor ablation procedures (fig. 15.108). MRI offers several imaging parameters that are dependent on temperature, such as T_1 relaxation time, diffusion coefficient and proton-frequency shift. The unique capacity of MRI to visualize thermal lesions in real time as they develop during therapy as well as immediately after treatment and during follow-up treatment has been demonstrated repeatedly [15.164, 15.165].

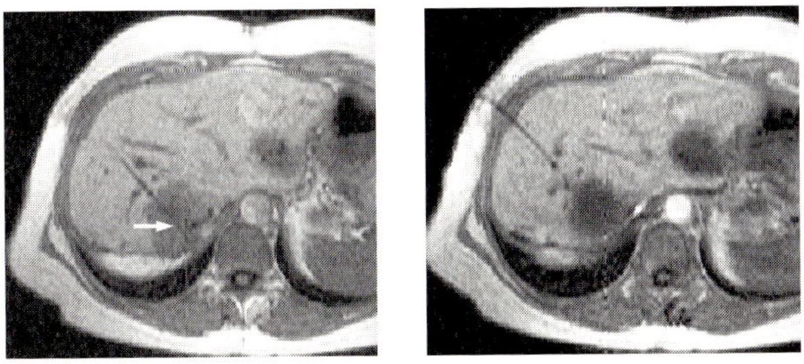

Figure 15.108
Unenhanced transverse T_1-weighted gradient echo MR images. **(a)** Baseline image obtained after placement of a laser applicator (arrow) inside the metastasis and before energy application. **(b)** Image obtained during application of laser energy (Nd:YAG laser at 1064 nm) shows a decrease in signal intensity within the lesion due to temperature increase.

Typical examples of the clinical and investigational application of MRI-guided ablation procedures include interstitial laser thermal ablation and radiofrequency thermal ablation involving the central nervous system, the neck, the liver, the kidney, the spine and the prostate. Most clinical thermal ablation procedures center on the application of laser and RF to liver tumors, although the clinical value of these methods is still under investigation. Initial single-center results of MRI-guided LASER ablation show average survival rates of 3.3 years in patients with colorectal liver metastases [15.164]. In addition to laser and RF, other ablation methods such as cryotherapy, focused ultrasound and alcohol injections can be controlled by MRI.

Many of the ablation studies performed under MRI guidance were not carried out with open magnets, i.e. with systems that provide the degree of access necessary for proper probe placement and excellent patient handling [15.165]. However, the therapeutic benefit of MRI thermometry for thermal-ablation guidance has encouraged some groups to use a dual imaging modality approach in which MRI is either combined with CT or US. New technical solutions that avoid such dual-modality approaches and nonetheless enable the performance of both puncture and thermal ablation entirely in a closed-bore MR system constitute an important step toward the wider use of MRI-guided thermoablation [15.166].

Vascular intervention

The use of MRI is not limited to a direct percutaneous approach. The unique ability of MRI to produce angiograms (MRA), cholangiograms (MRCP) and urograms (MRU) can be used for diagnostic purposes and to guide interventional procedures. The first endoluminal MRI-guided applications were cholangiographies involving drainage procedures and percutaneous nephrostomies. MRI offers a unimodal approach for both procedures [15.167], thereby replacing dual-guidance methods such as methods based on ultrasound and fluoroscopy. The first step in a percutaneous MRI-guided endoluminal intervention resembles that of a biopsy procedure. It is greatly facilitated by the above-mentioned multiplanar imaging capabilities of MRI. Once the bile ducts or the urinary tract have been accessed, MR cholangiography or urography sequences

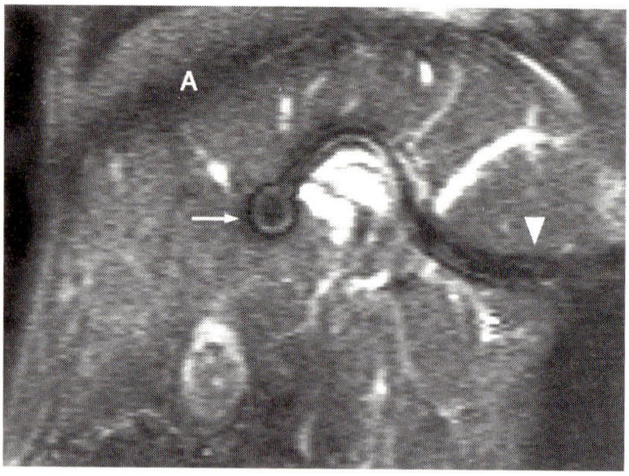

Figure 15.109
MR image extracted from a continuously acquired (every 1.3 s) T_2-weighted image series (trueFISP sequence) that controls guidewire insertion (arrow) and catheter (arrowhead) advancement. Note artifact (A) due to field inhomogeneities (from [15.167]).

are used to control and guide catheters and guidewires endoluminally (fig. 15.109). The absence of ionizing radiation represents a tremendous advantage because both procedures involve exposing the intervening physician to relatively high doses of radiation.

Although the avoidance of radiation exposure for patients and clinical staff is important, especially in the case of lengthy vascular procedures, the rationale for using MRI as a guidance tool when examining blood vessels is also based on its capacity to contribute therapeutically relevant information during interventional endovascular procedures. Unlike any other imaging modality, MRI is capable of displaying functional information (e.g. concerning flow, perfusion and diffusion) that can greatly influence treatment endpoints. MRI also contributes additional morphologic information during investigations of atherosclerotic arteries. Here, it visualizes not only the vessel's lumen as conventional angiography does, but also the vessel wall and the surrounding tissue. This is especially important in light of the mounting evidence that luminal appearance does not tell the whole story about atherosclerotic vessels, i.e. the correspondence between narrowing of the vessel lumen and the potential dangers associated with this devastating disease is not straightforward. In addition to the diagnostic benefits, MRI-guided endovascular procedures can also be performed without an iodinated contrast agent, which makes it an even more valuable imaging modality.

A number of proposed methods of tracking endovascular devices have proven valuable. Visualization according to the so-called passive approach is based on the local field distortions that are produced by paramagnetic rings or ferrite admixtures [15.168, 15.169] and that show up as areas of signal loss in gradient-echo images (fig. 15.110). Alternatively, paramagnetic contrast agents in the lumen [15.170] or doped onto the surface of a catheter can be used in combination with a T_1-weighted sequence. The main disadvantage of passive tracking is that it is image-based, thereby resulting

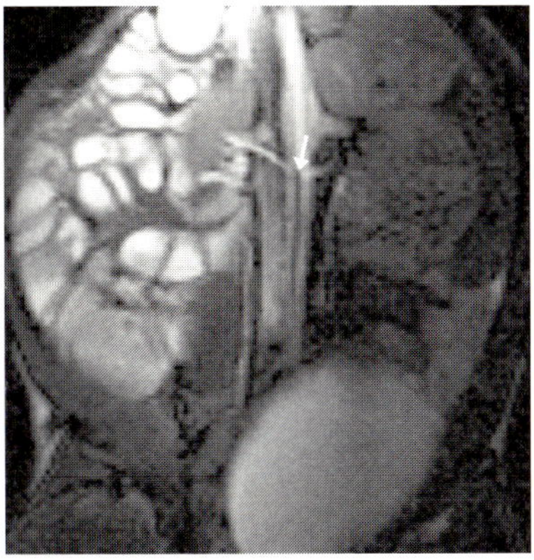

Figure 15.110
Unenhanced MR image from a dynamic series of coronal 2D trueFISP images acquired and displayed at 2.5 images per second during catheterization of the right renal artery prior to a balloon dilatation procedure. The susceptibility-inducing catheter (arrow) can be identified at the ostium of the right renal artery.

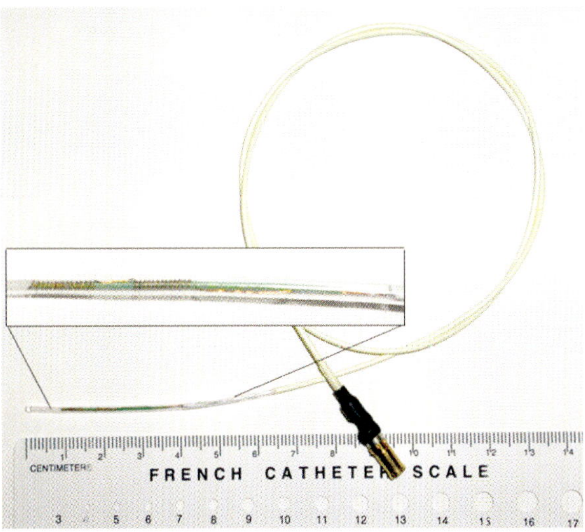

Figure 15.111
Angiographic catheter prototype equipped with an opposed-solenoid antenna with an independent miniaturized tune, match and decoupling circuit. The catheter can be used for tracking as well as for endovascular vessel-wall imaging. (Source: C.M. Hillenbrand and J.L. Duerk, Case Western Reserve University, Cleveland, Ohio, USA).

in a relatively time-consuming tracking scheme that makes it difficult to achieve fast and automatic scan-plane adjustments relative to the catheter tip. In contrast, the active approach [15.171] involves the use of small catheter-mounted receiver coils to determine the actual position of the catheter (fig. 15.111). Here, only three gradient readouts are needed for coil localization, making this method far more time efficient than the image-based method. The position of the device inside the body is determined without acquiring an image on the basis of the 3D localization data delivered by the coils. This localization data can be superimposed on MR roadmap images acquired prior to the intervention and on images acquired in real time during the procedure. Furthermore, the method enables the easy application of automated scan-plane adjustments based on the catheter position. However, one significant drawback to this active approach is the problem of the potential heating of the long connecting-signal cables [15.172]. It will be necessary to address this problem before introducing the active tracking technique (in high-field systems) to routine clinical practice [15.173]. Another tracking approach is based on low flip angle amplification [15.174]. A coil that is tuned to the Larmor frequency of the scanner, but is not connected to it will appear bright at low flip angles due to the resonance in the coils while the surrounding tissue will yield a relatively low signal. Such fiducial markers can be made switchable without raising safety concerns by detuning the resonant circuit using an optic fiber and a photoresistor within the circuit.

Most MRI-guided catheter-based endovascular experiments are initially performed in animal models to test device visibility and procedure feasibility. More complex procedures such as iliac and renal artery stenting, coil embolization, septal occluder placement and transjugular intrahepatic portosystemic shunting have also been performed recently in pre-clinical settings. Only a few reports on patient applications are currently available [15.175-15.176]. These clinical applications involve feasibility studies that fail to demonstrate the achievement of any clear additional benefits via MRI guidance. However, despite the fact that endovascular MR-guided procedures are still in their infancy, the possibilities inherent in the technology offer completely new paradigms for almost any kind of intravascular therapy based on immediate functional information and more detailed morphologic information (e.g. concerning direct vessel-wall pathology). The large manufacturers of MR scanners are well aware of the inherent potential in MRI for guiding interventional vascular procedures. Shorter and more open MR scanners equipped with more flexible software are being developed. The development and introduction of MR-compatible and MR-visible devices such as guidewires, diagnostic catheters, stents and other interventional instruments will represent a further crucial step in the evolution of interventional MR. Without such dedicated instruments, responsible physicians will refrain from taking the risk of performing the clinical studies that are necessary to verify the benefits of MRI guidance for patient and physician alike.

15.2.7 Clinical MR spectroscopy

MR spectroscopy (MRS) is an established method used in analytical chemistry and basic research to non-destructively identify molecules, analyze molecular structures and characterize molecular interactions. The use of MRS when conducting in vivo examinations of human organs is referred to as clinical MRS. The purpose of clinical MRS is to resolve and quantify concentrations of metabolites (i.e. molecular compounds involved in various metabolic cycles). The potential of clinical MRS rests on the chances that the MR-visible signals of cell metabolism reflect tissue degeneration or organ recovery earlier or more specifically than other contrast mechanisms, allowing for improved diagnosis, differential diagnosis or even prognosis of disease or therapy progress. In the present chapter, we describe clinical MRS in terms of its major requirements, methods and applications.

15.2.7.1 Principles, requirements and restrictions

An MRS experiment is easy to imagine within the macroscopic framework of the Bloch equations: a simple pulse-acquire experiment yields time-domain MRS data. The various chemical shifts of the ensembles of various nuclei detected give rise to signals of various frequencies. A frequency analysis of the time-domain data via Fourier transform yields the spectrum. Quadrature detection of the transverse magnetization results in complex time-domain and spectral data. The absorption spectrum is usually considered while the dispersion spectrum, exhibiting less advantageous signal properties, is ignored. The position of a signal within the spectrum determines its frequency, which in turn reflects its chemical shift. The area of the signal is proportional to the number of contributing molecules. The signal-to-noise ratio is defined as the signal amplitude versus the standard deviation for the values of a signal-free spectral range. Some molecules show various MR-visible signals of different chemical shift, and thus leave a characteristic “fingerprint” in the spectrum.

The detection of an MR signal within a period of time that is short enough to allow for a clinical examination requires a sufficient concentration of the metabolites of interest. This detection limit restricts in vivo MRS examinations to the few MR-visible nuclei that occur naturally in sufficient quantities in living tissue. The most commonly studied nuclei in the context of in vivo MRS examinations are ^{1}H and ^{31}P. Few studies record the spectra of naturally abundant ^{13}C compounds, due to their low abundance. ^{13}C, ^{19}F and ^{7}Li in vivo spectra have been recorded after the administration of enriched compounds or medication.

Certain minimum volumes and concentrations of metabolites are required to permit detection of metabolites during clinical MRS examinations. Given a 1 cm^3 measurement volume, a concentration of approximately 1 mM of a compound (e.g. containing a methyl group with three protons) will be required to detect a signal within 10 minutes of acquisition time on a clinical scanner. The required concentration will increase for detection of the other nuclei because the detected signal depends on the gyromagnetic ratio to the power of three.

The minimum achievable echo times restrict localized in vivo MRS to the observation of smaller liquid-phase molecules showing typical T_2 values of a few hundred milliseconds and signal linewidths of only a few Hertz. The larger macromolecules showing T_2 values of a few milliseconds give rise to broad signal humps. Bound molecules with microsecond T_2 values can only by detected indirectly via in vivo MRS, i.e. if they transfer magnetization to molecules in the liquid phase (magnetization transfer effect).

MRS benefits from high B_0 field strength, high field homogeneity and high field stability. The field strength range currently available for clinical MRS ranges from 1 to 7 T. Within this range, noise increases approximately linearly with B_0, while signal amplitudes increase quadratically. However, the expected linear net increase in signal-to-noise ratio (SNR) can only be observed if the same field homogeneity is reached. As susceptibility-based distortions increase along with B_0 field strength, many areas of the human body show a less homogeneous B_0 at high B_0 compared to low B_0 despite shimming. This is the major source of signal loss in the case of high fields. Given that T_1 increases and T_2 decreases as B_0 increases, one also observes a tendency for relaxation to counterbalance field-dependent *SNR* gain. However, the variation of in vivo relaxation properties is minor for many metabolites of interest in the context of ^{1}H MRS [15.177, 15.178]. Apart from *SNR*, the second user-relevant quantity positively affected by increased field strength is spectral resolution. The chemical shift dispersion Δf of a spectral line with respect to a reference line scales linearly with B_0. To allow for a comparison of spectra obtained from different B_0 scanners, the ordinate of the spectra is usually scaled by the relative dispersion with respect to B_0 in parts per million (ppm). Thus, while the spectral positions of two identical singlet lines remain identical at B_0 and $2B_0$, they appear half as wide or twice as distinct when separated at $2B_0$.

15.2.7.2 Localization techniques

The use of small surface coils in combination with the above-mentioned non-localized pulse-acquire experiment may provide sufficient localization, for instance, when studying calf muscle tissue or tumors close to the surface of the body. However, most MRS studies (e.g. involving the brain, prostate or heart) require additional localization: either a single spectrum from a defined location is recorded per experiment using single-voxel spectroscopy (SVS) or spectra from multiple voxels are acquired simultaneously using a chemical-shift imaging (CSI) technique. In both cases, the voxel locations are defined using anatomical MR reference images acquired beforehand. The described workflow also characterizes the role of clinical MRS: it is often deployed to further investigate the appearance of a dubious spot in the images, to add information for the sake of differential diagnoses and to increase diagnostic specificity.

While many localization techniques have been invented and tested since the introduction of MRS, only the most robust of these have prevailed in clinical practice. These are described below.

The STEAM (stimulated echo acquisition mode) single-voxel spectroscopy sequence detects the stimulated echo generated by three consecutively applied RF pulses, each with a flip angle of 90° (fig. 15.112) [15.179]. Each of the RF pulses is slice-selective. Given that their underlying gradient pulses are applied along mutually orthogonal directions, these pulses define a cuboid subvolume, i.e. the voxel. The first pulse selects a slice within the sample, the second orthogonal pulse selects a pencil-shaped cuboid from within the slice and the third pulse cuts the voxel out of the pencil shape. However, the three pulses not only generate the desired stimulated echo, they also lead to the population of seven other coherence pathways. The FIDs generated by each of the three pulses and the spin echoes generated by any two of the pulses need to be eliminated because the magnetization of these signals has not undergone complete localization. Two techniques have proven effective. First, spoiling gradients (shaded dark in figs. 15.112 and 15.113) can be used to dephase the unwanted signals during each acquisition. Here, the complete spoiling of the third pulse's FID immediately before acquisition is often critical. Second, if more than one acquisition is performed, then

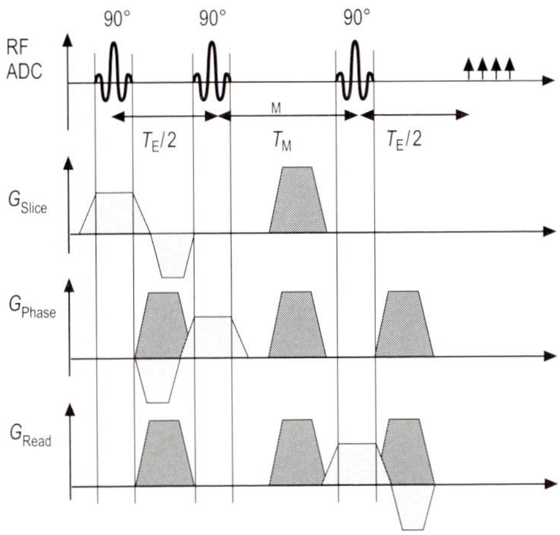

Figure 15.112
SVS STEAM sequence: spoiling gradient pulses are shaded dark, slice selection pulses are shaded gray; T_E: echo time, signal decay determined by T_2; T_M: mixing time, signal decay determined by T_1; signal acquisition starts upon the formation of the stimulated echo.

phase-cycling can be used to eliminate the unwanted coherences. The phases of the RF pulses and the data acquisition are modified for each accumulation so as to ensure that the unwanted echoes contribute deconstructively and the stimulated echo contributes coherently. At least eight phase cycles are required to select the desired echo of a three-pulse sequence.

As in the simple pulse-acquire experiment described above, no gradients are applied when recording the stimulated echo. This means that a 1D Fourier transform will lead from the time-domain data to the frequency-domain spectrum. It is essential to use precisely the echo peak as the first sample of the time-domain data. The amplitude of this sample depends solely on T_2, while any signal dephasing due to field inhomogeneity is rephased. Hence, the frequency domain signal area, which is correlated with metabolite concentration, becomes independent of field homogeneity. Secondary reasons for using the echo maximum as the first time-domain sample center on the fact that weakly coupled signals such as lactate exhibit a well-defined signal behavior as well as the fact that first-order phase correction is unnecessary during data post-processing.

The above discussion of localization and signal acquisition also applies to the spin-echo SVS sequence, also referred to as PRESS (point resolved spectroscopy). While half of the originally excited magnetization is dephased during the STEAM sequence, the 90°–180°–180° spin-echo sequence (fig. 15.113) utilizes the entire excited magnetization. Given that the currently available selection profiles for 90° and 180° pulses are of virtually equal quality and given that RF heating is usually not an issue in MRS due to the long T_R, the spin-echo sequence's two-fold sensitivity advantage makes it preferable to STEAM. The spin-echo sequence's lower sensitivity to diffusion (i.e. due to the shorter intervals between spoiling gradient pulses) represents a further minor advantage. However, the STEAM sequence does enjoy the advantage of shorter minimum echo times (during which magnetization decays by T_2). The stimulated echo's magne-

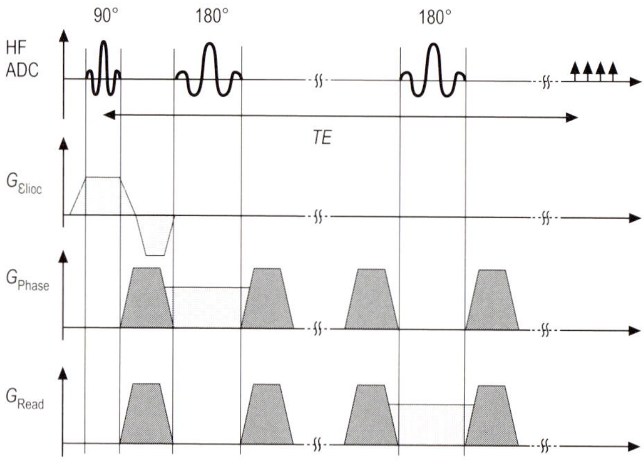

Figure 15.113
SVS spin-echo sequence: spoiling gradient pulses are shaded black, slice selection pulses are shaded grey; T_E: echo time, signal decay determined by T_2; signal acquisition starts upon the formation of the second spin echo.

tization is stored as longitudinal magnetization that decays only by T_1 during the second and the third RF pulse in the STEAM sequence (i.e. the mixing period). Furthermore, some coupled resonances show higher signals at intermediate echo times when detected by STEAM [15.180].

These SVS techniques are used in combination with a water suppression sequence module when applied in ^{1}H MRS. The water signal in the brain is 10^5 times more intense than typical metabolite signals. While one could remove a smooth water signal from the spectrum during post-processing, tiny water signal modulations may appear as severe distortions with respect to the metabolite signal scale. Hence, the water signal is suppressed experimentally, usually by chemical-shift-selective (CHESS) excitation in combination with dephasing. The optimization of CHESS-pulse flip angles to minimize the sensitivity of water suppression to B_1 and T_1 variations is referred to as water suppression enhanced through T_1 effects (or WET).

CSI sequences usually involve the phase-encoding procedures commonly used in imaging sequences designed to resolve metabolite concentrations from multiple voxels. The phase-encoding gradients in conventional CSI experiments are incremented upon each acquisition, while the readout period is again reserved solely for resolving the spectroscopic dimension. The 3D-CSI sequence shown in fig. 15.114 represents an extreme example. It involves the achievement of spatial resolution along all spatial dimensions via phase encoding. The spatially resolved spectra are obtained from the *k*-space data via 4D Fourier transform. Unlike the position of a slice-selection profile, the position of a CSI grid realized by phase encoding can be modified retrospectively, at least up to the size of one voxel. Due to the cyclic behavior of the Fourier transform, a larger grid shift will lead to the same results as those obtained from the corresponding inner-voxel shift. One spatial dimension is often selected using a slice-selective RF

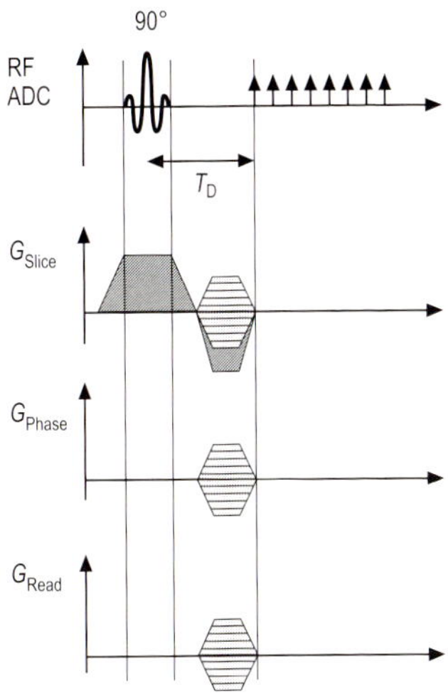

Figure 15.114
CSI FID sequence: the slice selection pulse is shaded grey. The delay T_D (during which the signal decays by T_2^*) is minimized. The experiment is repeated to complete each of the $N_x N_y N_z$ phase-encoding steps (i.e. assuming full *k*-space acquisition).

pulse, while phase encoding is performed only for the other two dimensions (2D-CSI). In order to minimize the above-mentioned quantitation errors, it is necessary to minimize the delay T_D between the center of the pulse (when the echo maximum is formed) and the start of the acquisition. Such 2D or 3D-CSI sequences that involve only a short sampling delay are especially useful for avoiding heavy T_2 weighting in non-proton applications where the T_2 values are often low.

Hybrid CSI sequences have been used effectively in brain ^1H MRS. Phase encoding is added to an SVS sequence during a period of transverse magnetization, yielding a 2D or 3D hybrid CSI sequence. The volume selected by the slice-selective pulses covers a region of interest in the inner brain that is further resolved by phase encoding while allowing to avoid the selection of intense subcutaneous or bone-lipid signals. The fact that the field of view (FOV) defined by phase encoding can be made small without the risk of signal folding (as long as the selection profile is sufficient to effectively suppress any outside signals) represents another advantage to hybrid CSI sequences.

The minimal measurement time for a conventional CSI experiment of the sort discussed so far is defined by the number of phase-encoding steps along each direction times T_R (i.e. $T_A = N_x N_y N_z T_R$). 3D CSI, in particular, can take too long, depending on the desired resolution. The goal of fast CSI techniques is to reduce the minimum measurement time. The conventional CSI experiment is difficult to surpass in terms of sequence sensitivity (i.e. the *SNR* reached per unit of measurement) [15.181]. The fast sequences that come close to matching the sensitivity of the conventional sequence include those that use an echo-planar readout module designed to simultaneously encode spectral and spatial dimensions during signal acquisition (fig. 15.115).

The CSI measurement time can also be significantly reduced by applying a reduced phase encoding procedure that covers a spherically or elliptically shaped inner portion of *k*-space only. This strategy is advantageous, for instance, when a spherically

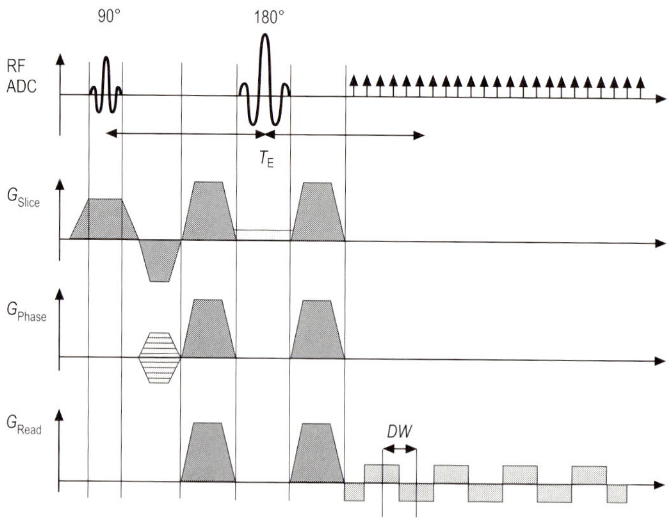

Figure 15.115
2D-CSI sequence with an EPI readout module. If data are acquired during both negative and positive symmetric readout gradient lobes, the dwell time determining the spectral bandwidth will be equal to the duration of a single gradient lobe. Note: due to the first half-negative gradient lobe, signals acquired at the center of the subsequent lobes will have undergone no gradient encoding because the effects of the positive and negative lobes cancel out. One can substitute the effect of the readout gradients in the case of non-central samples by assuming a phase-encoding gradient applied before readout. However, the samples acquired during negative readout lobes reach the same *k*-space positions as those acquired during positive lobes in reverse order. Hence, an additional time reversal of one half of the data is required to process EPI-CSI data.

symmetric Hamming *k*-space filter is applied to reduce voxel-bleeding effects. It is important to control voxel bleeding so as to avoid signal contamination in each spectrum of the CSI dataset, especially when the low-intensity metabolite signals are surrounded by disturbing signals, i.e. such as lipid signals whose intensities are several orders of magnitude higher (fig. 15.116). The price that one pays for reduced voxel bleeding is a concomitant reduction in spatial resolution. The effective voxel size of filtered CSI data is approximately 1.5 times larger along each CSI dimension than the nominal voxel size obtained when one divides the FOV by the number of phase-encoding steps, with the precise value depending on the shape of the filter function. However, spatial resolution in the filtered case is determined by the filter function and not by the decision as to whether a full or an elliptical portion of *k*-space is to be phase-encoded. In this case, the most efficient encoding technique establishes the filter function during data acquisition to avoid attenuating the outer *k*-space during the filtering step and thus wasting measurement time. Acquisition weighting represents one example of such a technique. Here, the innermost portion of *k*-space is acquired four times during an experiment of 4 averages, while the outer portions are acquired only once. The number of averages for the intermediate *k*-space portions is determined by an apodization function (e.g. a Hamming function). The same SNR – for in-

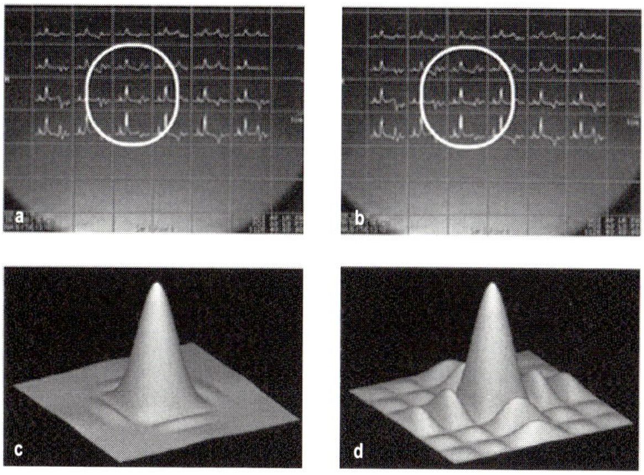

Figure 15.116
The effect of voxel bleeding: only citrate and choline signals within the phantom container are visible in the case of *k*-space filtering using a spherical Hamming filter **(a)**. The point-spread function shows only minor side lobes **(c)**. Lipid signals from another outside container appear in the unfiltered case **(b)**. The point-spread function shows significant contributions originating from outside areas **(d)**.

stance, that of a 3D-CSI experiment involving 8 phase encoding steps along each direction ($N_A = 4$, $T_R = 1.5$ s) and requiring more than 50 minutes using conventional encoding – is then obtained in less than 10 minutes.

The question whether to use an SVS or a CSI technique depends among many factors on the size and the spatial distribution of the pathology. Generally speaking, however, CSI techniques are more efficient than SVS techniques because they involve the simultaneous coverage of multiple voxels without thereby incurring any major sequence-sensitivity losses (i.e. the only source of CSI signal losses – and these amounting to no more than a few percent – is inner voxel dispersion). However, the question whether a CSI technique can be applied will depend critically on whether sufficient field homogeneity can be reached across larger volumes of interest.

15.2.7.3 Matrix spectroscopy

One can substantially increase the sensitivity of clinical MRS by using parallel-acquisition channels and multiple element-receive matrix coils. Advances continue to be made in the area of multi-channel hardware for ^{1}H detection. These can also be transferred to the detection of other nuclei. The problem of combining the data from the individual receive elements is more difficult in the case of complex MRS data than for magnitude imaging data. Avoiding signal cancellation is a matter of making sure that the data from the various channels are in phase before combination. Reference scan methods and methods based on the data themselves have been suggested as ways of achieving phase coherence. Furthermore, as pointed out by Roemer et al., the best *SNR* of the combined data is achieved via an additional weighting of the data with their

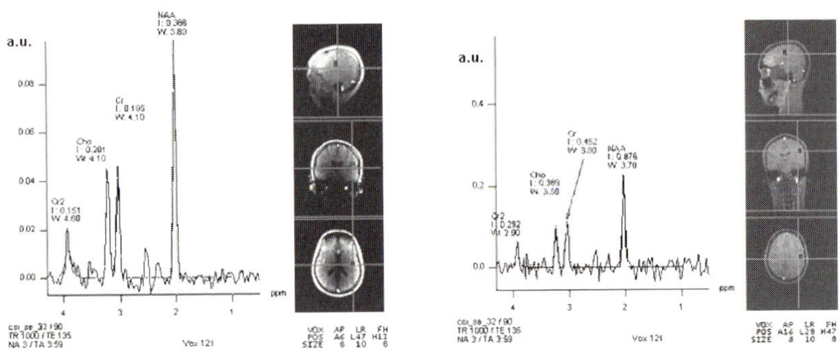

Figure 15.117
Upon the coherent, appropriately weighted combination of each channel's data, the multiple-array brain coil increases the signal-to-noise ratio, especially in the case of cortical voxels **(left)**. This can be compared to a single-array head coil **(right)**.

signal intensity [15.11]. This self-weighting property exhibited by the combination algorithm leads to an additional advantage in that the contributions made by low SNR data are virtually negligible, thus facilitating the selection of coil elements. A normalization of the signal amplitudes across all locations is to be carried out for CSI data after signal combination. Data-inherent procedures commonly used in the area of imaging (e.g. sum-of-squares normalization) can also be applied to spectroscopy. However, even better homogeneity can be achieved when the sensitivity profiles of the selected coil elements are compared in a pre-scan imaging experiment to the profile of the large and homogeneous body coil. This pre-scan data enables one to normalize the CSI data to the body coil's reception profile.

Fig. 15.117 shows a comparison of a multiple-array brain coil and a single-element receive coil. The 23-channel coil enables one to triple the sensitivity of an MR examination of cortical and white matter voxels. The clinical potential of matrix ^{1}H spectroscopy appears high when one considers its possible realization at very high field strengths such as 3 T or 7 T.

15.2.7.4 Multinuclear techniques

Nuclear Overhauser enhancement (NOE) and proton-decoupling methods have been introduced to clinical practice in order to increase signal intensity, especially in the case of ^{31}P and ^{13}C experiments. NOE enhancement involves the irradiation of ^{1}H RF pulses prior to signal excitation with a frequency of ^{31}P or ^{13}C. As explained above, the upper limit of enhancement is determined by the ratio of the gyromagnetic ratios of the irradiated and the detected nuclei. A signal gain of up to 50% has been observed in the case of in vivo ^{31}P MRS. Irradiating ^{1}H RF pulses during ^{31}P or ^{13}C-signal detection leads to the saturation of the transitions between the different energy levels (i.e. due to coupling between the X-nuclei and the protons). The effect of such decoupling pulses on the spectrum is one of simplification as multiplet signals collapse into singlets. While successful decoupling causes the multiplet signal intensity to condense in a sin-

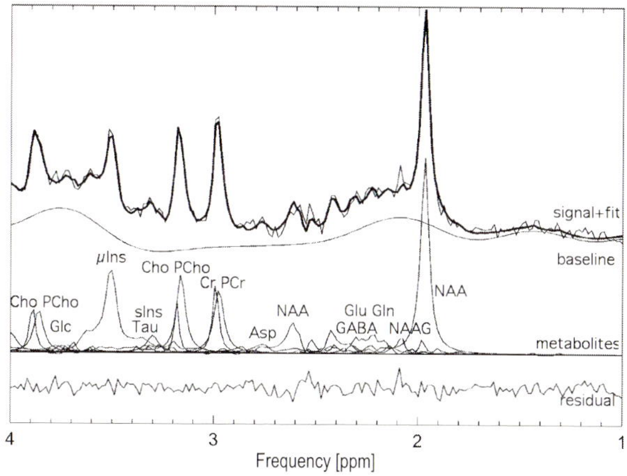

Figure 15.118
Typical metabolite signals made visible via short T_E brain MRS. The signal properties are detailed in [15.182]. The quantification of signal areas remains challenging owing to the multitude of partially overlapping signals in the presence of a slowly varying baseline.

gle line, decoupling may cause a concomitant NOE enhancement. Decoupling is of special importance in ^{13}C spectroscopy, where most signals show a coupling with protons.

15.2.7.5 Post-processing

The purpose of MRS post-processing is mainly to evaluate relative metabolite concentrations and to display results. Given the number of parameters that are not typically determined during a clinical MRS examination (e.g. T_1 and T_2 values for metabolite signals in pathological tissue) and given the absence of a basis for verifying in vivo results, the task of devising a general purpose algorithm for absolute metabolite quantitation would appear to be scarcely manageable. An intensity value in arbitrary units is thus usually obtained for each metabolite signal via a fitting procedure based on prior knowledge. This value can be compared to the other intensities in the same spectrum. The quantitation of short T_E ^1H clinical spectra that exhibit a large number of partially poorly resolved signals and that may contain artificial lipid signals represents one of the biggest challenges in the development of MRS post-processing (fig. 15.118).

15.2.7.6 Main applications

^1H MRS of the brain is currently the most common type of MRS examination. The most common disorders that are studied with the use of MRS include tumors in adults and children, epilepsy, stroke, neurodegenerative diseases, psychiatric disorders and congenital disorders. The relative importance of CSI techniques compared to SVS techniques has increased in light of technical developments such as acquisition weighting and various readily available post-processing and display functions. Furthermore, a

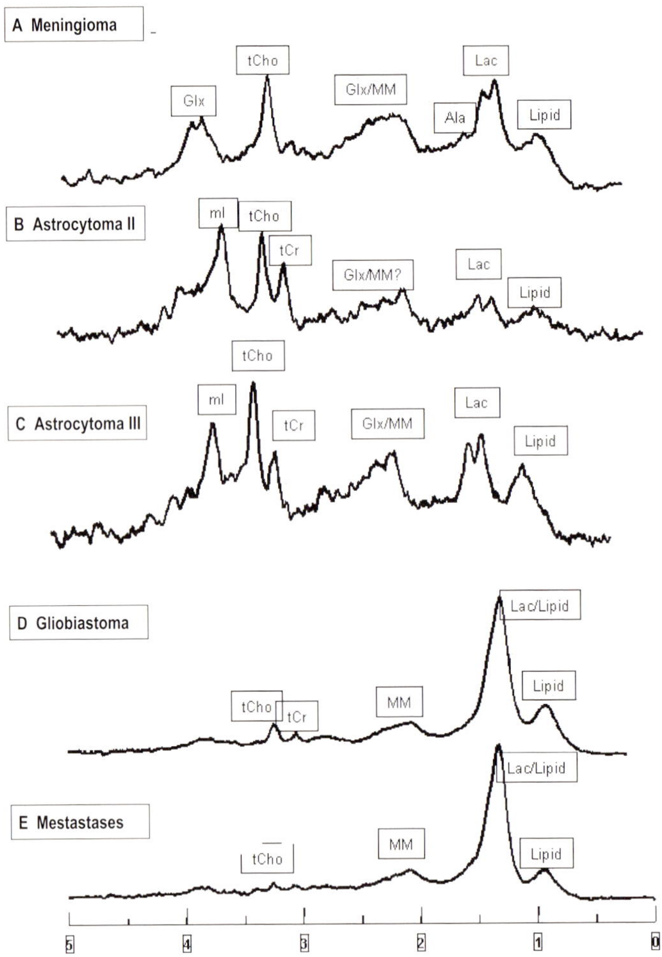

Figure 15.119 Short T_E ^1H average spectra for various brain tumor types

number of multicenter studies designed to generate large disease-specific databases are currently underway. Examples include the EC-funded projects INTERPRET and its successor eTumour. Both of these are aimed at providing tools to assist clinicians with tasks involving brain-tumor classification (fig. 15.119).

It has been shown that combining MRI with MRS significantly increases the diagnostic value of MR prostate examinations [15.183]. A typical MRS protocol uses 3D hybrid spin-echo CSI ($T_E/T_R = 120/650$ ms) to cover the entire prostate in a measurement time of less than 13 minutes. The procedure includes the use of acquisition weighting and the achievement of a nominal voxel size of 5 by 5 by 5 mm^3 [15.184]. Additional spatially and spectrally selective saturation pulses suppress lipid contamination. While the citrate signal at 2.6 ppm dominates in healthy prostate tissue and that of choline-containing compounds at 3.2 ppm is relatively low, these signal levels are significantly altered in cancer tissue. Hence, the ratio of tumor signals to citrate signals has been suggested as a pathologic marker. Nevertheless, the heterogeneity of the prostate also needs to be taken into account when interpreting the MRS results. Furthermore, the effects of various other diseases such as prostatitis may be confounding factors.

While contrast-enhanced MRI is currently capable of achieving a high degree of sensitivity when it comes to detecting suspicious masses in the breast, the use of the technique has yielded variable specificities. MR spectroscopy is capable of detecting metabolic changes in tissue and may provide an added measure of confidence in the characterization of breast lesions. In vivo investigations of phospholipid metabolism using ^{13}C or ^{31}P MRS appear to be restricted to cases of advanced cancer due to their low sensitivity. The much greater sensitivity of ^{1}H-MRS allows one to detect smaller carcinoma. In the context of in vivo ^{1}H MRS, the singlet signal of choline-containing compounds at 3.2 ppm appears to be an important factor in the detection of carcinoma. Other in vivo ^{1}H signals of breast tissue have their origin in water and lipid compartments. An additional lactose signal is seen in spectra of the lactating breast. While one used to assume that choline was only detectable in malignancies, high-field studies have shown that it also produces a weak signal at 3.2 ppm in healthy breast tissue. It is thus necessary to calibrate the detected choline signal. One suggested method involves using the unsuppressed water signal as an internal standard (i.e. estimating

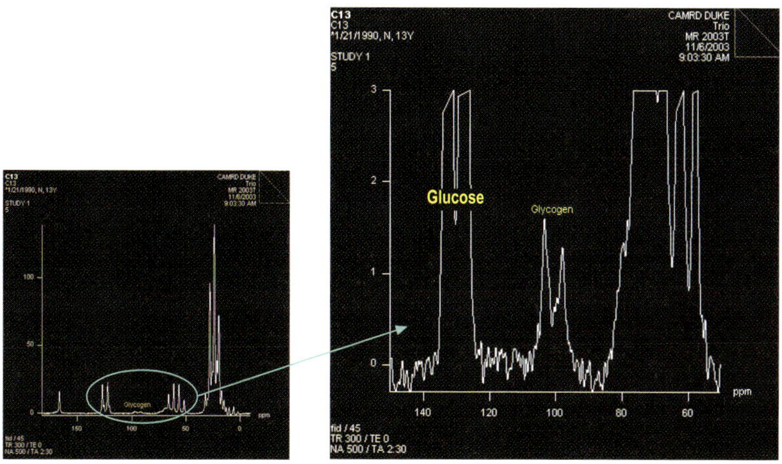

Figure 15.120
In Pompe's disease, the concentration of glycogen is increased. The ^{13}C spectrum of a 2 years old child's calf muscle clearly shows glycogen by detection of natural abundant ^{13}C (Magnetom Trio with $B_0 = 3$ T, acquisition time $T_A = 2{:}30$ min). In this application, non-invasive MRS has the potential of replacing biopsy, which is a tedious procedure for the usually young patients. (Source of case report: C. Charles, Duke University)

the concentration of choline in its solvent, water, and then correcting for the partial volume of adipose tissue). Other technical requirements for ^{1}H breast MRS include an effective suppression of the lipid signal and a correction for the signal variations induced by breathing. The application of MRS to the breast would appear to promise increased primary-diagnosis specificity, a method of monitoring the effects of cancer treatment and a method of checking for tumor recurrence.

Assessing the energy status of heart muscle via ^{31}P MRS represents a challenging application on account of the motion of the heart and the technique's low sensitivity [15.185]. A double-resonant $^{31}P/^{1}H$ surface coil is used for RF transmit and signal reception. Nuclear Overhauser effect (NOE) enhancement and ^{1}H decoupling are used for maximizing SNR. ECG-gating is used for reducing signal loss induced by motion. Usage of 3D CSI and acquisition weighting is advantageous in order to maximize the *SNR* gained per unit acquisition time.

Fig. 15.120 shows a clinical application of glycogen detection, based on the detection of natural abundant ^{13}C.

15.2.8 Hyperpolarization

Hyperpolarization can increase the signal intensity of a magnetic-resonance-imaging or spectroscopy measurement by several orders of magnitude. This is of special interest in the case of non-hydrogen nuclei that exhibit a poor signal-to-noise ratio. However, the increased magnetization is only available for purposes of imaging for a period of time corresponding to the longitudinal relaxation time T_1. Useful applications include:

- Lung imaging involving the inhalation of ^{3}He gas
- MR angiography and perfusion measurements using hyperpolarized ^{13}C compounds in a liquid state to produce images of an injected agent without an inherent background signal
- MR metabolic imaging using a substrate containing hyperpolarized ^{13}C that enters the metabolic pathways, whereas substrate and metabolic products may later be distinguished by their chemical shifts

^{3}He and ^{129}Xe gas can be polarized indirectly via optical pumping. Two different methods have been developed to produce various liquid compounds containing hyperpolarized ^{13}C: parahydrogen-induced polarization (PHIP) [15.186, 15.187] and dynamic nuclear polarization (DNP) [15.188, 15.189]. While polarization mechanisms have been studied and used in physics for many years, progress in their development for use in medical MR imaging has only been made recently. Except for the case of lung imaging with ^{3}He, this development is still a matter of ongoing research limited to animal models.

Hyperpolarization involves preparing a nuclear spin system in such a manner that its polarization

$$P = \frac{N_+ - N_-}{N_+ + N_-} \tag{15.65}$$

exceeds that of thermal equilibrium. Theoretically, a spin system could become 100% polarized. The presently available techniques for hyperpolarizing nuclear spins are applied ex vivo, with the spin system being prepared in a special polarizer. In order to be of use in medical imaging, hyperpolarized agents are required to exhibit longitudinal relaxation rates in tissue that are slow enough to permit (1) their administration and bio-distribution (possibly including involvement in metabolic processes) and (2) the carrying out of the relevant imaging procedures (i.e. before their polarization reverts to thermal equilibrium).

15.2.8.1 ^{3}He lung imaging

While ^{3}He has a gyromagnetic ratio of $\gamma/2\pi = 32.44$ MHz/T and a detection sensitivity of 0.443 of ^{1}H at the same field strength, its spin density is not sufficient for imaging, even when inhaled. This situation can be changed via hyperpolarization. A method of optically pumping Rb atoms to cause them to transfer polarization to ^{3}He or ^{129}Xe nuclei was demonstrated as early as 1960 [15.190]. Optical pumping became more efficient with the introduction of more advanced laser technology. Several methods have been successfully used to produce polarization levels of 15% to 60% for ^{3}He and ^{129}Xe gas. These methods can be used for MR imaging in conventional scanners.

Optical pumping involves the directing of circularly polarized light into an alkali metal vapour (fig. 15.121). The wavelength is selected so as to excite the single alkali valence electron from its ground state to the first excited state. The conservation of the angular momentum of the absorbed photon imposes the selection rule $\Delta m = +1$ on the excited electron, where m is the magnetic quantum number of the electron spin. This will depopulate the $m = -1/2$ ground state. Atoms in the excited state can decay to either ground state, but when they decay to the $m = +1/2$ state, they are no longer susceptible to the incident radiation and remain in that state. Eventually, nearly all of the atoms gather in the $+1/2$ state and the ensemble is magnetically oriented (fig. 15.122).

Such ^{3}He polarizers were refined with an eye to using them for medical purposes by MITI in Durham, NC, USA (later Amersham Health) and a group of researchers at the University of Mainz in Germany [15.191]. However, ^{3}He is a rare isotope that does not occur naturally in significant amounts. The various methods of polarization differ in terms of their technical complexity, polarization times and achievable polarization levels.

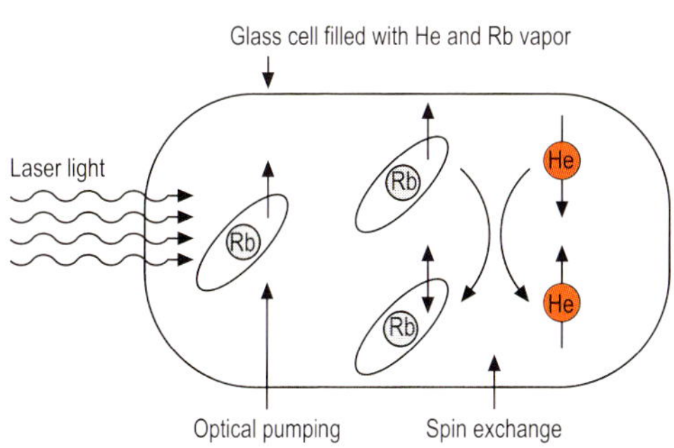

Figure 15.121
Setup for manufacturing hyperpolarized ^{3}He via optical pumping

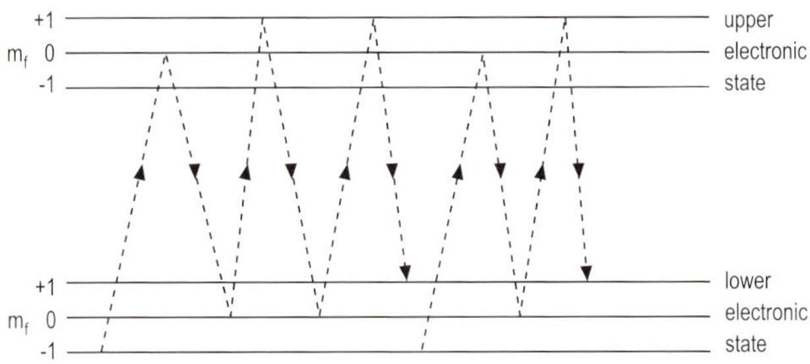

Figure 15.122 Transition history of alkali atoms undergoing optical pumping

The hyperpolarized ^{3}He gas can be kept in special glass containers for several hours (T_1 = 2 h) or in plastic bags for several minutes (T_1 = 10 min) before inhalation. The substance's T_1 relaxation rate is substantially reduced in the presence of oxygen. If high signal intensity and long relaxation times are required, then hyperpolarized helium gas can be mixed with nitrogen gas and then inhaled. The ventilation is accessed via the initial ^{3}He signal intensity, while the rate at which the signal intensity decays may be correlated to perfusion and oxygen-gas exchange [15.192]. Some lung research studies aim at measuring partial oxygen pressure via its effect on the T_1 relaxation of ^{3}He.

Given that there is no background signal prior to inhalation, the distribution of the gas through the major airways to the alveoli can be followed dynamically during inhalation using fast imaging [15.193]. Studies indicate that airway branching up to the seventh generation can be visualized [15.194].

Another approach uses ^{3}He diffusion imaging to assess the lung microstructure, i.e. based on a connection between the calculated apparent diffusion coefficient (ADC) maps and the airway size [15.195] (fig. 15.123). As with conventional diffusion imaging, a set of at least two images is acquired nearly simultaneously (interleaved, line-by-line), one without diffusion sensitizing gradients and the other with a pair of diffusion sensitizing gradients that dephase the gas signal that can freely diffuse in larg-

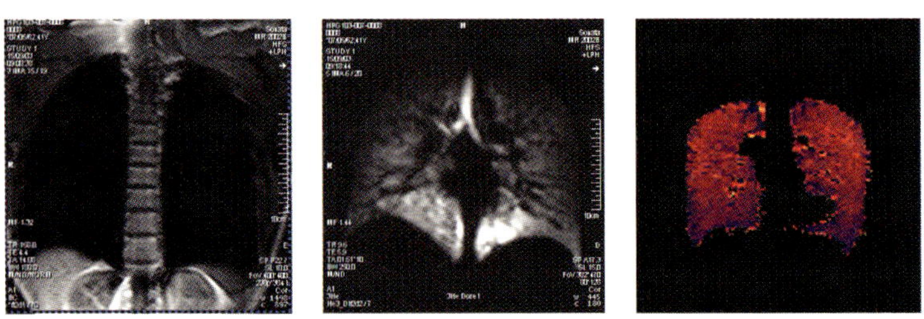

Figure 15.123
Hyperpolarized ^{3}He lung imaging: **(a)** ^{1}H localizer image, **(b)** ^{3}He lung image, **(c)** ^{3}He apparent diffusion coefficient (ADC) map of lung (the trachea have been removed from the image)

er structures. Studies have shown that the ADC histograms of healthy subjects show a fairly narrow distribution of ADC values over the lung area (excluding the trachea) while the ADC histograms of lung emphysema patients show a wide distribution. The generally larger ADC values have been interpreted as indicating distal air spaces of increased size and altered morphology [15.196].

15.2.8.2 Parahydrogen-induced ^{13}C polarization

The hydrogen molecule H_2 is a system that is comprised of two nuclei with nuclear spin 1/2 and that is capable of assuming 4 different states. The system exhibits a total nuclear spin of $I = 1$ in the parallel orthohydrogen configuration (triplet state) or $I = 0$ in the antiparallel parahydrogen configuration (singlet state). At room temperature, all of these 4 states are equally populated so that hydrogen gas normally consists of 25% parahydrogen and 75% orthohydrogen. According to the Pauli principle, the rotational ground state of parahydrogen is $J = 0$ while the rotational ground state of orthohydrogen is $J = 1$ (fig. 15.124). Given that the energy level at $J = 0$ is lower than that at $J = 1$, the Boltzmann distribution will favour the antiparallel state of the nuclear spins at low temperatures. At liquid nitrogen temperature (77 K), for instance, most H_2 consists of parahydrogen. The transition rates between the para and ortho states are very slow, so that it takes a long time (several days) for an excess of parahydrogen to develop. However, paramagnetic catalysts can be used to significantly increase the transition rate and achieve reasonable production rates. Parahydrogen gas can be kept in normal pressurized gas bottles at room temperature for several days or weeks after being removed from the catalyst.

Parahydrogen-induced polarization (PHIP) occurs when two protons from the same parahydrogen molecule are transferred to an organic molecule during a chemical reaction in which the nuclear spin correlation is maintained. If the parahydrogen's two ^{1}H nuclei attach to different sites in the molecule and these can be distinguished by chemical shift, then the non-Boltzmann populations at these sites can result in enhanced absorption and emission lines in the NMR spectrum (fig. 15.125). Given that this situation persists only for the duration of the longitudinal relaxation time, it will be helpful to ensure that this time is sufficiently long. Therefore the polarization is transferred from the ^{1}H nuclei with a short T_1 relaxation time to the ^{13}C nuclei with a substantially longer T_1. PHIP is used for imaging purposes observing the strong NMR signal emitted by the labelled ^{13}C molecules.

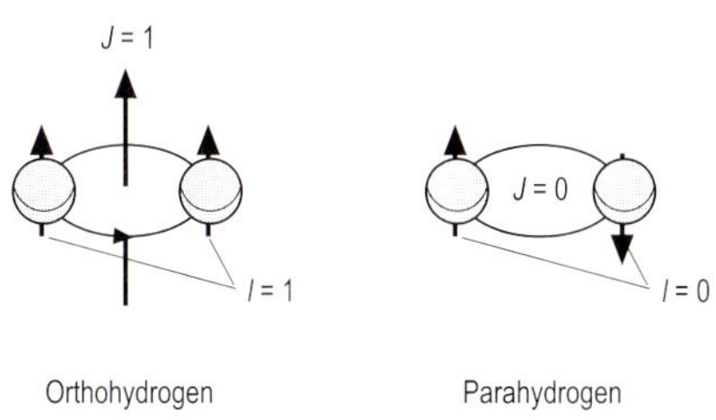

Figure 15.124
Electronic configuration of ortho and parahydrogen

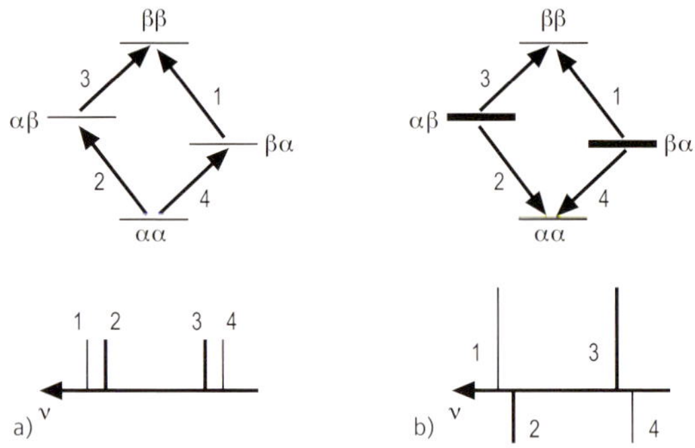

Figure 15.125
NMR spectrum of two proton spins A and B, showing **(a)** occupation of energy levels and transitions at normal NMR and **(b)** occupation of energy levels and transitions at parahydrogen-induced polarization NMR

This method of producing hyperpolarized agents is attractive because it can be run very efficiently. A hyperpolarized ^{13}C-containing agent can be produced in a rapid chemical reaction from stored parahydrogen immediately before administration. However, the choice of ^{13}C-labelled agents is limited because the agents will be required to (1) react chemically with H_2 gas, (2) allow the polarization transfer from the ^1H to the ^{13}C nuclei and (3) possess (ideally) a long T_1 relaxation time.

Given that the transfer of polarization from the ^1H to the ^{13}C nuclei is due to the J-coupling of the nuclei, the gradient echo sequences, including EPI, will be subject to a rapid dephasing of the ^{13}C signal from PHIP-produced agents. It is difficult to apply ^1H decoupling in combination with fast imaging sequences. Inversion pulses on the ^{13}C nuclei will allow for signal rephasing. TrueFISP sequences [15.197] with $\alpha/2 = 90^\circ$ pre-pulses and $\alpha = 180^\circ$ flip angle pulses enable fast imaging with high sensitivity [15.198].

Parahydrogen-induced polarization has been used to obtain MR angiograms and perfusion studies in animal models [15.199-15.201]. The absence of a background signal enables projection imaging and/or a reduction in the field of view without aliasing artifacts. Regional saturation can eliminate signal that is incapable of recovering. This may be useful in perfusion studies (figs. 15.126, 15.127).

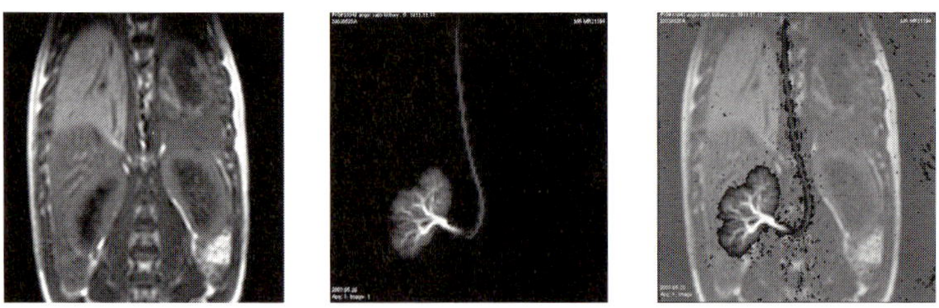

Figure 15.126
Pig with catheter in renal artery: **(a)** coronal slice generated via ^1H imaging, **(b)** radial trueFISP ^{13}C image with a contrast agent hyperpolarized via parahydrogen polarization depicting the renal arteries, **(c)** image fusion of **(a)** and **(b)**

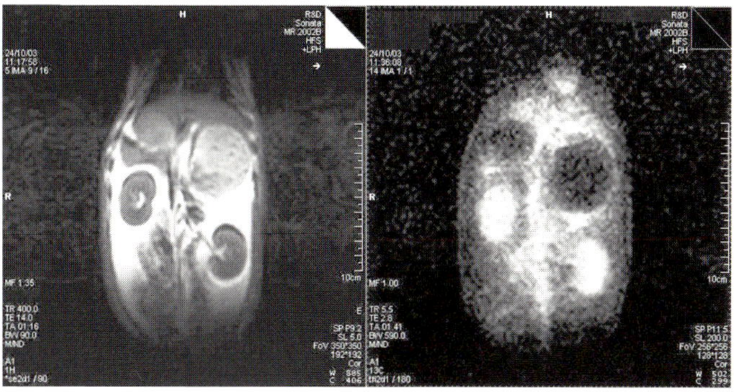

Figure 15.127
(a) Coronal slice through a rabbit generated via ^{1}H imaging, **(b)** ^{13}C image of the same slice acquired 20 s after injection of an endogenous ^{13}C-enriched contrast agent hyperpolarized via dynamic nuclear polarization (Overhauser effect)

15.2.8.3 Dynamic nuclear ^{13}C polarization

The dynamic nuclear polarization (DNP) method involves the application of spin refrigeration and the Overhauser effect to enhance nuclear magnetization beyond thermal equilibrium. A chemical compound enriched with ^{13}C is doped with a small number of paramagnetic ions viz. free radicals. This mixture is cooled, preferably to temperatures in the ~ 1 K range, and then exposed to a strong magnetic field in a superconducting magnet. While the electron spins of free radicals under such conditions become nearly 100% polarized, the nuclear spins of ^{13}C remain less than 1% polarized. Irradiating with an RF field at the electron spin resonance (ESR) frequency will then transfer electron-spin polarization via hyperfine coupling to the nuclear spins that are to be used for NMR. Given that the gyromagnetic ratio of the electron spin (2.8025 GHz/T) is much larger than that of the nuclear spin, the electronic thermal equilibrium polarization extends that of the nuclei by several orders of magnitude. When the power of the RF field for the ESR is increased until the electron spin resonance is saturated (i.e. the two electron spin states exhibit equal populations), the ESR signal vanishes and the following nuclear polarization arises:

$$P = P_0\left(1 + \xi \frac{\gamma_S \, I(I+1)}{\gamma_I \, I(S+1)}\right) \tag{15.66}$$

P_0: Thermal equilibrium polarization of the nuclear spins, S: Electron spin
γ_S: Electronic gyromagnetic ratio, I: Nuclear spin, γ_I: Nuclear gyromagnetic ratio
$\xi < 1$: Factor taking the relaxation mechanisms into account

The Overhauser effect may be used with dedicated contrast agents in MRI. In vivo application would require very low field imaging instruments (~ 0.01 T) to enable the ESR-RF field to penetrate the body. The loss in NMR signal intensity will then have to be compensated for by the enhanced polarization of the contrast agent. Given that the usefulness of such low field instruments is restricted to these particular agents, contrast agents that apply DNP for standard MRI equipment represent a better choice.

Work is currently underway on the development of dedicated contrast agents for ^{13}C NMR that are polarized in a solid state in the presence of a high magnetic field and at a low temperature with the Overhauser effect [15.202]. Such samples are then dissolved and rapidly brought to room temperature for administration. Endogenous substances that enter the metabolic pathway will be of particular interest as potential substrates [15.203].

15.3 References

[15.1] D.I. Hoult, C.N. Chen, V.J. Sank
The field dependence of NMR imaging II: arguments concerning on optimal field strength
Magn. Reson. Med. 3 (1986), 730-746

[15.2] P.A. Bottomley, T.H. Foster, R.E. Argersinger, L.M. Pfeifer
A review of normal tissue hydrogen NMR relaxation times and relaxation mechanisms from 1-100 MHz
Med. Phys. 11 (1984), 425-448

[15.3] M.A. Bernstein, X.J. Zhou, J.A. Polzin, K.F. King, A. Ganin, N.J. Pelc, G.H. Glover
Concomitant gradient terms in phase contrast MR: analysis and correction
Magn. Reson. Med. 39 (1998), 300-308

[15.4] P. Mansfield, B.L.W. Chapman
Active magnetic screening of gradient coils in NMR imaging
J. Magn. Reson. 66 (1986), 573-576

[15.5] S.C. Cripps
RF power amplifiers for wireless communication
Artech House, Boston 1999

[15.6] J. Halamek, P. Jurak, M. Kasal, M. Villa, P. Cofrancesco
Analog-to-digital-converter and dynamic range
J. El. Eng., 48 (1997), 183-189

[15.7] D.W. Alderman, D.M. Grant
An efficient decoupler coil design which reduces heating in conductive samples in superconducting spectrometers
J. Magn. Reson. 36 (1979), 447-451

[15.8] C.E. Hayes, W.A. Edelstein, J.F. Schenck, O.M. Mueller, M. Eash
An efficient highly homogeneous radiofrequency coil for whole-body NMR imaging at 1.5T
J. Magn. Reson. 63 (1985), 622-628

[15.9] J. Tropp
The theory of the bird-cage resonator
J. Magn. Reson. 82 (1989), 51-62

[15.10] J.T. Vaughan, H.P. Hetherington, J.O. Otu, J.W. Pan, G.M. Pohost
High frequency volume coils for clinical NMR imaging and spectroscopy
Magn. Reson. Med. 32 (1994), 206-218

[15.11] P.B. Roemer, W.A. Edelstein, C.E. Hayes, S.P. Souza, O.M. Mueller
The NMR phased array
Magn. Reson. Med. 16 (1990), 192-225

[15.12] J. Wang, A. Reykowski, J. Dickas
Calculation of the signal-to-noise ratio for simple surface coils and arrays of coils
IEEE Trans. Biomed. Eng. 42 (1995), 908-917

[15.13] W. Schnell, W. Renz, M. Vester, H. Ermert
Ultimate signal-to-noise-ratio of surface and body antennas for magnetic resonance imaging
IEEE Trans. Ant. Prop. 48 (2000), 418-428

[15.14] A. Reykowski, S.M. Wright, J.R. Porter
Design of matching networks for low noise preamplifiers
Magn. Reson. Med. 33 (1995), 848-852

[15.15] A. Reykowski
Theory and design of synthesis array coils for MRI
Texas A&M Univ., Dissertation 1996

[15.16] Magnetic resonance equipment for diagnostic imaging – determination of characteristics (Committee draft Nov 18th, 2004)
IEC Standard 62312-1

[15.17] NEMA Standard MS-1-1988 (R-1994)
Determination of signal-to-noise ratio
(SNR) in diagnostic magnetic resonance images
National Electrical Manufacturers Association, Washington DC, USA

[15.18] NEMA Standard MS-3-1989 (R-1994)
Determination of image uniformity in diagnostic magnetic resonance images
National Electrical Manufacturers Association, Washington DC, USA

[15.19] R.M. Henkelman, M.J. Bronskill
Artifacts in magnetic resonance imaging
Pergamon, New York 1987

[15.20] EN/IEC 60601-2-33
Particular requirements for the safety of magnetic resonance equipment for medical diagnosis

[15.21] F.G. Shellock
Reference manual for magnetic resonance safety
AMIRSYS, Salt Lake City 2003

[15.22] ISO/IEC 14971
Medical devices – application of risk management to medical devices

[15.23] Magnetom family – the perfection of care, safety video
Siemens Medical Solutions

[15.24] Magnetom Avanto system manual, part A: safety
Siemens Medical Solutions

[15.25] F.G. Shellock (ed.)
Magnetic Resonance Procedures: Health Effects and Safety
CRC Press, Boca Raton 2001

[15.26] M.V. Berry, A.K. Geim
Of flying frogs and levitrons
Eur. J. Phys. 18 (1997), 307-313

[15.27] L. Barregard, B. Järvholm, E. Ungethüm
Cancer among workers exposed to strong static magnetic fields
The Lancet (1985), 892

[15.28] F. Schmitt, W. Irnich, H. Fischer
Physiological side effects of fast gradient switching
in: F. Schmitt, M.K. Stehling, R. Turner (eds.)
Echo-planar imaging, theory, technique and application
Springer, New York 1998

[15.29] IEC 601-2-33 Ed. 2.0, 2002; Medical electrical equipment – part 2-33
Particular requirements for the safety of magnetic resonance equipment for medical diagnosis

[15.30] F.X. Hebrank, M. Gebhardt
SAFE model – a new method for predicting peripheral nerve stimulations in MRI
Proceedings Soc. Mag. Res. Im. conference 2000, p. 2007

[15.31] K.R. Foster, H.P. Schwan
Dielectrical properties of tissues
in: C. Polk, E. Postow (ed.)
Handbook of biological effects of electromagnetics fields
CRC Press 1996

[15.32] G. Brix, J. Griebel, M.V. Knopp, J. Bernhardt
Sicherheitsaspekte bei der Anwendung magnetischer Resonanzverfahren in der medizinischen Diagnostik
Zeitschrift für medizinische Physik (2000), 5-15

[15.33] J. Hennig, A. Nauerth, H. Friedburg, D. Ratzel
Ein neues Schnellbildverfahren für die Kernspintomographie
Radiologe 24 (1984), 579-580

[15.34] P. Reimer, T. Allkemper, G. Schuierer, P.E. Peters
Brain imaging: reduced sensitivity of RARE-derived techniques to susceptibility effects. Cine MR imaging: feasibility study
J. Comput. Assist. Tomogr. 20 (1996), 201

[15.35] B. Kiefer, J. Grässner, R. Hausmann
Image acquisition in a second with half-Fourier acquired single shot turbo spin echo
J. Magn. Reson. Imaging. 4 (1994), 86

[15.36] P. Margosian, F. Schmitt, D. Purdy
Faster MR imaging: imaging with half the data
Health Care Instrum. 1 (1986), 195

[15.37] D. Levine, P.D. Barnes
Cortical maturation in normal and abnormal fetuses as assessed with prenatal MR imaging
Radiology 210 (1999), 751

[15.38] J.S. Waugh
Sensitivity in Fourier transform NMR spectroscopy of slowly relaxing systems
J. Mol. Spectr. 35 (1979), 298

[15.39] W.A. Edelstein, J.M.S. Hutchison, G. Johnson, T.W. Redpath
Spin warp NMR imaging and applications to human whole-body imaging
Phys. Med. Biol. 25 (1980), 751

[15.40] A. Haase, J. Frahm, D. Mathaei, W. Haenicke, K.D. Merboldt
FLASH imaging. Rapid imaging using low flip-angle pulses
J. Magn. Reson. 67 (1986), 256

[15.41] H. Bruder, H. Fischer, R. Graumann, M. Deimling
A new steady-state imaging sequence for simultaneous acquisition of two MR images with clearly different contrasts
Magn. Reson. Med. 7 (1988), 35

[15.42] M. Deimling, G. Laub
Constructive interference in steady state (CISS) for motion sensitivity reduction
Proc. SMRM Book of Abstracts 2 (1989), 842

[15.43] P. Mansfield
Multi-planar image formation using NMR spin-echoes
J. Phys. C 10 (1977), L55

[15.44] M.E. Moseley, J. Mintorovitch, Y. Cohen, H.S. Asgari, N. Derugin, D. Norman, J. Kucharczyk
Early detection of ischemic injury: comparison of spectroscopy, diffusion-, T2-, and magnetic susceptibility-weighted MRI in cats
Acta Neurochir. Suppl. (Wien)51 (1990), 207

[15.45] P.A. Bandettini, E.C. Wong, A. Jesmanowicz, R.S. Hinks, J.S. Hyde
Spin-echo and gradient-echo EPI of human brain activation using BOLD contrast: a comparative study at 1.5 T
NMR Biomed. 7 (1994),12

[15.46] Y.P. Du, D.L. Parker, W.L. Davis, G. Cao
Reduction of partial-volume artifacts with zero-filled interpolation in three-dimensional MR angiography
J. Magn. Reson. Imaging 4 (1994), 733

[15.47] N.M. Rofsky, V.S. Lee, G. Laub, M.A. Pollack, G.A. Krinsky, D. Thomasson, M.M. Ambrosino, J.C. Weinreb
Abdominal MR imaging with a volumetric interpolated breath-hold examination
Radiology 212 (1999), 876

[15.48] P.J. Hore
A new method for water suppression in proton NMR spectra of aqueous solutions
J. Magn. Reson. 54 (1983), 539

[15.49] M. Wiesmann, T.E. Mayer, I. Yousry, R. Medele, G.F. Hamann, H. Bruckmann
Detection of hyperacute subarachnoid hemorrhage of the brain by using magnetic resonance imaging
J. Neurosurg. 96 (2002)), 684

[15.50] O.P. Simonetti, J.P. Finn, R.D. White, G. Laub, D.A. Henry
Black blood T2-weighted inversion-recovery MR imaging of the heart
Radiology 199 (1996), 49

[15.51] E.D. Becker, J.A. Ferretti, T.C. Farrar
Driven equilibrium Fourier transform spectroscopy
J. Amer. Chem. Soc. 91 (1969), 7784

[15.52] E.R. Melhem, R. Itoh, P.J. Folkers
Cervical spine: three-dimensional fast spin-echo MR imaging-improved recovery of longitudinal magnetization with driven equilibrium pulse
Radiology 218 (2001), 283

[15.53] A. Haase A, D. Matthaei, R. Bartkowski, E. Duhmke, D. Leibfritz
Inversion recovery snapshot FLASH MR imaging
J. Comput. Assist. Tomogr. 13 (1989), 1036

[15.54] D.J. Atkinson, D. Burstein, R.R. Edelman
First-pass cardiac perfusion: evaluation with ultrafast MR imaging
Radiology 174 (1990), 757

[15.55] J. Carr, F. Pereles, R. McCarthy, T. Dunphy, R. Omary, O. Simonetti, J. Finn
Delayed contrast-enhanced imaging of left ventricular myocardial scarring using single-shot inversion recovery (IR) trueFISP
Proc. Intl. Soc. Mag. Reson. Med. 11 (2003), 1612 abstr.

[15.56] J.P. Mugler, J.R. Brookeman
Three-dimensional magnetization-prepared rapid gradient-echo imaging (3D MP RAGE)
Magn Reson Med 15 (1990), 152

[15.57] J.P. Mugler, J.R. Brookeman
Theoretical analysis of gadopentetate dimeglumine enhancement in T1-weighted imaging of the brain: comparison of two-dimensional spin-echo and three-dimensional gradient-echo sequences
J. Magn. Reson. Imaging 3 (1993), 761

[15.58] K. Oshio, D.A. Feinberg
GRASE (gradient- and spin-echo) imaging: a novel fast MRI technique
Magn. Reson. Med. 20 (1991), 344

[15.59] T. Allkemper, P. Reimer, G. Schuierer, P.E. Peters
Study of susceptibility-induced artifacts in GRASE with different echo train length
Eur. Radiol. 8 (1998), 834

[15.60] J.W. Carlson
An algorithm for NMR imaging reconstruction based on multiple RF receiver coils
J. Magn. Reson. 74 (1987), 376-380

[15.61] M. Hutchinson, U. Raff
Fast MRI data acquisition using multiple detectors
Magn. Reson. Med. 6 (1988), 87-91

[15.62] J.R. Kelton, R.L. Magin, S.M. Wright
An algorithm for rapid image acquisition using multiple receiver coils
Proceedings of the 8th Annual Meeting of SMRM 1989, 1172

[15.63] D. Kwiat, S. Einav, G. Navon
A decoupled coil detector array for fast image acquisitions in magnetic resonance imaging
Med. Phys. 18 (1991), 251-265

[15.64] J.W. Carlson, T. Minemura
Imaging time reduction through multiple receiver coil data acquisition and image reconstruction.
Magn. Reson. Med. 29 (1993), 681-688

[15.65] J.B. Ra, C.Y. Rim
Fast imaging using subencoding data sets from multiple detectors
Magn. Reson. Med. 30 (1993), 142-145

[15.66] D.K. Sodickson, W.J. Manning
Simultaneous acquisition of spatial harmonics (SMASH): Fast imaging with radio-frequency coil arrays
Magn. Reson. Med. 38 (1997), 591-603

[15.67] P.M. Jakob, M.A. Griswold, R.R. Edelman, D.K. Sodickson
AUTO-SMASH, a self-calibrating technique for SMASH imaging
MAGMA 7 (1998), 42-54

[15.68] R.M. Heidemann, M.A. Griswold, A. Haase, P.M. Jakob
VD-AUTO-SMASH imaging
Magn. Reson. Med. 45 (2001), 1066-1074

[15.69] M.A. Griswold, P.M. Jakob, R.M. Heidemann, M. Nittka, V. Jellus, J. Wang, B. Kiefer, A. Haase
Generalized autocalibrating partially parallel acquisitions (GRAPPA)
Magn. Reson. Med. 47 (2002), 1202-1210

[15.70] K.P. Pruessmann, M. Weiger, M.B. Scheidegger, P. Boesiger
SENSE: sensitivity encoding for fast MRI
Magn. Reson. Med. 42 (1999), 952-62

[15.71] M.A. Griswold, P.M. Jakob, M. Nittka, J.W. Goldfarb, A. Haase
Partially parallel imaging with localized sensitivities (PILS)
Magn. Reson. Med. 44 (2000), 602-609

[15.72] W.E. Kyraikos, L.P. Panych, D.F. Kalcher, C.F. Westin, S.M. Bao, R.V. Mulkern, F.A. Jolesz
Sensitivity profiles from an array of coils for encoding and reconstruction in parallel (SPACE RIP)
Magn. Reson. Med. 44 (2000), 301-308

[15.73] D.K. Sodickson, M.A. Griswold, P.M. Jakob, R.R. Edelman, W.J. Manning
Signal-to-noise ratio and signal-to-noise efficiency in SMASH imaging
Magn. Reson. Med. 41 1999), 1009-1022

[15.74] M.A. Griswold, S. Kannengiesser, R.M. Heidemann, J. Wang, P.M. Jakob
Field-of-view limitations in parallel imaging
Magn. Reson. Med., 52 (2004), 1118-1126

[15.75] P. Kellman, F.H. Epstein, E.R. McVeigh
Adaptive sensitivity encoding incorporating temporal filtering (TSENSE)
Magn. Reson. Med. 45 (2001), 846-852

[15.76] M.A. Griswold, P.M. Jakob, Q. Chen, J.W. Goldfarb, W.J. Manning, R.R. Edelman, D.K. Sodickson
Resolution enhancement in single-shot imaging using simultaneous acquisition of spatial harmonics (SMASH)
Magn. Reson. Med. 41 (1999), 1236-1245

[15.77] B. Merlino, M. Salcuni, L. Salute, R. Marano, L. Bonomo
Total body MR angiography and atherosclerosis
Rays 26 (2001), 305-314

[15.78] M. Goyen, C.U. Herborn, K. Kroger, T.C. Lauenstein, J.F. Debatin, S.G. Ruehm
Detection of atherosclerosis: systemic imaging for systemic disease with whole-body three-dimensional MR angiography – initial experience
Radiology 227 (2003), 277-282

[15.79] H. Kramer, S.O. Schoenberg, K. Nikolaou, A. Huber, A. Struwe, E. Winnik, B. Wintersperger, O. Dietrich, B. Kiefer, M.F. Reiser
Cardiovascular whole body MRI with parallel imaging
Radiology 44 (2004), 835-843

[15.80] H. Kramer, S.O. Schoenberg, H. Nikolaou, A. Huber, S. Struwe, E. Winnik, B. Wintersperger, O. Dietrich, B. Kiefer, M.F. Reiser
Cardiovascular screening with parallel imaging techniques and a whole body MR imager
Radiology 236 (2005), 300-310

[15.81] T.C. Lauenstein, S.C. Goehde, C.U. Herborn, M. Goyen, C. Oberhoff, J.F. Debatin, S.G. Ruehm, J. Barkhausen
Whole-body MR imaging: evaluation of patients for metastases
Radiology 233 (2004), 139-148

[15.82] L.J. Horvath, B.A. Burtness, S. McCarthy, K.M. Johnson
Total-body echo-planar MR imaging in the staging of breast cancer: comparison with conventional methods – early experience
Radiology 211 (1999), 119-128

[15.83] J. Barkhausen, H.H. Quick, T. Lauenstein, M. Goyen, S.G. Ruehm, G. Laub, J.F. Debatin, M.E. Ladd
Whole-body MR imaging in 30 seconds with real-time trueFISP and a continuously rolling table platform: feasibility study
Radiology 220 (2001), 252-256

[15.84] D.G. Kruger, S.J. Riederer, R.C. Grimm, P.J. Rossman
Continuously moving table data acquisition method for long FOV contrast-enhanced MRA and whole-body MRI
Magn. Reson. Med. 47 (2002), 224-231

[15.85] M. Sabati, M.L. Lauzon, R. Frayne
Space-time relationship in continuously moving table method for large FOV peripheral contrast-enhanced magnetic resonance angiography
Phys. Med. Biol. 48 (2003), 2739-252.

[15.86] N.A. Ghanem, H.P. Fautz, M. Weigel, O. Speck, J. Hennig, T. Bley, M. Langer
Whole Body-MR imaging with a continuously moving table platform in detection of metastatic disease in cancer patients: First results of a feasibility study
11th Ann Meeting ISMRM, Toronto (2003), 1333

[15.87] Y. Xu, E.M. Haacke
Partial Fourier imaging in multi-dimensions: A means to save a full factor of two in time
J. Magn. Reson. Imaging 14 (2001), 628

[15.88] J.L. Duerk, J.S. Lewin, D.H. Wu
Application of keyhole imaging to interventional MRI: a simulation study to predict sequence requirements
J. Magn. Reson. Imaging 6 (1996), 918-924

[15.89] X. Hu, T. Parrish
Reduction of field of view for dynamic imaging
Magn. Reson. Med. 31 (1994), 691-694

[15.90] L.W. Bartels, C.J.G. Bakker
Endovascular interventional magnetic resonance imaging
Phys. Med. Biol. 48 (2003), R37-R64

[15.91] Z.W. Fu, Y. Wang, R.C. Grimm, P.J. Rossman, J.P. Felmlee, S.J. Riederer, R.L. Ehman
Orbital navigator echoes for motion measurements in magnetic resonance imaging
Magn. Reson. Med. 34 (1995), 746-753

[15.92] E.B. Welch, A. Manduca, R.C. Grimm, H.A. Ward, C.R. Jack
Spherical navigator echoes for full 3D rigid body motion measurement in MRI
Magn. Reson. Med. 47 (2002), 32-41

[15.93] J.V. Hajnal, D.L.G. Hill, D.J. Hawkes
Medical image registration
CRC Press (2001)

[15.94] K.J. Friston, J. Ashburner, J.B. Poline, C.D. Frith, J.C. Heather, R.S.I. Frackowiak
Spatial registration and normalization of images
Hum Brain Map 2 (1995), 165-189

[15.95] S. Thesen, L.R. Schad, A. Bongers, E. Müller
Experimental determination of accuracy in image-based motion detection in fMRI
Book of abstracts ISMRM 2001, 1203

[15.96] C. Studholme, D.L.G. Hill, D.J. Hawkes
An overlap invariant entropy measure of 3D medical image alignment
Pattern Recognition 32 (1999), 71-86

[15.97] D. Atkinson, D.L.G. Hill, P.N.R. Stoyle, P.E. Summers, S. Clare, R. Bowtell, S.F. Keevil
Automatic compensation of motion artifacts in MRI
Magn. Reson. Med. 41 (1999), 163-170

[15.98] IBM Technical Disclosure Bulletin 31-2 (1988)

[15.99] S. Thesen, O. Heid, E. Müller, L.R. Schad
Prospective acquisition correction for head motion with image-based tracking for real-time fMRI
Magn. Res. Med. No.44 (2000), 457-465

[15.100] M. Unser, A. Aldroubi, M. Eden
B_spline signal processing: part I+II
IEEE Transactions on Signal Processing 41 (1993), 821-833 and 834-848

[15.101] A.L. Baert (foreword), I.P. Arlart, G.M. Bongartz, G. Marchal (eds.)
Magnetic resonance angiography
Springer, 2nd edition (2001)

[15.102] M.R. Prince, T.M. Grist, J.F. Debatin
3D contrast MR angiography
Springer, 3rd edition (2002)

[15.103] F.W. Wehrli
Time of flight effects in MR imaging of flow
Magn. Reson. Med. 14 (1990), 187-193

[15.104] P.M. Ruggieri, G.A. Laub, T.J. Masaryk, M.T. Modic
Intracranial circulation: pulse-sequence considerations in three-dimensional (volume) MR angiography
Radiology 171 (1989), 785-791

[15.105] D.L. Parker, C. Yuan, D.D. Blatter
MR angiography by multiple thin slab 3D acquisition
Magn. Reson. Med. 17 (1991), 434-451

[15.106] C.L. Dumoulin, S.P. Souza, M.F. Walker, et al.
Three-dimensional phase-contrast angiography
Magn. Reson. Med. 9 (1989), 139-149

[15.107] J.F. Debatin, R.H. Ting, H. Wegmuller, et al.
Renal artery blood flow: quantification with phase-contrast MR imaging with and without breath holding
Radiology 190 (1994), 371-378

[15.108] J.L. Creasy, R.R. Price, T. Presbrey, et al.
Gadolinium-enhanced MR angiography
Radiology 175 (1990), 280-283

[15.109] F.R. Korosec, R. Frayne, T.M. Grist, C.A. Mistretta
Time-resolved contrast-enhanced 3D MR angiography
Magn. Reson. Med. 36 (1996), 345-351

[15.110] J.F.M. Meaney, J.P. Ridgeway, S. Chakraverty, et al.
Stepping-table gadolinium-enhanced digital subtraction MR angiography of the aorta and lower extremity arteries: Preliminary experience
Radiology 211 (1999), 59-67

[15.111] G. Laub
Displays for MR angiography
Magn. Reson. Med. 14 (1990), 222-229

[15.112] F. Calamante, D.G. Gadian., A. Connelly
Quantification of perfusion using bolus tracking magnetic resonance imaging in stroke
Stroke 33 (2002), 1146-1151

[15.113] S. Ogawa, T.M. Lee, A.S. Nayak, P. Glynn
Oxygenation-sensitive contrast in magnetic resonance image of rodent brain at high magnetic fields.
Magn. Reson. Med. 14 (1990), 68-78

[15.114] J.A. Detre, J.S. Leigh, D.S. Williams, A.P. Koretsky
Perfusion imaging
Magn. Res. Med. 23 (1992), 37-45

[15.115] T.P.L. Roberts
Physiologic measurements by contrast-enhanced MR imaging: expectations and limitations
J. Magn. Reson. Imaging 7 (1997), 82-90

[15.116] M.V. Knopp, H. von Tengg-Kobligk, F. Floemer, S.O. Schoenberg
Contrast agents for MRA: future directions
J. Magn. Reson. Imaging 10 (1999), 314-316

[15.117] R. Weissleder, D.D. Stark, B.L. Engelstad, et al.
Superparamagnetic iron oxide: pharmacokinetics and toxicity
AJR 152 (1989), 167-173

[15.118] M.S. Albert, G.D. Cates, B. Driehuys, W. Happer, B. Saam, C.S. Springer Jr, A. Wishnia
Biological magnetic resonance imaging using laser-polarized ^{129}Xe
Nature 370 (1994), 199-201

[15.119] Golman K., O. Axelsson, H. Jóhannesson, S. Månsson, C. Olofsson, J.S. Petersson
Parahydrogen-induced polarization in imaging: subsecond ^{13}C angiography
Magn. Reson. Med. 46 (2001), 1-5

[15.120] L. Østergaard, R.M. Weisskoff, D.A. Chesler, C. Gyldensted, B.R. Rosen
High resolution measurement of cerebral blood flow using intravascular tracer bolus passages - part I: mathematical approach and statistical analysis
Magn. Reson. Med. 36 (1996), 715-725

[15.121] L. Østergaard, A.G. Sorensen, K. Kwong, R.M. Weisskoff, C. Gyldensted, B.R. Rosen
High resolution measurement of cerebral blood flow using intravascular tracer bolus passages - part II: experimental comparison and preliminary results
Magn. Reson. Med. 36 (1996), 726-736

[15.122] F. Calamante, D.L. Thomas, G.S. Pell, J. Wiersma, R. Turner
Measuring cerebral blood flow using magnetic resonance imaging techniques
J. Cereb. Blood Flow Metab. 19 (1999), 701-735

[15.123] R.L. Evans
Two comments on the estimation of blood flow and central volume from dye-dilution curves.
Journal of Applied Physiology 14 (1959), 457

[15.124] J.R. Keys, P.S. Hetzel, E.H. Wood
Revised equations for calculation of blood flow and central blood volume from indicator-dilution curves
Journal of Applied Physiology 11 (1957), 385-389

[15.125] H.K. Thompson, C.F. Starmer, R.E. Whalen, H.D. McIntosh
Indicator transit time considered as a gamma variate
Circulation Research 14 (1964), 502-515

[15.126] P.S. Tofts
Modeling tracer kinetics in dynamic Gd-DTPA MR imaging
J. Magn. Reson. Imaging 7 (1997), 91-101

[15.127] R.M. Weisskoff, D. Chesler, J.L. Boxerman, B.R. Rosen
Pitfalls in MR measurement of tissue blood flow with intravascular tracers: which mean transit time?
Magn. Reson. Med. 2 (1993), 553-559

[15.128] L.J.M. Kroft, A. de Roos
Blood pool contrast agents for cardiovascular MR imaging
J. Magn. Reson. Imaging 10 (1999), 395-403

[15.129] D. Le Bihan
Looking into the functional architecture of the brain with diffusion MRI
Nature Reviews Neuroscience 4 (2003), 469
www.nature.com/reviews/neuro

[15.130] K.D. Merboldt, W. Haenicke, J. Frahm
Self-diffusion NMR imaging using stimulated echoes
J. Magn. Reson. 64 (1985), 479

[15.131] R. Turner, D. LeBihan, J. Maier, R. Vavrek, L.K. Hedges, J. Pekar
Echo-planar imaging of intravoxel incoherent motion
Radiology 177 (1990), 407

[15.132] M.E. Moseley, J. Kucharczyk, J. Mintorovitch, Y. Cohen, J. Kurhanevicz, N. Derugin, H.S. Asgari, D. Norman
Diffusion-weighted MR imaging of acute stroke: correlation with T2-weighted and magnetic susceptibility-enhanced MR imaging in cats
AJNR 11 (1990), 423

[15.133] S. Warach, D. Chien, W. Li, M. Ronthal, R.R. Edelman
Fast magnetic resonance diffusion weighted imaging of acute human stroke
Neurology 42 (1992), 1717

[15.134] C.G. Cleveland, D.C. Chang, C.F. Hazlewood
Nuclear magnetic resonance measurements of skeletal muscle. Anisotropy of the diffusion coefficient of the intracellular water
Biophys. J., 16 (1976), 1043

[15.135] P.J. Basser, J. Matiello, D. LeBihan
MR Diffusion tensor spectroscopy and imaging
Biophys. J., 66 (1994), 259

[15.136] C. Pierpaoli, P. Jezzard, P. Basser, A. Barnett, G. Di Chiro
Diffusion Tensor MR imaging of the human brain
Radiology, 201 (1996), 637

[15.137] T.E. Conturo, N.F. Lori, T.S. Cull, E. Abdukak, A.Z. Snyder, J.S. Shimony, R.C. McKinstry, H. Burton, M.E. Raichle
Tracking neuronal fiber pathways in the living human brain
PNAS USA , 96 (1999), 10422

[15.138] E.O. Stejskal, J.E. Tanner
Spin diffusion measurements
J. Chem. Phys. 42 (1965), 288

[15.139] D. Porter, E. Mueller
Multi-shot diffusion-weighted EPI with readout mosaic segmentation and 2D navigator correction
Proc. Intn. Soc. Magn. Reson. Med. (2004), 442

[15.140] R. Turner, D. LeBihan, C.T.W. Moonen, D. Despres and J. Frank
Echo-planar time course MRI of cat brain deoxygenation changes
Magn. Reson. Med. 22 (1991), 159

[15.141] L. Pauling, C.D. Coryell
The magnetic properties and structure of hemoglobin, oxyhemoglobin and carbonmonoxyhemoglobin
Proc. Natl. Acad. Sci. USA 22 (1936), 210

[15.142] K.K. Kwong, J.W. Belliveau, D.A. Chesler, I.E. Goldberg, R.M. Weisskoff, B.C. Poncelet, D.N. Kennedy, B.E. Hoppel, M.S. Cohen, R. Turner, H.M. Cheng, T.J. Brady, B.R. Rosen
Dynamic magnetic resonance imaging of human brain activity during primary sensory stimulation
Proc. Natl. Acad. Sci. USA 89 (1992), 5675

[15.143] C.S. Roy, C.S. Sherrington
On the regulation of the blood-supply of the brain
J. Physiol. 11 (1890), 85

[15.144] P.T. Fox, M.E. Raichle
Focal physiological uncoupling of cerebral blood flow and oxidative metabolism during somatosensory stimulation in human subjects
Proc. Natl. Acad. Sci. USA 82 (1986), 1140

[15.145] R. Turner, A. Grinvald
Direct visualization of patterns of deoxygenation and reoxygenation in monkey cortical vasculature during functional brain activation
Proc. Soc. Magn. Reson. 1 (1994), 430

[15.146] D. Malonek, A. Grinvald
Interactions between electrical activity and microcirculation revealed by imaging spectroscopy – implications for functional brain mapping
Science 272 (1996), 551

[15.147] S. Thesen, G. Krueger, E. Mueller
Absolute correction of B0 fluctuations in echo planar imaging
Proc. Intn. Soc. Magn. Reson. Med. (2003), 1025

[15.148] P.A. Bandettini, E.C. Wong, R.S. Hinks, R.S. Tikofsky, J.S. Hyde
Time course EPI of human brain function during task activation
Magn. Reson. Med. 25 (1992), 390

[15.149] W.H. Press, B.P. Flannery, S.A. Teukolsky, W.T. Vetterling
Numerical recipes in Pascal – the art of scientific computing
Cambridge University Press (1989)

[15.150] K.J. Friston, A.P. Holmes, K.J. Worsley, J.B. Poline, C.D. Frith, R.S.J. Frackowiack
Statistic parametric maps in functional imaging: a general linear approach
Human Brain Mapping 2 (1995), 189

[15.151] R.S.J. Frackowiack, K.J. Friston, C.D. Frith, R.J. Dolan, J.C. Mazziotta
Human brain function
Academic Press (1997)

[15.152] Human Brain Mapping Conferences
www.humanbrainmapping.org

[15.153] C.T.W. Moonen, P.A. Bandettini
Functional MRI
Springer (2000)

[15.154] WHO Guidelines Subcommittee: 1999 World Health Organization – International Society of Hypertension
Guidelines for the management of hypertension
J. Hypertens. 17 (1999), 151-183

[15.155] WHO Task Force: Report of the WHO Task Force on Stroke and other Cerebrovascular Disorders
Recommendation on stroke prevention, diagnosis and therapy
Stroke 20 (1989), 1407

[15.156] The National Institute of Neurological Disorders and Stroke rt-PA Stroke Study Group
Tissue plasminogen activator for acute ischemic stroke
N. Engl. J. Med. 333 (1995), 1581

[15.157] O. Jansen, P.D. Schellinger, J.B. Fiebach, W. Hacke, K. Sartor
Early recanalization in acute ischemic stroke saves tissue at risk defined by MRI
Lancet 353 (1999), 2036

[15.158] J.B. Fiebach, P.D. Schellinger with K. Sartor, S. Heiland, S. Warach, W. Hacke
Stroke MRI
Springer (2003)

[15.159] A. Lardo, Z.A. Fayad, N.A.F. Chronos, V. Fuster (eds.)
Cardiovascular magnetic resonance: established and emerging applications
Martin Dunitz, Ltd, (2004)

[15.160] W.J. Manning, D.J. Pennell (eds.)
Cardiovascular magnetic resonance
Churchill Livingstone, (2002)

[15.161] C.B. Higgins, A. de Roos (eds.)
Cardiovascular MRI and MRA
Lippincott Williams & Wilkins Publishers (2002)

[15.162] J. Bogaert, A. Duerinckx, F. Rademakers
Magnetic resonance of the heart and great vessels
Springer Verlag (2000)

[15.163] J.S. Lewin, J.L. Duerk, V.R. Jain, C.A. Petersilge, C.P. Chao, J.R. Haaga
Needle localization in MR-guided biopsy and aspiration: effects of field strength, sequence design, and magnetic field orientation
Am. J. Roentgenol. 166 (1996), 1337-1345

[15.164] T.J. Vogl, R. Straub, K. Eichler, O. Sollner, M.G. Mack
Colorectal carcinoma metastases in liver: laser-induced interstitial thermotherapy – local tumor control rate and survival data
Radiology 230 (2004), 450-458

[15.165] F.K. Wacker, K. Reither, J.P. Ritz, A. Roggan, C.T. Germer, K.J. Wolf
MR guided interstitial laser-induced thermotherapy of hepatic metastasis combined with arterial blood flow reduction: technique and first clinical results in an open MR system
J. Magn. Reson. Imaging 13 (2001), 31-36

[15.166] M. Wendt, F. Sauer, A. Khamene, B. Bascle, S. Vogt, F.K. Wacker
A head-mounted display system for augmented reality: initial evaluation for interventional MRI
RöFo 175 (2003), 418-421

[15.167] F.K. Wacker, S. Faiss, K. Reither, T. Zimmer, M. Wendt, K.J. Wolf
MR imaging guided biliary drainage in an open low-field system: first clinical experiences
RöFo 172 (2000), 744-747

[15.168] C.J. Bakker, R.M. Hoogeveen, J. Weber, J.J. van Vaals, M.A. Viergever, W.P. Mali
Visualization of dedicated catheters using fast scanning techniques with potential for MR-guided vascular interventions
Magn. Reson. Med. 36 (1996), 816-820

[15.169] F.K. Wacker, K. Reither, G. Branding, M. Wendt, K.J. Wolf
Magnetic resonance-guided vascular catheterization: feasibility using a passive tracking technique at 0.2 Tesla in a pig model
J. Magn. Reson. Imaging 10 (1999), 841-844

[15.170] O. Unal, F.R Korosec, R. Frayne, C.M. Strother, C.A. Mistretta
A rapid 2D time-resolved variable-rate k-space sampling MR technique for passive catheter tracking during endovascular procedures
Magn. Reson. Med., 40 (1998), 356-362

[15.171] C.L. Dumoulin, S.P. Souza, R.D Darrow
Real-time position monitoring of invasive devices using magnetic resonance
Magn. Reson. Med., 29 (1993), 411-415

[15.172] W.R. Nitz, A. Oppelt, W. Renz, C. Manke, M. Lenhart, J. Link
On the heating of linear conductive structures as guide wires and catheters in interventional MRI
J. Magn. Reson. Imaging 13 (2001), 105-114

[15.173] M.E. Ladd, H.H. Quick
Reduction of resonant RF heating in intravascular catheters using coaxial chokes.
Magn. Reson. Med., 43 (2000), 615-619

[15.174] M. Burl, G.A Coutts, I.R. Young
Tuned fiducial markers to identify body locations with minimal perturbation of tissue magnetization
Magn. Reson. Med. 36 (1996), 491-493

[15.175] C. Manke, W.R. Nitz, B. Djavidani, M. Strotzer, M. Lenhart, M. Volk, S. Feuerbach, J. Link
MR imaging-guided stent placement in iliac arterial stenoses: a feasibility study
Radiology 219 (2001), 527-534

[15.176] R. Razavi, D.L Hill, S.F. Keevil, M.E. Miquel, V. Muthurangu, S. Hegde, K. Rhode, M. Barnett, J. van Vaals, D.J. Hawkes, E. Baker
Cardiac catheterisation guided by MRI in children and adults with congenital heart disease
Lancet 362 (2003), 1877-1882

[15.177] R. de Graaf
In vivo NMR spectroscopy
Wiley, Chichester 1998

[15.178] T. Ethofer, I. Mader, U. Seeger, A. Ludolph, W. Grodd, U. Klose
Comparison of metabolite T1 relaxation times in different brain regions at 1.5 and 3 Tesla
Proc. ISMRM (2003), 434

[15.179] J. Frahm, K.D. Merboldt, W. Hänike,
Localized proton spectroscopy using stimulated echoes
J. Magn. Reson. 72 (1987), 502-508

[15.180] J. Hennig
Coupling effects in volume selective 1H spectroscopy of major brain metabolites
Magn. Reson. Med. 21 (1991), 82-96

[15.181] R. Pohmann, M. v. Kienlin, A. Haase
Theoretical evaluation and comparison of fast chemical shift imaging methods.
J. Magn Reson. 129 (1997), 145-160

[15.182] V. Govindaraju, K. Young, A. Maudsley
Proton NMR chemical shifts and coupling constants for brain metabolites
NMR Biomed. 13 (2000), 129-153

[15.183] J. Scheidler, H. Hricak, D. Vigneron, K. Yu, D. Sokolov, L. Huang, C. Zaloudek, S. Nelson, P. Carroll, J. Kurhanewicz
Prostate cancer: localization with three-dimensional proton MR spectroscopic imaging – clinicopathologic study
Radiology 213 (1999), 473-480

[15.184] T. Scheenen, D. Klomp, S. Röll, J. Fütterer, J. Barentsz, A. Heerschap
Fast acquisition-weighted three-dimensional proton MR spectroscopic imaging of the human prostate
Magn. Reson. Med. 52 (2004), 80-88

[15.185] S. Neubauer
High-energy phosphate metabolism in normal, hypertrophied and failing human myocardium
Heart Failure Rev. 4 (1999), 269-280

[15.186] C.R. Bowers, D.P. Weitekamp
The transformation of symmetrization order to nuclear spin magnetization by chemical reaction and nuclear magnetic resonance
Phys. Rev. Lett. 57 (1986), 2645

[15.187] C.R. Bowers, D.P. Weitekamp
Parahydrogen and synthesis allow dramatically enhanced nuclear alignment
J. Am. Chem. Soc. 109 (1987), 5541

[15.188] A. Abragam, M. Goldman
Principles of dynamic nuclear polarisation
Rep. Prog. Phys. 41 (1978), 395-467

[15.189] M. Goldman
Spin temperature and nuclear magnetic resonance in solids
Oxford Univ. Press, Oxford 1970

[15.190] M.R. Bouchiat, T.R. Carver, C.R. Varnum
Nuclear polarization in 3He gas induced by optical pumping and dipolar spin exchange
Phys. Rev. Lett. 5 (1960), 373-375

[15.191] M. Ebert, T. Grossmann, W. Heil, E.W. Otten, R. Surkau, M. Leduc, P. Bachert, M.V. Knopp, L.R. Sachad, M. Thelen
Nuclear magnetic resonance imaging with hyperpolarized ^{3}He
Lancet 347 (1996), 1297-1299

[15.192] B. Eberle, N. Weiler, K. Markstaller, H.U. Kauczor, A. Deninger, M. Ebert, T. Grossmann, W. Heil, L.O. Lauer, T.P.L. Roberts, W.G. Schreiber, R. Surkau, W.F. Dick, E.W. Otten, M. Thelen

Analysis of intrapulmonary 02 concentration by MR imaging of inhaled hyperpolarized helium-3
J. Appl. Physiol. 87 (1999), 2043-2052

[15.193] D.S. Gierada, B. Saam, D. Yablonskiy, J.D. Cooper, S.S. Lefrak, M.S. Conradi
Dynamic echo planar MR imaging of lung ventilation with hyperpolarized ^{3}He in normal subjects and patients with severe emphysema
NMR Biomed. 13 (2000), 176-181

[15.194] A.C. Tooker, K.S. Hong, E.L. McKinstry, P. Costello, F.A. Jolesz, M.S. Albert
Distal airways in humans: dynamic hyperpolarized ^{3}He MR imaging – feasibility
Radiology 227 (2003), 575-579

[15.195] D.A. Yablinskiy, A.L. Sukstanskii, J.C. Leawoods, D.S. Gierada, G.L. Bretthorst, S.S. Lefrak, J.D. Cooper, M.S. Conradi
Quantitative in vivo assessment of lung microstructure at the alveolar level with hyperpolarized ^{3}He diffusion MRI
PNAS 99/5 (2002), 3111-3116

[15.196] M. Salerno, E.E. de Lange, T.A. Altes, J.D. Truwit, J.R. Brookeman, J.P. Mugler
Emphysema: hyperpolarized helium-3 diffusion MR imaging of the lungs compared with spirometric indexes – initial experience
Radiology 222 (2002), 252-260

[15.197] M. Deimling, O. Heid
Magnetization prepared true FISP imaging
Proc. Soc. Magn. Res. Med., Scientific meeting San Francisco (1994), 495

[15.198] J. Svensson, S. Månsson, E. Johansson, J.S. Petersson, L.E. Olsson
Hyperpolarized 13C MR angiography using trueFISP
Magn. Reson. Med. 50 (2003), 256-262

[15.199] J. Svensson
Contrast-enhanced magnetic resonance angiography – development and optimization of techniques for paramagnetic and hyperpolarized contrast media (doctorial dissertation)
Dept. of Radiation Physics, Lund University (2002)

[15.200] S. Månsson
Hyperpolarized nuclei for NMR imaging and spectroscopy – methodology and model studies of lung and vascular function (doctoral dissertation)
Dept. of Experimental Research, Lund University (2002)

[15.201] L.E. Olsson, K. Wicklow, C.M. Chai, O. Axelsson, M. Karlsson, J.S. Petersson, K. Golman
MR coronary angiography in pig with intra arterial injections of hyperpolarized C13 forthcoming

[15.202] J.H. Ardenkjaer, B. Fridlund, A. Gram, G. Hansson, L. Hansson, M.H. Lerche, R. Servin, M. Thaning, K. Golman
Increase in signal-to-noise ratio of >10,000 times in liquid-state NMR
PNAS 100-N18 (2003), 10158-10163

[15.203] K. Golman, J.H. Ardenkjaer-Larsen, J.S. Petersson, S. Mansson, I. Leunbach
Molecular imaging with endogenous substances
PNAS 100/18 (2003), 10435-10439

16 Ultrasound imaging systems

16.1 Introduction

The term ultrasound, defined rigorously, means sound at such a high frequency that people cannot hear it. Conventionally, this is defined as frequencies above 20 kHz. Diagnostic ultrasound, as used in medicine, has frequencies varying from approximately 1 to 15 MHz (some special purpose ophthalmic and intravascular imaging systems, which are not discussed in this chapter, use higher frequencies).

Ultrasound has been used for imaging in medicine since the middle of the 1950s. Over these 50 years, the technology contained in these systems has progressed dramatically, and we now have imaging systems that range from handheld systems weighing less than 2 kilograms to large high-performance systems that can weigh over 100 kilograms. All of these systems are considered portable, in that they can be moved to the patient (on wheels in most cases) and they all operate on conventional electrical power found in most institutions.

Another common characteristic of all modern ultrasound systems is that they produce images in real time.

Portability and real-time imaging are the primary characteristics that distinguish ultrasound from other imaging modalities such as MRI and CT.

In fig. 16.1 a number of ultrasound imaging systems are shown.

16.1.1 Operation

When producing images with ultrasound, the clinician holds the transducer (a device that converts electrical signals into sound waves and back) in his or her hand and places the transducer face (the surface that emits and receives sound) against the patient's skin in order to make images. This skin contact is critical because at the frequencies used for diagnostic imaging, ultrasound will not propagate in air.

In order to insure good contact between the transducer (or probe, as it is sometimes called) and the patient, a high viscosity water-soluble gel is used.

All ultrasound imaging systems assume that sound propagates through the body with a uniform velocity, and that all received acoustic waves are the result of propagation to a point from which a wave is directly backscattered.

Unfortunately, as the sound propagates into the patient, there are many opportunities for this assumption to be violated. Multiple scattering can occur, and different tissues have different velocities of sound. These deviations from the assumed model often

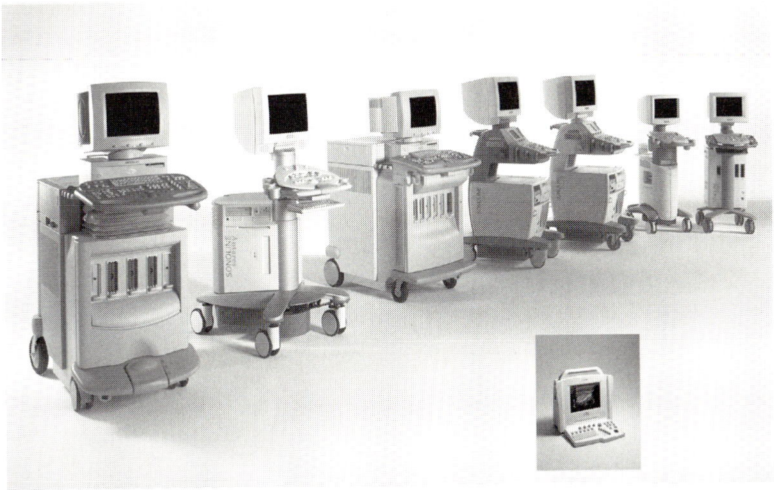

Figure 16.1
Typical ultrasound systems. The small system in the lower right can be easily carried to remote locations. All other systems can be rolled to a patient's bedside.

cause a degradation in image quality. Specific examples for that, such as excessive clutter, will be discussed later in this chapter.

Much of the distinction between different ultrasound manufacturers is in the features offered to reduce this image degradation. Because this degradation is patient dependent, it is important that the performance of any ultrasound system be evaluated on the patient population with which it will be used. Images of subjects that are easy to image can mislead the clinician into expecting better image quality than will be achieved on real patients.

Because of the dramatic dependence of image quality on the specific patient, there are many image optimization controls on all ultrasound systems. Different manufacturers provide different controls that reflect the different architectures of their systems, although all systems have basic settings such as control over imaging depth, gain, dynamic range, variable gain with range (DGC), Doppler frequency scale, Doppler gain, and others.

The discussion that follows describes the basic principles relevant to all ultrasound imaging systems.

16.1.2 Typical modes

Ultrasound systems operate in three major modes: B-mode, spectral Doppler, and Doppler flow imaging. B-mode is primarily used to image soft tissue structure, spectral Doppler provides precise measurements of blood flow at a single location, and Doppler flow imaging (commonly called color flow, because the velocity information

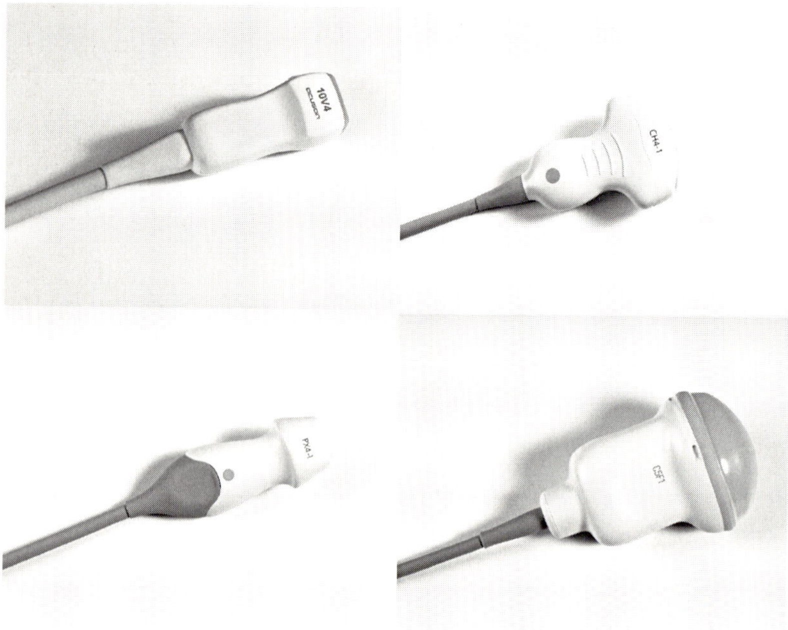

Figure 16.2
Typical ultrasound transducers (probes). Clockwise from upper left: high-frequency pediatric sector probe, curved probe for adult abdominal imaging, mechanically scanned curved array for 3D imaging, and an adult sector cardiac probe.

is presented as a color overlay on the B-mode image) allows visualization of blood flow.

Currently, ultrasound systems produce two-dimensional images and three-dimensional images in some modes.

The transducers used to make both B-mode and flow images and to measure Doppler spectra are typically one-dimensional arrays (exceptions will be discussed later) in which the element sizes vary between 150 and 600 μm in width and have heights between 6 and 18 mm. Typically, these transducers have between 64 and 256 elements, resulting in apertures that range from 14 to 60 mm in width (azimuth), with heights (elevation) equal to the height of the elements. Fig. 16.2 illustrates a selection of typical transducers.

16.1.2.1 Structure imaging (B-mode)

In fig. 16.3, two B-mode images (one of a heart, one of a liver) are shown. These images are produced by launching a short pulse of ultrasound into the body and then receiving echoes and displaying the amplitude of these echoes. Regions filled with fluid (usually blood) appear black in these images, while soft tissue has a gray textured appearance.

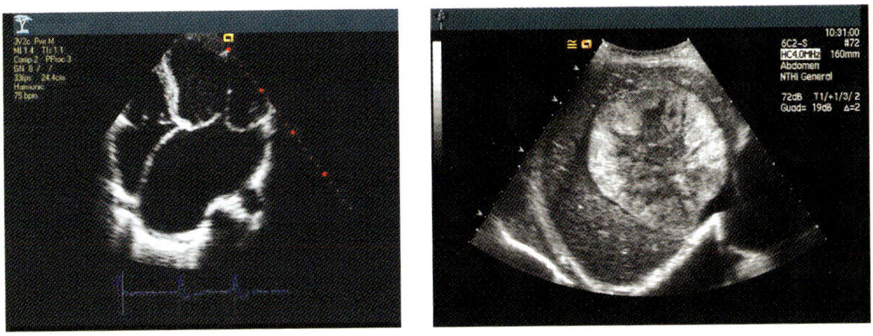

Figure 16.3
Typical B-mode images. The image on the **left** is of a heart with an enlarged atrium, and is made with a 2.5 MHz sector probe. The image on the **right** is of a liver with a large tumor, and is made with a 3.5 MHz curved probe.

The texture of soft tissue in ultrasound images is one of the most obvious differences between ultrasound images and other imaging modalities, especially MRI and CT. Texture is a consequence of the scattering of sound waves by microscopic tissue inhomogeneities (scattering sites) and is due to the constructive and destructive interference of echoes originating from many scattering sites within a resolution volume. Burckhardt [16.1] presents an early discussion of the physics behind the creation of speckle in ultrasound images.

Resolution

The short pulses of ultrasound used in B-mode imaging are characterized by center frequency and bandwidth. Any time domain signal (such as the typical B-mode imaging pulse shown in fig. 16.4) can also be represented by a spectrum which shows the frequencies that make up the short pulse.

The bandwidth of a pulse is frequently characterized as the ratio of the width of the spectrum to the center frequency of the spectrum; in the case of the pulse shown in fig. 16.4, the fractional bandwidth (*FBW*) is 66%. In general, longer pulses have a narrower bandwidth (see the 25% bandwidth pulse in fig. 16.5).

Axial (along the direction of the ultrasound beam) resolution Δr is determined by the bandwidth and the wavelength (λ_c, at the center frequency) of the ultrasound pulse as follows:

$$\Delta r = \frac{\lambda_c}{2FBW}\,. \tag{16.1}$$

Using the relationship between frequency and wavelength ($\lambda = c/f$ where c is the velocity of sound) axial resolution can be expressed as:

$$\Delta r = \frac{c}{2f_c\,FBW}\,. \tag{16.2}$$

Clearly higher bandwidth transducers enable finer axial resolution (smaller Δr), as do higher frequency transducers.

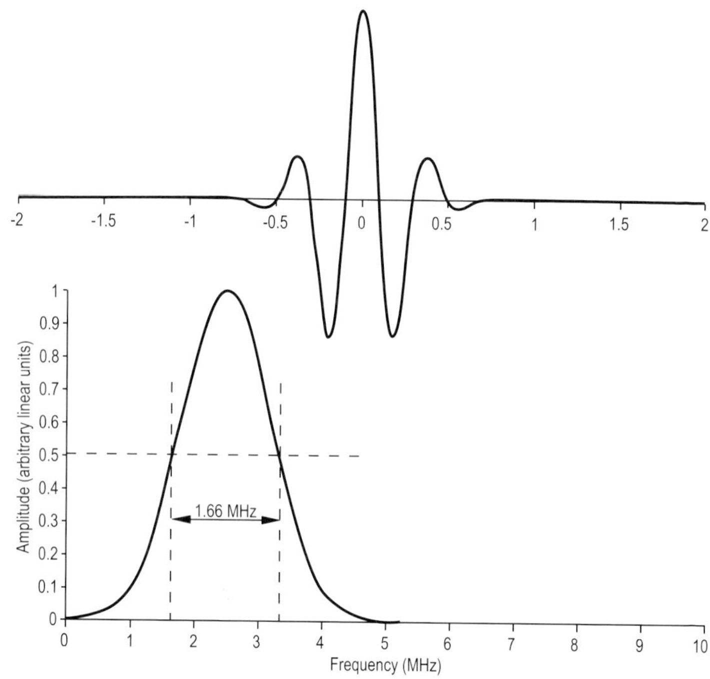

Figure 16.4
Typical B-mode imaging pulse. The upper graph represents the instantaneous pressure of the acoustic pulse as a function of time, with the horizontal axis labeled in microseconds. The lower graph shows the frequency content of this pulse. The full width of the spectrum at half the peak amplitude is 1.66 MHz. Dividing this by 2.5 MHz (the center frequency of the pulse) yields a fractional bandwidth (*FBW*) of 66%.

It is interesting to note that other transducer parameters (such as size) do not affect axial resolution. Note that eq. (16.2) is the same as eq. (8.27b), given that $f_c FBW = 1/\Delta t$.

Unlike axial resolution, azimuthal (across the beam) resolution is determined by the size of the transducer as well as the center frequency of the transducer. In fig. 16.6, a typical azimuth beam profile for a focused transducer is shown.

The width of the main lobe determines the azimuthal resolution (Δx) and this width is given by:

$$\Delta x = \frac{c}{f_c} \frac{2r}{w \cos\theta} \tag{16.3}$$

where r is the distance from the transducer to the imaging range, w is the width of the transducer, and θ is the angle (as defined in fig. 16.13b) to the imaging location.

From eq. (16.3), one can see that azimuthal resolution improves (smaller Δx) as frequency increases and degrades as range increases. Somewhat counterintuitively, resolution improves as the transducer aperture increases.

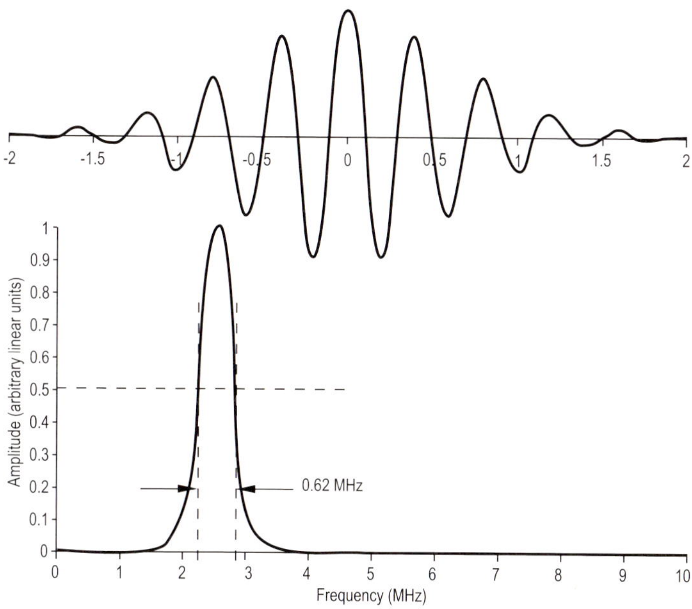

Figure 16.5
Typical flow imaging pulse. Note how the longer pulse (in comparison to the B-mode pulse of the previous fig.) results in a narrower spectrum. In this case, the full width of the spectrum at half the peak amplitude is 0.62 MHz. Dividing this by 2.5 MHz (the center frequency of the pulse) yields a fractional bandwidth (*FBW*) of 25%.

Clutter

Clutter refers to low-level signals that are displayed in inappropriate locations in the image. For example, frequently the “noise” that is seen in a ventricle of the heart, or in the large vessels of the liver, are in fact low-level echoes from the myocardium or liver parenchyma. The beam profile illustrated in fig. 16.6 shows how this clutter occurs.

The system must reconstruct images assuming that signals that arrive simultaneously are scattered from the same region of the body, specifically the region defined by the main lobe of the beam profile. As can be seen in fig. 16.6, although the beam profile is strongly peaked at the central angle, there is some sensitivity to signals scattered from other directions. Although this sensitivity is very low (typically 0.1% of the sensitivity of the main beam) modern ultrasound systems are capable of displaying signals over a wide range of amplitudes, and therefore these erroneous signals are visible in the image.

Many parameters of a system affect clutter levels, but the most important parameters are beamformer accuracy and the number of system channels. Since neither of these parameters is reliably available to the end user, evaluation of clutter levels must be performed through clinical experience.

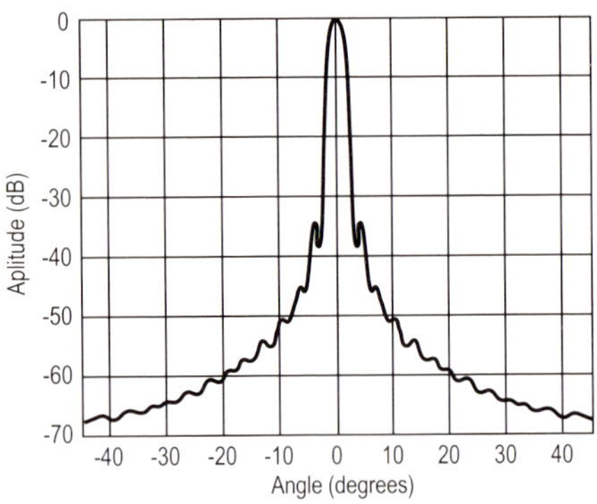

Figure 16.6
Typical ultrasound beam profile. Note that the vertical axis is logarithmic, so the greater than 60 dB suppression of signals more than 20° off the beam axis means that echoes from these directions have an amplitude that is more than 1000 times less than echoes from the main beam.

Noise

As discussed in chapter 8, the human body inherently generates acoustic noise due to thermal energy (see eq. (8.28)). In practice, current imaging systems have electronic noise levels that are slightly higher (typically 3 dB, or a factor of 1.4 in amplitude) than this fundamental limit. To place this 3 dB in perspective, consider that current ultrasound systems display signals over a range of approximately 120 dB (a factor of one million in amplitude).

For most imaging conditions, the electronic noise of the imaging system is insignificant, with this noise becoming visible at a depth of approximately 350 wavelengths (about 15.5 cm at 3.5 Mhz).

Because attenuation of ultrasound increases proportionally with frequency, the range at which the returned echoes become comparable to the noise is at about the same number of wavelengths. This is why high frequency (around 15 MHz) transducers can be used for shallow scans (breast and testicles) while somewhat deeper scans require lower frequencies (the liver is often imaged at approximately 2.5 MHz).

A common value used for the attenuation of tissue is 0.5 dB/cm·MHz, but the exact attenuation of tissue varies significantly, see table 8.1 for several values of attenuation. The depth to which an image is not dominated by noise is referred to as the penetration.

Summary of B-mode imaging

B-mode imaging is the primary imaging mode for most ultrasound exams. It is the mode in which the clinician visualizes the structures in the body and usually first notes anomalies. B-mode also allows the clinician to guide other modes (such as blood flow measurement) to appropriate regions.

Frequently, B-mode images are degraded by clutter (which is often mistakenly identified as noise), but the technique of harmonic imaging (discussed later) provides significant clutter reduction. If true noise limits the ability to visualize deep structures, then switching to a lower frequency transducer should provide better penetration (with some reduction in resolution).

On some systems, more subtle trade-offs between resolution and penetration are possible on one transducer, so different system settings may provide sufficient noise suppression to allow a diagnostic image.

16.1.2.2 Spectral Doppler

Before describing Doppler signal processing, the concept of a baseband signal should be introduced. Since ultrasound signals have limited bandwidth, it is convenient to think of a signal $f(t)$ as a combination of a slowly varying amplitude envelope $a(t)$ and a radio frequency (RF) "carrier" signal:

$$f(t) = a(t)\cos(\omega_0 t + \phi) = a(t)\left(\frac{e^{i(\omega_0 t + \phi)} + e^{-i(\omega_0 t + \phi)}}{2}\right) \tag{16.4}$$

(Note, the "carrier" frequency ω_0, is often the center of the useful frequency range for the ultrasound imaging conditions).

The useful information (for an ultrasound imaging system) in this signal is contained in the envelope and the phase of the carrier. This information can also be represented in a baseband signal. The baseband signal $b(t)$ is a complex function that can be determined by first multiplying the RF signal by $e^{-i\omega_0 t}$ and then filtering to eliminate the $2\omega_0$ component.

$$\begin{aligned} f(t)e^{-i(\omega_0 t + \phi)} &= a(t)\left(\frac{e^{i(\omega_0 t + \phi)} + e^{-i(\omega_0 t + \phi)}}{2}\right)e^{-i\omega_0 t} \\ &= a(t)\left(\frac{e^{i\phi} + e^{-i(2\omega_0 t + \phi)}}{2}\right) \Rightarrow a(t)\frac{e^{i\phi}}{2} = b(t) \end{aligned} \tag{16.5}$$

where the symbol $\Rightarrow$ has been used to indicate applying a filter that suppresses signals around the frequency $2\omega_0$. This is usually achieved by using a low pass filter with a cut-off frequency around ω_0.

The baseband signal includes both the amplitude of the signal $b(t)$, which is of limited interest for Doppler processing, and the phase of the signal Φ. Changes in this phase, due to motion of the blood, are the source of the Doppler effect.

Blood flow velocity can be measured using ultrasound via the Doppler effect. The fundamentals of Doppler blood flow measurements are discussed in section 8.3.4. Here some basic principles are reviewed before discussing implementation in a system.

In the simplest approach, a continuous signal is transmitted from one half of the transducer at a frequency f_0, and, as described in eq. (8.21) in chapter 8, the signal received on the other half of the transducer has a frequency of approximately $f_0\left(1 + 2\frac{v_b}{c}\cos\theta\right)$, where v_b is the velocity of the blood, c is the velocity of sound and θ is the angle between the direction of propagation of the sound and the direction of blood flow.

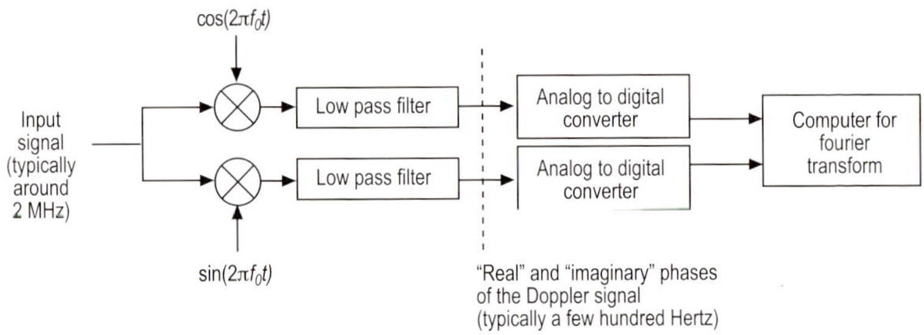

Figure 16.7
Simplified Doppler signal processing elements. The processing elements to the left of the dotted line shift the received signal down so that the original transmitted frequency is shifted to zero (DC). This means that the frequency change due to blood flow appears as an audio frequency signal that can be sampled and digitized to high accuracy for analysis.

In order to determine the blood velocity from this signal, the processing illustrated in fig. 16.7 is used to extract the baseband (or Doppler) signal.

The Doppler signal (shown in fig. 16.8) is a complex signal with both real (or in-phase) and imaginary (or quadrature-phase) components.

It is important to retain both components of the Doppler signal because this allows one to determine if the Doppler signal is positive (was originally shifted to a higher frequency, indicating blood flow towards the transducer) or negative (was originally shifted to a lower frequency, indicating blood flow away from the transducer).

When the imaginary component of the Doppler signal crosses zero with a positive slope at an earlier time than the real component does (the case in fig. 16.8), the Doppler frequency is negative.

When the reverse is true, the Doppler frequency is positive.

The Doppler signals shown in fig. 16.8 would result if all the blood insonified were moving at the same speed. In fact, even when blood flow is laminar, many velocities are present and the signals are much more complicated than those illustrated here.

In order to visualize these complex signals it is easiest to view them in the frequency domain rather than the time domain.

Since different velocities result in Doppler signals of different frequencies, by decomposing the Doppler signal into separate frequencies, one is determining the different velocities of blood flow in the region insonified.

Ultrasound systems perform this decomposition by selecting approximately 128 sequential samples (this is referred to as the flow sample count, and typically represents about 50 ms of signal, but this varies significantly with system setting) of the complex Doppler signal and then using the Fourier transform [16.2] to determine the frequency components (referred to as the Doppler spectrum). This spectrum is recalculated

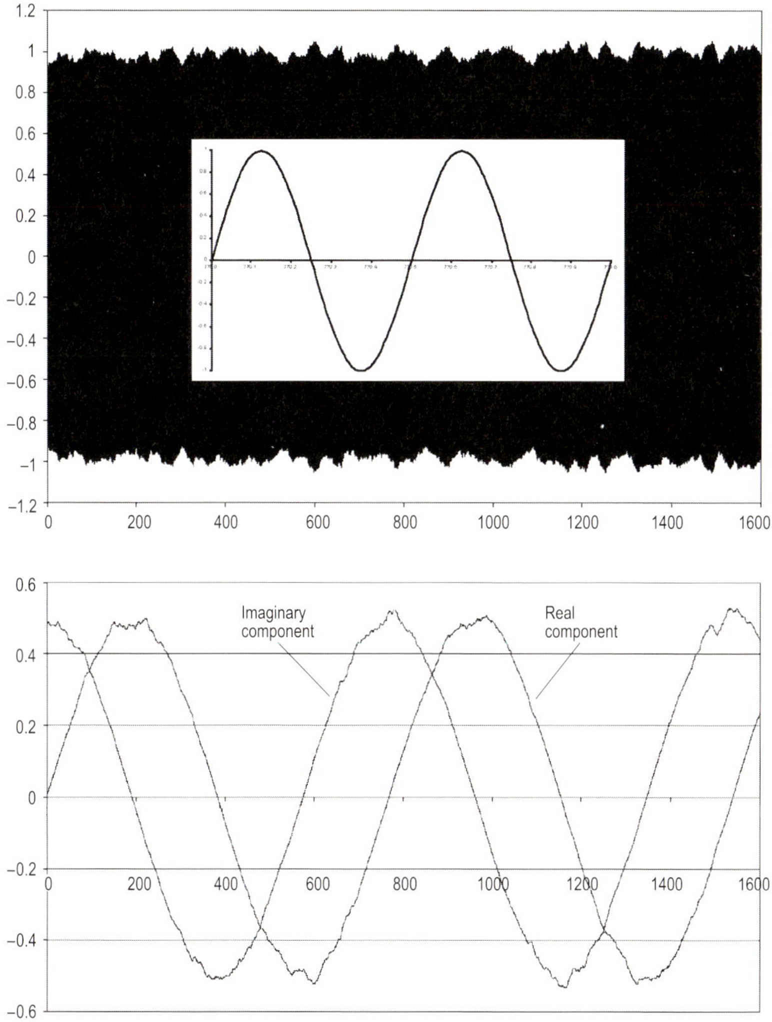

Figure 16.8 Continuous wave Doppler signals.
The **top panel** shows the input signal. This 2 MHz signal has approximately 3,200 oscillations in the 1,600 μsec timescale shown here, so the individual oscillations cannot be seen. Inset into the top panel is an expanded time scale (specifically from 770 μsec to 771 μsec) plot of the input signal. This inset shows that the input signal looks like a 2 MHz wave, although it has actually been shifted to 1.9987 MHz by the motion of the blood.
The **lower panel** shows the real and imaginary components of the Doppler signal. These signals were simulated with the signal processing shown in fig. 16.7 and the following conditions: transmitted frequency = 2 MHz, blood velocity = 50 cm/sec, and $\theta = 0$. The lowpass filter has a bandwidth of approximately 400 kHz, which is much higher than a typical ultrasound system would use, but sufficient for illustrating the concept.

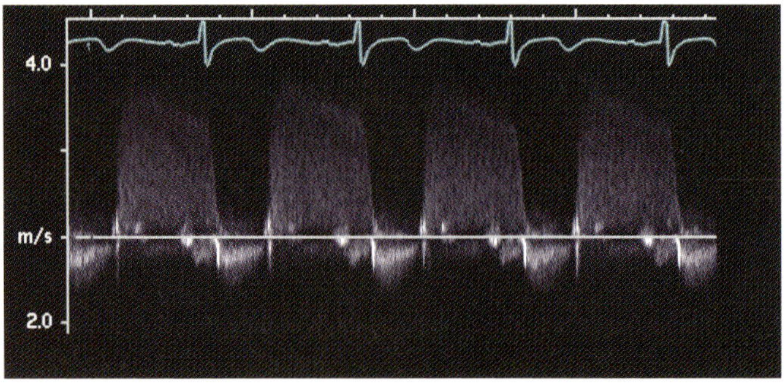

Figure 16.9 Typical CW Doppler spectrum.
The velocity range is from −2 m/s to 4 m/s. In this case, the Doppler gate has been placed in the opening of the aortic valve, where the blood exits the ventricle and flows into the aorta during systole. This spectrum was obtained using an apical view, so blood flow away from the transducer (negative velocity) is the normal expulsion of blood from the ventricle. This systolic outflow normally has a peak velocity of approximately one meter/second. In this case the aortic valve does not close completely during diastole, and a high velocity (approximately 3.5 meters/second) flow back into the ventricle occurs. The electrocardiogram signal at the top of the display provides a reference for the timing of the cardiac cycle.

approximately every millisecond or two, so that changes in the Doppler signal during the heart cycle can be observed.

The Doppler spectra are displayed as shown in fig. 16.9. In this display, the velocity is displayed on the vertical axis, while the time at which the Doppler spectrum was calculated is displayed on the horizontal axis. The brightness in the Doppler display is proportional to the signal amplitude of each frequency component, which correlates with the amount of blood moving at each velocity displayed.

Pulsed wave Doppler

The Doppler signal processing described above is referred to as Continuous Wave (CW) Doppler, because the transmitter is emitting one continuous signal.

While very useful, especially in situations where high velocity flow is present, one problem with CW Doppler is that the range at which the measurement is obtained is indeterminate. When range selection is important, Pulsed wave (PW) Doppler can be used. In this case, a short burst (typically about 10 microseconds long, although this is also very dependent on system settings) of sound is transmitted repeatedly. During reception, a gating circuit is used to select signals that arrive from the desired range.

Typically, approximately 128 pulses (flow sample count) will also be used for a single PW Doppler spectrum.

In fig. 16.10, typical PW Doppler signals are shown. Note that, if the analog to digital converter (see fig. 16.7) samples the Doppler signal during the time that the Doppler gate is open, then the PW Doppler signals are indistinguishable from the CW Doppler signals.

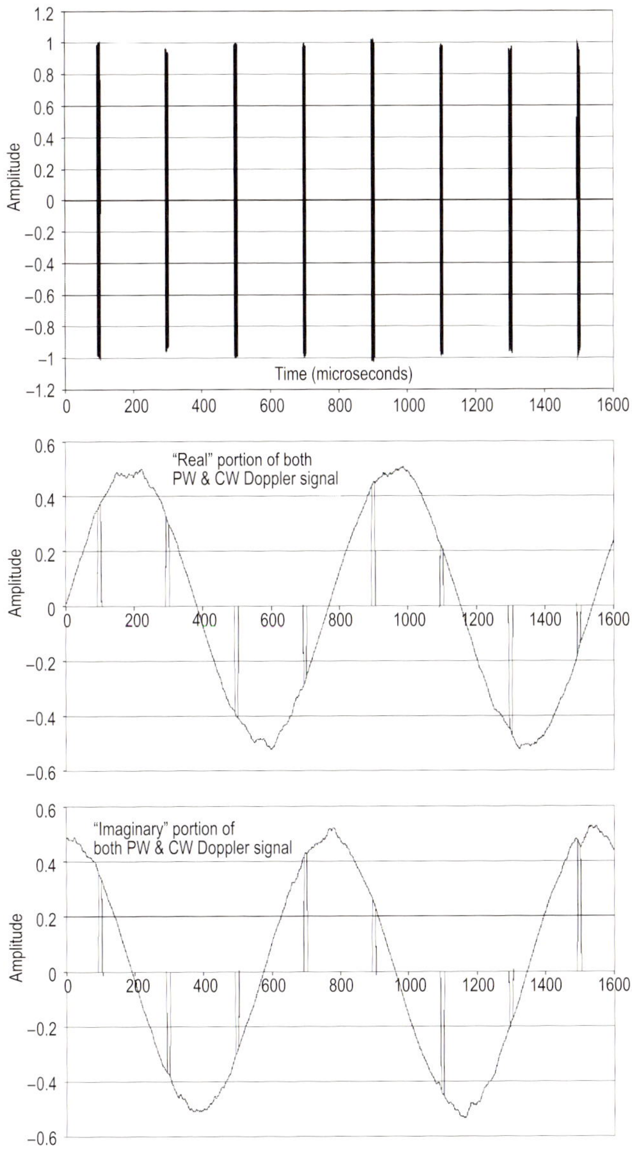

Figure 16.10 Pulsed wave Doppler signals.
The **top panel** illustrates a sequence of short (10 microsecond) bursts of 2 MHz sound with a 200 microsecond pulse repetition interval. This signal is the same as the signal used in the previous CW Doppler fig., except that the signal is only gated on for short bursts. The **lower two panels** depict both the CW Doppler signals from the previous fig. and the PW Doppler signals that result when the pulsed signal is processed by the exact same processing as that used in the CW Doppler fig. Note that during the time the Doppler gate is on the PW Doppler signals are identical to the CW Doppler signals.

The Fourier transform processing for CW Doppler and display proceeds in the same manner as that for PW Doppler.

The important difference between PW and CW Doppler is that PW Doppler is fundamentally a sampled signal.

Since the entire goal of PW Doppler is to isolate signals from a particular range, the system must wait long enough for the transmitted signal to travel out from the transducer to the region of interest and then back to the transducer before transmitting the next pulse.

This limits the rate at which the Doppler signal is sampled to $\Delta\tau = 2r/c$ where r is the range of the Doppler gate and c is the velocity of sound. ($1/\Delta\tau$ is frequently referred to as the pulse repetition frequency, or PRF).

Practically, this means that Doppler signals are typically sampled at around 5 kilohertz, which means that Doppler shifts between plus and minus 2.5 kilohertz can be measured with pulsed wave Doppler. (See discussion on aliasing in chapter 9 in order to understand the limitations of a sampled system to accurately characterize broadband signals)

At typical ultrasonic frequencies used for Doppler measurements (2 MHz), this means that velocities up to almost one meter/second can be measured in a pulsed system without aliasing. This is sufficient for almost all blood velocities found in the body, with the exception of regurgent jets in the heart, where CW Doppler is frequently used to insure that no aliasing occurs.

16.1.2.3 Flow imaging (color Doppler)

Although Doppler spectra such as those shown in fig. 16.9 provide detailed information about flow at a particular location, sometimes visualization of the spatial distribution of flow is also desired. In such a case, signal processing very similar to PW Doppler is used, with three important exceptions.

First, although short bursts of ultrasound are transmitted, the returned echoes are continuously received so that velocity can be measured at a number of ranges; secondly, in order to interrogate a large area, instead of transmitting approximately 128 pulses in one direction for a velocity estimate, only 4 to 12 pulses are typically used; and finally, rather than displaying an entire spectrum, only one "average" velocity for each position is displayed.

These "average" velocities are displayed as a color, with shades of red indicating flow in one direction and shades of blue representing flow in the other direction. In fig. 16.11, a color Doppler display is shown. The "average" value used is actually the centroid of the spectrum, which corresponds to the center of mass of the spectrum. This is not necessarily the velocity at which most of the blood is flowing (although it is usually close to this), nor is it the average velocity between the maximum and the minimum velocity.

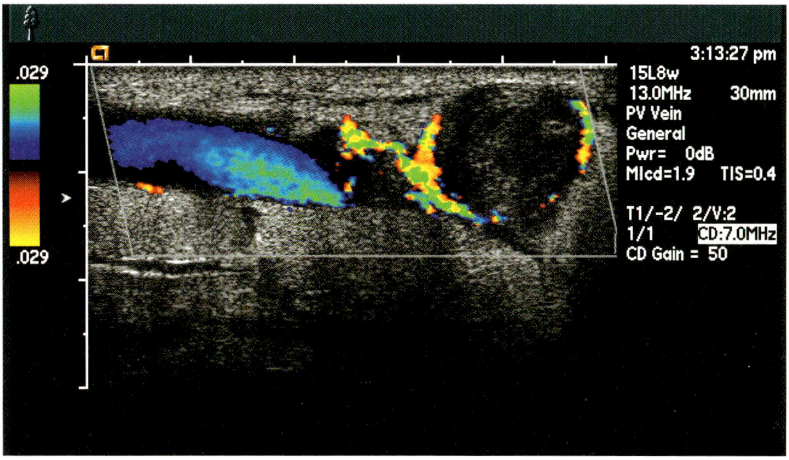

Figure 16.11 Color flow image of a varicosity in the leg.
In this case, flow around a large clot on the right of the image can be seen. In this image, the flow velocity information is overlaid as a color on top of the grayscale B-mode image. Since the flow is largely parallel to the surface of the transducer in this case, the color flow beams have been steered to the right so that flow toward the left of the image (or up towards the transducer) appears in blue-to-green hues and flow to the right (or downward away from the transducer) appears in red-to-yellow hues. The color bar on the left of the display indicates this color scale, with the colors at the top of the bar indicating flow toward the transducer, and those on the lower half of the color bar indicating flow away from the transducer. The maximum velocity the system can display in this case is 0.029 m/sec (29 mm/sec) either toward or away from the transducer. In color flow images this color bar is almost always presented on the screen because many color maps are available to the user.

Intuitively, if one were to graph the Doppler spectrum and cut it out, the centroid is the velocity at which the resulting graph would balance. Fortunately, this centroid is easy to calculate using eq. (8.40a), which is reproduced here in a slightly different form:

$$f_c = \frac{1}{2\pi\Delta\tau}\arg\left(\sum_{i=1}^{N-1} a_i^* a_{i+1}\right), \tag{16.6}$$

where $\Delta\tau$ is again the pulse repetition interval, and a_{i+1} and a_i^* are the samples and complex conjugate, respectively, of the Doppler signals, N is the flow sample count (4 to 12 typically), and the arg function means to take the phase of the complex value resulting from the summation.

16.2 System architecture

When thinking about the signal processing required for ultrasound imaging, it is convenient to divide the system into 3 components: beamformer, midprocessor, and display.

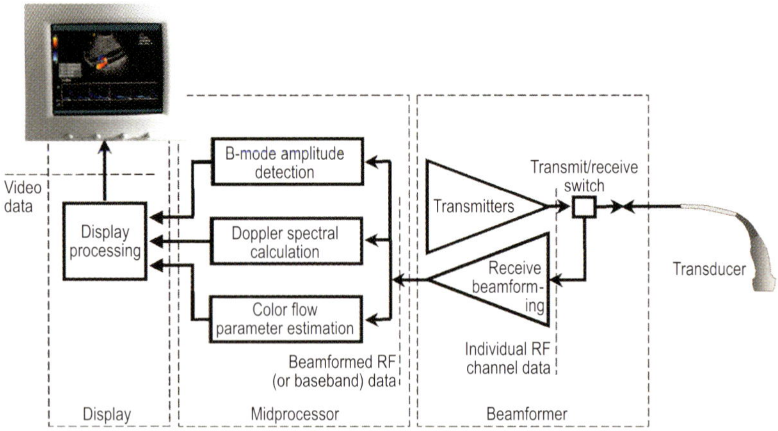

Figure 16.12
Block diagram of an ultrasound imaging system showing the three major components and some of the functions contained in these components

The flow of information during reception is from the transducer to the beamformer, through the midprocessor and to the display. As the data moves through the system, the data rate is reduced from approximately 200 gigabits per second at the input to the beamformer to approximately 200 megabits per second at the output of the display.

16.2.1 Beamformer

Originally, ultrasound images were produced using a large (typically 1.0 to 1.5 cm diameter) transducer that generated a beam of ultrasound directed perpendicular to the transducer face. Images were formed by mechanically wobbling the element from side to side in order to direct the beam to different regions of the body. Currently, however, arrays of small transducer elements are used, and by transmitting on the small elements at slightly different times, the ultrasound beam can be steered and focused to different regions of the body.

The beamformer is responsible for generating appropriately focused beams during both transmission and reception.

16.2.1.1 Coherent beamforming in general

To illustrate how array beamforming works, in figs. 16.13 the signal timing for focusing during transmission is shown.

By transmitting with the outer elements first, and then with precise timing transmitting slightly later with more interior elements, a focused wave front can be emitted. The focusing can be understood by considering that each individual element emits an approximately cylindrical wave front that propagates at the speed of sound away from the element. (Note, the wave front has a cylindrical shape because the element that

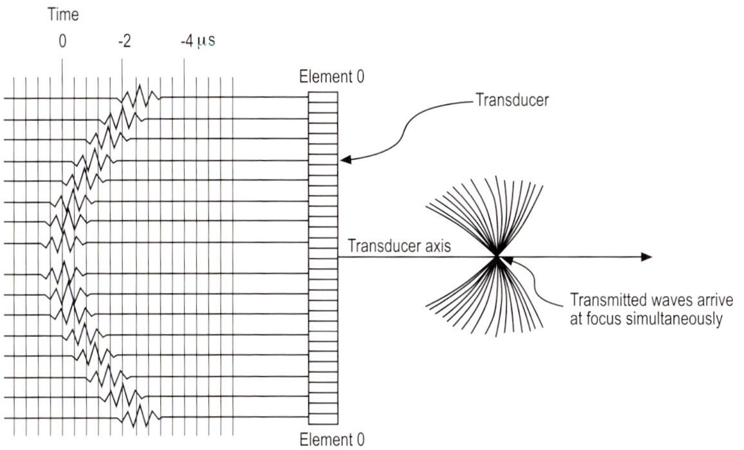

Figure 16.13a
Illustration of signal timing for focusing using a one-dimensional array at a range of 9.8 mm from the transducer and along the axis of the transducer: The pulses are typical 2.5 MHz imaging signals and the transducer has 32 elements with a spacing of 0.616 millimeters (one wavelength). Note that these conditions are for illustration purposes only. In reality, this transducer could not use the entire aperture at this range due to the angular response of the elements.

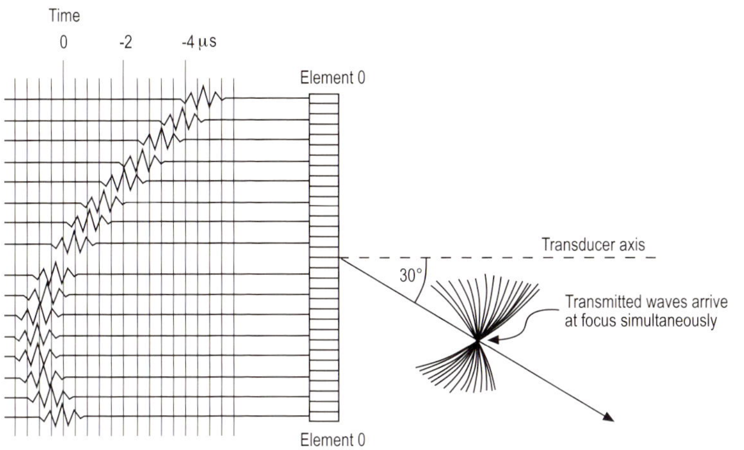

Figure 16.13b
Illustration of signal timing for focusing steered 30 degrees from the axis of the transducer: All parameters are the same as in fig. 16.13a, except for the steering angle.

emits the wave is very tall, producing an approximately plane wave in the vertical direction, but very narrow, producing a curved wave front in the horizontal direction).

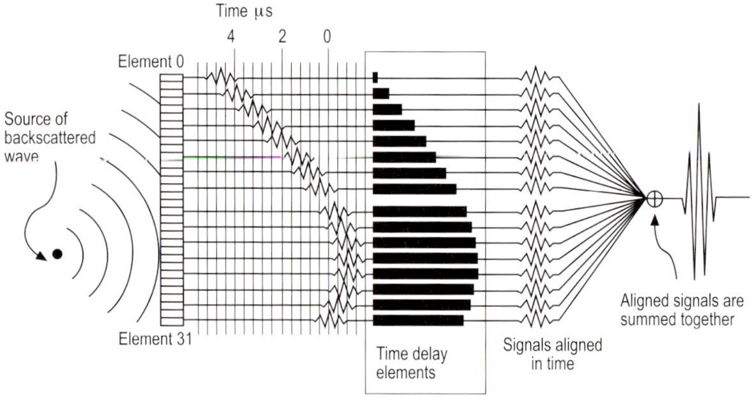

Figure 16.14a
Receive focusing at a range of 9.8 millimeters and an angle of 30 degrees from the transducer axis. Signals that arrive at the transducer first are delayed the longest, so that a coherent sum of signals from the focal zone can be performed.

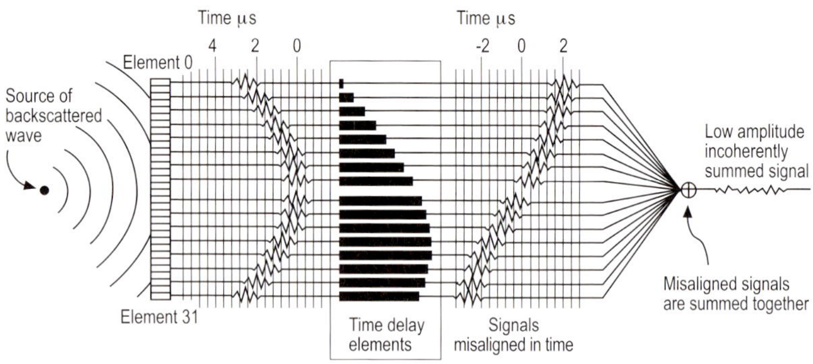

Figure 16.14b
Receive focusing when the source is not in the focal zone. This source is at a range of 9.8 millimeters and at an angle of 0 degrees from the axis of the transducer, while the focus delays are appropriate for a source at the same range but an angle of 30 degrees.

The curved lines in figs. 16.13a and 16.13b show the locations of the emitted wave fronts from the elements. As is shown in the figs., at the desired focal range and angle, the wave fronts arrive simultaneously, resulting in constructive interference and a high amplitude acoustic wave. Away from the focal zone, the wave fronts arrive at different times, resulting in destructive interference and a low amplitude acoustic wave.

Figs. 16.14 illustrates the focusing process during reception. Signals from the focal zone are received by individual elements, with arrival times determined by the distance from the location of the source to the individual element. These electrical signals are delayed (using at least one of several techniques discussed later) such that the signals are aligned in time. These electrical signals are then added together to produce one large signal that is proportional to the acoustic signal emitted from the focal zone.

Fig. 16.14b illustrates how signals that arise from regions other than the focal zone are suppressed. In fig. 16.14b, the electrical time delays are the same as in fig. 16.14a, but the source has been placed at a different location. Since the arrival times of the acoustic signals do not match the electrical delays, the electrical signals are not aligned in time before summation and consequently the output of the summation is a very low amplitude signal due to destructive interference.

For an array imaging system to function properly, the timing for both transmission and reception must be calculated precisely.

Referring to fig. 16.15, a location in the image is specified by an angle, θ, and a range, r. Since this is a one-dimensional array, the element positions are given by their location on the x-axis.

The distance from an element to the imaging point is given by:

$$r' = \sqrt{r^2 + x^2 - 2rx\sin\theta}. \tag{16.7}$$

In order to focus at this location, the element located at x would have to transmit at a time

$$\Delta t = \frac{r - r'}{c} \tag{16.8}$$

relative to transmission at the center of the array.

Note that positive times indicate transmission after the center of the array, while negative times require transmission before the center of the array.

Even though there may not be an element exactly at the center of the array, it is convenient to use the center as the reference point for calculating all time delays. The same timing is used during reception, with a positive time indicating that signals should be delayed relative to the center of the array while negative times indicate that signals should be advanced.

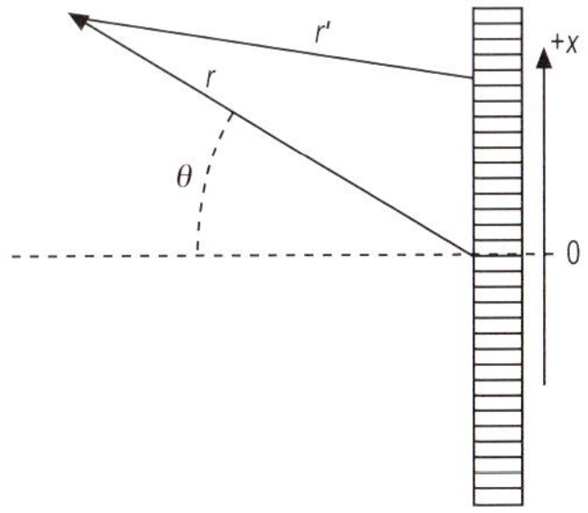

Figure 16.15
Geometry for calculating focusing time delays

By expanding the square root in the expression for r' and substituting into eq. (16.8), the following useful approximation can be obtained:

$$\Delta t \approx \frac{x\sin\theta}{c} - \frac{x^2\cos^2\theta}{2rc} \tag{16.9}$$

While this approximation is not accurate enough to use for focusing in an imaging system, it is useful for estimating certain design parameters of systems.

Grating lobes

One of the major issues faced by designers of array imaging systems is the problem of grating lobes. Grating lobes cause signals to be transmitted to and received from regions other than the focal zone.

In fig. 16.16, the conditions that result in a grating lobe are illustrated. In this case, the intended transmit angle is 30° from the axis of the transducer. Taking the approximation for Δt in eq. (16.9) to the limit where $r \to \infty$, we get a transmit time delay between elements equal to one-half of a pulse period. At −30°, the combination of the one-half period delay plus the propagation delays means that the signals from adjacent elements arrive approximately one period apart. While these signals do not arrive exactly simultaneously (as they do at 30°), they do add constructively to create a significant source of artifact.

Continuing to use eq. (16.9) with $r \to \infty$, we can determine the conditions to create a grating lobe by requiring that the difference between time delays for adjacent ele-

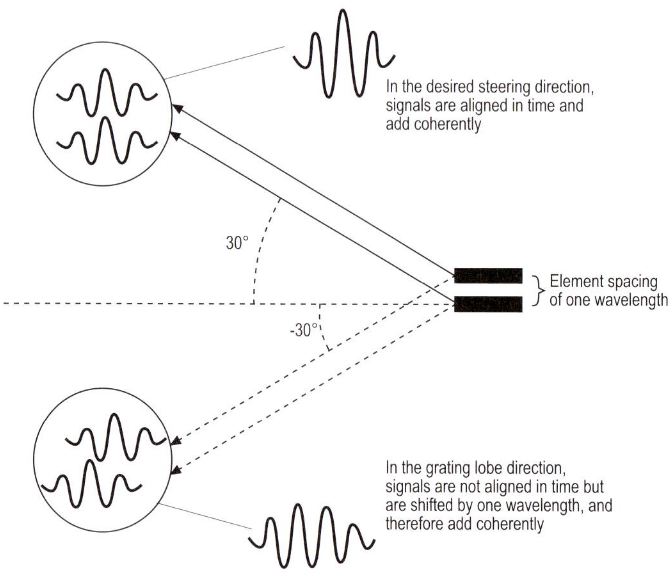

Figure 16.16 Illustration of conditions leading to a grating lobe

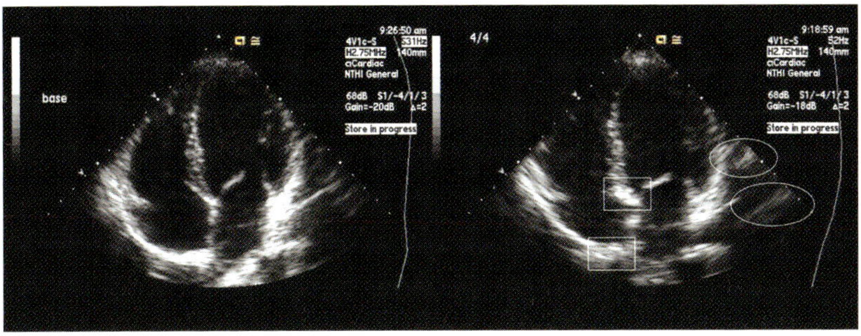

Figure 16.17
Images with and without a grating lobe. The grating lobes in the right hand image are located in the elliptical regions. These echoes are due to sound that is really backscattered from the regions surrounded by the rectangles. The element spacing in the right hand image is 1.2 λ, which means that at 45° steering angle, the system is also sensitive to echoes coming from scatterers located at –7 degrees (see table 16.1). In the left hand image, the element spacing is 0.3 λ.

ments applied for a desired steering angle θ_s and the propagation delays to a grating lobe angle θ_g equal one period.

$$\frac{\Delta x \sin\theta_s}{c} - \frac{\Delta x \sin\theta_g}{c} = \frac{\lambda}{c}$$

$$(\sin\theta_s - \sin\theta_g) = \frac{\lambda}{\Delta x} \qquad (16.10)$$

Using eq. (16.10), table 16.1 presents the approximate grating lobe angle for a range of element spacing (in terms of the wavelength λ of sound) and steering angle.

Usually grating lobes are not obvious in an image, since system designers avoid the conditions that lead to grating lobes; however, in fig. 16.17 a system has been modified to produce very clear grating lobes while imaging a heart.

Element directivity

For the purposes of calculating appropriate time delays and grating lobe angles, one can usually think of an individual element as a point. However, when considering real system performance, the physical size of the element is important. This is because a non-point element is limited in the directions in which it can transmit and receive sound.

If we consider an element as a simple piston moving back and forth in an infinite baffle, the amplitude of radiated sound as a function of angle is given by:

$$D(\theta) = \cos\theta \sin\left(\frac{d \sin\theta}{\lambda}\right) \qquad (16.11)$$

where d is the width of the element, λ is the wavelength of sound, and θ is the angle to the axis of the transducer.

Eq. (16.11) is called the directivity function of an element.

Table 16.1
Grating lobe angle (in degrees) for a range of element spacing and steering angle. Empty cells in the table indicate conditions for which there is no grating lobe. Because there is no reason to place elements any closer together than required to suppress grating lobes, most systems are designed such that they operate under the conditions indicated by table cells with a gray background. The entry for an element spacing of 1.2 λ and a steering angle of 45 degrees (marked with a bold border) is the condition under which grating lobes are observed in fig. 16.17.

Element Spacing (Wavelenght) \ Steering Angle (degrees)	0	5	10	15	20	25	30	35	40	45
0.5										
0.6										–74
0.7							–68	–59	–52	–46
0.8				–82	–65	–56	–49	–43	–37	–44
0.9			–70	–58	–50	–44	–38	–33	–28	–24
1.0	–90	–66	–56	–48	–41	–35	–30	–25	–21	–17
1.1	–65	–55	–47	–41	–35	–29	–24	–20	–15	–12
1.2	–55	–48	–41	–35	–29	–24	–19	–15	–11	**–7**
1.3	–50	–43	–37	–31	–25	–20	–16	–11	–7	–4
1.4	–45	–39	–33	–27	–22	–17	–12	–8	–4	0
1.5	–42	–35	–30	–24	–19	–14	–10	–5	–1	2

In fig. 16.18 the directivity function is presented for elements with a width of $\lambda/2$ and λ. Note that the smaller elements can easily transmit and receive sound at angles of 45° while the larger elements are limited to a range of approximately 30°.

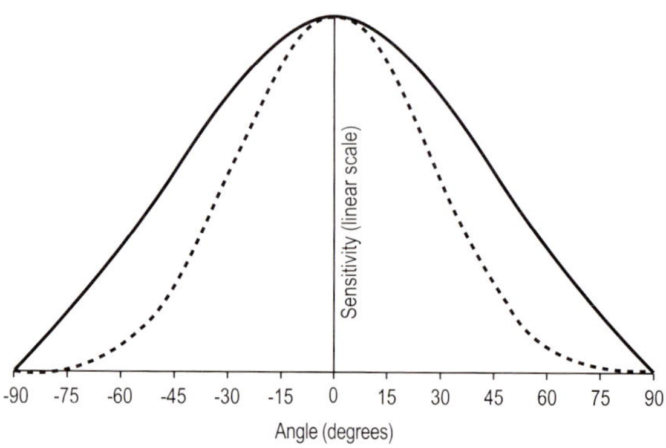

Figure 16.18
Directivity functions for an element with a width of one-half wavelength (solid line) and an element with a width of one wavelength (dashed line). Transducers that use the smaller elements can easily steer beams to ±45°, while the larger elements only allow steering to less than ±30°. (Note, even this ±30° limit based on directivity factor may be further limited by grating lobes.)

Clearly, for transducers that must steer to large angles (such as most cardiology probes) small elements are critical.

16.2.1.2 Transmit beamforming

The purpose of the transmit section of the beamformer is to apply electrical signals to the transducer elements with the desired shape and appropriate timing to create a focused acoustic wave in the body. Usually the waveform transmitted on all elements has the same shape, with the exact timing varying from element to element in order to compensate for the different propagation times to the desired focal point.

Most systems have simple transmitters that can only produce 3 voltage levels during a pulse, a positive high voltage, zero voltage, and a negative high voltage. These systems have limited ability to control the shape of the transmitted waveform, but acceptable images can be produced with these simple transmitters.

High performance systems usually have programmable waveforms that can be applied to each element, providing greatly improved control of the transmitted waveform. This is especially important during harmonic imaging, where controlling the transmitted energy in the harmonic band is critical.

Sequential focus

A transmitted beam can be focused at only one range; however, ultrasound images usually cover significant depth. One common solution to this problem is the sequential focus technique in which a single line of an image is constructed from several ultrasound transmissions focused at different ranges. Fig. 16.19 shows two images, one using four different focal zones and a similar image created with only one focal zone.

Of course, building up an image from several different transmissions reduces the imaging frame rate. This is acceptable in many applications, such as imaging of the liver,

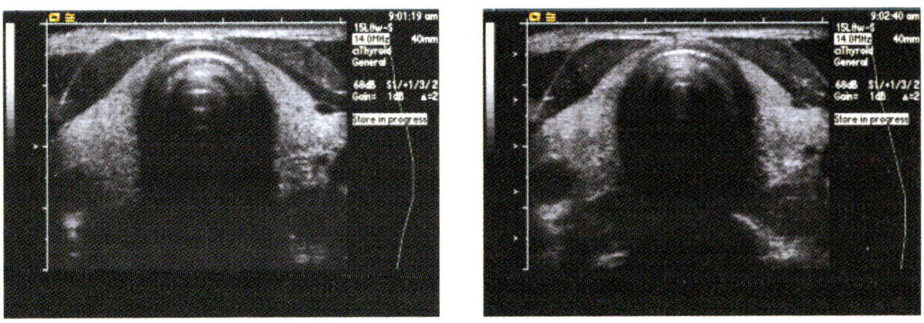

Figure 16.19
Demonstration of sequential focus (Source: Sara Good and Kathy Quiroz, Siemens Ultrasound). The **left** image is produced with only one transmit focal zone, while the **right** image uses 4 different focal zones. The **right** image has a significantly lower frame rate, but for many applications, this lower frame rate is preferred to gain the improvements in image quality. Note in particular how deeper structures in this thyroid can be seen in the right image, but are only vaguely apparent in the **left** image.

where the sequential focus technique is commonly used, but in other applications (such as imaging the heart) this reduction in frame rate is unacceptable.

Compound transmit focus

A significant improvement in transmit beam focusing can be achieved by simultaneously transmitting waves focused at several different ranges. This produces a more collimated beam, without the degradation in frame rate that is inherent in the sequential focus technique. This technique of focusing at several ranges simultaneously is referred to as a "compound transmit focus."

In fig. 16.20 we show an example of the transmit waveforms used to produce a compound transmit focus at two ranges. Note that although for some channels this looks like just pulsing the element twice, for some elements the two pulses overlap.

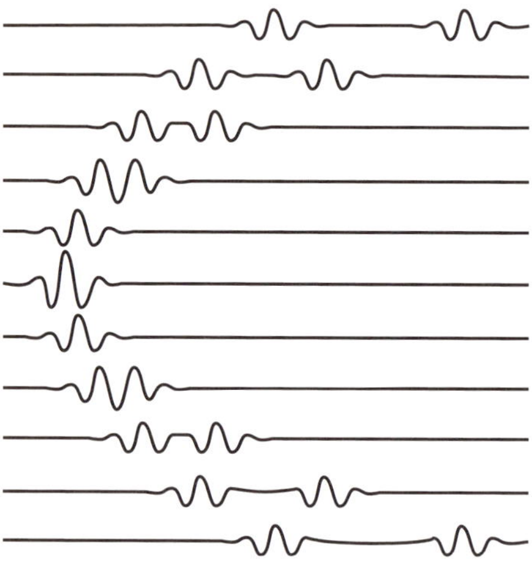

Figure 16.20
Illustration of typical pulses used for compound focus. For the outer elements of the array (the top and bottom waveforms), the two pulses corresponding to two different focal ranges appear as distinct pulses in time. For elements closer to the center of the array, the two pulses overlap to form more complicated waveforms. At the very center of the array (the middle waveform), the two pulses are launched at exactly the same time, so the transmitted waveform appears as a single pulse with twice the amplitude of the individual pulses.

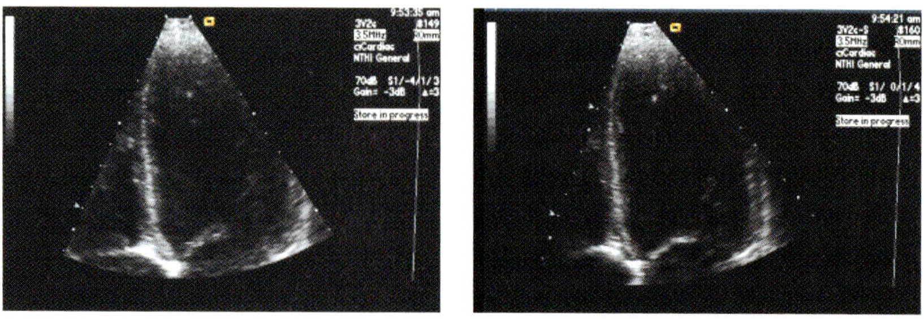

Figure 16.21
Demonstration of compound focus. The **left** image is produced with only one transmit focal zone, while the **right** image uses 2 simultaneously transmitted focal zones. Note how the clutter (noise in the ventricle of the heart) near the apex of this left ventricle (the top of the images) is greater in the **left** image than the **right**.

In order to accurately transmit these precise pulses, precise control over the transmitted waveform is required. Fig. 16.21 shows cardiac images produced using both conventional single transmit focus and compound transmit focus.

16.2.1.3 Receive beamforming

The most important difference between transmit and receive beamforming is that during reception, signals from different ranges arrive at different times. This allows the system to dynamically adjust the receive time delays as a function of range to maintain the focusing at all ranges.

The output $b(t)$ of the receive beamforming process can be described with the following equation:

$$b(t) = \sum_{i=1}^{N} a_i s_i(t - \Delta t(r)) \tag{16.12}$$

where $s_i(t - \Delta t_i(r))$ are the individual channel signals delayed by Δt (as given in eq. (16.8), which is a function of r), N is the number of channels in the system, and a_i is an apodization factor that is often equal to one.

When beamformers used analog components like tapped delay lines and mixers to achieve this dynamic time delay, there were many artifacts that could result from the constant changing of the time delays required, and many signal processing tricks were required in order to suppress these artifacts.

Digital beamformer

Fortunately, due to the rapid advances of digital electronics, even very low cost ultrasound imaging systems now use digital beamformers.

In a digital architecture, each active element is connected to a receiver amplifier that provides some gain such that the signal amplitude is matched to the input range of the subsequent analog to digital converter (ADC). This ADC converts the analog signal into a digital representation, and digital electronics are used thereafter for all signal processing. The sampling rate for each channel of a system may be as low as 20 MHz, and as high as 80 MHz.

Most ultrasound systems use application specific integrated circuits (ASICs) to implement eq. (16.12). In the simplest model for beamforming, the output of the ADC would write into memory, a processor would calculate which data from all the channels should be summed together, these data would be read from memory, summed, and output to the mid-processor.

Unfortunately, since the ADC samples the data on a regular sampling interval, and since the time delays required (the Δt in eq. (16.12)) must be much more precise (typical required accuracy is approximately 5 ns) than the sampling interval (typically 25 ns) and these time delays are changing with range, usually there is no sample of the input signal at the desired time for beamforming. Therefore, appropriate samples for beamforming must be generated by interpolating the ADC data.

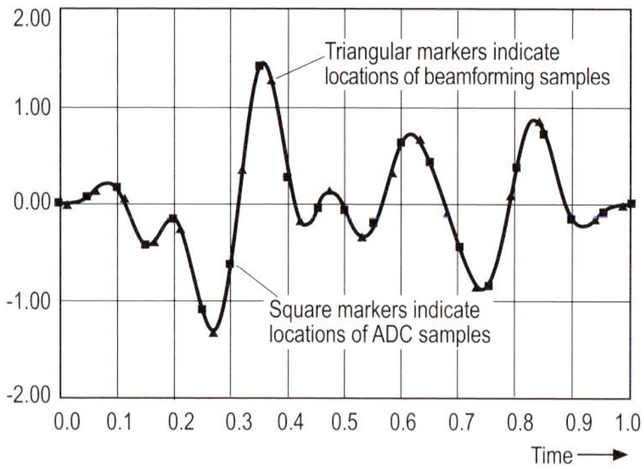

Figure 16.22
Illustration of digital sampling and beamforming samples. The line graph represents a typical analog signal received on a single channel. The regularly spaced square markers show the times at which the analog to digital converter (ADC) samples the analog signal. For beamforming, samples at the times indicated by the triangular markers are required. Note that the triangles are not only at different times than the squares, but the relative timing of the squares and triangles changes with time. Early in this signal, the beamforming samples (triangles) are only 10 nanoseconds after the ADC samples (squares). As time progresses, the beamforming samples are increasingly delayed relative to the ADC samples, until at the end of this trace the beamforming samples (triangles) are 40 nanoseconds after the ADC samples. Interpolating the ADC samples to generate the beamforming samples is the primary function of the beamformer subsystem.

Fig. 16.22 shows a representative analog signal along with typical timing of the ADC samples as well as the data used for beamforming.

Time delay beamforming

The most direct method for generating appropriate samples for beamformation via summation is to interpolate the ADC data. Many different algorithms for interpolation have been used in the industry; the two most common techniques are interpolation with functions of various orders (linear, quadratic, and cubic) and interpolation with a truncated sinc function. Other approaches convert the signal to baseband first, then the closest complex baseband sample is selected and a phase shift is applied. (For example, if a 5 MHz signal is to be delayed by 10 nanoseconds, a phase shift of 18 degrees produces largely the same effect as interpolation).

Regardless of the specific interpolation method used, generating the desired samples and summing these samples with those from other channels is the primary task the beamformer performs.

Multiple receive beams

All ultrasound imaging modes involve launching focused pulses and then receiving echoes from along the direction in which the pulse was launched.

After echoes from the maximum depth of interest are received, another pulse can be launched (usually in a slightly different direction) and echoes from that new direction

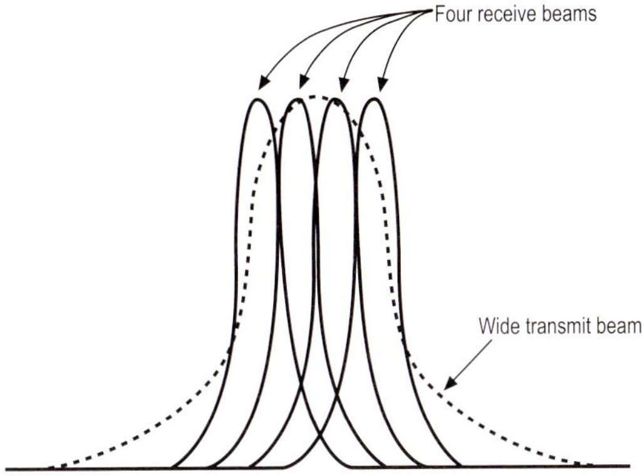

Figure 16.23
Representation of 4 simultaneous receive beams. Clearly, the sensitivity of the outer beams will be significantly reduced (due to the decreased intensity of the transmitted beam). These sensitivity variations can be reduced with a variable beam gain, but intensity variations that result from simultaneous receive beamforming usually inhibit the use of this technology in B-mode imaging unless coherent image formation technology is available.

are received. This pulse-echo process determines the time to acquire one line (or beam) of an image, and the resolution of the aperture determines the spacing of the beams. Therefore, the time required to acquire one frame is simply the propagation delay to the maximum depth of interest (and back) times the number of beams required to form the image.

The only way to significantly increase the frame rate is to reduce the number of pulse-echo cycles required to form the image. Therefore, in order to increase the frame rate, most ultrasound systems provide the capability to form multiple receive beams simultaneously. This requires that some portions of the beamforming hardware are replicated.

Commonly, high performance imaging systems use at least four simultaneously formed receive beams when producing color Doppler flow images. An illustration of how these four receive beams are arranged is shown in fig. 16.23. Clearly, the outer beams in the set of four simultaneous beams receive signals from areas insonified with lower amplitude ultrasound than the inner beams, and this can result in image artifacts. For imaging of flow, these artifacts are easily managed, and the benefits of forming multiple simultaneous beams are largest for flow imaging because of the multiple pulses that must be transmitted on each beam in order to measure flow.

For these reasons, many systems use simultaneous receive beams for flow imaging, but at present (2004) only the Siemens Sequoia uses simultaneous receive beams for B-mode.

Synthetic line

If only two simultaneous receive beams are used, in theory these two beams could have identical gain; however, in practice, variations in the body make this impossible.

High end ultrasound imaging systems like the Siemens Sequoia ultrasound imaging system use two simultaneous receive beams and a technique known as synthetic line to effectively increase frame rates without compromising image quality. The synthetic line technique is illustrated in fig. 16.24.

The important feature is that pairs of receive beams are combined with appropriate phase shifts in order to retain the full resolution capability of the system while eliminating the artifacts due to subtle variations between the two receive beams. This phase sensitive summation is critical to maintaining resolution. If the beams were averaged together after amplitude detection, then artifacts would be reduced significantly, but resolution would also be reduced.

16.2.2 Mid-processor

The output of the beamformer is an RF, or the equivalent complex baseband, signal that represents the echoes received after transmission and reception along a particular direction in the body. Although these signals (called RF A-lines) were used by early

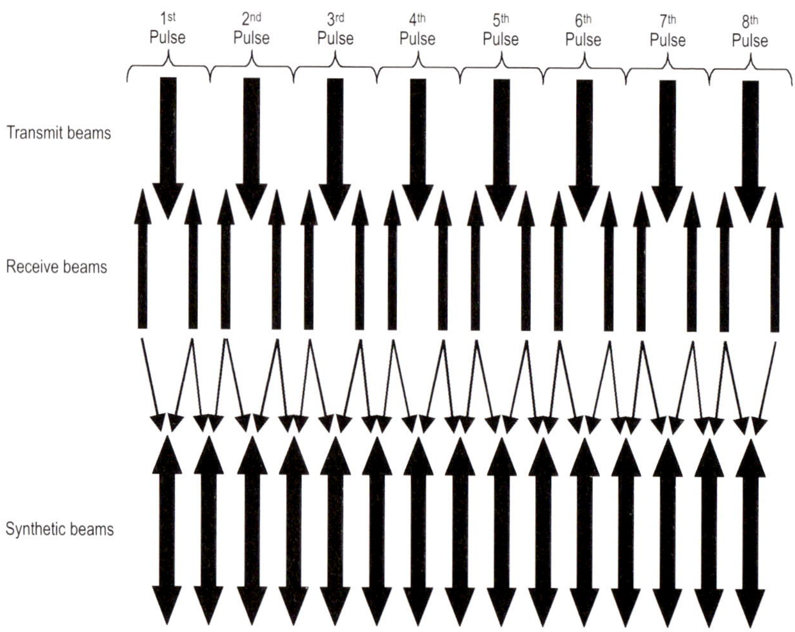

Figure 16.24
Schematic representation of the use of two simultaneous receive beams and synthetic line generation to eliminate simultaneous beamforming artifacts for B-mode imaging

ultrasound pioneers, contemporary systems process these signals to extract either amplitude information that is reconstructed into an image (B-mode), Doppler spectra that represent flow at a single location, or Doppler images, in which a spatial image of flow velocities is reconstructed. Extracting these parameters is the function of the midprocessor.

The hardware that makes up a midprocessor usually includes field programmable gate arrays (FPGAs) and digital signal processors (DSPs).

In some cases, custom integrated circuits (ASICs) may be used when cost and power constraints are critical and the flexibility of programmable devices is not needed.

16.2.2.1 Amplitude Detection

B-mode images are simply images of the post-beamformation received echo amplitude. This amplitude can be obtained from the baseband signal as follows:

$$a(t) = \sqrt{b(t)b^*(t)}. \tag{16.13}$$

This is a straightforward process that is performed digitally with minimum hardware.

The dynamic range of ultrasound echoes is typically 60 or 80 dB (a factor of 1,000 to 10,000 in amplitude), while the dynamic range of the eye is less than 40 dB (a factor of 100 in amplitude). For this reason, rather than display the amplitude of the received echoes, the logarithm of the amplitude of the received echoes is usually used.

The mid-processor in most systems also performs this logarithmic compression. Therefore, the processing usually required of the midprocessor for amplitude detection reduces to:

$$\log(a(t)) = \frac{1}{2}\log(b(t)b^*(t)) \tag{16.14}$$

where the division by two is not usually performed since other scaling factors will be applied during the display process.

Although a pure logarithmic amplitude scale is often available on most ultrasound systems, the most useful images are frequently obtained when the exact mapping of echo intensity to image brightness is slightly distorted, usually in such a way that low level echoes and high level echoes are slightly compressed so that the dynamic range used for mid-range echoes can be expanded.

This modification of the pure logarithmic mapping is controlled by the user when a particular gray scale map or post processing curve is selected.

Bandwidth increase with detection

One of the consequences of the processing described in eq. (16.14) is that the bandwidth of the signal increases. This increase in bandwidth means that a signal that is barely sufficiently sampled can become undersampled due to the frequency increase that takes place during amplitude detection.

In a B-mode image, this aliasing results in changes in the appearance of the speckle pattern seen from soft tissue. This can be demonstrated by imaging a relatively stationary organ (such as the liver) or a phantom and then moving the transducer in and out so that there are small changes in range.

If no aliasing occurs, then the speckle pattern will simply move slightly with the transducer motion.

If there is some aliasing, then the speckle pattern will change with the motion of the transducer. The speckle will reconfigure, appearing to sparkle or wiggle with very small motion by the transducer.

Although a small amount of aliasing will not reduce the diagnostic value of an image, severe aliasing will make subtle lesions difficult to detect.

When a system uses a minimally sufficient sampling rate for the output of the beamformer, then care must be taken to avoid aliasing during amplitude detection. Usually this is achieved by interpolating the samples to increase the sampling rate by approximately a factor of two.

An alternative is to simply oversample the signal. Depending on the details of the system architecture, retaining an oversampled signal out of the beamformer may be more cost-effective than optimally sampling the signal and then interpolating just before amplitude detection.

Analytic line interpolation

Just like the aliasing in the range direction (discussed in the previous section) that can occur due to amplitude detection, a similar problem can occur across beams. If the beams that are used to make up an image are optimally spaced, and conventional amplitude detection is used, then aliasing in the lateral direction will occur. This can be detected by sliding a transducer sideways while imaging a relatively uniform speckle target. (Again, the liver, or a phantom, is a good choice.) If lateral aliasing exists, the speckle will again reconfigure as the transducer is translated.

Lateral aliasing effects often produce much more severe artifacts than axial aliasing. People often describe the effects of lateral aliasing as looking as though the image is being viewed through a window screen.

Lateral aliasing is often a much more severe problem because oversampling (placing the beams that make up the image closer together) the image laterally results in reducing frame rate. The optimal solution to this problem is to interpolate the beams (before amplitude detection) to create additional beams (just like the additional samples created when the signal is interpolated in range). Once these beams are created, conventional amplitude detection can proceed.

At this time (2004), only the Siemens Sequoia ultrasound system is capable of interpolating beams before detection. Other systems must find the correct trade-off between placing the beams very close together (to avoid lateral aliasing effects) and spreading the beams apart to increase frame rate.

16.2.2.2 Doppler signal processing

The fundamentals of the Doppler processing carried out by the midprocessor have already been described in earlier sections of this chapter. However, there are some important aspects of how this processing is achieved that will be discussed here.

All Doppler signals include echoes from tissue other than blood. Even when the ultrasound beam is focused in the middle of a large vessel or a ventricle of the heart, sidelobes allow low-level echoes from the surrounding tissue to be included in the received signal.

The combination of sidelobe sensitivity and the relatively weaker scattering from blood versus tissue means that frequently the echoes from surrounding tissue are one hundred times (40 dB) stronger than those from blood.

Clutter filter

The case of CW Doppler has an even more difficult problem with echoes from surrounding tissue because echoes from tissue immediately in front of the transducer arrive at the same time as echoes from the region of interest. (This is because the transmitter is on continuously, so there is no opportunity to reject echoes based on arrival time).

Fortunately, tissue is usually moving much slower (if at all) than blood, so the echoes from tissue can be rejected based on frequency. This rejection is usually achieved during CW Doppler by placing a high-pass filter just before the analog to digital converters.

Since echoes from tissue have little or no Doppler shift, they show up in the baseband signal at zero (or DC) frequency, therefore a filter that rejects DC suppresses echoes from tissue.

FFT windows

In order to display the complicated mix of velocities present in typical blood flow, the Fourier transform is used to decompose the Doppler signal into individual velocities. It is important to note that the Doppler signal is sampled, and therefore the Fourier transform can produce artifacts if the Doppler signal is not appropriately windowed before applying the Fourier transform.

Frequently a Hanning window ($\sin^2(\pi t/\tau)$) is sufficient, but choice of a specific windowing function is dependent on details of the measurement conditions.

Auto Doppler measurement

Doppler measurements of blood flow are frequently used to determine physiologic parameters (such as pressure change across a stenotic valve via an approximation to the Bernoulli equation). Therefore, extracting information such as the peak velocity of the blood is important.

Historically these measurements were made by the clinician using a cursor to indicate the location of the peak velocity on the Doppler spectrum, and the system would re-

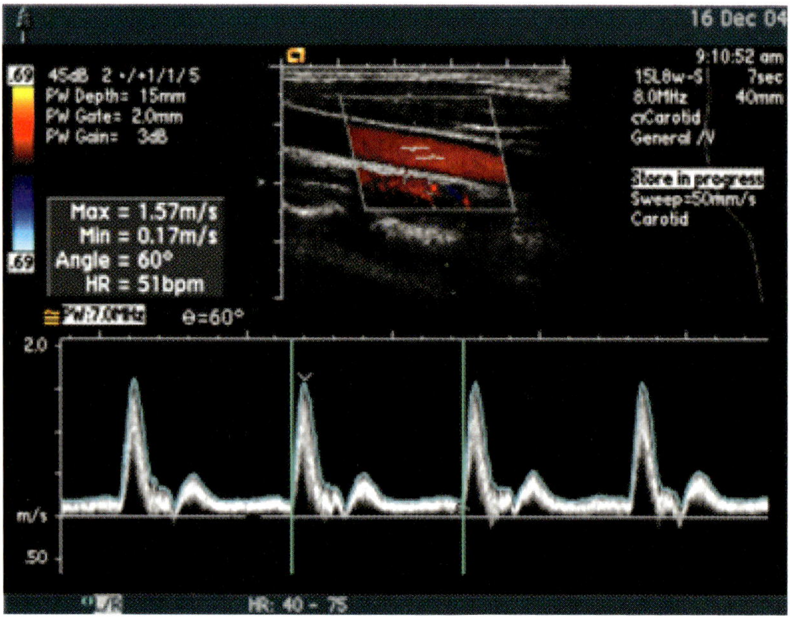

Figure 16.25
Spectral Doppler display showing automatic detection of the velocity and heart-rate. This Doppler spectrum was obtained from the carotid artery, and shows normal flow. In real-time, the imaging system detected the upper border of the Doppler spectrum. Using these data the heart rate as well as the maximum and minimum blood velocity were determined automatically. The angle (60°) between the direction of the ultrasound beam and the direction of blood flow was determined by the operator placing a marker on the upper image that was parallel to the walls of the artery.

port the velocity corresponding to that location. Fortunately, now, most ultrasound systems can automatically determine the peak velocity and report this information automatically. In fig. 16.25, a spectral Doppler display with automatic velocity detection is shown.

Automatic optimization of PW and CW Doppler

The ability of systems to automatically detect features of the Doppler spectrum (such as peak velocity) enables automatic optimization of these Doppler controls: gain, dynamic range, scale, and offset. In fig. 16.26, on the left, is shown a suboptimal spectral Doppler display, while the automatically optimized spectral Doppler display is shown on the right. Note how the velocity scale has been adjusted to match the velocities in the signal. In addition, the display gain and dynamic range has been adjusted so that the noise is suppressed, but useful signal is still displayed.

The ability to automatically detect critical features of images or spectra, combined with an improved understanding of the algorithms used by clinicians to optimize images or spectral displays, has allowed a significant growth in features that automati-

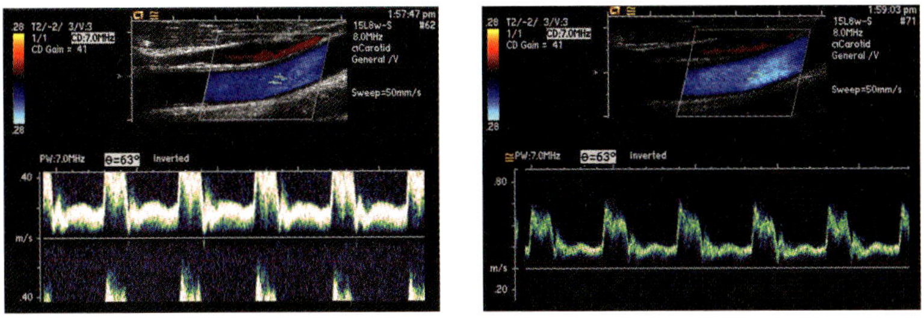

Figure 16.26
Automatic optimization of Doppler acquisition parameters. Both of these images use a display mode where the flow image is displayed in the top half of the screen for reference while the Doppler spectra are displayed in the lower half of the screen. In the **left image** the Doppler gain is set too high (noise is obvious), Doppler dynamic range is set too low (spectra appears very white, with limited subtle variation in intensity), the velocity scale is too limited (signal is aliasing, with high velocities wrapping around to be displayed as high negative velocities), and the Doppler baseline is set to the middle of the screen, which is unnecessary because there is no negative flow (towards the transducer) in these spectra. In the **right image**, all these problems have been corrected automatically.

cally optimize images or spectral displays. These capabilities allow the clinician to focus on more critical aspects of the exam, leaving the optimization of controls to the system.

16.2.2.3 Color Doppler

Producing an image of flow uses essentially the same signal processing as PW Doppler; however, due to the computational demands of estimating velocity at every location in the image, flow imaging (often called color flow, or color Doppler) is usually implemented differently from PW Doppler. Unlike PW Doppler, where as many as 128 pulses may be transmitted along a single line in order to measure velocity, for flow imaging far fewer pulses are typically used.

The reason so few pulses are used is that so there is time to sample along other directions in order to build up a full image. (Frequently the region over which a flow image is formed is reduced, or limited to a region of interest (ROI), in order to decrease the time required to form one frame of the image, thereby increasing the frame rate).

Most flow imaging systems start by digitizing and storing all the baseband echoes from the several pulses transmitted along a scan line. Once the final sequence of echoes is stored, the data can be read out across the pulses, generating a sequence that is equivalent to the data generated in PW Doppler.

Clutter filter

The baseband signals that are read out of memory are then filtered by a high pass digital filter that removes any echoes from slow moving or stationary scatterers, and then the velocity estimate is performed (see eq. (16.6)). This digital clutter filter (sometimes called a wall filter) is critical to the performance of the velocity estimate.

If the filter fails to eliminate the signals from tissue, then the velocity estimate will be dominated by echoes from tissue. If the clutter filter is too aggressive, then it can eliminate low velocity blood flow.

Extensive effort is put into determining exactly the optimal clutter filter parameters (finite impulse response (FIR) versus infinite impulse response (IIR) filters, and the specific coefficients used for these filters) for each flow imaging condition.

The performance of the clutter filter is the primary determinant of flow imaging performance. This is because with only a few samples of the flow signal the echoes from tissue and the echoes from blood overlap in the Doppler spectrum. Therefore, the clutter filter must be carefully positioned in order to eliminate enough of the signals from tissue to allow a useful estimate of the blood velocity.

Adaptive clutter filter

If tissue were stationary, an optimal clutter filter could be designed for the imaging conditions and applied to all locations in the flow image. Unfortunately, tissue is not stationary (respiration or motion of the transducer can cause motion of the tissue relative to the transducer) and therefore an optimal adaptive clutter filter cannot be designed a priori.

For applications other than imaging the heart, tissue motion is a problem only when trying to image very low velocity blood flow (velocities less than 5 mm/sec). In these situations, it is important to measure the properties of the clutter signal and then dynamically adjust the clutter filter parameters on a pixel-by-pixel basis to more effectively eliminate the clutter.

The simplest version of this approach uses the same processing (eq. (16.6)) to estimate the velocity of the tissue, and then adjusts the clutter filter parameters to shift the filter (in frequency) such that it is centered on the clutter signal. This allows the clutter filter to be as narrow as possible, thereby eliminating most of the clutter signal while retaining most of the flow signal for further analysis.

For cardiac imaging, the motion of the heart is too fast to allow the adaptive clutter filter technique to work. Therefore, heart wall motion limits the ability to visualize low velocity flow.

Color power estimator

Flow imaging usually displays the velocity of blood flow, but sometimes the clinician is only interested in visualizing where blood is flowing, not the direction of flow. In this case, rather than using the velocity estimator shown in eq. (16.6), the energy in the flow signal (after the clutter filter has removed the echoes from tissue) is displayed.

The energy can be calculated using:

$$E = \sum_{i=1}^{N} a_i a_i^*. \qquad (16.15)$$

(Note, eq. (16.15) is a non-normalized version of eq. (8.39). The normalization is usually ignored because of the scaling that will occur during display)

As in B-mode imaging, this energy is usually displayed on an approximately logarithmic scale with all the usual B-mode controls such as gain and dynamic range, as well as various post-processing curves for optimizing the appearance of the flow.

16.2.3 Display

After the midprocessor extracts the desired information from the beamformed signal, this information must be displayed in a usable format.

Most imaging systems use cathode ray tubes (CRTs) for display, but increasingly, systems are being designed with flat panel displays.

Flat panels have the advantage of being both lighter and thinner, thereby offering more options to achieve an ergonomic and attractive industrial design.

When using a CRT, images are best viewed in a dark room, so that the full dynamic range of the display can be used.

Flat panels are brighter than CRTs, so they can be used with some ambient light without loss of diagnostic information. The disadvantages of flat panels are that they do not display true black (some light is emitted by all pixels) and the appearance of the image depends on viewing angle. Each generation of flat panel displays improves these deficiencies, so eventually the inherent brightness and better physical properties will make these displays the universal choice of designers.

Regardless of the actual display device used, all of these displays use a raster scan. This means that the pixel in the upper left corner of the display is illuminated first, followed by the adjacent pixel to the right, continuing on across the top of the screen before returning to the left side of the screen to start displaying the second line in the image.

Since the acoustic data is not collected in this format, scan conversion is necessary.

Scan conversion

As data pass through the beamformer and midprocessor, they are organized in a format that conforms to the acoustic scanning geometry. For example, the first sample to exit the midprocessor is the shallowest sample from the first beam in the image, the second sample is the next deeper sample, continuing until the deepest sample from the first scan line is produced. Then the system transmits a pulse along the second scan line and reception along this direction results.

Eventually, the deepest sample from the last scan line exits the midprocessor before the sequence repeats.

These scan lines may not be parallel (as for example in the case of a sector transducer) and even if they are parallel, it is unlikely that the beams are appropriately spaced for the raster display, especially since the acoustic beams are usually displayed vertically while the raster lines run horizontally.

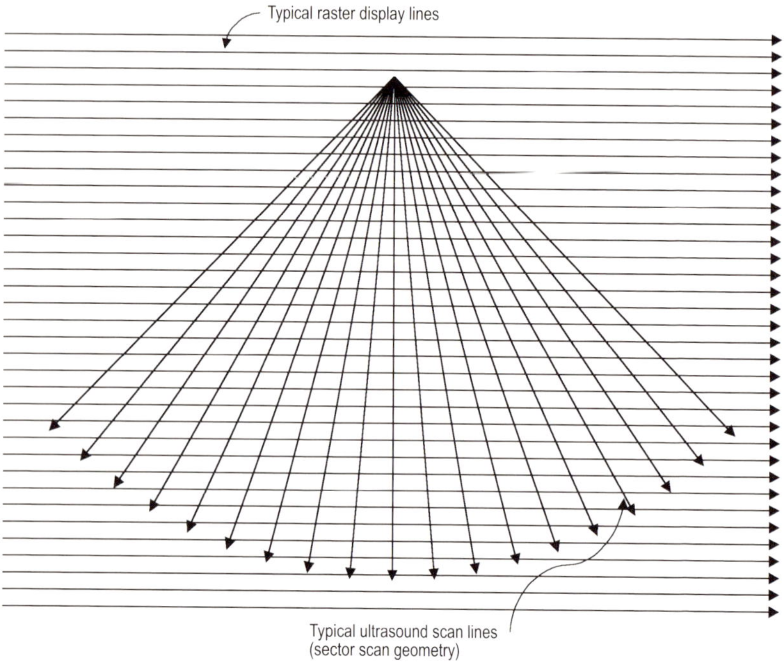

Figure 16.27
Geometry of typical ultrasound scan lines and display raster scan lines. The scan converter component of the display subsystem is responsible for reformatting the data from the acoustic grid to the display grid. Even if the acoustic scan lines were parallel, they would probably run at right angles to the display lines, so scan conversion is still necessary.

A typical geometry for the acquisition of acoustic data is shown in fig. 16.27 superimposed on a typical raster scan.

In order to generate the data necessary for display, the process called scan conversion must interpolate the acoustic data to generate display data. Two types of interpolation are typically used: bilinear, in which the four acoustic samples nearest the desired display point are used to determine the display value (see fig. 16.28), or bicubic interpolation, in which 16 samples are used.

Rarely can scan conversion artifacts be observed if bicubic interpolation is used, but bilinear scan conversion is often used, with some artifacts resulting.

It is possible to perform bicubic interpolation using a very small ASIC for even the most demanding ultrasound systems.

Alternatively, since there is usually a general-purpose central processing unit (CPU) that is responsible for responding to keyboard input and overall control of the imager, this CPU can often be used for scan conversion. (In some cases where the CPU is used

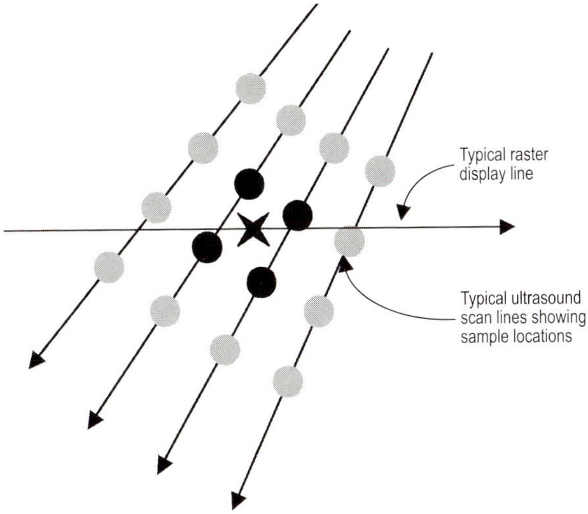

Figure 16.28
Geometry for scan conversion. Bilinear scan converters use the 4 acoustic samples (dark black circles) closest to the desired display sample (shown as a four point star) to calculate the display value. Bicubic scan converters use 16 acoustic samples (the 4 dark black circles plus the 12 gray circles) instead.

for scan conversion, only bilinear interpolation may be possible, depending on the speed of the CPU and the other tasks that it must perform).

Recently, three-dimensional ultrasound scanning systems have become available. These systems still require scan conversion and additional rendering in order to display the three-dimensional information on a flat screen. Often these systems use dedicated hardware to perform the initial scan conversion, followed by a high performance CPU to render the volumes.

Graphics processors

Graphics processors, such as those available from nVidia or Matrox, have become important elements in high performance ultrasound display systems. These graphics processor cards are capable of performing all scan conversion and rendering necessary for viewing ultrasound images (in some cases, even three-dimensional images) in real time. This relieves the CPU of this task while providing higher quality rendered images.

In the same way that ASICs have become the critical technology that drive improvements in beamforming, graphics processors are expected to drive improvements in ultrasound displays [16.3].

16.3 Transducer types (from a system perspective)

Ultrasound images are usually presented in one of three geometries, as determined by the type of transducer used.

When the acoustic "window" is limited in size, such as when imaging the heart through the chest wall between the ribs, the arrays are small and a sector (or vector) geometry is used. For applications where the acoustic window is larger and a modest field of view is required, a linear geometry scan is used. When the acoustic window is large and a very large field of view is necessary, such as imaging the lower abdomen, a curved linear geometry is used.

All of these three scan geometries are illustrated schematically in fig. 16.29.

16.3.1 Sector and vector transducers

Sector scans are produced by arrays with relatively small apertures and closely spaced elements. (These are also sometimes called "phased" arrays).

These elements are typically spaced by one-half wavelength, allowing steering to 45°. For example, a typical phased array used for imaging the heart may have a center frequency of 3.5 MHz, and an element spacing of 220 μm. If this transducer has 64 ele-

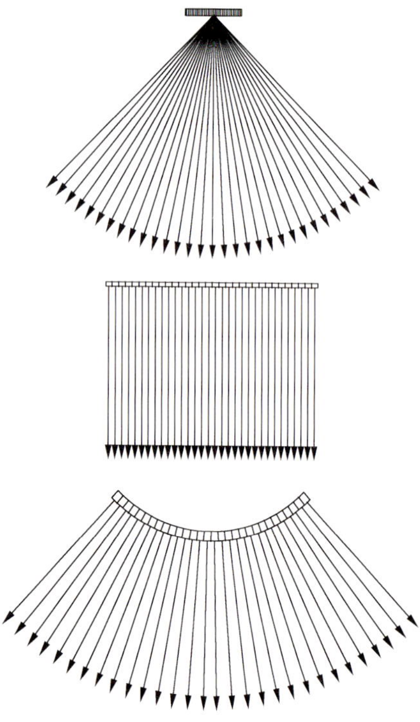

Figure 16.29
Schematic drawings of the three major scan geometries. **Top:** sector, **middle:** linear, and **bottom:** curved

ments, then the aperture width will be 14 mm, which is a good size for imaging the heart by placing the transducer between the ribs.

As can be seen from table 16.1, if the maximum steering angle a transducer will be used for is 45°, then an element spacing of one-half wavelength insures that grating lobes are impossible.

Even at a pitch of 0.6 wavelengths, grating lobes only occur at large steering angles, where the individual elements have a weak response (see eq. (16.11)). Therefore, for systems with a small number of channels, even a sector probe may have an element spacing of 0.6 wavelengths.

For higher performance systems, where the aperture size is limited by anatomy to be imaged, elements even smaller than one-half wavelength may be used in order to improve the off-axis sensitivity. (For larger steering angles, the individual element response increases significantly, as described by eq. (16.11), as element size is reduced).

The distinguishing feature of a sector transducer is the ability to steer beams to large (typically 45°) angles.

In a sector scan, all the beams originate at a point on the transducer's surface. This geometric choice somewhat simplifies the control requirements for the beamformer. Unfortunately, this also means that the lateral field of view is zero at the skin surface, and very small for the shallow ranges. A nice solution to this limited field of view is to place the origin of the beams behind the transducer, such that the beams on the edge of the scan intersect the end elements of the array.

When the scan line origin is offset, the scan geometry is referred to as a vector (rather than sector) scan. On a typical sector transducer this increases the field of view by 1.5 to 2 cm. As an example, in fig. 16.17 a sector scan is used, while the left image in fig. 16.3 is a vector scan.

16.3.2 Linear transducers

In situations where the transducer size is not limited by anatomy (for example, imaging the breast, carotid artery, or vessels in the arms or legs) then the aperture should be as large as possible.

One way to increase the aperture (without a similar increase in system channels) is to increase the element spacing and reduce the allowed steering angles.

Referring to table 16.1, for a transducer with an element spacing of one wavelength, grating lobes can be avoided by not steering the ultrasound beams at all. This leads to the linear scan format, where the transmit and receive beams are directed perpendicular to the transducer face, allowing elements to be spaced as widely as one wavelength and still produce images free of grating lobes.

The advantages of a transducer designed to operate in the linear mode over a sector mode transducer is a wider field of view at the skin surface and better resolution deep in the image (due to the larger aperture).

Because Doppler flow measurements require that the flow not be perpendicular to the ultrasound beam, even a linear transducer must be steered (typically to 15° or 20°) during Doppler measurements. Usually this is accomplished by performing Doppler measurements at a lower frequency, so that the element spacing is approximately 0.8 wavelengths at the frequency used for Doppler.

16.3.3 Curved transducers

The limited field of view that is provided by the linear scan format can be corrected by using a curved-linear (usually referred to as just "curved") array.

In a curved array geometry the transducer elements are arranged along a convex surface. By using groups of elements, but still not steering the beam relative to the local orientation of the transducer face, the transmit and receive beams can cover a sector-like region.

Clearly, not all the elements in a curved array can be used on every beam, which results in a reduced aperture and consequently lower resolution compared to an equivalent linear array, but for many applications the increased field of view deep in the image is more valuable than the lost resolution.

16.3.4 Intra-cavity transducers

Several transducers can be used to image from within the body. These include transducers that can be inserted into the esophagus for imaging the heart and transducers that can be introduced into the heart via a catheter. These trans-esophageal transducers and intra-cardiac transducers are both special cases of sector probes.

There are also transducers that are small enough to be placed inside a coronary artery via a catheter. These intraluminal probes are a special case of a curved array; in this case the array is curved into a complete circle.

Transducers that can be used from inside the rectum or vagina are either very small, tightly curved arrays, or small linear arrays.

All of these intracavity probes follow the same principles as the three basic probe types: sector, linear, and curved.

16.3.5 Multi-row arrays (1.25 and 1.5 dimensional arrays)

The previous discussion of different array types and scan geometries ignored the issue of the elevation direction.

Usually a transducer is provided with a fixed focus, achieved using a silicone rubber lens in the elevation direction; however, manufacturers are increasingly providing probes that allow some electronic focusing, or at least aperture control in the elevation direction.

The simplest approach to improving the elevation resolution is to have an adjustable aperture size. When imaging at deep ranges, the full elevation aperture is used, allowing the lens to produce good resolution in the focal zone. When imaging at shallower ranges (in front of the fixed lens focus) the aperture size can be reduced, which does not change the focal range of the lens, but does limit the off-axis sound and improves the resolution in front of the focal range.

This aperture limiting approach to improving the elevation focus is achieved by dividing the elements into several smaller elements in the elevation direction and using electronically controlled switches to either connect the outer elements to the inner elements (for imaging at deep ranges) or leaving the switches open and using only the inner elements.

Since these switches can only be changed while not receiving ultrasound, using this aperture control approach requires transmitting and receiving several times to obtain information at all depths along a beam; however, this is not a disadvantage if multiple transmit focal zones are already in use, since the narrow elevation aperture can be used with shallow transmit focal zones, and the elevation aperture is increased for deeper focal zones.

In cases where the imaging system has more processing channels than the transducer has elements, such as a sector array for transthoracic cardiac imaging, these extra channels can be used with separate elevation elements, and focusing can proceed in a manner very similar to focusing in the azimuth direction. Since these elevation elements are usually quite large, these transducers cannot be steered in the elevation direction, but improvements in elevation focusing can be achieved.

A good detailed discussion of these various strategies for controlling elevation beamwidth can be found in [16.4].

16.3.6 Hanafy lens approach to control elevation beamwidth

Another approach (that does not require the same complexity as expanding aperture or elevation focusing techniques described above) to improve the elevation beamprofile is to use different frequencies to focus at different ranges.

By making the transducer thickness vary in the elevation dimension, so that the transducer element is thick at the top and bottom of the element, and thin in the middle, the transducer bandwidth can be increased, while allowing reduced beamwidth in the near field. (This varying thickness transducer element is called a Hanafy lens, after Amin Hanafy, the inventor).

While a broadband pulse is transmitted, producing acoustic signal from all regions of the transducer, a time-varying filter is used during reception that selects only the higher frequencies from shallow echoes and lower frequencies from deeper echoes. This is similar to the expanding elevation aperture technique described above, in that only signals originating from the center of the transducer are used for imaging at shallow depths, while signals from the entire aperture are used deeper.

The advantage of the Hanafy lens is that only one pulse needs to be transmitted, thus maintaining frame rate. The complexity of hundreds of switches in the trans-

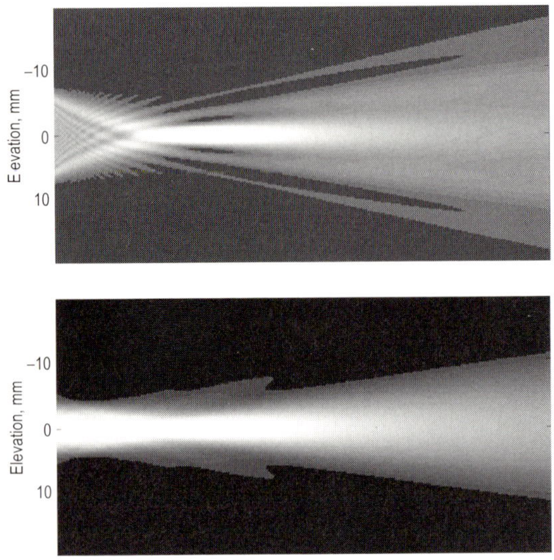

Figure 16.30
Elevation beamprofiles of a conventional and a Hanafy lens transducer: The horizontal axis of these images covers a range from zero (the transducer face, on the left side of the images) to 250 millimeters on the right side of the images. In these simulated image of acoustic beams, higher intensity regions are shown as lighter shades of gray while lower intensity regions are darker. The acoustic field radiated by a conventional transducer focused at 80 mm is shown in the upper image while the lower image illustrates the acoustic field from a Hanafy lens transducer. Note the reduced width of the acoustic field close to the Hanafy lens transducer.

ducer is replaced by a filter (often one that already exists) in the midprocessor of the imager.

In fig. 16.30, images of the elevation beam profile of a conventional transducer and a Hanafy lens transducer are shown.

16.3.7 Summary of different transducer types

In general, sector probes are used when the anatomy limits the area through which sound can be transmitted. This typically occurs when imaging through the ribs.

Linear transducers are used when a larger area can be used for access and a wide field of view deeper in the body is not required. Typically, this occurs when imaging larger blood vessels, the breast, or testicles.

Curved arrays are used when both resolution and field of view are important. This is usually the case when imaging in the abdomen, and especially when imaging a fetus.

Intra-cavity transducers are more invasive than external probes, but these arrays provide superior image quality due to the close proximity of the transducer to the organs imaged.

Multi-row arrays and the Hanafy lens are important advances to limit the elevation beamwidth of transducers, however, the most important advance in ultrasound transducers is the two-dimensional array used for three-dimensional imaging. These arrays are discussed later in the section on three-dimensional imaging.

16.4 B-mode imaging

The purpose of B-mode imaging is to visualize structure and detect abnormalities. Sometimes these abnormalities are only seen as subtle variations in echo strength due to slightly different compositions of the tissue.

One of the major impediments to visualizing these subtle variations is clutter. Clutter results when echoes from directions other than the steering direction are received by the imager.

High clutter levels can occur either because the velocity of sound in the body is inhomogeneous, which degrades the quality of the transmit focus, decreasing the energy in the main beam and transmitting more energy into sidelobes, or multiple scattering, which allows sound to follow a path through the body other than straight out from and straight back to the transducer.

The most powerful tool available today to reduce clutter is harmonic imaging.

16.4.1 Harmonics for clutter reduction

When sound propagates in tissue, the velocity of propagation varies slightly with pressure, and since sound is itself a pressure wave, the higher pressure portions of the sound wave travel slightly faster than the low pressure portions. This effect is illustrated in fig. 16.31.

This distortion of the sound wave can be thought of as the increasing presence of harmonic frequencies (that is, sound that has a frequency that is an integer multiple of the original fundamental frequency) as the sound propagates through the body.

Assuming an initial pulse of the form:

$$p(t,r=0) = a(t)\sin(\omega_0 t) \tag{16.16}$$

at some range r, the pulse shape can be well approximated by:

$$p(t,r) = a(t)\sin(\omega_0 t) + a^2(t)\alpha_2 \sin(2\omega_0 t) + \ldots \tag{16.17}$$

where the term α_2 is a parameter that increases with increasing pulse amplitude that accounts for conversion of energy from the fundamental frequency ω_0 to the harmonic frequency $2\omega_0$. (Even higher harmonics at $3\omega_0$, $4\omega_0$, etc. are generated, but for diagnostic imaging these higher order harmonics are small enough to be ignored).

Harmonics are important for clutter suppression because higher amplitude sound waves create disproportionately higher amplitude harmonics. Therefore, if a side lobe is a factor of 10 weaker than the main ultrasound beam, then the harmonic signals

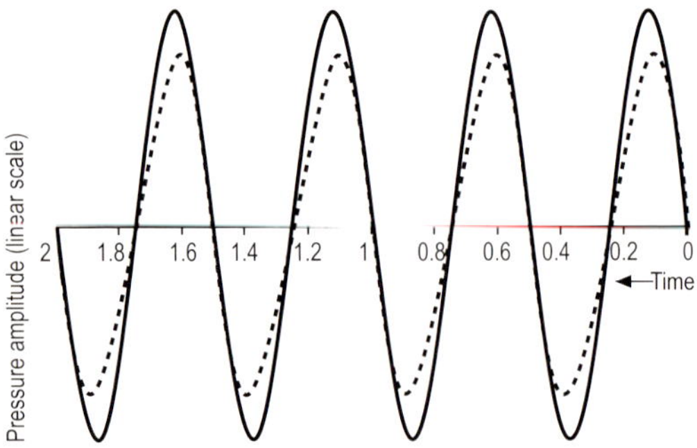

Figure 16.31
Undistorted (solid line) and distorted by harmonic generation (dashed line) waveforms. Note how the high pressure regions of the distorted waveform have moved earlier in time (to the right in this graph), while the low pressure regions are lagging. This distorted waveform has components at integer multiples of the initial frequency. The further sound propagates in the body, the more distorted the waveform becomes. Moreover, high amplitude waveforms distort more (generate more harmonics) than low amplitude waveforms. This is an important mechanism for clutter reduction in harmonic imaging.

generated by the side lobe will be between 20 to 50 times weaker than the harmonic signals generated by the main beam.

Similarly, a signal that has been scattered several times will always have a lower amplitude than the directly reflected wave, and therefore even lower amplitude harmonics.

Pulse shaping (for filtered harmonics)

The most direct method for detecting harmonics is to use a filter to select the higher frequency components in the received signal.

If the transmitted pulse is centered around 2 MHz, then the harmonic signal will be centered around 4 MHz, and a filter that suppresses frequencies below 3 MHz will eliminate the fundamental frequencies, and consequently the higher clutter from the higher sidelobes, while retaining the harmonic signals that have lower sidelobes and therefore lower clutter. In fig. 16.32, a fundamental image and harmonic image are presented for comparison.

There is one critical requirement for the filter method of harmonic imaging: the transmitted pulse cannot initially contain any signals in the frequency range selected by the filter. If this does occur, then these signals transmitted in the harmonic frequency range will be detected as harmonics even though no nonlinear harmonic conversion has occurred.

The biggest effect of this limitation is on the imaging bandwidth. Consider a pulse containing signals from 1.25 MHz to 2.75 MHz: this pulse will generate harmonics from 2.5 MHz to 5.5 MHz, but the lower end of this bandwidth is useless because the original pulse has frequency components as high as 2.75 MHz.

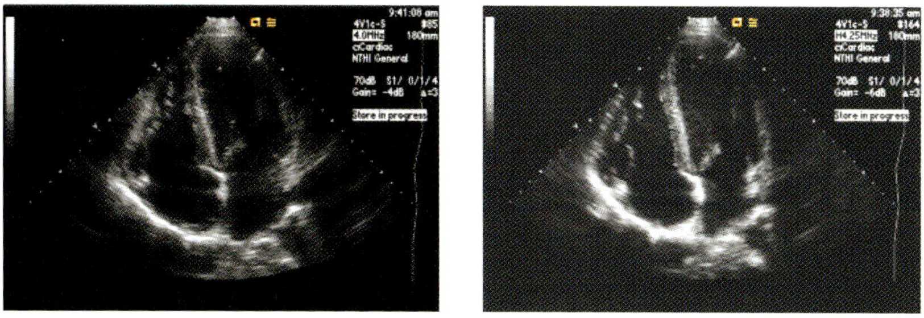

Figure 16.32
Fundamental and filtered harmonic images. Note the high levels of clutter in the valve plane (approximately two-thirds of the image height from the top of the images) in the fundamental image on the **left**, while the harmonic image on the **right** has no clutter in the valve plane. The dim echoes in the ventricle are scattering from blood. This visualization of blood without the aid of a contrast agent is not common, but is seen on occasion.

For practical design reasons, filtered harmonics can not be used with an imaging bandwidth of greater than 40%.

Pulse inversion

By using two pulses in quick succession, the bandwidth limitations of filtered harmonics can be avoided.

If a first transmit pulse is used to generate echoes with a form:

$$a(t)\sin(\omega_0 t) + a^2(t)\alpha_2 \sin(2\omega_0 t) + \dots, \tag{16.18}$$

and then a second pulse transmitted with the opposite sign is used to generate echoes of the form:

$$-a(t)\sin(\omega_0 t) + a^2(t)\alpha_2 \sin(2\omega_0 t) + \dots \tag{16.19}$$

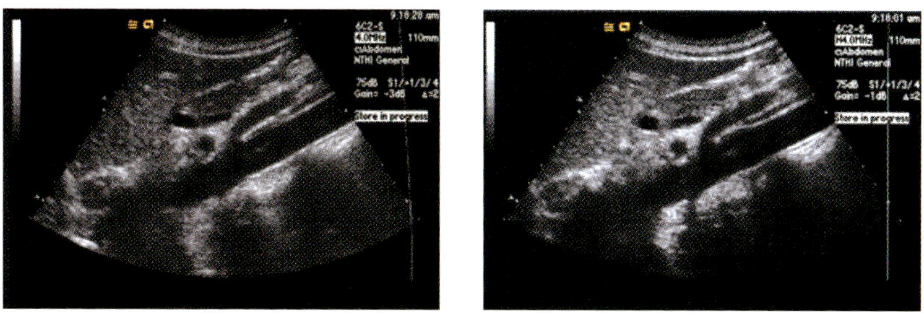

Figure 16.33
Fundamental and pulse inversion harmonic images. In the **left** image, note the higher clutter levels (the slightly brighter gray levels) in the fundamental image of the abdominal aorta (the dark structure running diagonally from the **right** edge of the image). The pulse inversion harmonic image on the right has a clearer aorta.

(the first negative sign is because the original transmit pulse is inverted, but the second harmonic is proportional to the square of the transmit pulse, so it always has a positive sign) when the two received signals are added together, the fundamental terms (those proportional to $a(t)$) cancel, while the harmonic terms (those proportional to $a^2(t)$) add constructively.

While pulse inversion requires two transmissions per beam, in many imaging situations the increased bandwidth, and therefore the increased axial resolution (see eq. (16.2)) allowed by pulse inversion is more important than the frame rate reduction accompanying this technique. Fig. 16.33 shows a fundamental and a pulse inversion harmonic image for comparison.

16.4.2 Transmit pulse coding

There are two limitations on how much acoustic power can be transmitted into the body: one is the limit on the maximum rarefractional pressure allowed (this limit is reflected in the mechanical index, or MI) and the other is the limit on the total power dissipated in the body at one location (this limit is referred to as "intensity, spatial peak, temporal average, or ISPTA).

For B-mode imaging, where very short pulses are usually used, the MI limit is in most cases reached well before the ISPTA limit is encountered. Therefore, if a longer pulse could be used, a better signal to noise ratio could be achieved.

Longer pulses are in general undesirable, since this reduces the axial resolution of the system. However, if a longer pulse can be processed to recover axial resolution, then the signal to noise improvements inherent in a long pulse can be achieved without loss of axial resolution.

Long signals that can be processed to recover axial resolution are called codes.

Chirp coding

Referring to eq. (16.1), one can see that the axial resolution of an image depends on the bandwidth of the ultrasound pulse. Figs. 16.4 and 16.5 suggest that longer pulses have narrower bandwidths, but this is not strictly true. A wide bandwidth pulse, where the phase of the frequency components varies, will be longer than a pulse where each frequency component has the same phase. In fig. 16.34, a short pulse and a long pulse with the same bandwidth are shown.

Echo signals from tissue that is insonified with a chirp pulse can be compressed in order to retain the full axial resolution inherent in the bandwidth of this pulse. This compression is achieved by convolving the received signals with a pulse that is similar in shape to the transmitted pulse. The convolution causes a phase shift in the different frequencies such that all frequency components now have the same phase, and axial resolution is preserved. The chirp pulse after convolution is also shown in fig. 16.34.

When a chirp code undergoes harmonic distortion, the second harmonic signal is also a chirp, and an appropriate filter can be created to compress the harmonic signal from a chirp also.

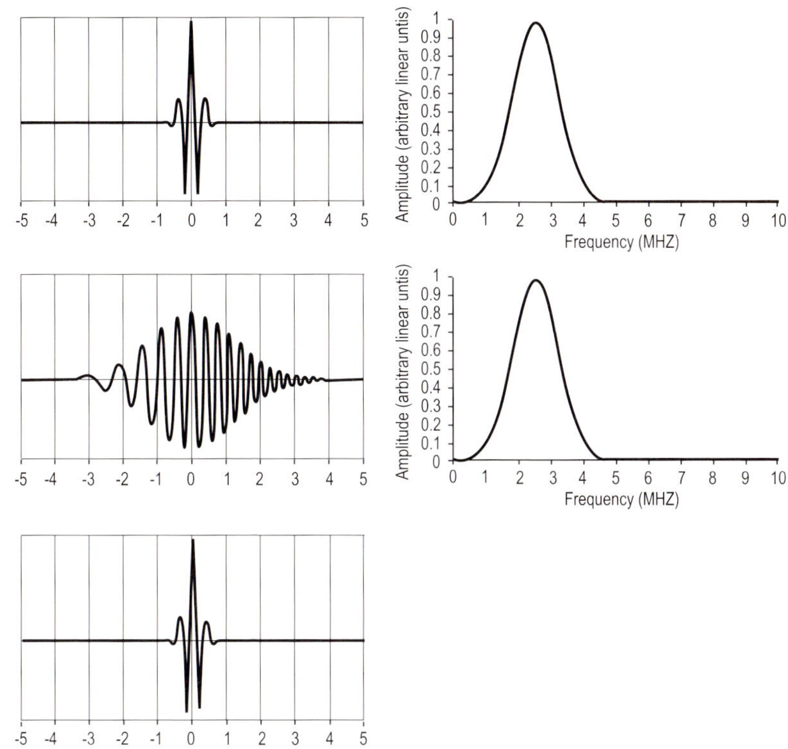

Figure 16.34
Illustration of chirp coded pulses. The **top panels** show a typical imaging pulse waveform **(left)** and the frequency spectrum of that pulse **(right)**. The **middle panels** show a chirp waveform and the frequency spectrum of that chirp. Note that even though the chirp waveform is quite long in duration, the bandwidth is very similar to the bandwidth of the short pulse. This chirp has 7.5 dB more power than the short imaging pulse. At 2.5 MHz, this increased power produces approximately a 3 cm increase in penetration. The **lower panel** shows the result of convolving the chirp with an appropriate reference waveform to recover the short duration desired for imaging.

Golay codes

Although chirp codes have the very desirable property that they can be used during both fundamental and harmonic imaging, transmitting a chirp requires a very flexible transmitter.

Many systems use very simple transmitters that are capable of providing only three voltage levels, $+V$, 0, and $-V$. For these systems, the Golay code pair is most useful.

As an example, consider transmitting a sequence of pulses with the following amplitudes:

1, 1, 1, −1, 1, 1, −1, 1

If this sequence of pulses were correlated with itself (i.e. the same sequence), the result would be:

1, 0, 1, 0, 3, 0, −1, 8, −1, 0, 3, 0, 1, 0, 1

While this sequence of pulses does have a strong peak at the center, there are range lobes (the pulses with amplitudes of −1, 3, and 1 that are not at the center of the sequence) that would be unacceptable for B-mode imaging.

However, if a second sequence of pulses with this form:

1, 1, 1, −1, −1, −1, 1, −1

is transmitted and then correlated with itself, the resulting sequence is:

−1, 0, −1, 0, −3, 0, 1, 8, 1, 0, −3, 0, −1, 0, −1

The desirable property of this second sequence is that the range lobes are exactly the same size, but with opposite sign, as the range lobes of the first pulse.

Therefore, if the two result sequences are added together, the following sequence is achieved:

0, 0, 0, 0, 0, 0, 0, 16, 0, 0, 0, 0, 0, 0, 0

This illustrates how Golay code pairs can be used even with very simple transmitters to generate long pulses that can be compressed to recover axial resolution.

Golay codes do require two transmissions, thus reducing frame rate. Because the received signals from the two transmissions must remain coherent for the range lobes to cancel, Golay codes require that the tissue being imaged does not move significantly between the two transmissions. For this reason, Golay codes are not used for Doppler modes.

The range lobe canceling property of Golay code pairs also does not survive harmonic conversion, thus harmonic imaging with Golay codes is not practical. (There are four code sequences that can be used for harmonic imaging; these are essentially a combination of Golay codes and pulse inversion).

Barker codes

Chirp codes can be used for either B-mode or Doppler flow imaging.

Golay codes can only be practically used for B-mode imaging, since the blood is moving too fast for the range lobe canceling properties of Golay codes to work. For systems with simple transmitters that require codes for Doppler flow imaging, Barker codes are currently preferred.

Barker codes require only transmitting at two levels (like Golay codes) but have the property that all range lobes have amplitude one or less. The 13 element Barker code is:

1, 1, 1, 1, 1, −1, −1, 1, 1, −1, 1, −1, 1

When this sequence is correlated with itself, the result is:

1, 0, 1, 0, 1, 0, 1, 0, 1, 0, 1, 0, 13, 0, 1, 0, 1 0, 1, 0, 1, 0, 1, 0, 1

Although regular rangelobes do occur in this result, they are all are more than 20 dB lower than the main pulse (with amplitude 13). For some systems, these range lobes are considered acceptable for Doppler flow imaging.

Unfortunately, the Barker code shown above (with 13 elements) is the longest known, so if longer codes are required for Doppler flow imaging in order to increase signal power without increasing signal amplitude, more sophisticated transmitters and chirps must be used.

Pulse coding summary

All three forms of coded transmission discussed here can be used to improve signal to noise ratio (and therefore penetration) while imaging.

Systems with sophisticated transmitters that are capable of generating chirps can use these chirps for both fundamental and harmonic B-mode imaging as well as Doppler flow imaging.

When simpler transmitters are present, Golay codes may be used during fundamental B-mode imaging, and Barker codes for Doppler flow imaging, but the Golay code pairs must be extended to four transmissions when Golay codes are used for harmonic imaging.

To the clinician, the use of codes is transparent since all signal processing is automatically provided by the imaging system; however, the increased resolution (due to the use of higher frequencies) and improved penetration that modern systems exhibit is in part due to the development of coded transmission techniques.

16.4.3 Compounding

Speckle is inherent in a coherent imaging system that relies on scattering. When trying to detect subtle lesions that have scattering properties very similar to the surrounding tissue, speckle can obscure these subtle variations.

Compounding is a technique that allows suppression of speckle, while making some sacrifice in either axial or lateral resolution (or both).

Speckle arises because there are many scattering centers within the resolution cell of any ultrasound imager. These scattering centers produce reflected waves that have random phases (depending on the precise round-trip distance from the transducer to each scattering center). When these random phases align (are coherent), high-intensity echoes result; when the phases do not align, a low amplitude signal is produced. (This is similar to the coherent and incoherent summation that occurs in the beamformer, but in this case, the constructive or destructive interference is taking place in the body as the scattered waves interact).

A small change in frequency, or a small change in the location of the imaging transducer, will change these precise relationships, resulting in a complete change in the speckle pattern.

This strong dependence of the speckle pattern on both ultrasound frequency and transducer position is the basis for speckle reduction via compounding.

Frequency compounding

One method for reducing speckle is frequency compounding. This approach involves breaking the received signals up into separate frequency bands (using a filter on the post-beamformation signal) and producing independent images from these separate bands. These images are then averaged together to produce one image with reduced speckle.

For example, if a wide-band pulse with frequency content from 1 MHz to 3 Mhz were transmitted, and two images were formed, one using signals from 1 MHz to 2 MHz, and the other from 2 MHz to 3 MHz, then these two images could be averaged together to reduce the speckle in each, while preserving all other structure. (Note, in a real system the frequency ranges would overlap to insure that no information was lost).

Of course, the initial 1 MHz bandwidth images have less axial resolution than would have been achieved if the full 2 MHz bandwidth had been preserved, but in some cases this loss of axial resolution is acceptable in order to reduce speckle.

Aperture compounding

Similar to frequency compounding is receive aperture compounding. This technology uses the entire transducer aperture to transmit sound into the body, but instead of summing the signals from all elements together into one beam, several subapertures are summed to produce independent beams from the same location. (This is achieved by applying the same time delays as if a single beam were going to be formed, so all beams are focused to the same locations, but each beam is produced from an independent aperture.

For example, if a transducer has a 2 cm wide face, the left 1 cm could be used for one beam, while the right 1 cm is used for another beam. As with frequency compounding, in a real system these apertures would be overlapped in order to insure no loss of information). The detected images formed with each subaperture are then averaged to produce a speckle reduced image.

As with frequency compounding, receive aperture compounding results in some loss of resolution, in this case lateral resolution.

In a more extreme form of aperture compounding, the different subapertures are used for both transmission and reception. Using different apertures on both transmit and receive increases the independence of the images formed, therefore allowing for more speckle reduction when these images are combined. Because these different subapertures must transmit at different times, a reduction in frame rate occurs, but a more important negative consequence of aperture compounding (either receive only, or full transmit-receive aperture compounding) is the loss of clinical markers.

Clinical markers are really artifacts that occur in an image and indicate the presence of an abnormality that is between the transducer and the artifact. An example of a clin-

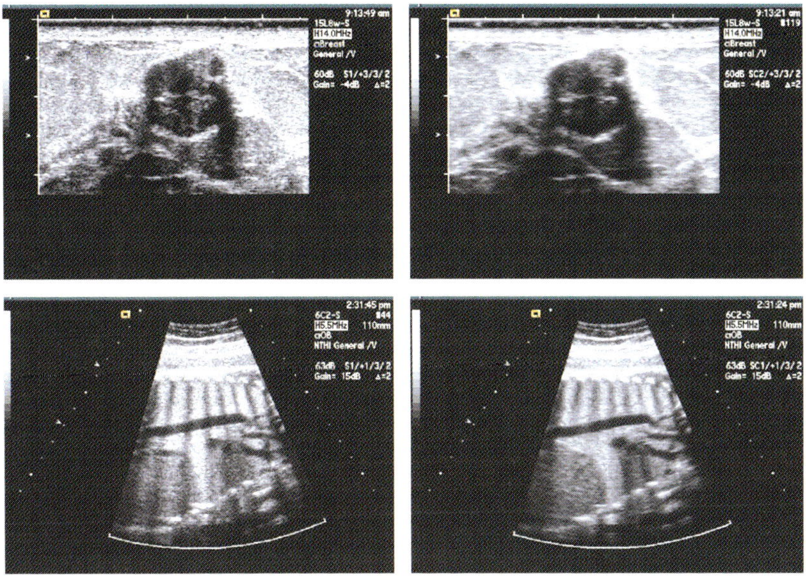

Figure 16.35
Images illustrating compounding. The images on the **left** are without compounding, those on the **right** use compounding. The top pair of images are of a breast, the lower two images are a fetal abdomen, including the ribs. Note how the speckle in the compound images is less distinct. This reduction in speckle allows clinicians to visualize subtle variations in tissue brightness. Compounding also produces more continuous images of the connective structures in the breast. In the fetal images the ribs create long dark shadows that obscure the organs below. Transmit-receive aperture compounding suppresses these shadows, which helps visualization of fetal organs. However, in some cases these shadows are the only indication of a highly attenuating lesion, and therefore loss of these shadows can reduce diagnostic information. This is a good example of how the operator's knowledge of both the anatomy of interest and the principles behind each image enhancement function is critical to obtaining diagnostic information with ultrasound.

ical marker is the shadowing that occurs when a highly attenuating lesion is present. The image distal to the lesion appears darker than the surrounding tissue because the incident sound has been attenuated by the lesion.

When aperture compounding is used, the shadow can be reduced or eliminated when sound propagates at an angle from behind the lesion to the transducer.

Receive aperture compounding produces less reduction in clinical markers than full transmit-receive aperture compounding.

Frequency compounding does not result in any loss of clinical markers.

Fig. 16.35 shows images produced with several compounding schemes. Frequency and aperture compounding may be combined in order to uniformly reduce resolution in both the axial and lateral dimensions while achieving the maximum speckle reduction.

16.5 Contrast agent imaging

Like other imaging modalities, ultrasound also uses contrast agents to improve image quality or to allow quantification of important quantities such as perfusion.

Almost all ultrasound contrast agents are microscopic gas bubbles (typical diameter around 8 microns) stabilized by a shell. Usually the gas is a high molecular weight gas (such as octafluoropropane or perfluoropropane) in order to slow diffusion of the gas across the shell.

In almost all cases where contrast agents are used, a special imaging mode that emphasizes echoes from the contrast agent over echoes from tissue is required.

Specificity, defined as the ratio (usually expressed in decibels, or dB) of echoes from contrast agent to echoes from tissue, is a useful measure of the performance of a contrast agent imaging technique.

16.5.1 Brief discussion of the physics of contrast agents

Bubble contrast agents have two properties that are used to allow selective imaging of contrast agents.

One property is that the shell of the bubbles can be broken, or disrupted, by the pressures used (typically around 1 MPa) in diagnostic imaging. This means that a contrast agent detection technique can be based on the changes in backscattered signals between successive pulses due to the bubble shell being disrupted by earlier pulses.

The second property is that bubbles are highly nonlinear. The nonlinear scattering from bubbles is much greater than the generation of nonlinear signals (harmonics) by tissue.

The echo from a single contrast agent bubble can be modeled using a power series:

$$s(t) = \alpha_1 p(t) + \alpha_2 p^2(t) + \alpha_3 p^3(t) + \alpha_4 p^4(t) + \ldots \tag{16.20}$$

where $p(t)$ is the acoustic pulse incident on the bubble and α_n is an amplitude weighting factor that can be determined experimentally or via more extensive modeling.

In general, higher order terms in the power series have lower amplitudes than lower order terms, but even at very low transmit pulse amplitudes the third order scattering (the cubic term with an amplitude of α_3) from microbubble contrast agents is observable with a good signal-to-noise ratio.

These two properties (easily disrupted at typical imaging pressures and highly nonlinear scattering) mean that microbubble detection schemes fall into two broad categories: high transmit amplitude techniques that rely on disrupting the bubbles and low transmit amplitude techniques that preserve the bubbles and rely on the nonlinear scattering properties.

16.5.2 Destructive contrast agent detection techniques (disruption)

The most direct technique for imaging bubbles selectively by disrupting the bubble shell is to use a sequence of two identical imaging pulses and then subtract echoes due to the second pulse from echoes due to the first pulse. (Note: Effective bubble disruption occurs when the mechanical index is higher than one, and some bubble disruption will occur even at mechanical indices as low as 0.2).

Assuming no tissue motion occurs between the two imaging pulses, then the subtraction results in canceling echoes that are unchanged (such as from tissue) while preserving echoes that change (such as from disrupted microbubbles). This approach, illustrated in fig. 16.36, produces images that are highly specific to contrast agent.

In fig. 16.37 an image based on bubble disruption of contrast agent in the liver is shown. Note that there are almost no echoes from tissue displayed. (Of course, in some circumstances, the clinician may prefer to see both contrast agent and tissue displayed in the same image. In this case, an image generated with a single pulse is combined with the contrast agent image in much the same manner as color flow images are combined with B-mode images).

While the specificity of bubble disruption techniques is exquisite, the disadvantage of this approach is that once the bubble shells are disturbed, the gas bubble dissolves and the ultrasound contrast effect is lost. This means that bubble disruption (high amplitude) imaging techniques cannot be used for applications where monitoring the contrast agent continuously (even if only for a fraction of a second) is required. In this case, a low amplitude detection scheme is needed.

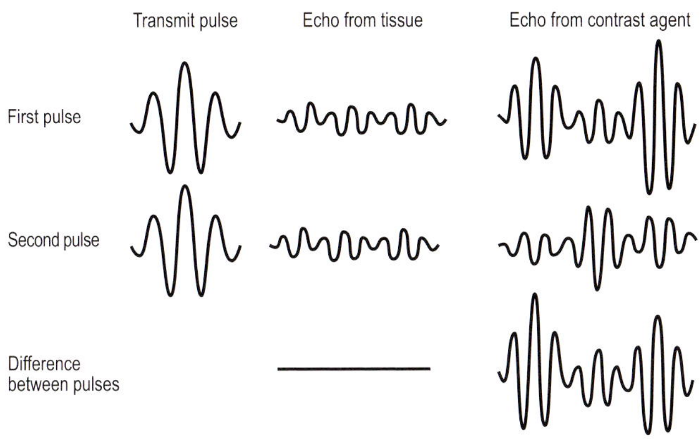

Figure 16.36
Illustration of the use of bubble disruption to detect contrast agent while suppressing echoes from tissue. The echoes from tissue are unchanged from pulse one to pulse two, while echoes from contrast agent are very different due to breaking (or disrupting) the bubble shell with transmit pulse one. Therefore, when the received signals resulting from pulse two are subtracted from those resulting from pulse one, the echoes from tissue cancel, while the bubble echoes retain significant amplitude.

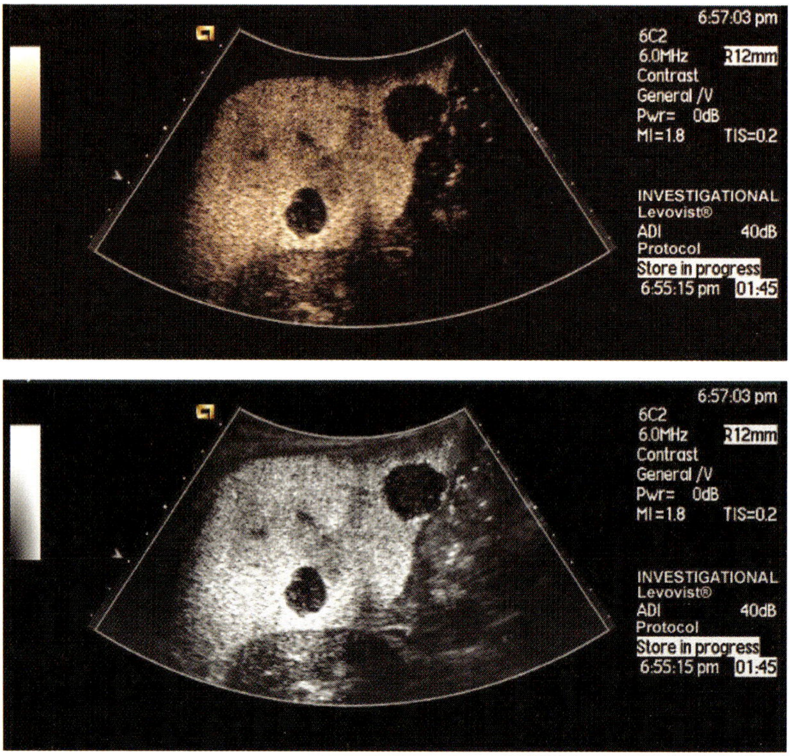

Figure 16.37
Contrast agent images in the liver produced using the bubble disruption technique.
The **top image** is of the contrast agent only signal. In this case, the contrast agent Levovist was injected and then allowed to circulate until most of the agent had been removed from the circulatory system. Healthy liver cells tend to accumulate Levovist, providing enhancement of the image long after contrast agent has stopped circulating. This image shows two liver cancer lesions as dark circular regions because the cancer cells do not accumulate the contrast agent.
The **lower image** is a combination of contrast agent signals and tissue signals. Note that the time stamps for the two images are identical (6:57:03 pm). This is because the two images are generated virtually simultaneously by interleaving imaging pulses in a manner similar to the pulses transmitted for B-mode and Color Flow. Upon review the clinician can choose to display either just the contrast agent, just the tissue, or a mixture of both.

16.5.3 Pulse inversion as a nondestructive contrast agent detection technique

An early nondestructive low transmit amplitude technique used for imaging contrast agents was pulse inversion.

Pulse inversion for contrast agent imaging is no different than pulse inversion for harmonic imaging of tissue, except for the amplitude of the transmitted pulses. Instead of transmitting high amplitude pulses that generate significant harmonics while propagating through tissue, a low amplitude pulse (typically with a mechanical index, or MI, that is less than 0.2) is used.

At these transmitted amplitudes, only a weak harmonic signal is generated in the tissue, but the highly nonlinear scattering from contrast agents generates significant harmonics. These harmonic signals are detected using pulse inversion in exactly the same manner as pulse inversion is used for tissue harmonics.

Unfortunately, even at low transmit power, some harmonics are generated by the tissue, and these tissue harmonic signals can be confused with contrast agent signals. Fortunately, better techniques exist.

16.5.4 Third order scattering for nondestructive contrast agent detection

The best method for imaging contrast agents nondestructively is to use the third order (the $\alpha_3 p^3(t)$ term in Equation 16.20) nonlinear response of the agent. Tissue has a very weak third order response, and therefore, tissue signals are effectively eliminated.

The most conceptually straightforward way to detect third order scattering would be to use the higher order harmonic frequency. Assuming a transmit pulse given by $p(t) = a(t)\cos(\omega_0 t)$, the third order response looks like:

$$p^3(t) = a^3(t)\cos^3(\omega_0 t) = \frac{a^3(t)}{4}\{3\cos(\omega_0 t) + \cos(3\omega_0 t)\} \tag{16.21}$$

Therefore, if one transmits a signal centered around 2 MHz, the third order response of the contrast agent produces signals at 6 MHz (the $\cos(3\omega_0 t)$ term in Equation 16.21).

As appealing as simply detecting the presence of signals at three times the transmitted frequency would be, many practical limitations make this approach unattractive.

A better approach is to use a multiple pulse technique (similar to pulse inversion, but involving amplitude changes as well) to cancel the linear response of tissue, and use the third order signals that are at the original transmitted frequency (the term in Equation 16.21 proportional to $\cos(\omega_0 t)$).

Consider the following example where three pulses of amplitude –1, 2, and –1 are transmitted and the resulting received signals are all added together. The received signals from these three pulses can be written as:

$$\begin{aligned}
s_1(t) &= -\alpha_1 p(t) + \alpha_2 p^2(t) - \alpha_3 p^3(t) + \alpha_4 p^4(t) - \ldots \\
s_2(t) &= 2\alpha_1 p(t) + 4\alpha_2 p^2(t) + 8\alpha_3 p^3(t) + 16\alpha_4 p^4(t) + \ldots \\
s_3(t) &= -\alpha_1 p(t) + \alpha_2 p^2(t) - \alpha_3 p^3(t) + \alpha_4 p^4(t) - \ldots
\end{aligned} \tag{16.22}$$

Adding these three received signals gives:

$$s_1(t) + s_2(t) + s_3(t) = 6\alpha_2 p^2(t) + 6\alpha_3 p^3(t) + \ldots . \tag{16.23}$$

Note that Equation 16.23 has no terms proportional to α_1. Therefore, fundamental signals are suppressed by this approach.

Note also that according to Equation 16.21, $p^3(t)$ has frequency components at the original transmitted frequency, $\cos(\omega_0 t)$. Therefore, using this three pulse technique, a signal at the original transmit frequency, which is a result of the third order scattering by contrast agent, can be extracted.

In fig. 16.37, two images illustrate the effective suppression of signals from tissue and the excellent sensitivity to contrast agent that this three pulse technique provides.

16.6 Quantification

Since the beginning of diagnostic ultrasound, clinicians have measured and quantified the information presented on the imager screen.

Usually this quantification is either a distance determined interactively by placing two markers on the screen or a velocity again obtained interactively.

Increasingly, manufacturers have developed the capability to identify interesting features either automatically or with minimal user interaction and to provide measurements based on these features. Examples include automatically determining fetus head diameter or femur length and calculating gestational age, extracting maximum blood velocity from Doppler spectra and estimating pressure drop across a valve, and automatic border detection of the heart ventricle and calculation of ejection fraction.

Perfusion estimation

A major new extension of quantification is to determine parameters that provide better characterization of the condition of the tissue imaged. A good example of this approach is estimating perfusion based on the wash – in of contrast agents.

In this technique, contrast agent is infused into the patient via a peripheral vein. Once a uniform concentration of contrast agent has been established in the blood, a short burst of high amplitude sound is used to rupture the bubbles in the region of interest, then low amplitude imaging is used to follow the flow of blood into the region of interest. Areas that are poorly perfused show delayed uptake of new contrast agent.

The sets of images in fig. 16.38 show how the inflow of contrast agent can be monitored using ultrasound. This technique is currently used to study both the heart and the liver.

Strain rate

A second important new quantification technique is calculation of strain rate in the heart. Strain characterizes how much muscle fibers shorten during systole; strain rate is a measure of how rapidly the muscle fibers shorten. (Strictly, strain rate is the temporal derivative of strain). Strain rate can be determined by calculating the difference between Doppler velocity measurements at two different points.

In order to determine strain rate over a large enough area to be interesting, Doppler imaging must be used to acquire velocity data at a number of locations. Only recently have Doppler imaging methods become accurate enough to provide useful estimates of strain rate. This technique is discussed in detail in [16.5].

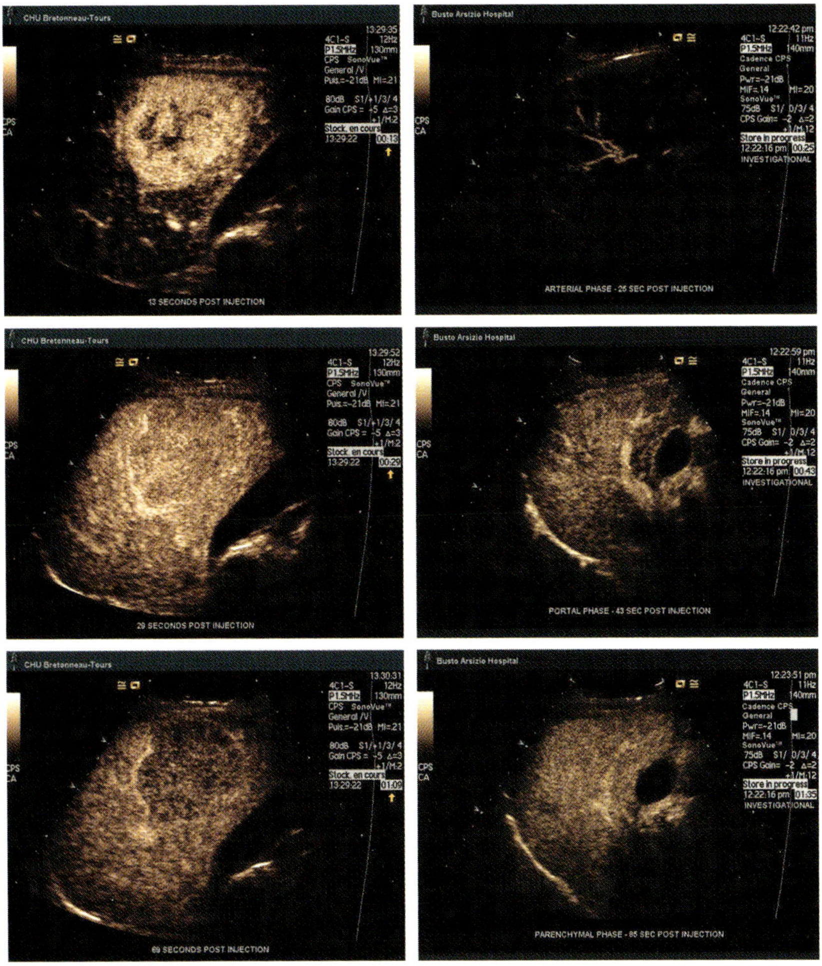

Figure 16.38
Contrast agent images using the third-order scattering from the agent.
The three images on the **left** are of a hypervascular metastasis. In the **top image**, taken 13 seconds post injection of contrast; the agent is primarily in the cancer due to the extensive vascularization of the cancer. By 29 seconds post injection **(middle panel)** both the cancer and surrounding parenchyma are equally infused with agent. At 69 seconds post infusion, the bolus of agent has begun to pass through the cancer, but is still enhancing the parenchyma.
On the **right side** are images that clearly show the arterial phase (**top Panel**, 25 seconds post injection) where the agent has just entered the hepatic artery, the portal phase (**middle panel**, 43 seconds post injection) where contrast agent has reached the portal vein, and the parenchyma shows some enhancement, and finally the parenchymal phase (**lower panel**, 85 seconds post injection) where contrast agent has spread throughout the parenchyma.

16.7 3D imaging

Until 2004, almost all diagnostic ultrasound imaging systems produce two-dimensional images that are portions of slices into the body.

For a decade, some systems have produced three-dimensional images, but only recently have these three-dimensional images become clinically useful. Three-dimensional imaging uses two distinctly different technologies for two different applications: mechanical wobbling one-dimensional arrays for obstetric imaging and electronically steered two-dimensional arrays for cardiac imaging.

16.7.1 Wobblers

For making three-dimensional images of the fetus, current systems use a conventional curved array attached to a small motor that wobbles the transducer up and down to scan in the elevation direction. The entire curved array is covered by a thin plastic shell that is filled with oil to allow the transmission of sound from the wobbling transducer to the body. (One of these probes is shown in fig. 16.2).

These systems usually produce volume images at a rate of approximately eight volume images per second (with wide variations depending on the size of the area scanned). In fig. 16.39 typical obstetric images are presented.

Since wobbler transducers are conventional one-dimensional arrays (with a motor) they place minimal new requirements on the imaging system; therefore, many systems can support this kind of imaging if the display system (back end) has the capa-

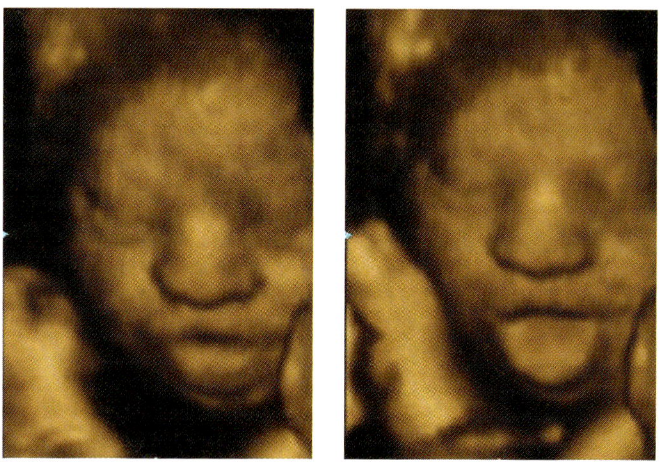

Figure 16.39
3D images of a late-term fetus. In the image on the **left** the baby is just opening his or her mouth, seconds later, in the **right** image the baby sticks out his or her tongue. In addition to the obvious family photo album value, 3D images have been used to diagnose developmental problems *in-utero*, especially in the fetal heart.

bility to render the three-dimensional data onto the two-dimensional screen of the imager. As graphics hardware becomes less expensive, this is less and less of a problem.

16.7.2 2D arrays

For three-dimensional imaging of the heart, the slow volume rates provided by wobblers are unsatisfactory.

In addition, since the acoustic windows to the heart are small (between the ribs), the large areas of skin surface covered by mechanical wobbler transducers are unavailable. Therefore, several manufacturers have recently introduced two-dimensional arrays for three-dimensional cardiac imaging.

A two-dimensional array has small elements arranged in a checkerboard-like grid. These two-dimensional arrays allow the ultrasound beam to be focused and steered in both elevation and azimuth, providing a pyramid-shaped volume to be imaged.

A typical cardiac two-dimensional array contains approximately 3000 elements, far more than the typical number of channels (128) an ultrasound imaging system has. Therefore, instead of connecting each element to only one channel, the two-dimensional array must use electronics in the transducer to combine signals from several elements (typically 20) before passing the summed signals on to the imaging system.

This subarray beamforming technique works because for a very small subarray (only a few wavelengths on a side) the signal processing required to combine the signals from individual elements is quite simple.

For transmission, the easiest solution is to place thousands of very simple transmitters in the transducer. All this electronics in the transducer makes 2D arrays transducers larger and heavier than conventional one-dimensional arrays, but these 2D arrays can still be held in the hand.

In fig. 16.40 a typical two-dimensional array transducer for real-time three-dimensional cardiac imaging and a representative three-dimensional image are presented.

Two-dimensional cardiac arrays do present one major new challenge to the ultrasound imaging system. To fully sample a 90° by 90° pyramid requires approximately 64 by 64 beams, for approximately 4000 beams. (Some beams in the corners can be left out without loss of useful information).

For sound to travel from the transducer, to a depth of 15 cm, and back to the transducer, requires approximately 200 µs.

$$4000\frac{\text{beams}}{\text{volume}}\times 200\frac{\text{microseconds}}{\text{beam}} = 0.8\frac{\text{seconds}}{\text{volume}} \Rightarrow 1.25\frac{\text{volumes}}{\text{second}} \tag{16.24}$$

A useful cardiac system must produce at least 20 volumes per second. Therefore, to achieve the frame rates required by the beating heart, the imager must transmit a rather wide beam and receive simultaneously several receive beams from the one transmitted beam.

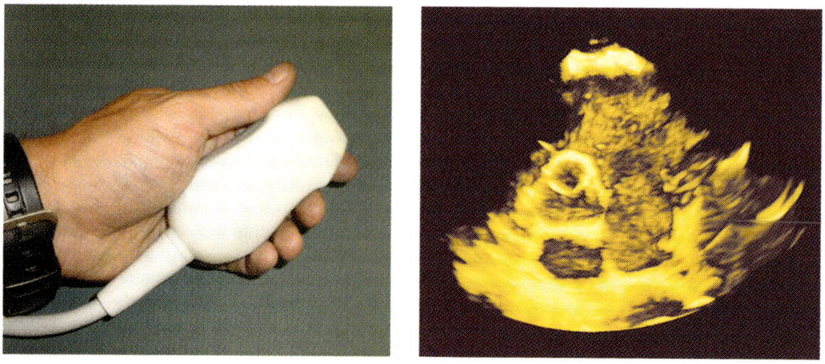

Figure 16.40
2D array and cardiac 3D image. In the right image the aorta is located approximately in the middle of the image and slightly to the left of center and is pointing at the viewer. The septum of the ventricle can be seen curving away from the viewer behind of the aorta and extending up and to the right. These three-dimensional images are much easier to interpret when the heart is beating and the viewing angle can be changed to confirm the location of structures.

To achieve 20 volumes per second requires the system to form approximately 16 simultaneous receive beams. Many systems do not have the processing capability to do this and so they use a compromise. One common approach is to form four simultaneous receive beams and reduce the size of the volume to be imaged.

This is an area that will develop rapidly in the coming years, and one should eventually expect any premium imaging system to provide full three-dimensional cardiac images at reasonable volume rates.

16.7.3 3D transesophageal imaging

One of the earliest approaches to making 3D images of the heart is the use of gated acquisition with a transesophageal transducer. Transesophageal transducers are small sector probes that are placed near the heart by passing them down the esophagus.

The sector probe can typically be rotated such that the sector scan rotates about the axis of the transducer. This produces a sequence of sector scans that when combined result in a scan that fills a cone-like volume.

Since the heart beats much faster than the transducer can be rotated, the current approach is to acquire images at one location for one heart cycle, then advance to a new location and acquire images for another heart cycle.

After imaging at approximately 30 positions, the entire cone-like volume has been sampled. Although these image positions are all gathered during different heart beats, the motion of the heart is usually repetitive enough that the images from one position during one phase of the heart cycle can be grouped with images from another position during the same phase of the heart cycle. In this way, the images from

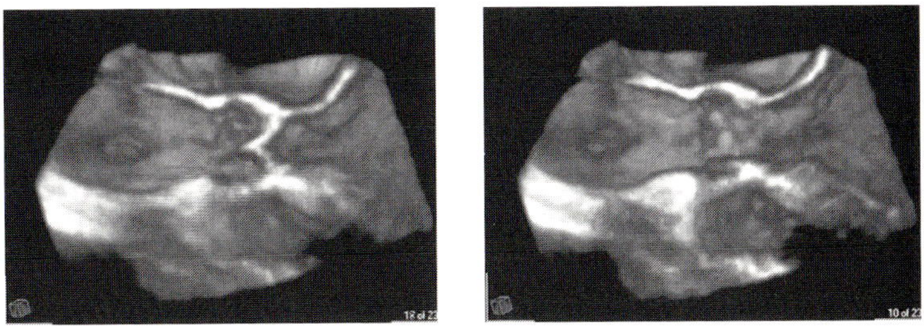

Figure 16.41
3D images of the heart obtained with a transesopheageal transducer. This is a side-view of the aortic valve. In the **left** image the valve is closed; in the **right** image the ventricle has just started to contract and the valve is open.

30 heart cycles can be combined to form a sequence of 3D images that span one heart cycle.

In fig. 16.41 a pair of 3D transesophageal images is shown. Although these images appear to have been formed at two unique instants in time (when the aortic valve is closed, and when it is open), in fact each image is the compilation of many images gathered over approximately 30 seconds.

16.8 Conclusion

Ultrasound has existed as a diagnostic imaging mode since the mid 1950s. Over that time progress in transducers, analog electronics, and now digital electronics has allowed systems to progress from simple a-scans and bi-stable 2D images to complex detailed images which accurately display echoes that vary over a factor of 1000 in amplitude.

With 3D imaging, almost life-like images of the fetus are possible and surgeons planning procedures on heart valves can now precisely visualize the defects to be corrected.

Despite all this progress, ultrasound has remained an imaging modality that critically depends on the skill of the operator.

Acoustic windows into the body vary greatly from patient to patient. System controls are myriad and complex, therefore only an experienced operator can produce images with diagnostic value. (For example, when unacceptable clutter levels are present, the operator has the option of adding more transmit focal zones, switching to harmonic imaging, or trying to find a better acoustic window. Choosing between these options requires knowledge and experience).

3D imaging in real time is relatively new in ultrasound and will probably drive technology advances for many years.

Ultrasound systems still typically have a few hundred channels for acquiring data from the transducer, but to fully acquire all the information necessary for 3D imaging requires thousands of channels. Improvements in electronics and transducer technology will allow systems to have more channels and to produce more simultaneous beams.

Expect dramatic improvements in 3D image quality as system technology improves.

Although the ultrasound images produced today look nothing like those produced 25 years ago, the process of acquiring these images has remained essentially unchanged for approximately the entire lifetime of ultrasound imaging.

Clinicians still apply handheld transducers to patients and look at the images in real time.

In 25 years ultrasound will produce images that can not be imagined by today's technologists, but the process for producing those images will probably look very familiar, even to those ultrasound pioneers who 50 years ago first applied single element transducers to patients' bodies and tried to understand the echoes returned.

16.9 Methods and applications in sonography

While clinicians today have access to sonographic equipment that enables them to examine and display almost any region of the human body, bones and air spaces within the body continue to represent a limitation for various applications.

Frequencies ranging from 2 MHz to 50 MHz are used for medical imaging. The standard frequencies of 3.5 MHz, 5.0 MHz and 7.5 MHz to 13 MHz are suitable for most cases. Special applications such as intraluminal and dermatological ultrasound imaging use frequencies of up to 30 MHz.

The velocity of the sound depends on the type of tissue through which the sound is to travel. All ultrasound systems assume an average sound velocity of $c = 1540$ m/s for the various types of tissue found in the human body for distance measurements. While this is sufficiently exact for soft tissue applications, some tissue types (e.g. bone) exhibit very different velocities that need to be accounted for by the clinician.

16.9.1 2D-imaging

The ultrasound transducer is an ultrasound transmitter and receiver. An electric impulse excites the transducer elements (pulse length of approx. 1 µsec) and these excite a mechanical wave that propagates into the tissue. The wave is reflected by tissue boundaries. This reflection or echo generates an electric signal in the transducer elements. The time elapsed between transmission and reception is a measure of the distance between the sound element and the reflecting object (see section 8.3.1).

The portion of the reflected ultrasound energy depends on the difference in the acoustic impedance (density × velocity of sound) of the tissue layers involved. The impedance of soft tissue is similar to that of water and very different from that of air and bone, which reflect ultrasound energy almost completely. Objects lying behind such interfaces cannot be detected. Stones in the gallbladder and kidney are characterized, for instance, by a typical shadow. Shadows of air in the intestines can make ultrasound imaging difficult or even impossible. However, in the case of small impedance differences, the penetrating sound beam retains sufficient ultrasound energy to produce further reflections from yet deeper boundaries.

A-mode (A for amplitude) is the oldest image acquisition technique in ultrasound. The echo signals reflected by the body are demodulated (i.e. rectified) and displayed as a function of depth. Today, the use of A-mode is restricted to a small number of special applications such as examinations of the paranasal sinus where it enables one to detect fluid very easily.

In B-mode (B for brightness) the signal amplitude of the echo is transformed into the brightness of a picture element. These pixels are addressed laterally by the moving position of the sound-emitting transmitter elements and longitudinally by the echo's time of flight (see section 8.3.3). B-mode is the standard mode for almost all applications.

In M-mode (also referred to as time-motion mode or TM mode), the echo intensities generated by a series of transmit pulses from a transducer at a fixed position are recorded according to their time of flight as a function of time. This technique is used to detect and evaluate fast organ movement (e.g. cardiac wall and valve movement) in echocardiography. It is also used to document prenatal life during the very early stages of pregnancy.

B-mode is used to create 2D images. The process involves the scanning of a sectional plane of the body using a sequence of transmit pulses that are shifted laterally. Each pulse generates an image line. When utilizing a linear array transducer, the image consists of parallel lines (parallel scan). The transducer signals are written into an electronic memory base (scan converter) and displayed as a geometrically correct gray-value image on a monitor.

The scanning procedure is repeated continuously, with the previously stored images being replaced, thus enabling one to render moving structures for visual inspection in real time on the monitor. Among other factors, the frame rate depends on the image depth (travel time) and the number of lines per image (see section 8.3.3).

The three principal scanning techniques (fig. 16.42) are parallel, sector and convex scanning.

A parallel scan involves the deployment of a linear array (of transducer elements) that is advanced step by step to create a rectangular image based on parallel ultrasound lines. Given that the image format close to the probe is wide, the linear array is the preferred choice for imaging superficial organs and structures (e.g. thyroid, breasts, testicles, muscles).

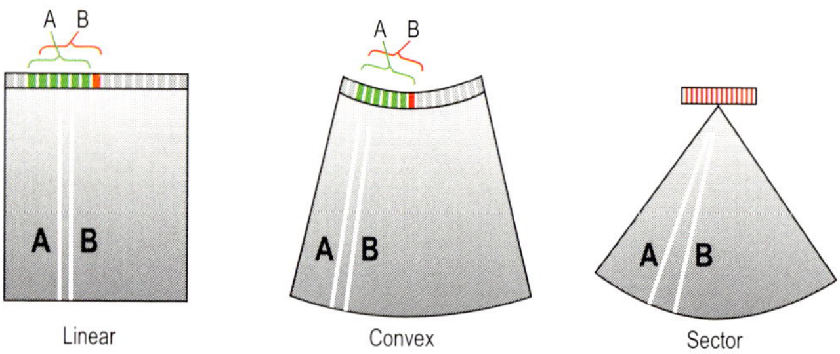

Figure 16.42 Principal ultrasound scanning techniques

A sector scan involves the generation of a sector image based on an ultrasound line that swivels around a pivot point on or above the contact area. Today, this is done primarily by utilizing phased (linear) array transducers that perform the beam steering electronically. Mechanical sector scanners outfitted with one or more individual transducer elements that rotate or oscillate around an axis are also available. The fact that the transducers have a small footprint makes sector scanning the preferred method for examinations that are limited by anatomical conditions (echocardiography, transcranial sonography).

A *convex scan* involves the use of a convex array so to combine the advantages of sector scanning in deeper body regions (large scanning width) and parallel scanning (large scanning width in superficial regions). Convex arrays are the preferred transducer types for abdominal and obstetric examinations. The convex array is in fact a curved linear array with a point of origin at a distance above the contact area that is determined by the radius of the curvature.

16.9.2 Doppler imaging

B-mode imaging is based on the reflection and scatter of ultrasound at interfaces and intrinsic organic structures. The information carriers that make Doppler sonography possible are the red blood cells (erythrocytes) inside the vessels, which either move towards the transducer or away from it at various speeds. The Doppler Effect is named after the physicist Christian Johann Doppler (1803-1853). Doppler offered a physical explanation and mathematical expression for the following phenomena: starlight moving towards the earth undergoes a shift towards blue (shorter wavelength) and starlight moving away from the earth undergoes a shift towards red (longer wavelength).

Sound waves reflected by moving erythrocytes in blood undergo a similar frequency shift with regard to transmit frequency (see eq. (8.21) in section 8.2.2.5). The frequency shift depends on the magnitude and direction of the blood flow velocity v. The scatter echoes from within the vessels are weaker (by a factor of 100 to 1000) than the signals obtained from organs and tissue interfaces. The detection and processing of these echoes relies on a dedicated system technique (see section 16.2.2.2). The sound shadows of structures are more critical in Doppler-mode applications than in normal B-mode. So e.g. shadowing caused by calcifications of plaques sometimes result in missing Doppler signals in the vessel behind.

The frequency shift measured by Doppler techniques (also referred to in the following as Doppler frequency or Doppler shift) is a direct measure of the velocity of blood. Given that the frequency shift is proportional to the transmit frequency, it is advisable to investigate areas involving slow blood velocities (e.g. in peripheral veins) using higher transmit frequencies. High velocities in deep-lying vessels are evaluated at lower transmit frequencies (e.g. in echocardiography).

The Doppler shift also depends on the angle of incidence. The shift is at its highest when the incident sound beam is directed parallel to the vessel axis. No Doppler signal is obtained at perpendicular incidence. It is necessary to measure the angle between the vessel direction and the sound beam in a B-mode or color-Doppler image to calculate the velocity from the Doppler frequency. The application of Doppler modes must take account of this angle dependency. The accuracy of quantitative Doppler is significantly higher when a small Doppler angle is applied.

The echo-signal frequency also contains information on the direction of flow (bi-directional Doppler). In order to evaluate the echo signals, the flow velocities towards the transducer are usually displayed on the positive axis in the spectral Doppler curve and encoded e.g. red when color Doppler is used. The flow velocities away from the transducer are displayed on the negative axis and encoded e.g. blue in color Doppler (see below).

The Doppler frequencies that occur in the ultrasound frequency range of 2 to 10 MHz and at physiological flow velocities ranging from several mm/s to 1 to 2 m/s are in the audible range between 50 Hz and 16 kHz and are thus directly accessible to the human ear as audio signals.

CW Doppler

While CW (continuous-wave) Doppler and PW (pulsed-wave) Doppler differ in terms of their mechanisms of signal acquisition, they show similarities with respect to signal processing and the presentation of results. In the case of CW Doppler, the piezoceramic elements of the (phased array) transducer are divided into two groups. One of these transmits continuously while the other one receives the incoming signals. In the case of pencil probes, the transducer element is divided into two parts. Due to the continuous operation, it is not possible to assign a point of origin to an echo. On the other hand, CW Doppler enables one to unambiguously analyze very high flow velocities (e.g. in the case of high-grade valvular stenosis). In simple Doppler units that are not equipped for duplex operation (i.e. without B-mode imaging support), CW Doppler is helpful for easy detection of vessels supplied with blood.

PW Doppler

PW Doppler meets the requirements for measuring flow in user-selected areas of interest. A single group of array elements is used both for receiving and transmitting.

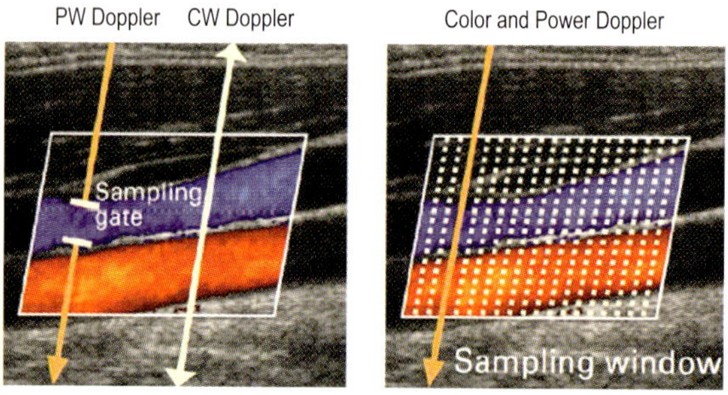

Figure 16.43
Doppler sampling locations

These elements transmit sequences of short pulses into the body, just as in B-mode imaging. Once a pulse has traveled to the selected sample site and back, the sampling gate is opened for a short period of time to receive the echo (fig. 16.43). The Doppler spectrum is derived with the help of a Fourier transform from the time course of the signal samples collected with the pulse repetition frequency (*PRF*) (see section 8.3.4.2). PW Doppler is therefore also referred to as spectral Doppler. The position and width of the sampling gate can be controlled and adjusted on the monitor in the case of B-mode imaging (duplex imaging). The shape of the Doppler spectrum characterizes the vascular resistance distal to the sampling site. Spectral Doppler provides a detailed qualitative and semi-quantitative or quantitative evaluation of hemodynamic changes in tissue.

The pulse travel time determines the shortest possible time interval between two successive transmit pulses at which the Doppler signal can be attributed unambiguously to depth. The term 1/(pulse travel time) defines the maximum pulse repetition frequency. Since the applicable pulse repetition frequencies (*PRF*) are in the range of the Doppler frequencies, depth discrimination when using PW Doppler is achieved at the price of an ambiguous determination of higher flow velocities due to aliasing effects.

Aliasing is proportional to the maximum *PRF*. The distant end of the gate limits the maximum detectable velocity without aliasing (fig. 16.44). Aliasing in the Doppler spectrum can be recognized by the fact that positive frequencies above the Nyquist limit (i.e. half the pulse repetition frequency) reappear as negative frequencies at the bottom part of the spectral measuring range. Shifting the reference axis for the flow direction up or down (baseline shift) can extend the measuring range for one direction up to twice the Nyquist limit. Doing so, however, will mean that the other direction cannot be represented.

Color Doppler

While spectral PW Doppler is used to calculate the velocity distribution at a preselected sample site, Color Doppler techniques are used to analyze the flow velocity at many sample sites distributed across the entire 2D image or a part of it (fig. 16.43). Color Doppler is also a PW technique that is subject to the restrictions relating to the pulse repetition frequency. The result is the spatial distribution of the mean flow velocity

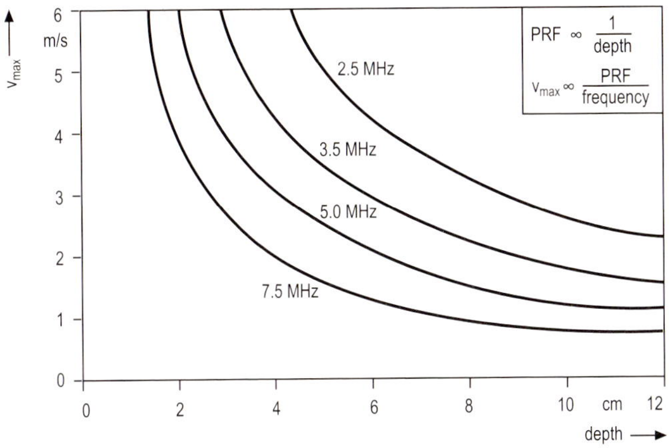

Figure 16.44
The maximum velocity that can be detected using PW Doppler as a function of the depth of the field of view and the applied frequency

and the flow direction in the perfused vessel in a temporal sequence determined by the frame rate.

While the Fourier transform is used for spectral Doppler, most manufacturers use autocorrelation algorithms for flow imaging based on color Doppler. FFT analysis involves sampling the Doppler signal from the sample volume 64 or 128 times for each time interval in the spectrum. In autocorrelation mode, the echo signals from one transmit pulse are compared (correlated) to those from the previous one (see section 8.3.4.3). Autocorrelation is repeated across 4 to 16 pairs of samples in order to increase the reliability of the measurement.

Several types of color-encoding scales are currently in use. A red-white/blue-white color scale has been commonly used in vascular diagnostics, with red-white generally marking the flow direction towards the probe and blue-white the direction away from the probe. The user may also select an inverse color coding in order to encode flow in arteries red-white and blue-white in veins. The user may also specify either a linear or a nonlinear color scale in order to facilitate the detection of pathological features in the flow profile. Other color scales, for instance, consisting of red-yellow and blue-turquoise (a scale that is commonly used today) can be selected by the user. The degree of turbulence in the flow may also be displayed by adding green.

Velocity derived in color-Doppler mode is influenced by the angle of insonation (fig. 16.45). The use of a linear probe to examine vessels running parallel to the skin requires the application of electronic beam steering or a wedge-shaped water path device so as to avoid the perpendicular incidence of the ultrasonic beam.

Color Doppler supplements B-mode imaging of organ anatomy and tissue structures by offering a superimposed depiction of blood flow in vessels and aiding in the iden-

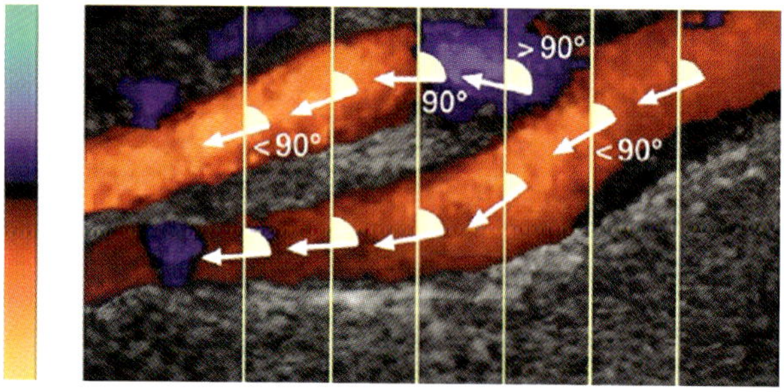

Figure 16.45 Influence of angle in color Doppler imaging

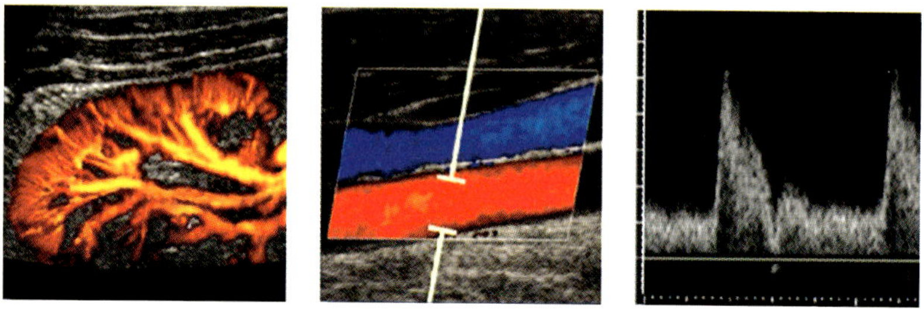

Figure 16.46
Doppler modes: power-Doppler **(left)** displays the distribution of flow without velocity information. The spatial distribution of the flow velocity is displayed with color Doppler **(middle)**. The velocity distribution within a region of interest as a function of time is displayed in the Doppler spectrum. The spectral intensity (equivalent to the number of scatters at a certain frequency) is encoded as gray level **(right)**.

tification of these vessels. It enables one, for instance, to localize and identify vessels and vascular stenoses, to rule out the occurrence of vascular occlusion, to more quickly detect angiopathies and vascular abnormalities and to arrive at an initial evaluation of hemodynamic conditions. Color Doppler also facilitates the setting of sampling gates for further examinations involving PW and spectral Doppler (fig. 16.46).

Power-Doppler

The power-Doppler mode (see section 8.3.4.3) involves the superimposition of the moving blood cells (irrespective of their velocity) onto the B-mode image in a single color as a spatial distribution of flow. While the power-Doppler image does not contain information about flow velocity and the direction of flow, it provides a complete and clear view of vascular structures (even very small structures) and pathological changes. It also enables the physician to rule out vascular occlusion and to differentiate between blood-carrying vessels and other fluid-related occurrences. The evaluation of hemodynamic properties such as the pulsation of flow is limited owing to the fact that the image frame rate is usually low.

Power-Doppler is the most sensitive Doppler mode. It enables one to detect even extremely slow or weak blood flow. Augmenting power-Doppler with the direction information of color Doppler leads to what is known as directive power-Doppler, a mode that exhibits properties that are similar to those of power-Doppler with respect to sensitivity and temporal averaging effects.

Hemodynamics and Doppler signal evaluation

Spectral Doppler is utilized to assess the perfusion of organs, to detect stenoses and sites of occlusion and to evaluate the functioning of the heart. Spectral Doppler investigations center on the measurement of volume flow. Given that the volume flow is not accessible for direct measurement, it is assessed directly or indirectly from the Doppler spectrum.

In order to evaluate flow dynamics and to enable further quantitative processing, the following typical velocities are deduced from the Doppler spectrum and displayed on a time axis: $v_{max}(t)$ is the envelope of the spectrum and displays the highest velocity detected that corresponds to the axial flow velocity at laminar flow (fig. 16.47).

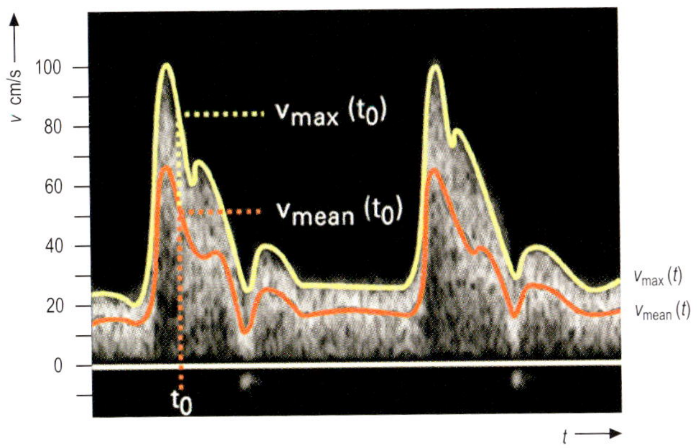

Figure 16.47 Evaluation of the Doppler spectrum

The momentary mean velocity curve $v_{mean}(t)$ represents the sum of all velocities weighted with their respective frequency of occurrence $a(v)$:

$$v_{mean}(t) = \int a(v)\, v(t)\, dv \tag{16.25}$$

The mode velocity $v_{mode}(t)$ is the most frequently observed velocity in the spectrum, however, it is not often used in practice and therefore not indicated in fig. 16.47.

The time-averaged velocities TAV_{mean} and TAV_{max} are obtained by time averaging $v_{mean}(t)$ or $v_{max}(t)$ over one complete cardiac cycle T:

$$TAV_{\substack{max \\ mean}} = \frac{1}{T}\int_{t}^{t+T} v_{\substack{max \\ mean}}(t)\,dt \tag{16.26}$$

TAV_{mean} originates from a double averaging, i.e. the amplitude-weighted averaging over all instantaneous flow velocities registered in the sample volume and temporal averaging over a cardiac cycle. TAV_{mean} is the basis for the direct quantitative calculation of the volume flow Q:

$$Q = A\,TAV_{mean} \tag{16.27}$$

$A = \pi r^2$ is the cross section of the vessel at the sampling site obtained from the vessel diameter measured in the B-mode image. When interpreting these values with regard to the volume flow Q, two critical sources of error must be considered: first, the limited measuring accuracy of the vessel diameter (especially in the case of very small vessels) and second, the angle correction error, which depends on the angle of incidence.

The time-averaged maximum velocity cannot be used to determine the volume flow because it would overestimate it. TAV_{max} is often used for the indirect evaluation of organ perfusion.

The volume flow in a vessel is analogous to Ohm's law in that it depends on the blood pressure P and the vascular resistance R:

$$Q = \frac{P}{R} \tag{16.28}$$

Vascular resistance, which is inversely proportional to volume flow, can be indirectly evaluated via indices derived from the Doppler spectrum. These indices are dimensionless relations of flow velocities, which are therefore independent of the Doppler angle correction.

The resistance index (RI), also referred to as Pourcelot Index, is calculated from the maximum systolic peak velocity $v_{Systole}$ and the end diastolic velocity $v_{Diastole}$ (fig. 16.48):

$$RI = \frac{v_{Systole} - v_{Diastole}}{v_{Systole}} \tag{16.29}$$

The numerical values for RI range from 0 to 1. A low value is indicative of low vascular resistance and a value close to 1 is indicative of high resistance. RI is commonly used in the evaluation of vessels that usually exhibit low vascular resistance (e.g. the carotid and renal arteries).

The pulsatility index (PI) or Gosling index is also frequently used to identify low resistance vessels. In contrast to RI, the time-averaged velocity TAV_{max} is part of the calculation:

$$PI = \frac{v_{Systole} - v_{Diastole}}{TAV_{max}} \tag{16.30}$$

Values of $PI < 3$ are indicators of low vascular resistance and values of $PI > 3$ are indicators of high vascular resistance. Like the RI, the PI is angle-independent.

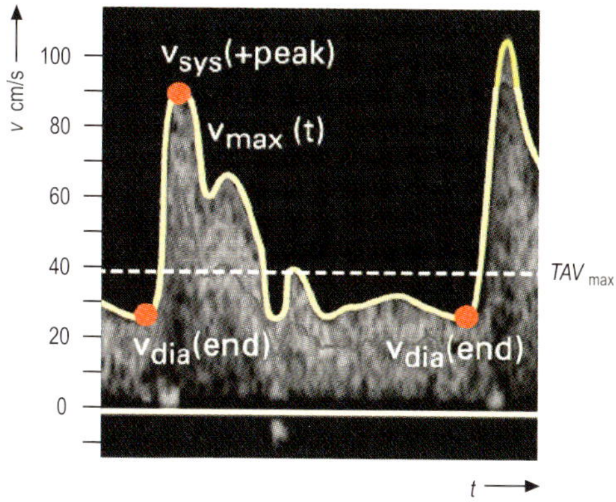

Figure 16.48
Maximum velocities at systole and diastole

While the resistance index *RI* is based on only two measuring values on the Doppler spectrum and may be of limited value (i.e. depending on the complexity of the waveform), the calculation of the *PI* takes the entire curve into account, including the *TAV* value. When analyzing complex waveforms, it is therefore advisable to use the *PI* instead of the *RI* value.

16.9.3 Harmonic imaging

The occurrence of non-linear effects as the ultrasound signal propagates within the tissue (see section 8.2.2.6) or when it is scattered by contrast-enhancing microbubbles means that echo signals will consist of more than just fundamental frequencies (echo frequency = transmit frequency). These signals also exhibit multiples of the transmit frequency (2nd, 3rd, etc. harmonics) utilized in harmonic imaging.

Harmonic imaging techniques

Two methods are available for separating fundamental and harmonic echo signals (fig. 16.49). Second-harmonic imaging separates the harmonic components (mainly the strongest second harmonic) from the fundamental components using a high-pass filter. It is necessary to give the transmit pulse a narrow bandwidth to obtain an efficient separation. This leads to some reduction in axial resolution. Nevertheless, second harmonic contrast is still influenced by the unavoidable overlap with fundamental signal components.

Wide-band harmonic imaging applies phase inversion to the transmit pulse so as to enable one to use the transducer's full bandwidth. Fundamental signals are significantly reduced compared to signals from harmonic frequencies. The smaller degree of overlap enables one to select a wider transmit frequency spectrum.

The phase inversion technique (fig. 16.50) requires an ultrasound system with fully-digital signal-processing capability. The technique involves the transmission of two consecutive pulses into the body. Given that the phase of the second pulse is inverted

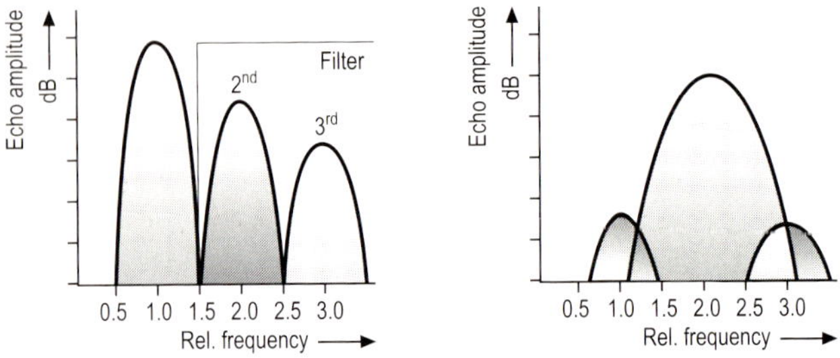

Figure 16.49
Harmonic imaging: Narrow-band harmonic imaging involves the application of a long transmit pulse and the suppression of the fundamental frequency in the echo using a high pass filter **(left)**. Wide-band harmonic imaging involves the application of two short phase-inverted transmit pulses and the suppression of all uneven frequencies via the addition of the two resulting echoes **(right)**.

by 180°, the phases of the fundamental echoes from the first and second transmit pulses are also shifted by 180° while remaining the same for the second harmonic echo. This is because the second harmonic echo amplitude is proportional to the square of the transmit pulse amplitude. Thus, when the echo signals from the two transmit pulses are added, the fundamental components cancel out, while the second harmonic echo signals add up. As a result, the fundamental and odd harmonic components are suppressed, while the even harmonic components, especially the second harmonic frequency components, are retained. The second harmonic B-mode images that are obtained thus exhibit significantly enhanced contrast.

The side lobes of the ultrasound beam are reduced significantly compared to conventional imaging. The narrower width of the second harmonic main lobe results in better lateral resolution. Wide-band harmonic imaging also preserves the axial resolution. The images appear sharper and exhibit higher contrast resolution and less noise.

Wide-band harmonic imaging can be used with transducers that cover a wide frequency range, and thereby enable e.g. low-frequency transcranial applications or high-fre-

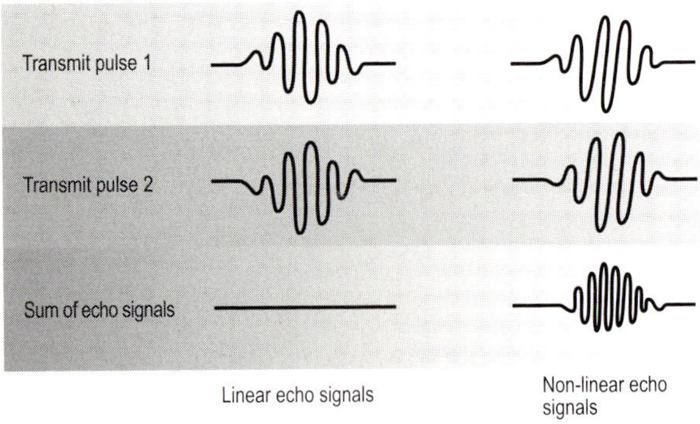

Figure 16.50
Phase inversion technique

quency vascular and small-parts applications. Tissue harmonic imaging utilizes only the higher harmonic signal portions for imaging in order to ensure higher contrast. The enhancement of contrast and spatial resolution is advantageous in the case of obese patients and other patients who are difficult to image and cannot be scanned at a higher frequency. However, this technology also contributes to greater definition and accuracy in various diagnostic examinations, including examinations of the gall-bladder, kidneys, vascular structures, the fetal heart, gynecologic anatomy, the brain, the pancreas, the liver and the uterus.

Contrast harmonic imaging

Contrast agents are used to enhance the signal amplitude for blood flow. These agents enable one to better visualize vascular structures and detect low velocities. They can also be used to permit one to evaluate perfusion textures and perfusion time courses in tissue regions (e.g. tumor parenchyma).

Contrast agents are used in ultrasound to:

- Differentiate among types of tissue in the liver (hemangioma, metastases, focal nodular hyperplasia, hepato-cellular carcinoma, etc.)
- Evaluate heart functioning (filling of ventricle, wall perfusion)
- Enhance signal in transcranial applications (vessels, brain tissue)
- Detect reflow of urine from bladder to kidney in children

Other applications such as breast imaging are currently under investigation.

Contrast agents are comprised of gas-filled microbubbles (with diameters of $< 10\ \mu m$). The microbubbles react to the pressure amplitudes of the transmit pulse by oscillating (expanding and contracting). The oscillating amplitude of the microbubbles at low ultrasound intensities is linearly proportional to the excitation pressure.

This dependency becomes nonlinear at larger oscillating amplitudes as the bubbles begin to oscillate at fundamental and higher harmonic frequencies. This effect does not depend on depth (in contrast to tissue) and occurs upon each interaction between a signal and a microbubble.

If the negative pressure amplitude exceeds a certain threshold value, the microbubbles will burst and the gas they release (e.g. air or perfluoride) will dissolve in the blood. In certain circumstances, this can be a useful tool in the context of ultrasound imaging (e.g. for stimulated acoustic emission or *SAE*). Ultrasound contrast agents of the first generation were mostly used in what is referred to as high mechanical index (*MI*) mode. The mechanical index is defined as follows:

$$MI = \sqrt{\frac{P_-}{f}} \tag{16.31}$$

High *MI* technologies are still in use today. Sonovist (Schering), for instance, has liver tissue specific properties that enable one to differentiate between liver tissue and other types of tissue.

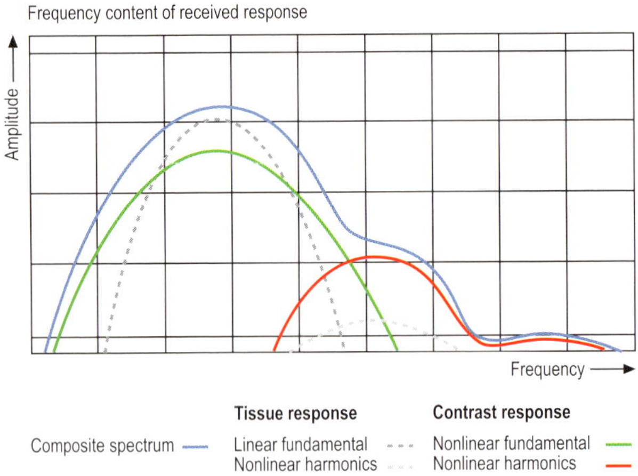

Figure 16.51 Schematic frequency content of the echoes received from tissue and contrast agent

One disadvantage associated with this technology is that all of the bubbles are destroyed during a single sweep (e.g. through the liver), making it impossible to perform real-time evaluations. Second generation ultrasound contrast agents (e.g. SonoVue®, Definity®, Optison™, and Imagent) are used at a low *MI* so that the bubbles do not burst and can be observed over a longer period of time. This longevity forms the basis for hemodynamic studies of the various perfusion behaviors that are associated with specific tissue properties.

Contrast harmonic imaging shows the harmonics of the echoes sent out by the oscillating microbubbles.

Traditional technologies involving contrast agents and ultrasound imaging (e.g. second harmonic imaging) have focused on the second harmonic properties of the contrast agents and tissue. While these techniques have proven helpful, it has become

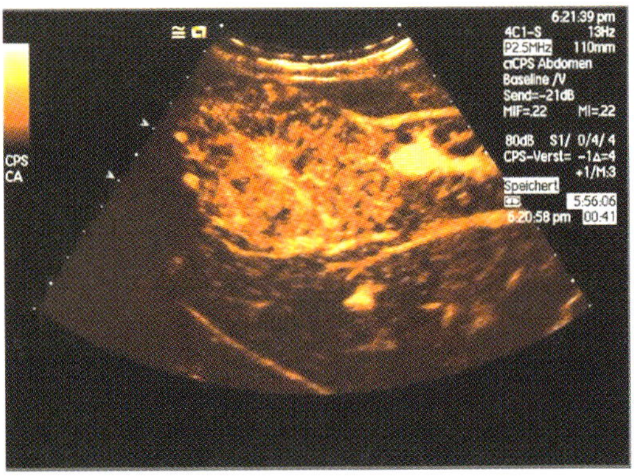

Figure 16.52
CPS study of a liver lesion (FNH – Focal Nodular Hyperplasia) demonstrating the central arterial supply with pronounced portal venous enhancement

clear that the second harmonic signals do not arise from the contrast agent alone, but also from tissue (fig. 16.51). This means that the contrast is diminished. Third-order harmonic imaging enables one to nondestructively image the contrast agent only (see section 16.5.3). This technique centers on the detection of nonlinear bubble expansion and contraction that is proportional to the third power of the exciting ultrasound pressure wave and contains both fundamental as well as third-order frequency components.

Contrast harmonic third-order imaging, also referred to as cadence contrast pulse sequencing (CPS), can be facilitated by applying at least three transmit pulses with different amplitudes and phases in succession. The resulting echoes can be combined to yield either an image with signatures that are unique to contrast agents or unique to tissue or both together. The specificity of the contrast agent to the tissue is significantly increased, thereby providing improved performance even at low *MI* power levels (fig. 16.52).

16.9.4 Compounding technologies and applications

Synthetic aperture

Digital beamformer technology was introduced to ultrasound imaging in the form of high-end systems in the middle of the 90s. The technology then became more broadly available around 5 years later, leading to dramatically increasing the performance of mid-range systems. Digital beamformer technology so enables one to improve spatial resolution by synthetically enlarging the receiving aperture.

While one can achieve optimal lateral focusing when receiving echo signals from deep regions by using the full width of the array, beamformers with a number of channels covering the total aperture are often too costly. Synthetic aperture technology is well known in the field of radar. The area of the transducer array is divided into subapertures that can be processed sequentially. The number of hardware processing channels can thus be kept manageable.

If one starts with 2 subapertures, the synthetic aperture technique will involve the application of two consecutive transmit pulses. The echo signals are processed after the first transmit pulse by one-half of the array elements in the beamformer and electronically stored. The echo signals of the second transmit pulse are received by the other half of the array elements, processed again in the beamformer and then added phase correctly to the previously stored information to form an image line. One thereby brings about the effect of twice the number of processing channels. The transmit pulse is excited from a group of elements (with half the total element number in the present case) that is always located in the same position in the middle of the active array area.

The synthetically enlarged aperture increases both sensitivity and lateral resolution in deeper body regions. However, it does so at the expense of the frame rate. The introduction of synthetic aperture technology to mid-range systems enables one to achieve nearly the same detail resolution capabilities associated with high-end systems (although with lower frame rates).

Spatial compounding

Ultrasound images are characterized by an interference pattern (speckle) that is determined by the frequency used. Methods of speckle reduction help one to achieve a more homogenous tissue presentation and with it a clearer rendering of differences in tissue properties. The methods of speckle reduction include spatial compounding and frequency compounding.

Spatial compounding involves the acquisition of images from different points of view. These images are then added together in a geometrically correct manner without considering phase effects. In most cases, the result is an attractive and smooth looking image.

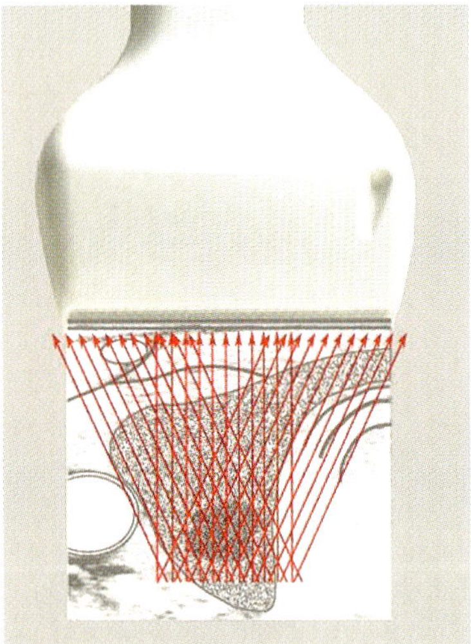

Figure 16.53
Spatial compounding via receiving subapertures (SieClear)

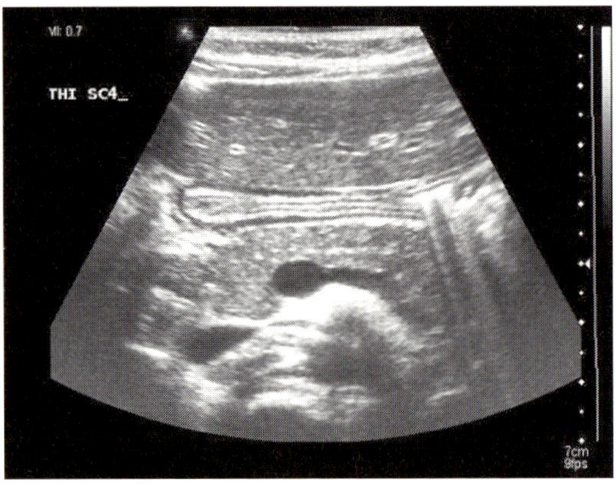

Figure 16.54
SieClear spatial compounding image of the pancreas

There are various approaches to spatial compounding (SC):

1. Transmitting in one direction only while receiving from different aspect angles (SieClear):
   This can be performed using different subapertures and a fixed transducer location. No movement of the transducer is necessary (figs. 16.53 and 16.54).
2. Transmitting and receiving from different aspect angles.
   This can be performed using different transducer apertures and a fixed transducer location.
3. Acquiring images by shifting the transducer manually (freestyle spatial compounding) in cutting-plane direction (figs. 16.55 and 16.56).
   This procedure can be also used to enlarge the field of view (panoramic imaging).

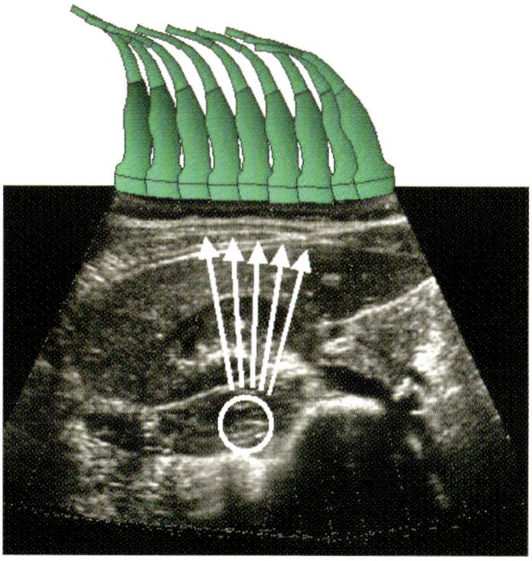

Figure 16.55
Freestyle manual shift of the image sampling location

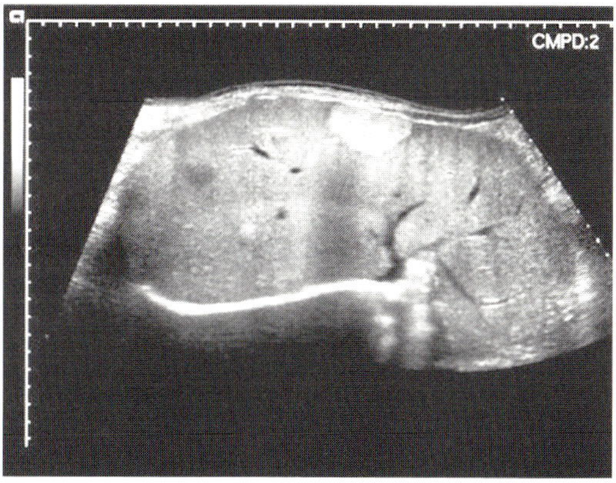

Figure 16.56
Liver mass imaged using freestyle spatial compounding

The various approaches are associated with following results:

1: Curved boundaries are more pronounced and show less angle dependency. Diagnostically relevant artifacts used as landmarks such as the shadowing behind strong reflectors (e.g. stones, microcalcifications) are still present. Areas are presented more homogenously. Tissue differences appear more striking.

2: Curved boundaries are enhanced (as in 1 above) and areas appear smoother. Diagnostically relevant artifacts often disappear, especially in the case of small structures.

3: Similar effects as in 2 above. The method is used in panoramic imaging to extend the field of view.

Frequency compounding

Compound images can be calculated from images that were acquired at the same geometrical site using different frequencies. The different frequencies correspond to different speckle patterns. The superimposition of these images leads to a more homog-

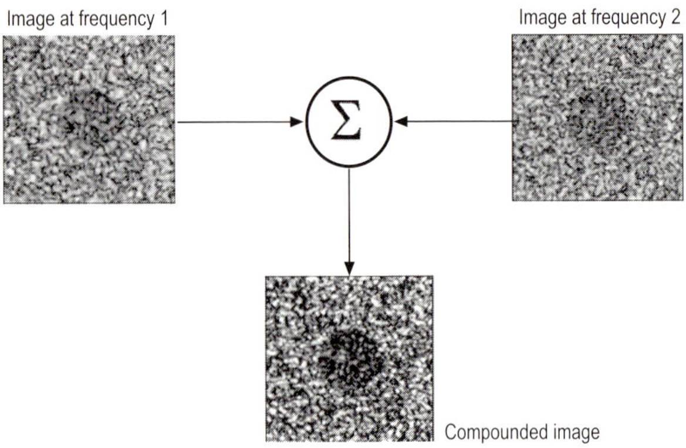

Figure 16.57
Frequency compounding

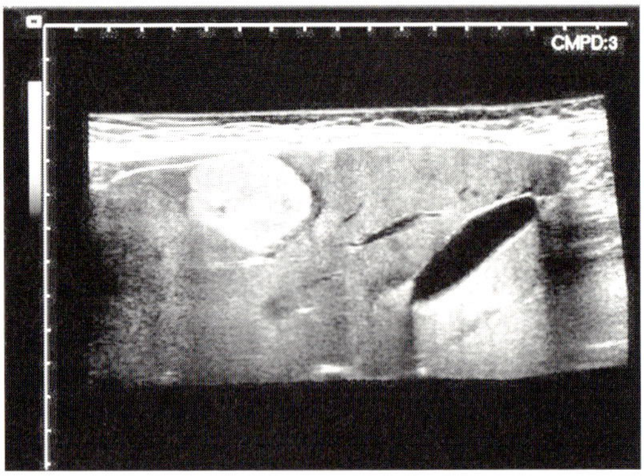

Figure 16.58
Liver mass rendered using frequency compounding

enous display of areas characterized by homogenous fine tissue (figs. 16.57 and 16.58). Given that the angle dependency of sound reflection still applies, the organ borders appear as they do in normal 2D imaging.

Panoramic imaging (SieScape)

Panoramic images (SieScape) are images calculated from many real-time images sampled by manually shifting the transducer in the scan-plane direction.

The calculation of the transducer's position in the absence of position sensors constitutes a special challenge for SieScape imaging (B-mode, fig. 16.59) and Color SieScape (power-Doppler mode, fig. 16.60). Such calculations are based on the similarity of consecutively scanned images.

A 2-dimensional panoramic image is obtained by guiding the transducer freehandedly across the sectional plane (x,y). The move from position 1 to position 2 can be described by two translational movements in x and y direction and a rotational move-

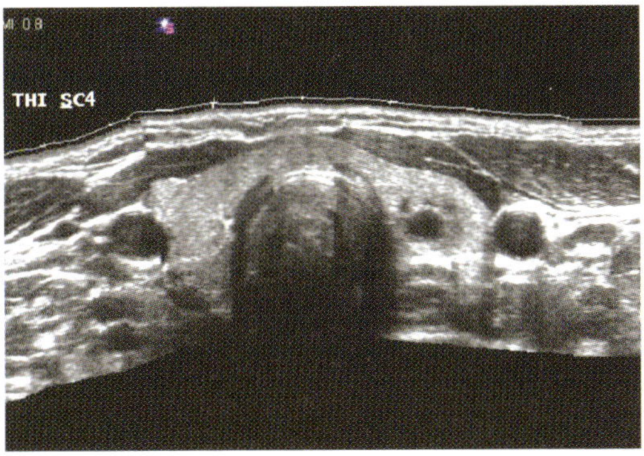

Figure 16.59
Panoramic image of the thyroid

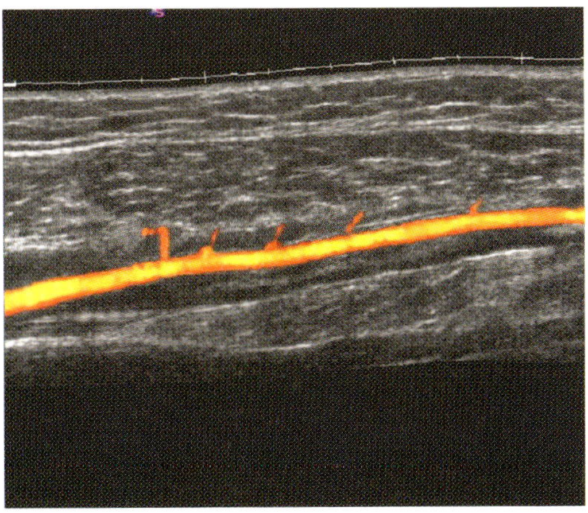

Figure 16.60
Panoramic power-Doppler image of the tibial artery

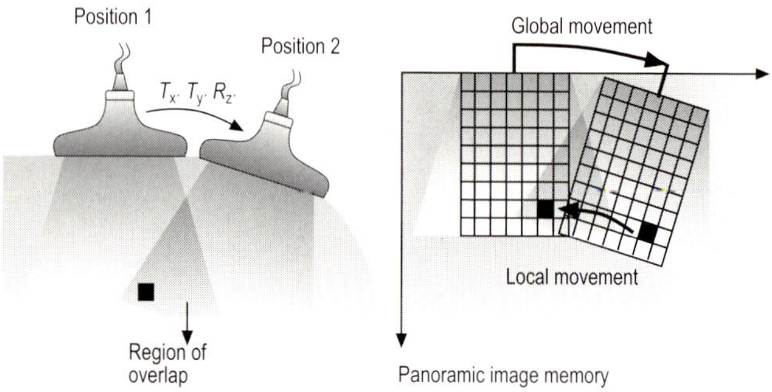

Figure 16.61 Position calculation using SieScape™

ment around the z axis perpendicular to the x-y plane. A direct move of the transducer in the z direction is not allowed.

The calculation of the transformation matrix is based on the similarity or equality of the image contents within overlapping regions. The images are first divided into segments and the local movement of the image content is calculated for each segment (fig. 16.61). The estimated global movement is obtained by analyzing the local movements. The calculation becomes more and more precise as an iterative comparison with actual image information is applied and as the movement parameters are corrected. The panoramic image is ultimately assembled from the original images (fig. 16.62). The precision of the image assembly enables one to apply the usual geometrical measurements in the panoramic image to even longer distances.

FreestyleDynamic (fig. 16.63) is a panoramic imaging technology that includes dynamic color clips of vessel perfusion, i.e. the dynamic color clips show the direction of blood flow and the hemodynamics within the panoramic image.

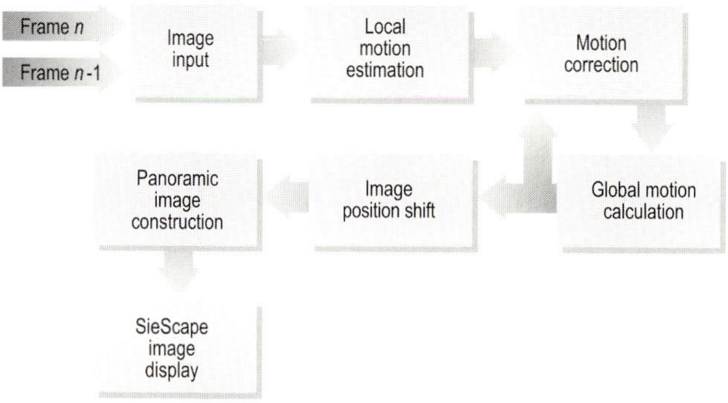

Figure 16.62 SieScape™ image reconstruction

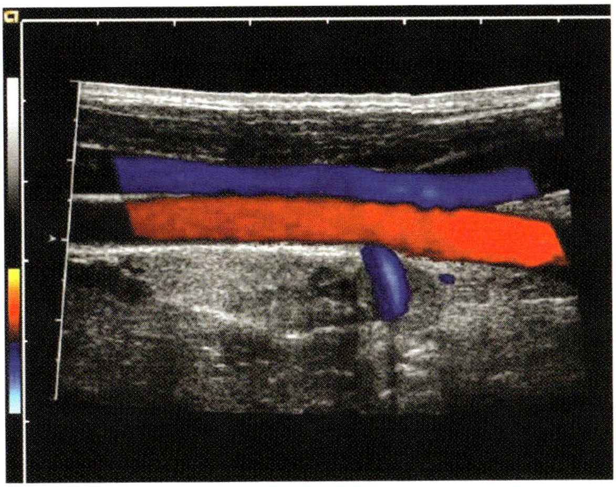

Figure 16.63 Arteria communis and vena jugularis rendered using panoramic imaging

The advantages of panoramic imaging technologies include:

- The creation of overviews of prolonged areas of up to 60 cm including precise distance measurements
- Overview image resolution that equals the resolution of individual high frequency images
- More precise comparison of different tissue textures in large organs

3D imaging

The high performance of the image processor and the motion correction procedures developed especially for SieScape imaging are the key to the acquisition of 3D images in real time. In order to acquire 3D images in B-mode and power-Doppler mode, one moves the transducer (freehandedly) parallel to z (i.e. perpendicular to the sectional plane), around the y-axis using rocket motion or around the center of the transducer using rotational motion. While position sensors are not required, they can be employed to achieve higher geometric accuracy.

Algorithms that are similar to those used in SieScape and based on echo information from adjacent layers are used to register the images for the sake of aligning the image data and determining the position of the transducer. 3D data sets for B-mode and power-Doppler mode are stored with isotropic voxels so as to enable standard post-processing at a later time.

The application of 3D real time puts the user in direct control of the quantity and quality of the image data, given the fact that a real-time mid-sagittal panoramic image is displayed on the monitor during image acquisition. The user can then immediately reconstruct and interactively depict organic and vascular structures at high resolution and in any orientation in addition to obtaining surface and volume-rendered views

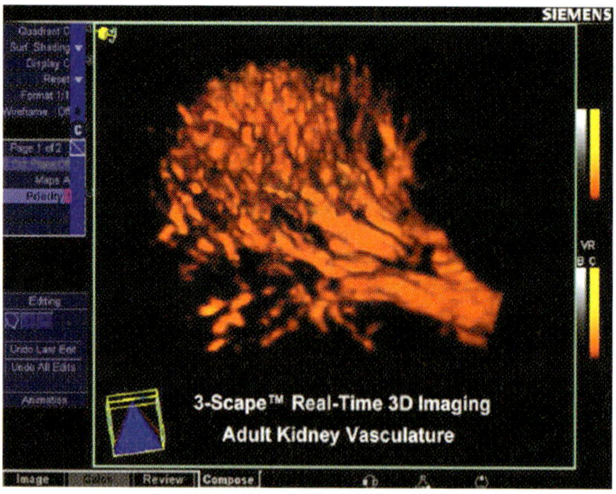

Figure 16.64
3D ultrasound image showing kidney vasculature

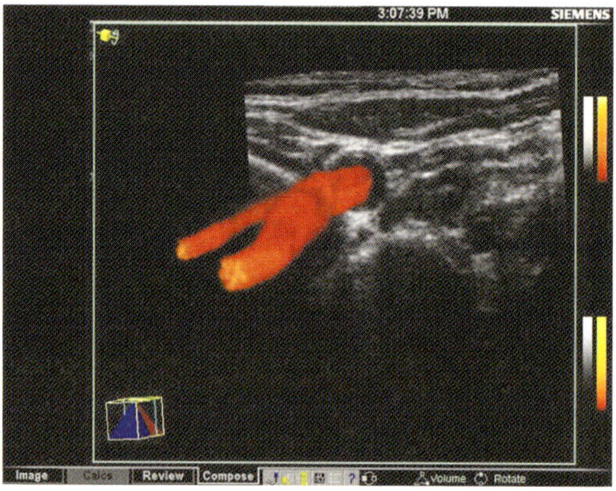

Figure 16.65
3D image of the carotid arteries

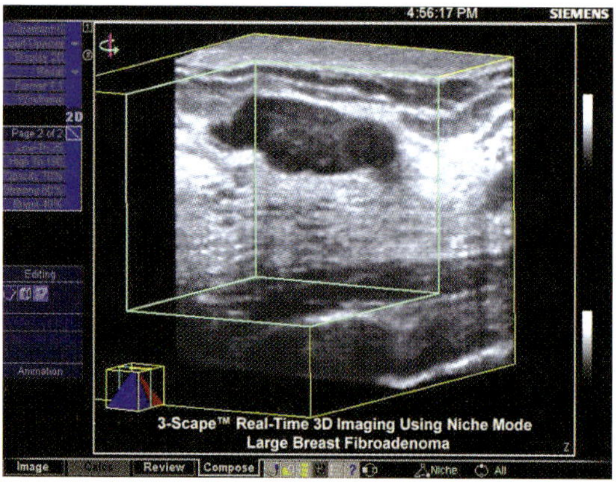

Figure 16.66
3D image of a breast fibroadenoma

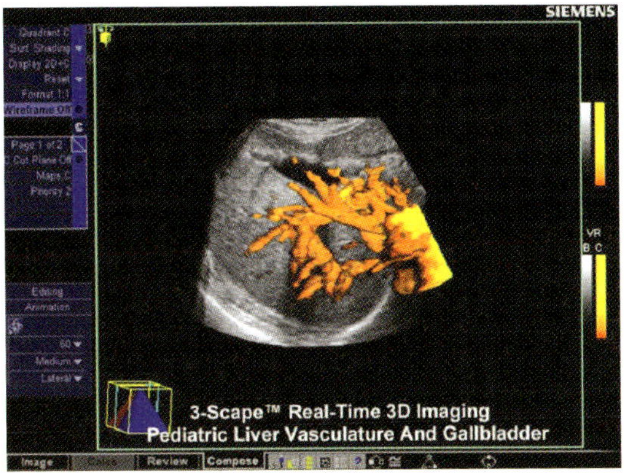

Figure 16.67
Pediatric 3D image showing liver vasculature and gallbladder

(e.g. maximum intensity projection) from any angle. B-mode and power-Doppler-mode data can also be selected (figs. 16.64 to 16.67).

4D imaging

3D volume presentations including the surface rendering of anatomic details (e.g. the fetal face) lead to impressive 3D images. One can augment the 3D presentation of parts of the fetal face or other details by refreshing the volume image at short intervals in order to show fetal movement. This defines 4D imaging. Several volumes can be presented per second (with maximum volume rates of 4 to 20 frames/s) in the case of obstetrics (fig. 16.68).

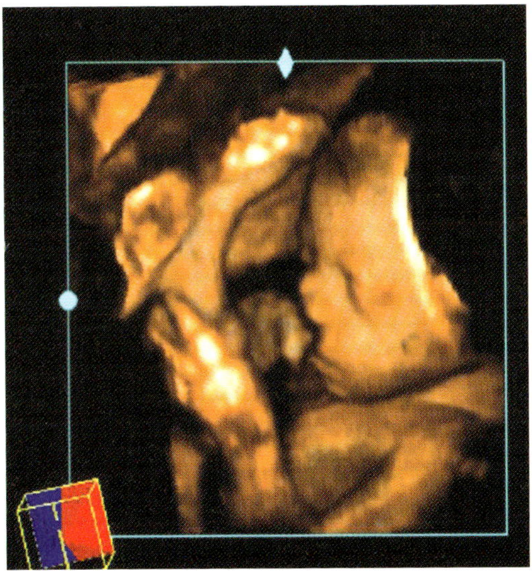

Figure 16.68
Fetal face from a 4D investigation

16.9.5 Workflow-improvement and standardization technologies

Tissue equalization technology (TEQ)

Intelligent image processing algorithms enable one to optimize the image parameters in the ultrasound system and keep them updated at the press of a button, tasks that would otherwise have to be performed manually (e.g. depth-gain control). TEQ™ technology (tissue equalization technology) makes use of the RF data of the echoes before the image is formed. Information acquired within a grid covering the field of view is analyzed via comparison with different tissue models (fig. 16.69). This is important when it comes to avoiding the overenhancement of hypoechogenic regions such as cysts and applying optimal noise filtering.

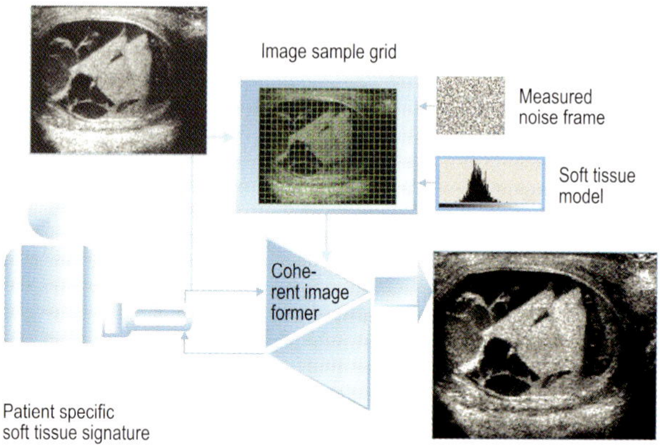

Figure 16.69
Tissue equalization technology (TEQ)

The receiver gain is automatically set in both image directions so that tissue presentation is optimal in both dimensions over the total image width and depth. This is equivalent to a 2D DGC (depth-gain control). Moreover, the gray level (i.e. the brightness and contrast) of fine tissue presentation (e.g. liver) is set in the same way that an ultrasound expert would set it. This accomplishment requires the implementation of artificial intelligence.

TEQ thus helps the system user to work faster and achieve standardized and reproducible results.

Autotracking contrast quantification (ACQ)

The technology that enables panoramic imaging can also be applied to other procedures such as automatic contrast quantification. It is often necessary to measure the inflow and outflow of contrast agents in areas of interest for longer acquisition periods (e.g. 2 min). This can be accomplished (even despite breathing activities) using automatic tracking (fig. 16.70).

Heart examinations involving the tracking of an area of interest represent a similar situation (see strain imaging below).

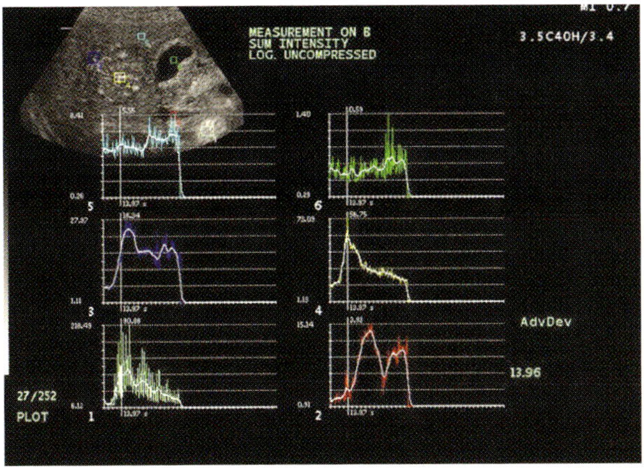

Figure 16.70
Autotracking contrast quantification. The contrast wash in / wash out curve is displayed for 6 areas of interest that have been tracked automatically.

16.9.6 Special cardiac transducers and evaluations

Transesophageal probes (TEE transducers)

Transthoracic cardiac imaging of structures in the atria is often hindered by chest walls that are too thick. The transesophageal approach is advantageous for various specific diagnostic purposes. An electronic sector probe offers the clinician a full spectrum of imaging modes (fig. 16.71). Turning the probe around the axis of the esophagus enables one to obtain 3D images of the beating heart using 4D technology (fig. 16.72).

The shorter distance to the heart permits one to use higher frequencies, and thus to obtain enhanced spatial resolution. This procedure is applied to investigate atrial defects, general atrial masses, valve functioning (fig. 16.73) and the presence of thrombogenic masses in the left atrium in cases of stroke and stroke prevention.

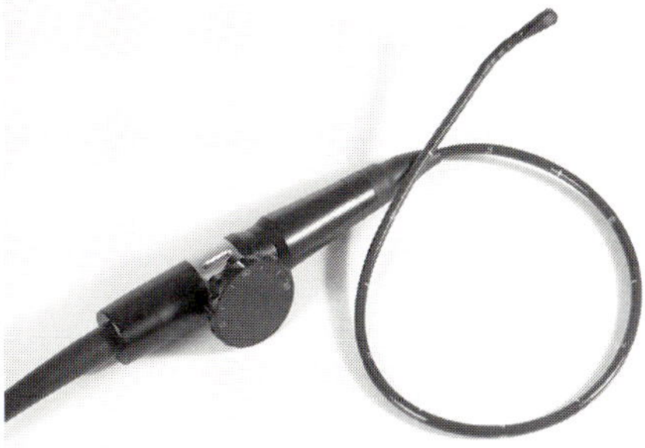

Figure 16.71
Transesophageal probe (TEE Transducer) for imaging the heart

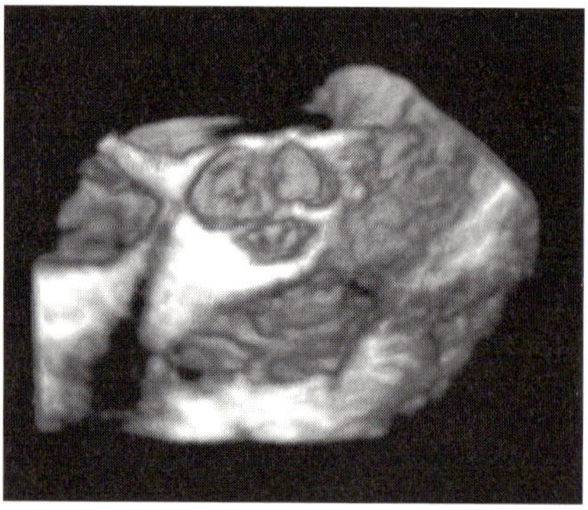

Figure 16.72
3D image of a heart from a 4D TEE series

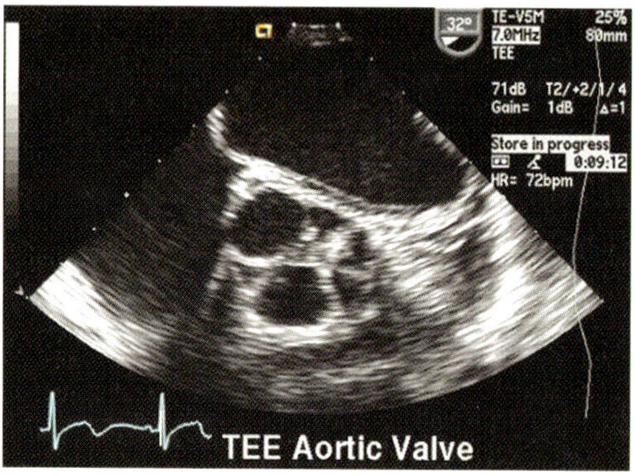

Figure 16.73
TEE image of the aortic valve

Intracardiac probes

In the case of electrophysical procedures, it is very helpful to be able to acquire images directly from the inside of the heart. AcuNav is a phased-array transducer set within a 10 or 8 French catheter (fig. 16.74). Introduced via the venous system, it is located in the right heart and can be applied, for instance, to bring about the exact placement of patent foramen ovale (PFO) closure devices. Simultaneous quality control can be performed using color Doppler (fig. 16.75) or spectral Doppler. Many other applications involving different locations in the body are possible. So as an example direct intrahepatic portal caval shunt (DIPS) placement (or the placement of other intrahepatic stents) can be monitored from the vena cava (fig. 16.76).

Special cardiac evaluation technologies

Application technologies such as the stress-echo method, Doppler tissue imaging (DTI), strain imaging (SI) and the coronary flow reserve (CFR) method are used to evaluate heart functioning on the basis of an investigation of the moving heart wall that is conceived to detect deficiencies in coronary blood flow support at a very early stage.

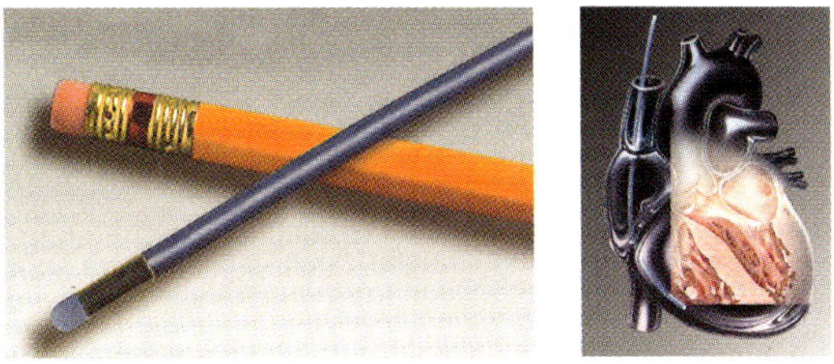

Figure 16.74
AcuNav catheter for ultrasound imaging from within the heart or large vessels. The catheter has a diameter of 3.3 mm (10 French). It employs 64 transmit and receive elements for an electronic sector scan.

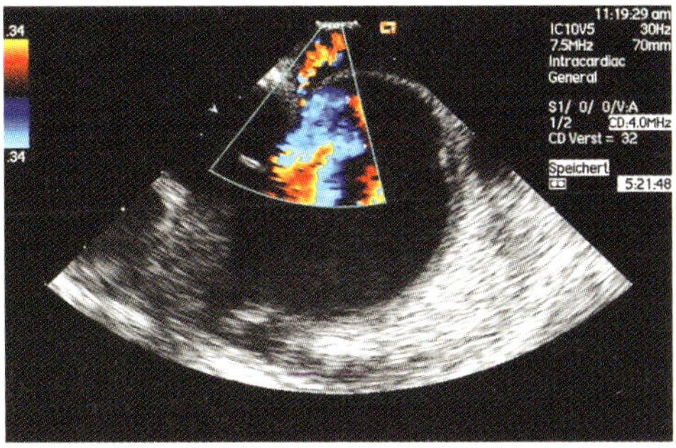

Figure 16.75
Color-flow image from a septum defect obtained with AcuNav from within the heart

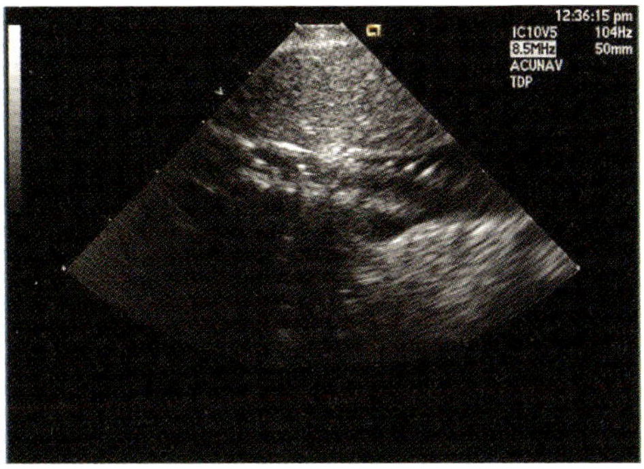

Figure 16.76
View from the vena cava with AcuNav showing a stent

The stress echo technique is used to compare heart wall thickness in different heart phases and different stress applications (mechanical or drug-induced stress) from single 2D images. This technique is especially effective in the diagnosis of coronary artery disease (CAD), which shows decreased wall contractility. A further application centers on the analysis of scarred myocardium.

Stress can be induced via exercise or the administration of e.g. dobutamine. Ultrasound images are usually acquired during 4 stages (rest, stage 1, stage 2, post stress).

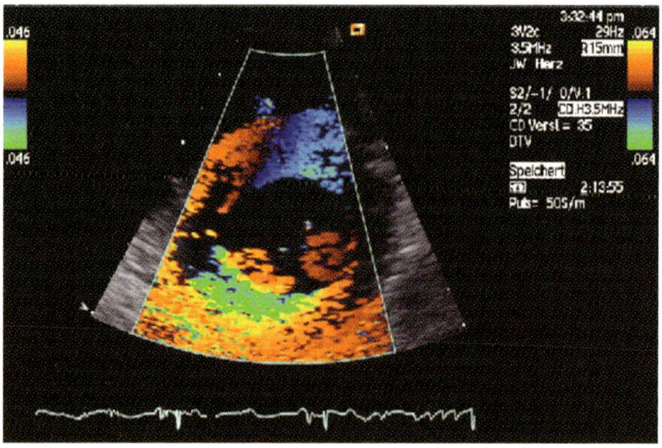

Figure 16.77 Doppler tissue imaging of the heart

The four most common views of the heart include parasternal long axis (PLAX), short apical axis (SAX), apical four chamber (A4C) and apical two chamber (A2C). Images are shown on a quad screen that compares one view from all of the stages (ECG gated) in order to ascertain changes in wall motion.

Doppler tissue imaging (DTI) is deployed to detect differences in wall velocities under different conditions (fig. 16.77). In the case of DTI, the Doppler information concerning tissue motion is displayed as an image. However, the fact that the color-coded result is angle-dependent makes interpretation difficult and even impossible in regions that move perpendicular to the insonification direction.

While the stress-echo technique is commonly used in clinical routine, strain imaging is regarded more as a research tool.

While similar to the stress-echo technique, strain imaging (fig. 16.78) involves a subtraction of the absolute movement of the heart. The values for the temporal development of strain across the heart cycle

$$\varepsilon(t) = \frac{L(t) - L(t_0)}{L(t_0)} \tag{16.32}$$

and the strain rate

$$\dot{\varepsilon}(t) = \frac{\mathrm{d}\varepsilon(t)}{\mathrm{d}t} \tag{16.33}$$

are derived.

Regional contraction can thus be assessed in order to discriminate between actively contracting and passively tethered myocardium.

The coronary flow reserve technique is designed to detect Doppler flow (spectral Doppler) at a distinct coronary artery branch (e.g. LAD, RCA) in the absence of and under drug-induced stress by transthoracic ultrasound (fig. 16.79). The Doppler spectrum is

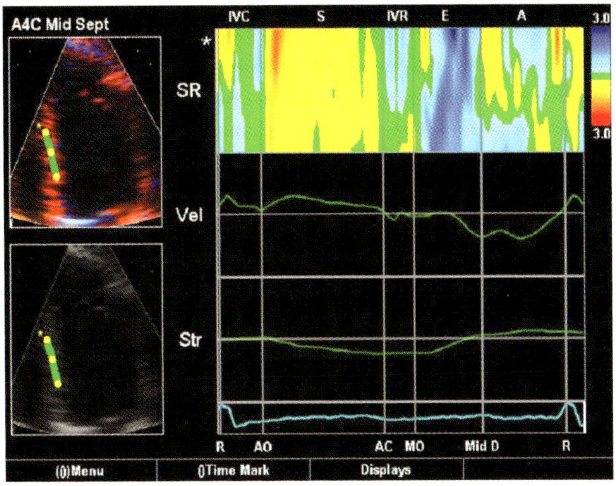

Figure 16.78
Quantitative strain imaging. Areas of interest are located at the ventricular septum in the color-flow **(upper left)** and B image **(lower left)**. The curves show velocity, strain and ECG. The **upper right** map displays the strain rate as a function of time.

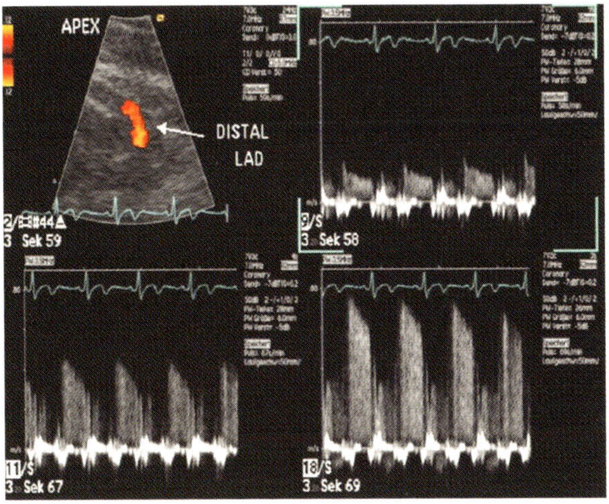

Figure 16.79
Study of coronary flow reserve. The **upper left** power-Doppler image shows the descendent left coronary artery at which a Doppler spectrum is obtained at rest **(upper right)** and at exercise (**lower left** and **right**).

measured at rest and at exercise (e.g. following the administration of adenosine). The ratio of the signals is identical to the ratio of volume flows and may indicate the presence of a stenosis, which may give cause for intervention. The technique is also applied as a follow-up examination to coronary intervention.

16.10 References

[16.1] C.B. Burckhardt
Speckle in ultrasound B-mode scans
IEEE Transactions on Sonics and Ultrasonics SU-25 (1978), 1-6

[16.2] R.N. Bracewell
The Fourier transform and its applications
McGraw-Hill, Inc., New York 1986

[16.3] T. Sumanaweera
Applying real-time shading to 3D ultrasound visualization
In R. Fernando (ed): GPU Gems, programming techniques, tips, and tricks for real-time graphics
Addison-Wesley, 2004

[16.4] C.M.W. Daft, D.G. Wildes, L.S. Smith, L.J. Thomas, W.M. Leue, and K.W. Rigby
Elevation beam profile control with bias polarity patterns applied to microfabricated ultrasound transducers
Proceedings of 1994 IEEE Ultrasonics Symp., 1491-1496

[16.5] J.I. Jackson, L.J. Thomas
Application of ultrasound-based velocity estimate statistics to strain-rate estimation
IEEE Trans. Ultrasonics, Ferroelectrics, and Freq. Control.50 (2003), 1464-1473

17 Special and hybrid systems

17.1 Imaging for radiation therapy

17.1.1 Introduction

Radiation therapy is a common form of cancer therapy; over half of all patients diagnosed with solid tumors will receive radiation therapy as part of their treatment. The most prevalent apparatus for delivering external beams of therapeutic radiation to the patient target is a linear accelerator, or linac, since the energies required are in the megavoltage (10^6 eV) range, primarily for reasons of penetration and skin-sparing.

Portal imaging is best understood in the context of its role in the radiotherapy process. A typical radiation treatment workflow begins with a CT scan, which allows the 3D definition of relevant target and healthy tissue structures (fig. 17.1a). Increasingly, images from other modalities such as MR and PET are also employed in this process. The next step is virtual simulation and treatment planning, in which advanced 3D or 4D (respiratory) visualization, optimization, and evaluation techniques are employed to select various treatment parameters such as beam energy, direction, shaping as well as spatial intensity modulation. The goal is to achieve adequate dose coverage of the target volumes with acceptable sparing of the neighboring healthy tissue, as shown in fig. 17.1b). At the end of the planning process, the treatment parameters are exported to the control system of the accelerator along with a set of digitally reconstructed radiographs (DRRs), constructed from the CT data. This is demonstrated in fig. 17.1c. The DRRs simulate X-ray projection images corresponding to the planned directions and shapes of the radiation beams.

Immediately before treatment, the patient is placed in the planned position on the table of the linear accelerator (linac) delivery system, shown in fig. 17.1d, usually by aligning lasers to tattoo marks on the skin. A portal X-ray image is acquired using the megavoltage photon beam. The cross section of the beam forming components is illustrated in fig. 17.1e. The image is captured on a deployable detector opposing the source. The point of the portal image is to confirm the placement of the radiation field with respect to the patient anatomy. The field shown in fig. 17.1f is indeed in agreement with the planned placement as reflected by the corresponding DRR shown in fig. 17.1c. Image registration techniques are often used to evaluate the correlation between the portal images and the DRRs and to determine required corrective measures.

Thus success of the therapy strongly depends on accurate alignment of the patient's target with the linac beam. All on-line imaging is motivated by the need to ensure that alignment. There are a variety of different types of portal images, taken at different points in the treatment process and with different exposures. A "pre-port" image tak-

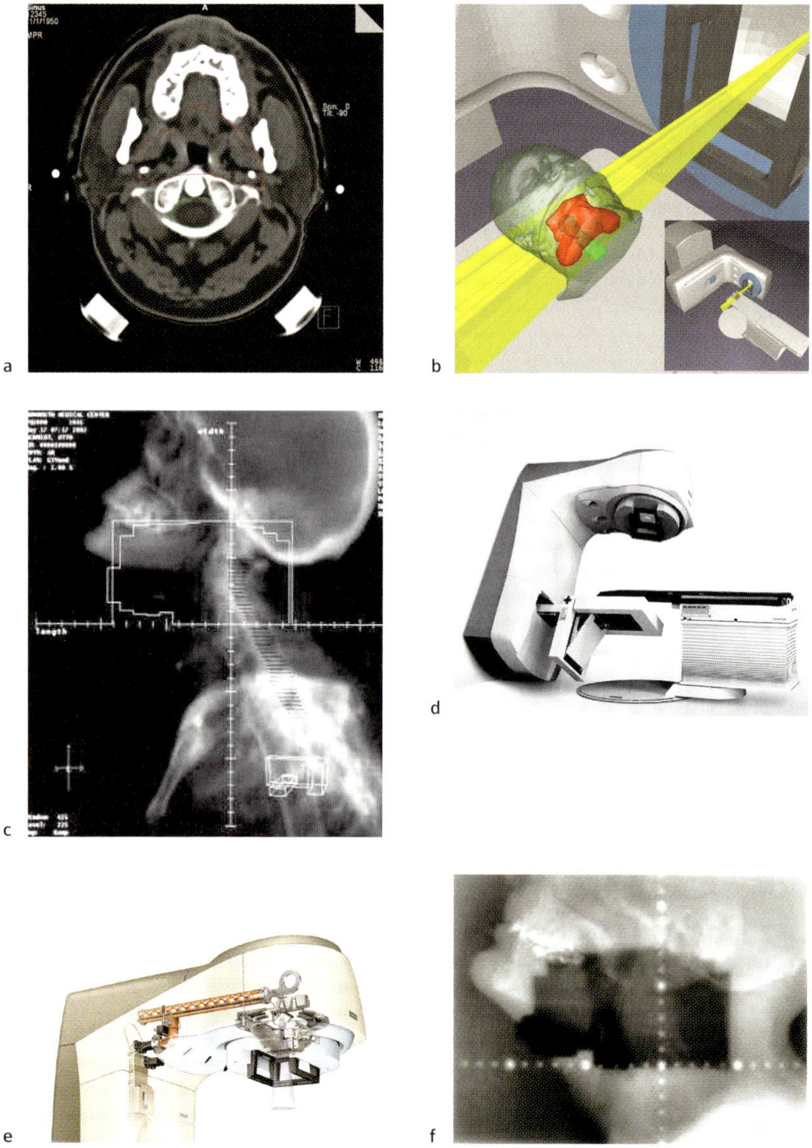

Figure 17.1 Various components of radiation therapy planning, delivery and verification systems. CT data is commonly used for localization and definition of target and critical structure volumes **(a)**. Virtual simulation and planning is performed to generate optimal treatment parameters in terms of beam directions and shapes **(b)**. Digitally reconstructed radiographs (DRRs) with superimposed radiation field outline are generated to serve as reference images for patient alignment prior to treatment **(c)**. Medical linear accelerator (linac) delivery systems are employed to generate megavoltage ionizing beams for external beam therapy **(d, e)**. Portal images of the patient in treatment position are acquired with the actual treatment beam and compared to DRRs for target positioning verification **(f)**.

en prior to starting the therapy, as described above, must be accomplished with the lowest dose that will yield sufficient quality for DRR registration (generally one monitor unit, or 1 MU[1]). In addition, a second type of portal image may be accumulated throughout the treatment delivery as a means of quality assurance of the entire process, resulting in a „verification image", also called a "port during" image of 50 MU or more. In more advanced applications, volumetric imaging is achieved by reconstructing many „projection images" from varying angles, each having 0.1 MU or less in order to keep the total patient imaging dose as low as possible. Thus it is generally difficult to optimize the system for any single purpose because of the wide range of applications desired.

17.1.2 The portal imaging beam

The linac system used for portal imaging is designed foremost for its therapeutic properties, and used only secondarily for imaging. Due to the different and sometimes conflicting requirements for these two operations, the beam itself is quite suboptimal for imaging. Several key aspects of the beam deserve discussion since they will have a significant impact on the image quality. The components are illustrated in situ in fig. 17.1e and in a magnified view in fig. 17.2.

The beam is formed when electrons are emitted from a gun and accelerated with microwaves through a multichambered waveguide which is over a meter long. The electrons gain energies of several MeV before reaching a magnetic bending sector, which allows desired energies in a narrow band (a few percent about the center energy) to pass through. The electrons then exit the vacuum and are incident on a thin high atomic number (gold or tungsten) target, as shown in fig. 17.2, which produces photons in a bremsstrahlung process. The spot size of the photon beam is approximately the same as the electron beam width at the target, about 2 mm typically and up to 4 mm.

The photons that exit the target have a broad spectrum, covering the entire range between almost negligible energy and the full energy of the electron beam (fig. 17.3). Since the photon angular distribution is forward peaked, most of the intensity is released in the center in the beam. Traditionally most radiation therapy prescriptions called for large flat fields across the tumor. For this reason, a flattening filter is commonly used to preferentially absorb the intensity in the central region of the beam such that the dose rate is forced to be equal across the maximum treatment field size of 40 cm by 40 cm about the isocenter[2]. Other elements on the beamline include a

---

[1] In a machine with standard calibration, 1 MU is equal to 1 cGy at a depth of maximum dose (e.g., d_{max} = 1.5 cm for 6 MV) at the linac isocenter.

[2] The isocenter is a point 100 cm from the target on the beam axis. Beams from multiple gantry angles will overlap at the isocenter, thus the patient is generally positioned such that the isocenter is central to their treatment volume.

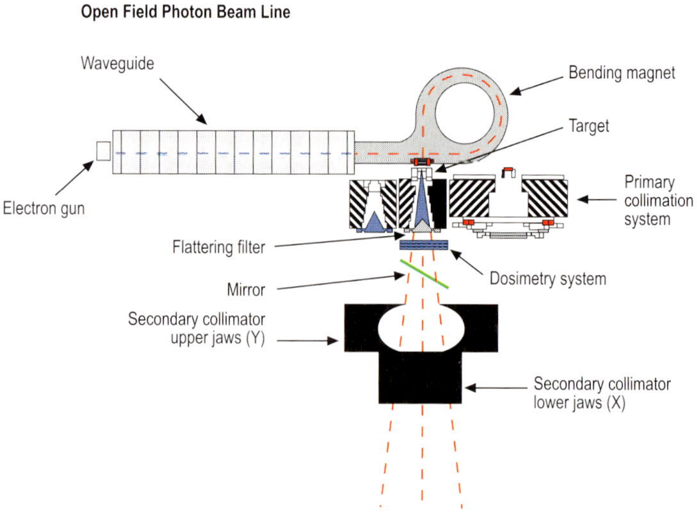

Figure 17.2
Cross-sectional view of a photon beamline. Electrons are emitted by the gun at left, accelerated through the multi-chamber waveguide, and steered through a 270-degree curve before impinging on a target. Approximately 1% of these electrons form bremsstrahlung photons (the rest are absorbed). The photons travel through the primary collimator, a flattening filter, a pair of ion chambers, a mirror (used to project a light field through the beam shaping devices onto the patient), and the lower variable jaws, which may include a multileaf collimator for conformal shaping of the radiation field to the target.

dose chamber for monitoring dose rate and field flatness/symmetry, and a mirror to direct a light field used for patient positioning.

By the time the beam reaches the patient, the average energy of the photons is significantly less than the energy of the incident electron beam, depending primarily on the filtration of downstream components, especially the flattening filter. For example, a typical clinical 6 MV beam has an average energy of approximately 2 MeV, and essentially all photons below 200 keV are absorbed before reaching the patient and the imager. The hardened beam traverses the patient, often including the table and/or immobilization devices, which are designed to as transparent as possible, and then reaches the imager typically at 140 cm to 160 cm from the source.

Due to these beam properties, typical portal images suffer from poor contrast and spatial resolution, especially in comparison to their counterparts acquired with kilovoltage X-rays. The gap in image quality mainly arises from the difference between the ways in which photons in these two energy ranges interact with biological tissues (fig. 17.3). At megavoltage energies, Compton scattering is the dominant mode of interaction, although the pair production process plays a minor role. The Compton process is free-electron interaction in nature, and therefore independent of the atomic number to first order. Thus any contrast of tissues in portal images is primarily deter-

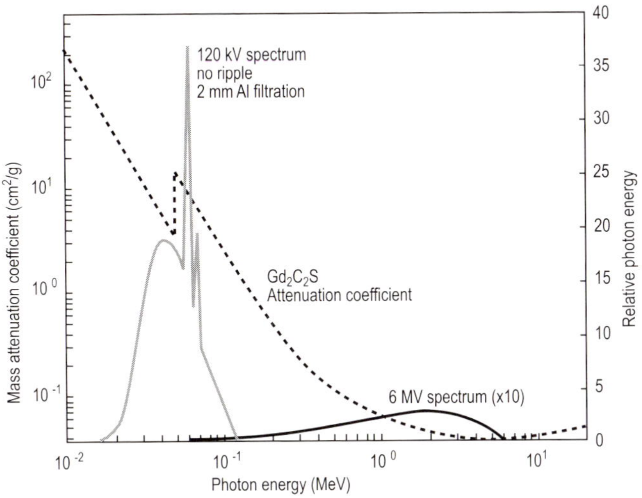

Figure 17.3
Energy dependence of the mass attenuation coefficient of Gd_2O_2S phosphor superimposed with the photon spectra of a kilovoltage (120 kV) and a megavoltage (6 MV) linac radiation sources. The magnitude of the 6 MV spectrum is multiplied by a factor of 10 for better visualization.

mined by difference in electron densities, and is nearly independent of the tissue composition when imaged with acceptably low doses. Hence it is challenging to differentiate tissues of similar densities but different compositions. On the other hand, for kilovoltage photons in diagnostic energy range, both Compton scattering and photoelectric effect take place. The attenuation coefficients are much larger (by approximately an order of magnitude) and the photoelectric process is strongly dependent on the atomic number, permitting much higher contrast differentiation at a comparable dose level.

17.1.3 Portal imaging detectors

Although in some cases external imaging devices may be available in the treatment room, it is desirable to treat and image from the same hardware without moving the patient.

Historically film cassettes with a build-up plate and phosphorescent screen were used. Although the quality of film systems was generally adequate for this purpose, using film is inconvenient. This is not only due to the usual limitations of hardcopy format, but also due to the time delay involved in processing the films, since linac time is extremely valuable. In fact, the total appointment time per patient daily, including set-up, imaging, corrections in positioning if required, and delivery of the treatment, is often constrained to approximately 15 minutes. Thus efficiency and streamlined workflow are very important aspects to the process. EPIDs (electronic portal imaging devices) offer a workflow improvement, but the camera and image intensifer systems used initally suffered from inferior image quality compared to film.

More recently, amorphous silicon (a-Si) flat panel imagers have been shown to compare favorably with film, and have become increasingly available for clinical use. A typical a-Si flat panel imager for therapy is substantially similar to those used for diagnostic imaging. It consists of a housing, a build-up plate, a scintillator and a photodiode array with associated electronics to read it out. However, each of these components is subject to unique constraints due to the application.

Buildup plates of various materials and thickness are used with the scintillator screen [17.1] to capture more megavoltage photons and help the charged particles to reach equilibrium at the detector. However, the improvement in the detection efficiency usually comes at the expense of decreasing spatial resolution [17.2, 17.3].

A scintillator screen on a typical flat panel imager, such as the Kodak Lanex screens, has a much larger probability to intercept kilovoltage photons than megavoltage ones. Consequently the imager has higher detective quantum efficiency (*DQE*) when used in conjunction with the diagnostic energy photons [17.4, 17.5] than it does in the therapy regime.

Finally, because much of the megavoltage beam will pass through the detector, the radiation sensitive electronics must be moved out of the primary beam path to the periphery of the panel, which may be as large as 40 cm $\times$ 40 cm at the isocenter. The additional lead lengths introduce more electronic noise than seen in diagnostic panels.

As in other imaging modalities, scattered photons cause image degradation in electronic portal images by increasing the noise in the image and decreasing the spatial resolution. This problem has been mitigated in diagnostic imaging by placing a divergent grid of an attenuating material over the detector. Radiation that has undergone significant scattering is absorbed and thus rejected from the image. Unfortunately this physical approach can not easily be applied to megavoltage imaging because of the unwieldy thickness that an effective grid would require. However the scatter cross sections at megavoltage energies are lower than those at kilovoltage, the average energy of the scattered photons is higher and the angular distributions are more forward peaked. Thus the scatter can be improved somewhat by increasing the distance between the patient and the detector, allowing fewer scattered photons, particularly those generated in the patient, to intercept the detector. Increasing the air gap also decreases the field of view, however; the tradeoff must be weighed in the larger clinical context.

In addition to the inherent decrease in subject contrast, a major factor for the poor image quality of megavoltage images in comparison to kilovoltage ones is the dramatic drop in the photon detection efficiencies of the existing detectors as the energy of the imaging beam approaches the megavoltage range. Fig. 17.3 illustrates the energy dependence of the mass attenuation coefficient of Gd_2O_2S phosphor superimposed with the photon spectra of kilovoltage (120 kV) and a megavoltage (6 MV) linac radiation sources. (Gd_2O_2S is often used in combination with photodiode amorphous silicon arrays in digital X-ray imaging systems). Fig. 17.3 also demonstrates that, while the interaction properties of Gd_2O_2S are quite well matched with the typical kV X-ray spectrum, the megavoltage spectrum spans an energy range in which the Gd_2O_2S X-ray interaction probability approaches its minimum. Thus, for the same photon fluence impinging on the X-ray detector, the overall probability of X-ray interaction for a megavoltage beam is more than two orders of magnitude smaller than that for a kilovoltage beam and therefore there is at least tenfold deterioration in the image signal-to-noise ratio.

In order to augment the photon detection efficiency, portal-imaging detectors are designed with a high-density "build-up" metal plate on the top of the scintillating material. In this case, besides the direct detection of X-ray photons within the phosphor, there is an additional mechanism to photon detection and image formation.

For a typical portal detector with a 1 mm copper "build-up" plate, Compton recoil electrons generated by photons with energy above 1 MeV interacting within the body of the metal plate have a sufficient range to reach the phosphor where their remaining energy is converted to light. This mechanism further enhances the detection efficiency of the portal-imaging detector. The magnitude of the enhancement depends on numerous factors such as the photon energy, phosphor thickness and composition, as well as metal plate thickness and composition. Furthermore, there is a compromise between the detection efficiency of the detector and the additional image blur introduced by the spread of the recoil electrons. A detailed discussion and evaluation of these effects is given in [17.6-17.8].

17.1.4 Advanced techniques

Megavoltage beamline optimization

There are several ways to improve the existing beamline of a therapeutic accelerator for imaging.

For example, in place of the usual bremsstrahlung target, a low atomic number target may be employed to preserve the soft part of the initial bremsstrahlung spectrum and minimize the photoelectric absorption of the kilovoltage photons in the target [17.5, 17.9-17.11]. A copper (or aluminum) target of millimeter thickness may be used in a special mode on the linac to produce portal images of higher contrast and resolution. The flattening filter may also be removed in the imaging mode, to further increase the influence of diagnostic energy X-rays and reduce scatter.

X-ray sources

One obvious way to improve the image quality is to use a separate X-ray source specifically for imaging. This may be achieved by making a diagnostic imaging modality available in the treatment room, such has been done with CT scanners on rails that slide it toward the linac for imaging, portable C-arm imagers or kV tubes mounted directly on the linac gantry.

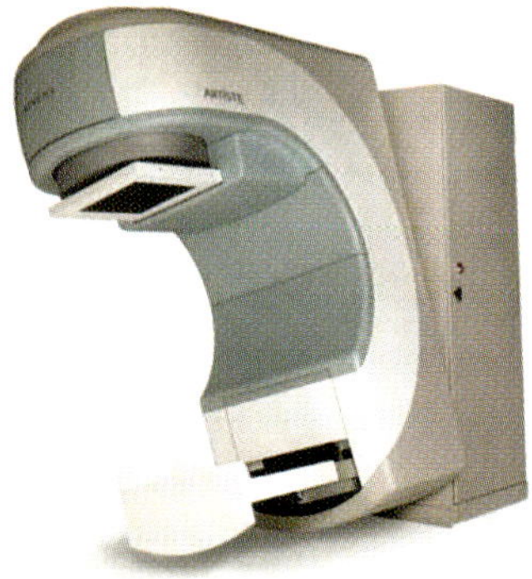

Figure 17.4
A linac design concept which incorporates a diagnostic X-ray tube in a retractable lower shelf (shown extended) which projects onto a flat panel imager in the accessory tray of the linac. For treatment, this detector may be retracted if not being used. Alternatively if it is desirable to obtain kV images interspersed with the treatment pulses, the MV beam is allowed to pass through the upper panel from the backside before reaching the patient. In this case the MV beam undergoes minor attenuation which is accounted for in the treatment.

An advantage of this approach is that they can also be used in a fluoroscopic mode, which is particularly useful to monitor respiratory motion. This technique is most effective when the treatment beam and the new source are co-linear, such that the motion in the treatment “beam's eye view“ can be accounted for. An example of this kind of machine is shown in fig. 17.4.

New detectors

Imaging detectors designed for kilovoltage applications have inherent low detection efficiencies when used for portal imaging applications. For this reason there has been a continuous research effort toward the design of high detection efficiency dedicated to megavoltage imaging applications such as for instance linac-based cone beam computed tomography (CBCT).

Two different approaches have been pursued. In the first, the thickness of the energy conversion layer (i.e., amorphous selenium or phosphor screen) is increased to compensate for the inherently low interaction probability of phosphor materials at megavoltage energies (fig. 17.3). This, however, will significantly decrease the spatial resolution mainly due to X-ray scatter in the thick conversion layer (and also the spread of optical photons in the case of phosphor screens). In order to have a high-detection efficiency while maintaining resolution, the energy conversion layer of flat panel systems must be redesigned. Possible examples of the redesign for the conversion layer include the use of segmented phosphor (e.g., CsI) with reflective layers in between segments that can be straight [17.12] or focused [17.13] toward the X-ray source of the linear accelerator (linac). The use of the segmented phosphor is to reduce the spread of optical photons generated by X-rays by multireflecting optical photons within each phosphor segment and collecting them on the same pixel element.

The second approach enhances the conversion of the build-up plates by involving high-density-material (HDM) converters (e.g., W) [17.14, 17.15] in air or in organic liquid with electrostatic focusing in which the electric field lines are focused toward the X-ray source. X-rays are converted first into energetic secondary electrons primarily in the HDM converters and then into ions in the air or organic liquid. The range of energetic electrons generated by megavoltage X-rays is much larger than that generated by diagnostic imaging X-rays, about 1.7 mm for Cu and 0.7 mm for W for a 6 MV photon beam. If the size of the HDM converters is smaller than the electron range, most of the energetic electrons generated in the converters will escape and generate ions in the air or organic liquid. These ions can then be driven by the electric field lines where they are collected on electrodes and read out by an active matrix. Further details on these new detectors can be found in [17.12-17.15].

Volumetric image reconstruction

Although a pair of orthogonal images has been commonly used to locate the isocenter of the treatment plan relative to the patient's anatomy, full three-dimensional imaging with the „cone beam" is also possible. This is achieved by sweeping the linac gantry in an arc having an extent of at least 180 degrees plus half the fan angle. Note that the fan angle is variable depending on the placement of the imager. The MV linac (or external kV source) is then triggered to pulse every degree (or few degrees) of rotation. The imager is read out between two pulses to obtain each projection image. The projection images can then be backprojected and reconstructed using a Feldkamp-based algorithm.

The rotation of the linac gantry is currently limited by regulatory agencies to 1 rpm, and the mechanical precision of the isocenter is ±1 mm. Thus the acquisition is slower than diagnostic modalities, and the orbit is slightly eccentric but is accounted for using a correction matrix obtained during a calibration run at each projection [17.16].

The MV- or kV-cone beam CT reconstructed image can then be fused with the planning CT either manually or automatically [17.17]. Once the vector offset between the fused CTs has been established, if it is above a critical threshold the patient table is shifted along its x, y, and z axes to approximate this vector and bring the target into better alignment before the treatment begins.

Dosimetry

Another recent trend is to use the imager not only as a tool for assessment of anatomy and positioning but also as a quantitative dosimeter. The flat panel responds linearly to the amount of megavoltage irradiation received by it. For each detector pixel, a ray is traced back to the source through the patient and other attenuating material in the beampath. A CT scan is used to provide this information (note that for a CT scan taken at kilovoltage energies the attenuation coefficient different than that experienced by

Table 17.1
ICRU compact bone and soft tissue mass attenuation coefficients (μ/ρ) and corresponding radiographic contrast C (1 mm thick bony structure in tissue) at 50 keV and 1 MeV.

Energy (MeV)	$(\mu/\rho)_{bone}$ (cm^2/g)	$(\mu/\rho)_{tissue}$ (cm^2/g)	C (%)
0.05	0.4242	0.2264	5.5
1.00	0.0656	0.0700	0.5

the megavoltage beam, see table 17.1). Knowing the incident spectrum, the radiographic attenuation can then be used to approximate the energy left behind, most of which is absorbed by the patient as dose.

17.1.5 Summary

In summary, there are a number of challenges in conventional portal imaging, especially when compared to diagnostic imaging sytems:

- High beam energy (low interaction cross sections and low contrast)
- Broad energy bandwidth
- Large spot size
- Large area detector
- No anti-scatter grid feasible for megavoltage photons
- Large source to detector distance required
- Large dynamic range required for various applications
- Limited time for imaging, reconstruction and analysis

Some of these challenges have been mitigated by having other dedicated imaging modalities available in the treatment room such as CT scanners, X-ray tubes on board the gantry or portable C-arms. To be most useful, the kV source should be co-linear with the treatment beam in order to monitor the tumor from the beam angles that are most relevant to the therapy. Nonetheless, there are advantages to imaging with the treatment beam directly, either to obtain the true beam's eye view through the treatment port of the anatomy, or as a verification mechanism of the total treatment, either qualitatively or quantitatively using exit dosimetry.

At present, although imaging with the megavoltage treatment beam is challenging, many improvements are anticipated, including optimization of the beamline for a softer spectrum; optimization of the detector to increase the response to the incident beam; and volumetric reconstruction. Workflow improvements provided by integrated software will make it convenient to incorporate these images into clinical decision making, including adaptation of the treatment to dynamic patient anatomy. The new era of radiotherapy promises to have an unprecedented level of image guidance.

17.2 Hybrid systems: PET/CT and SPECT·CT

Functional imaging with PET and SPECT provides detailed information on metabolic activities in patients. While FDG imaging provides some anatomical landmarks, more specific tracers make the task of anatomical registration more difficult. Moreover, FDG uptake is sometimes very difficult to localize and characterize.

The need for combined functional and anatomical imaging has led to the introduction of combined PET/CT and SPECT/CT systems such as the Siemens biograph (fig. 17.5) and the Siemens TruePoint SPECT·CT technology (fig. 17.11).

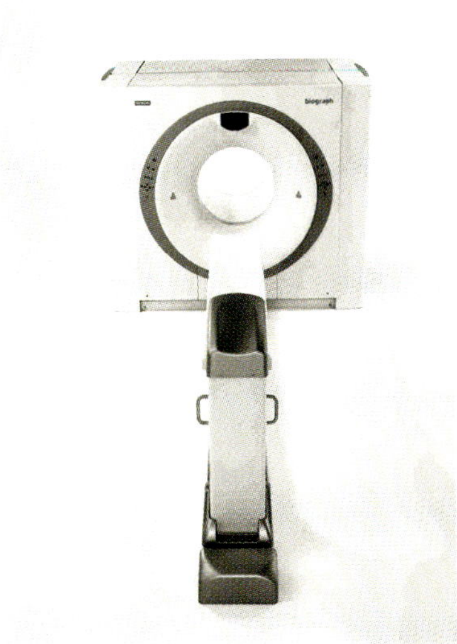

Figure 17.5
Combined PET/CT system (Siemens biograph)

17.2.1 Clinical benefits of combined functional and morphological imaging

Combining anatomical and functional imaging in a single clinical setting offers several advantages:

- The quick and interactive topogram provides an easy and effective means of positioning the patient for both the spiral CT and a PET or SPECT scan.
- The subsecond rotation of the CT tube enables a fast whole-body spiral CT. This can be used to calculate the attenuation map [17.18] for the attenuation and scatter correction of a PET or a SPECT scan.
- The high statistical quality of the attenuation map generated by the CT enables shorter emission scan times.
- A perfect match between the patient position in the CT and the emission scan allows for the anatomical localization and quantification of tracer uptake.
- Anatomical and functional information are available at the same time to support the physician when it comes to arriving at a diagnosis.
- The short combined scan improves patient comfort.

17.2.2 Design criteria for PET/CT systems

The biograph PET/CT system combines the anatomical information generated by the CT scan with the information on metabolic activity generated by PET. Combined systems are required to enable the highest degree of flexibility for both applications.

- The PET/CT system enables diagnostic CT studies that reflect currently available degrees of quality and flexibility. It is also to enable low dose applications for the calculation of attenuation maps whenever a diagnostic CT is not needed.

- The PET/CT system is to enable the full spectrum of PET applications.
- A patient handling system is required to operate on the basis of an identical patient position for PET and CT scanning.
- PET and CT applications have to to be integrated for easy PET/CT scanning and processing.

The standard CT components in the biograph enable diagnostic CT imaging with 2, 6, 16, and 64 CT slices of the highest quality. The standard LSO detector technology of the ECAT ACCEL is used for PET, either with the standard 8 × 8 block or the new high-resolution 13 × 13 block. The patient handling system exhibits a completely new cantilever design that enables precise patient positioning (all patients up to 204 kg) for CT and PET.

The integration of PET and CT acquisition, reconstruction and processing is accommodated by the *syngo* platform. Post-processing and clinical applications are performed at a workstation (Siemens Leonardo) that provides an interface to the full spectrum of multimodality applications (including virtual simulation and radiation therapy).

17.2.3 PET/CT applications

Drawing upon experiences gained between 1996 and 1998 with the first prototype of a PET/CT system, Siemens introduced the biograph in 2001 [17.19]. Since this time, the clinical and research applications enabled by the system have been fully exploited and increases in sensitivity and specificity as well as changes in patient management have been reported [17.20, 17.21].

PET/CT has become the ideal tool for pharmacological research and molecular imaging. While specific tracers only highlight certain areas and structures in the body, the anatomical information contributed by the CT enables one to localize and quantify their uptake.

Oncology

As with dedicated PET, most PET/CT studies are related to oncology (fig. 17.6). In addition to the typical functions associated with dedicated PET, PET/CT systems enable a much better differentiation between normal tissue and tumor uptake. This is especially true for areas exhibiting high anatomical-structure density such as the head, neck and abdomen. Uptake due to inflammation and muscle activity can be clearly localized.

Oncology patients whose investigations require the use of extended axial scan fields benefit considerably from the shorter acquisitions times (fig. 17.7).

PET/CT can help one to ascertain the best location for biopsy and interventional procedures. PET/CT information can be used for radiation therapy. In addition to the standard CT information on tumor localization and size, the PET dataset provides insight into the metabolic activity of the cancer. This may lead to a redefinition of the treatment plan. Today's planning systems (e.g. coherence workplaces) allow for the integration of PET and CT for optimized radiation therapy.

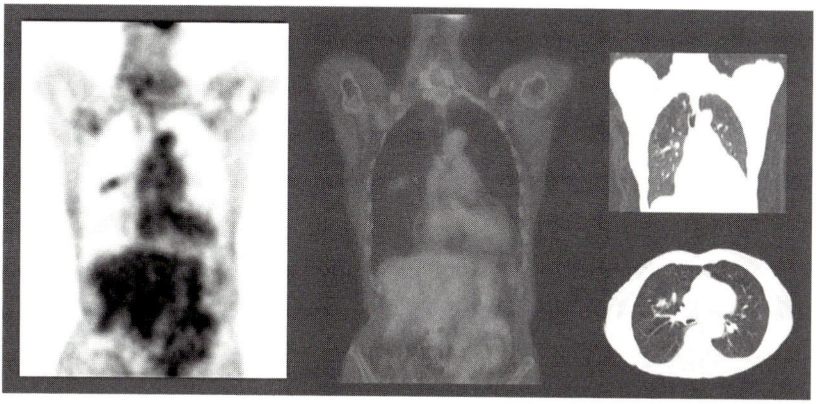

Figure 17.6 Pulmonary nodule (Source: CCF, Cleveland, OH, USA)

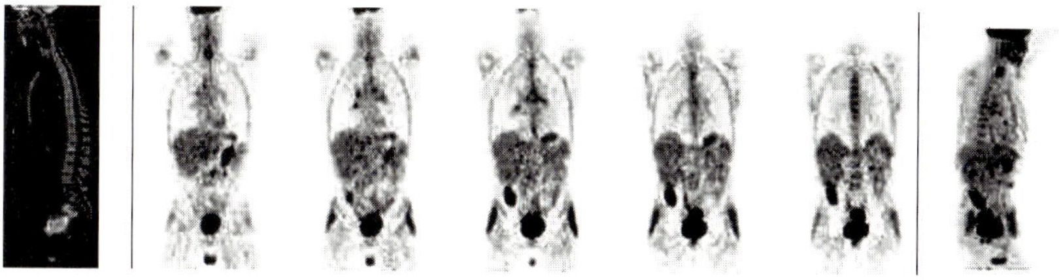

Figure 17.7
A biograph whole-body study performed in less than 10 minutes (Source: UTMC Knoxville, TN, USA)

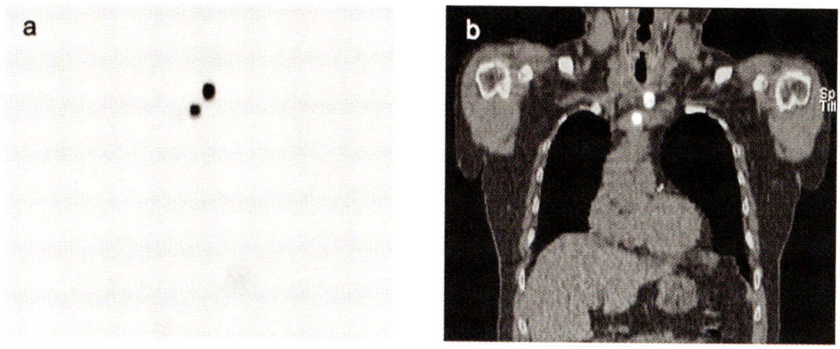

Figure 17.8
I-124 uptake in a patient with thyroid cancer in PET **(a)** and in the fused study **(b)**. The CT information is needed to correctly diagnose the patient (Source: University Essen, Germany)

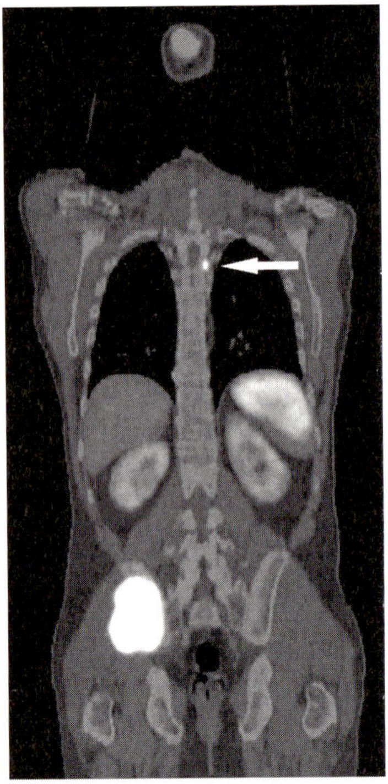

Figure 17.9
Specific uptake of ^{68}Ga-DOTATOC, see also fig. 14.26 (Source: MHH, Hannover, Germany)

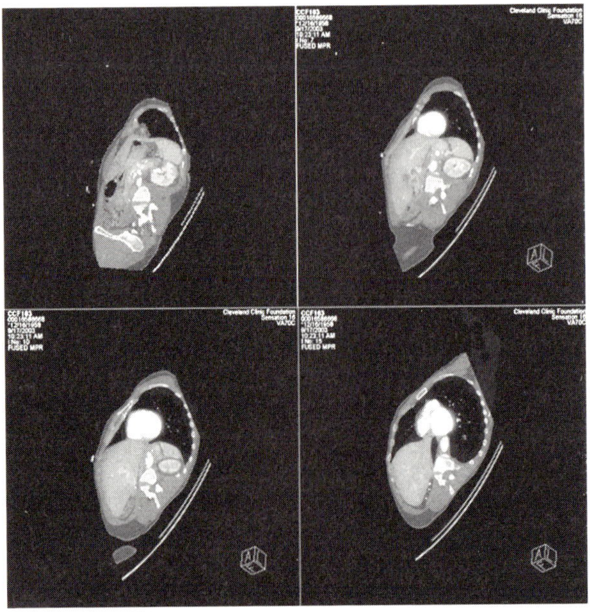

Figure 17.10
Cardiac FDG scan with IV contrast CT (Source: CCF, Cleveland, OH, USA)

The additional anatomical information is necessary for correct diagnosis in the case of highly specific tracers such as ^{124}I for thyroid cancer (fig. 17.8) and ^{68}Ga-DOTATOC for neuroendocrine tumors (fig. 17.9).

Cardiology

For cardiology, the PET/CT can provide the full spectrum of PET and CT examinations in a single clinical setting (fig. 17.10). Myocardial perfusion and metabolism can be combined with the high spatial and temporal resolution of modern spiral CT systems. Calcium scoring and angiographic CT procedures can be combined with PET information to enable improved cardiac examinations. Gating the CT or the PET scan will enhance the diagnostic possibilities even further.

17.2.4 SPECT and CT

In the time since PET/CT scanners first became available around the year 2000, it has become clear that these hybrid scanners offer synergistic possibilities that go well beyond what can be achieved with two stand-alone modalities. The improvements in clinical workflow and diagnostic accuracy that are made possible by PET/CT devices have inspired the development of a similar combination involving SPECT and CT. The functional information provided by new and highly specific SPECT tracers, which are currently being developed to include a high target-to-background ratio for application in oncology and cardiology, can thus be combined with morphological image information.

Clinicians have used software to combine SPECT images with CT images for many years. CT is used with SPECT to provide data both for attenuation correction in image reconstruction and for image fusion. Siemens TruePoint SPECT·CT unifies state-of-the-art SPECT with comprehensive multislice CT (fig. 17.11). The accurate attenuation contributed by CT significantly improves the image quality of the SPECT reconstruction (fig. 17.12). Accurate diagnostic information available at the molecular and anatomical level can be captured with a single scan and displayed in a single image (fig. 17.13).

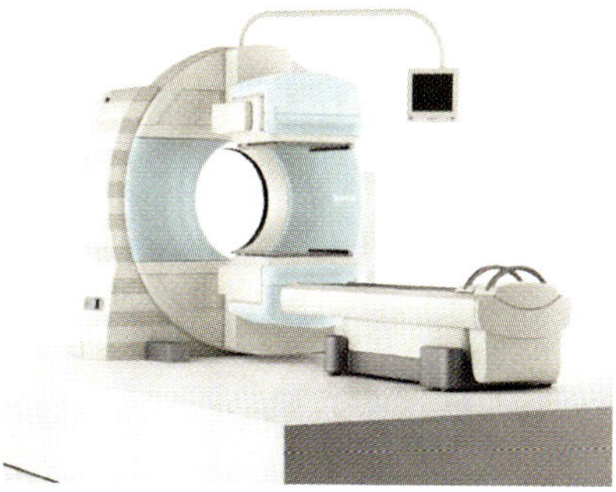

Figure 17.11
TruePoint SPECT·CT hybrid imaging system (Siemens Symbia)

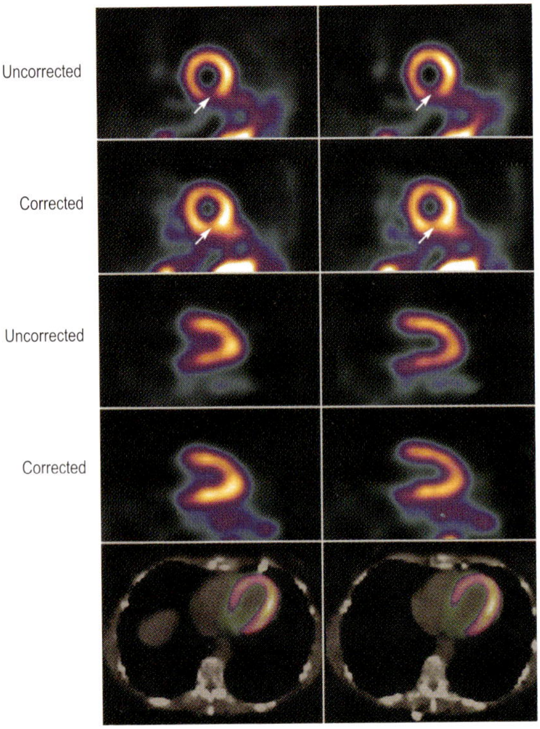

Figure 17.12
Comparison of SPECT images with and without attenuation correction from a myocardial perfusion study. Attenuation data are taken from a diagnostic multi-slice CT study. Attenuation correction decreases the risk of false positives, and thereby increases specificity.

SPECT/CT enables one to plan treatment more effectively and provides better feedback on the efficacy of treatment. The treatment of lymphoma with ZEVALIN® (ibritumomab tiuxetan), a substance used in radionuclide therapy, offers a good example. The protocol calls for a pre-treatment scan with an imaging radionuclide surrogate. The patient has the same uptake with the surrogate and the therapy agent. The surrogate images are used to estimate the treatment dose that is to be applied to the tumors and to the patient's organ systems. Anatomic images are used to improve the accuracy of the dose estimate.

17.3 Combining imaging modalities for interventional procedures

Many cases in medicine require imaging information from more than one diagnostic modality. During interventional procedures in particular, clinicians rely on continual access to such information. However, the use of well-established diagnostic equipment is subject to the rather strict condition that rules out repositioning of the pa-

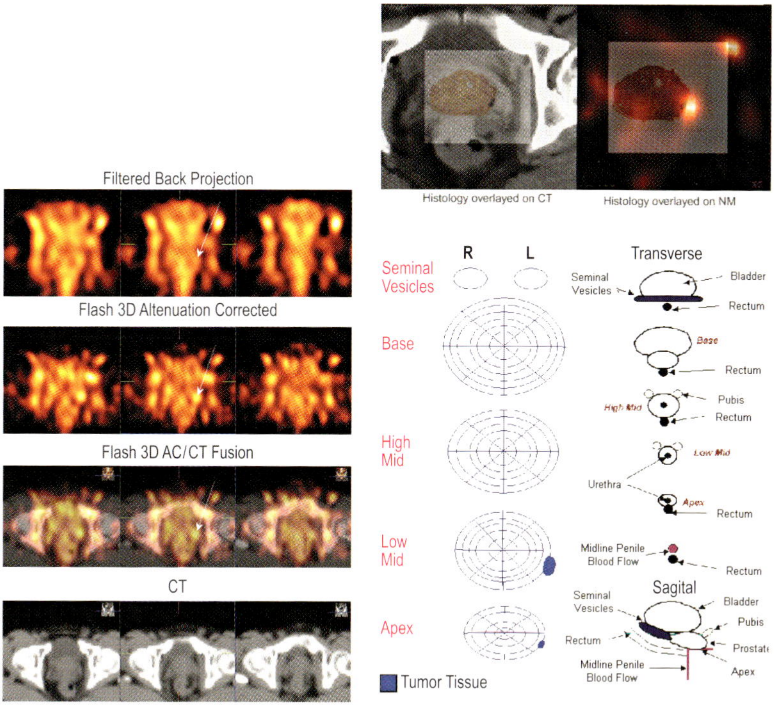

Figure 17.13 SPECT-CT imaging of prostate cancer

tient. This condition can be met either by deploying a mobile form of one of the modalities or by ensuring the convenient, fast and smooth transfer of the patient between the modalities [17.22]. Applications involve the combining of CT and MR systems with interventional X-ray systems to combine the advantages of low contrast resolution, 3D tissue information and real time information with high spatial resolution.

17.3.1 Interventional angiography combined with CT imaging

Specific cases in which low contrast CT information can be used to support interventional angiography procedures include:

- Chemoembolization of hepatic tumors. The procedure can be controlled thanks to the CT's capacity to detect tumors (fig. 17.14).
- Percutaneous biopsy of the spine. CT provides detailed anatomical information when it comes to determining the biopsy route. Angiography enables the real-time control of the needle insertion.

The Siemens Angio-CT Miyabi (miyabi is the Japanese word for elegance) represents an example that allows the use of the two modalities in a combined procedure without repositioning the patient (fig. 17.15). The relatively high incidence of hepatic cancer

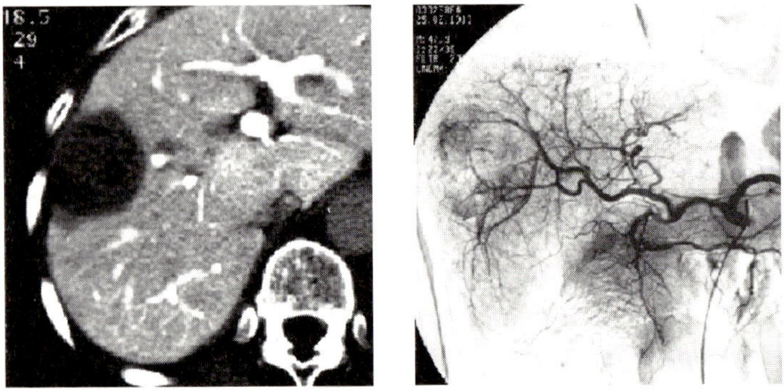

Figure 17.14
Hepatic cellular carcinoma in the right lobe **(a)**. Celiac arteriography reveals a hypervascular tumor and shows the supporting vascular tree through which the embolization will be performed **(b)**. (Source: Dr. Ishijima et al., Department of Diagnostic Radiology Gunma Univ. School of Medicine, Maebeshi, Japan)

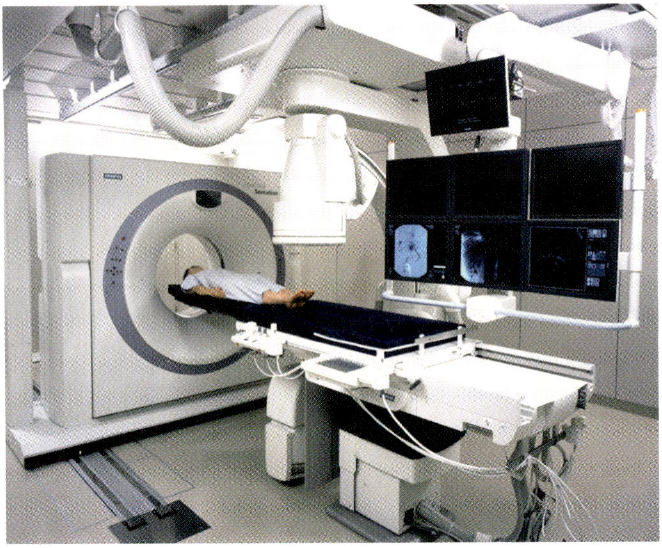

Figure 17.15
Angio-CT Miyabi: CT sliding gantry in park position combined with ceiling-mounted angiography system

in the Japanese population is one of the reasons why combined Angio-CT procedures were first introduced in Japan. The tumor is located via CT and the chemical embolization (with alcohol) is performed using catheters that are advanced (under fluorescence control) via the vascular tree.

The technical implementation includes a standard angiographic unit and a CT gantry on floor rails. The rails allow one to slide the CT gantry from a parking position to the angiography table, where spiral CT investigations can be carried out when the C-arm X-ray unit is swiveled to the side.

17.3.2 Interventional angiography combined with MRI imaging

Owing to its capacity to deliver high soft-tissue contrast, MR has come to play an increasingly important role in interventional procedures. However, angiography is often still requested as an immediately accessible imaging modality for crucial support at interventional MR procedures. Cases in which angiography is required as an emergency imaging alternative or as a means of handling certain difficulties at MR interventions include:

- Valve repair
- Transcatheter injection and localization of labeled stem cells (fig. 17.16) [17.25, 17.26].

On the other hand, there are specific applications in which MRI can be used to support interventional angiography, neurological and cardiovascular procedures include (see section 15.2.1.4):

- Controlled chemo and thermoembolization
- Local thrombolysis monitored by MR perfusion

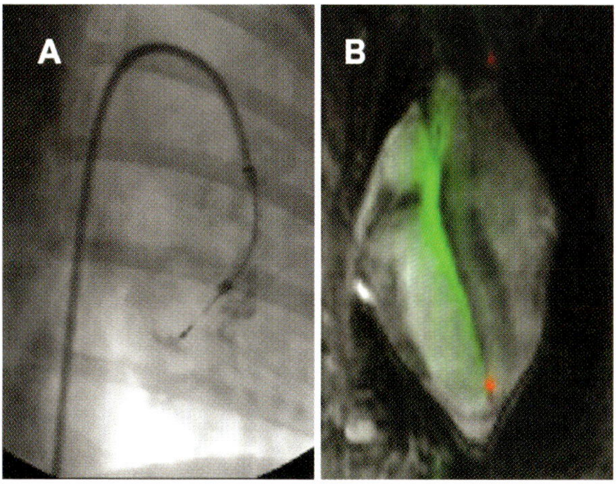

Figure 17.16
Animal study of an interventional procedure with the Miyabi: angiography image showing a catheter ready for the injection of stem cells into the heart **(a)**. MRI image showing the position of the catheter within the ventricle **(b)**. The catheter is visible in MR because it acts as an active antenna (green). A passive micro coil ensures the visibility of the catheter's tip (red). (Source: Dr. Robert Lederman, National Institute of Health, Washington).

- MR-controlled stent placement [17.23]
- 3D MRA to support the treatment of congenital heart disease [17.24]

However, combinations involving X-ray angiography and MR require to overcome several technical problems:

1. Special attention is needed if the X-ray unit is placed close to the MR system to make sure that magnetic fringe field will not affect the operation, even as today's X-ray imaging systems are equipped with flat panel detectors.
2. The fact that the MR modality has to be placed in an RF-shielded room makes installing ceiling-mounted C-arms and/or rails difficult. Furthermore, an X-ray system placed inside the cabin has to be turned off completely during MR examination in order to avoid RF interference. A necessary reboot time of several minutes would gravely hinder a fast transfer from MR to Angio imaging.
3. Independently performed X-ray investigations must not interfere with MR examinations conducted at the same time.
4. Special patient tables are required to be MR and X-ray compatible.
5. The MR coils placed under the patient must not affect the X-ray examination during combined procedures.

The Angio-MR Miyabi is a system that meets these challenges (fig. 17.17). The angiography and the MR suites are positioned side by side, with their respective modalities being arranged in a line (fig. 17.18, left). An RF-shielded door enables one to transfer the patient between the two imaging systems. The standard rail-based angiography ta-

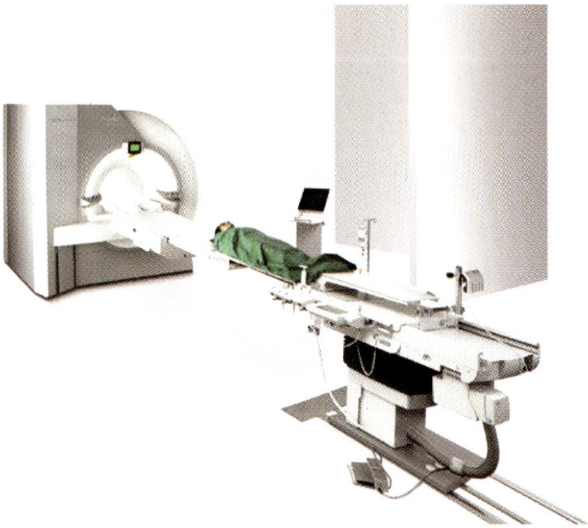

Figure 17.17
Angiography table in docking position with the MR table, patient on a shell moved from the angiography to the MR table top.

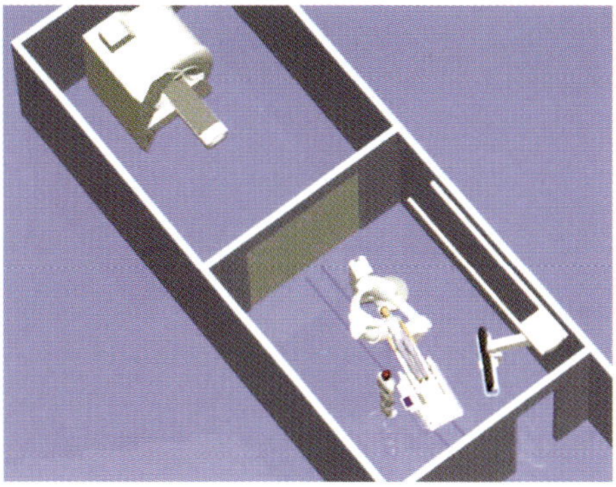
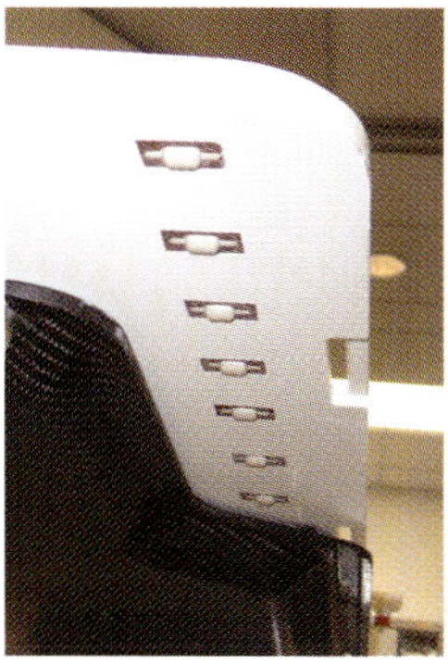

Figure 17.18
Left: Top view of an MRI and angiography suite separated by a sliding door for combined or dedicated operation. **Right:** Shell with micro bearings riding on the table top. Micro rails provide longitudinal guidance (seen from below).

ble can be moved with the help of an electric motor from the angiography position to the open RF-shielded door. The table top is then pulled out through the door opening so that it docks on the MR table top.

The transfers between the angiography and the MRI lab must be smooth and rapid and are to involve no repositioning of the patient. The patient is therefore placed on a dedicated thin shell manufactured of MR and X-ray-compatible materials. The shell is supported by many plastic micro bearings (fig. 17.18, right) that enable low-friction movement and can also be locked onto the angiography or MR table top. The table tops are retrofitted with covers furnished with mini grooves that help to guide the shell when it is moved from the angiography to the MR table or vice versa. It will be necessary to move any mobile patient-monitoring and anaesthetic equipment at the same time as the patient is being transported.

Patient transfer with the shell provides unrestricted angiography imaging thanks to the fact that it is largely radiolucent and therefore permits unattenuated X-ray transmission even at extreme angulations. The option of using the coil arrays embedded in the MR table is retained, although with some slight image degradation owing to the slightly larger distance between coil and patient. The head part of the shell fits into the standard MR head coil.

The angiography and MRI suite can be used for both combined and dedicated procedures. This is an important aspect when it comes to the cost effectiveness of the Miyabi combined angiography-MR system. But the patient on a shell concept is not restricted to combined Angio-MR treatments. With aid of a special designed trolley the shell can be smoothly transferred without patient repositioning to any image modality and even to an operation table using the same docking procedure. The system can be easily retrofitted requiring only little modifications at existing modalities. Thus it may be a step to a significant improvement of workflow in a hospital.

17.4 Imaging in the operating room

The significance of intraoperative image acquisition continues to grow within the main areas of therapeutic intervention. This trend is a part of an ongoing evolution in the operating room (OR) and within the various surgical disciplines towards less traumatic, minimally invasive surgery (MIS). This evolution is characterized by the following two facts:

First, the general complexity of surgical treatment is increasing due to the growing prevalence of microsurgical procedures. Second, minimally invasive methods are associated with restrictions relating to the surgeon's field of view and capacity to maneuver in the focused region. The significance of the surgeon's hand-eye coordination, a central aspect in open forms of surgery, has diminished in proportion to the rise in the significance of intraoperative imaging. Indeed, the very goal of establishing effective form of minimally invasive intervention presupposes the use of image-guided procedures. Imaging modalities play an essential role in image-based surgery when it comes to accessing the region of intervention, detecting and displaying specific structures, guiding instruments, controlling therapeutic procedures and documenting treatment results.

In addition to intraoperative imaging modalities such as ultrasound, X-ray, computed tomography and magnetic resonance, endoscopy occupies an important position in MIS. Endoscopy opens the surgeon's view to organ surfaces, enables true-color examinations and represents reliable means of anatomical orientation. These characteristics enable one to accurately monitor and control the use of instruments in the therapeutic region.

The increasing complexity of the surgical environment (including imaging modalities and surgical devices) has also increased demands for smart OR-system solutions. The use of information technology (IT systems) in the OR with the aim of providing the greatest functional versatility and comprehensive data management offers a necessary unburdening of the surgeon and OR staff.

The seamless integration of imaging technology in a modern OR framework enables one to effectively deploy information technology so as to:

- Control a multitude of OR components via a single user interface, and thereby manage the spatial separation and the diverse functions of the various components
- Manage preoperative and intraoperative data as well as image data in a patient-oriented way for the sake of visualization, documentation and database administration.

17.4.1 Intraoperative imaging

Intraoperative imaging modalities generally aim to compensate for the restrictions in the surgeon's field of view and to introduce a third dimension. The main imaging modalities that offer intraoperative support for endoscopy include X-ray imaging (mobile C-arms), ultrasound, computed tomography and magnetic resonance imaging.

17.4.1.1 X-ray imaging

The intraoperative application of X-ray imaging is often necessary to provide answers to a wide array of questions. This is especially true, for instance, if the surgeon needs to look behind the surfaces of bones and into their inner (trabecular) structures or needs to visualize the morphology of blood vessels or the biliary tract. Apart from the application of X-ray imaging in various surgical disciplines to assist in the placement of cardiac pacemakers, stents and guide wires, this imaging modality is used in orthopedic traumatology to enable the position monitoring of implants, protheses, screws and nails.

One important aspect in this context is checking the position of screws that are relatively close to joints, vessels or nerves. X-ray imaging is also an indispensable surgical tool for joint reconstruction and the repositioning of dislocated bone fragments.

Computed tomography and mobile C-arm technology can be used to support image-guided surgery (figs. 17.19, 17.20). The use of mobile C-arms in operating rooms predominates because they are less costly than CT scanners, they can be used for more than one operating room, they can be positioned closer to common patient tables

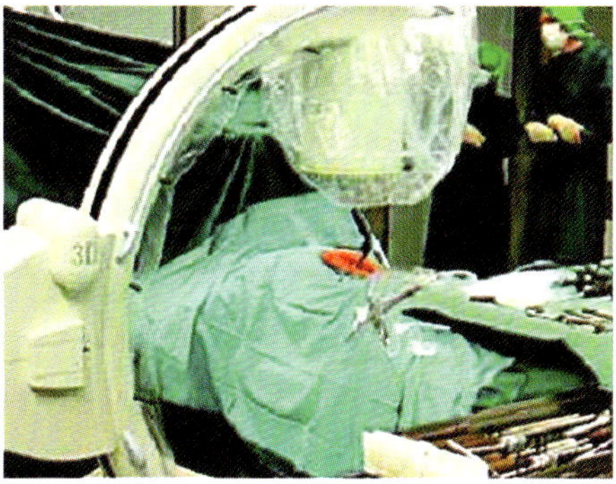

Figure 17.19
Intraoperative imaging by mobile C-arm

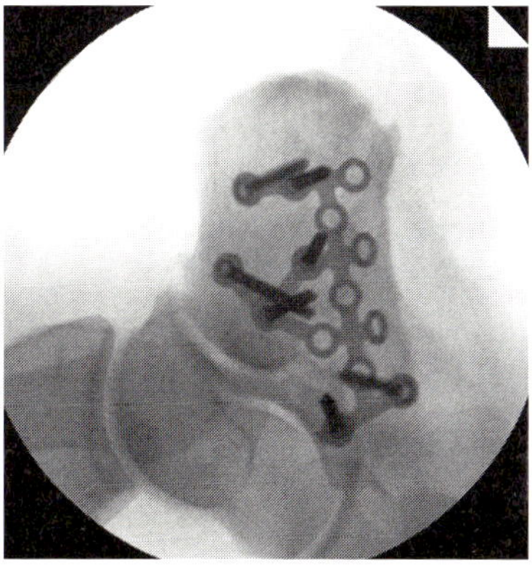

Figure 17.20
Reconstruction of a bone fracture

(which can thus remain in place) and they occupy less space in the vicinity of the surgical table.

CT technology used to enjoy an advantage over 2D fluoroscopy in that it was capable of generating real 3D data. This advantage has essentially been compensated for by the latest developments in fluoroscopy, which include the use of isocentric C-arm technology to enable the acquisition of true 3D-volume data.

The application of adequate signal processing and reconstruction algorithms (e.g. filtering and backprojection) enable one to derive (reconstruct) a 3D-voxel volume of a region within the patient's body from a given number of fluoroscopic 2D-projection images. The basic principle is similar to that of CT filtering and backprojection. However, one can use the true cone-beam reconstruction technique after adapting it to the isotropic 2D area of the detector (image intensifier or flat detector).

This true 3D imaging can be used by the surgeon as an important source of additional information to help guide and improve the reliability of the therapeutic procedure.

17.4.1.2 Computed tomography (CT)

Computed tomography (CT) essentially reveals features that can be used to support surgical procedures and that open the door to a more widespread application of CT in the ORs of the future:

- Complete and continuous acquisition of large body regions (even isotropically as real volume datasets)
- Dynamic imaging of moving organs
- Optimized contrast and spatial resolution
- High geometric accuracy

CT imaging enables one to display anatomical structures and objects of pathological degeneration for intraoperative use in ORs of diverse disciplines, including traumatology, orthopedics and neurosurgery. Solutions are available today that improve the interaction between intraoperative imaging and surgical procedures in the OR and also improve the surgeon's access to the patient during the procedure. These are among the main reasons for the increasing importance of computed tomography in interventional therapy. Technically, this is based on three essential construction variants, including mobile CT-gantry units, patient support systems that allow for CT examination and therapy away from the gantry on common moving tables that eliminate the need to physically transfer and reposition the patient and virtually open CT that features enlarged inner gantry diameters and that enables surgical procedures directly within the gantry.

The application spectrum for CT-guided surgery is manifold and comprises a wide array of tasks:

- Placement and position monitoring of implants, prostheses, screws and nails
- Reconstruction and repositioning of dislocated bone fragments
- CT-guided osteosynthesis of the posterior pelvic ring

- Plate implantation on the anterior pelvic ring
- Tumor resection in neurosurgery
- High-precision positioning of probes for the thermal ablation of tumors and for pain therapy.

This opens new fields of application, especially for neurosurgery, but also for interventional procedures (biopsies, HFTT-needle placement in tumors, etc.) under CT-imaging surveillance.

17.4.1.3 Magnetic resonance imaging (MRI)

Diagnostic imaging with high-field MRI is set to become the gold standard in neurosurgery when it comes to providing surgeons with detailed anatomical and functional information during interventional procedures in the OR. Intraoperative scanning delivers current information about the patient, thereby enabling the surgeon to control the surgical result during the procedure. An MR imaging modality can be effectively used in a wide range of clinical applications to achieve improved patient care. The benefits include:

- Improved resection control with high selectivity
- Less invasive surgery and lower complication rates
- Reduced need for repeat surgery

When used in combination with a specifically designed, movable surgical table (fig. 17.21), MR imaging enables one to treat patients outside of the magnetic field and to control the surgical process without unnecessary patient transfers.

The scope of intraoperative MR imaging today includes various neurosurgical applications:

- Brain biopsies (fig. 17.22)
- Tumor resections (fig. 17.23)
- Functional neurosurgical procedures (thalamotomy, deep-brain stimulator placements, unilateral cingulotomy, bilateral cingulotomy)

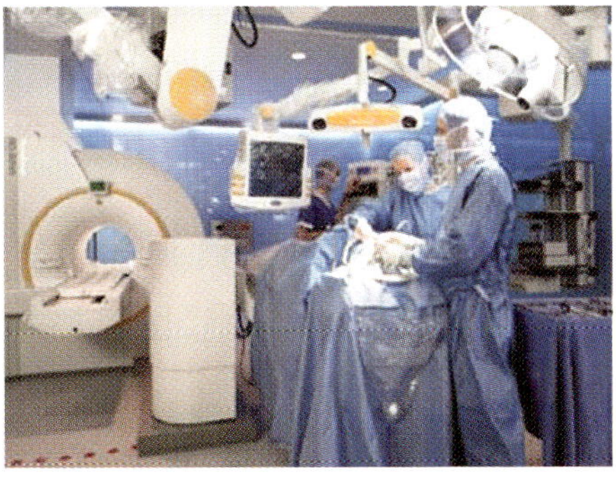

Figure 17.21
Intraoperative MR in the OR (Siemens Magnetom)

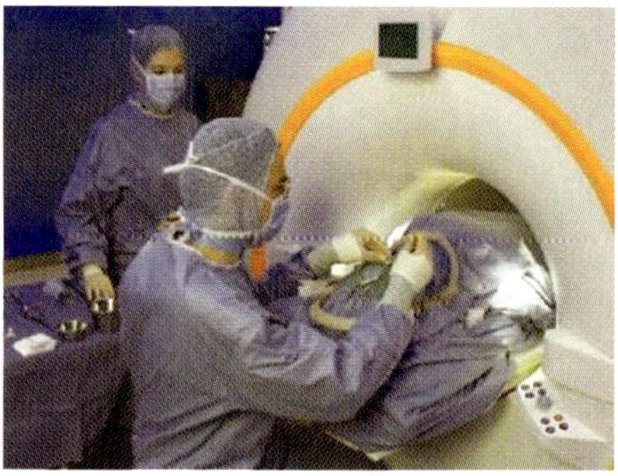

Figure 17.22
MR-guided brain biopsy

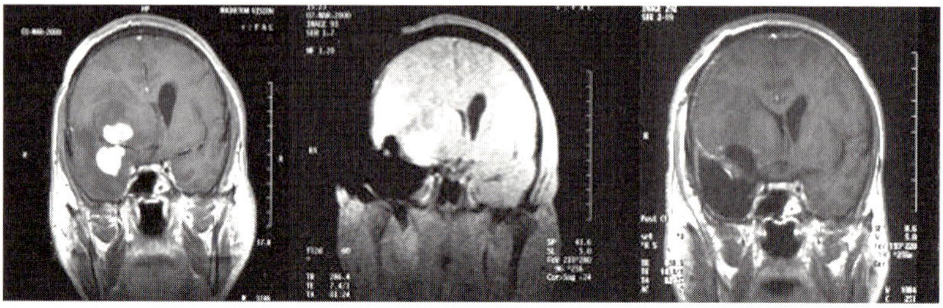

Figure 17.23
MR-guided tumor resection: **(a)** preoperative, **(b)** intraoperative, **(c)** postoperative (Source: G. Rubino, UCLA)

- Cyst drainage
- Shunts
- Laminectomies

Further improvements can be achieved by combining high-field intraoperative MR imaging with navigational systems for image-guided neurosurgery. All of these applications have been demonstrated to be safe forms of routine intracranial intervention.

17.4.1.4 Ultrasound (US)

The use of intraoperative ultrasound image acquisition (B-mode) and Doppler methods is becoming increasingly prevalent in the area of visceral surgery. Owing to its capacity for soft-tissue rendering, its immediately available results (real-time display) and the fast localization of tissue and vessel variations and deformations that it enables, US has emerged as a very competitive technique that is especially well-suited to and frequently used in examinations of the liver, pancreas, bile and biliary tract, stomach, intestine, heart and brain.

The major fields of application for US include:

- Biopsy/puncture (controlled via ultrasound visualization)

- Accurate placement of high-frequency (HF) ablation needles
- Drainage laying
- Navigation to the locations of metastases
- Determination of resection borders
- Resection monitoring and control
- Vessel localization
- Inspection of interior vessel walls

The biggest advantage of intraoperative ultrasound over transcutaneous ultrasound applications is that it enables one to apply higher ultrasound frequencies. This leads to a significantly improved discriminatory capacity for detecting tissue changes and malformations (i.e. important additional information for the surgeon during interventional procedures). Various ultrasound probes (applicators) have been designed for this purpose.

Various types of probes are available today for use in special surgical areas. These include rigid ultrasound laparoscopes (fig. 17.24), flexible ultrasound endoscopes (fig. 17.25), ultrasound catheters and micro-probes (handheld) for open surgery.

Rigid ultrasound laparoscopes are used in examinations of the liver (fig. 17.26a), pancreas (fig. 17.26b), bile ducts, etc. Flexible ultrasound endoscopes are used in examinations of the stomach, intestines and esophagus. Ultrasound catheters enable one to examine the interiors of blood vessels and heart chambers (fig. 17.27).

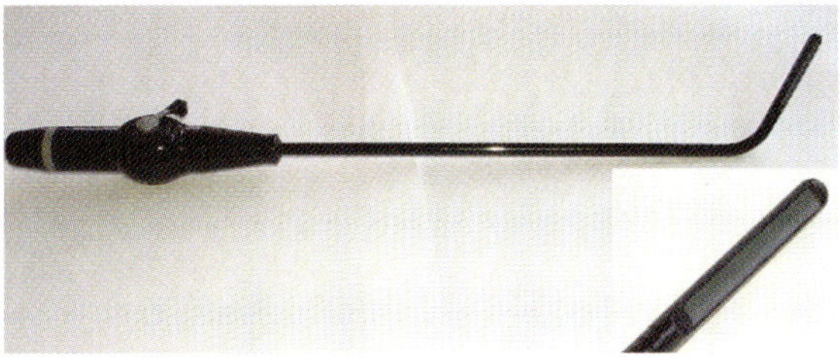

Figure 17.24
Ultrasound laparoscope (bottom right: zoomed view of the transducer at the instrument tip)

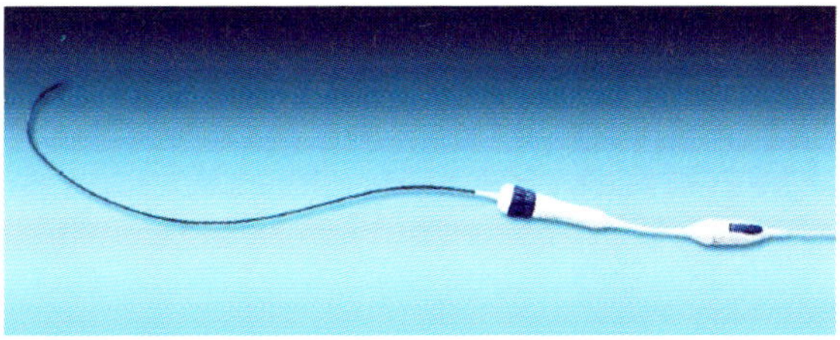

Figure 17.25 Flexible ultrasound catheter (Acunav, Siemens)

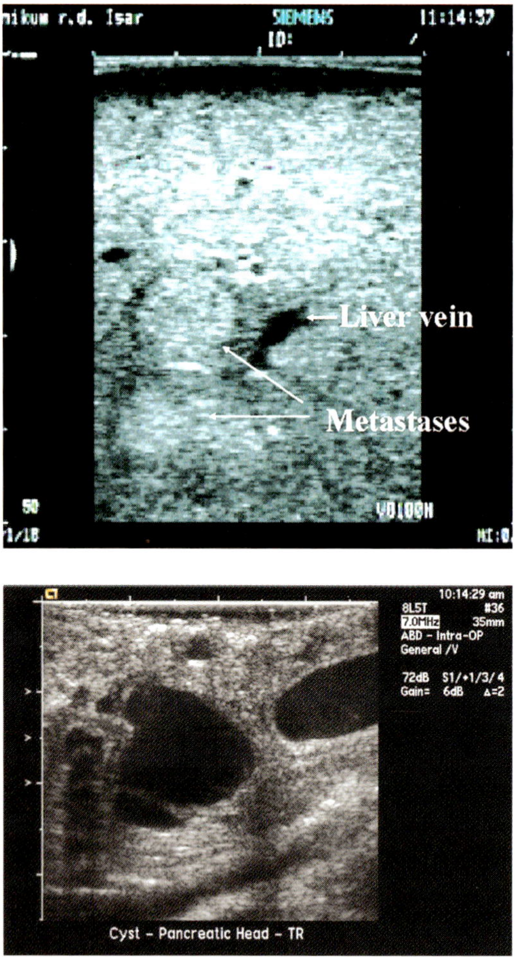

a

b

Figure 17.26
Liver metastases **(a)** and pancreas cyst **(b)** imaged with a rigid ultrasound laparoscope

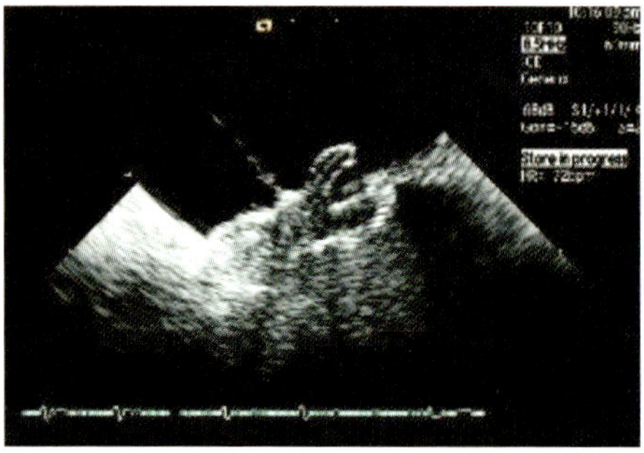

Figure 17.27
Septal occluder placement monitored with intracardiac ultrasound catheter

In addition to the imaging of anatomical structures, the ultrasonic Doppler method can be used to provide insight into the functioning of moving organs, the perfusion of tissue regions and the flow characteristics and fluid dynamics within blood vessels.

17.4.1.5 Endoscopy

In addition to the common radiological imaging modalities, endoscopy plays an especially important role as an intraoperative imaging method in the OR. The term endoscopy stands for imaging on an optical basis. An endoscope is a medical instrument for optical image acquisition and transmission whose length is a multiple of its diameter. The diameters of endoscopes range from 0.5 mm to 15 mm. Endoscopic images are acquired at the tip of the instrument, which may be positioned deep inside the body of the patient and directly in front of the region to be examined.

The advantages of endoscopic imaging include:

- True-color rendering of tissue and organs
- The capacity to assess organ surfaces with respect to their condition
- The direct visual control of interventional procedures with minimal traumatic impact even in regions situated deep within the body

Images are acquired using two basic types of instruments:

- Rigid endoscopes, including laparoscopes, arthroscopes and cystoscopes (fig. 17.28)
- Flexible endoscopes, including gastroscopes, duodenoscopes and colonoscopes (fig. 17.29)

The selection of a particular instrument is made by the physician in light of the relevant access path into the body. Flexible instruments are used for natural access paths

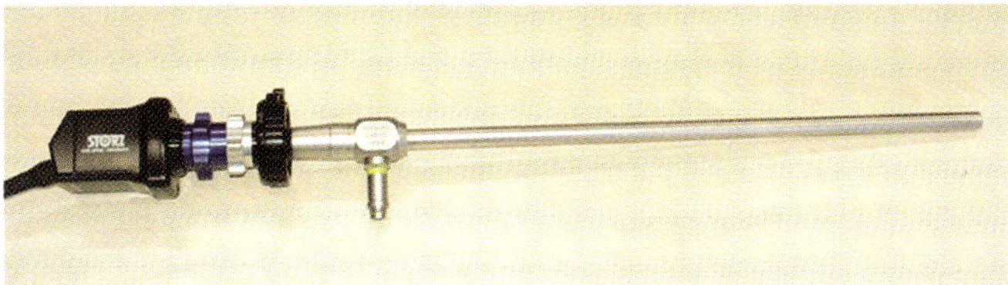

Figure 17.28
Laparoscope (including video camera) (Source of figures 17.28 to 17.34: Karl Storz, Tuttlingen)

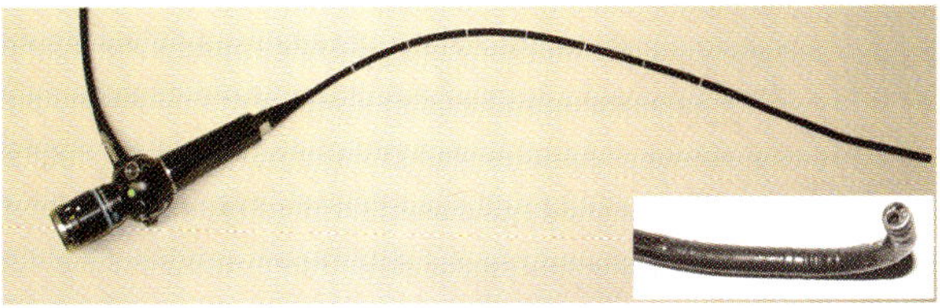

Figure 17.29
Flexible endoscope

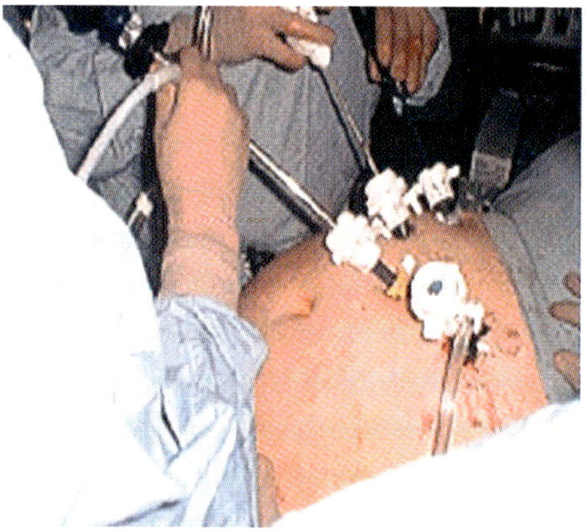

Figure 17.30
Typical laparoscopic intervention

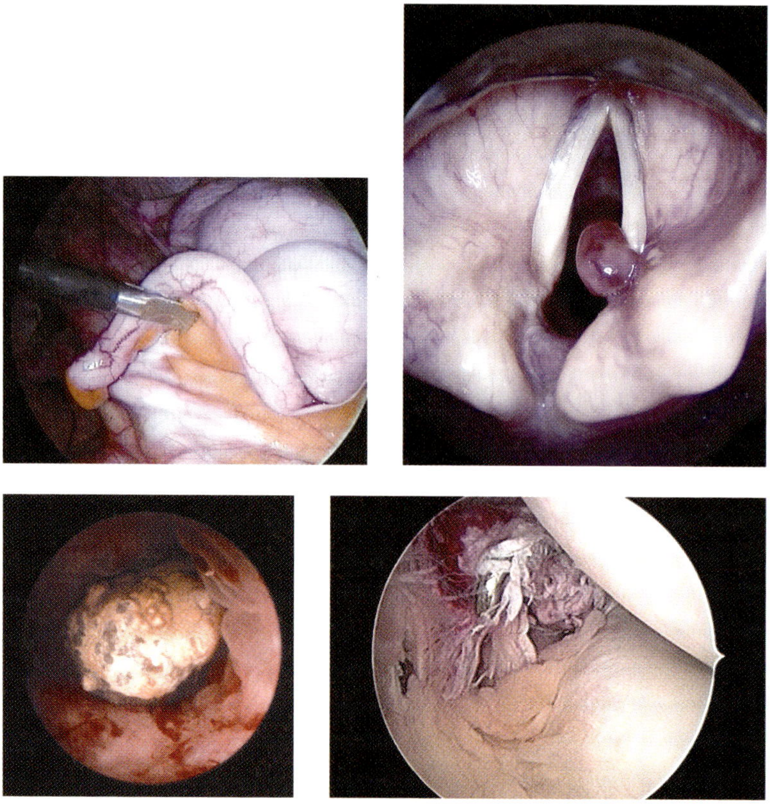

Figure 17.31
Endoscopic images: **(upper left)** laparoscopic appendix, **(upper right)** intubation granuloma at the left vocal resection chord for laser resection, **(lower left)** renal concrement, **(lower right)** arthroscopy of a posterior cruciate ligament rupture (dorso-medial access)

such as the esophagus and colon. These instruments enable one to reach and examine organs such as bronchi, the esophagus, the stomach and the intestines. Some of these instruments are outfitted with channels (working channels) that enable one to deploy miniaturized therapeutic instruments to the tip of the endoscope for the sake of performing surgical procedures (e.g. the resectioning of polyps and other mutated tissue).

In contrast, rigid instruments require artificial access (small transcutaneous incision) to the body (fig. 17.30). Such instruments come in various forms depending on the surgical discipline involved. Their primary application is intraoperative imaging. The laparoscope, for instance, is a rigid endoscope that is frequently used for gastrointestinal surgery. Fig. 17.30 shows a typical laparoscopy scenario. Figures 17.31 show various images obtained during endoscopic examinations.

The first report of a laparoscopic examination was submitted by Georg Kelling of Dresden, Germany in 1901. The first surgical laparoscopic procedures were performed in the area of thorascopy in 1959 by Raimund Wittmoser and in the area of gynecology (as endoscopic abdominal surgery) by Kurt Semm (around 1980). Two technical inventions made between 1960 and 1970 helped to bring about the establishment of laparoscopy as a standard surgical procedure:

- The development of the cold-light source (Karl Storz, Tuttlingen, Germany)
- The development of the rod-lens endoscope (Harold Hopkins, London 1954) and its product integration (Karl Storz, from 1963).

The final breakthrough for laparoscopy in the surgical disciplines came with advancements in the miniaturization of video techniques.

Laparoscope design

A standard laparoscope is a rigid endoscope with a diameter of 10 mm, a viewing direction of 30° or 0° and a field of view (FOV) of about 80° (fig. 17.32). Laparoscopes are used for minimally invasive surgery of the abdomen. They consist of an optical channel for image transmission and a fiber-optic light channel for illuminating the intracorporal region. As illustrated in fig. 17.32, modern image transmission systems are based on the Hopkins rod lens and are different from conventional endoscopic transmission systems based on achromats. The rod lens transmission system enables significantly increased light transmission and better image quality. Contrary to operating laparoscopes, which include a channel for performing simple operations via instruments that are manipulated in the viewing direction, standard laparoscopes are not equipped with a working channel. Laparoscopes are inserted through the abdominal wall by means of a trocar and an obturator.

The transmission of images along the instrument (i.e. from the instrument's tip to its back end) is usually performed optically. Electrical endoscopes whose tips are equipped with micro CCDs or wireless endoscopes are available, but currently these do not have a widespread practical importance. In flexible endoscopes such as e.g. colonoscopes as they are also known, light and images are transmitted via a combina-

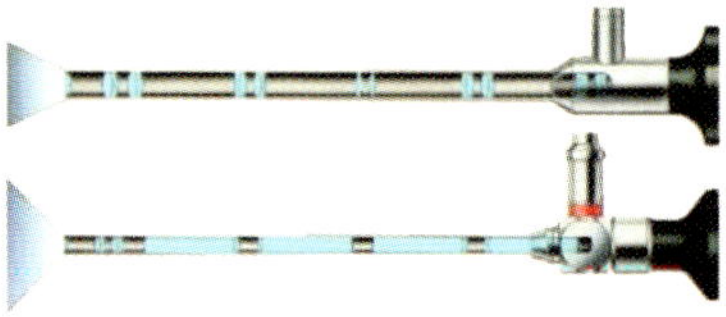

Figure 17.32
Laparoscope design: **top:** conventional laparoscope, **bottom:** Hopkins rod-lens laparoscope

tion of back and front lenses and micro glass fibers bundled into a highly flexible light cable. The manufacturing challenge centers on the accurate sorting and packing of the fibers at the cable's distal and proximal interfaces.

In the rigid tube of a laparoscope, high-quality lens optics transmit lighting and images between the distal end (instrument tip) and the proximal end (camera mount). The rod lens plays an especially important role here.

Laparoscopy components

In addition to the laparoscope, a number of other devices are necessary to carry out a laparoscopic examination. As illustrated in fig. 17.33 the standard configuration for laparoscopy includes:

- Cold-light source
- Video camera system
- Gas insufflator
- Suction/irrigation unit
- Monitor and documentation unit

Light source

A light source to illuminate the endoscopic examination area and to ensure proper image quality represents an important prerequisite for laparoscopy. The best choice is a cold-light source that generates light at a sufficient intensity and that exhibits reproducible and excellent spectral quality. With spectral characteristics close to those of sun light (a color temperature of about 6,000 Kelvin), xenon light sources represent the current state of the art. The light is bundled by a lens system and transmitted via a fiberglass cable to the tip of the laparoscope where it provides complete illumination for the field of view.

Camera system

In combination with the instrument lenses, the quality of the applied video camera (analog/digital) and the quality of the camera control unit are important prerequisites for the examination of organ surfaces. A reliable white balance adjustment is needed to generate the true-color image display of tissue. Here, the camera system's color display is adjusted to the color temperature of the cold-light source.

Single and three-chip cameras are available. The 1-CCD (charge-coupled device) variant processes all three colors on one chip by means of a micro mask. The 3-CCD variant splits the light by means of 3 optical prisms onto three separate chips, allowing for better color separation and more brilliant colors. A 3-CCD camera outfitted with sensors gives video images a degree of sharpness and contrast that is far superior to what is achievable with a single-CCD camera.

Different endoscopes produce images in different sizes. Most cameras are outfitted with a zoom objective to compensate for this difference. Optical zooms are preferable because they improve image quality whereas electronic zooms merely magnify pixels without increasing definition.

Most modern endoscopic cameras can be soaked completely and their cleaning becomes much more convenient. Such cameras can be draped completely using single-use sterile drapes. Special camera heads capable of withstanding the autoclave process are also available.

Monitors and documentation units

High quality color monitors that guarantee true-color tissue rendering are generally used for image display. Laparoscopic images are usually documented as video sequences using standard video cassette recorders (e.g. S-VHS, Hi-8, Mini-DV). Video

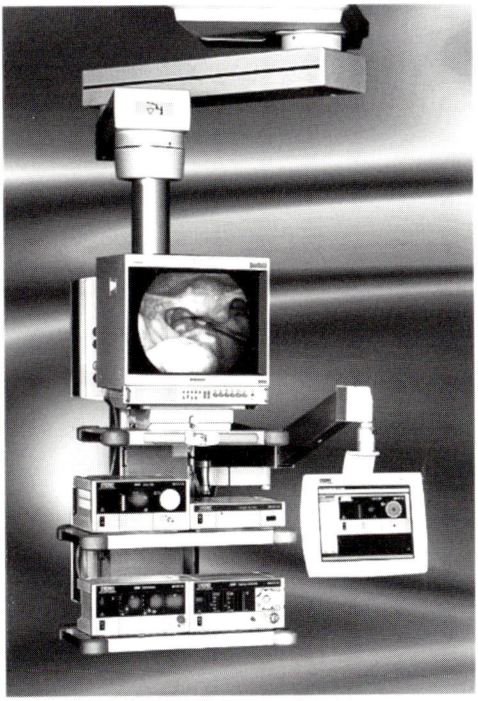

Figure 17.33
Ceiling-mounted laparoscopic equipment

printers are also used for documentation. Given the increasing prevalence of digital imaging systems, standard on-line real-time recording is used in the OR (AVI, MPEG, JPEG, TIFF).

Insufflator

Standard laparoscopic examinations of the gastrointestinal region begin with the creation of a pneumoperitoneum. This procedure involves inflating the abdomen with CO_2 gas so that the abdominal wall lifts away from the internal organs, thereby creating a safer working space for surgical procedures. This enables one to view the inside of the abdomen with the instrument from an optimal distance.

Suction/irrigation

The suction/irrigation unit represents an important auxiliary component used to support laparoscopic procedures. It is frequently necessary to suction and clean organ surfaces to secure a clear view (e.g. extracting blood from the abdomen). The front lenses are cleaned via irrigation and a dilution is used to improve suction conditions.

Photodynamic diagnosis, autofluorescence and molecular imaging (future prospects)

Apart from its application in the optical imaging of organ surfaces, this method can be used to discriminate malignant tissue from normal tissue at an early stage. Methods of photodynamic diagnostics (PDD) and autofluorescence (AF) enable the surgeon to visualize and detect changed cell areas by means of blue light and specially tuned endoscopes. These areas are not visible via conventional illumination. It is necessary to use light of a special spectral composition. This light is transmitted to the region of intervention within the patient's body using an endoscopic light conductor (e.g. fiber optics).

The core of a PDD unit is its D-light system. D-light generates the diagnosis light for endoscopic tissue characterization. After the instillation of a tumor marker substance (induced fluorescence), the fluorescence mode is used to make malign tissue appear different from benign tissue. The stimulation of the D-light system causes tumorous

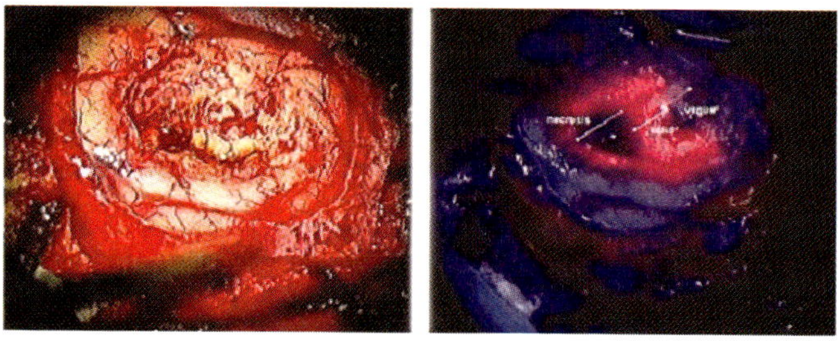

Figure 17.34
Intraoperative images of a tumor cavity viewed with the use of conventional white light **(left)** and violet-blue illumination **(right)**. Note the different qualities of tumor fluorescence (necrosis, solid, vague). (Source of figures 17.28 to 17.31: KARL STORZ, Tuttlingen)

areas to appear a fluorescent red. This enables one to easily detect flat neoplastic lesions (such as dysplasias and carcinoma in situ that may be hidden in normal or non-specifically inflamed mucosa) and small papillary tumors. As it cannot achieve this sort of differentiation, the use of pure white light will reduce the likelihood of early detection (fig. 17.34).

The autofluorescence method is based on the existence of substances below the mucosa that can be stimulated and temporarily lifted to a higher energy level via light of a specific wavelength. Upon falling back from the higher level, this energy is re-emitted in the form of a visible light that has a different wavelength than the irradiated light. As this phenomen involves no substances administered from the outside, it is referred to as autofluorescence. When using this imaging technique, evidence of pathology appears in the form of dark spots.

Molecular imaging (primarily an optical procedure) represents a further method of acquiring specific information about physiological and pathological changes in human tissue. Optical tissue differentiation can be achieved using an endoscope and marker substances combined with fluorescence (i.e. to reveal tumor-specific accumulation).

The principal challenge that faces these optical imaging methods is to effectively prevent the recurrence of tumors via the detection and the complete and reliable removal of the smallest areas of mutated cells during tumor resection.

17.4.2 Integrated surgical workplaces

General aspects

The initial impact of embedding intraoperative imaging modalities in the surgical workflow represents an increase in the complexity of the operating room infrastructure and an increase in the complexity of the tasks faced by surgeons and clinical staff. This difficulty can be expressed in terms of the following factors:

- Confrontation with a variety of device interfaces (user interface panels) that are placed at different locations around the surgical table
- Different locations for accessing and visualizing image data and other information
- User intensive data management (e.g. documentation).

Furthermore, minimally invasive surgery (MIS) relies upon image-guided surgical procedures due to the restricted or entirely absent direct view of the intervention region. This makes it necessary to integrate both well-defined navigation and image processing sequences into the image-guided surgical procedure. The interaction of these two functional components represents an important instrument for the surgeon because the components are essential for hand-eye coordination.

The assessment of the overall situation in the operating room reveals a clear demand for integrated OR solutions as a basis for the most effective and ergonomic work at the surgical table. Furthermore, information technology (IT) plays an important role in the integration of the diverse functions in the operating room. Information technology takes over control and data management tasks in the OR. It also provides the general platform for all integration tasks in the OR. For the surgeon, such an OR system solution means:

- Control over all instruments and devices in the OR at a single man-machine interface implemented as a central user interface whose functions are executed according to a common operative design.
- Centralized visualization of all relevant image data in an ergonomically optimized (i.e. eminently reachable) location.
- The integrating platform takes over essential tasks relating to OR data management without burdening the OR staff in any way.
- Partial processes are embedded in global workflow sequences, thus minimizing the number of necessary tasks and interactions for the surgeon and the OR staff.

This concept makes all of the functions that are necessary for the therapeutic process available to the surgeon at a central location in the sterile area of the operating room. If desired, certain functions can also be accessed during the planning or preparation phases of the interventional procedure or for assistance from an operating console outside the sterile area.

Apart from integration tasks within the operating room, it is also necessary to integrate the operating room itself into the clinical therapeutical process. This includes the following aspects:

- Providing relevant preoperative data and information in the OR
- Providing therapy planning data
- Involving and integrating the pathology department directly during therapy by means of information technology (IT)
- Recording intraoperatively acquired image data and OR process documentation in archival systems
- Quality assurance for the therapeutic process on the basis of the complete online documentation

The integrated OR workplace

The OR system solution known as *syngo*OR/OR1 (fig. 17.35) that was developed jointly by Siemens and Karl Storz is an example of such an integrated workplace. *syngo*OR is an IT platform that was conceived to meet the requirements of an operating room. It enables the integration of the most diverse OR functions, instruments, devices and intraoperative imaging modalities. It provides interfaces to all hospital IT systems (PACS, HIS, RIS). This integrated OR solution features a central user interface that provides the surgeon and clinical staff all of the integrated system's functions. All of the functions made available by the integrated OR solution can be intuitively controlled from within the sterile and nonsterile units of the OR via touch screen or voice control.

Intraoperative image data (e.g. endoscopic images) are displayed on a flat panel screen that can be ergonomically positioned in the surgeon's field of view. A second

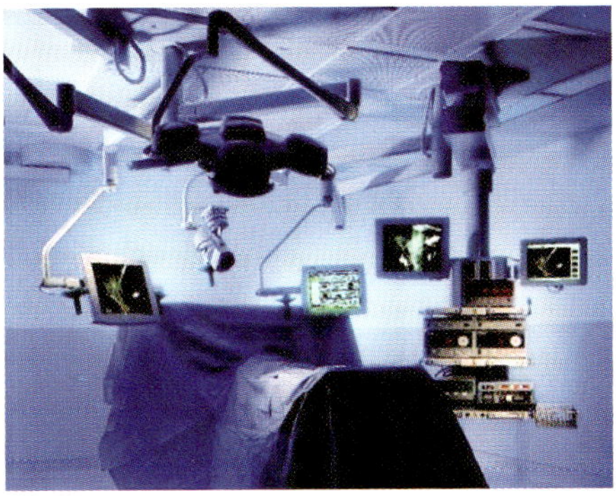

Figure 17.35
The *syngo*OR/OR1 operating theatre

flat panel display functions as a digital light box for the parallel visualization of preoperatively acquired image data (e.g. CT, MR, PET). This makes all of the relevant image information available to the surgeon (at a central location) during the surgical procedure.

The following key features are supported by the *syngo*OR/OR1 platform:

- Interdisciplinary device management (video camera control, light source, suction/irrigation, insufflation, HF surgery, etc.)
- Integration of nearly all OR facility functions, including the surgical table, room light, etc.
- Integrated intraoperative imaging (endoscopy, ultrasound, X-ray)
- Administration and archiving of all image data generated by the medical imaging modalities
- Local, OR-specific network technology for image and patient data
- Optional local-image archive (PACS) for the OR
- Online interface to hospital IT systems such as PACS, HIS and RIS (Sienet from Siemens)
- Multimedia tools for telecommunication with various operating rooms and external locations, also for teleconsulting and (prospectively) telesurgery.

The functionality of the OR platform allows one to centrally register and store intraoperative images from endoscopic, ultrasound and X-ray examinations in DICOM 3 standard during the treatment phase. These intraoperative images are also made available as reference images (in the same way as preoperative images) immediately after their acquisition. They can be included in the surgical report or archived in a patient-oriented manner together with the report in the hospital archiving system.

Furthermore, the integrated network technology of *syngo*OR offers a multitude of basic functions in the area of clinical OR management. This concerns the functioning of image display, basic reporting, the distribution of pre- and intraoperative image data, improved workflow via study management and enhanced viewing functions (e.g. for images from nuclear medicine). The *syngo*OR also enables one to tailor and enhance PACS functionality to meet the requirements of the surgical field. *syngo*OR can play the role of an OR-specific local network and offer the advantage of a local archiving system attached to the individual OR. This enables one to administer and provide all relevant patient-oriented data from a central repository. All workstations in the domain of the OR thus have access to the stored data. A teleradiological module allows for the automation of fast image distribution, standby call staffing and the solicitation of second opinions.

The concept of integrated device management ensures the holistic functioning of the OR workplace. The integration of therapeutic systems, imaging modalities and telemedicine allows one to achieve a consistent, workflow-based optimization for the surgeon and the OR staff.

The bus-system central control allows one to individually preset the startup configurations for the entire system per surgeon and intervention. The completely integrated telemedical applications have been conceived to take account of future developments in surgical workflow and provide for a direct connection between the sterile area in the OR and external workplaces. This enables data transfer, video conferencing and the live broadcasting of surgical procedures for purposes of consultation, teaching and research.

Given the system's thoroughly modular design, it can be easily adapted and expanded to meet current and future operating room specifications. The system solution for OP workplaces comes in various packaging modules for use in visceral surgery, urology/gynecology and orthopedics/traumatology.

Neurosurgical workplace

BrainLAB has designed a special workplace for neurosurgery (BrainSUITE) that includes the Siemens Magnetom as a core element (fig. 17.36). This OR concept provides and integrates all of the relevant surgical and diagnostic tools that are used in the handling of complicated neurosurgical cases. This solution includes an MRI imaging modality with an integrated operation table for neurosurgical demands, BrainLAB Vector-

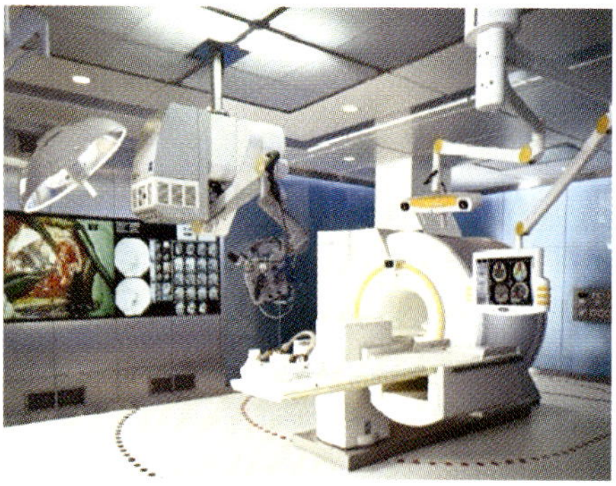

Figure 17.36
Neurosurgical workspace featuring intraoperative MR imaging (BrainSUITE)

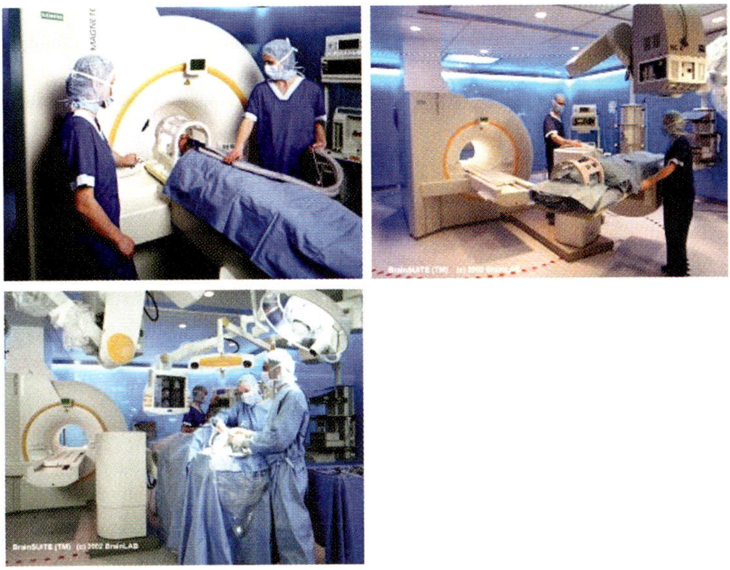

Figure 17.37
Integrated OR table for intraoperative MR imaging: **upper left:** table position for intraoperative imaging, **upper right:** rotation of the table into operating position, **bottom:** table in operating position (outside the magnetic field)

VISION navigation technology, a Zeiss OMPI multivision microscope, basic room functionality and a wall-mounted screen for the central visualization of all relevant information, including images from the MR scanner and other imaging data, online video images from the microscope and pre- and intraoperative patient data.

The system's workplace configurations have been designed for flexibility and convenient use. With regard to the positioning of the magnet and the surgical table, the operation field is outside of the 5-Gauss line. This means that standard instruments and equipment can be used. The table can be tilted around a roll and pitch axis and can thus be brought into optimal position for surgical intervention (fig. 17.37). One section of the MR head coil is integrated in the table. The patient's head is fixed by an MR-compatible head clamp. The table can be easily turned on an axis towards the opening of the MR for the intraoperative imaging process. The table itself (with the patient) is then moved straight into the MR gantry from this position. The related patient-monitoring and anaesthesia equipment does not need to be moved during this procedure.

17.5 References

[17.1] C. Kausch, B. Schreiber, F. Kreuder, R. Schmidt, O. Dössel
Monte Carlo simulations of the imaging performance of metal plate/phosphor screens used in radiotherapy
Med. Phys. 26 (1999), 2113-2124

[17.2] G. Cho, H.K. Kim, Y.H. Chung, D.K. Kim, H.K. Lee, T.S. Suh, K.S. Joo
Monte Carlo analyses of X-ray absorption, noise, and detective quantum efficiency considering therapeutic X-ray spectrum in portal imaging detector
IEEE Trans. On Nucl. Sci. 48 (2001), 1423-1427

[17.3] J.P. Bissonnette, I.A. Cunningham, P. Munro
Optimal phosphor thickness for portal imaging
Med. Phys. 24 (1997), 803-814

[17.4] A.E. Schach von Wittenau, C.M. Logan, M.B. Aufderheide III, D.M. Slone
Blurring artifacts in megavoltage radiography with a flat-panel imaging system: comparison of Monte Carlo simulations with measurements
Med. Phys. 29 (2002), 2559-2570

[17.5] D.W. Mah, D.M. Galbraith, J.A. Rawlinson
Low-energy imaging with high-energy bremsstrahlung beams: analysis and scatter reduction
Med. Phys. 20 (1993), 653-655

[17.6] D.A. Jaffray, J.J. Battista, A. Fenster, P. Munro
Monte Carlo studies of X-ray energy absorption and quantum noise in megavoltage transmission radiography
Med. Phys. 22 (1995), 1077-1088

[17.7] T. Falco, B.G. Fallone
Characteristics of metal-plate/film detectors at therapy energies. II. Detective quantum efficiency
Med. Phys. 25 (1998), 2463-2468

[17.8] T. Falco, B.G. Fallone
Characteristics of metal-plate/film detectors at therapy energies. I. Modulation transfer function
Med Phys. 25 (1998), 2455-2462

[17.9] D.M. Galbraith
Low-energy imaging with high energy bremsstrahlung beams
Med. Phys. 16 (1989), 734-746

[17.10] O.Z. Ostapiak, P.F. O'Brien, B.A. Faddegon
Megavoltage imaging with low Z targets: implementation and characterization of an investigational system
Med. Phys. 25 (1998), 1910-1918

[17.11] S. Flampouri, P.M. Evans, F. Verhaegen, A.E. Nahum, E. Spezi, M. Partridge
Optimization of accelerator target and detector for portal imaging using Monte Carlo simulation and experiment
Phys. Med. Biol. 47 (2002), 3331-3349

[17.12] E.J. Seppi, P. Munro, S.W. Johnsen, E.G. Shapiro, C.Tognina, D. Jones, J.M. Pavkovich, C. Webb, I. Mollov, L.D. Partain, R.E. Colbeth

Megavoltage cone-beam computed tomography using a high-efficiency image receptor
Int. J. Radiat. Oncol. Biol. Phys. 55 (2003), 793-803

[17.13] M.A. Mosleh-Shirazi, P.M. Evans, W. Swindell, J.R.N. Symonds-Tayler, S. Webb, M. Patridge
Rapid portal imaging with a high-efficiency, large field-of-view detector
Med. Phys. 25 (1998), 2333-2346

[17.14] J. Ostling, M. Wallmark, A. Brahme, M. Danielsson, C. Iacobaeus, P. Fonte, V. Peskov
Novel detector for portal imaging in radiation therapy
Proc. SPIE 3977 (2000), 84-95
in J.T. Dobbins, J.M. Boone (eds.), Medical Imaging 2000: Physics of Medical Imaging

[17.15] G. Pang, J.A. Rowlands
Development of high quantum efficiency flat panel detectors for portal imaging: intrinsic spatial resolution
Med. Phys. 29 (2002), 2274-2285

[17.16] J. Pouliot, A. Bani-Hashemi, J. Chen, M. Svatos, F. Ghelmansarai, M. Mitschke, M. Aubin, P. Xia, O. Morin, K. Bucci, M. Roach, L. Verhey, P. Hernandez, Z. Zheng, D. Hristov
Low-dose Megavoltage cone-beam CT for dose-guided radiation therapy
Int. J. Radiation Oncology Biol. Phys. 61(2005), 238-246

[17.17] M. Svatos, J. Pouliot, A. Bani-Hashemi, S. Diliplane, A. Khameni, F. Sauer, M. Aubin, F. Ghelmansarai
Correlation of MV cone beam CT to a planning CT for patient alignment
Med. Phys. 30 (2003), 1471

[17.18] P.E. Kinahan, D.W. Townsend, T. Beyer, D. Sashin
Attenuation correction for a combined 3D PET/CT scanner
Med. Phys. 25 (1998), 2046-2053

[17.19] T. Beyer, D.W. Townsend, T. Brun, P.E. Kinahan, M. Charron, R. Roddy, J. Jerin, J. Young, L. Byars, R. Nutt
A combined PET/CT scanner for clinical oncology
J. Nucl. Med. 41 (2000), 1369-1379

[17.20] G. Antoch, L. Freudenberg, A. Nemat, T. Beyer, A. Bockisch
Preoperative staging of non-small cell lung cancer with dual-modality PET/CT imaging: a comparison with PET and CT
J. Nucl. Med. 44 (2003), 172P

[17.21] T.M. Blodgett, C.C. Melzer, D.W. Townsend, J.T. Yap, B. McCook, D.E. Heron, K. Gerszten, A. Sit, R. Edwards, J. Comerci, H. Gallion
PET/CT in staging and re-staging patients with cervical carcinoma
J. Nucl. Med. 43 Suppl. (2003), 309P

[17.22] T.J. Vogl, J.O. Balzer, M.G. Mack, G. Bett, A. Oppelt
Hybrid MR interventional imaging system: combined MR and angiography suites with single interventional table. Feasibility study in vascular liver tumor procedures
Eur. Radiol. 12 (2002), 1394-1400

[17.23] C. Manke, W. Nitz, B. Dyavidani, et al.
MR imaging guided stent placement in iliac arterial stenoses: a feasibility study
Radiology 219 (2001), 527-534

[17.24] R. Razavi, D.L. Hill, S.F. Keevil, M.E. Miquel, V. Muthurangu, S. Hegde, K. Rhode, M. Barnett, J. van Vaals, D.J. Hawkes, E. Baker
Cardiac catheterization guided by MRI in children and adults with congenital heart disease
Lancet 362 (2003), 1877-1882

[17.25] A.J. Dick, M.A. Guttman, V.K. Raman, D.C. Peters, J.M. Hill, S. Smith, G. Scott, E.R. McVeigh, R.J. Lederman
Magnetic resonance fluoroscopy allows targeted delivery of mesenchymal stem cells to infarct borders in swine
Circulation 108 (2003), 2899-2904

[17.26] R.J. Lederman, M.A. Guttman, D.C. Peters, R.B. Thompson, J.M. Sorger, A.J. Dick, V.K. Raman, E.R. McVeigh
Catheter-based endomyocardial injection using real-time magnetic resonance imaging
Circulation 105 (2002), 1282-1284

18 Molecular imaging

18.1 Introduction

The past decade has seen an immense growth of knowledge in the field of molecular biology, leading to a better understanding of pathologic processes at the molecular level. New genetic tests have been among the first translations of these discoveries into diagnostics. These tests can be used for prevention screening, provide prognostic information and predict disease in progeny. However, in vitro diagnostics in general does not provide anatomical information on the actual localization of the event. Imaging procedures will be necessary to localize abnormalities identified by in vitro diagnostics. Identifying e.g. the presence of blood in the stool through in vitro tests requires pinpointing the lesion for diagnosis by virtual or real colonoscopy. Obtaining a non-invasive diagnosis of preclinical or even pre-malignant disease states is highly desirable and could be achieved with molecular imaging (MI), which is capable of detection and visualization of molecular disease markers in vivo via specific probes. While conventional imaging yields anatomical maps or a rendering of physiologic functions, molecular imaging provides additional information on the distribution and (in some cases) amount or activity of specific molecular markers in vivo and will thus expand the emphasis of radiological imaging beyond the anatomical and functional level to a molecular one. Since changes on the molecular level always precede anatomical restructuring which can be detected in conventional imaging, molecular imaging methods enable diagnosis at an earlier stage in the course of a disease and therefore also an earlier treatment start. Obtaining a non-invasive diagnosis of preclinical or even reversible states of serious diseases is highly desirable and may be achieved with molecular imaging.

There are hundreds of potential molecular imaging targets and a variety of probes currently under development. Among the existing imaging modalities PET, SPECT and also MRI are particularly suited for molecular imaging. A new technology is in vivo near infrared imaging (NIR), so far in preclinical use. MRI integrates best tissue characterization at high spatial resolution with biochemistry, though concepts have to be developed to further increase the sensitivity of this modality. Beside hardware adaptations, there is a need for dedicated post-processing tools for quantification, image fusion and parameter mapping for MI. The most successful probes for a defined disease as well as the most appropriate imaging modality for any clinical application, will finally be determined by its sensitivity and specificity and the compatibility with clinical workflow.

This chapter aims to provide an overview on some of the most promising MI concepts also including a brief discussion of relevant imaging modalities.

18.2 Imaging probes

In order to visualize specific cellular and molecular events non-invasively in living subjects, appropriate imaging probes need to be designed [18.1]. In general, imaging probes can be categorized into three main groups [18.2]: nonspecific, targeted, and activatable probes as illustrated by fig. 18.1. Nonspecific probes are currently the most commonly used imaging probes and do not interact with a specific molecular target. They accentuate dissimilarities between tissues such as differences in permeability or perfusion. These probes are helpful to characterize physiological processes such as blood volume, flow, or perfusion, all representing late changes in disease processes. Characterization of early changes in disease development by imaging necessitates visualization of specific biological processes at the cellular or molecular level. Thus, imaging probes need to interact specifically with targets on these levels, leading to the development of targeted or activatable probes. In principle, targeted probes are used to localize biomolecules and to reveal their distribution. Such probes are detectable regardless of their interaction with the target. Therefore, background noise can initially be high, but tends to decrease over time as the probe remains bound to the target and remaining unbound probe is eliminated.

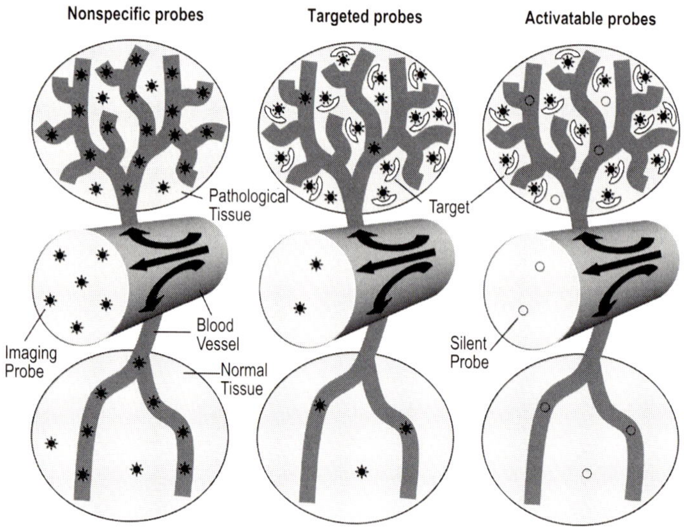

Figure 18.1
Imaging probes. Nonspecific probes do not interact with a specific molecular target. They can be used to image dissimilarities between pathological tissues (e.g. tumors) and normal tissues such as differences in permeability or perfusion. Targeted probes and activatable probes are directed specifically to cellular or molecular targets, allowing for visualization of specific biological processes at the cellular or molecular level. In contrast to targeted probes, activatable or "smart" sensor probes do not give a signal in their native injected state (silent probe), but become detectable after activation through the target (from [18.3]).

Activatable or "smart" sensor probes do not give a signal in their native state. Since these probes become detectable only upon interaction with their designated target, the signal-to-noise-ratio is significantly increased. Smart probes can be activated through interaction with ions or through cleavage by enzymes. Thus, smart probes also allow visualization and localization of the molecular functions [18.4]. A combination of targeted and activatable probes are so-called smart MRI probes. They are detectable in their native form, but upon interaction with their target they undergo a change in relaxivity ("activation") resulting in different signal characteristics: higher T_1 or lower T_2 signal [18.5].

Designing probes for molecular imaging

The design of target specific imaging probes is challenging since numerous key issues must be addressed. Namely 1) identification of a suitable molecular target by target screening, 2) finding a ligand that binds to this molecular target with high specificity by ligand screening, 3) labeling this ligand with a signal molecule for visualization depending on the imaging modality, 4) overcoming biological delivery barriers for the probe on its way to the target in vivo, and 5) finding strategies for signal amplification in order to increase sensitivity. After these conceptual challenges have been overcome pre-clinical studies have to prove effectiveness as well as bio-compatibility, then clinical trials have to verify clinical benefit.

Identification of suitable targets for molecular imaging

Finding an appropriate target proves to be the first barrier in designing an imaging probe. To find novel targets for drug development, the pharmaceutical industry undertakes screening tests in the magnitude of millions of samples. Technologies such as recombinant techniques, phage display, proteomics, robotics, and high throughput screening have increased the effectiveness of this procedure considerably. Using high throughput screening, thousands of samples can be evaluated simultaneously, quantitatively and rapidly to shorten the time between development and final patent filing. At present, therapeutic drugs are directed against approximately 500 different molecular targets, of which 45% are receptors, 30% are enzymes and 25% are other molecules. Triggered by the human genome project at least ten times more potential targets will become accessible in the future. More recently, screening technologies are also being extended to identify targets for molecular imaging [18.6 and references mentioned herein].

Potential molecular targets are primarily nucleic acid sequences (DNA and mRNA) or proteins, but can also include any other specific cell structure such as carbohydrates or lipids (fig. 18.2). Several features of these biomolecules need to be considered, including the localization of the target molecules (on the cell surface or within the target cells) and the amount of copies of the same molecule in a single cell (quantity). The number of DNA-sequences encoding for genes per cell is usually only two. Furthermore, DNA usually takes on a supercoiled form, surrounded by organizing proteins such as chromatin. Therefore, the target sequence might be shielded and hidden. Additionally, a DNA-directed probe upon reaching its target cell, must overcome two bar-

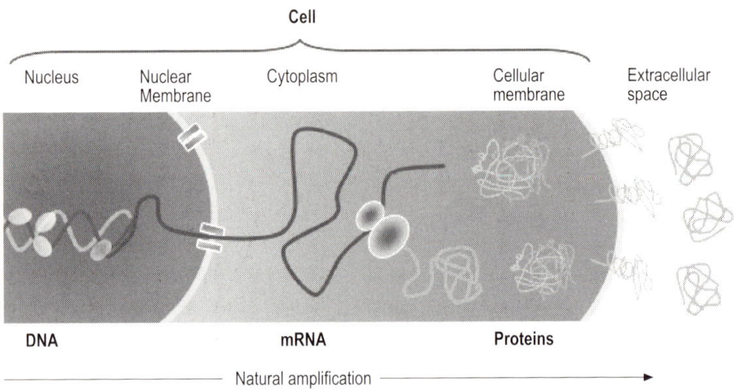

Figure 18.2
Potential targets for molecular imaging and their localization. While the DNA is located in the nucleus, mRNA can be located in the nucleus and the cytoplasm. Proteins are either localized intracellularly, on the cell surface, or secreted into the extracellular space. The flow of genetic information via DNA transcription (generally only 2 copies per cell) into mRNA (approximately 50 to 1.000 copies per cell) and translation of the mRNA into proteins (approximately 100 to 1.000.000 copies per cell) comprises a "natural amplification" process. Since the number of copies per cell increases in this process, selecting a "downstream" target of gene expression is much more feasible. (adapted from [18.3])

riers to finally reach the DNA: the cell membrane and the nuclear membrane. Imaging the message of a gene "downstream" of the DNA on the mRNA or protein level, is therefore much more feasible. This strategy, referred to as "downstream imaging", utilizes the flow of genetic information via transcription of the DNA into mRNA (about 50 to 1.000 copies per cell) and translation of the mRNA into proteins (about 100 to 1.000.000 copies per cells). In consequence, the "natural amplification" process provides significantly more copies of the target molecule thereby allowing detection with much higher sensitivity by a specific imaging probe.

Identifying and labeling a ligand that binds to a molecular target

Once a suitable target has been identified, a molecule (ligand) that specifically binds to this target has to be identified. These can be small molecules, such as receptor ligands and substrates for enzymes, or larger ones such as recombinant proteins or monoclonal antibodies. Identification of a suitable ligand is usually performed using libraries of molecules, phage display or in silico (ligand screening). Depending on the imaging modality, a detectable signal molecule (label) has to be bound to the ligand. For nuclear imaging, a variety of appropriate radioisotopes are available and already in clinical use, simplifying potential clinical applications. Numerous labeling techniques assist in probe design, whereby radioisotopes are either chelated or covalently coupled to the ligand [18.7]. For MRI, paramagnetic metal cations such as chelated gadolinium or dysprosium (or other Lanthanides), or superparamagnetic nanoparticles based on crystalline iron-oxide can be used for labeling [18.8, 18.9 and references mentioned herein]. For optical imaging, organic fluorochromes or anorganic compounds such as quantum dots for fluorescence optical imaging, as well as substrates for bioluminescence optical imaging are available [18.10 and references mentioned herein]. Perfluorocarbon emulsion nanoparticles, acoustically reflective liposomes, and stabilized perfluorocarbon gas microbubbles are under investigation as ultrasound contrast agents [18.11]. For CT, high-atomic number atoms that absorb X-rays such as iodine or bismuth are being evaluated [18.12].

Delivery of the probe

To be detectable in living subjects, imaging probes must have the ability to reach the intended target at a sufficient concentration and sufficient time. Fig. 18.3 illustrates the major biological barriers for imaging probes on their way to their target. After administration, imaging probes are subject to pharmacokinetic precepts: absorption, distribution, metabolism, and elimination. In order to leave the vascular system, the vascular wall needs to be traversed. Imaging probes below a certain cut of molecular weight can extravasate and be distributed in both target and non-target tissues, the latter leading to background signal. However, extravasation can be challenging, especially in the brain when the blood-brain-barrier is intact [18.13]. In tumors or inflammatory processes, the vasculature is “leaky” and therefore easier to traverse [18.14]. Once the probe crosses over into the interstitial space of the target tissue, it needs to reach the target cells. Additional barriers may be present, e.g. if the target is located

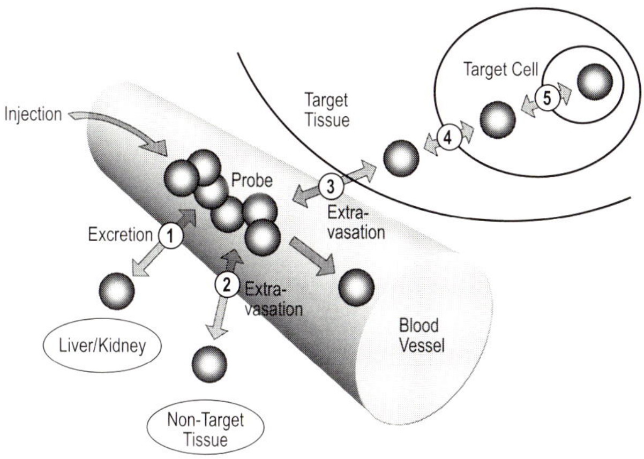

Figure 18.3
Major biological delivery barriers for imaging probes on their the way to the target. The liver and kidneys, major excretory organs, are very efficient in eliminating “foreign” molecules **(1)**. The imaging probe can extravasate and distribute in non-target tissues **(2)**. To reach the target cell, the probe has to be able to extravasate into the target tissue **(3)**. Once the target tissue is reached, the imaging probe needs to find the target cell. For intracellular targets the cellular membrane is another barrier that needs to be crossed **(4)**. If the target is located in intracellular compartments such as the nucleus, another hurdle (in this case, the nuclear membrane) needs to be overcome **(5)** (figure according to [18.1], adapted from [18.3]).

in the cytoplasm of the target cells, or situated in intracellular compartments such as the nucleus. The "fate" of a compound in vivo depends on properties of the probes such as molecular size, water solubility or binding characteristics. The main process by which the body eliminates "foreign" substances is excretion. Hydrophilic materials are eliminated by the kidneys, whereas lipophilic compounds usually are metabolized by the liver, the principal organ for metabolism [18.15]. Lipophilic compounds are also redistributed into faty tissue.

18.3 Signal amplification strategies

Adequate visualization of biological processes in vivo requires a sufficient level of imaging signal per unit level of target and probe interaction. To increase the signal and therefore improve sensitivity, signal amplification strategies need to be considered. This is especially important for imaging modalities with relatively poor sensitivity or when imaging on the DNA- or mRNA-level where the number of targets per cell is limited to a few copies. In this respect, the strategy to image proteins or protein function ("downstream imaging") is much more viable because of much larger number of targets per cell. A number of signal amplification strategies for molecular imaging have been developed. Target concentration can be improved by means of pre-targeting [18.16], by avidin-biotin amplification [18.17], by improving kinetics [18.18], or by trapping of converted ligands [18.19]. Labelling with a high number of signal generating compounds may be applied to increase the payload of the probe. The binding avidity to a particular target can be increased by coupling more than one ligand to the probe (e.g. several antibody fragments can be coupled to a nano-sized probe). Another strategy is to design the imaging probe in a way that the probe changes its physical properties after target interaction. Examples include, activatable smart sensor probes for imaging of enzyme activity based on fluorescence dequenching, or so-called smart MRI probes based on changes of magnetic relaxation upon assembly of paramagnetic or superparamagnetic particles, resulting in a higher T_1 or lower T_2 signal, respectively (see below).

18.4 Imaging modalities

Academia and pharmaceutical companies are increasingly expressing interest in small animal imaging (SAI), because small animal models constitute an established research tool for molecular imaging and for the biological validation of new therapies. SAI allows for repetitive studies on the same animal and therefore enables the evaluation of disease progression or treatment response over time. It furthermore aids in target identification and early prioritization of candidate drug compounds. Imaging instrumentation used for SAI includes those modalities already used in clinical radiology with the important addition of optical imaging. Dedicated scanners for SAI are today available for all different modalities. While animal scanners for MR imaging have been around for decades, micro-PET became commercially available around

1997, followed by micro-SPECT in 2001. Commercial optical systems utilizing bioluminescence or fluorescence imaging were developed in the early 1990s. Planar ultrasound transducers for high-resolution imaging are also used to examine mice. All these dedicated systems are specifically designed for the needs of SAI and, if compared with clinical systems have a much smaller sampling volume and provide higher spatial resolution. However, since dedicated systems are expensive and clinical systems, are usually available in larger hospitals, there is also a trend to adapt clinical scanners (mainly MRI) to the needs of SAI by using dedicated animal coils, sometimes also in combination with dedicated high field gradient systems [18.20]. Most of the systems today are tomographic, whereas optical systems are usually designed for planar imaging, although tomographic optical systems are available as prototypes today.

18.4.1 Nuclear imaging

Nuclear imaging has always been at the forefront of molecular imaging. Many of the clinical probes have already been designed to detect molecular mechanisms, e.g. radiolabeled annexin to image apoptosis [18.21]. Nuclear techniques include planar scintigraphy, PET and SPECT. All of these systems have a lower resolution (1 to 2 mm) than MRI and CT, but are highly sensitive and inherently quantitative. Picomolar concentration of isotopes can be detected with no depth limit. However, like optical imaging, nuclear imaging provides only limited anatomical information. The output is merely a map of activity in the animal, the exact anatomical location of which can only be derived from the shape of the accumulated activity, if at all possible. This makes combinations with other modalities that deliver good anatomical information such as CT or MRI very valuable. PET and SPECT are currently the most advanced methods to image molecular events in patients.

For PET, positron-emitting isotopes are needed (^{15}O, ^{13}N, ^{18}F, ^{124}I, $^{94m}T_C$, ^{11}C). Most of these isotopes are produced in a cyclotron and have short half lives (e.g. ^{18}F has a half life of 110 minutes), thus cannot be transported over long distances, require rapid chemical synthesis of the radio-labeled probe and ideally a cyclotron on side. As a result probes for PET imaging are relatively expensive and cumbersome to use. On the other hand, the short half-life allows for repetitive experiments within shorter time cycles. Small molecules are widely used as probes, which are recognized by enzymes, receptors or other targets (39). ^{18}F-fluorodeoxyglucose (FDG) is the most widely used tracer molecule for PET imaging in clinical studies to detect metabolically active tumors (fig. 18.4). This glucose analog is transported into the cell by a specific transporter molecule, over-expressed in many cancers, which leads to an accumulation of the tracer within the tumor cells. FDG might serve as a surrogate marker to assess treatment response after chemotherapy, challenging the more widely used CT [18.23]. PET has further been applied to study multi-drug resistance, apoptosis [18.24] and also gene expression in animal studies using reporter genes [18.25]. Reporter genes are used to study the expression of either generic or transfected genes by coupling the expression of the reporter gene to the expression of the gene of interest. This is achieved by placing the reporter and the gene of interest under the control of the same promotor. To study gene expression with PET, herpes simplex thymidine kinase (HSV-TK) is

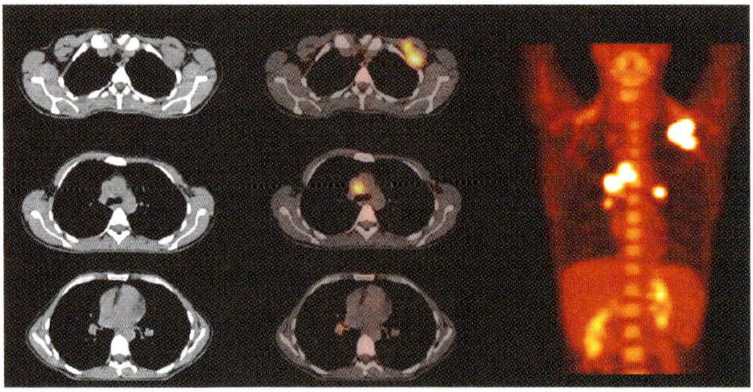

Figure 18.4
CT/PET with image fusion technique of a 37 year old female patient with history of metastatic breast cancer. Multiple areas of increased FDG uptake consistent with metastatic disease in the mediastinum, bilateral pulmonary hila, left upper lateral chest wall.

utilized as a marker gene. If HSV-TK is expressed, nucleoside analogs are phosphorylated and become trapped within the cell due to the associated change in charge. The accumulation of activity is therefore an indicator of HSV-TK presence and consequently successful transfection. Those marker genes can also be utilized for tracking of transfected cells in vivo [18.26].

SPECT utilizes gamma-emitting nucleotides (^{99m}Tc, ^{111}In, ^{123}I, ^{131}I), which are produced in generators without needing a cyclotron. These isotopes are generally cheaper and have a longer half-life than the positron emitting nucleotides used for PET imaging (e.g. ^{111}In has a half-life of 2.8 days). This makes SPECT easier to work with and facilitates imaging of probes with slow kinetics such as antibody fragments. However, unlike PET scanners, SPECT requires the presence of lead collimators to correct for scattering, which is done electronically in PET imaging. This requirement decreases both the detection efficiency and sensitivity of current SPECT scanners as compared with PET, which is about one order of magnitude more sensitive. However, these disadvantages could be overcome in the future through new technical developments such as increasing the numbers of detectors, using multiple-pinhole collimators or allowing data multiplexing (i.e. overlapping images) to allow more counts to be registered.

The decay of all isotopes utilized in PET results in the emission of 2 photons of the same energy (511 keV). Since it is not possible to distinguish different isotopes with PET scanners, the imaging of two different molecular probes simultaneously is impossible with this technology. Different probes have therefore to be injected sequentially. Isotopes suitable for SPECT imaging on the other hand emit gamma rays of different energies, which allows for the simultaneous detection of several isotopes, e.g. simultaneous imaging of different molecular targets. SPECT has been used to track cells or molecules such as radiolabeled annexin-V to image apoptosis [18.21] or tumor specific peptides [18.27, 18.28 and references mentioned herein] in vivo (fig. 18.5). It has also been deployed to image oncogene expression. Preliminary reports show that SPECT imaging

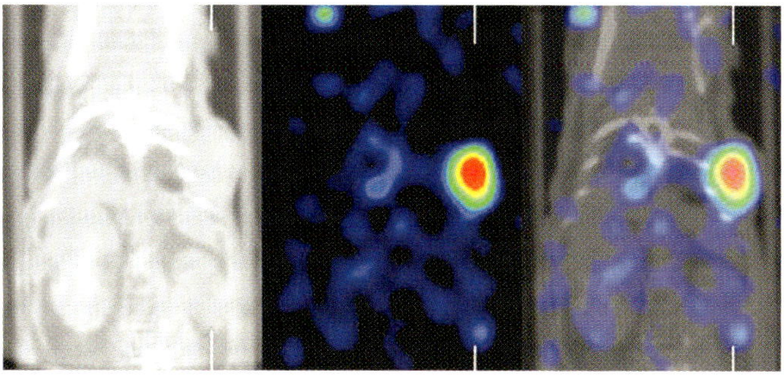

Figure 18.5
SPECT-CT of a nude mouse bearing a CEA-positive LS174T human colon cancer xenograft 23 hours after injection of a I-123 labeled minibody (antibody fragment) targeting CEA [18.28]. The accumulation of the labeled minibody in the tumor is clearly detectable. (Source: Dr. Anna Wu, Crump Institute, UCLA)

might play a role as surrogate marker after chemotherapy as well [18.29]. Combinations of nuclear imaging modalities with other techniques are discussed below.

18.4.2 Magnetic resonance imaging (MRI)

MRI offers several advantages over nuclear or optical imaging techniques: it has a high spatial resolution, unlimited depth penetration and offers good soft tissue contrast along with spatial anatomical orientation in conjunction with the information retrieved from the molecular probe. Unlike optical or nuclear imaging, where only the activity of the probe is extracted and presented in the images, MRI simultaneously shows the event and its anatomical localization. On the other hand, MRI is less sensitive than those modalities, being in the order of milli- to micromole (compared to nano- to picomole or even lower for optical and nuclear probes). As a result higher quantities of probe have to be injected, and a sufficient signal amplification strategy has to be employed. Magnetic resonance spectroscopy (MRS) can furthermore be used to identify metabolites critical in a variety of diseases, such as tumors of the brain or prostate [18.30].

Clinically approved MR contrast agents [18.31 and references mentioned herein] can be modified for the needs of molecular imaging, but these modifications have not yet been approved for clinical imaging. For MRI two groups of contrast agents exist, paramagnetic and superparamagnetic agents. For all these probes signal amplification can be obtained by inducing an increase in relaxivity. The most prominent T_2 contrast labels are iron-oxide nanoparticles, which consist of a crystalline iron-oxide core with a dextran or polyethyleneglycol coating. Each of these particles contains thousands of iron atoms, which by itself increases the local iron concentration and in consequence the relaxivity considerably. Therefore, detection of even low concentrations of nanoparticles (micro- to nanomols of iron) is possible.

Lanthanide chelates such as gadolinium-DTPA and derivatives are typical T_1-contrast agents. Since there is only one lanthanide atom per chelate, the concentration necessary to image on a molecular level is considerably higher than it is for iron-oxide particles (in the order of milimols). T_1-contrast probes can be activated by different mechanisms. An enzyme-mediated polymerization of paramagnetic substrates into oligomers with higher relaxivity (due to an increase in the rotational correlation time of the lanthanide) is one approach. Another method utilizes conformational changes in the chelates, allowing access of bulk water to the inner sphere of the chelated lanthanide upon cleavage or binding of calcium [18.32]. Packing a large quantity of chelates into liposome-like nanoparticles is a third approach [18.33]. Chemical exchange saturation transfer has been used e.g. to sense glucose concentration with MRI [18.34].

Similarly to PET imaging, MRI can be used to image gene expression by exploiting marker genes such as the transferrin-receptor [18.35], tyrosinase [18.36] or ß-galactosidase [18.39]. The transferrin receptor binds to iron-loaded (or even specially labeled) transferrin, mediates the accumulation of superparamagnetic iron oxide within the cell and therefore induces a signal decrease in T_2-weighted images [18.37]. Tyrosinase catalyses the synthesis of melanin, which has a high iron binding capacity, resulting in a high signal intensity of melanin containing cells (such as melanoma cells) in T_1-weighted images [18.38]. Smart or activatable contrast agents have also been used to detect marker genes. In one example, a carbohydrate-modified Gadolinium chelate was used to image the activity of the enzyme ß-galactosidase as marker gene. The enzyme cleaves the carbohydrate residue from the chelate, inducing an increase in relaxivity by allowing access of water to the gadolinium [18.39].

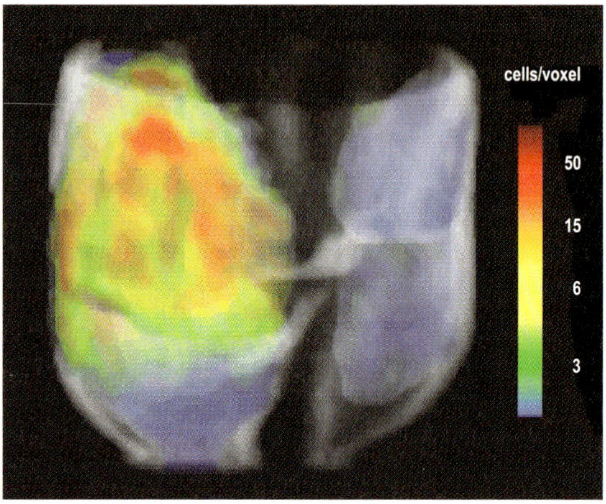

Figure 18.6
Antigen-specific lymphocyte tracking to tumors in vivo [18.45]. **Left** ovalbumine-producing tumor, **right** control tumor (both B16) after injection of ovalbumine-sensitive CD8-pos. T-cells. The image shows the color-encoded number of cells per voxel, derived from a MRI-T_2 map. The high number of tumor-infiltrating lymphocytes and their distribution within the tumor can be seen. (Source: Dr. Moritz Kircher, CMIR, Boston)

The principle of the magnetic relaxation switch can be utilized to obtain activatable MR contrast agents. Upon interaction with the target, iron particles change their physical properties by aggregation, resulting in a change of their relaxivity. This principle has been used to detect viral particles [18.40], enzymes [18.41], DNA or mRNA sequences [18.42] or telomerase activity [18.43] in crude biological samples. The combination of this method with the high throughput evaluation of thousands of samples with MRI [18.44] could offer a completely new method for rapid screening of large numbers of sample in proteomics or clinical laboratories (e.g. the evaluation of 10752 samples in seven stacked 1536 well plates in about 10 minutes within a clinical MR scanner).

A specific population of cells can be labeled with magnetic nanoparticles and followed in vivo using MRI, so called "cell tracking". This method has been used to study in vivo the spatial distribution of immuno-competent cells into tumors over time (fig. 18.6) [18.45], to map neuronal stem cell migration after stroke [18.46], to image injected myocardial stem cells [18.47] as well as to study the fate of hematopoietic stem cells in vivo [18.48].

High resolution MRI is furthermore well suited to screening transgenic mice for tumors and other abnormalities [18.49] and can be applied non-invasively to follow up new experimental treatment strategies.

18.4.3 Optical imaging

Optical imaging is a rapid and inexpensive way to image molecular events. Optical imaging techniques have been used for some time in molecular biology in the form of fluorescence and confocal fluorescence microscopy or benchtop fluorescent readers for the analysis of test kits. Transferring these optical techniques into imaging of living animals has to overcome the challenge that mammalian tissues are not well penetrated by light due to strong absorption and scattering effects. Therefore, the detectors have to be very sensitive and the emission spectrum of the probe has to be optimized for sufficient tissue depth penetration and quantum yield. On the detector side recent developments have resulted in very sensitive detectors such as cooled CCD chips. Since hemoglobin and water have the lowest absorption in the near infrared spectrum (700 to 900 nm), they provide an optical window in tissues. Using fluorochromes such as Cy5 or Cy7 with emission spectra in that region or even beyond, maximizes tissue penetration and minimizes autofluorescence [18.50]. However, relative variations in tissue structure as well as the contribution of varying pigmentation and the presence of melanin can significantly impact absorption and scattering properties of photons. The use of activatable optical probes further minimizes background fluorescence. These probes do not provide a signal in their native injected state, but become detectable after activation through interaction with the target. This new concept makes optical imaging in small animals feasible, however, the much larger dimensions of human patients require much deeper penetration into and through tissues and are so far limiting the application of optical fluorescence imaging in clinical settings. Applying optical methods only to the more accessible or superficial parts of the human body may circumvent these limitations. Dedicated handheld scanners to detect skin cancer or diagnose arthritic alterations in small joints in the hand are under development, as are scanners for minimally invasive surgery, intraoperative or endoscopic optical imaging.

In optical imaging today, two main practical principles are being exploited for molecular imaging: bioluminescence and fluorescence. Common to both methodologies is that a signal with a specific signature is generated at the tissue site of interest and then recorded by windowing the detection range specific to the signal generated from the target. Bioluminescence is an oxygen and ATP-consuming biological process, catalyzed by the enzyme luciferase that oxidizes its substrate luciferin, thereby emitting light. Luciferase is a naturally occurring enzyme found in insects, mainly in fireflies. In order to exploit this system the gene has to be expressed in the cells transgenically and its substrate luciferin has to be injected. Since this process requires genetic alterations of the target tissues, it can easily be applied in model animal studies but it is not likely to be transferred into clinical settings. Fluorescence on the other hand is a physical process in which the fluorochrome is excited by a specific wavelength to emit light shifted to a longer wavelength. These fluorochromes can be cyanine derivatives or fluorescent proteins such as the jellyfish protein GFP (green fluorescent protein) and its variations. Amplification of the signal can usually be obtained by accumulation of the probe (e.g. within cells) or by activation of smart sensor probes, which become activated only upon interaction with the target. This represents a more likely approach for clinical settings, since only the fluorochrome coupled to the molecule recognizing the target needs to be introduced into the tissue. However, the challenges of light scattering properties of tissues remain, possibly obstructing the penetration of the exciting signal as well as the emitted signal from the probe.

Similar to MRI and MRS, reflectance optical imaging can evaluate tissue composition due to the variation of chemicals present within tissues resulting in different spectral properties. In contrast to other well-established modalities, this method is still very young and currently in the clinical development phase. Among others, the most advanced applications relate to spectroscopic optical analysis of response to chemotherapy [18.51] or neuroimaging [18.52] based on tissue hydration and oxygenation by spectroscopy. However, similar to the other optical imaging modalities tracing photons within a highly light-scattering medium presents similar challenges for signal reconstruction and location of structures deep within tissues.

Bioluminescence imaging (BI) shows very little background since there is no excitation light necessary, which makes it useful to detect very low levels of targets. It is surface weighted and has limited depth penetration and resolution (several mm). So far the light emission of luciferin has been confined to green light, which provides very limited tissue penetration, and undergoes substantial signal attenuation with depth of tissue traversed. However, novel red-shifted luciferases with better tissue penetration may improve BI. Similar to the principle of SPECT imaging, scanner settings with rotating CCD cameras would allow tomographic BI studies. BI has successfully been used to non-invasively image tumors and their response to treatment approaches [18.53].

A

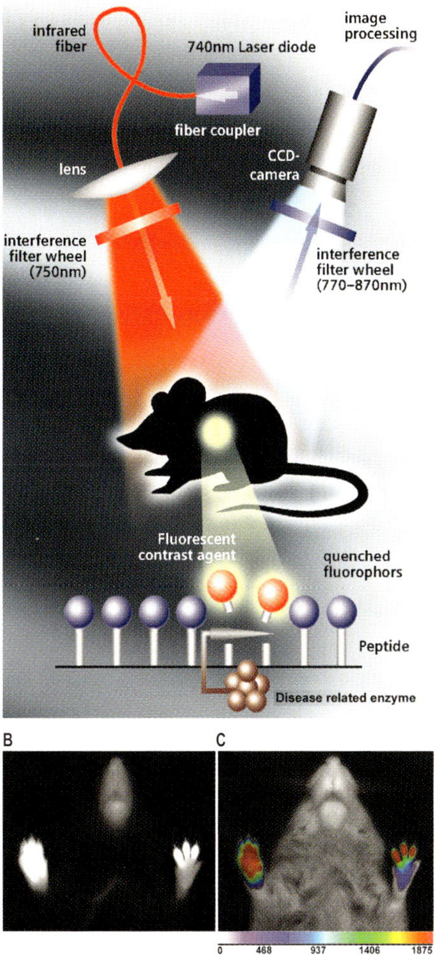

Figure 18.7
Principle of fluorescence reflectance imaging (FRI) using a near-infrared fluorescence (NIRF) smart sensor probe as a molecular reporter. The molecular reporter consists of a backbone bearing multiple bound fluorochromes and several cleavage sites for a disease-related enzyme. Due to interactions between the fluorochromes, fluorescence quenching occurs. Enzymatic cleavage releases these fluorochromes and results in activation of fluorescence that can be detected in vivo. Fluorescence is excited by laser light and fluorescence images are acquired using a CCD camera equipped with an appropiate filter to separate fluorescence from laser light **(A)**. NIRF image **(B)** and color-coded NIRF image from B superimposed on a white light image **(C)** of a mouse with arthritis affecting the left front paw and three toes of the right front paw, 24 h after injection of an activatable smart sensor probe. The imaging probe can be cleaved by Cathepsin B which is involved in the destruction of arthritic joints resulting in high fluorescence intensity in affected extremities. (Taken from [18.3], adapted with permission from [18.74])

The luciferase gene can be used as a marker gene for gene expression [18.54], sometimes together with the HSV-TK [18.55] for combined optical and nuclear imaging. Nevertheless, if small animal imaging is seen only as a step in development to clinical applications, BI represents major challenges due to the simultaneous introduction of genetic engineering to the human body (luciferase gene) and a foreign chemical luciferin for signal generation.

In case of *fluorescence optical imaging* several modi are available. In *fluorescence reflectance imaging (FRI)*, the animal is illuminated with light at the appropriate wavelength to excite the fluorochromes. The resulting light emission is then recorded with a sensitive, high resolution CCD camera (fig. 18.7). Multi-channel imaging of several wavelengths at the same time is also possible using filter wheels [18.56]. Opposed to the requirement of luciferin for bioluminescence imaging no substrate is needed, and FRI can also be utilized for imaging of fixed tissues [18.57]. Similar to bioluminescence, FRI is surface weighted and limited to targets relatively close to the surface. Targets deeper inside the body appear less bright even if the total concentration of the fluorochrome is as high as in those structures relatively close to the surface. This phenomenon is caused by scattering and absorption in tissues [18.58]. The resolution is furthermore confined to 1 to 2 mm. However, the use of multi-modality molecular probes detectable by MR, SPECT and optical imaging would add FRI as additional methodology to the analysis. Furthermore, pathology on tissue thin sections could utilize FRI to confirm targeting of a specific probe by fluorescence microscopy.

To overcome the challenges of tissue depth penetration mentioned above in reaching deeper targets, *fluorescence mediated tomography (FMT)* has been developed (fig. 18.8). In this system, spatially encoded sources or a laser scanning across the animal provides the excitation light. The emission is captured by a high resolution CCD camera. The image is mathematically reconstructed, taking photon propagation through tissues and interfaces into account. Targets several centimeters deep in the body can be detected and resolved, depending on the optical properties of the surrounding tissues: targets in lungs and breasts are detectable even deeper inside (around 7 to 10 cm) than e.g. in muscles, and resolution can reach sub-milimeter levels [18.59]. This approach is inherently quantitative and very sensitive (nanomolar to femtomolar concentrations of probe). Recent developments use pulsed lasers for time resolved imaging whereby early and therefore less scattered photons are exploited to achieve even higher image resolution. This time-domain optical imaging shows some advantages in localizing a target area within complex tissue structures such as animals [18.60]. Since ultra-fast pulsing lasers (mainly in the femto-second range) generate a dynamic source of radiation, the signal passes in a timely manner through the target area. Signal delays caused by either scattering or different tissue densities can be accounted for in the detection process and filtered from solely originating form the target. In order to do so, the complex temporal point spread function (TPSF) of photons traveling through tissue is applied and solved to exploit the "time-of-flight" information for signal reconstruction. Depending on the arrangement of the source and the detection components in such imaging platforms, optimal 3-dimensional reconstruction of small target areas can be achieved. However, two restrictions have made it difficult to

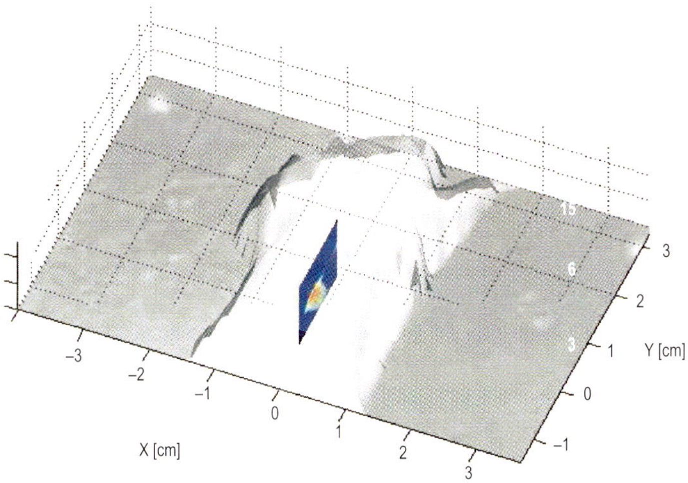

Figure 18.8
FMT image of a nude mouse, implanted with a Lewis lung carcinoma tumor within the lung after injection of a cathepsin-B activatable optical probe. The blue square indicates one of the planes, calculated from the original dataset. The tumor is shown color-encoded, red showing the highest amount of photons. (Source: Prof. Vasilis Ntziachristos, CMIR, Boston)

create commercial platforms. Ultra-fast laser systems are still under development for commercial use and the signal strength achievable with time-domain optical imaging is relatively low for molecular imaging applications. Nevertheless, time-domain optical imaging is in the process of developing into a methodology for molecular imaging. Other new developments include optical coherence tomography (OCT), which, analagous to ultrasound, uses reflections of coherent light, resulting in resolutions of about 10 µm. OCT is mostly applied in retinoscopy [18.61] and artherosclerosis [18.62].

Similar to nuclear imaging methods, FRI and FMT images depict only the spatial location of the source without any anatomical reference, making a combined imaging modality with CT or MRI desirable. Fluorescence imaging has been used for receptor targeted [18.63] or antibody mediated imaging of tumors [18.64]. Smart sensor probes are being developed to image enzyme activities associated with cancer (fig. 18.8) or rheumatoid arthritis (fig. 18.7). A cathepsin-B activatable probe could show the invasiveness of tumors in breast cancer, by correlating activity and invasiveness [18.65]. Matrix metalloproteinase (MMP) inhibitors have been reported to slow tumor progression in vivo [18.66]. Using a smart MMP-activated probe, a clear reduction in MMP activity after treatment with inhibitor has been shown [18.67]. Annexin-V labeled with Cy5.5 has been used to image apoptosis after chemotherapy treatment [18.68]. These and other studies show the feasibility of molecular imaging for assessment of prognosis and treatment efficacy. New developments include the use of NIR fluorescence imaging in combination with endoscopy and laparoscopy to detect intraperitoneal or intraluminal tumors, which may later help guide surgeons to suspect lesions.

18.4.4 Computed tomography

In CT images are generated based on the differential X-ray absorption of tissues. The physical characteristics of the high energy X-rays (120 kV) used in clinical CT scanners are considerably different from those for small animal imagers (around 50 kV). Therefore the image characteristics are not comparable to clinical scanners. While there is very low soft tissue contrast there is a good contrast between calcium-containing structures (such as bone) and soft tissues, comparable to mammographic equipment with similar voltage settings. To be able to distinguish organs, the application of iodinated contrast agents is necessary. Since these usually have only a short plasma half-life, long-circulating contrast agents are under development. The spatial resolution of scanners for SAI depends on the detector resolution and geometry as well as the focus size of the X-ray tube, and can be as low as 50 μm. The applied radiation dose to a mouse is relatively high (5 cGy or about 0.5% of the lethal dose LD50). To detect molecular events with CT, the required concentration of iodinated label to detect X-ray attenuation would need to be very high (in the millimolar range) which makes CT currently not suitable for molecular imaging. Furthermore, specific iodinated CT-probes need to be developed, probably based on a polymeric design to achieve a high ratio of iodine per label molecule. However, due to its very high resolution and fast imaging time it is currently used to screen phenotypes and to evaluate tumor treatment response. Since imaging of lung or osseous processes does not require contrast enhancement, CT is an ideal method to image bone structures. In order to localize a nuclear or optical signal anatomically, the combination of CT with PET, SPECT or optical modalities is very desirable and has already been applied clinically in PET-CT (fig. 18.4).

18.4.5 Ultrasound

Ultrasound is used extensively in clinical examinations. The resolution depends on the frequency of the transducer. SAI frequencies in the 7 to 20 MHz range can be used to produce images with a spatial resolution of less than 0.5 mm [18.69]. A technique called ultrasound bio-microscopy is even capable of resolutions below 100 μm in living tissues by applying high frequency pulses of 20 to 200 MHz [18.69]. The application of ultrasound in SAI reflects its clinical use: cardiac, abdominal, vascular and obstetric imaging are the most frequent application settings. It is used to screen for phenotypes, to measure blood flow with Doppler ultrasound and to image developing mouse embryos [18.69]. Real time imaging capabilities provide guidance during invasive procedures, similar to clinical applications. The development of contrast agents for ultrasound diagnostics is a challenging task, since it is not as simple a process as the attachment of a marker molecule to a target. Tissue contrast can only be detected by ultrasound, if the ultrasonic wave is reflected back from the interface between two different types of tissues. Contrast agents therefore have to provide a surface structure that can create a reflective interface between the contrast agent and the surrounding tissue to be detectable by ultrasound. In the last decade clinical contrast agents for ultrasound have been developed, consisting of lipid micelles around inert gas, thereby providing the difference in density needed for the ultrasonic detection. These micro-bubbles are applied to enhance vascular imaging but also increasingly help with delineation and characterization of tumors [18.70] and have expanded the usage of ultrasound into molecular imaging. Attachment of target specific molecules to micro-bubbles as a logical next step enabled the development of targeted ultrasound contrast agents. This new concept additionally provided a new drug delivery system. Micro-bubble contrast agents targeted to endothelial surface markers can be applied to image tumor angiogenesis and also deliver and release substances into specific tissues, by utilizing ultrasound-targeted microbubble destruction [18.71]. A second group of ultrasonic contrast agents under development is based upon non-microbubble technology, mainly split into two general types: 1) nongaseous acoustically reflective liposomes and 2) perfluorocarbon emulsion based nanoparticles. In the case of nongaseous liposomes, reflectivity is achieved by filling them with many very small vesicles instead of gas bubbles, thereby creating a new reflective microenvironment. However, to improve the lifetime of the contrast agent and increase the ultrasonic reflectivity from the background, emulsion nanoparticles with special properties have been developed. These new types of contrast agents not only have a much longer lifetime, but also generate reflective contrast only when accumulated in the target area due to specific binding [18.72]. Initial studies indicate that localized accumulation of target-directed nanoparticles significantly enhances the ultrasonic backscattering and generates an effect best described as "acoustic staining". However, ultrasound has just entered the initial phase of molecular methods and is currently not as widely used for molecular imaging as other imaging modalities.

18.4.6 Combined systems

To obtain the ideal combination of high-resolution anatomical localization with very sensitive detection of the molecular probe, new developments are currently leading to combined systems such as SPECT-CT (fig. 18.5) and PET-CT. Still under development are combinations of PET or optical systems with MRI. These systems are much more technically challenging, since all components must be designed to work in the high magnetic field environment of a MR scanner without interfering with image quality. Dual probes for optical and MR imaging with the same contrast agent have also been developed [18.73], allowing for true *multi-modality imaging*. Image fusion of CT with PET (fig. 18.4) is also being used in clinical medicine with PET-CT combinations. Ongoing developments in imaging software and computing hardware facilitate image fusion and enable online fusion.

18.5 Outlook

Molecular imaging is increasingly used for research purposes to facilitate the examination of metabolic functions, patterns of gene expression, or pharmacological questions in the living organism. Encouraging advances have already been achieved in animal research in the past decade. The ultimate goal, however, is the translation of these achievements into the clinic and the human scale. Molecular imaging has the potential to transform the practice of medicine and become a mainstay of patient management. It is expected that molecular imaging will allow earlier detection of disease, more efficient treatment planning and near-real-time treatment monitoring. Thus it will improve patient care by assisting the physician in providing highly efficient treatments tailored to each patient. Emerging molecular diagnostic methods such as genomics, proteomics and metabolomics will add complementary diagnostic data. MI and modern in vitro tests are two complementary emerging molecular diagnostic procedures of future medical practice. Raw molecular diagnostic data are highly complex. Large-scale integration of MI and in-vitro diagnostic data in conjunction with multidimensional data analysis must be applied to interpret the increasing amounts of data. The resulting patient specific patterns ("finger prints") need to be supplemented by medical knowledge bases to yield treatment guidelines in accordance with evidence-based medicine.

Molecular imaging is an emerging field and it will take some time and efforts to achieve so that its full potential in the clinical environment. Cost effectiveness is a general issue in molecular medicine, however, more diagnostics may lower overall healthcare costs. Some molecular imaging probes are highly specific and target pathologies are present only in a small number of patients, those probes might not be economically viable. Mechanistic probes, which target general processes such as apoptosis or angiogenesis might be more profitable. Existing imaging devices must be adjusted to the requirements of clinical molecular imaging, and workflow-compatible protocols as well as comprehensive post-processing tools must be created. If these requirements are fulfilled, molecular imaging will serve as an essential supplement to other imaging and diagnostic procedures.

18.6 References

[18.1] T.F. Massoud, S.S. Gambhir
Molecular imaging in living subjects: seeing fundamental biological processes in a new light
Genes. Dev. 17 (2003), 545-580

[18.2] R. Weissleder
Scaling down imaging: molecular mapping of cancer in mice
Nat. Rev. Cancer 2 (2002), 11-18

[18.3] J. Grimm, A. Wunder
Molekulare Bildgebung: Stand der Forschung.
RöFo, Fortschritte auf dem Gebiet der Röntgenstrahlen (2005); 177: 326-337.
Abb. 2, 3, 5, 6

[18.4] M. Funovics, R. Weissleder, C.H. Tung
Protease sensors for bioimaging
Anal. Bioanal. Chem. 377 (2003), 956-963

[18.5] J.M. Perez, L. Josephson, T. O'Loughlin, D. Hogemann, R. Weissleder
Magnetic relaxation switches capable of sensing molecular interactions
Nat. Biotechnol. 20 (2002), 816-820

[18.6] M.A. Lindsay
Target discovery
Nat. Rev. Drug Discov. 2 (2003), 831-838
Ave. Rev. Biochem. 72 (2003), 783-812

[18.7] U. Haberkorn, A. Altmann
Radionuclide imaging in the post-genomic era
J. Cell. Biochem. Suppl. 39 (2002), 1-10

[18.8] S. Aime, C. Cabella, S. Colombatto, S. Geninatti Crich, E. Gianolio, F. Maggioni
Insights into the use of paramagnetic Gd(III) complexes in MR-molecular imaging investigations
J. Magn. Reson. Imaging 16 (2002), 394-406

[18.9] L. Josephson, C.H. Tung, A. Moore, R. Weissleder
High-efficiency intracellular magnetic labeling with novel superparamagnetic-Tat peptide conjugates
Bioconjug. Chem. 10 (1999), 186-191

[18.10] R. Weissleder, V. Ntziachristos
Shedding light onto live molecular targets
Nat. Med. 9 (2003), 123-128

[18.11] P.A. Dayton, K.W. Ferrara
Targeted imaging using ultrasound
J. Magn. Reson. Imaging 16 (2002), 362-377

[18.12] E.L. Ritman
Molecular imaging in small animals – roles for micro-CT
J. Cell. Biochem. Suppl. 39 (2002), 116-124

[18.13] D.J. Begley, M.W. Brightman
Structural and functional aspects of the blood-brain barrier
Prog. Drug Res. 61 (2003), 39-78

[18.14] R.K. Jain
Transport of molecules, particles, and cells in solid tumors
Annu. Rev. Biomed. Eng. 1 (1999), 241-263

[18.15] M.J. Ratain, R. Mic
Principles of Pharmacokinetics and Pharmacodynamics
In: R.L. Schilsky, G.A. Milano, M.J. Ratain (eds.)
Principles of antineoplastic drug development and pharmacology
Marcel Dekker, Inc., New York 1996; 123-142

[18.16] J. Barbet, P. Peltier, S. Bardet, et al.
Radioimmunodetection of medullary thyroid carcinoma using indium-111 bivalent hapten and anti-CEA x anti-DTPA-indium bispecific antibody
J. Nucl. Med. 39 (1998), 1172-1178

[18.17] S.F. Rosebrough
Two-step immunological approaches for imaging and therapy
Q.J. Nucl. Med. 40 (1996), 234-251

[18.18] P. Hu, J.L. Hornick, M.S. Glasky, et al.
A chimeric Lym-1/interleukin 2 fusion protein for increasing tumor vascular permeability and enhancing antibody uptake
Cancer Res. 56 (1996), 4998-5004

[18.19] J.G. Tjuvajev, R. Finn, K. Watanabe, et al.
Noninvasive imaging of herpes virus thymidine kinase gene transfer and expression: a potential method for monitoring clinical gene therapy
Cancer Res. 56 (1996), 4087-4095

[18.20] P. Foster-Gareau, C. Heyn, A. Alejski, B.K. Rutt
Imaging single mammalian cells with a 1.5 T clinical MRI scanner
Magn. Reson. Med. 49 (2003), 968-971

[18.21] C. Van De Wiele, C. Lahorte, H. Vermeersch, et al.
Quantitative tumor apoptosis imaging using technetium-99m-HYNIC annexin V single photon emission computed tomography
J. Clin. Oncol. 21 (2003), 3483-3487

[18.22] R. Haubner, H.J. Wester, W.A. Weber, et al.
Noninvasive imaging of alpha(v)beta3 integrin expression using 18F-labeled RGD-containing glycopeptide and positron emission tomography
Cancer Res. 61 (2001), 1781-1785

[18.23] W.A. Weber, V. Petersen, B. Schmidt, et al.
Positron emission tomography in non-small-lung cancer: prediction of response to chemotherapy by quantitative assessment of glucose use
J. Clin. Oncol. 21 (2003), 2651-2657

[18.24] Y. Murakami, H. Takamatsu, J. Taki, et al.
18F-labelled annexin V: a PET tracer for apoptosis imaging
Eur. J. Nucl. Med. Mol. Imaging (2003), tbp

[18.25] L.A. Green, C.S. Yap, K. Nguyen, et al.
Indirect monitoring of endogenous gene expression by positron emission tomography (PET) imaging of reporter gene expression in transgenic mice
Mol. Imaging Biol. 4 (2002), 71-81

[18.26] G. Koehne, M. Doubrovin, E. Doubrovina, et al.
Serial in vivo imaging of the targeted migration of human HSV-TK-transduced antigen-specific lymphocytes
Nat. Biotechnol. 21 (2003), 405-413

[18.27] B. Rogers, M.E. Rosenfeld, M.B. Khazaeli, et al.
Localization of iodine-125-mIP-Des-Met14-bombesin (7-13)NH2 in ovarian carcinoma induced to express the gastrin releasing peptide receptor by adenoviral vector-mediated gene transfer
J. Nucl. Med. 38 (1997), 1221-1229

[18.28] P.J. Yazaki, L. Shively, C. Clark, et al.
Mammalian expression and hollow fiber bioreactor production of recombinant anti-CEA diabody and minibody for clinical applications.
J. Immunol Methods 2001; 253:195-208.

[18.29] C.H. Kao, J.F. Hsieh, S.C. Tsai, Y.L. Ho, J.K. Lee
Quickly predicting chemotherapy response to paclitaxel-based therapy in non-small cell lung cancer by early technetium-99m methoxyisobutylisonitrile chest

single-photon-emission computed tomography
Clin. Cancer Res. 6 (2000), 820-824

[18.30] S.J. Nelson
Multivoxel magnetic resonance spectroscopy of brain tumors
Mol. Cancer Ther. 2 (2003), 497-507

[18.31] M. Taupitz, S. Schmitz, B. Hamm
Superparamagnetic iron oxide particles: current state and future development
RöFo Fortschr. Geb. Röntgenstr. Neuen Bildgeb. Verfahr. 175 (2003), 752-765

[18.32] W.H. Li, G. Parigi, M. Fragai, C. Luchinat, T.J. Meade
Mechanistic studies of a calcium-dependent MRI contrast agent
Inorg. Chem. 41 (2002), 4018-4024

[18.33] A.M. Morawski, P.M. Winter, K.C. Crowder, et al.
Targeted nanoparticles for quantitative imaging of sparse molecular epitopes with MRI
Magn. Reson. Med. 51 (2004), 480-486

[18.34] S. Zhang, M. Merritt, D.E. Woessner, R.E. Lenkinski, A.D. Sherry
PARACEST agents: modulating MRI contrast via water proton exchange
Acc. Chem. Res. 36 (2003), 783-790

[18.35] R. Weissleder, A. Moore, U. Mahmood, et al.
In vivo magnetic resonance imaging of transgene expression
Nat. Med. 6 (2000), 351-355

[18.36] R. Weissleder, M. Simonova, A. Bogdanova, S. Bredow, W.S. Enochs, A. Bogdanov Jr
MR imaging and scintigraphy of gene expression through melanin induction
Radiology 204 (1997), 425-429

[18.37] D. Högemann, L. Josephson, R. Weissleder, J.P. Basilion
Improvement of MRI probes to allow efficient detection of gene expression
Bioconjug. Chem. 11 (2000), 941-946

[18.38] W.S. Enochs, P. Petherick, A. Bogdanova, U. Mohr, R. Weissleder
Paramagnetic metal scavenging by melanin: MR imaging
Radiology 204 (1997), 417-423

[18.39] A.J. Lonie, M.M. Huber, E. Ahrens, et al.
Math. Biotech. (2000), 8-32

[18.40] J.M. Perez, F.J. Simeone, Y. Saeki, L. Josephson, R. Weissleder
Viral-induced self-assembly of magnetic nanoparticles allows the detection of viral particles in biological media
J. Am. Chem. Soc. 125 (2003), 10192-10193

[18.41] M. Zhao, L. Josephson, Y. Tang, R. Weissleder
Magnetic Sensors for Protease Assays
Angew. Chem. Int. Ed. Engl. 42 (2003), 1375-1378

[18.42] J.M. Perez, L. Josephson, R. Weissleder
Magnetic nanosensors for DNA analysis
European Cells and Materials 3 (2002), 181-182

[18.43] J. Grimm, J.M. Perez, L. Josephson, R. Weissleder
Novel nanosensors for rapid analysis of telomerase activity
Cancer Res. 64 (2004), 639-643

[18.44] D. Högemann, V. Ntziachristos, L. Josephson, R. Weissleder
High throughput magnetic resonance imaging for evaluating targeted nanoparticle probes
Bioconjug. Chem. 13 (2002), 116-121

[18.45] M.F. Kircher, J.R. Allport, E.E. Graves, et al.
In vivo high resolution three-dimensional imaging of antigen-specific cytotoxic T-lymphocyte trafficking to tumors
Cancer Res. 63 (2003), 6838-6846

[18.46] M. Modo, K. Mellodew, D. Cash, et al.
Mapping transplanted stem cell migration after a stroke: a serial, in vivo magnetic resonance imaging study
Neuroimage 21 (2004), 311-317

[18.47] J.M. Hill, A.J. Dick, V.K. Raman, et al.
Serial cardiac magnetic resonance imaging of injected mesenchymal stem cells
Circulation 108 (2003), 1009-1014

[18.48] M. Lewin, N. Carlesso, C.H. Tung, et al.
Tat peptide-derivatized magnetic nanoparticles allow in vivo tracking and recovery of progenitor cells
Nat. Biotechnol. 18 (2000), 410-414

[18.49] J. Grimm, A. Potthast, A. Wunder, A. Moore
Magnetic resonance imaging of the pancreas and pancreatic tumors in a mouse orthotopic model of human cancer
Int. J. Cancer 106 (2003), 806-811

[18.50] V. Ntziachristos, C.H. Tung, C. Bremer, R. Weissleder
Fluorescence molecular tomography resolves protease activity in vivo
Nat. Med. 8 (2002), 757-760

[18.51] D.B. Jakubowski, A.E. Cerussi, F. Bevilacqua, et al.
Monitoring neoadjuvant chemotherapy in breast cancer using quantitative diffuse optical spectroscopy: a case study
J. Biomed. Opt. 9 (2004), 230-238

[18.52] Y. Hoshi
Functional near-infrared optical imaging: utility and limitations in human brain mapping
Psychophysiology 40 (2003), 511-520

[18.53] A. Rehemtulla, D.E. Hall, L.D. Stegman, et al.
Molecular imaging of gene expression and efficacy following adenoviral-mediated brain tumor gene therapy
Mol. Imaging 1 (2002), 43-55

[18.54] C. Guo, B.N. Armbruster, D.T. Price, C.M. Counter
In vivo regulation of hTERT expression and telomerase activity by androgen
J. Urol. 170 (2003), 615-618

[18.55] P. Ray, A.M. Wu, S.S. Gambhir
Optical bioluminescence and positron emission tomography imaging of a novel fusion reporter gene in tumor xenografts of living mice
Cancer Res. 63 (2003), 1160-1165

[18.56] U. Mahmood, C.H. Tung, Y. Tang, R. Weissleder
Feasibility of in vivo multichannel optical imaging of gene expression: experimental study in mice
Radiology 224 (2002), 446-451

[18.57] D.J. Spergel, U. Kruth, D.R. Shimshek, R. Sprengel, P.H. Seeburg
Using reporter genes to label selected neuronal populations in transgenic mice for gene promoter, anatomical, and physiological studies
Prog. Neurobiol. 63 (2001), 673-686.

[18.58] R. Weissleder
A clearer vision for in vivo imaging
Nat. Biotechnol. 19 (2001), 316-317

[18.59] E.E. Graves, J. Ripoll, R. Weissleder, V. Ntziachristos
A submillimeter resolution fluorescence molecular imaging system for small animal imaging
Med. Phys. 30 (2003), 901-911

[18.60] R.R. Alfano, S.G. Demos, P. Galland, et al.
Time-resolved and nonlinear optical imaging for medical applications
Ann. N. Y. Acad. Sci. 838 (1998), 14-28

[18.61] D. Thomas, G. Duguid
Optical coherence tomography – a review of the principles and contemporary uses in retinal investigation
Eye 2004, tbp

[18.62] G.J. Tearney, H. Yabushita, S.L. Houser, et al.
Quantification of macrophage content in artherosclerotic plaques by optical coherence tomography
Circulation 107 (2003), 113-119

[18.63] A. Becker, C. Hessenius, K. Licha, et al.
Receptor-targeted optical imaging of tumors with near-infrared fluorescent ligands
Nat Biotechnol 19 (2001), 327-331

[18.64] H.W. Kang, R. Weissleder, A. Bogdanov Jr
Targeting of MPEG-protected polyamino acid carrier to human E-selectin in vitro
Amino Acids 23 (2002), 301-308

[18.65] C. Bremer, C.H. Tung, A. Bogdanov Jr, R. Weissleder
Imaging of differential protease expression in breast cancers for detection of aggressive tumor phenotypes
Radiology 222 (2002), 814-818

[18.66] D.R. Shalinsky, J. Brekken, H. Zou, et al.
Broad antitumor and antiangiogenic activities of AG3340, a potent and selective MMP inhibitor undergoing advanced oncology clinical trials
Ann. N. Y. Acad. Sci. 878 (1999), 236-270

[18.67] C. Bremer, C.H. Tung, R. Weissleder
In vivo molecular target assessment of matrix metalloproteinase inhibition
Nat. Med. 7 (2001), 743-748

[18.68] E.A. Schellenberger, A. Bogdanov Jr, A. Petrovsky, V. Ntziachristos, R. Weissleder, L. Josephson
Optical imaging of apoptosis as a biomarker of tumor response to chemotherapy
Neoplasia 5 (2003), 187-192

[18.69] D.H. Turnbull, T.S. Bloomfield, H.S. Baldwin, F.S. Foster, A.L. Joyner
Ultrasound backscatter microscope analysis of early mouse embryonic brain development
Proc. Natl. Acad. Sci. U S A 92 (1995), 2239-2243

[18.70] D.B. Ellegala, H. Leong-Poi, J.E. Carpenter, et al.
Imaging tumor angiogenesis with contrast ultrasound and microbubbles targeted to alpha(v)beta3
Circulation 108 (2003), 336-341

[18.71] R. Bekeredjian, S. Chen, P.A. Frenkel, P.A. Grayburn, R.V. Shohet
Ultrasound-targeted microbubble destruction can repeatedly direct highly specific plasmid expression to the heart
Circulation 108 (2003), 1022-1026

[18.72] G.M. Lanza, S.A. Wickline
Targeted ultrasonic contrast agents for molecular imaging and therapy
Prog. Cardiovasc. Dis. 44 (2001), 13-31

[18.73] L. Josephson, M.F. Kircher, U. Mahmood, Y. Tang, R. Weissleder
Near-infrared fluorescent nanoparticles as combined MR/optical imaging probes
Bioconjug. Chem. 13 (2002), 554-560

[18.74] A. Wunder, J. Grimm, U. Muller-Ladner
Molecular imaging in rheumatoid arthritis
Z. Rheumatol. 62 (2003), II33-II36

Part V – Information Processing and Distribution

19 Software platform for medical imaging

19.1 Overview

The significance of software as a system component in the medical environment is growing. In the present chapter, we offer a sketch of the technical concepts that are used to create software platforms designed to support workstations in the medical imaging domain. The specific contents featured in this chapter include:

- An overview of the typical diagnostic imaging workflow: this overview includes a description of the problem domain for which the described software platform is designed and the key requirements that need to be met by such a platform (section 19.2).
- A brief explanation of a number of important software terms (section 19.3) to help the reader gain a better understanding of the component platform concepts presented later (section 19.4). In addition to the notion of runtime management, various components and communication models are introduced.
- A description of the business object model for medical imaging as defined by the DICOM standard: this model forms the basis of data modeling within the platform (section 19.5).
- An introduction of the notion of services, i.e. common functions used in all of the applications supported by the platform (section 19.6).
- A description of the tool support made available to programmers to assist them in writing platform-compliant components so as to ensure the easy development of platform-based applications (section 19.7).
- A brief discussion of the integration (enterprise application integration) of platform products with other systems (section 19.8).

In what follows, we are first concerned to familiarize readers with the various aspects of clinical workflow and the associated software applications for medical imaging systems. The technical terms that describe the software-platform architecture – which forms a base for the applications that support the described workflow – are presented in the second half of the chapter.

19.2 Introduction to medical imaging software domain

A medical professional requires a clear understanding of the disease that a patient is suffering from in order to determine a proper course of treatment. The diagnosis is usually based on various observations, including body temperature, blood pressure and blood picture. Advanced diagnostic procedures may be required in more complex cases.

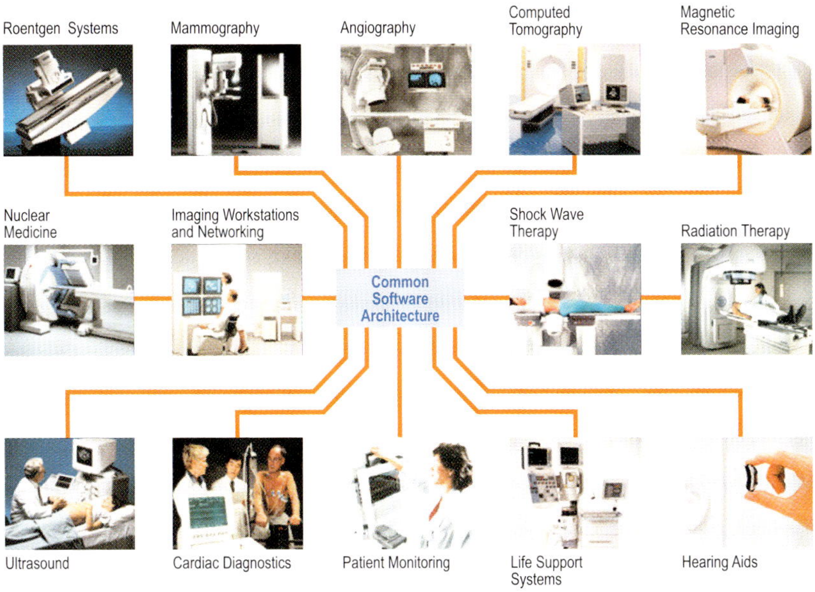

Figure 19.1 Medical imaging and waveform devices with common software architecture

One of these advanced diagnostic procedures is medical imaging – acquiring and processing information about structures and dynamics in the patient's body using procedures that are usually no more than minimally invasive. Depending on the information required, the doctor will choose from a variety of diagnostic imaging and waveform procedures, including ultrasound, CT, MRI, angiography, PET, ECG, EEG and many others (fig. 19.1). Waveform procedures capture and visualize physical processes in a patient's body (e.g. heart beat, blood pressure and brain waves).

Most of these systems are capable of acquiring, displaying, post-processing, printing and archiving images. In light of these common capacities, it would be very advantageous to be able to extensively reuse a particular software across all of the various imaging systems. The benefits of a common software architecture for medical imaging systems are obvious:

- *Know one – know all*: A user who has learned how to operate one type of medical imaging system built on a given platform will be able to operate other systems built on that same platform because the systems will have an identical look and feel. It is important in medical environments to ensure that the user can concentrate on the patient rather than on differences in software handling. The deployment of common software in different imaging systems also permits greater flexibility when it comes to operator planning because each operator will be able to handle a variety of systems.

- *Enhanced workflow*: An efficient workflow supported by intuitive and easy-to-use software is essential in critical care situations. Platforms that include an established style guide (i.e. a standard look and feel for all applications) make for a more efficient and intuitive cross-system workflow. The time saved can then be dedicated to the patient.
- *Stability*: Common software applications are tested in a variety of environments to ensure seamless serviceability in all situations. The detection and correction of a problem in one system will mean the elimination of similar problems in all of the systems that deploy the same software. It follows that the stability of the software platform will grow as the number of systems supported by the platform increases.
- *Corporate identity*: Different imaging systems are recognizable as being produced by the same manufacturer.
- *Costs*: Sharing software helps to reduce research and development costs and thus reduces the cost of medical imaging devices.

However, common software platform architectures also introduce challenges. These challenges will have to be met in order to enable one to fully exploit the potential associated with the reuse of software. It is very rare in real life that one size fits all: reusable software is required to be adaptable to the needs of different workplaces. This adds complexity to software design. These adaptations will have to be executed with respect to both the availability and behavior of software applications. Furthermore, a common software platform is required to enable various business units (or divisions) that may be in the process of developing systems at different locations around the world to add new applications to the set of shared applications. These new applications

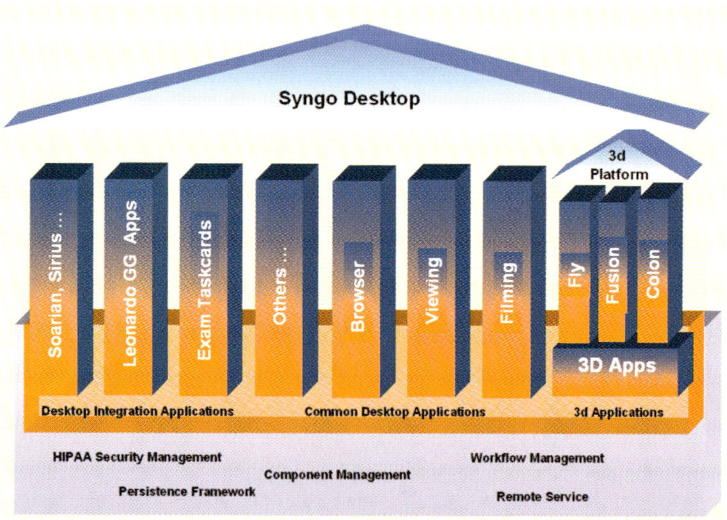

Figure 19.2 Common software applications developed for the *syngo* platform

need to be seamlessly integrated into the aggregate of existing applications. The principle involved is shown in fig. 19.2.

Software applications built on a common platform can be broken down into three categories:

- *Common workflow applications* that can be reused on almost any medical imaging system (e.g. an application for printing the images displayed on the monitor). Common applications behave as defined in the style guide.
- *Exam applications* that are bound to one type of system only (e.g. the image acquisition software used in a CT scanner). Such software usually depends on modality-specific hardware (e.g. the CT scanner itself) for proper functioning. System-bound applications should also conform to the style guide for the sake of seamless workflow integration.
- *Specific applications* that are tied to a certain modality, but are not tied to a modality-specific hardware. These types of applications usually involve post-processing (e.g. an application that calculates the bone density in a CT image for the sake of diagnosing osteoporosis). While such an application will work only on CT images (modality-specific), it will not rely on a connected CT scanner. This permits the reuse of the application on any machine where CT images are available. Modality-specific applications should also conform to the style guide for the sake of seamless workflow integration.

It is important to gain a full understanding of the problem domain for which a solution is needed before undertaking to design a technical solution. It follows from our discussion so far that a common style guide for medical imaging software will be indispensable. Other topics such as the adaptability and classification of application reusability will be explained with reference to a simplified workflow for acquiring diagnostic images from a patient.

19.2.1 Aspects of a common style guide

A common style guide is implemented to help secure a seamless workflow across all applications and to support the efficient usability of functions within an application. Such a style guide is required to account for the situations in which the applications will be used. It is important to enable users in medical environments to switch easily between different applications (tasks), to locate needed functions quickly (i.e. without having to navigate through an arbitrarily complex hierarchy of user interfaces) and to visualize function selectors via intuitive icons. It is also essential for diagnostic imaging that most of the monitor area remains available for the display of images. The color and brightness of other elements in the user interface will need to be defined carefully to ensure excellent image visibility.

The medical workflow is represented in fig. 19.3 using a task-card metaphor where each card corresponds to a task that the user is to perform for the patient. The various tasks are brought to the foreground by clicking on the relevant task-card tab.

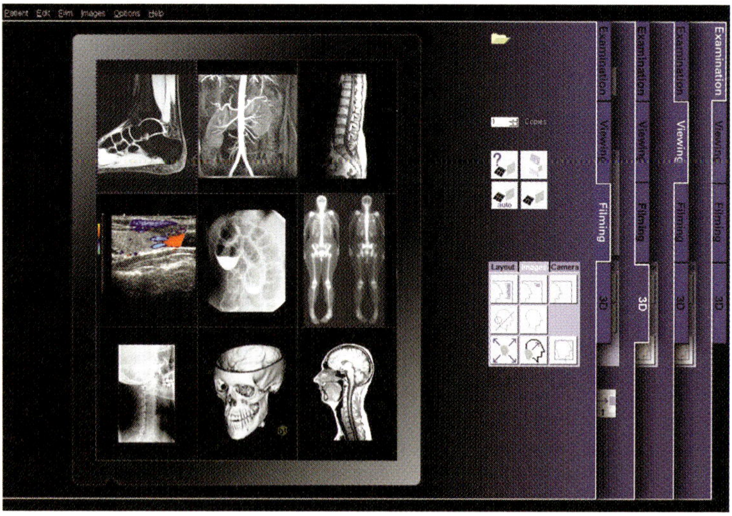

Figure 19.3 The task-card concept

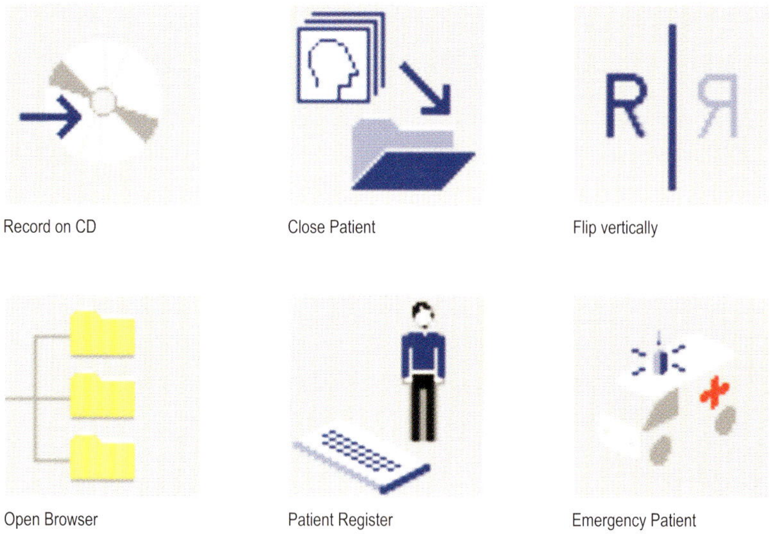

Figure 19.4 Intuitive icons

The layout of a task card's contents is well-defined: the left most area is reserved for displaying images. A tools area located immediately to the right of the task card enables the user to trigger functions for the active task. Intuitive icons (especially designed for medical users) incorporated in the tools area represent the available operations. The concept of task cards can also be deployed in the tools area for grouping sets of related operations (e.g. one group includes tools for controlling the layout while another group includes tools for manipulating images).

In addition to the task-card-based applications described above, the style guide also includes pop-up applications (i.e. applications that appear on top of the task cards when they are selected). This type of application is usually selected to initiate a workflow sequence or to control background activities. While task-card applications can be brought to the top of the card stack by clicking the associated tab, pop-up applications follow a different activation scheme. One method of activating them is to click on a corresponding icon. Another method is to select the application from a menu list. A yet further method is to enter a specific keyboard combination.

A common style guide requires the identical representation of functions throughout all of the applications that are built on the common software architecture. Fig. 19.4 shows a number of icons that are intuitive in a medical environment.

The next section includes a description of a sample medical imaging workflow. Various applications are introduced at the various workflow stages. These applications are classified in terms of their sharing category (common application, system-bound application, modality-specific application) and appearance (task card, pop-up).

19.2.2 A sample workflow

Before any scanning takes place, it will be necessary to register the patient's demographic data. This is important to ensure the correct display of the patient's name in the context of diagnosing the patient. The patient-register application is designed for recording a patient's demographic data.

Patient register application

Given that the patient register application is needed on all scanner systems (fig. 19.5), it is regarded as a common application that is to be reused across all acquisition systems. It will also have to be highly configurable because the various scanner systems require different demographic data. The patient register application is used as a pop-up application – so that it can be selected at any time without interfering with clinical procedures (i.e. regardless of which task-card application is currently active).

Scheduling an examination (scheduled procedure step)

Medical institutions that are equipped with several scanners often make use of software to schedule examinations for specific examination systems. The scheduling procedure involves entering the patient's demographic data, identifying a time slot and communicating this time slot to the patient. Once the patient shows up for the examination, the operator is afforded immediate access to the scheduling information and the patient's demographic data and will not be required to re-enter the patient's demographic data, a procedure that is time consuming and could lead to clerical errors subsequent confusion.

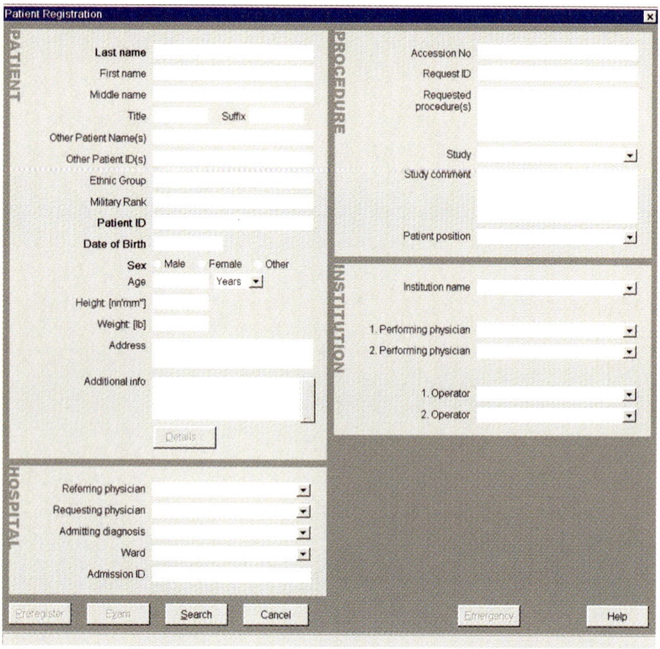

Figure 19.5 Patient register pop-up application (common application)

Entering a medical institution represents the initial step for the patient in a sequence of activities in the diagnostic workflow. The major steps in this workflow include patient registration, examination, the evaluation of measurement results, diagnosis, diagnosis review and the drafting of a report. Depending on the size of the institution, this workflow may extend to treatment and the continuous monitoring of the patient's condition until the disease has been cured and the patient's case is deemed closed.

A system that keeps track of completed and continuing procedures and schedules new procedures based on the results of previous ones is referred to as a workflow engine. A workflow engine requires notifications about completed procedures for the sake of scheduling subsequent procedures. A workflow engine may be part of a hospital information system (HIS) designed to collect all of the relevant information except for the medical images.

The establishment of seamlessly integrated workflow sequences in a hospital will require a link between the imaging systems and the HIS system.

Examination application

The acquisition parameters are set after the patient data have been entered and before the acquisition of diagnostic data is initiated. The examination application provides input fields for measurement parameters and protocols (fig. 19.6). It also provides for

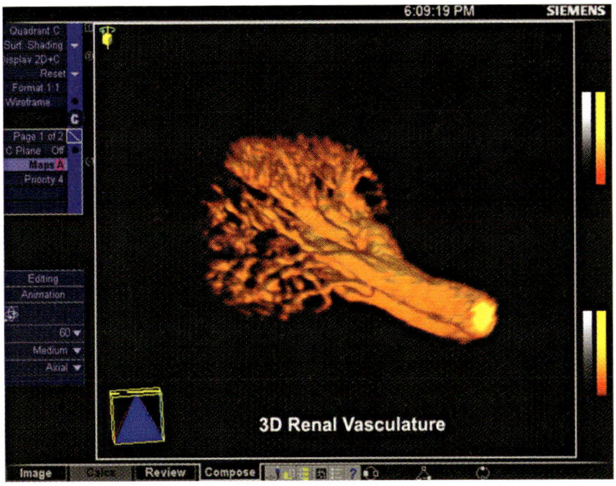

Figure 19.6 Examination task-card application (system-bound application)

graphical slice positioning (where applicable). The progress of a running acquisition is also usually indicated in this application. The examination is the first task-card application in the routine clinical procedure. Its tab is therefore located above all of the other tabs.

The examination application is entirely bound to a specific scanner type (i.e. this type of application cannot be shared with other imaging system types). However, the examination platform is also required to conform to the common style guide. Its behavior thus resembles that of all of the other applications built on the common software platform. The results of an acquisition are usually saved on the local system for purposes of review.

Modality-performed procedure step

If the examination scanner is connected to an HIS system, then it will retrieve patient data from the HIS system using a scheduled procedure step. Once the acquisition has been performed, the scheduled examination is finished and the scheduled procedure step will have to be closed in order to indicate its successful completion. This is done using the modality-performed procedure step (MPPS) application (fig. 19.7). The purpose of this application is to indicate to the HIS system that a scheduled procedure step has been successfully executed. The user can add information to the completion status of the examination. This information can then be used by the workflow engine to create and schedule subsequent work items that should trigger work on the data generated during the examination. Parts of the data supplied via the modality-performed procedure step are references to the acquired data. The MPPS application is a common application that is used on scanner systems for most of the modalities (i.e. if they are connected to an HIS system).

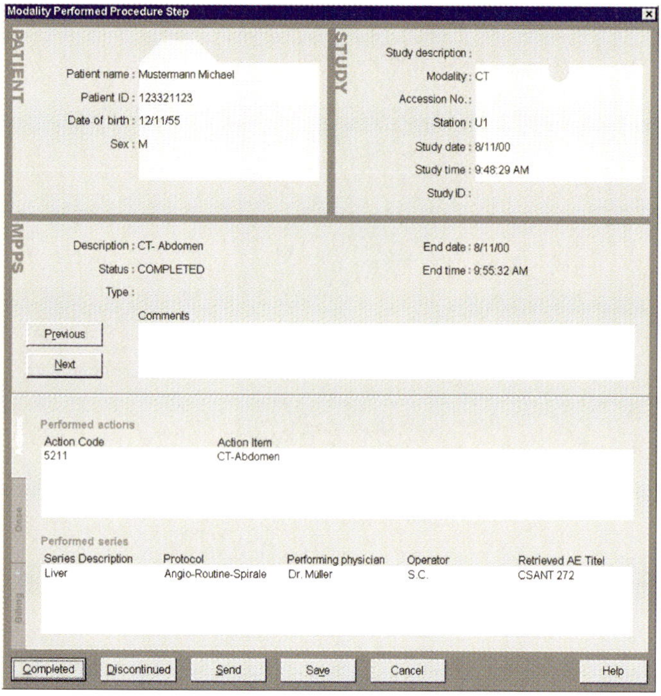

Figure 19.7 MPPS pop-up application (common application)

Patient-browser application

Scanner systems spend most of their operational time performing examinations involving the acquisition of data. Little time remains for them to perform tasks involving the post-processing of the acquired images. The initiation of a post-processing workflow sequence presupposes the prior selection of the relevant image data. The patient browser application provides a hierarchical view of the patient data and images that are available for post-processing (fig. 19.8). Users activate this application to select data and to initiate a processing session for that data.

The data model's hierarchy is defined by the DICOM standard (Digital Imaging and Communications in Medicine). The hierarchy basically consists of patient studies that are broken down into individual series that are (in turn) broken down into individual images (see section 19.5). Various patient data stores can be seen on the left side of the picture. The contents of each selected data store are shown on the right side. A close look at the screenshot reveals that the scheduled patient information can be viewed from the patient browser application when one is selecting the scheduler data store.

The user selects the desired data and the application task card where this data is to be processed next. Passing selected data to the target application is a matter of using the

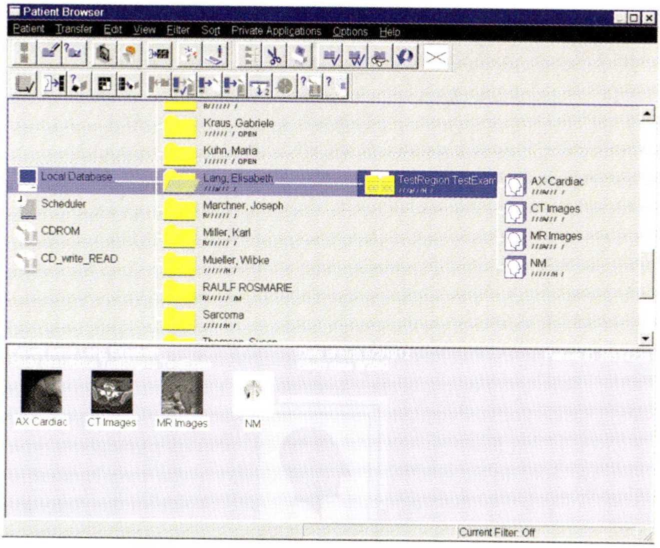

Figure 19.8 Patient browser pop-up application (common application)

drag-and-drop function or clicking on an associated icon (defined by the common style guide) displayed in the top area of the browser application. The browser application has been provided in the form of a pop-up application to secure its availability during any step in the workflow. In light of the fact that patient-selection functions are needed on all imaging systems, the patient browser function qualifies as a common application.

Viewing application

Once images have been loaded into the viewing application, the user is free to select an appropriate screen layout, i.e. determine the number of segments and images that can be viewed simultaneously (fig. 19.9). The user is afforded an opportunity to scroll through the set of loaded images, manipulate the contrast within the image view and zoom, rotate or move the image within its segment. The user also has the option of measuring distances in the image, calculating region statistics and adding graphics and text (e.g. to indicate conspicuous areas of interest). The image viewer is a frequently used application and is therefore considered a common application that is to be shared across all imaging systems.

3D application

Modern CT and MRI scanners generate a tremendous number of images during a single examination. It would be a tedious and time-consuming task to view all of these images with the standard viewing application discussed above. Treating a large number of images as a volume rather than as a set of individual images represents a more efficient approach to such data and enables the creation of computed views of diag-

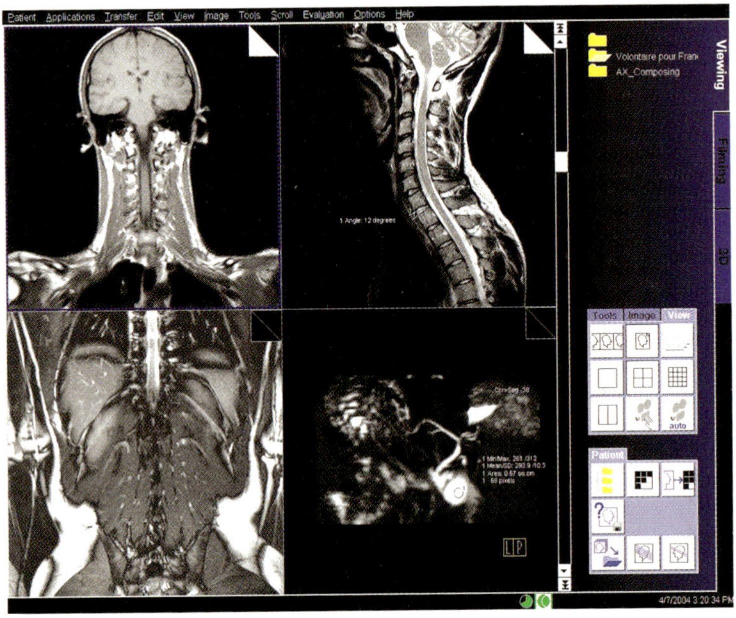

Figure 19.9 Viewing-task-card application (common application)

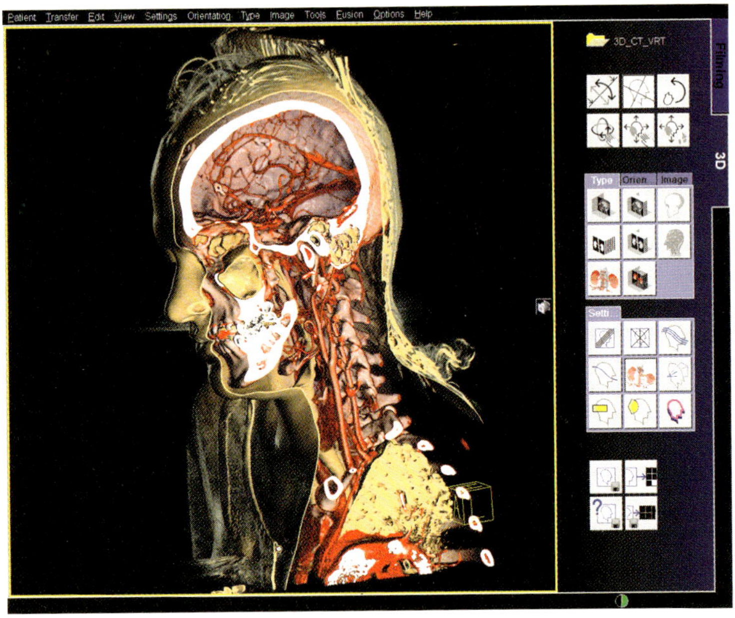

Figure 19.10 3D task-card application (common application)

nostically relevant cutting planes. A spatial representation of examination results is more intuitive for a doctor because it resembles the reality within a patient's head or body (fig. 19.10). 3D imaging encompasses many different post-processing modes, including displaying vessels without surrounding tissue, reconstructing the morphology of the esophagus or intestines, for instance, so as to permit the calculation of a virtual endoscopy, and creating shaded surfaces that can be viewed from various angles. Given that these modes exhibit many functions that could be described as 3D-specific, it would be advantageous to structure the 3D application itself as an extensible application capable of hosting new modes at runtime without requiring modifications in the base application. Many of the issues that apply to a common software platform also apply to the design of the 3D base application (see section 19.6.3).

The 3D application represents an option for some scanner systems and is a virtual must for those systems that create large numbers of images during a given acquisition. 3D applications thus also qualify as common applications that are to be shared across all imaging systems.

Filming application

After the images have been processed according to the diagnostic needs of the doctor, a selection of them is printed for documentary purposes (fig. 19.11). Such documentation is necessary for viewing the images at locations where no suitable computer is available (e.g. in a sterile environment or at a family doctor's office). Furthermore, many doctors are used to viewing images at a light box rather than on a computer monitor.

The filming application includes the task of composing the film sheet for the sake of printing. Even modifications of the image quality can be applied in a manner that is similar to that used in the viewing application. A look at the filming application reveals a new type of job: the background job. Once the user presses the expose button, the contents of the virtual film sheet are transferred to the connected camera or printer. Printing the data can be a time-consuming affair, depending on the number of images and concurrent print requests issued by other users and computers. However, the user on one system should be able to continue composing further film sheets without having to wait for the completion of a previous job. The actual printing takes place in the background while the user actively continues with the clinical procedure in the foreground. This scenario reveals an important challenge that is faced when creating medical imaging software: allowing the user to control the system at all times regardless of which activities have been initiated. This requirement is also expressed in the notion of providing a non-blocking user interface.

Background jobs need to be controllable all the time (e.g. users will want to know whether these jobs have been completed or how long it might take before work on them is begun). Users may also decide that a print job in the queue should be canceled, suspended, resumed or repeated.

Printing images is a common task across all imaging systems. The filming application therefore qualifies as a common application that is to be shared across these imaging systems.

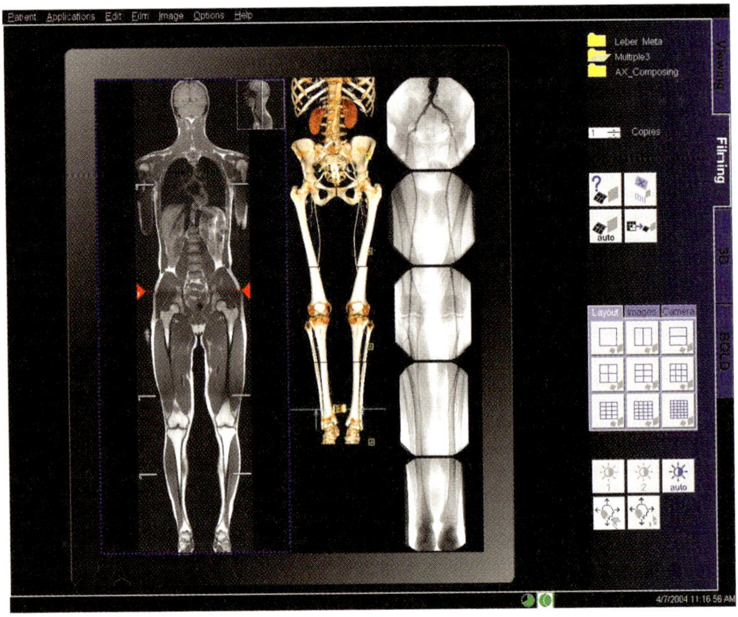

Figure 19.11 Filming-task-card application (common application)

Archiving and networking application

Finally, the images and results will need to be stored in electronic form for the long term. Depending on the institution and the data volume to be handled, this can be done either on removable media (MOD, CD, DVD, tape, etc.) or by passing the images on to dedicated image archives. Given that writing data to a removable medium or

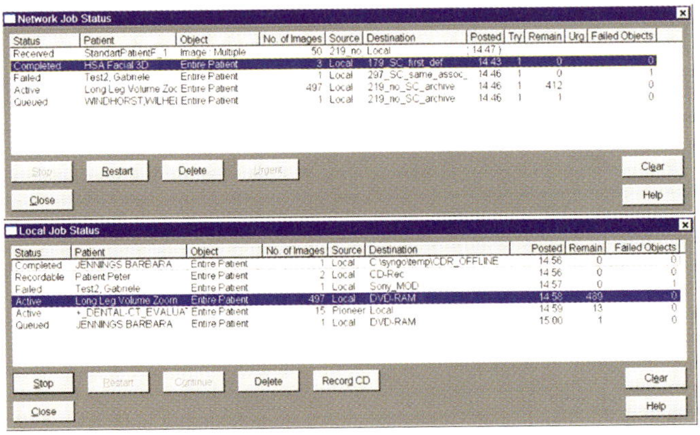

Figure 19.12 Archiving/networking pop-up job-control list (common application)

sending data across a network to an image archive can be rather time consuming, provision is to be made for their operation in the background. Therefore, this application is also required to provide job-control functionality that allows the user to continue foreground operations without having to wait for the completion of previous jobs (fig. 19.12). Once the data has been stored permanently, it can be deleted from the local machine (e.g. via the patient browser applications).

The archiving and networking application is needed on all imaging systems. It therefore qualifies as a common application that is to be shared by all of these systems.

Query/retrieve application

All of the acquired image data ultimately end up in an image archive where they remain until they are needed again or until the relevant statutory retention periods elapse. The image archive is thus a kind of central data storage facility where users can go to search for data. Data searches usually arise in connection with the need to post-process newly created images on a separate system or to compare acquisition results over longer periods of time (e.g. comparing images from last year with images from this year).

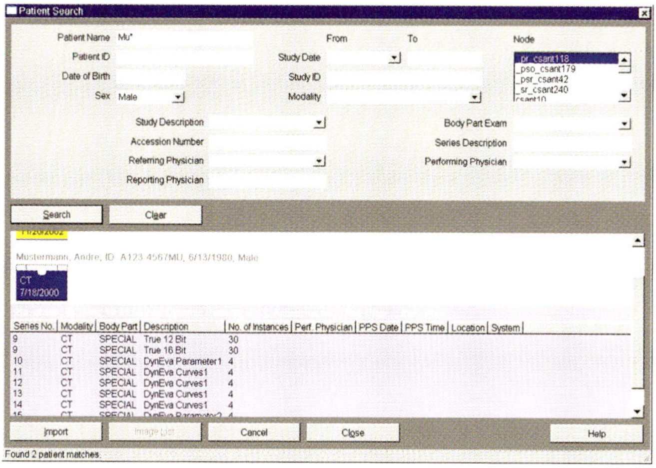

Figure 19.13 Query/retrieve pop-up application (common application)

The purpose of the query and retrieve application (fig. 19.13) is twofold:

- First, it enables the user to query an image archive for data belonging to a specific patient. Query results will indicate whether relevant data are available in the image archive at all and, if so, what attributes these data have. The user can then select data of interest (e.g. data still residing in a remote image archive) based on the query results.

- Second, it enables the user to retrieve selected data from the image archive. The retrieved data are copied from the image archive back to the local data storage medium (i.e. without being deleted from the image archive).

Once the data have been successfully retrieved, the user can select the data in the patient browser application and load them into a post-processing application.

The protocol used to query and retrieve data from an image archive is defined by the DICOM standard. The query/retrieve application can be used on all of the imaging systems that are connected to an image archive. It therefore also qualifies as a common application.

Note: The remote image archive is required to implement a DICOM service to handle the query and retrieve requests issued by the query/retrieve application. If the imaging system itself implements (or reuses) the same DICOM service for query/retrieve applications, then the imaging system can be queried for data by other systems as well. In addition to common applications, imaging platforms may include common services, i.e. the reuse aspect covers more than applications (see section 19.6).

Extended sample workflow, including modality-specific post-processing applications

The sample workflow that has been discussed so far is typical for almost any scanner system. The applications that have been introduced include either acquisition applications or common applications. All of the common applications can be reused on any medical imaging system. However, these systems may include other modality-specific applications. Modality-specific applications center on the post-processing of images from a specific modality (e.g. CT or MRI). In the remainder of the present section, we discuss two examples of this type of application.

CT calcium-scoring application

The purpose of this application is to detect and quantify coronary calcification on the basis of data volumes acquired using a CT scanner (fig. 19.14). This application is used at workstations with access to coronary CT data.

MRI/CT cardiac-evaluation application

This application is used by physicians to analyze and quantify ventricular functions (e.g. the ejection fraction rate) on the basis of vascular images generated by CT or MRI scanners (fig. 19.15). The application is used at workstations with access to cardiac images from MRI or CT.

These applications are only two examples drawn from a variety of modality-specific applications that center on particular diagnostic questions and evaluations relating to information contained in the images of a specific modality.

All of the modality-specific applications are also built in accordance with the common software architecture and the common style guide. This enables one to flexibly combine the various modality-specific applications with common workflow applications at

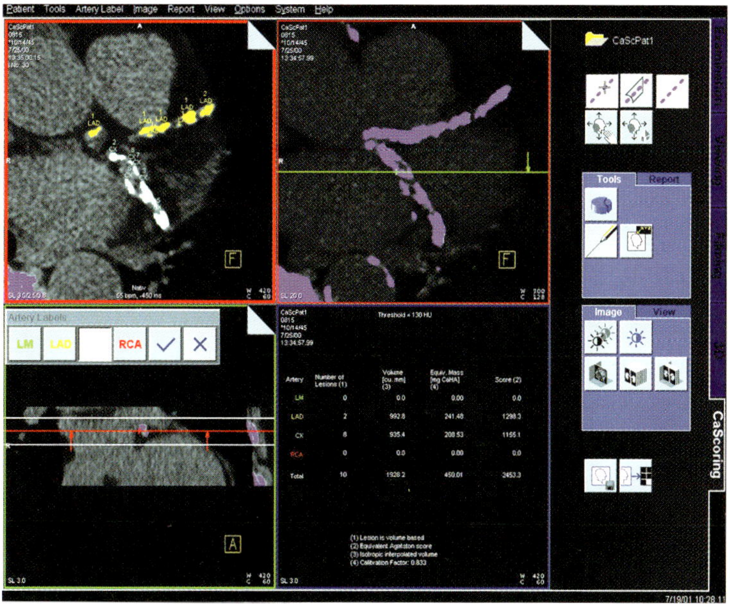

Figure 19.14 Calcium-scoring task-card application (modality-specific application)

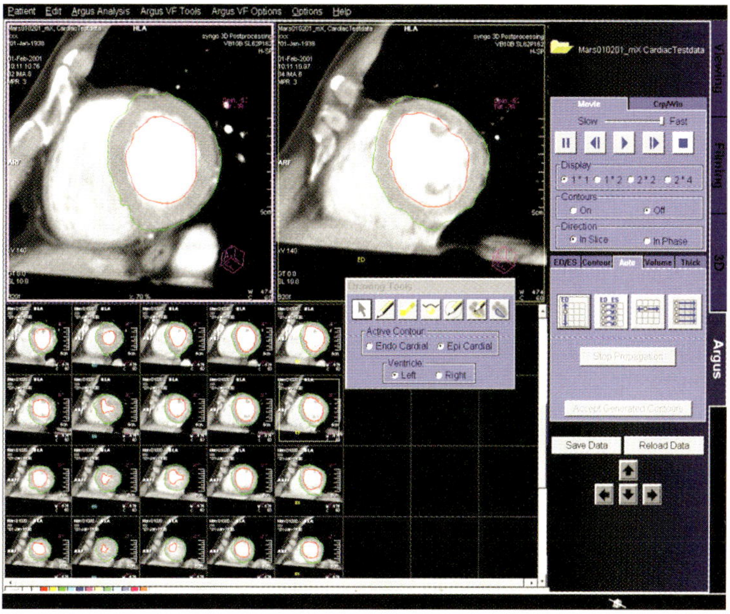

Figure 19.15 Cardiac evaluation task-card application (modality-specific application)

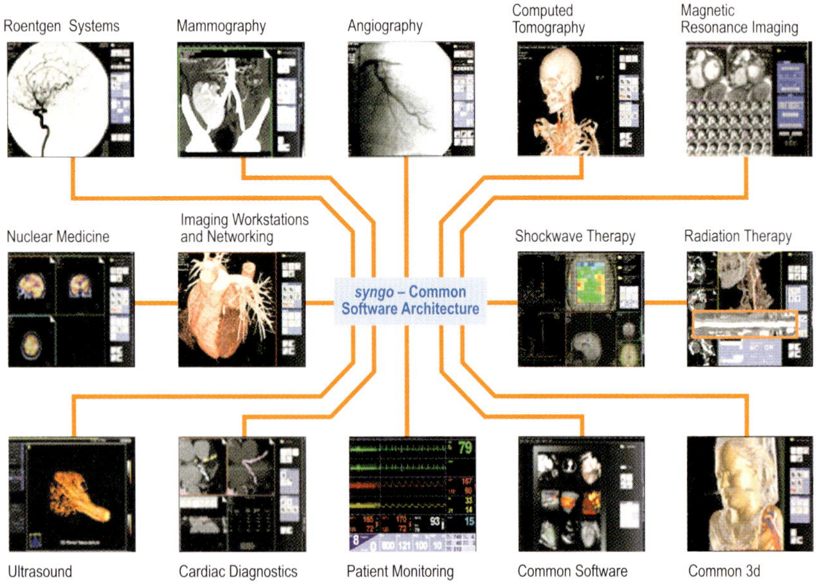

Figure 19.16
syngo multi-modality workstation: offers a synergy of multiple applications that were developed at different business units around the world. All these applications are based on the common *syngo* product-line architecture.

workstations where images generated by more than one modality are post-processed (i.e. multi-modality workstations) (fig. 19.16).

The definition, production and distribution of multi-modality workstations is a business in its own right (i.e. separate from the modality business). The set of applications installed on a multi-modality workstation usually depends on the department where the workstation is to be installed. For example, modality-specific cardiac-evaluation applications that are used with CT, MRI, US and angio images will be installed in cardiology departments.

A common software architecture and a common style guide support the creation of dedicated workstations (single-modality and multi-modality) that enable one to determine sets of applications on the basis of the diagnostic questions that are to be answered at the particular workstation. The style guide ensures efficient workflow within and between the various applications. The architecture of the common software platform ensures the seamless joining and exchangeability of applications. Furthermore, the architecture is required to be fully compatible with a variety of medical imaging systems, ranging from small portable devices for life-support functions (e.g. ECG monitors) and mobile scanners (e.g. ultrasound systems) to multi-modality workstations and large scale scanner installations such as CT, MRI and PET systems. These systems are typically deployed in different environments. Some of them are

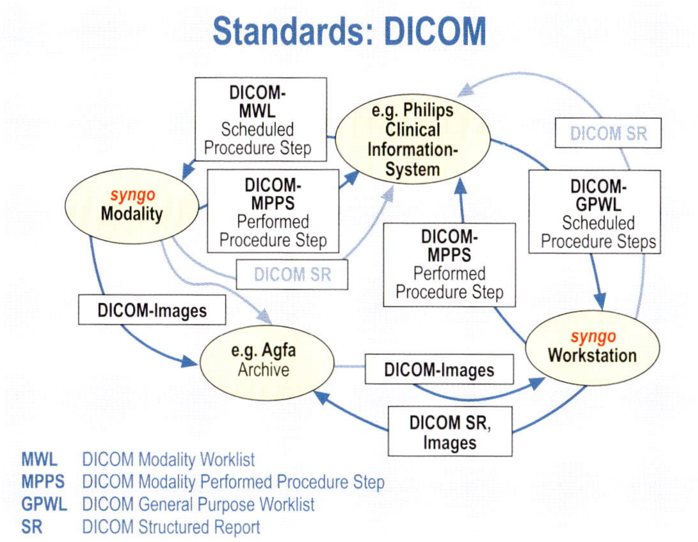

Figure 19.17
DICOM and IHE-defined workflow for medical-modality and multi-modality systems, PACS archives and departmental information systems. DICOM-defined work lists and medical reports, images etc. are also shown.

never connected to a network. Others are connected to and disconnected from the network at runtime. Others still remain continuously connected to the network. The number of monitors used to display patient data represents a further criterion for drawing distinctions between these systems. All of the screen shots shown so far were taken from a single monitor system. However, some applications and systems require the display of patient data on several monitors. All of these variations will need to be considered when defining the architecture for a common software platform that is to conform to the single-modality and multi-modality system workflow specifications that have already been well defined by industry standards such as DICOM and IHE (fig. 19.17).

19.2.3 Analysis of the problem domain

The creation of software systems with the functions discussed above requires a flexible software architecture that permits the integration of reusable applications that can be variously combined at different workstations. In contrast to DICOM-defined workflow sequences for connecting medical IT platforms, the focus here is more on enabling the seamless connection of a medical imaging system's inner workflow sequences to a department's outer workflow sequences.

A common software platform for medical imaging systems is required to provide a sound array of services for such applications:

- *Data management*: standardized data access and inter-application data sharing. This mechanism is also required to provide a means of avoiding or at least detecting simultaneous and conflicting manipulations of the same data from different applications.
- *Image processing*: standardized access to imaging algorithms and identical image quality across all applications. The typical quantity of medical image data has grown considerably and may exceed two Gbytes for a single examination. This requires efficient data sharing and efficient 2D, 3D and 4D imaging algorithms.
- *Connectivity*: standardized connectivity with the computer systems of other vendors to facilitate cross-system data exchange. This includes data exchange via a network as well as via removable media.
- *Security*: authenticating user identity and authorizing users to interact with the system. While this is primarily intended to ensure the privacy of patient data, there is a point at which security concerns should not be allowed to hamper the clinical care process.
- *System runtime management/service software*: The workplace is assembled out of a set of applications built on top of the common software platform. It will be necessary to define the controlled startup and shutdown of applications and to determine what should happen in case of detected faults. Preventive maintenance and the quick remote analysis and remedying of problems requires the deployment of service software that supports qualified engineers in controlling the system remotely.

Applications that are built on top of these services can be variously combined to account for the needs of a variety of dedicated workplaces. The adaptation of both individual applications and the set of applications to the specifics of a given workplace requires considerable flexibility in terms of the design of the common applications and should be carried out in a way that avoids introducing dependencies. A common software architecture must provide a means for achieving such flexibility without adding complexity to the task of the developers who write the applications. The common software architecture will therefore be required to meet the following specifications:

- *Independent applications*: Given the aim of independent deployability, applications are required to be free of dependencies on other applications. However, in the interest of their seamless integration into the clinical workflow, the applications will need to share imaging algorithms and data.
- *Customizable and extensible applications*: Reusable (common) applications must be adaptable to the needs of different workplaces. These adaptations might be as easy as changing the configuration parameters for an application or as complicated as extending the application logic/user interface by including new runtime behavior.
- *Responsive, non-blocking user interface*: Even if a task is in the process of being completed and further user input related to it cannot be accepted, the user must be able to control the system (i.e. the system must be responsive at all times).
- *Separation of concerns*: Both the components that make up the applications and workplaces and the applications and workplaces themselves should be manageable.

Complexity can be estimated by the number of technologies involved, the variation rates of the technologies involved and the organizational boundaries that are involved in creating a piece of software.

- *Creating compliant applications*: The construction of a common medical imaging platform requires that the engineers involved in the construction adhere to stringent rules and recommendations. Tools and processes are needed to support the engineers who are involved in the building of the compliant components and applications for the platform.
- *Internationalization and localization*: The applications that are created for the common software platform must be usable in different countries (i.e. their user interfaces must be adaptable to different languages and formats).
- *Enterprise application integration*: It is obvious that not all applications will be written for a single medical imaging platform (e.g. software for handling billing information or lab results will be based on different concepts). However, in the interest of seamless workflow sequences, these different applications should be capable of sharing information (e.g. the patient's name). In such a case, it will be possible to view the billing information or lab results for a patient who has been selected in the patient-browser application.

19.2.4 From programming to software configuration

All of the challenges that have been identified so far point to the advisability of implementing an architecture comprised of small independent building blocks (components) that one can extend, customize and combine to form larger building blocks and full applications without the needing to do any re-writing. The final imaging system product would thus consist of a collection of selected applications.

Many domain-class libraries, frameworks and applications offer the manufacturer of medical devices much potential for software reuse. However, a common software architecture will only guarantee success if the business units fully exploit this potential by consistently reusing and extending these common building blocks. High configurability and extensibility at system, application and component level enable one to both increase programmer productivity and adapt software to different product lines. Application programmers will be effectively relieved of the task of implementing middleware and will therefore be able to concentrate on creating new applications. Furthermore, end users will benefit from higher innovation rates. This can be summarized best in the architectural vision: "from programming to the configuration of software".

The platform-architecture (or *syngo* architecture) is provided as an application template consisting of black-box frameworks and application servers that are supported by some code generators (wizards) and documentation. The application template supports both application components for user-interface development and application components for business-logic development. These two types of components are strictly separated according to *syngo* architecture principles. The application servers themselves are implemented as generic executables. Two types of executables are provided: one for hosting user-interface components and another for hosting business-logic components. Application servers represent the backbone of the implemented software architecture and are ready for use by the application developers. In the following sections, we deepen our discussion of the *syngo*-application template.

However, before moving on to a discussion of the key concepts of a common software architecture, we offer a brief explanation of the terms used in the remainder of this chapter.

19.3 Software terminology

Functions and data: Procedural languages such as FORTRAN and COBOL strictly separate functions (algorithms) from data (block data).

Object orientation: A modeling and programming technique that combines data structures and associated behavior into *classes* (abstract data types). Classes expose *interfaces* through which the functionality of a class can be used. The programmer using an instance of a class (or *object*) does not need to know the implementation details or data structures used internally in the class (data hiding). The interface represents a contract between the implementer and the user of a class. Immutable interfaces allow for the modification of implementations within classes without breaking code that uses instances of that class (as long as the behavior visible to the user of the class does not change). A variety of programming languages support the paradigm of object orientation (e.g. Smalltalk, C++, Java and C#). Classes are usually modeled on the basis of real-world entities (e.g. wheels, persons, bank accounts, patients, etc.). Programmers who create instances of classes reuse code that the implementer of the class has provided, i.e. they do not have to reinvent/model the wheel over and over again. Classes and objects are design-time entities. Classes can be aggregated to create more complex entities.

Objects can be characterized as follows:

- Objects are units of instantiation; they have a unique identity.
- Objects may have a state that can be observed externally.
- Objects encapsulate states and behavior.

A collection of classes can be packaged as a class library for further reuse. STL (Standard Template Library) is an example of a class library [19.1].

Idioms: Idioms are best-practice recommendations for using a particular programming language more efficiently. For instance, idioms for C++ give hints on when to declare a *copy constructor* an *assignment operator* or how to make a C++ class non-derivable. Idioms help programmers to express their intentions clearly via a specific programming language without incurring undesired side effects. Idioms thus represent a kind of programming-language-specific pattern [19.2].

Design patterns: Design patterns are textual descriptions of proven solutions for recurring design challenges. They originate when engineers document the best design solution for a given problem on the basis of experience and an analysis of the advantages and disadvantages of various solutions. Design patterns typically describe a well-defined interaction pattern between different classes, participants or roles. Design patterns can be compared to cookbooks: they describe how to make good designs, but the hard work of realization remains with the engineer [19.3].

Frameworks: Frameworks can be viewed as implemented design patterns. While design patterns appear as documents, frameworks are realized as a collection of classes that contain built-in interactions with other classes of the framework. Developers can make use of these pre-manufactured design patterns by instantiating either existing classes of the framework or classes derived from them. The design pattern implemented in the framework can be customized and adapted to a concrete problem by inheritance. If no additional customization and adaptation is needed, the framework is referred to as a black-box framework, i.e. the programmer does not need to look inside the framework itself. If the framework needs customization and adaptation by the programmer, then it is referred to as a white-box framework, i.e. these modifications require deep insight into the framework's classes. Examples of frameworks include MFC (Microsoft Foundation Classes) [19.4], ACE (Adaptive Communication Environment) [19.5] and the .NET class library [19.6]. In contrast to class libraries, frameworks usually take an active role, controlling the event dispatching loop, following the hard-nosed Hollywood principle: Don't call us, we'll call you.

Components: Software components were created to magnify the reuse idea presented by classes. A software component usually provides functionality that far exceeds the functionality covered within a single class. Like objects, software components expose interfaces (irrespective of programming language) that enable one to use their functionality. However, in contrast to classes, software components are binary units of independent production, acquisition, and deployment that interact to form a functioning system [19.7].

Software components include the following characteristics:

- They can be deployed independently of one another.
- They are units for third-party composition.
- They have no (externally) observable state.
- They utilize, but do not expose programming-language-based features (e.g. inheritance) to the outside.

Various component technologies are currently available, including J2EE [19.8], CCM [19.9] and ActiveX/DCOM [19.1].

Containers: At runtime, every component must be hosted by a so-called container process that provides the components a guaranteed execution environment. The relationship between a component and its associated container process is exclusively a matter of configuration. Container process technology depends on the chosen component technology. Such container processes are usually referred to today as *application servers*.

Component models (componentware and containerware): Every component technology is associated with a component model. In general, a component model proposes a set of interfaces and associated behavior types to enable the seamless interaction of components with the hosting container. While componentware is the product that results from the technology of building complex solutions from simple components, containerware focuses on providing rich containers that support the hosting of such complex solutions in a variety of environments. For instance, ActiveX is based on a presentation-logic component model while CMM and J2EE support business-logic component models.

Web services: The users of components typically need to concern themselves with the instantiation and invocation of methods relating to the components. For that, they utilize mechanisms of the associated component technology. Web services build a stateless façade around components, thereby relieving the client of instantiation and technology concerns. Interaction with Web services is entirely based on messaging. In contrast to component-interface parameters, the parameters passed between client and Web service do not have object semantics. Web services conceal the location and instances of a component from their clients and conceal the sharing of service with other clients.

In summary, object orientation is currently regarded as the latest programming paradigm. Software components appear to the outside as building blocks that are independent of specific programming languages and that are designed for flexible reuse and composition while their inner logic is mainly implemented using class libraries and frameworks.

A sufficiently flexible software platform architecture will need to deliver software components, frameworks and class libraries that also enable customers to build software components. The final product might then be composed of software components developed at a late point in time using configuration.

In the remainder of this chapter, we present more details on how the mechanisms explained so far are utilized in the construction of the highly configurable, extensible and adaptable *syngo* architecture for medical imaging workplaces.

19.4 Application architecture

The various requirements from medical business units have influenced *syngo*'s component architecture in terms of application design: applications can be plugged into or removed from the system very easily on a one-by-one basis. All of the system's individual components are configured according to configuration rules. The application template includes a bus system that allows one to connect and disconnect applications (fig. 19.18).

When defining the application template structure, *syngo* architects were inspired by the notion of hardware standardization and various other hardware principles. It is a fundamental aspect of this modular system for applications that the applications

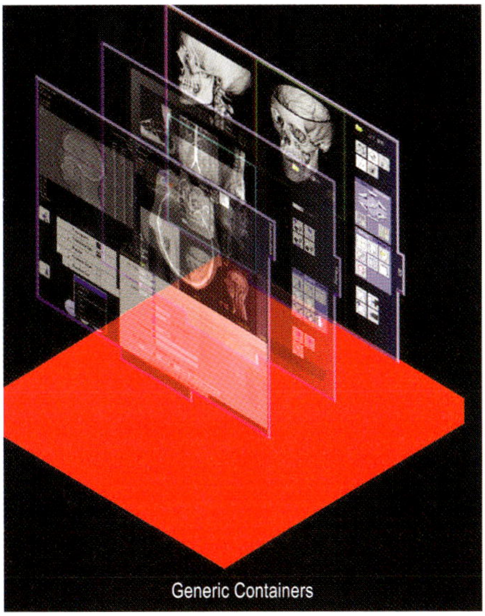

Figure 19.18
Reconfigurable plug-and-play architecture: plugging in of workflow-task cards into generic containers

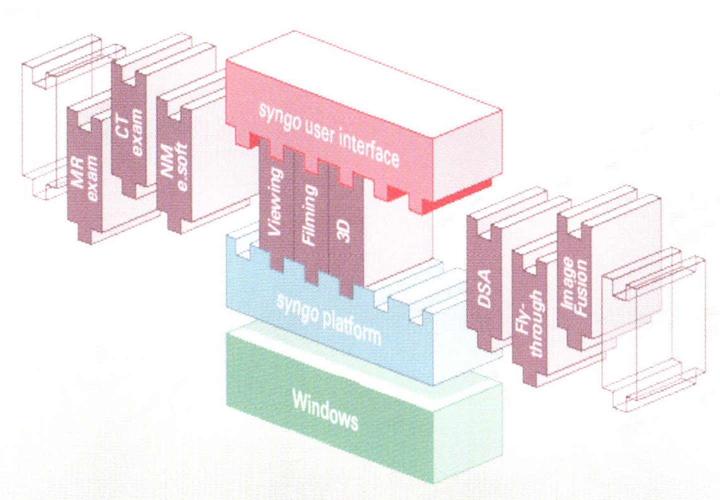

Figure 19.19
syngo architecture: application server for user interface and business logic as a framework for application components.

themselves are to be developed in a self-contained fashion so as to ensure their independence. They are exclusively based on the mechanisms offered by the *syngo* application template. The application template provides ready-to-use components and services, tools to allow the application developer to build new components and the backplane for the plugging in of these components. This backplane is provided in the form of purely semantic-free and generic containers. This generality allows for the use of the *syngo* application template outside of the medical domain. Furthermore, this principle even enables the exchange of applications across product and division boundaries.

The specific workflow for an individual product can be configured into generic containers accordingly. The rules for configuration are written in the form of ASCII configuration files and are read by the generic container at start-up time – or dynamically at runtime. The individual product is then constructed at runtime from the set of configured application components (fig. 19.19).

19.4.1 Three-tiered architecture model

syngo consists of many frameworks and common application packages that add up to many millions of source-code lines. These frameworks and applications are used by hundreds of developers within the divisions of *Siemens Medical Solutions* to produce end-user products for medical imaging. Common applications are therefore developed in strict adherence to the rules defined by the *syngo* application template. These rules apply to applications that are provided by *syngo* and to those provided by divisions or external suppliers.

Applications can be deployed in a generic container provided by the application template, an operation that resembles that of attaching a piece of Lego to a ground plate. This key concept enables one to use *syngo* as an open-software platform. While the variety of pre-manufactured design patterns, frameworks, generic components and application servers restricts developers in terms of diversity, it gives *syngo* the robustness that is necessary to enable its adaptation for different products.

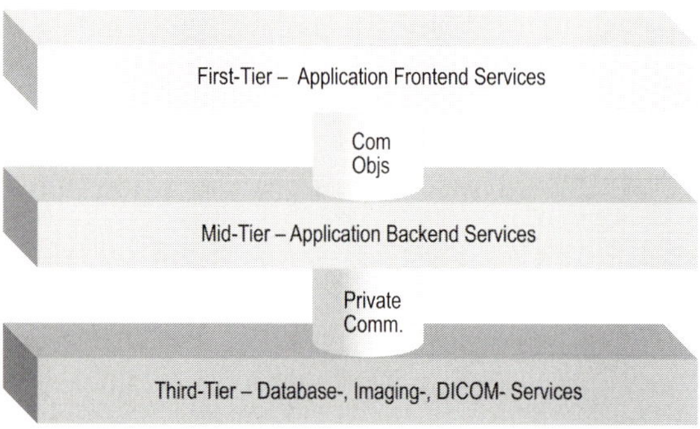

Figure 19.20
3 tier architecture model: the *syngo* architecture separates the user interface from business logic and business logic from the basic services.

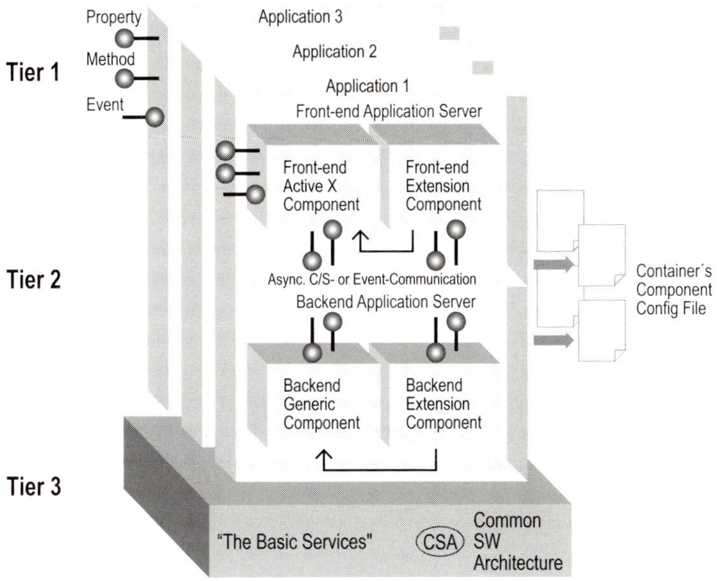

Figure 19.21
Application architecture: Application components are (re)configured with an arbitrary number of user interface, business-logic and extension components.

This flexibility and robustness is also the key concept when it comes to outsourcing application development to external suppliers. The external suppliers are required to use the application template framework and provide new applications in the form of components that conform to the application template. The application template guarantees the smooth integration of these new applications into the product – no matter where the applications have been programmed. The basic approach is thus well-suited to offshore development.

The configuring of applications represents a vertical sorting criterion. We will next have a look at a horizontal sorting criterion, i.e. the level of separation that is supported in the application template for an individual application.

As shown in fig. 19.20, the *syngo* architecture is three-tiered.

Component types are defined at each tier on the basis of the tier's characteristics.

The tiers are separated into the following key abstractions:

- Tier 1: User interface of an application (front-end component)
- Tier 2: Business logic of an application (backend component)
- Tier 3: Services infrastructure (libraries and service component)

As shown in fig. 19.21, the first two tiers form *syngo's* application architecture.

syngo offers different generic containers (application servers) for the deployment of the different component types at separate tiers:

- User interface components in the form of a front-end application server concept. The front-end application server supports runtime infrastructure for UI components such as status bars that enable applications to report status information to the user and menu bars that enable applications to make their respective menu entries. These convenient services that are provided by the generic UI container process make it easier to achieve compliance with a common look and feel.
- Business logic components in the form of a backend application server concept.

The business logic tier of the individual applications uses the services infrastructure as a part of the third architectural tier when necessary. The service components usually operate in backend application servers.

The strict separation of business logic and user interface represents one of the fundamental principles of *syngo* architecture. This separation offers the following advantages when it comes to application design (see fig. 19.22):

- User interface components (as parts of an application) can be easily replaced or adapted to a multi-monitor environment without requiring changes in the business-logic components.
- Customers are allowed to change the look and feel of applications by replacing the user interface component either completely or in part. This allows OEM (original equipment manufacturer) customers to utilize *syngo*'s business logic while maintaining their own look and feel.
- Developers and testers can specialize in the development of user interface components or the development of business logic components in accordance with their specific skills and interests.
- The user interface components and business logic components of all applications can be tested separately.
- The user interface components and business logic components can be developed using different development languages or even different frameworks.
- The user interface and business logic components interact with one another by means of messaging. This asynchronous decoupling supports flexible (configurable) execution architecture and it provides a sound basis for WebService utilization. Furthermore, the transmission of parameters between user interface and business logic does not involve the exposure of object semantics. This represents a further isolation factor that helps one to avoid development dependencies between the two components.

While the separation of presentation logic and business logic represents a basic principle, other technical aspects warrant mention:

- *Runtime extensibility* of delivered applications that is free of post-extension re-compiling and re-linking: The application template includes a built-in generic extension mechanism for components and a ready-to-use component skeleton that allows for the extension of applications even at runtime.

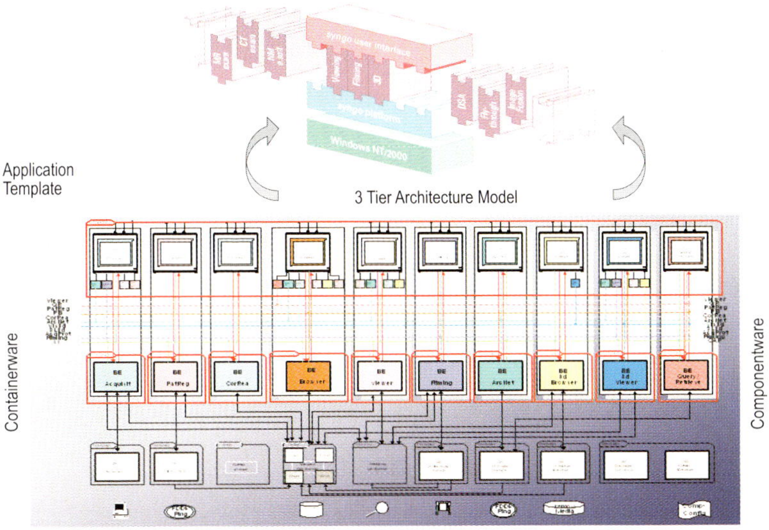

Figure 19.22
syngo application template: application support consisting of containerware and componentware with a common message bus

- *Flexible execution architecture* is needed to enable the configuration of a system consisting of both common applications and division-specific applications exclusively related to a dedicated medical product. The diversity of the medical product spectrum makes it necessary to provide for a configurable execution architecture and a rigid architecture model. The *syngo* application template does not force the use of fixed-execution architectures. On the contrary, it supports a very flexible execution architecture defined via the configuration of application components into application servers at server-start-up time or even at runtime.
- *Non-blocking user interfaces* are needed to provide appropriate support for mission-critical applications. The system will need to respond quickly to commands entered at the UI in time-critical situations. The *syngo* system provides mechanisms of asynchronous communication between front-end and backend components. This permits the activation of many parallel tasks and subsequent resynchronization.

19.4.2 Application architecture and component-runtime management

syngo applications consist of front-end components (implementing the applications' user interface) and backend components (implementing the applications' business logic) that together form a typical *syngo* application controlled by the component manager according to the design pattern of the *Model View Controller*. The services that are provided on the third tier are used within this business logic. Starting a *syngo* application first creates an empty hosting container. This is followed by the loading of the application components into the application server. A single application server is capable of hosting many components belonging to different applications. The association between a component and the hosting container process is strictly a matter of configuration description. The runtime execution architecture of applications is thus defined at the time of configuration. The runtime architecture in non-component-based systems is defined earlier, i.e. at the time of design and implementation. This precludes the implementation of late changes and makes it harder to adapt non-component-based systems to the needs of different systems with respect to runtime execution architecture.

The runtime infrastructure for front-end components is more demanding than that for backend components. This is due to the fact that front-end components need a well-defined UI area for the sending of status messages to the user (so-called status bar) and a location for the presentation of application-specific menu entries (so-called menu bar). Furthermore, the front-end application server also provides APIs for task-card management (i.e. the infrastructure for creating, selecting and removing different applications). The front-end application server is thus outfitted with a superset of the runtime services provided by the backend application server. This enables the front-end application server to host both front-end and backend components while

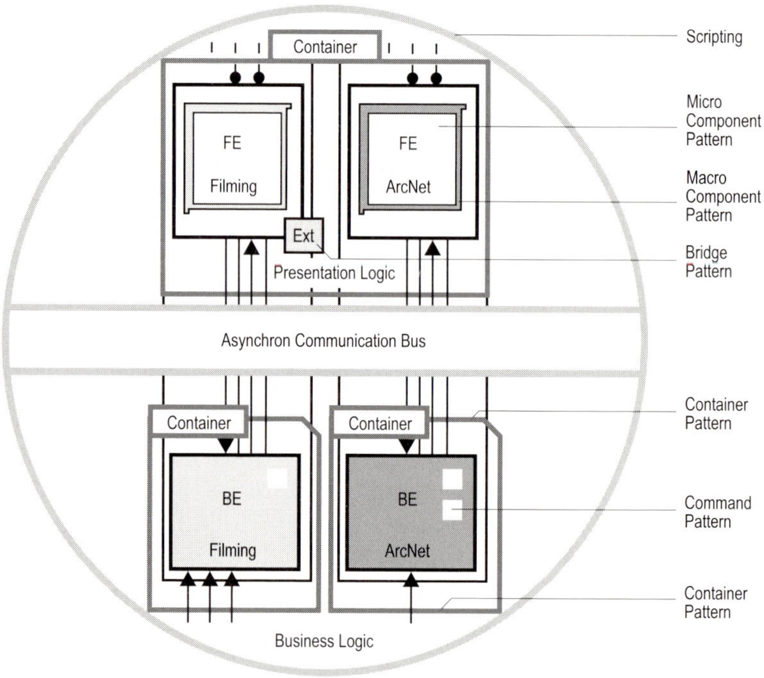

Figure 19.23
syngo's flexible runtime architecture: *generic containers* (executable programs) are configured via an arbitrary number of user-interface and business-logic components.

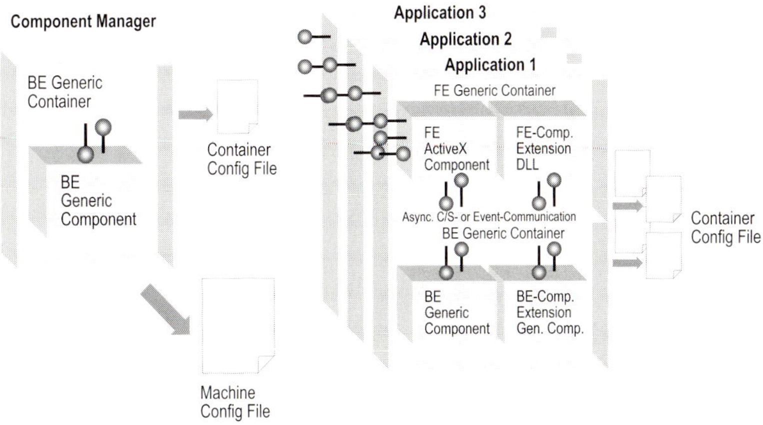

Figure 19.24 *syngo*'s component management service

the backend application server is only capable of hosting backend components. The process boundaries are less important at the time of design in component-based systems. Fig. 19.23 shows a sample excerpt from a typical *syngo* runtime configuration.

In the interest of maximum flexibility, *syngo* provides its container runtime infrastructure as a component. This enables one to use 3rd-party container processes for the hosting of *syngo* components. Adding the *syngo* container component to the 3rd-party application server creates a runtime infrastructure suitable for *syngo* components in the context of a foreign-application server.

A workplace that runs *syngo* will consist of many components that are all hosted in a specific application server (fig. 19.24). The runtime execution is controlled by means of a component manager that is itself a backend component that is executed within a generic backend container. The component manager reads an ASCII configuration file that lists the application servers along with their associated components. Upon request, the component manager starts the containers and the components that are to be deployed in these containers. Furthermore, the component manager allows for the grouping of components and the controlling of component groups (start, stop, suspend, resume) in a workflow-oriented way. The component manager is responsible for supervising the life cycle of components and removing running components from their containers or loading new components into running containers. For this reason, the component manager is assisted by a component-viewer user interface that allows one to drag and drop components from one container to another to support system tuning requirements.

The features of the component manager have been re-used at application level via a separate *syngo* design pattern: the MedDynamics concept. While this concept was initially used by another division to allow for the dynamic loading and unloading of applications at runtime, it has since been incorporated into the *syngo* application template as a generic design pattern so as to serve all divisions. This is a good example of software reuse on a large scale and how such reuse benefits from continuous improvement, not only within the *syngo* engineering group, but across all divisions.

Having presented the runtime execution architecture for component-based applications, we will now explore the essentials of creating front-end and backend componentware. The *syngo* application template provides separate black box frameworks for both types of components. These will now be presented.

19.4.3 Presentation-logic containerware and componentware

The common look and feel of front-end components in *syngo* enables users in clinical environments to easily identify and conveniently handle every product that is based on it. This is one of the reasons why *syngo* was distinguished in the year 2000 with an industry forum design award at the Hannover Trade Fair in Germany.

A common look and feel offers advantages to both the vendor and the end user. The advantages to *Siemens Medical Solutions* include an accelerated application development via a focus on reduced diversity and a facilitated process of company-wide know-how sharing among developers. End users can apply the knowledge they have gained concerning the operation of one medical device to other medical devices. The organizations they work for will also benefit from this added versatility.

The task-card concept for *syngo* was introduced to help optimize workflow in the area of medical imaging. The user interface part of an application is implemented as a task card and deployed as a front-end component within the front-end application server. For this purpose, *syngo* uses the Microsoft user-interface framework as the basic framework for all user-interface components of the medical imaging software. The application template extends this functionality by making it available to the *syngo* front-end developer community for reuse. front-end application components in *syngo* are also referred to as *Macro-Components*.

19.4.4 Business logic containerware and componentware

A *syngo* application that is designed in compliance with the presented architecture consists of a user-interface logic (front-end components) and a business logic (or backend components) that are strictly separated from one another. The *syngo* architecture helps to enforce this strict separation by providing different implementation criteria for front-end and backend frameworks inside the application template. The *syngo* application template's backend framework is neither dependent on medical domain frameworks nor on the underlying operating system. This independence is achieved by *syngo*'s consistent reuse of underlying state-of-the-art frameworks and design patterns. One example of this is the ACE framework (Adaptive Communication Environment) that was created by Douglas Schmidt [19.5] and later extended in the context of a joint venture between the *syngo* architecture team and Washington University (USA).

Given that they are UI-independent, backend components can essentially be developed for more than one operating system if necessary. The backend container and *syngo* component manager are *operating-system-independent*. This independence enables one to use the component viewer to control application components running on different machines and different operating systems. Some divisions have approved such procedures for the sake of coupling embedded real-time examination control systems to host systems.

19.4.5 Asynchronous communication: decoupling presentation and business logic

The front-end and backend components of a *syngo* application communicate with each other using an asynchronous communication model. *syngo* leverages many popular design patterns such as Command Object, Command Processor, Command Proxy, Adapter and Bridge as outlined in [19.11] and [19.3]. This *syngo* design provides a means for non-blocking and prioritized and queue-enabled processing.

The communication system detects potential communication deadlocks in typical re-synchronizing scenarios and resolves them. This enables one to avoid blocking situations in mission critical applications. Furthermore, the *syngo* communication model enables commands to respond to a request with no reply (one way request), or to issue multiple replies. Re-synchronization for clients upon the completion of a request is supported as well. Once started, each function can be suspended, resumed or canceled.

In addition to the 1:1-client-server mode, the asynchronous communication model also supports m:n-event mode, which can be used either with push or pull behavior. Every *syngo* component, including front-end, backend and extension components, features two built-in event channels that are implicitly created and named via configuration entries for correspondence with their host components. These event channels connect automatically to an event bus system that identifies each connection point by its configured name. Every event that is sent by a named channel is received by all components using the same connection name. Two channels are provided so as to enable one to use one channel for event communication between components belonging to the same application (application scope) while using the other channel to connect all of the components in a workplace. This allows one to group components to applications and workplaces more easily, i.e. via configuring and not programming.

The applications may consist of an arbitrary number of front-end, backend or extension components and they may be deployed within a single front-end container or in different front-end and backend containers on the same or on different machines. This enables user-interface and business-logic components to operate on different machines while still belonging to the same application. The communication protocol for internal use (e.g. sockets, shared memory, etc.) is absolutely transparent for the developer and is optimized for the configured deployment at runtime, i.e. the communication topology optimizes in a transparent manner for the configuration/deployment topology.

Once a command object is executed in *syngo* business logic, its implementation creates a group of domain business objects responsible for performing the domain tasks necessary for medical imaging applications.

These business objects create, read and modify data that represent patient imaging information. This data is shared in medical workflow sequences between different applications developed by different modalities or even vendors. It is therefore important to include a well-defined data model in the software platform concept so as to provide support for seamless data exchange. A standardized data model is available for the medical imaging domain. This model is used as the basis for data modeling within *syngo*.

19.5 Business objects for medical imaging

Compliance with the international standards that are applied in the field of medical imaging represents an important objective for *syngo*. One such standard for medical imaging that all major vendors support is DICOM (Digital Imaging and Communications in Medicine).

One of the goals of *syngo* was to build a common software architecture that would enable the development of business logic class libraries using the DICOM standard as the fundament for the domain object model.

The DICOM object model defines a coarse hierarchy based on patients (person-specific), studies (disease-specific), series (modality-specific) and instances (images, reports, waveforms, etc.).

The center of this entity-relationship model is the patient with all related study series, image and waveform objects that are used in various products from different divisions of Siemens Medical Solutions or other vendors. Helper objects are arranged around these main entities to distinguish images coming from different modalities (e.g. CT, NM, AX). Other objects are deployed to support medical imaging with different pixel-depth formats, ranging from 8-bit grey-scale to 32-bit colored formats. Medical images also vary with respect to resolution and image matrix sizes range from 128×128 pixels to $4{,}096 \times 4{,}096$ pixels for a single image. Furthermore, different modalities group different numbers of images into a series object (e.g. computer tomography creates more than 10,000 images within a single series). On the other hand, the typical number of series objects created by MR in a single study is increasing.

The data model represents one infrastructure aspect that enables applications (built from front-end and backend components) to share data with other applications (by reusing the same data model). Beyond this, there are more infrastructure services that represent logic so as to make it (re-)usable for various applications. *syngo* includes many services that support the implementation, servicing and deployment of the domain object model for medical imaging.

19.6 Services for medical imaging

The third tier of *syngo* architecture comprises services. These provide the basic domain infrastructure that is used from within business objects running in the business logic of application backends.

19.6.1 Data management services

Data management services in *syngo* are responsible for establishing data access to persistent data stores. *syngo* uses Versant OODBMS for data-persistence implementation.

syngo data management services are optimized for acquisition system scenarios rather than for the query scenarios typically associated with databases. The difference is that acquisition systems typically involve more demanding insertion requirements than query requirements. Data storage on scanner systems is more a matter of short-term storage, while long-term data storage capacities are provided by PACS (picture archiving and communication systems).

Most of the business objects shown in the DICOM data model are managed locally using data management services that help to ensure object persistence. Other DICOM communication services are needed whenever it becomes necessary to transfer these objects from the local machine.

19.6.2 DICOM work list, storage, query and print-management services

The data transfer management services in *syngo* are responsible for implementing the DICOM standard transfer protocol with the help of a DICOM toolkit. *syngo* uses MERGE as the underlying DICOM toolkit.

syngo data transfer management services implement *modality work list* functionality (*general purpose work list* will be added in the future) and the corresponding workflow sequences defined by the DICOM standard. DICOM storage primitives such as C-Store are provided for the sake of transferring image data to image archives. DICOM query primitives such as C-Find are provided for the sake of locating information within an archive. The DICOM toolkit is also used to handle the sending of images to a DICOM-compatible printer. These basic services are typically implemented on the basis of the SCU/SCP model (i.e. service-class user and service-class provider model) as defined by the DICOM standard. *syngo* includes the following concrete services:

- Study-transfer service (network transfer of DICOM-composite objects used by the archiving and networking application)
- Image-manager service (retrieval and storage of DICOM-composite objects using removable media such as CD, MOD, etc. used by the archiving and networking application)
- HIS/RIS-manager service (obtaining scheduled procedure steps and sending progress messages to a HIS/RIS used by the MPPS application)

- Hardcopy services (sending composed images and data to a printer used by the filming application)

While *syngo* uses the specified form of data representation when communicating DICOM data to the outside world, it uses a more efficient form of representation for internal communication. As a consequence, the incoming and outgoing data have to be transformed from the DICOM format into the *syngo* internal format and vice versa. A set of different division-specific filters can be applied during the transformation process. One example of such a transform/filter combination involves the receiving of data in a format that DICOM has retired. A filter detects the retired format and then updates the data representation to make the transformation process less complex. *syngo* applications are then no longer required to consider retired data formats in terms of their business logic.

However, it is not sufficient to make provision for the local and remote handling of DICOM data. A medical imaging platform is also required to make provision for the sophisticated display and manipulation of the images that are received and stored. These services are referred to as image-processing services and are mostly utilized by viewing applications.

19.6.3 2D/3D/4D image processing services and framework

Image processing services in *syngo* implement the DICOM standard formats for 2D, 3D and 4D image processing. 2D image processing is applied to individual images or to individual image series, with each image being treated as a single slice independent of the others. 3D image processing involves combining sets of 2D images into volumes and applying advanced image calculation algorithms to the volumes. Such algorithms include surface-shaded display or SSD (for reconstructing the surface of objects within the volume), multi-planar reformatting or MPR (for calculating 2D slices with various orientations in the volume) and maximum-intensity projection or MIP (for locating and visualizing the areas of highest signal intensity within the volume, such as contrast agent in a vessel). Finally, 4D image processing is applied to 3D volumes so as to account for time as a fourth dimension. This enables one to visualize dynamic processes in a volume over time.

In addition to basic 2D and 3D class libraries, *syngo* offers advanced volume rendering toolkits and image-pipeline engines.

In response to the steadily growing list of functional requirements in the area of 3D applications (volume rendering, surface shading, virtual endoscopy, fusion, etc.), different operating modes were introduced to expand the capacity of the *basic* 3D application. The selection of an operating mode involves the application of mode-specific algorithms to the loaded data volume and the generation of corresponding results. Switching between modes causes other algorithms to be applied to the loaded data and is thus a convenient way of continuing to work on the results of the previous mode without having to reload the data over and over again. The *basic* 3D application is thus required to provide the functions and services needed by all of the modes, along with mechanisms for dynamically loading and activating the various modes that operate as *plug-ins*. Modes can thus be regarded as sub-applications using services provided by the base 3D application or *framework*.

While the *syngo* application template provides a rich generic infrastructure for all types of component-based applications, the 3D framework enhances this infrastructure specifically for 3D-application semantics. This sub-application concept allows for a high degree of reuse in the area of 4D-CAD (computer-aided diagnosis).

19.6.4 Security management services

Security management services in *syngo* are responsible for extending the *syngo* application template with respect to HIPAA (Health Insurance Portability and Accountability Act) demands. The main intention of HIPAA is to ensure the privacy of patient data by restricting its access to authorized users and by subjecting such access and any manipulation of patient data to auditing procedures. Such functionality requires a reliable procedure of user authentication and well-defined rules outlining the privileges of each user. Furthermore, it will be necessary to secure the audit trail against manipulation because the trail represents legally relevant evidence. Providing consistent security for patient data in distributed systems as well as in systems where applications from different vendors are deployed is a major challenge.

The *syngo* software platform includes a security subsystem to enable one to satisfy these security requirements. The security subsystem handles the following two tasks:

- Providing security services to *syngo* based on non-*syngo* applications running on a *syngo* desktop machine.
- Hiding the complex enterprise security infrastructure from the applications using *syngo* security services. This enables one to adapt *syngo* to various enterprise security systems without changing the *syngo* applications themselves.

The *syngo* security service includes:

- *Support for user authentication*. Every user is required to log in at the desktop using the *syngo* login point application (LPA) to gain access to the software. Various user repository technologies are available to enable system administrators to store information about valid users. *Active Directory* is one of these technologies. The *syngo* SecServer hides the concrete user repository technology from applications running on the *syngo* desktop.
- *Enterprise-wide notion for a currently logged in user*. Applications can issue queries concerning the privileges and permissions granted to a given user. The SecServer utilizes an enterprise service referred to as A&A (Authenticate & Authorize) for this purpose. The capacity to share user identities across machines is important for web-based applications that present their user interfaces on the *syngo* desktop, but execute their business logic on a remote web-server machine. User identity sharing is implemented in the *global session management* or GSM service (yet another enterprise security service used by SecServer). The local sharing of user identities between applications developed by different vendors is supported by the *syngo* medi-

ator. The purpose of the mediator is to offer services to external applications without requiring them to show compile-time or link-time dependencies to *syngo* code.

- *Collection of audit trail messages*. HIPAA singles out the patient as the rightful owner of all medical data relating to the patient. Patients thus have the right to restrict access to their data to certain people and to be offered proof that no other persons have viewed their data. For this purpose, all access to patient data is audited within the applications. These audit trails must be securely stored and protected against manipulation so as to ensure non-repudiation. The *syngo* SecServer unburdens the *syngo* applications in this regard in that the applications pass the audit messages to the SecServer that then assumes the task of consistently and securely storing the data in a central audit-trail repository.

The *syngo* platform implements a role-based security model that differentiates between a user's functional privileges and data-access authorization. For example, users will only be able to delete data if they are generally authorized to do so *and* if permission to delete has been granted to them for the data in question.

Beyond the services described so far (i.e. specific to the medical imaging domain) other basic services are available to provide assistance when it comes to installing and maintaining a *syngo*-based system.

19.6.5 Basic services

Once a system has been assembled at the customer's site, its computing hardware and software are installed. The software typically consists of an operating system, device drivers for controlling specific devices connected to the computing system, and the *syngo* software, including division software.

The purpose of installation software is to make this bootstrap procedure as easy and secure as possible. The software is therefore grouped into packages that either do or do not have to be installed in a pre-defined order. The installation software displays a user interface to the technician. This interface solicits information from the technician concerning the packages that are to be installed. The corresponding software is then appropriately installed in accordance with the technician's input.

Once the software is available in the system, it will need to be configured according to the customer's requirements. Configuration offers a convenient way of customizing the appearance of *syngo* applications according to user preferences (e.g. whether the patient browser operates in list view or tree view and which data attributes are to be displayed). Many of these settings can be controlled by the users themselves. Once the desired environment has been established, the configuration is saved so that the system looks the same after each system boot. The configuration service is responsible for maintaining these user settings and making them available whenever the user logs on.

After installation and configuration, the user works on the system and tunes the applications for best usage via configuration. The user creates image-acquisition protocols to establish efficient scan initiation and optimal diagnostic output. These protocols need to survive system rebooting in the same manner as the acquired image data.

New versions of *syngo* are released periodically to take account of new functions. Simply installing the new software will leave the user with a blank system, as in the beginning (i.e. no protocols, no acquired images, no customized application settings). However, the *syngo* platform is equipped with a backup/restore service that enables one to avoid this loss of data. The service allows for the creation of backup copies for selected data. Once the new software has been installed, the restore function restores all of the data, protocols and user settings contained in the previously created backup data set.

Obviously all of these basic services need to be extensible in order to cover the needs of all divisions:

- The installation software must be capable of installing division-specific software (including device drivers) along with the *syngo* platform.
- The configuration service must be capable of managing configuration entities defined by the division software along with *syngo* configuration entities.
- The backup/restore service must be capable of including division-specific data along with data specified by the *syngo* platform at backup and restore points.

Finally, it warrants pointing out that the backup/restore service faces an inherent challenge: the data being backed up have been generated by an older version of *syngo* and the restored data will be consumed by a newer version of *syngo*. It is therefore important to back up data in a version-independent format.

Creating user accounts, granting permissions and privileges to users and installing and configuring software properties are important aspects when installing a *syngo* workplace in a clinical environment. *System management service* is the environment used by a service technician to perform most of these tasks.

19.6.6 Systems management service

When installing a *syngo*-based product, the service engineer will configure the machine using *syngo*'s system management service. Part of this configuration involves assigning IP addresses and establishing connections to other DICOM nodes for the sake of data exchange. Another step in this procedure involves naming the system and configuring the name of the organizational unit for display on images shown on the screen as well as on printed copies. One further important task involves creating roles and user accounts, and specifying permissions and privileges for them.

However, the purpose of the system management service exceeds installation issues. The system management service provides the means for service technicians to gain diagnostic information about the system to enable them to carry out preventive maintenance and problem analysis. The system management service can be accessed from a remote location via a web-based technology that grants service personnel fast access to the system without requiring them to be physically present at the system's location. Special security features have been built into the system to restrict remote access to qualified personnel only and to ensure that such access does not interfere with local system activities (e.g. examinations).

The system management service is obviously required to permit its extension by the various divisions for the sake of managing product-specific devices and division-specific software. *syngo* uses CA-Unicenter as a management infrastructure for the underlying system.

19.7 Tool support for *syngo*'s product-line architecture

The information presented so far offers a rough overview of the structure of a common software architecture for medical imaging systems. This overview also extends to the applications and services that are established in accordance with the component-based architecture. The *syngo* software architecture has been conceived to facilitate the large-scale reuse of software, i.e. a reuse that spans many divisions and product families. In the present section, we present tools that help programmers to write architecture-compliant components.

Idioms, design-patterns and frameworks are useful for the definition of horizontal, architectonic abstractions (presentation logic, business logic, service logic). Vertical, architectonic borderlines can be adequately defined using component technologies (front-end component, backend component, extension component, service component). The combination of both horizontal and vertical borderlines forms the basis for defining a software architecture and, in turn, identifying relevant design entities. The success of large-scale software projects strongly correlates with a broad compliance with the defined software architecture. Rigid software architectures enforce the reuse of well-established design patterns and discourage the creation of a variety of individ-

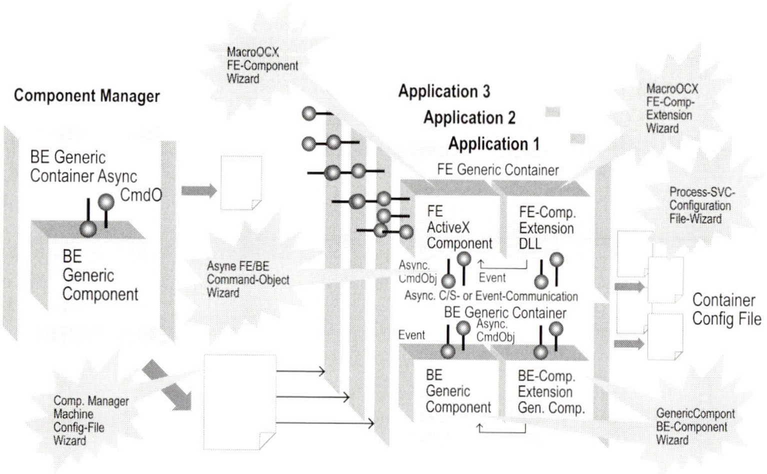

Figure 19.25
syngo application template wizards: ensuring correct reuse and increasing productivity in the development of *syngo* applications

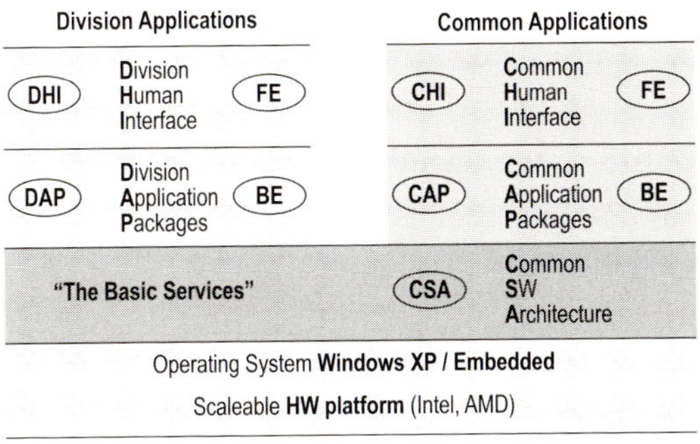

Figure 19.26
Integration of common and modality-specific medical imaging applications via the open *syngo* platform architecture (FE front-end, BE backend)

ual solutions that are incapable of working in concert. This is even more important in the case of projects that involve the development of software at different locations around the world.

Software development based on a software platform thus represents a step towards more automation in software development and away from individual solutions that are difficult to maintain. However, this introduces a further challenge: ensuring that developers create architecture-compliant components right from the beginning. The use of wizards (fig. 19.25) as helpers for automatic source-code production (model-drive architecture or MDA) can help one meet this challenge. Starting with wizard-generated code helps one to avoid excessive development cycles and increases developer productivity.

The *syngo* application wizards generate the complete project for an application component including configuration and deployment files and scripts. The generated code can be compiled and immediately started as an empty application component using the *syngo* component manager. The component developer then fills the generated component frame with the required presentation/business logic.

Using the same code generator at all development locations will help one to achieve components that consistently reuse architectural patterns and that are fully compliant with the given software architecture. This means the production of components that can be combined seamlessly in all product families.

The *syngo* platform aspect shown in fig. 19.26 offers a summary of what makes *syngo* more than just an architecture for medical imaging systems.

Only a platform will ensure that the application architecture is sufficiently sophisticated to allow for the extensive development by various divisions of platform-compliant applications with release cycles that are different from the release cycle of the platform. It is essential in the case of such architectures to define more than the layering (e.g. n-tiered models) and extension points for plug-in mechanisms because only the successful combination of both aspects will guarantee a product-line architecture comparable to *syngo*.

19.8 Medical enterprise application integration (EAI)

In the present section, we address future workplace needs by presenting medical solutions for clinical users that exceed the functions covered by a single platform architecture. Medical imaging is only one aspect in the complex workflow of treating patients. Other aspects include viewing lab results, scheduling physiotherapy sessions or planning patient medication regimes – typically covered by clinical information systems. Financial systems need to track and account for the treatments administered to a patient. Today, these systems are separately developed and mostly accessible from different computer systems. Furthermore, different standards and protocols exist in these various domains, with HL7 and DICOM being the most prominent.

It is advisable to make all of these functionalities accessible from a single workplace so that the clinical user no longer needs to move between separate computers to access specific information. Such workplaces help to enhance the clinical workflow.

Most of the relevant clinical and financial software is accessible via a web-based interface. Therefore, from a *syngo* perspective, enabling access to clinical and financial systems is identical to embedding a browser interface within a *syngo* front-end component, which is a straightforward task. Another important aspect is sharing the notion of the active user to provide a consistent set of functions across the different platforms based on the permissions and privileges granted to the user. Section 19.6.4 above offers a presentation of a corresponding infrastructure. Finally, it is also important to share the patient context across the different software platforms to ensure seamless

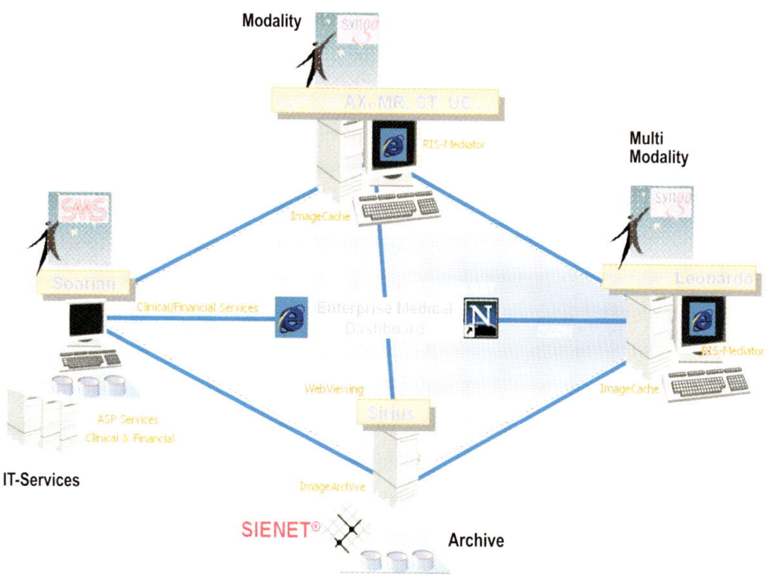

Figure 19.27 Integration of medical platforms for clinical systems and imaging systems

workflow support. CCOW (Clinical Context Object Working group) is a standard that defines sharing contexts and also introduces negotiation protocols for changing this shared context.

Reference to future workplaces again highlights the benefits of a common software platform architecture. Integration with other platforms can be achieved at platform level. All products based on the platform thereby clearly benefit from the extended capabilities. Enterprise application integration is just another example of achieving a high degree of reuse when creating a common software platform.

19.9 References

[19.1] D.R. Musser, G.J. Derge, A. Saini
The STL tutorial and reference guide: C++ programming with the standard template library
Addison-Wesley (1996)

[19.2] J.O. Coplien
Advanced C++ programming styles and idioms
Addison-Wesley (1992)

[19.3] E. Gamma, R. Helm, R. Johnson, J. Vlissides
Design patterns: elements of reusable object-oriented software
Addison-Wesley (1994)

[19.4] G. Shepherd, S. Wingo
MFC internals: inside the Microsoft foundation class architecture
Addison-Wesley (1996)

[19.5] S. Huston, U. Syrid, J. Johnson
The ACE programmer's guide – practical design patterns for network and systems programming
Addison-Wesley (2003)

[19.6] J. Richter
Applied Microsoft .NET framework programming
Microsoft Press (2002)

[19.7] C. Szyperski
Component software: beyond object-oriented programming
Addison-Wesley (1999)

[19.8] J. Bambara, P.R. Allen, M. Ashnault, Z. Dean, T. Garben, S. Smith
J2EE unleashed
SAMS Publishing (2001)

[19.9] J. Siegel
CORBA 3 fundamentals and programming
Wiley (2000)

[19.10] K. Brockschmidt
Inside OLE
Microsoft Press (1995)

[19.11] D.C. Schmidt, M. Stal, H. Rohnert, F. Buschmann
Pattern oriented software architecture: patterns for concurrent and networked objects
Wiley (2000)

20 Computer-aided detection and diagnosis (CAD)

20.1 Introduction

The increased amount of information available to a physician has correspondingly increased the complexity of physician tasks. This information ranges from clinical information, patient history, and laboratory tests to imaging tests that need interpretation by radiologists. Additionally, the context in which the physician deploys the information could range from prevention to early detection to diagnosis to therapy planning and monitoring (fig. 20.1). The rapid increase in image information, both morphological and functional, through better technologies that allow higher spatio-temporal resolution for all modalities (X-ray, CT, MR, US) has placed immense demands on radiologists' practice of shifting through all the data to diagnose any abnormalities. The need for combining information from multiple modalities or comparing current data with prior exams further strains the efficiency and accuracy of radiologist's interpretation of image data.

Decision support systems such as automated computer-aided detection systems can greatly improve the efficiency and accuracy of radiology readings if they have high sensitivity and specificity to the required task. The term 'detection' is typically used when a CAD system only marks a suspicious finding. The term 'diagnosis' is used for a CAD system capable of assigning probability of malignancy or a disease. The fact that

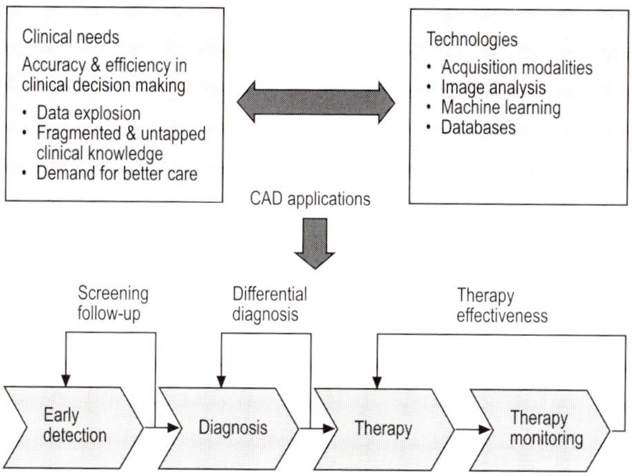

Figure 20.1
Computer-aided diagnosis and therapy: Supporting physician's decision making in entire workflow

Table 20.1 Diseases for potential application of CAD

Breast	Lung	Bone	Abdomen	Cardio-vascular	Neuro
Cancer	Cancer COPD Emphysema Pulmonary embolism Pulmonary fibrosis	Metastasis Scoliosis Bone age, densitometry	Acute pain Colon cancer Liver cancer/mets Oesophagus/ stomach cancer Inflammatory bowel diseases	Coronary artery disease Ischemic heart disease Cardio-myopathy Stenosis – plaque burden, vulnerable plaque Aneurysm	Cancer Alzheimer's MS Stroke

Whole Body

Screening: for diseases in asymptomatic high risk population
Diagnostic: Cancer detection and staging, Detection of metastatic disease in bones, liver, lung

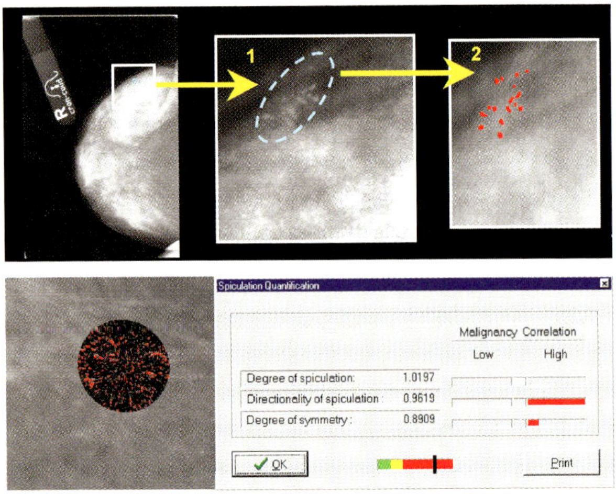

Figure 20.2
Computer-aided detection and diagnosis in mammography. **Top row:** Detection of microcalcifications by CAD. **Bottom row:** Analysis of a suspicious mass by a computer-aided classification system [20.5]. The color bar indicates that the likelihood of malignancy of the mass is high.

any automated system, just as a human, will miss some findings (less than 100% sensitivity, i.e., false negatives), and will point to spurious findings (less than 100% specificity, i.e., false positives) restricts the current clinical use of imaging CAD systems is currently accepted only as a second reader. The second reader workflow requires the physician to complete his review of the images prior to viewing the CAD findings. Other workflows include CAD as a first reader (physician reading only cases identified as

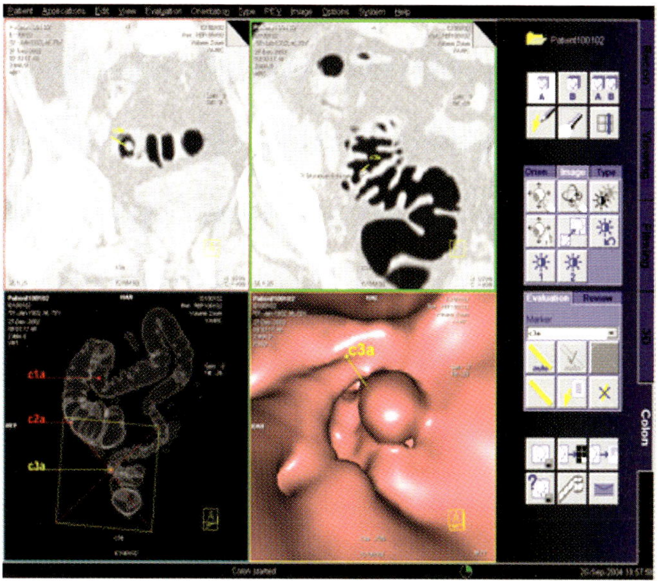

Figure 20.3 Computer-aided detection of polyps in CT colonography [20.6]

positive by CAD) and physician reading concurrently with CAD marks. Due to the possibility of missing positive cases in the first-reader workflow, and due to the possible distractions to the physicians in the concurrent reading workflow, more research is needed in studying the clinical benefits in the context of a specific CAD system before these workflows will become practical for CAD deployment.

Detection and diagnosis of cancer in breast and lung in 2D X-ray images has traditionally been the most researched area of CAD [20.1, 20.2], though there is an increased interest in applying CAD methods to 3D modalities, and other diseases and organs, particularly cardiovascular and brain (table 20.1) and [20.3]. Over the last decade, computer-aided detection (CAD) systems have moved from the sole realm of academic publications, to robust commercial systems in mammography and chest imaging that are used by physicians in their clinical practice to help detect early cancer from medical images. The growth has been fueled by the United States' Food and Drug Administration's (FDA) decision from 1998 onwards to grant pre-market approval for CAD systems that can identify structures of interest in medical images. Most of these approved commercial CAD systems focus on detection of breast cancer lesions for mammography [20.4] (fig. 20.2), though approved systems only exist for cancer detection in chest X-ray and nodule detection in lung CT. The applications that will constitute the next wave of clinically useful CAD systems are detection of colon cancer (fig. 20.3) and of lung cancer (fig. 20.4) from 3-dimensional computed tomography (CT) volumes. To be successful colon CAD and lung CAD systems must be efficient, have extremely high sensitivity, and introduce very few false positives per volume. As with

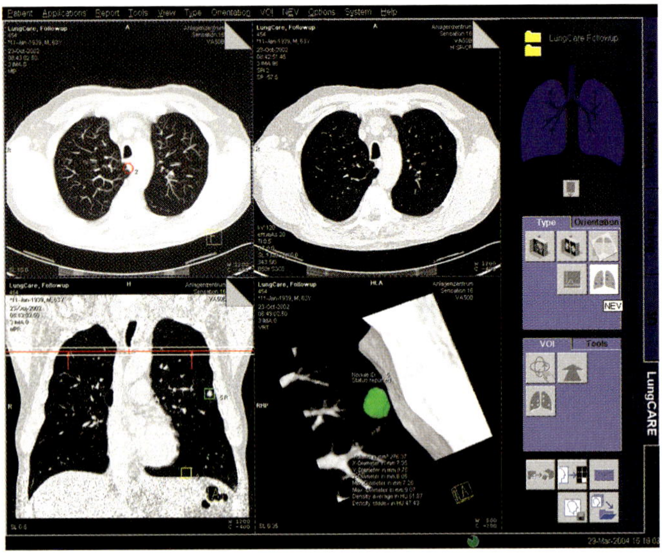

Figure 20.4 Computer-aided detection of nodules in lung CT exams

breast CAD, this superior performance must be demonstrated to the FDA in clinical trials, on new patient cases.

20.2 Performance measurement of CAD systems

Performance of CAD systems is measured in terms of the various possible operating points (sensitivity and specificity) of the system in a CAD-alone or CAD-assisted scenario. Since a user has the final say in the accepting or rejecting a CAD system's findings, the prospective clinical use of the system is the ideal way to measure CAD performance. However, a CAD system can also be developed and validated for clinical use on a retrospectively collected database using accepted statistical techniques of ROC analysis [20.7]. More sophisticated methods for studying CAD performance include multi-reader multi-case (MRMC) analysis that allow one to account for reader variability, patient variability, scanning device and parameter variability [20.8].

20.3 Computer-aided detection dataflow

The typical data-flow for CAD consists of the following steps (fig. 20.5): Pre-processing to extract the organ or a larger region of interest in the image, candidate generation, feature extraction, candidate pruning or filtering, and result visualization. Depending on the complexity of the detection algorithm, some steps might be eliminated or combined.

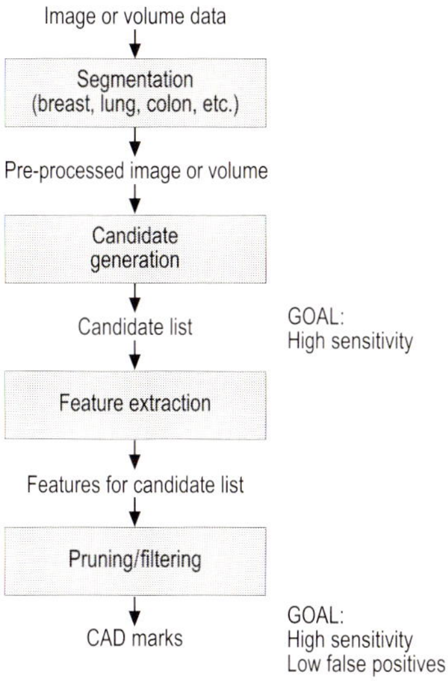

Figure 20.5
An overview of the data flow for computer-aided detection and diagnosis

Pre-processing

Even if the input data to the algorithm is nominally uniform, in the real world there are many reasons that introduce variability in image data. No two patients are alike, the positioning of the patient in the scanner will vary from one session to another, there might be extraneous objects in the scan (pace makers, tubes, patient tables, etc), scanner characteristics and acquisition protocols vary (tube current, slice thickness, pixel spacing, etc.) etc.

In order to simplify the succeeding steps, a pre-processing step is usually required that reduces the search area for the algorithm, identifies the orientation, and transforms the data into a standardized form. For example, a mammography CAD system will extract pixels corresponding only to the breast tissue, a colon or lung CT volume may be reduced to the voxels corresponding to the colon or the lung respectively. Even if the further CAD processing is not limited to the extracted organ of interest, the final display of the CAD marks can be limited to the extracted region to reduce the number of false positives shown to the user.

Candidate generation

Most medical images, particularly image volumes generated by high-resolution computed tomography (CT), are very large. Typically, a very efficient image processing algorithm considers each pixel (or voxel) in the image as a potential candidate "seed", and selects a small fraction of the seeds as candidates. Even this small fraction is necessarily very large, in order to maintain high sensitivity. High sensitivity (ideally very close to 100%) is essential, because any cancers missed at this stage can never be found by the CAD system.

The goal of any CAD system is to get as close as possible to the operating point of 100% sensitivity and 0 false positives. The goal of candidate generation step (CG) are 100% sensitivity, a minimal number of non-positive candidates, and computationally light-weight processing. Any positives that are lost in the CG step cannot be recovered in later steps. Having too many non-positives candidates will only raise the bar for the filtering capability of the candidate-pruning step, while increasing the overall computational time. And an efficient CG is required because the search space after pre-processing would still contain millions of potential detection locations.

These constraints are usually satisfied by image processing algorithms that characterize the essential qualities of the object being sought after. For instance, a lung nodule in a CT study is a roughly spherical structure that is often adjacent to other structures such as the pleural surface or a vessel. Therefore a fast filter whose weights are carefully chosen in order to yield a measure of "spherical-ness" is essential. A suitable threshold of the measure is selected that defines a compromise between the CG sensitivity and the number of candidates.

Feature extraction

Unlike the previous step, the image processing algorithms to extract the features may need to be computationally expensive. Thus, sparse feature selection (while building the classifier) is important in order to ensure a relatively small number of features in the deployed CAD system. Every candidate location obtained from the previous CG step is run through a battery of feature extractors. In general, each feature extractor's purpose is to quantify one characteristic that separates the positives from the negatives.

In the context of computer-aided detection of colonic polyps from CT data, the polyps are characterized by the roughly spherical protrusions from the colon surface, and by the inherent homogeneity of the polyps. Thus while one feature would measure the "spherical-ness" of the candidate, another feature would measure the variation of intensity values in the "polyp-like" region around the candidate. The "spherical-ness" feature would help in the discrimination of real polyps from folds, while the intensity feature would help discriminate the real polyps from candidates that point to residual stool (which often contains small trapped bubbles of gas/air).

Classification or candidate filtering

A previously trained classifier is used to label each candidate. The issues with classifier training are addressed later in the chapter. A classifier is a function that maps candidates to positive or negative, and the assumption is that the positivs will indeed correspond to the structures of interest for the physician.

Display of CAD findings

Typically, the CAD system will display a digitized image with overlaid marks to enable the physician to easily find and inspect the positive candidates. In the second-reader workflow for digital imaging modalities, the CAD marks are presented to the user on the diagnostic quality images after the initial diagnosis is made. Sometimes only the additional marks not originally found are presented (lung CT CAD). Alternatively, all CAD marks can be presented along with all of physician's findings. In order to not reduce a physician's true-positive rate (defined as the ratio of true-positives found to the total true-positives), the user is not expected to revise his/her original marks after seeing CAD's marks.

20.4 Development and validation of CAD systems – databases, training and testing of classifiers

The choice of features and the classifier in the CAD system is critical to its success. The typical process for off-line training of the classifier used to prune candidates (fig. 20.5), is to gather a database of patient images, within which structures have been labeled by a panel of expert physicians (or preferably from pathology findings from biopsy of the tissue), generate candidates from these images with very high sensitivity (i.e., ideally there should exist candidates corresponding to each "positive" label, which may require generating a very large number of candidates per image), and finally generate features for each candidate to produce a training set. A classification algorithm (a subset of machine learning) is then used to learn or train the classifier, which is basically a mapping from candidates (not just the candidates in the training set, but all candidates) to positive or negative findings.

The key requirement of the CAD classifier is its ability to generalize well. Namely, it should correctly label candidates drawn from as yet unseen patient images. If the training set is a representative sample of the structures seen in images that will encounter in the clinical setting and the classification algorithm is robust, then the classifier should have good generalization. Although generalization is a fundamental problem of machine learning commonly encountered in all domains, the inherent nature of the data collection and feature extraction process makes this problem more challenging to deal with in CAD algorithms.

The biggest problem is the choice of features, both in the training set, and in the deployed classifier. Physicians detect cancers by visually extracting shape and texture based features, that are often qualitative, rather than quantitative, from the images (hereafter, "image" and "volume" are used interchangeably in this chapter). However, there are usually no definitive image-processing algorithms that exactly correspond to the precise, often subtle, qualitative features used intuitively by physicians. To achieve high specificity, CAD researchers must necessarily consider a very large number of experimental image processing features.

Therefore, a typical training dataset for a CAD classifier is both extremely unbalanced (significantly less than 1% of the candidates are positive) and contains a very large number of candidates (several thousand), each described by many features (100+), most of which are redundant and irrelevant. Because of the efficiency requirement of the deployed CAD system, as few features as possible should be used by the CAD classifier.

Classifier training and testing

It is well-known paradox that learning a classifier that performs extremely well on the training data, has poor generalization. For instance by learning a classifier that has a very large number of parameters (for example, the same number of parameters as the number of candidates in the training data), it is possible to fit the training data perfectly. Such a classifier is said to have zero (or low) training set error. However, because the classifier has overfit the training data, it will often have poor performance on as yet unseen data (also called 'test data').

Because we can build a very large number of different classifiers from the same training data (using hundreds of classification algorithms, each with adjustable parameters), the choice of the classifier is critical. The selected methodology for training classifiers should try to achieve a balance between performing well on the training data while generalizing well on new cases. One such approach is described below:

A. Set aside a randomly chosen test dataset for final evaluation.
B. Use Leave-One-Patient-Out (LOPO) cross-validation as the principal evaluation metric.
C. Use the least number of features in the final classifier. (This is also desirable to improve the computational efficiency.)
D. Assess that the chosen classifier has good LOPO performance on the training data, and similarly good performance on the unseen test dataset.

We can present experimental results to justify each of the above steps [20.9]. Additionally, we can show that although cross-validation is a good scheme to prevent overfitting, it is not perfect. (We can build classifiers with low LOPO cross-validation error that generalize poorly.) The only true test of generalization is the classifier performance on totally unseen data [20.10].

Feature selection is a key component of classification. Each additional feature increases the discriminative power of a classifier, but also increases the risk of overfitting the training data. It is critical, therefore, to use as few features as necessary. We use the "wrapper" method for feature selection [20.11]: the classifier is run iteratively on the training data using different feature sets – during each iteration, one or more features are added, until cross-validation error converges. Therefore, with "wrapper" feature selection, the classifier itself determines the relevant features.

Another key issue is selection of the test database. When a system performs badly on some data, there is a strong temptation to exclude that data from the test set – and often it is easy to retrospectively justify the reason for eliminating a given dataset (such as, poor image quality). Data should be selected based on objective previously defined inclusion criteria (image quality, clinical relevance), and addressing all the potential biases [20.12, 20.13] prior to running any experiments.

Finally, a completely sequestered test set is essential. Cross-validation, and specifically, LOPO is an excellent performance measure – for instance, we can conclude that poor LOPO guarantees poor generalization, and good LOPO performance usually means good generalization. However, good LOPO does not guarantee good generalization.

This was not an issue 10 years ago, when a single cross-validation run took days, but with advances in computer technology, each LOPO run now takes seconds. The ability to iteratively "wrap" feature selection around a LOPO performance evaluation, allows one to evaluate many algorithms-feature set combinations, some of which, by chance, may have superior LOPO. Therefore, exceptional cross-validation performance, particularly on small datasets with many features, should be viewed with some degree of skepticism, until backed up by similar performance on completely unseen test data.

A final note of warning: A common mistake is that of tuning the classifier by continuously observing the classifier performance on the test data until a desirable performance is achieved. When the classifier is tuned according to its performance on the test data, then the test results lose all their credibility since the classifier no longer simulates real-world clinical settings. More importantly, such a classifier loses its ability to generalize on new data, which is, as stated in the introduction, one of the critical characteristics of a CAD system.

20.5 Future directions in CAD

There is much interest and the future need in pushing the state-of-the art in CAD along a number of dimensions: from detection of structures in 2D images to 3D volumes; from computer-aided detection to providing diagnostic decision support in the entire workflow (fig. 20.1); from single disease in an organ to comprehensive CAD systems for differential diagnosis of multiple diseases; from oncology applications to neuro and cardiovascular diseases; from detection of diseases to risk assessment [20.15]; from analyzing a single image/volume to multi-modality studies and/or serial studies; from analyzing static images to analyzing temporal information for change detection (fig. 20.6) and even motion (in cardiac CAD applications); from using labeled databases for offline training to online database mining systems to show similar cases [20.14]; and eventually to integrate all available clinical, genomic, and proteomic patient information with image-based decision support (fig. 20.7).

The future of clinical application of CAD systems is bright and the scope is broader than ever for researching, developing and deploying clinical decision support systems. The fundamental aspect of clinical utility [20.16, 20.17] of a CAD system in improving outcomes by enhancing accuracy and efficiency in patient care drives its acceptance by the clinicians as well as regulatory bodies and eventually the payers. Systematic multi-disciplinary research and scientific validation methods on high-quality databases are essential to ensure development of robust CAD systems that live up to their promised capabilities in routine clinical use.

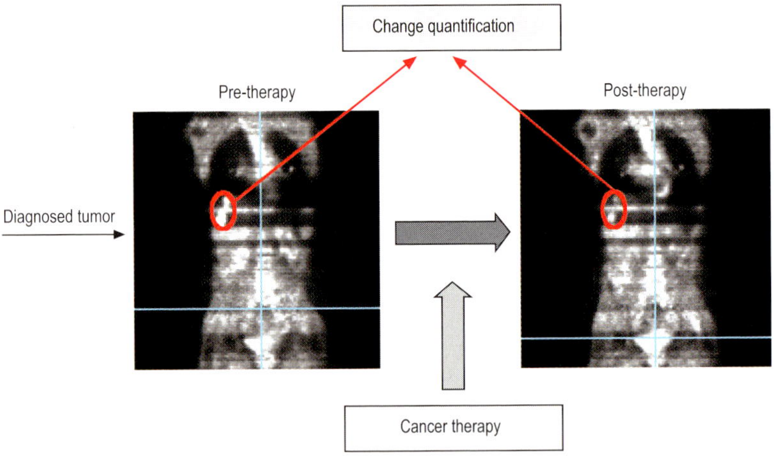

Figure 20.6
Change detection: Changes detected in longitudinal patient studies, subtle or obvious, are key for not only detection (in chest X-ray and mammography) and diagnosis (lung cancer in CT, Alzheimer's in brain MRI) of diseases, but also for detection of disease progression or regression after intervention or therapy. Statistically significant measurement of changes in morphology or function require understanding and accounting for all the other variables that may cause the changes (imaging conditions, scanner parameters, patient positioning, etc.).

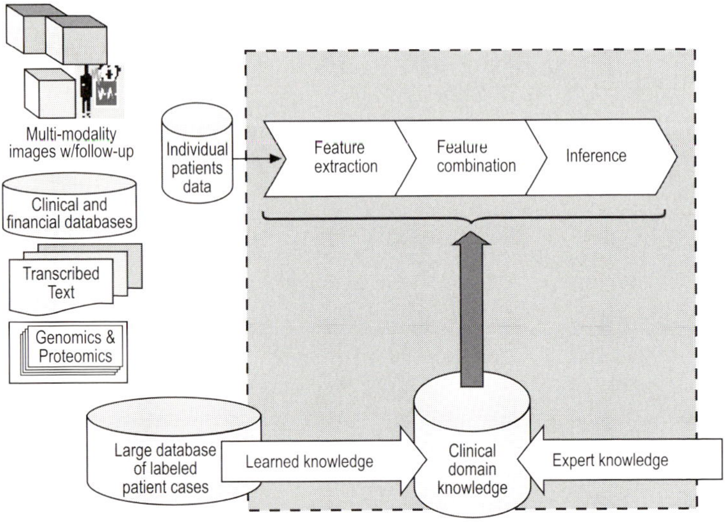

Figure 20.7
General representation of components of a decision support system. Large labeled databases and expert clinical knowledge are used offline by machine learning algorithms. The system is prospectively applied at the point of care with all relevant information available to the system. The online processing steps are the same as those in fig. 20.6.

20.6 References

[20.1] M.L. Giger, N. Karssmeijer, S.G. Armato III
Computer-aided diagnosis in medical imaging
IEEE Transactions on Medical Imaging 20 (2001), 1205-1208

[20.2] B. van Ginneken, R.B.M. ter Haar, M.A. Viergever
Computer-aided diagnosis in chest radiography: a survey
IEEE Transactions in Medical Imaging 20 (2001), 1228-1241

[20.3] R.M. Summers
Road maps for advancement of radiologic computer-aided detection in the 21st century
Radiology 229 (2003), 11-13

[20.4] TEC Assessment
Computer-Aided Detection (CAD) in Mammography
http://www.bcbs.com/tec/vol17/17_17.html

[20.5] S.S. Buchbinder, I.S. Leichter, R.B. Lederman, B. Novak, P.N. Bamberger, M. Sklair-Levy, G. Yarmish, S.I. Fields;
Computer-aided classification of BI-RADS category 3 breast lesions
Radiology 230 (2004), 820-823

[20.6] L. Bogoni, P. Cathier, M. Dundar, A. Jerebko, S. Lakare, J. Liang, S. Periaswamy, A. Laghi, M. Macari, T. Mang, D. Salovic, J. Wessling, M.E. Baker
Journal of Academic Radiology (2005), to appear

[20.7] N.A. Obuchowski
Receiver operating characteristic curves and their use in radiology
Radiology 229 (2003), 3-8

[20.8] X-H. Zhou, D.K. McClish, N.A. Obuchowski
Statistical methods in diagnostic medicine
Wiley (2002)

[20.9] P. Cathier, S. Periaswamy, A. Jerebko, M. Dundar, J. Liang, G. Fung, J. Stoeckel, T. Venkata, R. Amara, A. Krishnan, B. Rao, A. Gupta, E. Vega, S. Laks, A. Megibow, M. Macari, L. Bogoni
CAD for polyp detection: an invaluable tool to meet the increasing need for colon cancer screening
6th international workshop on computer-aided diagnosis, CARS. Chicago 2004

[20.10] M. Dundar, G. Fung, L. Bogoni, M. Macari, R.B. Rao
A methodology for training and validating a CAD system and potential pitfalls
6th international workshop on computer-aided diagnosis, CARS. Chicago 2004

[20.11] G.H. John, R. Kohavi, K. Pfleger
Irrelevant features and the subset selection problem
11th Intl. Conf. on Machine Learning, New Brunswick 1994

[20.12] N.A. Obuchowski
Special topics III: bias
Radiology 229 (2003), 617-621

[20.13] N.A. Obuchowski
One less bias to worry about (letter)
Radiology 232 (2004), 302

[20.14] I. El-Naqa, Y. Yang, N.P. Galatsanos, R.M. Nishikawa, M.N. Wernick
A similarity learning approach to content-based image retrieval: application to digital mammography
IEEE Transactions on Medical Imaging 23 (2004), 1233-1244

[20.15] M.L. Giger, Z. Huo, C.J. Vyborny, L. Lan, R.M. Nishikawa, I. Rosenbourgh
Results of an observer study with an intelligent mammographic workstation for CAD
Proceedings of the 6th International Workshop on Digital Mammography in Bremen (ed. H.O. Peitgen), 297-303
Springer 2003, Berlin

[20.16] D. Gur
Imaging technology and practice assessments: diagnostic performance, clinical relevance, and generalizability in a changing environment
Radiology 233 (2004), 309-312

[20.17] E.A. Krupinski;
Computer-aided detection in clinical environment: benefits and challenges for radiologists
Radiology 231 (2004), 7-9

21 Hospital information systems

The previous chapters of this book are largely devoted to discussions of various systems used in clinical settings for diagnostic purposes. These discussions have tended to focus on the physical and technical principles behind the systems as well as their specific areas of medical application. Some obvious questions relating to the larger clinical context have remained unaddressed:

- What becomes of the data once they have been evaluated (i.e. once the diagnosis has been finalized)?
- How can images and other data be distributed to other interested parties, such as referring doctors and the patients themselves?
- How might one go about organizing patient visits to hospitals, in particular, if the patients in question are to visit more than one clinic or specialist?
- How might one go about organizing the processes in a hospital so that physicians, nurses and other healthcare professionals can collaborate in an effective and efficient way?

The search for the answers to these and other related questions has led to the development of the general hospital information system (HIS). According to Degoulet and Fieschi [21.1], a hospital information system "may be defined as a computer system designed to ease the management of all of a hospital's medical and administrative information, and to improve the quality of healthcare." Haux et al. offer a broader definition, which includes the users (actors) of the HIS [21.2]. They describe a hospital information system as a "sociotechnical subsystem of a hospital, which comprises all information processing as well as the associated human or technical actors in their respective information processing roles." The authors go on to categorize the typical components of hospital information systems as "enterprise functions, business processes, application components, and physical data processing components."

In what follows, we construe the HIS as a "technical computer system" in the sense of [21.1] and [21.2], but without the sociological aspect suggested in [21.2].

The components of a typical HIS include, but are not limited to, planning and scheduling functions (i.e. the allocation of people, rooms and equipment for a patient at a certain time), a means of documenting clinical findings and treatment results, functions to handle the ordering of medication and other diagnostic and therapeutic procedures, archiving and retrieval services for patient data (including images) and billing and accounting functions for the sake of collecting payments from insurance companies and patients.

In the following sections, we first introduce the notion of an information system. We then offer a detailed description of the structure, functionality, technology and areas of application specific to hospital information systems. This description includes, in particular, a discussion of the relationship between the HIS and its various functions to the business processes in healthcare environments, and a characterization of how modern HIS applications can lead to improved outcomes based on workflow automation.

21.1 Information system basics

In general, an information system is "that part of an enterprise that processes and stores data, information and knowledge" [21.2]. Such systems can be described from various viewpoints, including their functionality, technology, logical implementation, deployment structure and usability. In the present context, we wish to concentrate on the layers of functionality that the systems exhibit, the service nature of their applications and their deployment within communication networks.

Information systems as layers of functionality

Fig. 21.1 offers an illustration of the various layers of hardware and software functionality contained in any information system.

The hardware layer is comprised of a computer and includes a central processing unit (CPU), input/output mechanisms, the storage memory for programs and data and controllers for all attached devices (keyboard, mouse, monitor, hard disk and other storage units, network access cards, etc.). Each software program is ultimately compiled into a sequence of instructions that can be understood and executed by the CPU.

The operating system (OS) enables one to use the hardware via application programs. For instance, a database application is for storing data on the hard disk, a graphics application is for displaying images on a monitor and an email application is for sending messages to other persons. All of these actions are organized by the operating system. Beyond this, the operating system is used to hide various configuration details and to optimize resources and access, for instance, with respect to the number of available CPUs (single vs. multiprocessor unit) and other components (e.g. hard disks), the number of users working simultaneously from the same computer (single vs. multiuser systems) and the number of applications running simultaneously on the same computer (single vs. multiprocess systems).

The most popular operating systems today include Windows for Intel-based computers (especially for desktop applications), various Unix implementations (mainly for

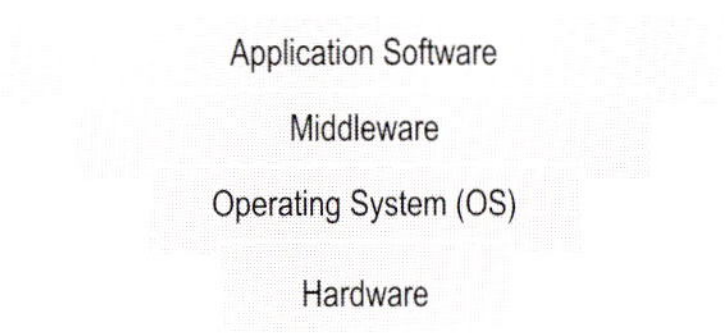

Figure 21.1
Layers of functionality in information systems

servers), including the Linux open source product, and the OS 390 for IBM mainframes and compatible clones.

The writing of application software that is to make use of system calls (i.e. that is to call operating system services) can be complicated and error prone. The suppliers of operating systems have therefore begun to provide higher level mechanisms to abstract the OS level and to make system programming more standardized. This higher level OS functionality is referred to as "middleware". Middleware can be used, for instance, to manage user sessions, security (authentication, access control lists, privacy), database transaction protocols and communication via various technologies (e.g. LAN, wireless, ISDN). The middleware can also optimize performance and scalability (e.g. via standardized caching/buffering mechanisms, load balancing and failover/recovery strategies).

The application software layer is ultimately the portion of a computer program that provides domain-specific functionality, such as factory automation, banking software and hospital-workflow management. One way of efficiently implementing various types of application software is to rely as much as possible on standardized off-the-shelf middleware and to avoid any proprietary mechanisms. This helps to ensure a high degree of portability and compatibility with respect to new technological developments.

Information systems as networks of communicating computers

Almost all of today's information systems rely on networks of communicating computers (servers and clients). Even so-called mainframes conform to the distribution approach (in terms of their logic) and are structured in virtual machines (VMs) that can also be referred to as servers.

Fig. 21.2 depicts the typical network structure of corporations today. They are all connected to each other via the Internet. The Internet is basically a conglomerate of wide area networks or WANs (i.e. dedicated networks and network servers provided by public or private organizations and made available worldwide).

Each organization requires one or more dedicated routers to access the Internet. In combination with a firewall server, the corporation can then connect its own local area network (LAN) to the Internet and give all of its employees access to the typical Internet services (email, WWW, etc.). If a corporation installs modern virtual-private-network (VPN) technology, its employees will be able to connect with the corporate LAN via the Internet with the same security provisions that apply within the corporate firewall.

WAN and LAN technologies are both mechanisms of communication. They typically differ only in terms of their bandwidth and associated costs.

As shown in fig. 21.2, the corporate LAN enables employees to access the connected application and database servers for the sake of performing enterprise resource planning (ERP), payroll and other employee services via their PCs. Furthermore, specialized servers give the employees access to the typical web services such as email, WWW

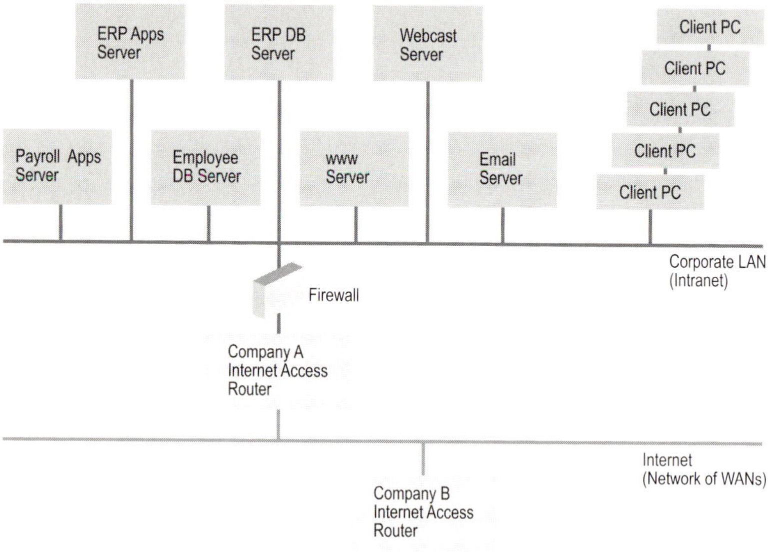

Figure 21.2 Distribution of functionality in networks of communicating computers

and webcasts. Multiple units of the various kinds of servers are typically clustered into server farms, with the size of the farms depending on the number of users and the volume of communication traffic.

In addition to the broad-based corporate applications made available by central servers, each client PC typically includes local software for tasks such as word processing and spreadsheet calculation.

Internet and Intranet applications are based on WAN/LAN technology:

- The http scheme (hypertext transmission protocol) is a message format and communication protocol used to send messages to Web clients. For example, the activation of http://www.google.com/search?q=Siemens will send a message to a Google Web server. Given the entry of the "Siemens" search parameter, the result will include a display of all pages that include the word "Siemens".
- The URL (uniform resource locator) addressing scheme defines the locations of documents in relation to a web server. For example, //www.smed.com/customer/index.php defines the location where users may go to find specific information for customers of the Siemens Health Services division. www.smed.com is the server address mapped to a TCP/IP number (Transmission Control Protocol/Internet Protocol) that can be looked up by means of the domain name service (DNS).
- The HTML (hypertext markup language) document format is a simple page/screen layout syntax that is understood by Web clients that are responsible for rendering the output format on the screen. DHTML (dynamic HTML) is a special variation of HTML that allows one to add output details or change screen displays at runtime.

Given that a predefined HTML page is typically loaded and combined with current data, it creates an output screen that reflects the current context of the application.

3-tier architecture for information systems

Fig. 21.3 depicts the 3 tiers of modern enterprise application software.

- The web server tier (tier 3, also referred to as the presentation tier) provides user access to the application's graphical user interface (GUI). This tier is responsible for handling security concerns relating to access through the company firewall (the upper firewall in fig. 21.3) and ensuring proper load balancing for all users connected via web clients. Presentation tiers are typically designed as thin clients, with no business logic (see tier 2) being included in the GUI code. Thin-client GUIs are accessed via web browsers such as Internet Explorer and Netscape.
- The application server tier (tier 2) runs the business logic, which is a technical term for data-processing algorithms. For example, business logic drives all of the data entry steps that are involved in the admission of a new patient into the hospital. A second firewall is often used to protect the application servers, in particular from unauthorized application code that may be executed on the web servers (virus protection). At the other end, the application tier communicates with the database tier via a specific access protocol such as open database connectivity (ODBC).
- The servers in the database tier (tier 1) are responsible for storing all of the data that are entered into or manipulated within the HIS. This tier is typically comprised of a commercially available relational database environment that is sometimes accessi-

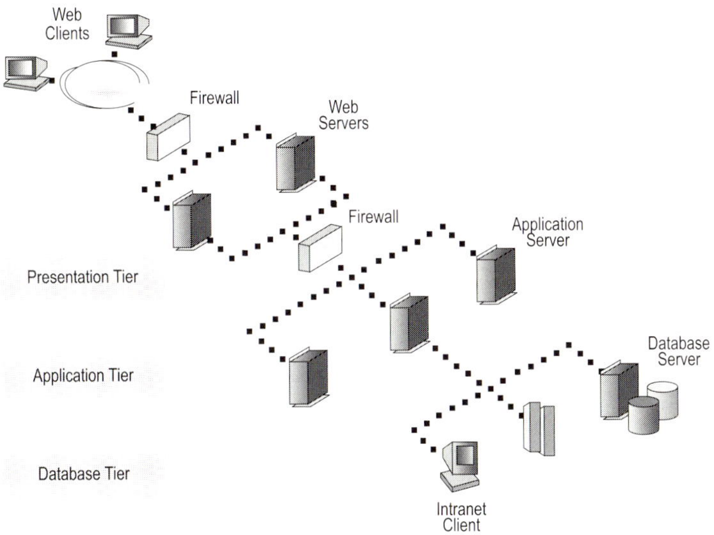

Figure 21.3 3-tier deployment architecture for enterprise application software

ble via an object layer so as to provide better support for the object-oriented modeling and programming style of the applications.

The actual storage of the data is handled by large hard-disk units that typically feature RAID technology (RAID = redundant array of independent disks) so as to prevent the loss of data. Multiple units of such RAID banks can be connected using modern SAN (SAN = storage area network) or NAS (NAS = network attached storage) concepts. SAN and NAS enable multiple database servers to share expensive RAID storage space.

RAID systems are usually also connected to long-term storage components for simple filing or back-up purposes. Examples of such components include large magnetic tape libraries and optical-disk jukeboxes (DVD, CD).

One clear advantage of 3-tier architectures is their scalable configurations, which can be flexibly adapted to the specific needs of the hospital. For example, an increase in users can be handled by making more web servers available at the presentation tier, and significant increases in the number of patients can be responded to by providing bigger database servers with more storage capacity at tier 1.

All of the servers can also be configured in a redundant manner, i.e. the servers can be implemented in pairs that provide a certain failover capacity whenever one of the servers of a pair is shutdown by technical problems. Alternatively, failover concepts might involve a more economical use of the machines on a farm by specifying fewer servers on the farm as redundancy machines for all of the others.

Application software as sets of services (SOA = service oriented architecture)

Application software is intended to take over human work. Human work is often provided as services. One example is an outsourced payroll service provider who administers a company's employee records, calculates the weekly paycheck, triggers a direct deposit for every employee, and sends the confirmation to the employees by electronic mail.

The same idea is used to structure the supporting software in terms of services. The presentation and application tiers described above interact via services, i.e. any activity (e.g. a user input) in the presentation tier involves the calling of a service from the application modules.

Fig. 21.4 illustrates the concept of an SOA in conjunction with a common service framework (see [21.4], [21.5]).

The common UI and service frameworks provide the mechanism of communication between the two tiers (see below). In addition, the framework ensures a consistent look and feel within all application modules.

Each application reveals its functionality via a service application programming interface (API) that can be used by any UI component. In fig. 21.4, for example, the patient management UI calls services from the electronic master person index (EMPI), patient-management and scheduling components. With respect to program implementation, this UI no longer qualifies as a strict vertical module for patient management.

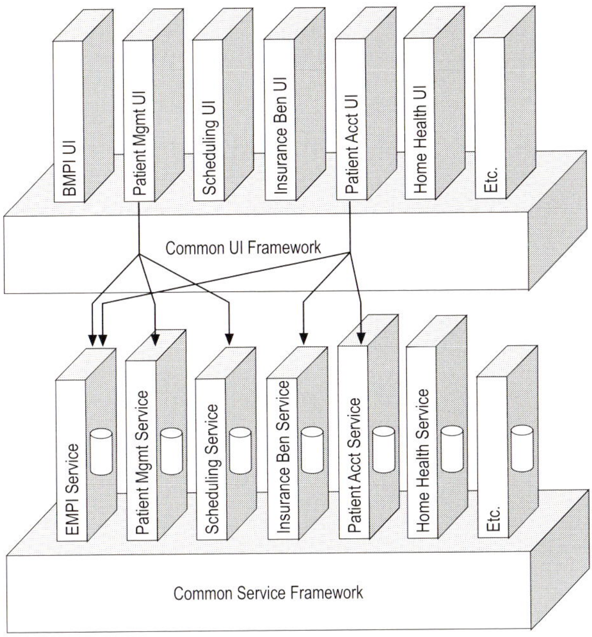

Figure 21.4
Concept of a service oriented architecture (SOA)

Instead, each application (e.g. patient management) can make use of services already available elsewhere.

The SOA approach is crucial for a general re-use strategy because the overall clinical workflow includes various sequences where the user needs access to the same or very similar services (e.g. *provide me the patient demographics*). The result will be identical, irrespective of whether it was called from the patient access module, the electronic-medical-record (EMR) viewer or a billing application.

The SOA approach thus represents a good balance between ones interest in modularizing large applications and optimizing the re-use of components (services). Providing a good SOA design leads to enhanced integration, unified behavior and faster programming cycles.

We will again refer to the SOA later in this chapter when we describe the service layers of an HIS.

21.2 Introduction to hospital information systems

Hospital information systems (HISs) have increasingly come to be regarded as enabler for better delivery of care. This notion is reflected in many national healthcare plans. Such systems were introduced in the early 1990s when they were more or less centered on the electronic health record and computerized physician order entry (CPOE).

Notable examples of such systems are deployed in the United Kingdom, France, the United States and Germany.

This enabling role is not different from that of information systems deployed in other industries where, for example, enterprise resource planning (ERP) systems support daily business routines in all areas, including human resource management, payroll administration, accounting, manufacturing, supply chain and customer-relations management. This highlights the role played by business processes and operational needs in driving the design and implementation of hospital information systems, while the systems themselves are best regarded as tools conceived to help generate better results.

The chief difficulty associated with the development of a good HIS as opposed to a good ERP system centers on the fact that doctors and nurses are generally expected to work directly with patients, and do not spend their whole time sitting at a desk in front of a PC. An HIS will thus need to be designed to supplement the daily routine of doctors and nurses and not to become their main tool. This emphasizes the importance of performance and ease of use for successful system deployment. Requirements concerning continuous safety and reliability represent a further difference between the two types of systems. After all, the life of a patient might depend on the faultless and continuously available functioning of an HIS. Furthermore, the designers of hospital information systems face the enormous challenges of accounting for both the complexity of medical knowledge – a complexity that is often occurring in clinical documentation – and low levels of standardization when it comes to the provision of care.

However, there are also many similarities. Just like ERP systems, hospital information systems have progressed through various developmental stages. The original HIS applications included data storage and retrieval. These were followed by further documentary applications whose main purpose centered on the management of information. Today, the list of applications includes mechanisms of knowledge-based workflow management [21.6, 21.7] that enable one to model the interaction between all of the disciplines in a healthcare institution, and that thus serve to automate the flow of information and tasks on the basis of established processes [21.5].

With respect to technology, hospital information systems have largely followed developments in computing. The accommodation of such systems was originally (and to some extent remains today) a matter of mainframes and batch applications based on terminal input. Interactive applications, usually in the form of PC-based frontends, were added. HIS technology then moved in the direction of client-server architectures, and is currently undergoing a slow transition to distributed web-based enterprise computing (i.e. via hospital Intranets) whose scope is often extended via VPN to associated practices and clinics.

21.3 Purpose and classification

The purpose of hospital information systems is to support clinical professionals in the context of their daily hospital routines, in particular by providing access to information and data management functions. The introduction of such systems goes hand in hand with the need to re-engineer hospital operations, i.e. to systematically change all of the necessary processes to be able to to achieve specific goals. These goals include improved:

1. Cycle time: shorter length of stay, shorter diagnostic cycles (from the order to the reception of the result), shorter general task-completion cycles, shorter bed turn-around times
2. Punctuality: increased percentage of examinations and surgical procedures that actually begin at the time they were scheduled to begin
3. Quality: reduced error rates (medication, transcription, others) and a reduction in the number of necessary follow-up treatment (e.g. re-stenosis removals)
4. Cost effectiveness: lower cost per surgical procedure, reduced IT spending per adjusted patient day, quicker payment of accounts receivable (A/R), increased market share
5. Satisfaction: with respect to all stakeholders, including patients, physicians, nurses, administrative staff, etc.

Hospital information systems support these goals by capturing data related to hospital operations, monitoring trend lines, offering helpful information, automatically forwarding information to the relevant people, reminding people to perform tasks at certain times and providing other useful assistance.

The hospital processes and their supporting information systems can be classified as follows:

- *Healthcare administration systems* enable the hospital staff to register and maintain all administrative patient data, and to bill for the services delivered. The main modules of such systems include:
  - Patient access and administration: registering patients and maintaining their core data (demographics, insurance information, billing status)
  - Appointment scheduling: inviting the patient to the hospital for a certain day and time, typically without further resource scheduling if not specifically requested (see the discussion on orders scheduling below under clinical information systems)
  - Revenue management: charging for the services delivered (sending bills to payers/insurers), collecting payments and maintaining contracts with employers and payers, etc. (One specialized function in this context is *physician revenue management*, i.e. making payments to associated physicians who are not employees of the hospital, but who provide services within the hospital.)
- *General administrative information systems* without direct reference to individual patients:
  - Management information system (MIS): an interactive application used by senior executives (CEO, COO, CFO) to analyze and monitor operational performance, fi-

nancial performance, staff performance, clinical performance (length of stay, number of medication errors), etc.

- General ledger systems to support the work of the CFO and accounting staff (accounting, finance, controlling, statistics and reporting)
- Human resources (HR) and payroll systems
- Supply-chain management (SCM) to support the purchasing department, e.g. to organize modern paperless orders of supply
- Customer relationship management (CRM): to provide regular information to patients, follow-up management, etc. (While this has long been a standard tool in other industries, it is relatively new to hospitals.)

- *Clinical information systems* (CIS) represent a main tool for nurses and doctors who *own* the patient. This typically involves the internal medicine department where patients first arrive and spend the most time. Patients are sent from this department to the various diagnostic and therapeutic service providers (e.g. radiology, orthopedics, oncology). Besides the electronic medical record (EMR) discussed below, the major modules of a clinical information system include:
  - Census management: the overview and updating of all patient data associated with a doctor, group of doctors, or hospital ward. Typical functions include the admission of new patients (their addition to the census), the transfer of patients to other clinics or wards (their removal from one census and addition to another) and the discharge of patients (their complete removal from all censuses). Further transfers may take place between outpatient (O/P) and inpatient (I/P) facilities.
  - Clinical documentation: the compiling of all observations, events and activities related to a patient. Documents can be broken down into various categories. General clinical documentation is standardized within a hospital. Department-specific documentation includes more details and often includes a considerable number of free-text elements. Disease-specific documentation provides the highest level of detail. With many numerical and categorical items, it is commonly used for clinical research, in particular in the context of controlled clinical trials.
  - Orders: the online entry of clinical procedures that have been ordered for purposes of diagnosis, therapy and patient care. This activity is particularly important in the case of medication orders due to their variety and amount (up to 100 orders per day for a single patient). Physicians typically write down orders on a notepad. These are then entered into the computerized order-entry screen by nurses.
  - Physician order entry (POE, also referred to as CPOE for computerized POE): a special extension of every orders module that enables the physicians themselves to enter orders directly via a computer form.
- The *electronic medical record* (EMR) is the core data repository in the clinical information system. This record encompasses information relating to all patient encounters, including diagnoses, orders, results, treatment plans, discharge instructions, etc. Given that the EMR is a legal document, the changes that are made to it are maintained on a long-term basis (as specified by the statutes of the specific country).

- *Departmental information systems* are dedicated software applications that cover the diagnostic and therapeutic workflow cycles for the various specialized departments in a hospital. Typical examples include:
  - Radiology information system (RIS) and picture archival and communication system (PACS)
  - Critical care information system (CCIS) for use in the intensive care unit (ICU), emergency room (ER) and operation room (OR)
  - Cardiology data management system (CDMS)
  - Other departmental systems are used in the areas of orthopedics and oncology, as well as in the hospital laboratory (Lab), hospital pharmacy, etc.
- Various *support tools and applications* that are not specific to the healthcare sector are increasingly used in combination with the HIS (e.g. office suites and portals).

21.4 Hospital workflow and integration

Fig. 21.5 shows a model of hospital processes [21.6]. The standard workflow starts with an administrative cycle where patients are scheduled before being admitted into an admission, discharge and transfer (ADT) system and (ultimately) discharged. This cycle ends upon the generation of a claim. The next cycle after admission is the clinical cycle where a physician order entry system (POE) may be used to enable doctors to give their orders online (the positive results of POE are quantified in [21.8]). Everything that happens to the patient during the clinical cycle must be documented for possible later use and for legal purposes. The procedure codes for all of the services

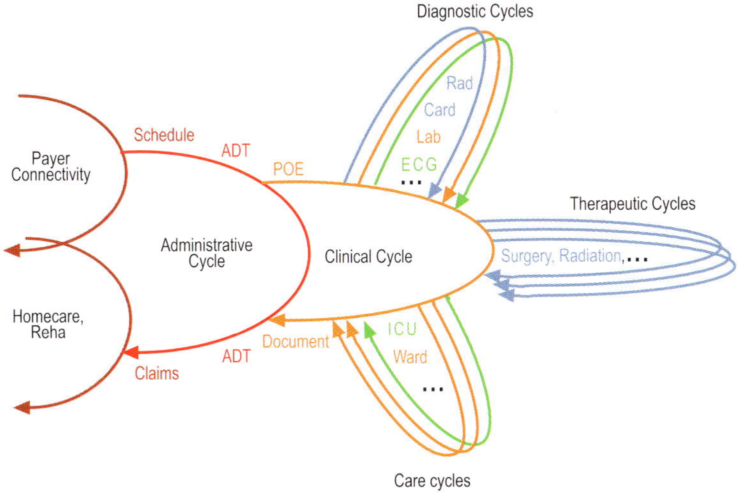

Figure 21.5 Process diagram of hospital operations

provided are sent back to the administrative cycle to enable the billing system to produce the insurance claim and the patient bill.

The physician first gathers information during the clinical cycle by sending the patient into the diagnostic cycles and then deciding on the best treatment. At this point, the patient enters the therapeutic cycle. Therapy may range from the simple administration of medication to surgery or to complex combined forms of treatment involving radiation and chemotherapy (e.g. for cancer patients).

The patient remains in the *care cycle* before, during and after treatment. This cycle may include days in intensive care or may be restricted to time spent in the general ward.

Current pain points in the hospital workflow include the various and highly disconnected process cycles.

- Example 1: Patients are registered more than once, in more than one place. Result: patient data are stored in multiple databases, leading to inconsistent data sets and, hence, to inconsistent documentation, claims and even inappropriate and dangerous treatment.
- Example 2: Physicians have limited access to the patient chart at the moment of placing an order. Risk: medication errors that could have been avoided: the Institute of Medicine (IOM) estimates that 7,000 deaths occur in the United States each year on account of erroneous medication and that 90,000 deaths occur each year as a result of adverse events [21.9].
- Example 3: The work of the various care providers in a hospital lacks sufficient coordination. Result: a diabetic patient is scheduled for a radiology exam at 11:30 a.m. The patient returns to find a cold meal in his/her room at 12:30 p.m. The person bringing the food was not aware of the examination and did not know to delay meal delivery.

The pain points described above provide us with a straightforward understanding of the term “hospital workflow”: the flow of patients, information and resources in a coordinated way.

21.5 HIS architecture

Fig. 21.6 shows the application architecture for an HIS. The diagram is directly correlated to the workflow cycle model shown in fig. 21.5. The core features include the applications for administrative and clinical workflow, sharing all patient information in the clinical data repository (the electronic medical record or EMR).

The grouping of applications in the administrative, clinical and departmental workflow also reflects hospital business practice (e.g. how and when the hospital makes purchasing decisions for the various applications). While these decisions are driven by different needs, they always reflect the desire to improve efficiency and lower the cost of operations. For example, the head of the radiology department might want to

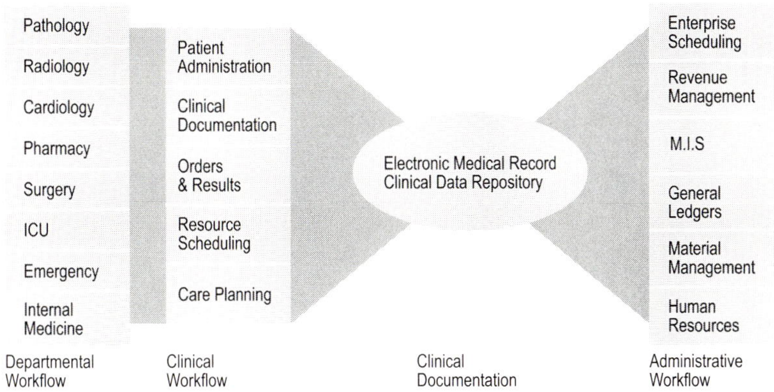

Figure 21.6 Application architecture for a complete hospital information system (HIS)

reduce the costs associated with the department's film archive and significantly increase the number of radiological examinations to be performed in the following year. With a radiology information system (RIS) already in use, the department head will now want to extend the department's automation via a PACS.

Two strategies are available when it comes to purchasing an HIS. There is the best-of-breed strategy according to which each department is allowed to purchase the best application on the market, independent of the choices made by the other groups and the single-vendor strategy based on the hope that one vendor can integrate first-rate applications with a consistent underlying architecture.

While the best-of-breed strategy usually leads to very high user-acceptance rates, it may well prevent hospital-wide optimization in terms of process support, technology bundling and deployment costs. On the other hand, it allows one to avoid total dependency on a single vendor.

The single-vendor or single-architecture strategy is thought to result in better TCO (total cost of ownership) figures, with reduced costs stemming from more comprehensive integration and thus reduced needs for interface engines, data mapping, interface maintenance and efforts to establish consistent database structures. Furthermore, partnering with one vendor typically enables one to demand volume discounts and reduced implementation charges.

Fig. 21.7 shows the concept of a modern HIS architecture that can be mapped onto the application architecture shown in fig. 21.6. The diagram is directly correlated to the workflow cycle model shown in fig. 21.5.

The architecture shown in fig. 21.7 conforms to a modern 3-tier approach (see fig. 21.3) that is particularly well-suited to web-based applications:

- The presentation tier (tier 3) provides the graphical user interface (GUI) that is responsible for rendering the windows with icons, forms, data entry fields and other

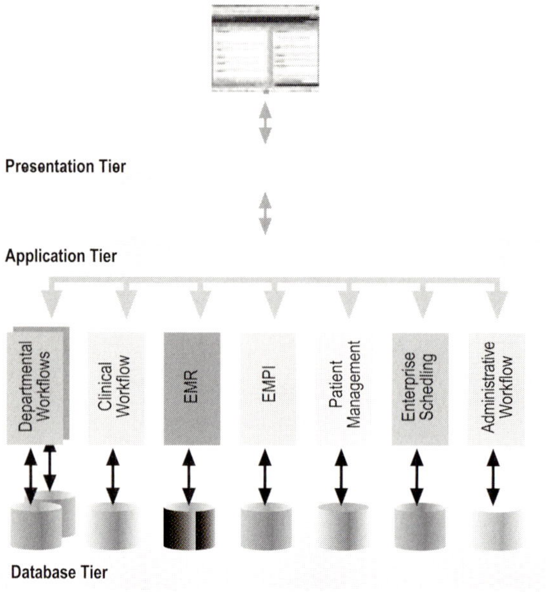

Figure 21.7 Hospital information system exhibiting a modular, three-tier architecture

control elements on the HIS user's computer screen. These elements can be manipulated via the keyboard and mouse.

- The application tier (tier 2) contains the so-called business logic, i.e. algorithms for data processing and other information manipulation (e.g. all data entry steps involved in the entry of a new patient into the ADT module). Each module publishes its interface in the form of services to the presentation layer (and within the applications), thus leading to the service-oriented architecture described above.
- The database tier (tier 1) represents a repository for all data that are entered or manipulated in the HIS.

Fig. 21.8 offers an illustration of the mechanisms used to access the application modules. Three scenarios are of special relevance in this context:

1. The user calls a function inside an application (e.g. a physician enters an order in the POE module of the clinical workflow). In this case, the UI framework creates a message that is handed over to the service broker (using the messaging API). This message is sent to one of the application services provided by the SOA interface (see above). The service responds accordingly and sends back the result. The call can be realized synchronously or asynchronously.
2. An external application calls a function (e.g. an external RIS needs certain patient data from the EMR). In this case, a standardized message is transmitted via the external communication engine (also frequently referred to as the interface engine or communication server). The typical standards include HL7 [21.10], DICOM [21.11] and XML-based structures [21.12]. The engine pushes the request to the

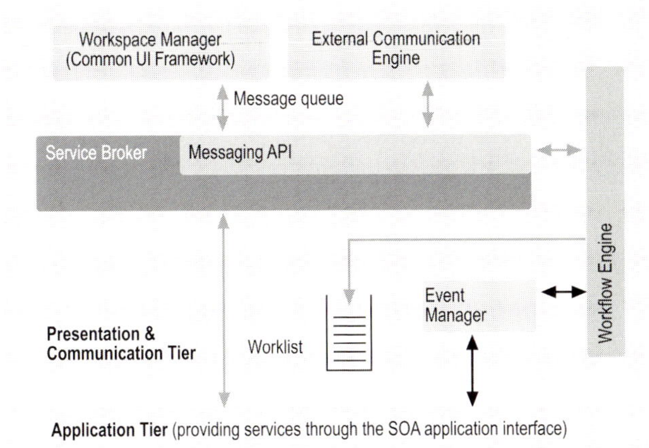

Figure 21.8 Communication mechanisms that enable one to use the HIS applications

HIS service broker and the service broker calls upon the EMR application to look up the needed data. The engine does not wait for the result (asynchronous communication)! Once the EMR application has found the requested data, it is sent back to the service broker, transferred to the communication engine and subsequently forwarded to the RIS.

3. The HIS's workflow management system (WfMS) invokes an application service. For instance, imagine the situation in which the WfMS wants to check the availability of a medication in the hospital's pharmacy in response to an urgent order for medication. If the medication is not available, the WfMS could automatically propose an alternative drug to the doctor. Technically, the WfMS sends SOA calls (requests for services) to the service broker. The service broker handles these calls like service calls from the user and the results are communicated the same way. A worklist is needed for the administration of the various tasks that are to be executed by the WfMS. The event manager is needed to administer the list of application services that can trigger a WfMS activity. Such services are required to *enroll* themselves as clients of the WfMS.

The concept of an integrated WfMS with an embedded workflow engine, first introduced in the form of the Soarian™ system by Siemens [21.6], is very new in the area of hospital information systems. Readers may wish to refer to a standard work for a good introduction to the technology behind workflow management systems [21.13].

It also warrants mention that the three communication cases may be heavily intertwined. A normal user request can trigger a WfMS sequence of activities, including calls to the communication engine to access external applications, and so on. The task of designing applications with automated workflow sequences carefully enough to avoid typical traps of cyclic repetition, deadlocks, unexpectedly long response times and other forms of unwanted behavior is very difficult. These types of problems are related to challenges faced in computer science with respect to the complexity of algorithms, the termination of programs and computability [21.14].

21.6 Patient administration and revenue management

21.6.1 Functionality

The HIS application architecture in fig. 21.7 depicts modules for administrative workflow (including revenue management), scheduling, patient management, and system-wide patient identification (by means of the electronic master person index EMPI). All four functions are needed for a complete patient administration system (PAS) and revenue management system as depicted in fig. 21.9.

Additional setup functions are necessary to make the patient-administration and revenue-management modules shown in fig. 21.9 work.

1. PAS configuration functionality

The configuration of a PAS requires the following preparatory steps:

- User administration and access rights distribution: The first stage in the setup involves the entry of user names and user access rights (read, write, delete, sign-off, etc.). User administration is typically based on commercially available tools (e.g. active directory) and is tightly coupled to the health professional masterfiles (see below).
- Masterfile setup: Masterfiles enable one to set up and execute decisions based on catalogue values and profiles. Given that hospitals tend to take a (slightly) different approach to the organization of their operations, the PAS's masterfile tool set must allow for flexible adaptations. A typical set of masterfiles includes:
  - Health professional master: A role-based description of the services provided by doctors, nurses and social workers, decision rights they have, what they are allowed to bill, etc. The connection to the location master can be used to define the clinics in which the various physicians work.
  - Location master: The description of all of the facilities a patient might enter.

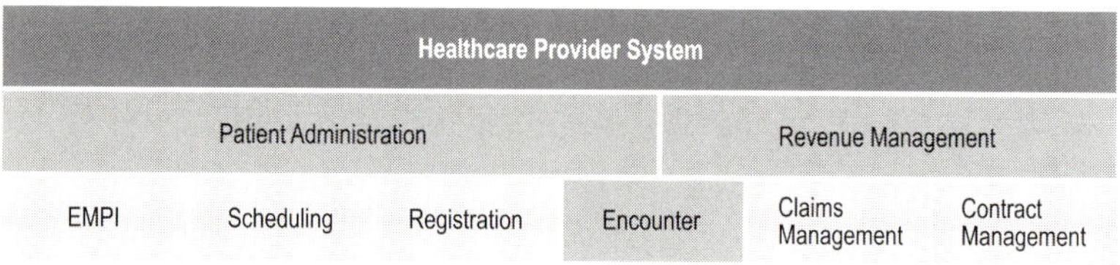

Figure 21.9
Function modules in a modern patient administration and revenue management system that is connected to payer organizations

  - Service master: The list of all of the services offered by the hospital, including price lists, charge codes (e.g. ICD-9, ICD-10, CPT-4) and charging rules.
  - Reimbursement master: The description of health plans, payer contracts, fee schedules, discount modifiers, diagnosis-related group (DRG) definitions, etc.
- Screen and form adaptation: Hospitals maintain different ways of organizing data entry on computer screens and different layouts for printed documents (e.g. bill forms, discharge letters, etc.). The setup functionality of a PAS enables flexible adaptation during the implementation phase.
- Data conversion and uploading: Once the masterfiles, screens and forms have been defined, they will need to be loaded with the live data for the hospital operations (e.g. the services provided in each clinic). If this data is already available in an older PAS, the data format will typically need to be converted before uploading. This process can be very difficult due to missing standards and varying degrees of data-format incompatibility.

2. Patient administration functionality

The major aspects of patient administration functionality (not including billing) cover patient registration, encounter management, transfer and discharge.

- Patient registration (or check-in): This step involves the admission of a patient to the hospital or health system. With the exception of emergency patients (quick check-in), the individual steps include entering the patient's demographics (name, address, etc.) and information about the patient's insurance coverage and benefit plans (regular check-in). If the patient has already been entered into the PAS, these data are at least validated. For various reasons (erroneous data entry, inconsistent data stored in different databases, external data collected), the data relating to a given patient may need to be merged into a single record. Special tools help the user to identify and join duplicate patient data and to split visits that belong to different patients.
- Appointment scheduling: Patients are typically registered when they need a service. Such services will then need to be scheduled (e.g. a time slot will have to be found for a certain diagnostic examination). Moreover, schedules may be repetitive (e.g. in the case of patients who are in need of regular physical therapy).

Fig. 21.10 shows a screen shot of a typical check-in screen. Demographic information (name, age, address, phone numbers) and insurance details appear on the left. A summary of the reasons for the encounter (e.g. chest pain), the diagnosis code (786.60) and various details (e.g. emergency case, commencement) and the name of the admitting physician (Dr. Barclay) appear on the right. Buttons on the bottom of the screen permit one to access more details.

- Eligibility and medical necessity check: Varying from country to country, the patient registration may also include a verification (e.g. online) as to whether the patient's insurance will cover a planned medical service (eligibility check) and even whether the service is medically necessary (medical necessity check). The latter is often no

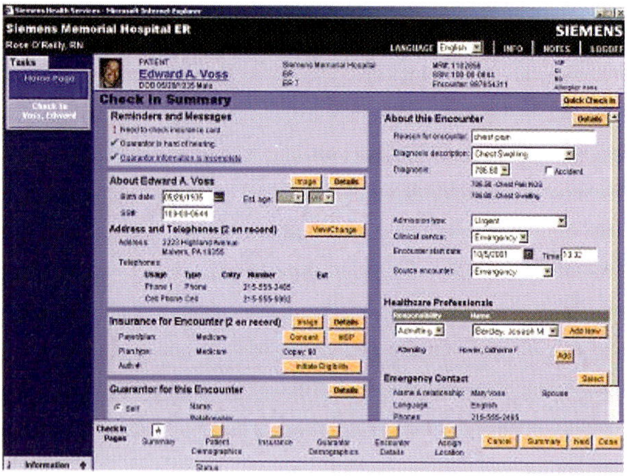

Figure 21.10
PAS check-in summary screen

more than information for the insurance company, seeing as how the final decision rests with the doctor. The medical necessity check is often not a part of the check-in, but of the order placement.

- Encounter management: Once the patient has been registered and admitted, the encounter-management function captures all of the services provided to the patient: who provided what and when, what supplies were consumed, how many hotel days were necessary for an inpatient, how the services are mapped to service charge codes, etc. A sophisticated implementation of the encounter-management function is crucial to capturing all service-related information in a way that allows for later snag-free reimbursement by the insurance company.
- Location management (ADT: admission, discharge, transfer): This part of a PAS involves a combining of various functions to enable the medical staff to document the movement of patients within a hospital or healthcare provider network.

3. EMPI setup

An electronic master person index (EMPI) is typically needed in healthcare provider network systems that include multiple facilities (inpatient, outpatient, associated practices) and often distributed HIS applications that do not share a central PAS. In this case, the EMPI toolkit generates one unique identifier for each patient (patient ID, PID). This identifier is usually related to the patient's demographics.

The identifier enables each HIS application at each facility to look up the identity of a patient before retrieving data from or entering data into the various databases. Using an EMPI helps one to avoid inconsistencies and the duplication of patient data, and thus to avoid dangerous situations (e.g. entering a critical drug prescription in the patient record of the wrong Peter Fisher who is undergoing treatment at a different location within a multi-entity provider network).

4. Revenue management

Modern revenue management systems are capable of modeling payer rules (What does a specific payer reimburse?) and contract rules (What specific options are covered by a patient's benefit plan?). The combination of such rules can lead to a high number of variations (around 800,000 in the United States). The the major components of a revenue management system are:

- Contract management: including ASC (ambulatory surgery classification) payment methodologies, DRG (diagnosis-related groups) contract calculations, early payment discount and late payment penalty rules, RUG (resource-utilization groups) payment methodology for skilled nursing facilities (SNFs), IRF (inpatient rehabilitation facility) PPS (prospective payment system) payment methodology, automatic percentage mark-up and expanded capabilities for contracts.
- Revenue management: including the collection of room and care charges for inpatients and ambulatory outpatients. This component supports across-the-board price increases and provides insurance billing and reimbursement management (i.e. it drafts, prints and then sends bills to payers). The billing module utilizes collection strategies (e.g. it determines which payers are to be billed first) to optimize processing cycle times and A/R days (accounts receivable days). A further module is the guarantor-processing and collection-letter subsystem that generates bills for the co-pay or private coverage of a guarantor (the patient and co-dependents).
- Claims management: this is of particular relevance in the United States where it originated from complex local health-benefit plans. Claims (insurance bills) are generated in a certain format (USA: ANSI X12 276). The healthcare provider can send claims electronically to the payer via electronic data interchange (EDI) transactions. The payer sends back a claim response (claims remittance). Discrepancies between claim and response may result from denials of eligibility or medical necessity, incomplete encounter documentation, or erroneous calculations. Hospitals may avail themselves of the claims-checking services offered by clearing houses before forwarding claims to the payer.

21.6.2 Technical realization of reimbursement workflow

Fig. 21.11 offers an illustration of revenue-management workflow sequences. The top of the figure depicts (from left to right) the five key workflow sequences:

- Collect data and generate claim: This sequence corresponds to the period during which the patient receives services. The relevant data are captured, the services provided are documented and billing codes (representing the charges) are produced with each procedure. The claim is then generated on the basis of the codes by the revenue management module.
- Edit claim: This sequence is for editing the generated claims (e.g. applying special multipliers to certain procedures that allow for higher payments). The editing can be performed manually (using a so-called *claim scrubber*) or automatically by the claims management module if the appropriate edit rules are available.

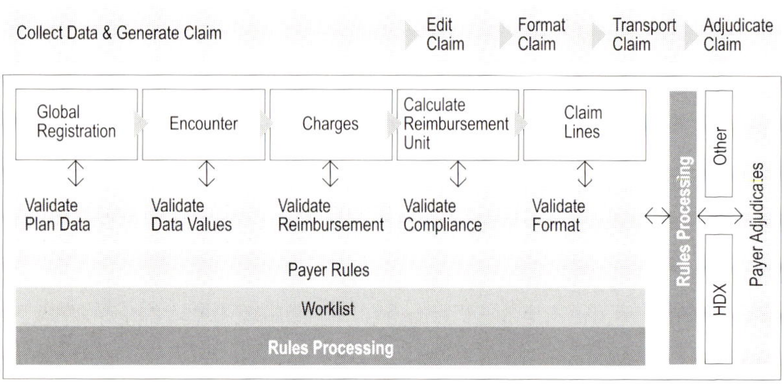

Figure 21.11 Workflow scheme and technical concept for a revenue management system

- Format claim: This sequence involves the formatting of the claim for compliance with relevant laws and regulations (e.g. HIPAA) or in order to meet specific payer requests. This sequence can be run manually (using the claim scrubber) or automatically by the claims management module.
- Transport claim: This sequence involves the sending of the final claim to the payer, either as a printed document or via electronic data interchange. One also has the option of first sending the claim to a clearing house (e.g. Siemens-HDX, WebMD or NDC) for additional editing so as to reduce the probability of denied or reduced payments.
- Adjudicate claim: This sequence involves the verification on the part of the payer. A fully adjudicated claim means that the payer accepts the claim and will reimburse the hospital accordingly. Otherwise, the payer sends a notification of non-adjudication citing the reasons for denial or reduction.

Recent studies suggest that around $30 to $50 billion could be saved in claims processing expenses in the United States if hospital information systems produced clean claims.

The lower part of fig. 21.11 maps the workflow sequences in the application architecture of the revenue and claims management modules:

- Rules processing is provided by a rules engine, i.e. an algorithm that is capable of interpreting the payer rules (defining what service is to be paid, how much, what co-payment is to be made by the patient, etc.) and calculating reimbursement values. The rules engine is also used for the various validation steps (e.g. determining whether a patient's benefit plan allows for a certain service). The validation steps (fig. 21.11) can be carried out during patient registration (validation of the plan), during the encounter when the doctor needs to order additional procedures (validation of data entered), when calculating the reimbursement unit (the one complete bill that may consist of different parts accumulated during the course of multiple visits and procedures making up the encounter) and in the context of all editing and formatting sequences.

- The payer-rules repository is a database containing all of the terms and conditions that apply to the payer as well as benefit plan information. The purpose of the repository is to ensure that the generated claims are accurate. Given the sheer diversity of payers and benefit plans in the United States (tens of thousands of variations), no system could accommodate all of them. While systems typically model only a few hundred benefit plans, these are selected so as to cover 95% or more of the total patients and procedures.
- Worklists are designed to collect all of the data sets that require manual processing by the staff of the hospital's business office. One prominent example is the A/R worklist (accounts receivable) that enables the office clerk to examine the details of each claim that has not yet been reimbursed (i.e. work on each item on the list). Other typical worklists include the late payment list (claims that have not been reimbursed by the expected or contracted date; the office worker might then call the payer for clarification) and the bad debt list (claims that are typically written off by an office worker with the authority to do so).

Fig. 21.12 shows the close relationship between a healthcare provider's system for patient administration and revenue management and a payer's administrative operations. In the case of the United States, this represents more a vision of the cost-efficient realization of e-business processes than a reflection of current conditions:

- e-Membership services: Patient administration in a hospital can be directly mapped to the membership management of an insurance provider or other payer. If both institutions share their EMPI information, they can avoid many of the problems (and costs) associated with mistakenly addressed patient bills.

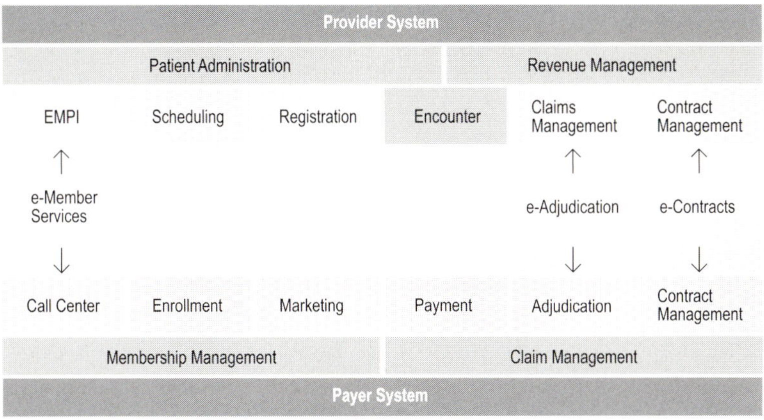

Figure 21.12
E-business concept for online data exchange between healthcare providers and payers

- e-Adjudication: The provider's claims management and the payer's adjudication represent the only processes today that utilize online connectivity for the sake of exchanging bills and remittance documents.
- e-Contracts: The online exchange of payer rules and contract structures would lead to additional time and cost benefits. However, even if online communication were to be established, the main problem would still remain: that lack of standards for broadly deployable contract models. All of the approaches today that make use of contract engines in revenue management systems require the manual entering and editing of such rules.

21.7 The electronic medical record (EMR)

21.7.1 Functionality

An electronic medical record (EMR) is the electronic version of the well known paper-based medical record or chart that contains all of the information relating to a patient's encounters at a healthcare service location. This information includes demographic data, patient and family history, diagnostic results, treatment plans and results and further important observations. The terms electronic patient record (EPR) and computerized patient record (CPR) are sometimes used instead of EMR.

The reference of the term "location" in the context of the electronic medical record may be much broader and include an entire healthcare network because the document can be much more easily shared between locations.

The EMR also qualifies as a legal document that is subject to various archiving requirements (as per legal statute), including the securing of its availability for audits (e.g. in case of a lawsuit). Confidentiality is a major issue relating to the EMR: access to identifiable patient data must be limited to the individual patient and the healthcare professionals who are directly involved in the treatment of the patient. All EMR systems must ensure compliance with legal regulations (e.g. HIPAA).

The collection of comprehensive patient information in a single EMR requires multiple interfaces to various hospital IT applications that feed the central data repository (unless a single HIS has been installed and all associated departmental IT systems use the EMR as their sole clinical repository). Typical data collected in the EMR include:

- Patient demographics and patient history
- Visitation information (date, time, duration, reason)
- Diagnostic data (lab results, radiology reports, ECG curves, etc.)
- Treatment plans, derived orders and observed results

A typical large hospital can be described as follows [21.3]: an institution that offers clinical services in one location, has around 1,100 beds, handles around 53,000 inpatient stays and around 230,000 outpatient visits per year, and its approximately 3,500 users created about 400,000 patient records in the last two years.

21.7.2 User interface and technical realization

Fig. 21.13 depicts a typical screen of a longitudinal EMR viewer (the term longitudinal is used if all patient data over time are accessible via the EMR interface). The layout is organized along the time axis on top (in blocks of weeks). Specific data, indicated by one of the icons, has been created for each day: vital signs, summary reports, lab results, radiology images and reports, surgery documentation and ECG flowcharts. The various sorts of information are organized in rows. Additional rows can be added as necessary.

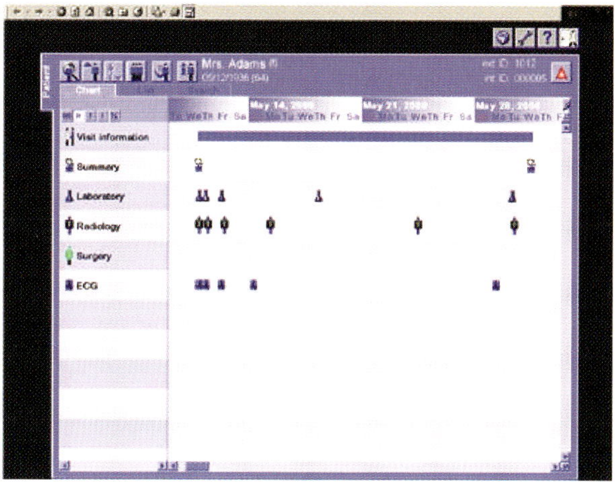

Figure 21.13 Graphical user interface for a longitudinal EMR viewer

Like all result-displaying tools, modern EMR viewers are web-based. This means that the data are accessed via a web browser and the user's navigation to the data proceeds via links.

Users access data by clicking on one of the icons (these essentially represent data links) in the figure. Doing so leads to the opening of a new window and the display of the relevant information. Fig. 21.14 shows the chemistry overview for the patient introduced in fig. 21.13. This overview appears when the user clicks on one of the lab-glass icons.

The use of web technology for results distribution is highly recommended because it enables global access (by means of the URL addressing scheme for establishing document links and by means of the universally available http transmission protocol). URL and http provide pull access to data: those who wish to view information are required to click on the link (icon, underlined text).

An alternative is to actively push information to a user, e.g. by sending a discharge summary or radiology report to the referring physician by email, fax or other means of communication.

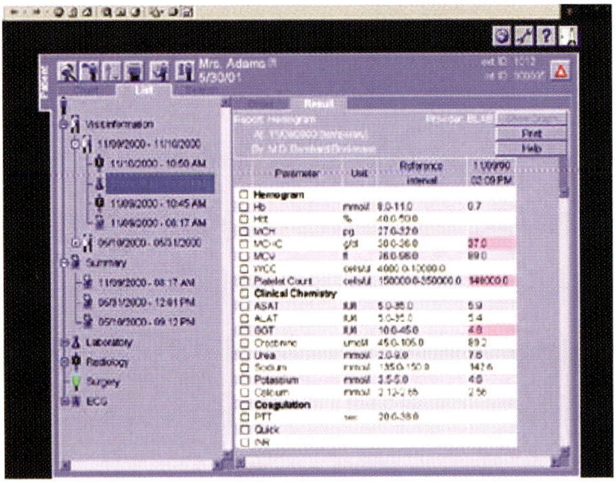

Figure 21.14
Patient chemistry overview as displayed in the EMR viewer

In any case, global access also requires special means of securing the confidentiality of patient data. Such patient privacy concerns are subject to legal statutes in virtually every country in the world (e.g. HIPAA in the United States).

Fig. 21.15 depicts the technical approach to connecting a hospital-wide (or enterprise-wide) EMR to all data-generating applications. The EMR server provides read and write access to the database and the application logic. These two tiers may reside on a single physical server in the case of small institutions. Any Internet Explorer or Netscape web browser can connect to the EMR application and look up data.

The communication engine transmits data from all data-collecting and data-generating applications (e.g. demographics changes in the ADT of the HIS, a new chemistry overview from the lab, a diagnostic report from the RIS, etc). While HL7 is the standard transmission protocol used by the communication engine, XML-based data exchange is becoming more popular.

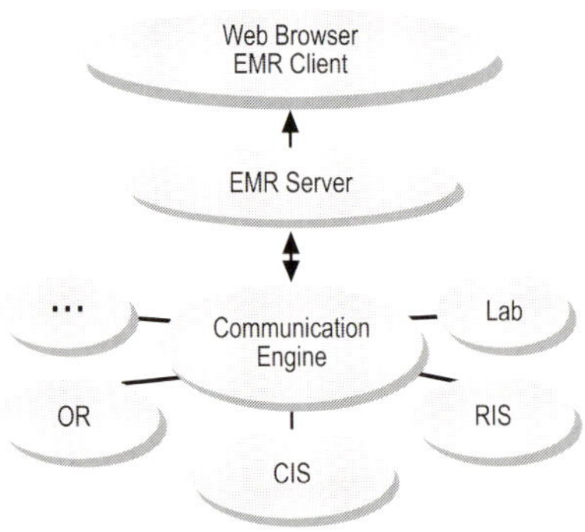

Figure 21.15
Technical realization of a centralized EMR

21.8 Clinical workflow applications

The typical users of clinical applications within an HIS include physicians, nurses, technicians (e.g. radiographers and lab specialists) and other clerical staff. The main activities that are supported by the clinical information system include diagnostic and therapeutic procedures and the documentation of all events, results, problems and improvements. While clinical applications cover the clinical cycle shown in fig. 21.5, they also overlap with departmental cycles involving diagnosis, therapy and care.

21.8.1 Functionality

Fig. 21.16 shows the typical modules of a clinical information system (CIS).

- Electronic medical record (as discussed in the previous chapter)
- Admission, discharge, transfer (ADT): While the admission (A) of a patient usually takes place in the check-in sequence in the administrative workflow, discharge (D) and transfer (T) to another clinic or service center usually take place in the context of the clinical workflow. After all, it is the physician who decides what to do next with, where to send and when to discharge the patient. In a deeply integrated HIS, the ADT is a module that is shared by administrative and clinical workflow applications.
- Clinical documentation: nurses or trained clerical staff are usually the ones who are responsible for collecting and updating patient data, for instance, patient problems, clinical notes and I&O (intake and output), documenting clinical assessments and charting results (e.g. vital signs, allergy progress, flowsheet data) and treatment plans. There are separate documentation forms for nurses and physicians.
- Order and results: clinical orders (diagnostic or therapeutic procedures) are given by physicians. The physicians either write down these orders in the form of notes that are later entered into the order-processing module of the HIS by a nurse or they enter the orders themselves into the POE module (see below).
  - Order processing starts with the provider census that is displayed in the list of patients a physician is taking care of and on whose behalf the physician can issue orders. In addition to the orders issued in his or her clinic (departmental orders), the physician can also issue consultation and referral orders (e.g. ask a colleague

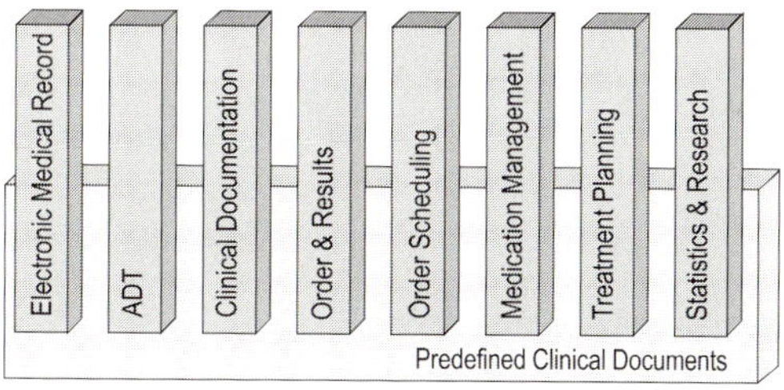

Figure 21.16
The application modules of a clinical information system (CIS)

for a second opinion or send the patient to another department for a special examination).

- The order-processing module includes interfaces for all departmental systems (e.g. to issue an order to the hospital pharmacy system to forward a medication). The possible orders are usually provided in catalogues or in the form of predefined order sets for standard treatment protocols. Nurses who use the order module usually do no more than enter the decisions made by physicians. They are not allowed to select from among order sets or sign off. Broad selection and sign-off capabilities are only available in the POE module (see below).
- The order-processing module must allow for recurring orders, avoid duplicate orders, make the connection to the charge codes (via the service masterfile) and support medical-necessity checking at the time of the order's entry. Everything that occurs while the order is being processed is documented in the CIS database to conform to legal requirements (e.g. the creation of audit trails specifying who entered or changed data and when).
- Results processing includes the monitoring of the outcome of the orders (e.g. the positive or negative result of a specific lab order). The entry screen for this module is again the census list containing all the patients for whom the physician is responsible. New patient results are highlighted in the results view window, e.g. via colored criticality indicators (see the red lab-glass icons on the right side of fig. 21.17). Results may include all sorts of data, images and flowchart information. If the CIS is connected to an enterprise-wide EMR, clicking on one of the criticality indicators shown in fig. 21.17 will activate the EMR results viewer as described above.
- Physician order entry (POE) [21.8] represents additional functionality for an order-entry module that is specifically designed for the online ordering by physicians (also referred to as computerized POE or CPOE). The POE application sup-

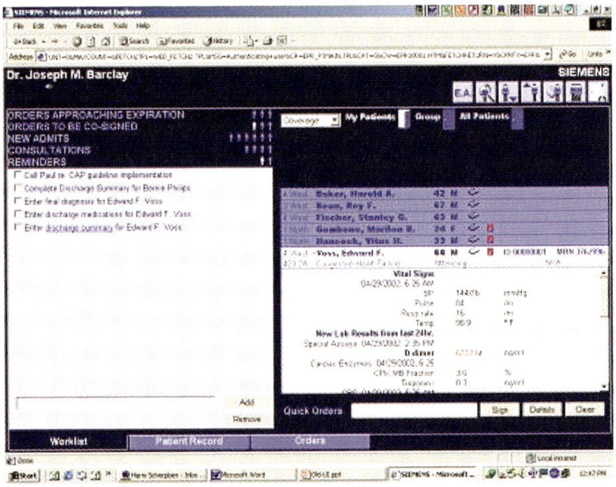

Figure 21.17
Physician worklist screen in a clinical information system, showing census list, results viewer and criticality indicators

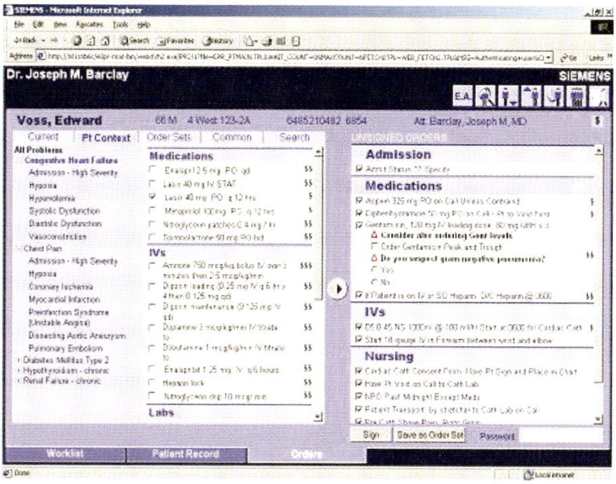

Figure 21.18 Physician order entry (POE) screen with generated medication alert

ports physicians by giving them access to all order catalogues and predefined order sets for standard treatment protocols and by its capacity to make intelligent proposals based on the patient and problem context (a type of artificial intelligence application). A sign-off button documents the physician's decision and commands the POE module to process the order (e.g. send a medication order to the hospital pharmacy).

Fig. 21.18 shows a typical POE screen. The five tab cards arranged on the left part of the screen correspond to the various ways of entering an order. *Current* displays the orders that are currently active for a patient. *Pt context* stands for patient context, and is a decision-support application that suggests orders based on the known patient problems. This corresponds to the active tab card in fig. 21.18 whose left side features a problem list detailing various issues relating to congestive heart failure. The remaining order tabs include *Order sets* (i.e. predefined combinations of orders that are considered standard protocols for certain diseases), and *Search* for looking up orders in the full catalogue.

- The physician uses the *Pt context* tab (fig. 21.18) to select medication, IV and other orders (i.e. by simply placing checks in the small boxes on the left side of each order). Dollar symbols on the right side of each order give an indication of the cost of each order. Once all of the relevant orders have been checked, the physician clicks on the *Accept* icon (circle in the middle of the screen) to add the selected orders to the list of all orders on the right side of the screen. The orders can be electronically signed off and forwarded for automatic processing by clicking on the *Sign* button below. Alerts and reminders help the physician to avoid errors.
- Alerts and reminders represent a sophisticated part of the POE application that warns physicians when one of their decisions might be sub-optimal or even wrong. A rules engine in the background relates the inputs made by the physician to the stock of patient information and a stock of general clinical information (in

particular, information about drug incompatibilities, patient allergies to specific drugs, incompatibilities with dietary needs, etc.). This represents an invaluable tool in light of the breadth and complexity of medical information, the fact that more than one physician may be issuing orders for a patient and the commonplace of human error [21.10].

Fig. 21.18 offers an illustration of a physician being alerted to the advisability of increasing gentamicin levels and the need to document a possible gram-negative pneumonia. If the latter is true, and the physician documents this finding now, then the reimbursement for the patient service will be higher. Fig. 21.18 also illustrates how an attempt is made to make it easier for the physician to react to an alert message: the screen also shows courses of action that the physician can initiate via a click.

- Order scheduling: When orders are given, in particular for diagnostic or therapeutic steps that require specific resources (people, room, special equipment), the order procedure is integrated into the scheduling function to allow for the necessary allocation of a time slot and the requested resources.
- Medication management refers to an automated workflow of ordering medications (best through POE), receiving the medication from the hospital pharmacy (verification and dispensing) and administering the medication to the patient. Fig. 21.19 depicts the four main steps of this process in a fully automated environment. In step 3, a dispenser robot picks up bar-coded medication packages from the storage area, thus avoiding errors of misreading.

  Barcodes also make the last step safer by allowing for a medication administration check (MAK). The nurse carries a barcode scanner and can scan both the patient ID and the barcode on the drug container. This enables one to assure the five patient rights of medication administration: right patient, right drug, right dose, right

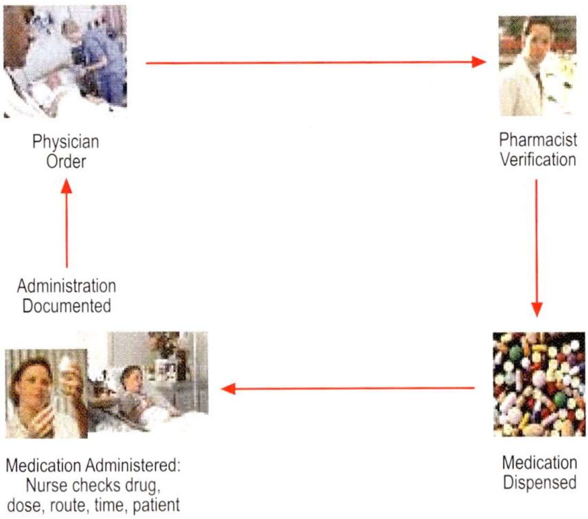

Figure 21.19
Automated medication management workflow based on POE, barcodes, and a dispenser robot system. (Model from Danville Regional Hospital, Danville, VA [21.15])

route, right time. Moreover, the MAK saves the nurse time because the administration of the medication is automatically documented after verification. The relevant legal document in the United States is the Med Administration Record (MAR).

- Care plans, treatment plans and protocols: All of these plans are standardized sequences for providing care to a patient with a certain problem. They can be regarded as a best-practice sharing approach according to which proven diagnostic and treatment sequences have been formalized and made available for broad re-use.
- Statistics and research: This module allows one to query the EMR, analyze data from multiple patients and encounters, de-identify personal records and copy data into external applications for further processing (e.g. into an Excel spreadsheet).
- Predefined clinical documents: These are the templates for forms that are to be filled out or printed. They often conform to standard layouts and even regulatory requirements.

21.8.2 Technical realization of system intelligence

The basic technical realization of a modern clinical workflow application system conforms to the architectural principles described above (see section 21.5). Key components for more workflow automation and smart behavior include an embedded workflow management system (WfMS) and various embedded decision-support capabilities or embedded analytics [21.6].

Workflow management system

A WfMS is typically designed around a workflow engine (see fig. 21.9 and subsequent explanations). The workflow engine is a rules engine that interprets a task sequence described graphically or in a script language. Siemens Soarian™ was the first clinical information system to include such a mechanism [21.3, 21.6]. With the embedded WfMS, Soarian™ provides the means of coordinating services between the departments of a given institution with the goal of making optimal use of human and material resources.

Soarian™ enables intentional and optimized workflow process designs by providing an intuitive graphical environment for designing reengineered workflow processes as depicted in fig. 21.20. The possible steps include making entries in worklists, sending messages (e.g. a reminder email), starting activities (e.g. an automated order renewal), etc.

Fig. 21.20 shows a workflow sequence for microbiological responsiveness that is designed to analyze patient lab data for potential MRSA and VRE incidents (caused by bacteria methacillin resistant staphyloccus aureus and vancomycin resistant enterococcus), and, in case of a positive result, prompt a nurse to validate the finding (the step). Subsequent steps might include the isolation of the patient (if the case is clear) and further lab examinations.

Workflow sequences can be triggered automatically (e.g. work allocation to housekeeping staff after the discharge of a patient) or via a specific user command (e.g.

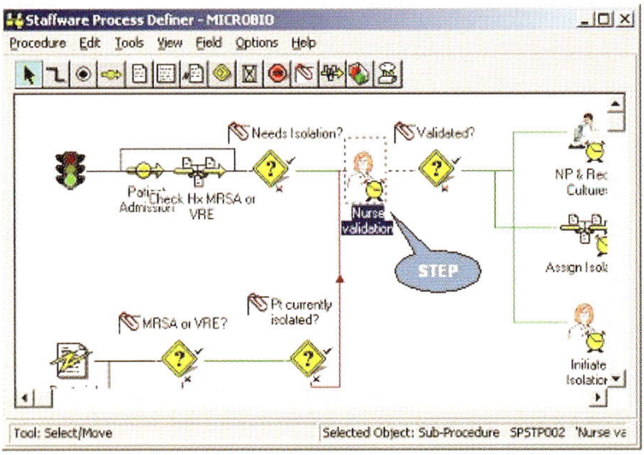

Figure 21.20
The graphical workflow design of the Soarian™ WfMS: processes are modeled as parallel-task sequences with branching conditions, including timers for starting, ending and reminding.

clicking on a sign-off button). Fig. 21.21 shows an example of a WfMS-generated alert box for the nurse Jane Gallant following the detection of a possible MRSA threat. The nurse may either remove the alert or initiate some or all of the suggested activities.

Further typical examples of automated workflow sequences in hospital environments include:

- ER stroke management: to streamline all activities needed for the optimal care of a stroke patient in the small time frame (1 to 2 hours) in which one can bring about the recovery of the affected brain areas.
- Bed turnaround management: to improve the bed turnaround time and optimize the utilization of available beds (cycle time improvements of up to several hours).
- Physician on-call management: to optimize the distribution and scheduling of the physicians on-call.

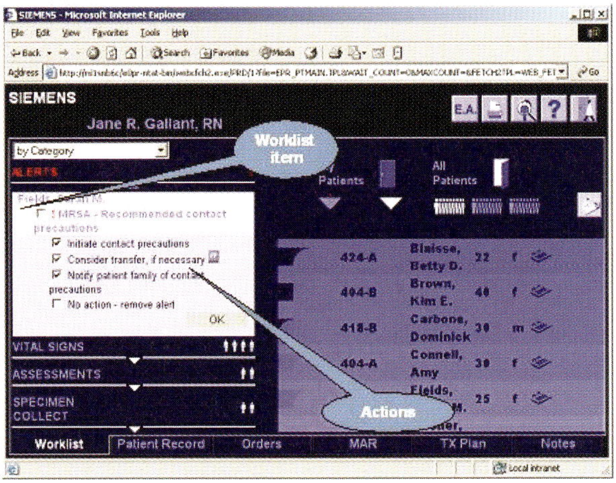

Figure 21.21
Alert box after the detection of a possible MRSA infection in Soarian™

- Diabetes management (in particular as part of a disease management program): to reinforce and monitor patient cooperation and health condition.
- Mammography management, including automatically triggered quality assurance procedures such as a mandatory second opinion.
- Epidemic disease surveillance: for population-wide infection control that statistically correlates findings (as in the example of the infection control workflow above) and offers predictions on potential outbreaks in certain regions (e.g. SARS surveillance in large cities such as Hong Kong and Shanghai, bioterrorism surveillance).

Embedded decision support (embedded analytics)

The embedded decision-support component in an HIS is intended to continuously track key business drivers, including all process metrics and their impact on clinical and financial outcomes. Examples include the cost of daily operations (cost of labor and supplies, cycle times), the quality of the healthcare services (avoided errors, optimal treatment, timely delivery) and the satisfaction of all stakeholders (patients, physicians, nurses, other staff). Monitoring these drivers helps one to identify opportunities for improvement.

Technically speaking, an embedded analytics component is a data-driven evaluation mechanism that can use sophisticated predefined queries with related thresholds to identify problems (OLAP or online analytical processing approach) or conduct proactive searches for data patterns (data-mining approach). An example of the first approach would involve the ascertainment by the embedded analytics component that the average length of stay for a given diagnosis-related group or DRG (e.g. pneumonia) is higher than expected where the expected length is defined by an industry or institution standard. Such findings can be utilized in a number of ways:

- *Automatic alerts*: When the embedded analytics component determines that a metric is outside of an acceptable performance range, an alert is pushed automatically to the appropriate end user. Typical push methods include email, SMS, TM and pager signals. The end devices that can be used to receive notifications include palm pilots, cell phones, pagers, as well as email and Internet browsers on wireless tablets.
- *Interactive analyses for quick understanding*: Corrective actions can only be initiated once the reasons are better understood. The critical information is therefore available in a simple, structured form (i.e. an OLAP cube). This enables one to interactively drill down and analyze the relevant data and to obtain a better understanding of the problem. The drill down may reveal that the longer stay for the pneumonia patient in our example above involves a failure to follow the defined protocol for the diagnosis and the selection of a suboptimal course of treatment. The main idea is that the length of stay for pneumonia patients is presented to the user. The situation can then be analyzed by the physician or payer to determine the reasons for the excessive length of stay.
- *Monitoring for continuous improvement*: As corrective action is taken to improve the situation, the embedded analytics component will monitor progress towards the de-

sired and defined goal. As explained above, alerts keep users informed of progress without their having to remember to check.

The underlying technologies for embedded analytics include the database (collecting the process metrics, as well as clinical and/or financial patient data), analysis and reporting tools and analysis services that generate the analytical cubes. Soarian™ features a web-publishing mechanism that gives authorized clinical users access to the reports and data cubes. This enables the provision of analytical and metrics-tracking information throughout the organization.

21.9 Departmental information system: radiology

As described above, departmental information systems support diagnostic, therapeutic and general care workflow sequences in hospital environments (see fig. 21.5). In the following section, we describe a complete radiology workflow based on the IT applications RIS and PACS.

21.9.1 The radiology workflow

The radiology workflow includes the following activities: patient referral, receipt of a specific diagnostic examination, the availability of the diagnostic results at the desk of the referring physician and the forwarding of a billing code to the revenue management system. The workflow is supported by computer workstations for a variety of activities:

- Patient registration at the radiology department (performed by nursing staff), with the registration being performed via the RIS or via the transmission of data from the hospital-wide order-entry system
- Performance of diagnostic examinations using modalities that generate digital images that are then forwarded to the PACS
- Quality assurance (QA) work: performed on dedicated PACS QA workstations where radiographers optimize radiographies before their interpretation by the radiologist (e.g. grey-level adjustment)
- Routine diagnosis (softcopy reading) of images from all modalities, performed by radiologists on PACS reading workstations
- Fast diagnosis of emergency cases on diagnostic workstations (often in the absence of certain patient information due to the emergency situation)
- Planning of interventions on PACS post-processing workstations, typically based on 3D reconstructions
- Interpretation of organ functioning (brain, heart) on PACS workstations, supported by the fusion of anatomical and functional data
- Daily clinical consultation involving radiologists and other physicians, with image studies being accessed on PACS workstations and projected onto large conference-room screens

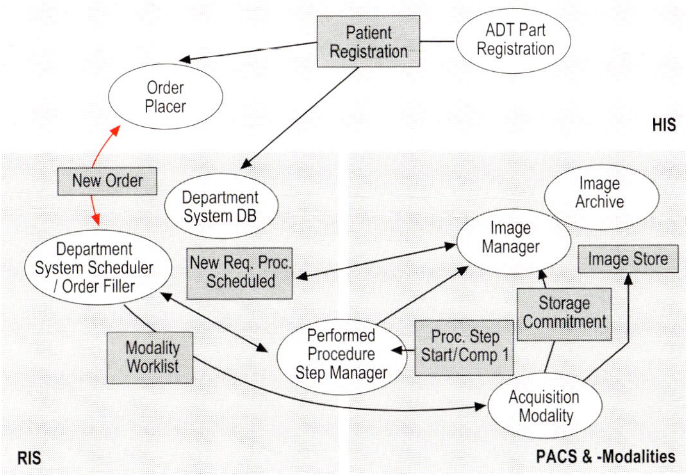

Figure 21.22
Formal IHE actor model of the radiology workflow [21.16]. The bubbles depict the actors, the boxes describe activities.

- Access to diagnostic results by the referring physicians on web-based result viewers (i.e. images and reports are available in digital form at the points where further medical decisions are made)
- Storing the digital images in and retrieving them from the PACS archive
- Training of various staff members involved in modern digital diagnostic imaging

All radiology workplaces are part of an organized process involving the application of diagnostic and therapeutic procedures. The IHE (Integrating the Healthcare Enterprise) consortium (a project sponsored by the RSNA and HIMSS societies [21.16]) has developed a workflow standard for radiology. The IHE model is *actor based*, i.e. the workflow is based on *acting entities* rather than technical components. One such actor is the *order placer*. The order placer may be a function of an HIS (as suggested in fig. 21.22) or a part of a stand-alone RIS with no connection to an HIS. However, independent of the technical realization and the vendor of the components, the IHE standard ensures that the *actor behavior* of all products in radiology is identical and that the interfaces allow for maximum interoperability in a mixed vendor environment.

21.9.2 The radiology information system (RIS)

Due to its independent development, the typical radiology information system (RIS) is a stand-alone application that is used to handle general processes in the radiology department of a hospital (or in an independent imaging center). While the RIS may be loosely connected to the HIS by means of HL7 protocols, many of its functions duplicate functions offered by the HIS. Given this overlap, we will restrict our discussion in the present section to a brief summary of RIS functions.

RIS functions

Patient management (overlap with HIS patient management)

- Registration and discharge of patients (only if they come to the radiology department)
- Instead of offering independent patient registration, the patient-management module in an RIS may simply import the patient demographics from an interfaced HIS (using HL7 messages) or enter them via a smart card reader.
- Patient searches (including phonetic search capacity)
- Creating and printing (barcode) labels for film jackets and films

Service management (overlap with HIS order and scheduling modules)

- Ordering examinations (radiology services such as a brain MRI or a heart CT) by selecting them from a service catalogue (also known as an order tree). The catalogue can also be set up in the HIS service master file.
- Scheduling examinations, e.g. by using graphical timetables to select the earliest possible time slot and allocate the necessary resources (personnel, equipment, rooms). This function could also be provided by the HIS enterprise scheduling module.
- Processing orders: First, the order is entered into the DICOM worklist of the modality that was selected in the ordering step (e.g. MRI, CT, ultrasound). If the RIS has a network connection to the modality, then the order can be entered automatically via a DICOM message.

  The second step is to add the order to the RIS worklist for the scheduled doctor and also to the PACS worklist if the doctor performs softcopy reading. Modern integrated RIS-PACS systems share the RIS worklist for this purpose.
- Documentation of examinations: After an examination has been performed using a specific modality, the radiographer (also called technician or rad tech) is required to document the procedure. Such documentation includes specifying the time taken, consumables used (e.g. contrast agents), radiation exposure (if required by law, as in the case of Germany) and other important information (e.g. allergic reactions on the part of the patient to contrast agents). The radiologist will add a report (including clinical findings) later.
- Supporting film-based workflow means using an RIS without a PACS by creating and printing (barcode) labels for the film jackets and films. These are needed for purposes of identification and tracking.

Administration and manipulation of reports

- Writing, editing, approving (signing off), printing and sending reports
- Additional reporting, second opinion, scanning of incoming reports
- Automated dictation, if possible with speech recognition that automatically transforms the dictated report into a digital text
- Flagging of interesting cases for a teaching repository

- Film archive management (in the absence of a PACS)

Billing (overlap with the HIS revenue management module)

- A complete billing module is often included in the RIS. The preferred way of billing within a hospital is to transmit a procedure code in an HL7 message via an interface to the external HIS billing system.

Administration and configuration (overlap with HIS administration module)

- User administration, including the defining of user roles and access rights and the defining of sign-off policies, etc.
- Maintenance of the radiology service catalogue (order tree)
- Definition and adaptation of screens, forms, report layouts and other site specific needs

Reporting and statistics (overlap with HIS research and statistics module)

- Defining and manipulation of lists, statistics, graphical display of evaluations, interface to spreadsheet applications for further processing (e.g. in EXCEL)

Materials management (overlap with the same module in an HIS or connected ERP system):

- Documentation of materials consumption and general inventory management

A description of the deep integration of RIS and PACS and their respective connections to the various modalities is offered in the following section.

21.9.3 The picture archiving and communication system (PACS)

Picture archiving and communication systems (PACS) were introduced in the late 1970s and early 1980s. The purpose of these systems was to support the diagnostic work of a radiology department by facilitating the acquisition, transmission, diagnosis, archiving and distribution of medical images. Reports have been drafted on the initial deployment of the PACS idea [21.17- 21.20] and excellent overviews of PACS history are also available [21.21, 21.22]. Technical standards for data formats and exchange protocols were defined early, ranging from ACR-Nema2 to DICOM 3.0 [21.11]. Today, the latter enables one to connect any modality to any PACS.

In addition to the establishment of broadly accepted standards, the networking technology behind such systems has reached a level (e.g. Gigabit Ethernet, 622 MB ATM, etc.) where bandwidth is no longer an issue when it comes to the implementation of large-scale PACS that enable the processing of millions of examinations per year.

PACS functionality

A PACS provides the following functionality for image-based diagnosis, mainly applied in radiology, but sometimes also used in other clinical disciplines such as cardiology, orthopedics and surgery:

- Diagnostic interpretation of medical images on PACS workstations (also referred to as softcopy reading)
- Distribution of images and related diagnoses (reports) to the clinical departments. The images and reports are typically accessible via web-based results viewers. The images that are compressed in the interest of greater transmission speed usually lose their diagnostic quality.
- Archiving of images and reports
- Support for clinical conferences involving radiologists and their colleagues. This may include support for multimedia interaction, e.g. online videoconferencing for complicated cases.
- Post-processing of original images, including 3D rendering functions (e.g. for virtual endoscopy), fusion algorithms (e.g. for fusing the anatomical and functional information of a PET/CT), CAD support (e.g. computer-aided diagnosis for automated tumor detection) and further interactive image manipulation packages (e.g. for intervention planning)
- Support for training and educational purposes (e.g. by providing access to case libraries for continuing medical education)

Technical implementation of the radiology workflow

Fig. 21.23 offers an overview of a typical filmless hospital. The radiology department has established its own high-speed network ring that connects all modalities and

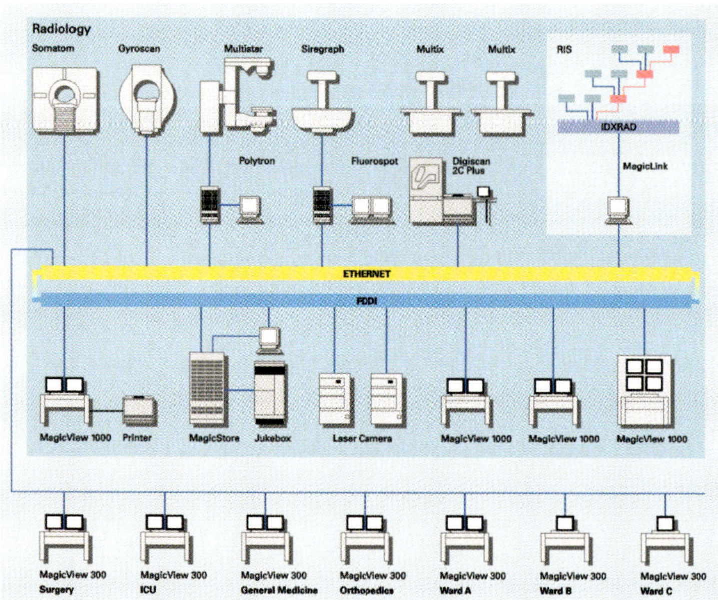

Figure 21.23 Schema for a filmless hospital

SIENET™ PACS components to the MagicStore archive (including OD jukeboxes) and the MagicView 1000 reporting workstations (including an attached MagicPrint film printer).

The blue LAN ring is connected to the yellow hospital-wide Ethernet. The link between the PACS and the RIS (here IDXRAD) is established via the Ethernet connections using a RIS-PACS broker (the SIENET™ MagicLink component). The hospital Ethernet connects the radiology department to all clinics (OR, ICU, orthopedics, wards), thus providing access to images and results on MagicView 300 or MagicWeb PCs.

A true filmless hospital is one in which radiology results can be distributed in digital form to all of the hospital's remaining departments.

21.10 Integrated workplaces

As summarized above in the section on radiology workplaces, the motivation for integrated workplaces is based on three main factors:

- Ergonomic usability to optimally support the users of the various applications (doctors, nurses, technicians) and to increase user acceptance of the applications
- Simplified technological integration (without creating a need for additional communication servers and message brokers) to reduce costs and enhance reliability
- Reduced TCO (total cost of ownership) via a reduction in the number of devices needed (integrated workplaces, in particular, enable one to significantly reduce the number of end devices such as PCs and monitors)

21.10.1 Integrated workplaces in radiology

One design goal for the interactive workplaces provided in the radiology workflow is to minimize the number of end devices and to integrate desktops. The key candidates for workplace integration are shown in fig. 21.24:

- Integration of examination applications with RIS and EMR access on a modality console (e.g. the monitors of a CT scanner): All three applications are typically used by radiographers, so that an integrated modality workplace involving one PC rather than three (as is the case today) would represent a cost-efficient and convenient solution.
- Integration of RIS, PACS and EMR at the reporting workplace of a radiologist: Operating all three applications (possibly enhanced by speech recognition and word processing) on a set of monitors (typically 2 to 4) with only one keyboard and one mouse provides an ergonomic environment that will lead to faster processing and enhanced acceptance.
- Integration of an EMR and PACS viewer on a clinician's desktop: This involves the typical integrated results-viewing application described above in the section on the EMR.

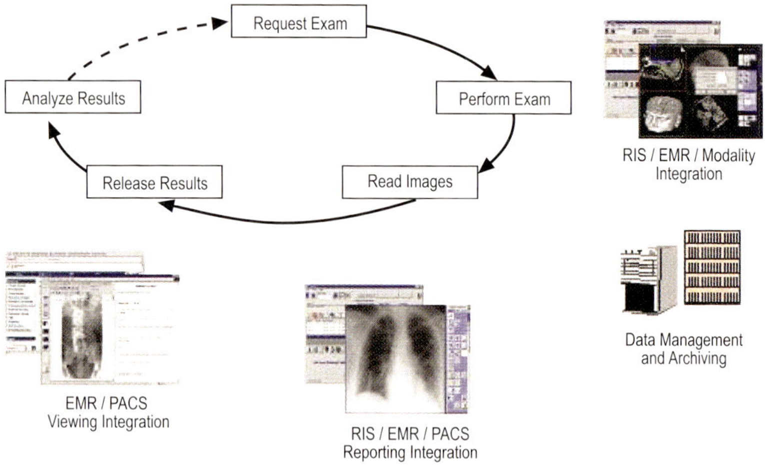

Figure 21.24 Integrated workplaces for the radiology workflow

Fig. 21.25 shows the Siemens Radiologist Command Center that provides RIS, PACS, and speech recognition on one workstation. Only one worklist (from the RIS) is used to open studies either on the RIS (right screen) or on the PACS (left two screens).

The desktop-integrated radiologist command center allows the radiologist to operate both applications across all screens with one keyboard and one mouse. Merely connected RIS-PACS systems (still the standard in many hospitals today) require one to operate two of each (mouse, keyboard), a quite inconvenient and unergonomic environment for efficient softcopy reading.

The basics for the technical integration of workplaces such as single sign-on and patient-context management will be described in the next section using examples from the field of cardiology.

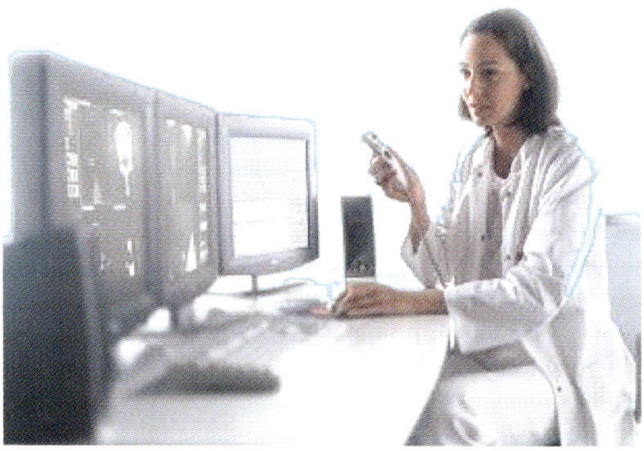

Figure 21.25 Desktop-integrated Siemens Radiology Command Center: RIS (right screen) and PACS (left screens) applications are operated with a single keyboard and a single mouse.

21.10.2 Integrated workplaces in cardiology

The fact that cardiology requires access to a broad number of different applications makes it a good subject of discussion in the context of workplace integration. Fig. 21.26 offers an illustration of the concept of an integrated cardiology examination workplace (ICEW). The ICEW provides cardiologists with access to all diagnostic information, patient data and reporting/documentation tools. These various items include:

- All image data and related reports (cath lab, echo, PET, etc.) as well as the applications needed to view and post-process the images
- All functional data, vital sign traces and related reports (ECG, EP, echo), including the applications for viewing, measuring and making other evaluations
- Access to the EMR and all other patient data
- Evaluation and reporting tools for the sake of compiling the final assessment for the patient, including quality assurance means such as ACS (American Cancer Society) and STS (Society of Thoracic Surgeons)-compliant documentation formats and filing
- POE (provider-order entry) capabilities (although rarely used by cardiologists today)

The immediate advantage of the ICEW is that it enables the cardiologist to access everything from a single workplace. This eliminates the need to work in the various labs (cath, echo, nuclear), write and print partial reports and then complete these reports later in the office.

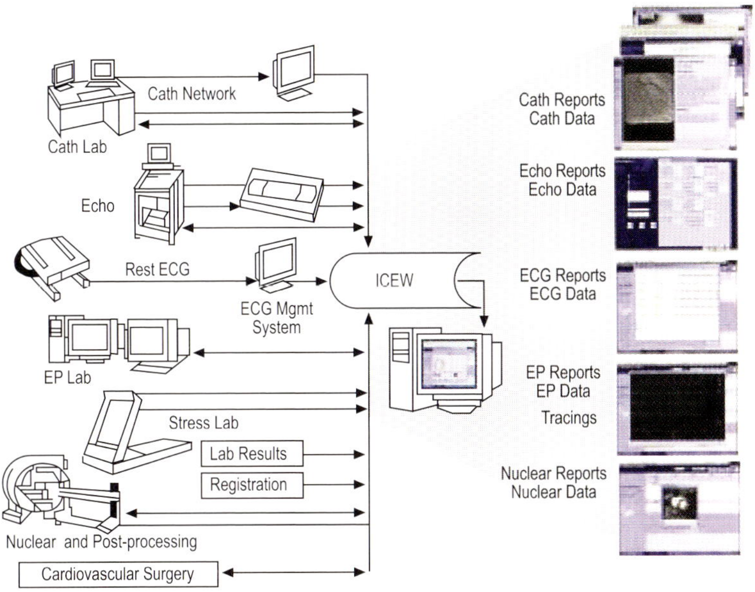

Figure 21.26 Concept of an integrated cardiology examination workplace (ICEW)

The requirements that apply to integrated workplaces can be best addressed with the following technical approach:

1. Establish a platform concept for the applications to enable the sharing of functions. The SOA (service oriented architecture) approach described in sections 21.1 and 21.5 provides a basis.
2. Introduce common components for consistent behavior with respect to access security, user administration, context management, workflow engine and UI concept.
3. Deploy 3-tier architectures with web-based presentation layers so as to allow for simple UI integration on any desktop device (desktop integration) and use only a small number of big application servers to provide the services.
4. Secure the two technical means that are necessary to establish a sufficient degree of integration comfort:
   - Single sign-on: A user login procedure that requests name and password only once and ensures access to as many applications (and databases) as are integrated in the workplace
   - Context sharing for the user and patient in all HIS applications (not only in the ICEW): First, this mechanism is required for the single sign-on (sharing of the same user credentials in all applications). Second, patient context sharing is necessary to ensure that all of the data accessed and manipulated in the various Web windows truly belong to the same patient. The inability to ensure this would represent a serious safety hazard and would prevent the deployment of desktop-integrated workplaces.

   The standard for desktop integration, including single sign-on and context sharing, has been defined by the Clinical Context Object Workgroup (CCOW) [21.23].

Fig. 21.27 offers a sketch of the Siemens approach to an ICEW. This workplace is based on three software platforms, including *syngo*™ (for all imaging applications), Soarian™ (for HIS/CIS applications) and SIENET™ (for image data management and archiving).

- The basis for the ICEW is any *syngo*™ workstation (e.g. the Siemens Leonardo™)
- The Web-based presentation layer gives the cardiologist access to all images, reports, tools and applications. The graphical user interface (GUI) for all applications conforms to the *syngo*™ style guide, thereby assuring maximum consistency and ease of use throughout all functions.
- The GSM (global session manager) and A&A (authorization and authentication) components allow for a single sign-on and ensure a patient context within the presentation windows and when accessing the databases.
- Three databases are involved: the Soarian™ EMR repository for all patient data and clinical information (see below), the SIENET™ PACS archive for images, and the Infinity Explorer™ server for real-time data monitoring.
- Images generated by the various modalities and measurements are sent to the PACS archive using the DICOM protocol and format. To save time, the images can be sent

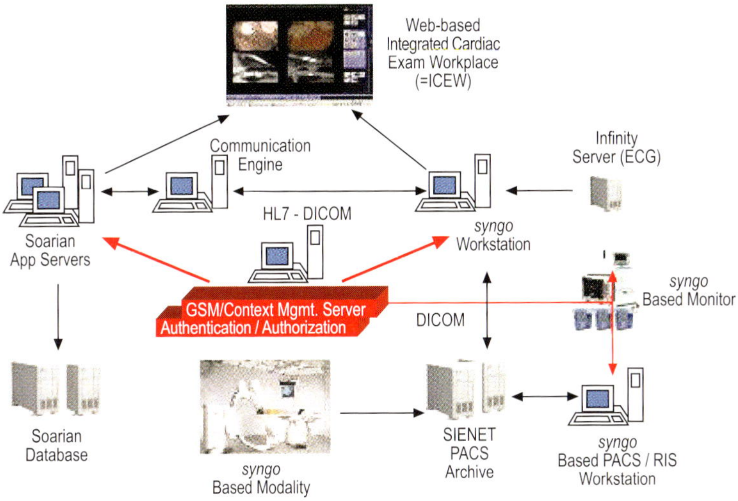

Figure 21.27
Technical realization of an ICEW based on the Siemens platforms *syngo*™, Soarian™, and SIENET™

directly to the workstation or the ICEW user can retrieve them from the PACS archive at a later time (i.e. as with any further image study that may be needed later).

- Measurement results on the ICEW can be added to the Soarian™ EMR by sending them via a communication engine that converts DICOM formats to HL7. The cardiologist can also use the communication engine to retrieve EMR data as needed.
- The *syngo*™ base of the Infinity Explorer™ patient monitor enables one to view waveforms and flowcharts directly at the ICEW workstation. Selected flowchart data can be entered into the EMR as described above.

Additional integrated workplaces – all based on the three Siemens platforms – are currently being developed. The workplaces have been conceived to create an operation room data management system (ORMS) including an anesthesia component, critical care information system (CCIS) components for ICU and ER and various other components.

Particular additions to the concept of the ICEW will be provided to account for the interventional nature of many of the applications.

21.11 The digital hospital and beyond – a vision

The digital hospital can be regarded as a goal-oriented vision of how to improve healthcare delivery and operations by means of modern medical and information technology. The driving forces behind the vision are the business needs of healthcare delivery organizations. These include the need to provide higher quality healthcare and the need to improve their economic situations (revenue, market share, expense growth, cash balance). These needs can be met via business re-engineering based on people (new roles) and processes that are supported by cutting-edge products (innovative technology) that can be combined to create new solutions such as the digital hospital [21.24, 21.25].

The systematic construction principle for role-based workplaces and complex workflows that is described above leads to very sophisticated forms of support both for individuals and entire healthcare teams. By way of presenting a basis, we have described a clear platform strategy for software applications that spans both medical and information technology.

Given the advantages of the platform-based system construction approach, it has become possible to provide more value-adding services in a digital hospital, i.e. in terms of helping to maximize the utilization of the technology investment. Examples of such services include the hosting of all software applications at a supplier's data center (application service providing or ASP concept), outsourcing the hospital's (information) technology to a technology partner and also outsourcing non-technological services such as the collection of accounts receivable and supply-chain management.

Hosting and outsourcing represent good examples of how one might implement a strategy of concentrating on core competences (the provision of medical care) that includes the buying of IT services from external providers.

Options for operating an HIS in a digital hospital

Arriving at an answer to the question of how one should operate an HIS is mainly a matter of considering costs. The task of achieving financial goals, in particular through the optimization of technology and non-medical activities, is not unique to hospital environments, and can thus can be approached as it is in other industries. The key idea behind fitnessing such non-core activities is the utilization of scale effects, with regard to the technology infrastructure (networks, servers, desktops) and the utilization of personnel, in particular coping with the needs of highly specialized experts. Three main options are available when it comes to the operation of information technology applications on the scale of an HIS.

Hospitals can outsource the task of operating their technological systems to providers who are capable of handling the task for less than what it would cost the hospital to have its own IT department handle the task. The cost advantages come from scaling effects associated with providing a service to many customers. For instance, one expert in billing software may provide consulting services at many locations within a specific territory.

Hospitals can outsource business processes to specialized providers who offer back-office services, including payroll management, collection of accounts receivable and supply-chain management. For instance, hospitals can save up to 50% by outsourcing their payroll services.

Hosting software applications is a special type of technology outsourcing where the servers and mainframes are located at a single facility run by the service provider and the client workstations located in hundreds of hospitals are connected via a data network. Hosting allows the provider to utilize the highest possible scale effect. A good example is the Siemens Health Services data center in Malvern, PA, where about 100 employees operate the software applications of more than 1,000 customers in a 24 by 7 mode (24 hours, 7 days a week, throughout the whole year). The customers would need an accumulated equivalent of 10,000 or more IT staff to provide the same services at the 1,000 individual sites.

Summary of the HIS approach described in this book

Supporting the concept of a digital hospital means utilizing the capabilities offered by technology (in this case a hospital information system) to improve the quality of care while lowering the cost of its delivery. The basis is to provide relevant information to end users as input for better clinical and operational decisions. This is only possible if the HIS is designed in the following way:

- Ease of use: Technology is for people and requires their acceptance. It is therefore necessary to make all user interaction with technology as convenient and brief as possible. Web-based UI technology in combination with desktop integration is the solution.
- Smart behavior: The software applications must interact intelligently with the user by exploiting concepts of anticipation (predicting what users need), feedback (proposing better alternatives) and automation (doing what is known). The sections on POE, including proposed order lists based on the patient context, alerts and reminders, and the section on DSS/embedded analytics offer a number of typical examples.
- Application support of teamwork: Teamwork support should maximize push technology so as to forward information and requests automatically to the persons responsible for the next workflow sequences. While the embedded WfMS described above represents a technical solution, well-modeled hospital processes are the basis for its efficient utilization.
- Consistent technology behavior: Independent of the specific tools and applications, technology should work consistently in all contexts, ranging from simple user login to complex surgical staff coordination. A consistent UI framework, together with the SOA approach to the optimal re-use of functions and a shared component strategy (e.g. for security, single sign-on, context management) represents a solution for this requirement.
- Scalability: Technological solutions should offer the same performance quality in all environments, ranging from small hospitals to complex university facilities. The proposed 3-tier architecture allows for scaling up and scaling out on each tier, depending on the workload involved. For example, high data volumes may require an extension of the database server farm, but not necessarily of the other tiers. While an increasing number of users would ask for more Web servers (and possibly more application servers as well), applications of high computational complexity (e.g. DSS) may only enlarge the application server farm.

- Portability and open standards: Hospital information systems will need to be designed to support various environments (e.g. write/read to operating systems and data bases) in order to be capable of responding quickly to technological developments. Open standards help one to keep pace with novel developments and ensure portability options often required by cost factors and standardization projects.
- Availability: Providing services in a healthcare environment requires the highest degree of technological availability, in particular when patients are undergoing critical interventional procedures. Server failover configurations, other hardware components and RAID technology for data storage and redundant network designs help one to achieve degrees of availability up to 99.99% and more. It is therefore crucial to build upon technologies that provide high availability.
- Connectivity: Connectivity is a prerequisite for supporting teamwork automation. The rigorous adherence to standards such as DICOM, HL7, EDI and others is crucial for establishing economic connectivity.
- Safety: The technology, in particular the applications that support workflow sequences, are required to work in a way that rules out any risk to the patients and hospital staff. Typical mechanisms for increasing patient safety at the application level include patient-context sharing, alerts and reminders, constant results monitoring via embedded analytics and the establishment of sign-off rights in the user master files.
- Consolidation: The consolidation of technology is needed to simplify today's complex configurations. Examples described in this book include multi-tiered networks run on stacked blade servers, multi-processor servers and mainframe computers for applications and databases, integrated storage networks (SAN, NAS) for long-term archiving and integrated desktops with web-based user access.
- Cost efficiency: While cost efficiency is partly a construction principle (e.g. scalable computers) for the digital hospital and partly a design goal, it is ultimately an outcome (e.g. reduced IT expenses per adjusted patient day). The biggest levers include a good process or workflow design that standardizes the core operations, the implementation of standards in tools and technologies, consolidation of infrastructure, the sharing of services (e.g. hosting) and outsourcing of non-core functions.

The digital hospital's new services and future role

Healthcare processes are not limited to (digital) hospitals. In more general terms, they include all of the activities relating to a person's health status, ranging from wellness and prevention activities to acute care encounters, subsequent convalescence, homecare and even assisted living. Utilizing modern technology for the entire span of health-related needs extends the idea of the digital hospital toward the notion of fully integrated digital healthcare environments. The following items will likely appear among the services offered by future enterprises:

- Seamless integration of inpatient and outpatient care: Communication services for family physicians and hospital doctors facilitate the planning and organization of hospital stays and help to coordinate follow-up activities to provide optimal treatment and care in a cost-efficient way.

- Support patient and family needs: One strategic goal of a digital hospital, in particular if it is competing for market share as many such institutions do in the United States, is to provide support for whole families – for the sake of prevention, acute care and recovery. Personalized web pages may provide relevant healthcare information such as customized dietary programs for at-risk patients and continuous support for individuals with chronic problems (e.g. disease management for diabetes, asthma or congestive heart problems).
- Screening services: regular screening may represent a more important means of prevention. Various screening procedures are widely used to detect cancer at an early stage (mammography, colonoscopy, lung screening), to identify individuals with diabetes who face an increased risk of developing diabetic retinopathy (can lead to blindness) and to detect calcification in the coronary arteries of at-risk patients at an early stage (to avoid a heart attack).
- Providing support to the family of a hospitalized patient via simple technological means is another target for the digital hospital of the future (especially in rural areas). The installation of a $50 web camera on each patient bed would allow the patient to talk to relatives face to face, allow the family to feel more comfortable and even help the patient to recover faster.
- Support business people: A specific variation of the web camera approach described above is the integration of a business office in every patient room. While the impact on the healing process would certainly need to be discussed for each particular case, access to video conferencing, email and other business office tools would probably persuade many business people (e.g. those with uncomplicated problems such as a broken leg) to select a digital hospital offering such services.
- Support the mobile citizen: The digital hospital will become a service provider for the mobile society. Chronically ill patients will be allowed to travel because traveling will no longer be incompatible with continuous monitoring. Doctors treating individuals who have had accidents abroad will be able to access patient data (history, digital images, etc.) provided by the digital hospital where the patient has subscribed for this service.
- Moreover, videoconferencing will enable doctors from the home digital hospital to consult with patients or physicians abroad or even assist in complicated surgical procedures via telesurgery.
- Connect to and serve the community: Besides offering services for individuals and their families, the digital hospital will also become an integral part of community life, thus forming a general digital healthcare environment based on the knowledge and skills of physicians and nurses. This is driven by the desire of individuals to avoid healthcare encounters because they are generally perceived as unpleasant and the need of the healthcare system to reduce healthcare encounters in order to limit healthcare expenditures.

Realizing this vision will certainly also entail changes centering on the responsibility of adults and children alike in matters of education, information and health awareness. Efforts will have to be made to make activities relating to healthcare and wellness a more important, interesting and convenient part of everybody's life, including prevention, rehabilitation, disease management and assisted living.

21.12 References

[21.1] P. Degoulet, M. Fieschi
Introduction to clinical informatics
Springer-Verlag (1997)

[21.2] R. Haux, A. Winter, E. Ammenwerth, B. Brigl
Strategic information management in hospitals
Springer-Verlag (2004)

[21.3] R. Haux, C. Seggewies, W. Baldauf-Sobez, P. Kullmann, H. Reichert, L. Luedecke, H. Seibold
Soarian – Workflow management applied for health care
Methods Inf. Med. 42 (2003), 25-36

[21.4] A.W. Brown
Large-scale, component-based development
Prentice Hall (2000)

[21.5] A. Brown, S. Johnston, K. Kelly
Using service-oriented architecture and component-based development to build web service application
Rational Software Corporation (2002)
http://www3.software.ibm.com/ibmdl/pub/software/rational/web/whitepapers/2003/TP032.pdf

[21.6] S. Bocionek, S. Brandt, J. Cseh, B. Haskell, D. Rucker, D. Thomas
Built for success – the new clinical and financial IT solutions from health services
electromedica 69 (2001), 76-81

[21.7] S. Bocionek
PACS 2000+ from networks to workflow and beyond
In W. Hruby (ed.), Digital (r)evolution in radiology, 1st edition
Springer, Vienna 2000.

[21.8] A. Ahmad, P. Teater, T.D. Bentley, L. Kuehn, R.R. Kumar, A. Thomas, H.S. Mekhjian
Key attributes of a successful physician order entry system implementation in a multi-hospital environment
J. Am. Med. Inform. Assoc. 9 (2002), 16-24.

[21.9] L.T. Kohn, J.M. Corrigan, M.L. Donaldson
To err Is human: building a safer health system.
Institute of Medicine, Committee on Quality of Health Care in America
National Academy Press, Washington, DC 2000

[21.10] http://www.hl7.org (HL7)

[21.11] http://medical.nema.org (DICOM)

[21.12] http://www.w3.org/XML (XML)

[21.13] S. Jablonski, C. Bussler
Workflow management: modeling concepts, architecture and implementation
International Thomson Computer Press (1996)

[21.14] P. Dadam, M. Reichert, K. Kuhn
Clinical workflows – the killer application for process-oriented information systems?
Proc. 4th Int'l Conf. on Business Information Systems (2000), 36-59

[21.15] W. Baldauf-Sobez, M. Bergstrom, K. Meisner, A. Ahmad, M. Häggström
How Siemens computerized physician order entry prevents the human error
electromedica 71 (2003), 2-10

[21.16] IHE Technical Framework (1998)
http://www.rsna.org/IHE/tf/

[21.17] M. Komori, Y. Nakano, K. Minato, I. Kimura, K. Okajima, T. Takahashi, M. Abe, J. Konishi, K. Satoh
Present status and performance of PACS at Kyoto University Hospital,
Comput. Methods Programs Biomed., 36 (1991), 77-84

[21.18] W. Hruby, H. Mosser, M. Urban, W. Rüger
The Vienna SMZO-PACS-project: the totally digital hospital
Eur. J. Radiol., 16 (1992), 66-68

[21.19] S.C. Horri, S.K. Mun, L.P. Elliott, B. Levine, B. Lo, B.S. Garra, R.K. Zeman, M. Freedman, C. Leftridge, D. Schellinger, et al.
PACS clinical experience at Georgetown University
Int. J. Biomed. Comput. 30 (1992), 275-280

[21.20] F.E. Lindhardt
Krankenhausweite Vernetzung in der Routine – ein Anwender berichtet
electromedica 63 (1995), 13-17

[21.21] E.L. Siegel, R.M. Kolodner
Filmless radiology
Springer, New York (NY) 1999

[21.22] W. Hruby (ed.)
Digital (r)evolution in radiology, 1st edition
Springer, Vienna 2000

[21.23] http://www.hl7.org/special/Committees/ccow_sigvi.htm

[21.24] E. Geisler, K. Krabbendam, R. Schuring
Technology, health care, and management in the hospital of the future
Quorum Books (2003)

[21.25] S. Bocionek, et al.
The digital radiology in the digital hospital of the future
W. Hruby (ed.), Digital (r)evolution in radiology, 2nd edition
Springer, Vienna 2004

Index

0th moment 646
180-LI 419, 453
1st moment 646
2D imaging 47
2D TOF 649
2nd moment 646
3 tier architecture 912, 947, 982
360-LI 418, 453
3D application 897
3D imaging 788, 811
3D TOF 649
^{3}He lung imaging 711
4D imaging 813

A

aberration 21
ablation therapy 694
absorption line 155
absorption spectrum 699
accommodation 21
acoustic absorption 187
acoustic impedance 186, 197
acoustic intensity 187, 192
acoustic lenses 190
acoustic pressure 185, 194
acoustic waves 185
action potential 30
active matrices 334
adaptation 29, 31, 248
ADC 332
AEC-sensor(s) 311
aliases 221
aliasing 223, 744, 760
A-mode 197
amorphous silicon 334, 826
analog digital converter 332
Anger camera 506
Anger localization 512
angiography 346, 353
angular momentum 144-145
anisotropic diffusion 672
anode 265, 272, 280, 395
anode temperature 289
antennas 541, 570
anti scatter grid(s) 311, 350, 396
aperture compounding 780
apodization 704
apparent diffusion coefficient 712
apparent diffusion tensor 163
application architecture 910, 915, 955
application programming interface 948
application server 907
application software 945, 948
application template 907
applications 893, 906
archiving application 900
area detector CT 488
array coils 619
arrays 202, 574, 734, 789
arterial spin labelling 670
artifacts 214, 428, 590
asynchronous communication 919
attenuation 738
attenuation coefficient 215
autocorrelation function 148, 164, 205, 225
autocorrelation time 150
autofluorescence 854
automatic exposure control 301, 310, 396
autotracking 814
axial resolution 198, 735
azimuthal 736

B

B_1 field 153
backend component(s) 913, 919
backprojection 239, 415
backup/restore service 925
barcodes 970
baseband signal 739
beam hardening 430
beam profile 737
beamformer 746
binomial excitation 613
bio heat equation 208
bioeffects 207
biological effects 135
bioluminescence 874
biopsies 693
birdcage 570
Bloch equations 146, 178
blood brain barrier 867
blood oxygenation level dependent contrast 679
blood velocities 194
B-mode 733, 759, 773, 794
BOLD 670, 679
BOLD imaging 643
Boltzmann statistics 145
breast tissue 394
bremsstrahlung 119, 823
bubble 782
build up plates 827-828
business logic 918

C

CAD system 931, 936
calibration 381
candidate generation 935
cardiac CT 470
cardiac function 484
cardiac transducers 815
cardiology 355, 534, 835
cardiovascular MR 688
C-arm 109, 353, 359, 378, 381
C-arm CT 393
cathode 265
cathode ray tube 244, 250
cavitation 195, 207
CCD 99, 329, 401, 853
center of gravity algorithm 512
centric elliptical encode order 665
cesium iodide 318, 336
characteristic radiation 120
charge converters 132
charge coupled device 326, 401
chemical shift 165, 699
chemical shift artifact 607

chemical shift imaging 700
chronaxie 596
cine phase contrast 659
circular polarized field 152
circular polarized high frequency magnetic field 574
CIS 358
classification 936
classifier 937
clinical information systems 952
clinical workflow 967
clutter 737
clutter filter 763
CMOS sensors 333
CMOS technology 349
coherent scattering 130
coil localization 697
coil losses 564
coil tuning 580
coincidence detection 526
collimator 359, 445, 506
collimator sensitivity 510
collimator(s) 508
color Doppler 206, 744, 763, 796
color encoding 797
color flow 733
color power *see* power color
combined systems 490
complex signal 205, 740
component architecture 910
component manager 917
component runtime management 915
componentware 910
compound scan 201
compound transmit focus 754
compounding 779, 805
Compton effect 127
Compton scattering 824
computed radiography 400
computed tomography 231, 413, 844, 878
computer aided detection 403, 931
computer aided diagnosis 931
concomitant gradients 555
cone angle 451
Cone beam CT 378
cone beam(s) 238, 460, 475, 828
configuration service 925
containers 909
containerware 910
contrast 178-180, 256, 428, 824
contrast agent(s) 151, 385, 602, 643, 670, 691, 782, 803, 871
contrast detail resolution 44
contrast enhanced MR angiography 660
contrast harmonic imaging 803
contrast resolution 27, 45, 323, 379, 584
contrast sensitivity 214, 246
contrast to noise ratio 214
coronary artery 818
coronary calcification 479
coronary CT 482
coronary imaging 692
correlation coefficient 682
correlation time 151
counting detectors 403
cross entropy 640
cross relaxation 167
cryostat 550
C-scan 202
CSI sequences 702
CT 231
CT angiography 482
CT detector 448
CT screening 486
customer relationship management 952
CW-Doppler 761, 795
cyclotrons 525

D

dark blood 616, 653
data flow 934
decision support systems 931
density 233
deoxyhemoglobin 678
departmental information system(s) 953, 974
depth gain control 198
detection 931
detective quantum efficiency 227, 343, 826
detector technologies 447
diagnosis 931
DICOM 920
DICOM standard 896
dielectric resonance 547
diffraction 190
diffusion 161, 174
diffusion encoding 673
diffusion imaging 672, 712
diffusion spectral imaging 674
diffusion tensor 672, 675
diffusion weighted EPI 618, 673
diffusion weighted imaging 688
diffusion weighted signal 673
digital beamformer 755
digital cine mode 354, 367
digital fluoro radiography 314
digital hospital 983
digital mammography 399
digital subtraction angiography 315, 368
digitization 332
direct conversion 334, 337, 400
dispersion line 155
dispersion spectrum 699
displacement propagator 161
display 244, 259, 765
DNA 135
documentation 377
Doppler effect 193, 739
Doppler flow 733
Doppler processing 761
Doppler spectrum 204, 742, 762, 799
Doppler tissue imaging 818
dose 301, 388, 468
dose modulation 476
dose profiles 432
dosimeter 829
dosimetric quantities 133
double resonance 166
double z-sampling 466
DQE 227, 334, 343
driven equilibrium 617
dual energy method 345
dual energy subtraction 403
dynamic equilibrium 158
dynamic nuclear polarization 710, 715
dynamic range 258, 341, 566, 569
dynavision 371

E

ECG gating 471
ECG triggering 471

echo planar imaging 611
echo sharing *see* shared echo
echo time 645
echoes 190, 734, 756
eddy current 556
effective dose 138
effective transverse relaxation time 155
electric power losses 546
electromagnetic radiation 124
electromagnetic spectrum 19
electromagnetic tracking 101
electron beam 275
electron beam CT 493
electron optical system 320
electron spin resonance 143, 715
electronic master person index 960
electronic medical record 952, 964
electronic patient record 378
element directivity 751
embedded decision support 973
emitter 265
endoscopy 842, 849
energy absorption 132
energy flux density 122
energy level 145
energy resolution 505
ensemble average propagator 162
enterprise resource planning 950
entrance dose 135
entrance surface air kerma 135
entrance surface dose 135
EPI 611, 672
equilibrium magnetization 147
Ernst angle 159
excitation pulse 152
exposure 371
exposure control 309, 312
exposure time 302
eye 19

F

fan beam 414
fast imaging with steady precession 161
fast low angle shot 160
FDK algorithm 239
feature extraction 936
Feldkamp algorithm 378
field emission displays 250
field stability 543
filament 269, 271, 306
filling factor 564
film 132, 316
film system(s) 350, 396, 825
filming application 899
filter kernel 236
filtered backprojection 235, 461, 519
filtration 122, 395
fine splitting 166
FISP 610
FLASH 160, 607
flat (panel) detector(s) 333, 340, 348, 351, 380, 389, 401, 489
flat panel imager 826
flatfielding 331, 338
flattening filter 823
flip angle 645
flow 163, 202
flow compensation 646
flow imaging 744
fluid attenuated inversion recovery 688
fluorescence 133
fluorescence optical imaging 876
fluoroscopic triggering 665
fluoroscopy 312, 316, 346, 352, 366
flying focal spot tubes 278
focal spot 272, 278, 300, 350
focal spot temperature 290
focus 190, 272
focusing process 748
focusing time delays 749
Fourier slice theorem 234
Fourier space 172, 234
Fourier transform(ation) 149, 155, 163, 172, 204, 217, 233, 415, 423, 638, 699, 740, 761
frame transfer CCD 329
frameworks 909
free induction decay 147, 153
frequency compounding 780, 808
fringe field 545
front end component(s) 913, 919
F-test 682
full frame CCD 329
functional imaging 678

G

gamma camera 506
gamma curve 364
gantry 439, 529
gating 635
Gauss Newton method 639
general administrative information systems 951
general ledger systems 952
general linear model statistics 682
generator 350, 359, 443
geometrical distortions 214
geometrical optics 21
ghosting 590
gradient coils 541, 557
gradient echo 599, 605, 646
gradient power supply 561
gradient strength 555, 559
gradient switching 595
gradient system 554
graphics adapters 59
graphics processors 767
grating lobes 750
gray matter 19, 602

H

Hanafy lens 771
hard copy 244
harmonic imaging 738, 753, 801
harmonics 773
healthcare administration systems 951
heat dissipation 295
high frequency generator 304
Hilbert transform 237
HIS 943
homogeneous coordinates 240, 382
hospital information system(s) 358, 894, 943, 949
hospital processes 951, 953
Hounsfield units 416
human resources systems 952

human visual system 244
hydrogen nuclei 147
hyperpolarization 710
hyperpolarized ^{3}He 712
hypertext markup language 946
hypertext transmission protocol 946

I

image contrast 215
image fusion 62
image intensifier 312, 316, 346
image intensifiers 389
image pick up tubes 327
image pre-processing 338
image quality 255, 386, 579
image reconstruction 231
image registration 639
image rendering 47
image sensor 324
image viewer 897
imaging chain 364
imaging probes 864
in phase 607
incoherent scattering 127
indicator dilution theory 672
indirect conversion 334-335, 400
input screens 318
installation software 925
integrated OR 856
integrated workplaces 979
integration 888
interline transfer CCD 329
intervention 107, 357, 842
interventional angiography 837, 839
interventional imaging 634
interventional MR 693
interventional procedures 354, 361, 836
interventional radiology 92
intracardiac probes 816
intraoperative imaging 96, 842
inversion recovery 157, 614, 691
inverter type generators 303
ionization chamber(s) 134
iron yoke magnets 552
iterative reconstruction 520

K

kerma 133, 300
kernel 236, 415
keyhole methods 633
Klein-Nishina formula 129
k-space 172, 610, 620, 632, 638, 642

L

Langmuir-Child relation 267
laparoscope 851
Laplace equation 549
Larmor frequency 146
late enhancement 690
layergram 236
layers of functionality 944
ligand 866
light emitting diode displays 250
line integral(s) 232, 414
line spread function 217
line width 155
linear accelerator 821
linear polarized field 152
linear system(s) theory 175, 216
lipids 865
liquid bearing 286
liquid crystal display 244, 250, 334
local area network 945
local illumination 56
local pick up coils 541
local receiver coils 619
localization 98
longitudinal magnetization 153
longitudinal relaxation 158
longitudinal relaxation time 147, 149
low contrast detectability 427
low contrast resolution 387
low radiation doses 140
luminance 246, 256
luminescence 132
luminescent screen 315

M

magnetic deflection 279
magnetic dipole moment 144
magnetic field 144, 152
magnetic field homogeneity 542
magnetic field inhomogeneities 155
magnetic forces 594
magnetic moment 145
magnetic resonance 143
magnetic resonance imaging 143, 170, 845, 871
magnetic resonance imaging system 540
magnetization 145
magnetization preparation 653
magnetization transfer 151, 648
main magnet 541
mammogram 394
mammography 312, 344, 393
matching network 573
matrix coil arrays 577
matrix coils 705
matrix spectroscopy 705
maximum intensity projection 53, 384, 435, 667
Maxwell gradients 555
mechanical index 210, 803
metabolites 699
microbubbles 803
Middleware 945
miyabi 837
M-mode *see* TM-mode
modality performed procedure step 895
modality specific post-processing applications 902
mode matrix 577
model based analysis 681
modulation transfer function 217, 273, 323, 342, 422
molecular imaging 536, 855, 863
molecular motion 148
motion artifacts 429
motion correction 635, 681
motional narrowing 149
move during scan 629
MR angiography 643
MR safety 592
MR spectroscopy 698
MR system 579
MTF 217, 342, 422
multi echo imaging 599
multi modality workstations 904
multi row arrays 770
multi slice CT 434, 438

multi slice linear interpolation 453
multi-planar-reformation 48, 434
multiple plane reconstruction 83, 462
multivariate data analysis 683
mutations 135
mutual information 71, 641

N

natural radiation 139
navigation 96, 348
navigator(s) 636, 674, 681
needle visualization 693
nerve cells 25
nervous system 19
network structure 945
networking application 900
networks 945
neural processing 36
neurology 534
neuron 19
neurosurgery 96
neurosurgical workplace 858
noise 44, 169, 198-199, 214, 224, 258, 331, 424, 738
noise equivalent count rate 530
noise equivalent quanta 425
noise figure 564
noise power spectrum 225, 343, 425
nominal air kerma rate 134
non rigid registration 74
nuclear imaging 869
nuclear magnetic resonance 146
nuclear medicine 88, 503
nuclear Overhauser effect 166
nuclear Overhauser enhancement 706
nucleic acid sequences 865

O

objects 908, 920
oncology 532, 832
operating room 842
operating system 944
opposed phase 607
optical illusions 38
optical image 315
optical imaging 873
optical imaging system 19
optical pumping 710-711
optical tracking 99
organ movement 96
orthohydrogen 713
output screens 322
Overhauser effect 715
over-operator 55
oxyhemoglobin 678

P

pair production 124
panoramic imaging 809
parahydrogen 713
parahydrogen induced polarization 710, 713
parallel imaging techniques 577, 619, 628, 676
paramagnetic ions 151
partial volume artifacts 429
particle velocity 186
patient administration system 958
patient browser 896
patient monitoring 356, 363
patient motion 674
patient table 360, 439
penetration 738
perfusion 194, 669
perfusion estimation 786
perfusion imaging 639, 690
perfusion weighted imaging 688
peripheral nerve stimulation 595
perivision 369
permanent magnets 552
PET 490, 516, 524, 869
PET detectors 527
PET/CT 492, 830
phase contrast angiography 655
phase cycling 701
phase dispersion 646
phase effect 643
phase encoding 620
phase sensitive detection 155
phase shift 655
photocathode 319-320
photodynamic diagnostics 854
photoelectric effect 124
photoelectrons 317
photomultiplier 504
picture archiving and communication system 977
piezoelectric effect 199
pile up effect 514
pitch 453
pitch factor 419
planar reformation 47
planigraphy 230
plasma display panels 250
point resolved spectroscopy 701
point spread function 217, 237, 422
Poisson distribution 505
Poisson equation 275
Poisson statistics 224
polarization 710, 715
portal imaging 821
positron emission 503
positron emitters 524
post processing 374
power color 206
power Doppler 798
power spectrum 425
precession 146, 152
presaturation 648
PRESS 701
preventive care 486
programming languages 908
projection matrix 383
projection reconstruction 237
projection(s) 171, 230, 233, 414, 610
projective coordinates 240
prospective methods 636
prostate examinations 708
proteins 865
proton decoupling 706
proton density weighted imaging 603
PSIF 610
pulse coding 779
pulse echo process 757
pulse height 504
pulse inversion 775, 784
pulse sequence 178, 541, 599
pulse sequence control unit 541
pulse shaping 774
pulsed gradient spin echo 161
pulsed wave Doppler 742
PW-Doppler 744, 795

Q

Q factor 564
q-space 164, 677
quality factor 169
quantum noise 424, 426
quenching 551
query/retrieve application 901

R

radial acquisition 610
radial sampling 633
radiation damage 135-136
radiation oncology 91
radiation output 134
radiation risk 136
radiation therapy 821
radio frequency coil 541
radiography 310, 316, 340, 344, 350
radiology information system 358, 975
radiology workflow 974, 978
Radon transformation 233
Rayleigh scattering 130, 189
real time imaging 631
receive path 568
receiver 568
receiver operating characteristic 42
reconstruction 384, 415
redundant array of independent disks 948
reflection 187
registration 62, 65, 104
regulations 207
relaxation 147-148
relaxation times 602
relay optics 326
repetition time 645
reporting 377
resistive magnets 552
resolution 736
resonator(s) 541, 570
retina 20, 25
retrospective gating 636
reusable software 890
revenue management 961
RF field strength 563
RF heating 597
RF losses 546
RF penetration 547
RF power 152, 169
RF pulse 153
RF system 563
rheobase 596
Richardson-Dushman equation 266
rigid transformation 66
RIS 358
road mapping 367
roadmap 633
ROC analysis 44
rotating anodes 283, 307
rotating envelope 278, 288, 297
rotating frame 152
rotation 638
runtime architecture 916

S

sampling 424
sampling theorem 173, 202, 222, 234
SAR 598
SAR reduction 627
saturation 151, 167, 612, 645, 706
saturation current 266
scan conversion 765
scattering 124
scintillation detector 504
scintillator 826
second quantum sink 323
security management 923
segmentation 48
segmented EPI 676
segmented k-space 651, 675
selective excitation 175
semiconductor γ-detectors 523
semiconductor sensor 311
sense organs 18
SENSE technique 622
sensitivity 33, 42, 934
sensitivity calibration 624
sensitivity encoding 622
sensitivity profiles 619
sequential focus 753
service oriented architecture 948
services 888, 921, 948
shared echo 604
shear-warp-factorization 52
Shepp-Logan kernel 237, 415
shielding 550
shim coils 541
shimming 553, 581
shock wave pulses 195
shock waves 194
shot noise 326, 331
signal coil 169
signal sampling 219
signal to noise performance 621
signal to noise ratio 168, 224, 326, 573, 588
silicon drift detectors 523
simplex algorithm 641
simultaneous acquisition of spatial harmonics 620
single photon emission 503
single voxel spectroscopy 700
skin contact 732
slew rate 555, 559
slice profile 177
slice sensitivity profile 433
slim algorithm 419
slip ring technology 417
slot scanning systems 402
SMASH technique 620
Soarian™ 957
soft copy 244, 403
software 888
software architecture 889, 904, 926
software components 909
software platform(s) 888, 905
software terminology 908
solid state detectors 360
sonography 404, 792
sound velocity 185
space charge 267
spatial compounding 806
spatial distortion 586, 589
spatial filtering 365
spatial resolution 26, 144, 174, 200, 214, 216, 255, 323, 364, 386, 508, 530, 583
specific absorption rate 598
specificity 43, 934
speckle 201, 735
SPECT 490, 503, 514, 870
SPECT/CT 492, 830
spectral density 149
spectral Doppler 733, 739
spectroscopy 165, 698
spectrum 699
spherical navigators 638
spin 146
spin coupling 166-167
spin echo 156, 599
spin echo imaging 602
spiral CT 417, 434
spiral interpolation 456
spiral sampling 633
spiral scan 453
steady state 158

steady state free precession 158, 607
STEAM 700
Stefan-Boltzmann law 289
stimulated echo 157
stimulated echo acquisition mode 700
stimulation monitor 596
stimulus presentation 680
storage phosphor 133, 316
strain 786, 816
stress echo 816
stroke 686
stroke protocol 687
style guide 891, 904
superconducting magnet 548
superparamagnetic nanoparticles 866
superparamagnetic substances 671
supply chain management 952
surface coils 574, 700
surface rendering 49, 668
surface shaded display 53, 384, 435
surgery 89, 107
surgical navigation 96
syncopation 652
syngo architecture 907, 913-914
syngo communication model 919
syngo platform 890, 927
syngo product line 904
synthetic line 758
system control 579
system dose 135
system management service 925
system theory 214

T

T_1 weighted imaging 602
T_2 weighted imaging 602
T_2^* relaxation 678
target 123
targets for molecular imaging 865
task card 891
t-distribution 682
television camera 324
temporal resolution 34
texture 735
texture mapping 59
TFT 334
thermal equilibrium 146
thermal index 209
thermionic emission 265
thermo monitoring 694
thin film transistor 334
third order scattering 785
three tiered architecture *see* 3 tiered architecture
three-dimensional vision 36
time delay beamforming 756
time gain control 198
time of flight 643
tissue ablation 151
tissue equalization 814
TM-mode 200, 793
TOF MR angiography 687
tomography 230
total imaging matrix 578
tracking 101
tracking endovascular devices 696
transducer(s) 199, 734, 768
transesophageal imaging 790
transfer function 56, 217
transition probabilities 167
transmit path 565
transmitter 565
transversal magnetization 154
transverse relaxation 157
transverse relaxation time 147, 149
treatment planning 91
triggering 635, 652
true FISP 161, 608
t-test 681
tumorous tissue 602
tungsten 123, 270-271, 284
tungsten filament 269
turbo spin echo 604

U

ultrasound 184, 363, 732, 846, 878
ultrasound impedances 200
ultrasound pulses 193
ultrasound transducer *see* transducer(s)
uniform resource locator 946
user interface 374, 891, 914, 965
user interface logic 918

V

valvular function 690
vascular intervention 695
vascular resistance 800
veiling glare 256, 323
velocity compensation 646
ventricular function 689
vessel tracking 668
viewing application 897
virtual private network 945
visual system 245
visualization 47, 62, 83, 97, 381, 384, 696, 868
volume data 434
volume flow 800
volume rendering 50, 59, 86, 385, 435

W

wall motion 689
water molecules 151
water suppression 702
wave optics 187
web based interface 928
web services 910
Wehnelt electrode 265, 276
Whitakker reconstruction 642
white matter 19, 602, 674
whole body contrast enhanced MRA 666
whole body imaging 628
wide algorithm 418
wide band harmonic imaging 802
Wiener spectrum 225
windowing 47, 365
workflow 888, 893, 953, 971
workflow management system 957

X

X-ray detectors 132
X-ray generator(s) 300
X-ray image 315
X-ray imaging 843
X-ray production 118
X-ray spectrum 300
X-ray tube(s) 123, 264, 280, 292, 305, 350, 359, 444

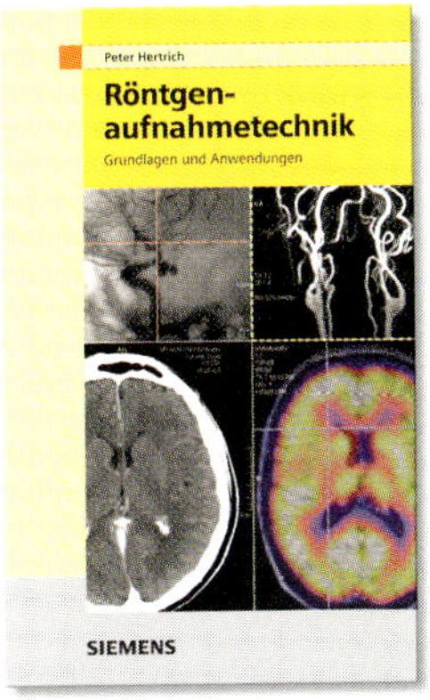

Hertrich, Peter

Röntgenaufnahmetechnik

Grundlagen und Anwendungen

2004, 344 Seiten, 222 Abbildungen,
14,3 cm × 22,5 cm, gebunden
ISBN 3-89578-209-2
€ 49,90 / sFr 80,00

MTRAs, Radiologen, Technikern, Entwicklern und Vertriebsingenieuren bietet dieses Buch eine einmalige Darstellung der Verfahren und Anwendungen der Röntgenaufnahmetechnik. Aufbauend auf den physikalischen Grundlagen und der Qualität und Wirkung von Röntgenstrahlen beschreibt das Buch Röntgensysteme für Diagnostik und Intervention, die Technik der Röntgenaufnahme, Bildqualität, das Patientendatenmanagement und die Datenarchivierung und -kommunikation mit PACS im Krankenhaus sowie zwischen Arztpraxen und Krankenhäusern. Alle Beschreibungen entsprechen dem technischen und diagnostischen Stand heutiger Forderungen an moderne, meist digitale Aufnahme- und Bildverarbeitungsverfahren und -systeme.

Inhalt

Medizin und Technik, Physikalische Grundlagen · Eigenschaften und Qualität von Röntgenstrahlen · Strahlenexposition, Dosis, Strahlenschutz · Röntgensysteme für Orthopädie, Trauma und Notfall, fahrbare Röntgensysteme für Bettaufnahmen, Röntgensysteme für die Mammographie, für universelle und spezielle Angiographie, Röntgensysteme mit Schwerpunkt Internistik, Röntgensysteme für die Urologie, für den OP, für Dentalaufnahmen, für die Computertomographie · Komponenten · Bildempfängersysteme · Bildbetrachtungsstationen · Röntgenaufnahmetechnik: Projektionen, Kontrastmittel, Aufnahmeparameter, Digitale Aufnahmetechnik · Bildqualität · Patientendatenmanagement · PACS.

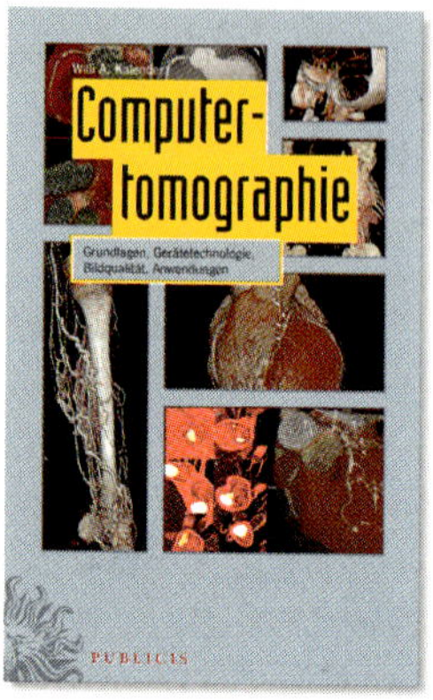

Kalender, Willi A.

Computertomographie

Grundlagen, Gerätetechnologie, Bildqualität, Anwendungen

2., überarbeitete und erweiterte Auflage,
ca. 310 Seiten, 130 Abbildungen,
18 Tabellen, 14,3 cm × 22,5 cm, gebunden
ISBN 3-89578-215-7
€ 49,90 / sFr 80,00
Geplanter Erscheinungstermin: Februar 2006

Das Buch stellt verständlich und benutzerorientiert die theoretischen und gerätetechnischen Grundlagen der Computertomographie (CT) für einen breiten Leserkreis dar, von der konventionellen Einzelschichtaufnahme bis zur Volumenaufnahme mit Kegelstrahl-CT. Es behandelt ausführlich die für die Bildqualität relevanten Einflussgrößen und die für die klinische Anwendung bedeutsamen Leistungsmerkmale. Leser erfahren so, wie ein jeweiliges CT-Gerät optimal eingesetzt werden kann. Dies schließt eine eingehende Diskussion des Dosisbedarfs und der Dosismessung sowie der Maßnahmen zur Dosisreduzierung bei CT ein.

Für die zweite Auflage wurden viele Inhalte aktualisiert und neue Themen wie Flächendetektoren, Kegelstrahl-, Mikro- und 16-Schicht-CT ergänzt.

Die beiliegende CD-ROM bietet attraktive aktuelle Anschauungsbeispiele, Animationen und interaktive Übungen zur Bildbetrachtung und -manipulation.

Zielgruppe des Buches sind alle, die tagtäglich, regelmäßig oder auch nur gelegentlich mit CT zu tun haben: Mediziner, MTRAs, Ingenieure, Techniker und Physiker. Am Ende des Buches befindet sich ein Glossar, in dem alle wichtigen Fachbegriffe zusammengestellt und erläutert sind.

Inhalt

Systemkonzepte · Systemkomponenten · Bildrekonstruktion · Spiral-, Mehrschicht-Spiral-, Kegelstrahl-, Dynamische CT · Quantitative CT · Bildqualität · Ortsauflösung · Kontrast · Bildpunktrauschen · Homogenität · Routine- und Spezialanwendungen · 3D-Darstellungen · Postprocessing · Qualitätssicherung.

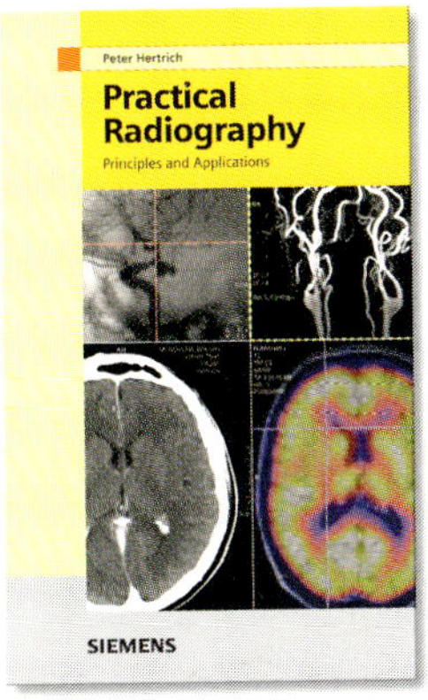

Hertrich, Peter

Practical Radiography

Principles and Applications

2005, 316 pages, 222 illustrations,
14.3 cm × 22.5 cm, hardcover
ISBN 3-89578-210-6
€ 49.90 / sFr 80.00

This book provides radiological technicians, radiologists, technicians, developers and sales engineers with a unique display of the methods and applications used in radiography. Building on the physical basis and the quality and effects of X-rays, the book describes X-ray systems for diagnostics and interventions, the technique behind a radiographic image, image quality, patient data management including data archiving and communication with PACS in the hospital as well as between a physician's practice and hospitals. All descriptions are in accordance with the technical and diagnostic requirements to be met by modern, frequently digital radiographic as well as image processing methods and systems.

Contents

Medicine and Technology, the physical principles · Characteristics and quality of X-rays · X-ray exposition, dose, radiation protection · X-ray systems for orthopedics, trauma, emergency and bedside exposures · X-ray systems for mammography, for universal as well as special angiography · X-ray systems with focus on internal medicine · X-ray systems for urology, for the OR, for dental images, for computed tomography · System components · Image receiver systems and viewing stations · X-ray exposure technique: projections, contrast agent, exposure parameters, digital exposure technique · Image quality · Patient data management · PACS.

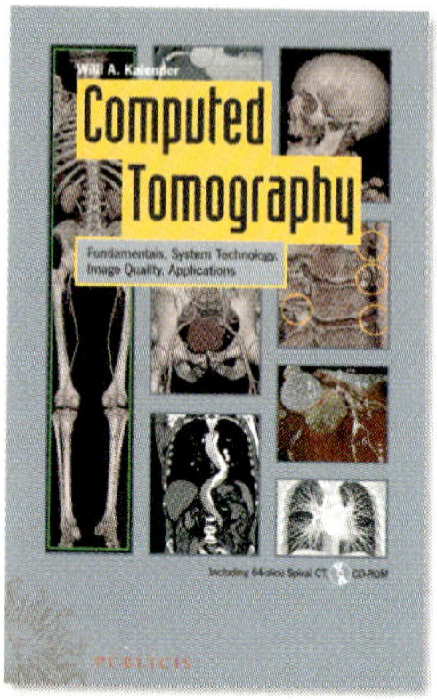

Kalender, Willi A.

Computed Tomography

Fundamentals, System Technology, Image Quality, Applications

2nd revised and enlarged edition, 2005,
306 pages, 130 illustrations, 18 tables,
14.3 cm × 22.5 cm, hardcover
ISBN 3-89578-216-5
€ 49.90 / sFr 80.00

The book offers a comprehensive and user-oriented description of the theoretical and technical system fundamentals of computed tomography (CT) for a wide readership, from conventional single-slice acquisitions to volume acquisition with multi-slice and cone-beam spiral CT. It covers in detail all characteristic parameters relevant for image quality and all performance features significant for clinical application. Readers will thus be informed how to use a CT system to an optimum depending on the different diagnostic requirements. This includes a detailed discussion about the dose required and about dose measurements as well as how to reduce dose in CT. All considerations pay special attention to spiral CT and to new developments towards advanced multi-slice and cone-beam CT.

For the 2nd edition many sections of this book have been updated. In particular, material on new X-ray technology, on 64-slice spiral and cone-beam CT scanning have been added.

The enclosed CD-ROM again offers attractive case studies, including many examples from the most recent 64-slice acquisitions, and interactive exercises for image viewing and manipulation.

This book is intended for all those who work daily, regularly or even only occasionally with CT: physicians, radiographers, engineers, technicians and physicists. A glossary describes all the important technical terms in alphabetical order.

Contents

System concepts · System components · Image reconstruction · Spiral CT · Multi-slice spiral CT · Dynamic CT · Quantitative CT · Image quality · Spatial resolution · Contrast · Pixel noise · Homogeneity · Routine and special applications · 3D displays · Post-processing · Quality assurance.